Medical-Surgical Nursing

An Integrated Approach

Lois White • Gena Duncan

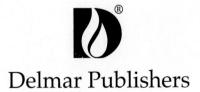

Delmar Publishers

an International Thomson Publishing company I(T)P®

Albany • Bonn • Boston • Cincinnati • Detroit • London • Madrid
Melbourne • Mexico City • New York • Pacific Grove • Paris • San Francisco
Singapore • Tokyo • Toronto • Washington

NOTICE TO THE READER

Cover Design: Brucie Rosch

Delmar Staff

Publisher: Susan Simpfenderfer
Acquisitions Editor: Dawn Gerrain
Developmental Editor: Jill Rembetski
Project Editor: William Trudell

Art and Design Coordinator: Rich Killar
Production Coordinator: John Mickelbank
Editorial Assistant: Sarah Holle
Marketing Manager: Katherine Slezak

COPYRIGHT © 1998
By Delmar Publishers
a division of International Thomson Publishing Inc.

The ITP logo is a trademark under license.

Printed in the United States of America

For more information, contact:

Delmar Publishers
3 Columbia Circle, Box 15015
Albany, New York 12212-5015

International Thomson Publishing Europe
Berkshire House
168-173 High Holborn
London, WC1V 7AA
England

Thomas Nelson Australia
102 Dodds Street
South Melbourne 3205
Victoria, Australia

Nelson Canada
1120 Birchmount Road
Scarborough, Ontario
Canada, M1K 5G4

International Thomson Editores
Campos Eliseos 385, Piso 7
Col Polanco
11560 Mexico D F Mexico

International Thomson Publishing GmbH
Konigswinterer Strasse 418
53227 Bonn
Germany

International Thomson Publishing Asia
221 Henderson Road
#05-10 Henderson Building
Singapore 0315

International Thomson Publishing—Japan
Hirakawacho Kyowa Building, 3F
2-2-1 Hirakawacho
Chiyoda-ku, Tokyo 102
Japan

1 2 3 4 5 6 7 8 9 10 XXX 03 02 01 00 99 98 97

Library of Congress Cataloging-in-Publication Data

Medical-surgical nursing : an integrated approach / [edited by]
    Lois White, Gena Duncan.
        p.   cm.
    Includes bibliographical references and index.
    ISBN 0-8273-6371-0 (alk. paper)
    1. Nursing. 2. Surgical nursing. I. White, Lois.
II. Duncan, Gena.
RT41.M484   1997
610.73—dc21   97-17371
                            CIP

DEDICATION

*To my mother, Norma Wacker,
for her love and support all these
years; and to my husband, John,
for his love, patience, understanding,
and valuable input to this book.*

Lois White

*This book is affectionately dedicated
to my husband, John, for his example of love, humor, wisdom, and
generosity.*

*I would also like to dedicate the
book to the contributors for their
long hours of work in writing their
chapters. Their expertise and dedication made this book possible.*

Gena Duncan

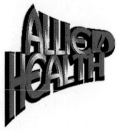

▶ CONTRIBUTORS

Joy E. Ache-Reed, RN, MS
Assistant Professor of Nursing
Indiana Wesleyan University
Marion, IN
**Chapter 7, Cultural Diversity
in the Workplace**

**Diane R. Behrens,
RNCS, MA, MSEd**
Instructor
Saint Francis College
Fort Wayne, IN
**Chapter 14, Fluid, Electrolyte,
and Acid-Base Balances**
**Chapter 24, Allergies, Immune,
and Autoimmune Disorders**

Susan L. Bredemeyer, RN, MS
Assistant Professor
Lutheran College of Health
Professions
Fort Wayne, IN
**Chapter 10, Nursing
Assessment**

Mary Jo Brock, RN, MSN
Clinical Nurse Specialist
St. Joseph Medical Center
Fort Wayne, IN
Chapter 4, Biomedical Ethics

Gyl A. Burkhard, RN, BSN, MS
Instructor
OCM BOCES
Syracuse, NY
Chapter 35, Urinary Disorders

Donna J. Burleson, RN, MS
Chair of Health Occupations
Cisco Junior College
Abilene, TX
Chapter 1, Critical Thinking

Diana L. Case, RN, MA, FNP
Neighborhood Health Clinic
Fort Wayne, IN
**Chapter 13, Perioperative
Nursing**

Gena Duncan, RN, MSEd, MS
Assistant Professor
Lutheran College of Health
Professions
Fort Wayne, IN
Chapter 20, Cardiac Disorders
Chapter 21, Vascular Disorders
**Chapter 22, Blood and Lymph
Disorders**
**Chapter 37, Critical Thinking
on Multiple Systems**

Mary Elias, RNC, BSN, CCE
Instructor
Practical Nursing Program
Ivy Tech State College
Fort Wayne, IN
**Chapter 31, Female
Reproductive Disorders**

Cheryl Erickson, RN, BSN, MA
Associate Professor
Lutheran College of Health
Professions
Fort Wayne, IN
**Chapter 10, Nursing
Assessment**

Michael A. Fiedler, CRNA, MS
Assistant Professor
Applied Health Sciences
University of Alabama
at Birmingham
Birmingham, AL
Chapter 11, Anesthesia

Cathy Greer, RN, MS
Instructor
Lutheran College of Health
Professions
Fort Wayne, IN
**Chapter 13, Perioperative
Nursing**

**Margaret L. Griffin,
RN, BSN, MS**
Instructor
Lutheran College of Health
Professions
Fort Wayne, IN
**Chapter 23, Integumentary
Disorders**

Susan Halley, RN, MS, FNP
Instructor of Nursing
Ball State University
Muncie, Indiana
**Chapter 3, Introduction to
Ethics**

**Beverly F. Hildebrand,
RN, BSN, MS**
Former Health Occupations
Coordinator
Washington, Saratoga, Warren,
Hamilton, & Essex Counties
BOCES
Saratoga, NY
Chapter 35, Urinary Disorders

Janet Leah Joost, RN, BSN
Instructor
Front Range Community College
Boulder, CO
**Chapter 19, Respiratory
Disorders**

Denise M. Jordan, RN, BSN, MA
Instructor
Practical Nursing Program
Ivy Tech State College
Fort Wayne, IN
**Chapter 2, Legal Aspects
of Nursing**

Janet E. Keith, RN, MSEd
Instructor
Practical Nursing Program
Ivy Tech State College
Fort Wayne, IN
**Chapter 26, Musculoskeletal
Disorders**

**Vicki L. Khouli,
RN, BSN, MA, IBCLC**
Instructor
Practical Nursing Program
Ivy Tech State College
Fort Wayne, IN
**Chapter 33, Sexually
Transmitted Diseases**

Mary E. A. Laskin, RN, MN, CS
Clinical Nurse Specialist
Surgical/Orthopedic Services
Kaiser Permanente
San Diego, CA
Chapter 12, Pain Management

**Celinda Kay Leach, RN, BS,
MPH**
Program Chair, Practical Nursing
Practical Nursing Program
Ivy Tech State College
Fort Wayne, IN
Chapter 15, Oncology Nursing

Sandra Liming, RN, MN
Nursing Instructor
North Seattle Community College
North Seattle, WA
**Chapter 32, Male Reproductive
Disorders**

Cheryl McGaffic, RN, PhD
Clinical Instructor
College of Nursing
The University of Arizona
Tucson, AZ
Chapter 25, HIV Disorders

**Robin Theresa McKenzie,
RN, MSN, CCRN**
Assistant Chairman
Navy Medical Center
San Diego, CA
Chapter 28, Sensory Disorders

**David K. Miller,
RNC, BSN, MSEd**
ICU/Medical-Surgical Manager
W.S. Major Hospital
Shelbyville, IN
Chapter 25, HIV Disorders

**Joan Fritsch Needham,
RNC, MS**
Director of Education
DeKalb County Nursing Home
De Kalb, IL
**Chapter 16, Caring for the
Older Adult**
**Chapter 17, Rehabilitation,
Home Health, and Long-
term Care**
**Chapter 18, The Dying Process/
Hospice Care**

**Raymond Phillips,
RN, MS, CCRN**
Clinical Nurse Specialist
Staff Development Coordinator
U.S. Naval Hospital
Rota, Spain
Chapter 28, Sensory Disorders

Martha Ann Rust, RN, BSN, MS
Instructor
Lutheran College of Health
    Porfessions
Fort Wayne, IN
**Chapter 27, Nervous System
    Disorders**

Russlyn A. St. John, RN, MSN
Associate Professor &
    Coordinator, Practical Nursing
St. Charles Community College
St. Peters, MO
**Chapter 29, Endocrine
    Disorders**

**Mary Kay Schultz,
    RN, MSN, ANP**
Instructor
Department of Nursing
Regis University
Denver, CO
Chapter 30, Diabetes Mellitus

Leslee R. Sinn, RN, BSN
Instructor
Front Range Community College
Boulder, CO
**Chapter 34, Digestive
    Disorders**

Susan Stranahan, RN, PhD
Chair, Nursing Department
Indiana Wesleyan University
Marion, IN
**Chapter 6, Cultural Aspects of
    Health and Illness**

**Diana S. Sullivan,
    RN, BSN, ET, MS**
Instructor
Lutheran College of Health
    Professions
Fort Wayne, IN
Chapter 36, Ostomies

Lois White, RN, PhD
Chairperson, Professor
Department of Vocational Nurse
    Education (recently retired)
Del Mar College
Corpus Christi, TX
**Chapter 5, Communication
Chapter 8, Health Maintenance
Chapter 9, Substance Abuse
Chapter 35, Urinary Disorders**

▶ REVIEWERS AND CONSULTANTS

Marilyn Adair, RN
Nursing
South Puget Sound Community
    College
Olympia, WA

Patricia D. Alft, RN, BSN
Coordinator, Practical Nursing
    Program
N.S. Hillyard, A.V.T.S.
St. Joseph, MO

**Linda Feeley Barber,
    RN, MS, MSN**
Associate Professor
School of Nursing
Union University
Jackson, TN

Wendy Baumle, RN, MSN
Clinical Nurse Specialist
Nursing Instructor
Lutheran College of Health
    Professions
Fort Wayne, IN

**Barbara J. Durkin, RN, BSE
    (retired)**
Licensed Practical Nursing
    Program
Albany County Boces
Albany, NY

**Sharon D. Elvidge-Kelly,
    RN, JD, PhD**
Van Ostrand Elvidge & Overturf
Attorneys at Law
Indianapolis, IN

**Captain Alston Kirk, CHC, USN
    (retired)**
Pastor
Trinity Lutheran Church
Corpus Christi, TX

Janice Levens, RN
Nursing Instructor, Practical
    Nursing
Minneapolis Community
    and Technical College
Minneapolis, MN

Mary S. Lewin, RN, BSN, MSEd
Nursing Instructor
Orleans Educational Center
Medina, NY

**Alice J. Longman,
    RN, EdD, FAAN**
Professor Emerita
The University of Arizona
College of Nursing
Tucson, AZ

Tina R. Monlezun, RN, MS
Nursing Instructor, Clinical Nurse
    Specialist
Louisiana Technical College-
    Jefferson Davis Campus
Jennings, LA

Kathleen A. Petet, RN, BSN, MS
Department Chairperson, Health
    Occupations
Skagit Valley College, Whidbey
    Campus
Oak Harbor, WA

**Barbara Gayle Talik,
    RN, BSN, MEd**
Instructor
Northwest Technical Institute
Springdale, AR

Harriet S. Tuyo, RN, MSN, ANP
Instructor
Vocational Nursing Program
Houston Community College
    Systems
Houston, TX

John M. White, PhD
Former Chairperson, Professor
    Biology Department
Del Mar College
Corpus Christi, TX

▶ CONTENTS

Section I

Chapter 5   Communication   68

Lois White, RN, PhD

Unit 2   Cultural Aspects   85

Chapter 6   Cultural Aspects of Health and Illness   87

Susan Stranahan, PhD, RN

Chapter 7   Cultural Diversity in the Workplace   97

Joy E. Ache-Reed, RN, MS

Chapter 32 Male Reproductive Disorders 914

Sandra Liming, RN, MN

Chapter 33 Sexually Transmitted Diseases 945

Vicki L. Khouli, RN, BSN, MA, IBCLC

Unit 11 Digestion and Elimination 963

Chapter 34 Digestive Disorders 965

Leslee R. Sinn, RN, BSN

▶ PREFACE

To face today's changing health care environment, nursing students rely on a solid foundation of accurate, essential information on which to build careers of effective client care. *Medical-Surgical Nursing: An Integrated Approach,* a new text for students of practical/vocational nursing, is designed to meet this aim.

A Focus on Critical Thinking

The ability to think critically is crucial for today's nurses whose roles are continually shifting and changing in the challenging health care environment. Unfortunately, the necessity to present vast amounts of information in a short time span often leaves instructors with little time to test their students' abilities to think critically. *Medical-Surgical Nursing: An Integrated Approach* has sought to address this area with an intense focus on the process of critical thinking throughout the text—

Chapter 1, Critical Thinking serves a dual purpose. First, it outlines the process of critical thinking in easy to understand terms, offering students tips and exercises on reading for comprehension, thus enabling them to study more effectively. Second, the chapter serves as the student's guide to the text itself, explaining the purpose and use of the various features, such as "Making the Connection" and "Learning Objectives." The chapter concludes with tips designed to help students work through the critical thinking exercises contained in the other chapters, namely the Case Studies and Review Questions. Thus, with careful study of Chapter 1, students will approach subsequent chapters in a thoughtful manner, with a complete understanding of the intentions behind the learning aids and enhanced ability to study effectively.

Making the Connection is each chapter's "quick reference," leading students from the chapter they are currently studying to related areas in the text. This helps them understand the interrelation of material and build upon their knowledge base.

Case Studies, in most chapters, provide real life scenarios with accompanying questions that guide students through the steps of the nursing process for the development of their own care plans and their future care of clients.

Chapter 37, Critical Thinking on Multiple Systems is a unique chapter containing a series of case studies involving multiple body systems. As students work through these case studies, whether alone or in the classroom, they will understand the complexity of human illnesses and that disorders are not text-book perfect and isolated to one body system. Their knowledge of all body systems will be challenged.

Text Organization

Medical-Surgical Nursing: An Integrated Approach contains 37 chapters that have been organized into 2 sections and 12 units.

Unit 1, Concepts Affecting Nursing Care, provides students with a solid understanding of the basic concepts underlying nursing. *Chapter 1, Critical Thinking,* explains the process of critical thinking in terms the student can understand, then illustrates how each feature of this text will challenge the students to think critically. Chapters 2 to 4 examine the legal and ethical issues involved in the care of clients. *Chapter 5, Communication,* discusses strategies for communicating effectively with clients, clients' families, and co-workers.

Unit 2, Cultural Aspects, contains two chapters on how culture and cultural identity affect health. *Chapter 6, Cultural Aspects of Health and Illness,* presents an overview of cultural beliefs and practices regarding health and illness, culturally appropriate health care, and illnesses associated with certain ethnic groups. *Chapter 7, Cultural Diversity in the Workplace,* expands on the material presented in Chapter 6 with discussions of how religious affiliation, language, and cultural responses to pain, grieving, and time/space orientation affect both the nurse and client's perceptions of health and illness.

Unit 3, Physical and Mental Integrity, begins with a chapter on health maintenance to establish the basics of good health promotion and concludes with a chapter on substance abuse, including special sections on geriatrics, co-dependency and the impaired nurse. There is also an emphasis on the impaired nurse in the legal chapter.

Section II begins with *Unit 4, Concepts of Medical Surgical Care,* which includes chapters on nursing assessment, anesthesia, pain management, perioperative nursing, and fluid, electrolyte and acid-base balances.

Unit 5, Special Topics of Medical Surgical Care, includes a separate chapter on oncology nursing, and two chapters focused primarily on older clients: *Chapter 16, Caring for the Older Adult and Chapter 17, Rehabilitation, Home Health Care, and Long-term Care.* The unit concludes with *Chapter 18, The Dying Process/Hospice Care.*

Unit 6 begins the traditional medical-surgical portion of the text and concludes with *Unit 11.* These units lead students through the nursing process of the most common disorders related to each body system. The text includes chapters on HIV, sensory disorders, diabetes mellitus, female reproductive disorders, male reproductive disorders, sexually transmitted diseases, and ostomies and provides students with complete, concise information about each.

The text concludes with *Unit 12, Integration of*

Body Systems, which contains **Chapter 37, Critical Thinking on Multiple Systems,** a unique presentation of a series of case studies related to many of the disorders covered within the other units. Each case study leads students through scenarios where the client experiences breakdown in multiple body systems. Whether used for self-study or as part of classroom discussion, this chapter will help students connect the concepts they have been learning throughout their course of study.

ANCILLARIES

Supplements for *Medical-Surgical Nursing: An Integrated Approach* include an instructor's guide, student study guide, and computerized testbank.

- *Study Guide to Accompany Medical-Surgical Nursing: An Integrated Approach* has been designed to further challenge students as they work their way through the text content. Each of the 36 chapters includes an introduction summarizing the main points from the text, plus learning objectives, multiple choice questions formatted to prepare students for the NCLEX-PN exam, and a crossword puzzle. Some chapters also include additional exercises, such as true/false, nursing process fill-in tables, short answer, and critical thinking questions as well as anatomy & physiology labeling exercises. Answers to all the exercises are included in the appendix.
- *Instructor's Guide to Accompany Medical-Surgical Nursing: An Integrated Approach* includes answers to the text's review questions and suggested responses to the case studies, plus a set of anatomy & physiology transparency masters. A guide for using Chapter 37, Critical Thinking on Multiple Disorders is also included to help the instructor integrate this chapter into the curriculum.
- *Computerized Testbank to Accompany Medical-Surgical Nursing: An Integrated Approach* includes approximately 2,000 multiple choice questions formatted to prepare students for the NCLEX-PN exam.

ACKNOWLEDGMENTS

We are deeply indebted to Jill Rembetski for keeping us on track, providing guidance, and the many hours of putting it all together. Her humor and sensitivity made this project pleasant. Sarah Holle cheerfully made arrangements and kept our working trips to Albany enjoyable and productive. We have learned much from all the contributors and reviewers without whom this book could not have been completed. The encouraging, supportive words of various contributors and friends were deeply appreciated. We thank the numerous manufacturers, Lutheran College of Health Professions and Lutheran Hospital for providing photos and forms. We would also like to acknowledge the Ivy Tech State College for providing us with many gifted, intelligent ,and hard-working contributors.

We are grateful to all these people and everyone who helped this book become a reality. Thanks!

ABOUT THE AUTHORS

Lois White

Working as an RN for 38 years, in both the clinical and educational arena, has provided Lois with a wide range of experiences in nursing. Her education began in a diploma nursing program and progressed through the AS and BSN degrees. These were followed by an MS, with the focus on nursing education, and culminated with a PhD.

During her professional career, Lois has served as a staff nurse, inservice director, assistant professor in an associate degree nursing program and later as a professor and chairperson of a vocational nursing program. As a faculty member of the two nursing programs, she developed and taught many of the courses in the curricula. Serving as an NLN site visitor has given insight into student and program needs which must be met to provide the best in nursing education. As a member of the Nursing Education Advisory Committee (NEAC) for the State of Texas, Lois participated in identifying and categorizing entry level competencies for all levels of nursing: vocational (practical), diploma, ADN and BSN.

It is her sincerest hope that this book will both mentally stimulate and educate future nurses.

Gena Duncan

Gena has been a maternal-child nurse, medical-surgical nurse, and assistant head nurse of a medical unit. She taught practical nursing students for 15 years and is presently assistant professor in an ADN and BSN nursing program at Lutheran College of Health Professions. As a practical nursing instructor, she was a member of the statewide curriculum committee for the Ivy Tech State College.

She obtained a MSEd and a MS in community health nursing. Her research thesis was entitled *An Investigation of Learning Styles of Practical and Baccalaureate Students*. The results of the study are published in the Journal of Nursing Education. She is a member of Sigma Theta Tau.

Critical thinking and sound nursing judgment are essential in the present health care system. Gena's desire in producing this book is that students will develop into caring, competent nurses.

KEY FEATURES

Each chapter includes a variety of learning aids designed to help students further their understanding of key concepts. These include:

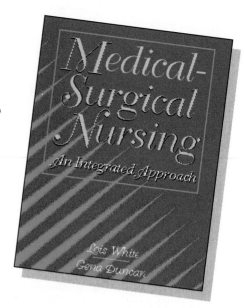

Medical-Surgical Nursing
An Integrated Approach

Lois White
Gena Duncan

CHAPTER
20
Cardiac Disorders

Gena Duncan

▶ **KEY TERMS**

angina pectoris
annulus
arteriosclerosis
ascites
atherosclerosis
automatic implantable cardioverter-
   defibrillator
cardiac catheterization
cardiac cycle
cardiac output
cardiac tamponade
depolarization
dyspnea
echocardiogram
ejection fraction
heart sound
hepatomegaly
hypertrophies
orthopnea
palpitation
paroxysmal nocturnal dyspnea
percutaneous balloon valvuloplasty
pericardial friction rub
pericardiocentesis
repolarization
stent
stroke volume
thallium scan
transesophageal echocardiography (TEE)

LIST OF DISORDERS

▶ Cardiac Dysrhythmias
Inflammatory Disorders
  ▶ Rheumatic Heart Disease
  ▶ Infective Endocarditis
  ▶ Myocarditis
  ▶ Pericarditis
  ▶ Valvular Heart Diseases
Occlusive Disorders
  ▶ Arteriosclerosis
  ▶ Atherosclerosis
  ▶ Angina Pectoris
  ▶ Myocardial Infarction
Decreased Function and Failure of Cardiac System
  ▶ Congestive Heart Failure
  ▶ Cor Pulmonale

LEARNING OBJECTIVES

Upon completion of this chapter the learner should be
able to:
• Define key terms.
• Describe the anatomy and physiology of the heart.
• Relate laboratory results to heart conditions.
• Describe basic heart dysrhythmias.
• Explain the pathophysiology of heart conditions.
• Describe nursing interventions in caring for clients
  with heart conditions.

CHAPTER 14 ▪ Fluid, Electrolyte, and Acid-Base Balances   267

COMMON DIAGNOSTIC TESTS

The following is a table of the commonly used diagnostic tests for clients who present electrolyte imbalances.

Test	Explanation/Normal Values	Nursing Responsibilities
Sodium (Na⁺)	Measure level of serum sodium 135–145 mEq/L. Function in the body: Major electrolyte in extracellular fluid Regulates fluid balance Stimulates conduction of nerve impulses Helps maintain neuromuscular activity	Explain to the client that blood will be drawn for this laboratory test. No food or fluid restrictions are required.
Potassium (K⁺)	Measure level of serum potassium 3.5–5.0 mEq/L	Explain to the client that blood will be drawn for this laboratory test. ...fluid restrictions are req...

▶ *MAKING THE CONNECTION*

Refer to the topics in the following chapters to increase your understanding of fluid, electrolyte and acid-base balance.

• **Chapter 13, Perioperative Nursing:** Postoperative, The Nursing Process in the Postoperative Care Unit, p. 247; Later Postoperative, p. 254.
• **Chapter 15, Oncology Nursing:** Oncological Emergencies, Hypercalcemia, p. 317.
• **Chapter 19, Respiratory Disorders:** Anatomy and Physiology Review, p. 388; Adult Respiratory Distress Syndrome (ARDS), p. 421; Acute Respiratory Failure, p. 423.
• **Chapter 20, Cardiac Disorders:** Congestive Heart Failure p. 455; Dysrhythmias, p. 456
• **Chapter 21, Vascular Disorders:** Anatomy and Physiology Review, p. 491.

• **Chapter 22, Blood and Lymph Disorders:** Anatomy and Physiology Review, Blood, p. 518.
• **Chapter 29, Endocrine Disorders:** Anatomy and Physiology Review, p. 780; Diabetes Insipidis, p. 800; Parathyroidism, p. 813; Adrenal Glands, p. 817; Addison's Disease, p. 819
• **Chapter 30, Diabetes:** Acute Complications of Diabetes, p. 840.
• **Chapter 34, Digestive Disorders:** Peritonitis, p. 992; Cirrhosis, p. 996; Pancreatitis, p. 1002.
• **Chapter 35, Urinary Disorders:** Anatomy and Physiology Review, p. 1015; Acute Renal Failure, p. 1039; Dialysis, p. 1048; Hemodialysis, p. 1048; Peritoneal Dialysis, p. 1049.
• **Chapter 36, Ostomies:** Pathophysiology of Bowel and Bladder, p. 1061.

KEY ABBREVIATIONS

The following abbreviations and acronyms are used in this chapter:

ABGs	arterial blood gases
ADH	antidiuretic hormone
Ca⁺	calcium ion
Cl⁻	chloride ion
CO₂⁻	carbon dioxide ion
ECF	extracellular fluid
H⁺	hydrogen ion
H₂CO₃	carbonic acid
H₂O	water
HCO₃	bicarbonate ion
ICF	intracellular fluid
K⁺	potassium ion
Na⁺	sodium ion
Mg⁺	magnesium ion
PCO₂ (PaCO₂)	partial pressure of carbon dioxide
pH	potential hydrogen, a scale that measures the acidity of a solution

Fluid Compartments

Approximately 60 percent of total human body weight is water, which is found in either intracellular compartments or extracellular compartments as shown in Figure 14-1. The majority of body fluid, or 65 percent, is located within cells and is known as intracellular fluid (ICF). The remaining body fluid, or 35 percent, is found outside the cell membranes and is called extracellular fluid (ECF).

ECF is divided into two subclassifications: interstitial fluids and intravascular fluids. Interstitial fluids are found in the spaces around cells. About three-fourths of all ECF is located in these interstitial compartments. Intravascular fluids are composed primarily of blood, plasma, and lymph located in blood and lymph vessels throughout the body. Tears, saliva, sweat, cerebrospinal fluid, digestive secretions, synovial fluid, aqueous humor, perilymph, endolymph, and serous fluid are sometimes classified as specialized extracellular fluids. A constant exchange of water occurs between the intracellular and extracellular compartments to maintain fluid balance.

Key Terms

1   Unfamiliar or critical vocabulary words are listed alphabetically at the beginning of each chapter and appear in bold on their first use within that chapter. These terms are later defined in a **Glossary** at the end of the text.

List of Disorders

All of the disorders discussed in Chapters 14 and 15 and 19 through 36 are listed in order of appearance at the beginning of each chapter for quick reference.   **2**

Learning Objectives

3   A series of student goals are presented at the beginning of each chapter to help students focus their study and use their time efficiently. The objectives are outcome-based to provide immediate feedback on progress.

Common Diagnostic Tests

These tables include the most common tests related to the disorders of each body system and appear in Chapters 14 and 15 and 19 through 36.   **4**

Making the Connection

5   This serves as each chapter's "quick reference," leading students from the chapter they are currently studying to related areas in the text. This helps them understand the interrelation of material and build upon their knowledge base.

Key Abbreviations

Lists of the abbreviations and acronyms used in each chapter, with meanings, are included for quick reference.   **6**

Sample Nursing Care Plans

7 Medical-surgical chapters include a sample nursing care plan that is based on a client scenario of a disorder discussed within that chapter. These serve as models for the students to refer to as they create their own care plans based on each chapter's case study.

Teaching Tips

8

Suggestions of the most effective ways to present information have been included in boxes throughout the text.

Case Study

9 Each chapter includes a client scenario and a list of accompanying questions to guide students through the development of a care plan.

Summary

10

Each chapter concludes with a bulleted list of the chapter's key concepts to help focus student study.

Review Questions and Critical Thinking Questions

11 A series of questions in standard format for the National Council Licensure Examination for Practical Nurses (NCLEX-PN) test student retention of each chapter's content. The NCLEX-PN format also helps familiarize students with the NCLEX-PN exam. Additional critical thinking questions help reinforce skills.

Medical Terminology

12

Common word parts related to medical-surgical chapters are included for quick reference.

News Flash

13 Real life events related to each chapter's content help students connect their course of study with the world of health care.

Glossary

14

A comprehensive glossary of the chapter terminology is included for reference.

References/Suggested Readings

15 This listing includes both the references used in each chapter and additional sources for further study. It is included at the end of the text for easy reference

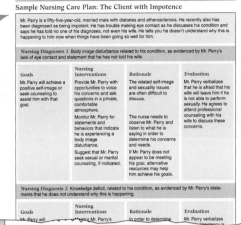

Sample Nursing Care Plan: The Client with Impotence

Mr. Parry is a fifty-five-year-old, married male with diabetes and atherosclerosis. He recently also has been diagnosed as being impotent. He has trouble making eye contact as he discusses his condition and says he has told no one of his diagnoses, not even his wife. He tells you he doesn't understand why this is happening to him now when things have been going so well for him.

Nursing Diagnoses 1 Body image disturbance related to his condition, as evidenced by Mr. Parry's lack of eye contact and statement that he has not told his wife.

Goals	Nursing Interventions	Rationale	Evaluation
Mr. Parry will achieve a positive self-image or seek counseling to assist him with that goal.	Provide Mr. Parry with opportunities to voice his concerns and ask questions in a private, comfortable atmosphere. Monitor Mr. Parry for statements and behaviors that indicate he is experiencing a body image disturbance. Suggest that Mr. Parry seek sexual or marital counseling, if indicated.	The related self-image and sexuality issues are often difficult to discuss. The nurse needs to observe Mr. Parry and listen to what he is saying in order to determine his concerns and needs. If Mr. Parry does not appear to be meeting his goal, alternative resources may help him achieve his goals.	Mr. Parry verbalizes that he is afraid that his wife will leave him if he is not able to perform sexually. He agrees to attend professional counseling with his wife to discuss these concerns.

Nursing Diagnosis 2 Knowledge deficit, related to his condition, as evidenced by Mr. Parry's statements that he does not understand why this is happening.

Goals	Nursing Interventions	Rationale	Evaluation
Mr. Parry will	Monitor Mr. Parry's	In order to determine	Mr. Parry verbalizes

▶ *Teaching Tip: Teaching the Client to Insert Vaginal Suppositories*

First, have the client wash her hands, then cleanse the vulva with a mild soap and warm water to remove any external discharge. Next, she should lie down in a supine position with her knees flexed. With one hand, the client can separate the labia and gently insert the suppository high inside the vagina. Once the suppository is in place, the client should remain supine for a minimum of thirty minutes to ensure adequate absorption of the medication through the vaginal mucosa.

▶ CASE STUDY

Mrs. Mary Keiver, a forty-year-old, African American school teacher, nullipara, was seen by her physician because of heavy menstrual bleeding. She stated that she had been saturating a sanitary pad every thirty minutes since early that same morning. She reported that her menstrual periods had been getting heavier for the past six months and were accompanied by severe cramping. She also noted that after her period she felt "physically drained." Other symptoms that Mary had observed included an increasing sense of heaviness in her pelvis and that her skirts and slacks were too tight around the abdomen, even though her weight had not changed significantly.

The following questions will guide your development of a nursing care plan for the case study.

1. List the clinical signs and symptoms manifested by this client that suggest that the heavy bleeding may be related to uterine fibroids.
2. List two reasons why a hemoglobin and hematocrit were ordered.
3. Describe what other diagnostic tests were ordered and why.
4. List the subjective and objective data the nurse should obtain during the assessment.
5. Write three individualized nursing diagnoses and goals for Mrs. Keiver.
6. Describe pertinent nursing actions/interventions to be taken in caring for this client prior to and following the D & C related to:
   - Bleeding
   - Cardiac output
   - Comfort/rest

SUMMARY

- Sexually transmitted diseases are among the most common infections occurring in the United States today.
- Despite massive education efforts, the number of new STD cases identified each year continues to grow.
- Early, intensive education regarding STDs is being utilized to help combat the high incidence of STDs, virtually an epidemic among young, urban-dwelling populations.
- Many STDs, such as gonorrhea, syphilis, and chlamydia, are treatable with antibiotics, but many others are caused by viruses and are not curable.
- The only solution to the problem of STDs is prevention.
- Identification of groups at risk for STDs and appropriate prevention teaching are the most effective weapons in the ongoing battle against STDs.

5. If a female client with chlamydia fails to complete treatment, complications that may arise in the future include:
   a. fever and headache.
   b. nausea, vomiting, and diarrhea.
   c. infertility and ectopic pregnancy.
   d. urinary retention.

Review Questions

1. When obtaining a health history from a client, the nurse asks the client to report on the presence of which of the following common symptoms of syphilis?
   a. nausea and vomiting
   b. fever, cellulitis, and diarrhea
   c. dysuria and mucopurulent discharge
   d. painless sore or ulcer in the genital area

2. The two most effective medications commonly used to treat chlamydia are:
   a. doxycycline and azithromycin.
   b. penicillin and podophyllum.
   c. erythromycin and acyclovir.
   d. doxycycline and penicillin.

3. The organism responsible for the spread of the sexually transmitted disease, syphilis, is known as a:
   a. bacteria.

Critical Thinking Questions

1. What would it be like to have syphilis or herpes vaginalis?
2. How would you tell your parents, boyfriend/girlfriend or spouse that you had an STD?
3. Develop a teaching plan for a client with multiple sexual partners. Consider the sensitivity of the information to be shared and the clients' receptivity.

Medical Terminology

cervic-	neck, cervix
cervicitis	inflammation of the cervix
condyl-	condyle, wart
condyloma	wart-like growth
cryo-	cold
cryosurgery	use of extreme cold in surgery
hyster-	uterus, womb
hysterectomy	surgical removal of the uterus
papill-	nipple-like protuberance or elevation
papilloma	nipple-like growth
papillomavirus	virus producing nipple-like growths
prostato-	prostate
prostatitis	inflammation of the prostate
salpingo-	uterine tube

294 **UNIT 4** ▶ Concepts of Medical-Surgical Care

5. A pH of 7.41 indicates:
   a. metabolic acidosis.
   b. impending coma.
   c. respiratory alkalosis.
   d. normal ph.

6. Respiratory acidosis develops as a result of:
   a. chronic obstructive pulmonary disease.
   b. diabetes mellitus.
   c. hyperventilation.
   d. nasogastric suctioning.

7. Diabetics who forget to take their insulin are prone to develop:
   a. metabolic alkalosis.
   b. respiratory alkalosis.
   c. metabolic acidosis.
   d. respiratory acidosis.

Critical Thinking Questions

1. How do you maintain fluid balance?
2. How would you feel having tube feedings?

MEDICAL TERMINOLOGY

Hyper-	an excess of

News Flash

The concentrated form of potassium chloride, supplied in 20 mEq per 20 mL vials, has been associated with more lethal medication errors than any other drug. Fatalities have occurred when it has been erroneously given IV push or added to an existing IV solution without thoroughly agitating the solution prior to administration. Government agencies, manufacturers, and hospitals have instituted guidelines to prevent potential dangers. Pharmaceutical companies have been mandated to package the concentrated form in black-capped vials. The print on the labels has been enlarged and includes the warning "Must Be Diluted." Based on regulatory agency recommendations, many hospitals have removed this concentrated form of potassium from nursing units. Instead, a 100 mL diluted solution is available. Physicians have been advised to avoid using the term "IV push" or "IV bolus" when ordering potassium intravenously. Hospital pharmacies have been given the sole responsibility of adding KCl to all IV solutions. Despite these changes, fatal errors continue to occur (Davis, 1995).

Nurses need to be especially cognizant of the inherent changes when administering potassium

SECTION

I

UNIT
1

Concepts Affecting Nursing Care

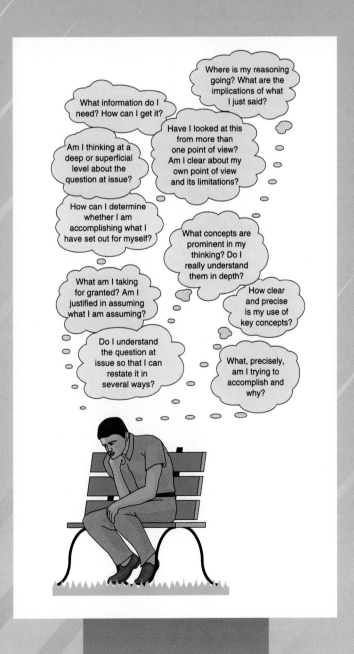

CHAPTER 1
Critical Thinking

Donna J. Burleson

► KEY TERMS

concept
critical thinking
discipline
disciplined
judgment
justify
logic
opinion
reasoning
reflectively
standard

LEARNING OBJECTIVES

Upon completion of this chapter the learner should be able to:
- Define key terms.
- Explain the relationship between critical thinking and the nursing process.
- State five characteristics of the person who uses critical thinking.
- Identify behaviors that illustrate the traits of a nurse who is a critical thinker.
- Assess own strengths and weaknesses in relation to critical thinking skills.
- Develop a personal plan for the enhancement of personal critical thinking and reasoning skills.

► MAKING THE CONNECTION

This chapter connects with every chapter in this text.

INTRODUCTION

Welcome to the continuing study of nursing. The purpose of this textbook is to help you and your instructors develop your ability to think like a nurse and to prepare you for nursing practice in the years to come. Ideally, you will view this text as a resource and use each feature to help you learn. Thinking as a nurse involves much more than gathering an assortment of facts and skills. Critical thinking in nursing education is not a separate component of the curriculum. It is "an approach to inquiry where both students and faculty examine clinical and professional issues and search for more effective answers" (Miller & Malcolm, 1990).

Nursing is part of a rapidly changing and increasingly complex society. Everyone who expects to have a successful career in nursing, at any level, must be able to compete effectively. This means that practical/vocational nurses must have good problem-solving skills and make quality decisions related to the client care they deliver. Over the last 15 years increasing attention has been paid to the need for graduates of educational programs at every level and in every **discipline** (branch of learning or field of study) to develop better thinking skills. Nurse educators have been among the leaders in the current movement to find ways to improve the thinking ability of their students. Nurses in clinical practice have also been challenged to improve their ability to reason clearly and logically. Because of these movements, you, as a beginning nursing student will find textbooks with activities planned to include "critical thinking skills." Take a moment now to review the study aids that are part of this and all chapters in this text.

The first features include a listing of **Key Terms**, action-oriented **Learning Objectives**, and a section called **Making the Connection**. Set a goal to accurately define and correctly use each of the key terms. Take the time to learn the exact way in which words and terms are used in nursing. The dictionary meaning often does not give the exact way a term is used by nurses. Understanding the meaning of terms, as they are used in nursing, will help you clarify the meaning of the material as you go along. Review the learning objectives before beginning your study period. The learning objectives tell you what you are expected to learn in each chapter and how you will know that you have learned it. You have mastered each objective when you can perform the action described in the learning objective. The section called Making the Connection appears in every chapter and is designed to help you understand how the chapter you are studying relates to the other chapters in this textbook and to your other courses. Often, other chapters will explore a topic in greater depth or with a different focus. For example, Chapter 5, Communication, discusses strategies for communicating effectively with clients. Chapter 6 explores communicating with clients who are from cultures different than your own. Thus, you can connect the information.

At the end of each chapter you will find one or more **Case Studies** or scenarios, a chapter **Summary**, **Review Questions**, **Medical Terminology**, **References and Suggested Readings**, and **Resources**. These features will also help you apply what you have learned and test what and how well you have learned. Do not neglect these activities or other similar activities your instructors have developed for you.

CRITICAL THINKING

The first step in improving your ability to think well is to develop an idea of what is meant by **critical thinking**. This involves much more than memorizing a simple definition of this process. The ability to think critically requires a great deal of effort and time. There are many definitions, all of which may be valuable, as you begin the process of learning to assess your own thinking and the quality of the thinking of others (see Figure 1-1). In fact, memorizing an exact definition of

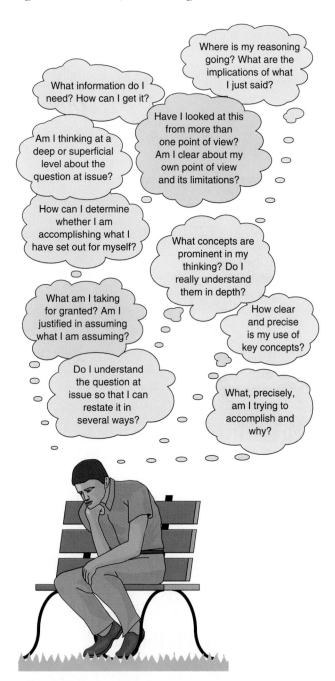

FIGURE 1-1 Assessing our own thinking. (*Courtesy The Foundation for Critical Thinking, Santa Rosa, CA*)

critical thinking would be detrimental to the full development of an understanding of this **disciplined** (trained by instruction and exercise) type of thinking. The **concept** of critical thinking includes the basic idea that one becomes a better thinker by developing specific attitudes, traits, and skills. A concept is a mental picture of abstract phenomena. Each person must learn to think **reflectively**, or introspectively, about his or her own thinking. Critical thinking was briefly described in this way in a workshop presented by Richard Paul (Paul & Willsen, 1993): "Critical thinking is that mode of thinking—about any subject, content, or problem—in which the thinker improves the quality of his or her thinking by skillfully taking charge of the structures inherent in thinking and imposing intellectual **standards** (or a level of degree of quality) upon them." To ensure integrity and consistency of the presentation in this chapter, the criteria, standards, and materials developed by the Center for Critical Thinking have been used as the organizing framework.

Penny Heaslip (1994), in a newsletter designed for nurse educators interested in the use of critical thinking within the nursing curriculum, presents a definition of critical thinking. This definition serves as a basis for your development of strategies and tactics as you begin the exciting experience of learning to think more clearly, and in a disciplined manner, about nursing. The definition is: "Critical thinking is the disciplined, intellectual process of applying skillful clinical **reasoning** (thinking to solve a problem) and self-reflective thinking as a guide to belief or action in nursing practice" (Heaslip, 1994; Norris & Ennis, 1989; Paul, 1990).

Table 1-1 contains some definitions of critical thinking. Review them and compare the elements that are common to all of them and the elements that are different.

Most of the authors who have written about critical thinking have addressed instructors. This chapter is written for you. This first chapter is designed to guide your process of thinking about and evaluating your own thinking. While your instructors want to help you with the process, you are ultimately responsible for your own thinking.

Barriers to Critical Thinking

Many students enter nursing programs unprepared to think critically. Many educators believe this inability may be the result of a lack of instruction in thinking. The result is similar to what would happen to you if you tried to play soccer without knowing the rules or having had a chance to learn the basic skills of the game. Quality thinking is like any skill; it takes practice and discipline to learn. This is a good time to do a self-evaluation related to your current ability to perform

Table 1-1

DEFINITIONS OF CRITICAL THINKING

"Reflective and reasonable thinking that is focused on deciding what to believe or do" (Ennis, 1985).

"An investigation whose purpose is to explore a situation, phenomenon, question, or problem to arrive at a hypothesis or conclusion about it that integrates all available information and that can therefore be convincingly justified" (Kurfiss, 1988).

"Critical thinking is the attentive commitment to a self-reflective process of examining one's thoughts ensuring that the thinking occurring meets intellectual standards" (Heaslip, 1993).

the four basic critical thinking processes: reading for meaning, writing clearly, listening critically, and speaking in a logical, coherent manner. If your basic education program did not emphasize all these skills, decide to develop these abilities.

New Information

The quantity of new information that you must be prepared to master is another barrier. Many students (and instructors) focus so intently on the content of a course that they allow little time to think about the material. The ability to think critically about the knowledge base of nursing is essential for learning the content of your nursing courses. The discipline of nursing has an organizing **logic**, or formal principles of a branch of knowledge, which serves to define the appropriate facts and methods required to produce effective nursing practice. This logic serves as a framework within which the student can construct a unique, meaningful system for the practice of nursing. Your nursing program probably has a philosophy and a statement of the main concepts that the nursing faculty uses to present the course material in a logical framework.

Activity

If you have not reviewed your program's philosophy and main concepts with the idea that they will help you understand your program of study, this would be a good time to do so. Most programs of nursing include the philosophy statement, organizing concepts and program outcomes in the student handbook or other document provided to students. To use these resources to help you use your own logic to discover the logic of nursing as presented in your program try the following activities:

1. Identify the major concepts (such as nursing, learning, caring) that provide structure for your program's philosophy and organization.
2. Discuss the components or parts of each major mental picture with your classmates and instructors.
3. Use your own words to see how your mental pictures of these ideas may be the same or different from those in your program materials.
4. Review the material you have already covered in your nursing program to identify how the major parts of each course relate to these concepts.
5. Look at the objectives for this course and the topics in this textbook to see how they will relate to the main ideas you have discovered in this activity.

The Nursing Process

The main process of applying the logic of nursing is the use of the nursing process. The nursing process is derived from the problem-solving process that is basic to every discipline. To use the nursing process effectively you must be able to develop the skills of critical thinking. These are the skills and attitudes you need to reason well and solve problems effectively.

Beginning nursing students must be careful to understand that the nursing process is not a set, rote formula. If it is not understood as a framework for problem-solving, it may actually become a deterrent to critical thinking. As you study each part of your medical-surgical course, use the nursing process as a framework. Seek to understand the use that will be made of each concept and principle related to the nursing process. If you can do this, the facts will become easier to acquire, understand, and apply.

Student Responsibility

Finally, many students find the process of becoming responsible for their own thinking to be painful. For many students the education processes that were part of their basic school preparation were based upon a very structured approach to acquiring selected facts and skills. Then the students' recall was tested by using "objective" tests. If this was your experience, you may view learning as the result of the teacher's actions in presenting what must be learned and devising "fair" tests. Your own input to the process may seem to be of less importance than that of the teacher. You, along with many other students, may find that you are uncomfortable when you are asked to decide what is important or to be able to defend your **opinions** (subjective beliefs) and **judgments** (conclusions based on sound reasoning and supported by evidence). You may prefer to be told, with no ambiguity, what you need to know. Nursing, however, does not take place in predictable, highly structured events.

Practical/vocational nurses are required to make decisions at many levels. Knowing how to make good decisions begins with developing the essential skills, traits, and attitudes associated with critical thinking.

THE SKILLS OF CRITICAL THINKING

Four basic skills are necessary for the development of higher level thinking skills. These skills are part of the process of developing and using thinking for problem-solving and reasoning. Your abilities in these four areas can be measured by the extent to which you are achieving the universal intellectual standards. These standards are discussed in the following section and are illustrated in Table 1-2. These four basic skills are critical reading, critical listening, meaningful writing, and coherent speaking.

Critical Reading Skills

Reading for meaning is basic to the acquisition of knowledge from textbooks and journals. The student who can read critically will also do better on tests. Study time will be reduced and retention of material will be enhanced. An exercise that can help build reading skills is to use a highlighter pen to mark the main idea of a sentence. Students who have not learned to read critically will find that they have

---

Table 1-2

THE SPECTRUM OF UNIVERSAL INTELLECTUAL STANDARDS

Clear	Unclear
Precise	Imprecise
Relevant	Irrelevant
Accurate	Inaccurate
Deep	Superficial
Significant	Insignificant
Consistent	Inconsistent
Broad	Narrow
Logical	Illogical
Realistic	Unrealistic
Sufficient	Insufficient
Appropriate	Inappropriate
Justifiable	Unjustifiable
Reasonable	Unreasonable
Rational	Irrational
Fair	Unfair
Insightful	Undiscerning

(*Courtesy The Foundation for Critical Thinking, Santa Rosa, CA*)

marked most of the text. Joining a study group may help you identify main ideas by comparing with others the various main ideas each of you have derived from the same material. During test reviews you can make sure to note when misreading or misinterpretation caused an error on the test. By making a conscious effort to identify your individual weaknesses, you will improve your critical reading skills. Another tactic you can try is to practice restating the main idea to yourself or to another student. As you read the text have a dialogue with yourself, which could go something like this: "What is the reason for studying this material? How does this relate to what I already know? This does not seem to fit. Did I misunderstand? Can I say this in my own words?" Worrell (1990) has developed a useful tool for guiding your dialogue. It is illustrated in Table 1-3.

Critical Listening

Communication skills, especially listening skills receive a great deal of emphasis in the nursing curriculum. Even so, many persons do not have effective listening skills. One reason is that many people have developed the habit of tuning in only occasionally to orally presented material. The result is that the meaning of the oral communication is lost. A way to improve your listening skills is to try to restate the points made in a discussion with another student and have that student give feedback about how accurately you have restated her position. Critical listening also requires that you carry on a mental dialogue with the speaker. For instance, as you listen, focus on what the speaker is saying, listen for key points, notice anything that seems confusing to you as well as those points you already understand.

Review the materials in your communication skills classes and in Chapters 5 and 6 of this text for more techniques to improve this area. Critical listening requires that you make a conscious commitment to focus on the topic of discussion. This means that you should actively attend to the words and meanings of the speaker. Your ability to recognize things that distract your attention is a valuable tool to increase listening skills. Some distracters for students are attempting to take word-by-word notes, focusing on the mannerism or appearance of the speaker, and daydreaming. As in all areas, a good thinker is not afraid to identify weaknesses and strengths in order to improve.

Critical Writing

The ability to state one's thoughts coherently, clearly, and concisely is basic to good thinking skills. Many students arrive at college unable to write well. The discipline required to state facts and judgments well improves the quality of thinking. Many students

Table 1-3

STRATEGIC READING LIST

The following questions serve as a guide for self-talk when you are learning from reading texts or journal articles. An effective reader is an active, strategic reader! Soon you will find yourself using these and other questions that you have developed automatically, no longer needing the checklist.

PREREADING QUESTIONS
1. Have I previewed (skimmed) the title, headings and subheadings, objectives, and overview?
2. Do the headings/subheadings identify main ideas?
3. What is the chapter about?
4. How is the content related to what I already know?
5. How has the author organized the material? How will this organization help me?
6. Will I need other resources as I read?
7. Based on previewing, what questions should I formulate to guide my reading?

QUESTIONS DURING READING
1. Does this make sense to me?
2. Do I need to look up any unfamiliar words?
3. Do I need to reread difficult material? Or will this be explained further if I read on?
4. Is the author using signal words (first, next, therefore, as a result, etc.)?
5. How is this information related to what I know?
6. How is this section linked to the previous section?
7. Can I summarize this section before going any further?
8. Can I answer my prereading questions? Can I formulate new questions?

QUESTIONS AFTER READING
1. Do I understand the main points?
2. Can I outline the content?
3. How is this related to previous learning?
4. How would I use or apply this information?
5. Are there points that I need to clarify? How will I do this?
6. What questions would likely be on an exam from this material?
7. Can I answer my questions, paraphrase the content, and link main points without looking at my notes or text?

From: Worrell, P. J. (1990). Metacognition: Implications for instruction in nursing education. *Journal of Nursing Education, 29*(4): 170–175.

(Courtesy Journal of Nursing Education, SLACK Incorporated, Thorofare, NJ)

are afraid to write down their thoughts, as though writing is too revealing. Writing also requires discipline. It is important for the improvement of thinking because it can be reviewed using the Universal Intellectual Standards to evaluate the quality of the thinking reflected in the writing. These standards are discussed in greater detail later in the chapter. You may also refer back to Table 1-2.

A technique for improving the quality of your thinking through writing might be to summarize, in your own words, the main idea in a reading assignment. Then use that main idea in relation to a client care problem from the material you are studying. Put the writing away until the next day and reread it. Can you understand it? Then submit it to a friend for critique. Could your friend understand what you meant to say? How could it be improved? Improving your writing skills may not seem like fun, but it is an effective and vital process for improving the quality of your own thinking.

Critical Speaking

Perhaps the most neglected skill is disciplined speaking. We do not hear many examples of clear, logical, accurate spoken communication. Oral communication is different from written communication. It is usually more spontaneous and must be carefully presented since the communication, unless recorded, is present only for the moment. Ambiguous statements are misleading. Personal biases influence what the other person hears. Practicing in a small group with feedback from the listeners can help a student assess and improve this skill.

STANDARDS FOR CRITICAL THINKING

The simple definition of critical thinking used in the previous section includes the provision that the assessment of your own thinking relies on the use of universal standards for quality thinking. As you begin to develop and apply critical thinking to nursing, the first requirement is to become familiar with these standards. The Spectrum of Universal Intellectual Standards developed by The Center for Critical Thinking is used for this presentation because it provides a valid and reliable measure for the quality of thinking. Whether you are reading the assigned material from a textbook, listening to an oral presentation, writing a paper, answering test questions, or presenting ideas in oral form, the following standards should be applied.

Clarity vs. Unclarity

Fundamental to quality thinking is the ability to think clearly. To think clearly means that you can place the facts and ideas of course content into a logical and coherent framework. The measure for the degree to which this is true is the degree to which you can state these relationships orally or in writing so others can understand your position. One tactic for increasing your clarity of thought is to pay particular attention to the exact meaning of the words encountered. The year that you spend in the practical/vocational nursing program is filled with many new terms and concepts. Time spent in practicing the appropriate use of these terms and in applying concepts appropriately will result in improved clarity of thought and increased retention of content. You can use small study groups to challenge one another to write and speak clearly as you review content together.

A review of the words used in the preceding paragraph may illustrate how the meaning of words can be misunderstood. For example, think about the word "clarity." When you look up the word in a dictionary, you find that there are several shades of meaning. Look up the word for yourself and decide which of the definitions applies to the use of clarity in describing a standard for critical thinking.

Think about some expressions you use every day. Would someone who is from another part of the country understand them? An example is the use of the term "this evening" which is common in some parts of the South. If someone told you they would visit you "this evening," when would you expect them? In some places, the person might arrive in the early afternoon, in other places, at night. When speaking to clients, families, and other health team members the nurse must be sure that the words used clearly express the intended message. When reading or listening, do not assume that you understand a term. Take the time to verify the meaning. Chapter 5 contains material that will provide more information about therapeutic communication. There are specific methods for ensuring clarity of communication.

Precision vs. Imprecision

Sometimes, we have a "ballpark" mentality. That is, we learn enough about a subject to be "in the ballpark," but not enough to hit a home run. The result is a general idea of the meaning of a fact or idea, but not enough understanding to apply it or to use the information for problem-solving or promoting communication of an idea to someone else. You may be making this mistake if you find yourself saying something like this: "I knew that, but on the test they stated it differently." Precision of thought means that the meaning of a concept is clearly understood with its relationship to other concepts and to its practical implications, so that the thought is exact, accurate, and definite (Paul & Willsen, 1993).

Specificity vs. Vagueness

Specificity means that the student can be concrete or exact in stating or applying a fact. An example of vagueness, which can be commonly ascribed to nursing students, occurs during the use of the planning phase of the nursing process when students do not write concrete nursing interventions. For example, a student may state that the nursing action will "provide support to the client and his family." It is difficult to explain exactly what this statement means, either in general or in relation to this client and this nurse. Appropriate planning involves deciding upon definite, well-stated nursing diagnoses, goals, and nursing actions. The use of the nursing process requires that the student learn the degree of specificity required for each nursing situation. State or itemize the nursing actions to be performed.

Accuracy vs. Inaccuracy

Accuracy means correct and within the proper parameters. Nursing students can readily understand the need for accurate calculation of a drug dose or the accurate measurement of blood pressure. In the same way the collection and interpretation of data must be accurate. Accuracy usually infers the use of some measuring instrument. In the case of blood pressure, this is easy to see. In the case of accuracy of thinking it may be harder to visualize. An example would be when the nurse uses the term hypertension to mean someone who is anxious and hyperactive instead of the actual meaning, an elevation of blood pressure above the accepted normal maximum. When dealing with more abstract concepts, accuracy of interpretation and understanding are equally important. Students can improve the accuracy of their thinking by trying to write new information in their own words and having another student interpret what this means. Inaccurate information will become evident. Accurate recording of findings during client care is essential to quality care. Accurate understanding of the concepts underlying each part of your medical-surgical course, plus understanding the ways in which each part of your nursing course relates to this client, will enable you to be more accurate in your thinking.

It is understood that there are degrees of accuracy. For example, you could measure a client's temperature with a thermometer that could measure 0.01 degree, but it is obvious that this degree of accuracy is unnecessary. On the other hand, when figuring a pediatric dosage a difference of 0.01 can be important. One of your challenges is to increase your awareness of the degree of accuracy required in nursing situations.

Relevance vs. Irrelevance

Relevance refers to the ability to separate needed information from information that is not needed at the moment. Students may spend time arguing for a position that does not matter. For instance, students may

get sidetracked from the purpose of an exercise by failing to limit their response to a question to the central issue or heart of the problem to be solved. It is also important to be able to recognize when sufficient relevant information is not available. An example of failing to recognize relevant information might involve ignoring the client's comment that his rash began the day after starting a new medication. On the other hand, the nurse may assume that a client is depressed about being in the hospital and so fail to ask him why he seems sad.

During the study process you can ask yourself how a particular concept is relevant to the application of the nursing process to client care. **Justify** (prove or show to be valid) your ideas to yourself and to another student.

Consistency vs. Inconsistency

Consistency means that principles and concepts are used appropriately for related applications. For instance, if you are using a particular nursing diagnosis based upon accepted indicators, it should be applied when those indicators are present and should not be used if the indicators are not present. Failure to follow this standard results in inconsistent use of a nursing diagnosis.

Consistency can also refer to the habit of recognizing and using basic concepts appropriately whenever they apply. For example, knowing the basic actions of epinephrine will enable the student to predict client responses to the administration of the drug or when a client situation triggers increased secretion of epinephrine and norepinephrine.

Logical vs. Illogical

To be logical means to build one idea upon another so that the conclusion is based upon a sequence of steps. Each step should be reasonable and related to the step before it and the step afterward. Many symptoms that clients exhibit can be understood logically, based upon your knowledge of normal physiology and the changes produced by the person's disease. The successful student will make more efficient use of study time by identifying the logical basis of the material being considered.

The author of a nursing textbook uses nursing logic to organize the content of the book. You must use your own logic to grasp the meaning of the material. Do this by discovering the logic of the author. In this way you will begin to think within the logic of nursing.

Depth vs. Superficiality

Busy students are tempted to determine how much material they need to master by relying on finding the answers to specific learning objectives and on the teacher's pre-test review. This may result in only a superficial understanding of basic processes and principles. Students can improve their ability to recognize the depth to which they must explore concepts and ideas. For some areas, time should not be spent on material that is not relevant. There is no easy way to do this, but knowing that different material requires different depth of study can assist the student. With time, these decisions will be easier to make. Your instructor and the learning aids within your textbook are useful guides. The more you use them, the better you will become at identifying relevant information and the appropriate depth of knowledge required to make good clinical decisions.

Completeness vs. Incompleteness

During the assessment phase of client care it is important for the nurse to know when the client data base is sufficiently complete. Proper nursing care is based upon identification of priority needs. The nurse will provide care only for those problems that have been identified. Although the physician orders treatments and nursing observations related to the medical diagnosis, these orders are not meant to direct all required care. Nursing care is essential to client well-being. Incomplete information or analysis of client needs will result in inappropriate or inadequate nursing care. Of course, your ability to identify and prioritize client care problems depends on the completeness of your knowledge base. This standard is related to accuracy. An incomplete data base leads to inaccurate conclusions.

Significance vs. Triviality

When making decisions or sorting out information it is important for the nurse to identify information that is necessary for good decision making. Recognition of irrelevant facts or data that are not helpful for the problem at hand is an important skill. It is easy for a student to view all the material in a textbook as equally significant. Learning to identify significant (important) concepts will help you avoid being distracted by trivial materials.

Adequacy vs. Inadequacy

In solving problems or exploring a subject, adequacy refers to the degree to which the available information is sufficient for the purpose and the amount of time and effort spent on the matter. When making clinical decisions, the nurse must be able to recognize when there is sufficient information upon which to base a decision. Premature closure of the process or the inability to decide because of fear that there is not enough information are equally detrimental to quality thinking.

As you study each chapter you will be given information that will help you identify the basic information required to care for each client problem. Knowing that good client care decisions are based on good preparation by the nurse can help you fit information into the logic of nursing.

Fairness vs. Bias

You, along with other students, come to the educational setting with a set of beliefs, opinions, and points of view. Each person is predisposed to believe that what they think is true must be true. The improvement of the quality of your thinking depends on your ability to identify the biases present in your thinking and the biases that are present in the thinking of others. Commitment to fairness will lead a person to challenge conclusions in the light of the presence or absence of personal bias. A nursing example would be the assessment of a person in pain. Each individual has learned a way to respond to pain: some become quiet, some complain loudly, some are stoic, some are emotional. When a nurse who has a stoic response to pain assesses a person who has an emotional response to pain it is possible to allow personal values to influence the assessment. This can lead to stereotyping of a client as a "cry baby" with the result that the nurse provides inadequate pain control for this person.

REASONING AND PROBLEM-SOLVING

Reasoning has been defined as the process of figuring things out by using critical thinking skills. Although reasoning involves thinking, all thinking is not reasoning. A human being is thinking when daydreaming, jumping to conclusions, stereotyping, or deciding to listen to music. None of these activities can be called reasoning. In order to use reasoning, to figure things out, or to problem-solve, the student must become familiar with the elements that comprise reasoning. These elements are purpose, a question at issue, assumptions, point of view, information, concepts, inferences and conclusions, implications and consequences (Paul & Willsen, 1993). Table 1-4 illustrates the elements of thought in reasoning.

Table 1-4

THE ELEMENTS OF THOUGHT IN REASONING

1. All reasoning has A PURPOSE.
   - Take time to state your purpose clearly.
   - Distinguish your purpose from related purposes.
   - Check periodically to be sure you are still on target.
   - Choose significant and realistic purposes.

2. All reasoning is an attempt TO FIGURE SOMETHING OUT, TO SETTLE SOME QUESTION, TO SOLVE SOME PROBLEM.
   - Take time to clearly and simply state the question at issue.
   - Express the question in several ways to clarify its meaning and scope.
   - Break the question into sub-questions.
   - Identify if it is a factual question, a preference question, or a question that requires reasoning.

3. All reasoning is based on ASSUMPTIONS.
   - Clearly identify your assumptions and check for their probable validity.
   - Check the consistency of your assumptons.
   - Reexamine your question at issue when assumptions prove insupportable.

4. All reasoning is done from some POINT OF VIEW.
   - Identify your own point of view and its limitations.
   - Seek other points of view and identify their strengths as well as weaknesses.
   - Strive to be fairminded in evaluating all points of view.

5. All reasoning is based on DATA, INFORMATION, AND EVIDENCE.
   - Restrict your claims to those supported by sufficient data.
   - Lay out the evidence clearly.
   - Search for information against your position and explain its relevance.

6. All reasoning is expressed through, and shaped by, CONCEPTS AND IDEAS.
   - Identify each concept that is needed to explore the problem, and precisely define it.
   - Explain the choice of important concepts and the implications of each.
   - Define when concepts are used vaguely or inappropriately.

7. All reasoning contains INFERENCES by which we draw CONCLUSIONS and give meaning to data.
   - Tie inferences tightly and directly from evidence to conclusions.
   - Seek inferences that are deep, consistent, and logical.
   - Identify the relative strength of each of your inferences.

8. All reasoning leads somewhere, has IMPLICATIONS AND CONSEQUENCES.
   - Trace out a variety of implications and consequences that stem from your reasoning.
   - Search for negative as well as positive consequences.
   - Anticipate unusual or unexpected consequences from various points of view.

(*Courtesy The Foundation for Critical Thinking, Santa Rosa, CA*)

Purpose

All reasoning is directed toward some specific purpose. This is one way in which it is different from daydreaming. In the case of the nursing student the purpose of reasoning is to effectively solve client care problems. During your formal education process you will use reasoning to discover the logic of the practice of nursing.

The Question at Issue

The reasoning process has as its purpose the solution to some problem. This problem must be clearly defined. At the beginning of each study period you must be able to state clearly the particular problems presented by this particular material. In the clinical setting, good clinical judgment begins with the clear statement of the problems presented by each client. One purpose of the nursing process is to arrive at significant client problems that are stated with sufficient clarity and simplicity to enable appropriate responses by the nurse.

Assumptions

Assumptions are those ideas or things that are taken for granted. In the process of reasoning, you must be aware of the assumptions that are made in contrast to the facts that are known. Assumptions are accepted as true without examination. Assuming certain things may be helpful in problem-solving but an attempt should be made to recognize the assumptions. An example of an assumption is the idea that nursing makes a difference in the outcome of a client's illness. It is evident that this is a necessary assumption for the nurse to engage in problem-solving related to client care needs, but it is also important for the nurse to examine this assumption from time to time. One of the issues in nursing today is the question of what nurses do and what preparation is necessary.

It is important to remember that assumptions that have proven reliable can help in decision making. It is just as true that faulty assumptions may cause you to make faulty conclusions and lead to poor problem-solving. Learn to recognize your own assumptions and those of others. Never be afraid to challenge your own assumptions or to ask others to clarify the assumptions they are using.

Point of View

Each person reasons using his own logic. This logic consists of previous experience, the quality of thinking acquired already, available information, and many other factors. These factors work together to give each person a unique way of thinking and a unique perspective. This unique perspective determines the individual's point of view. This can be visualized by thinking about what a person can see from a small window as compared to a view of the same landscape from an airplane. Each person will see things differently. They may both see a house, but may differ in what they see. In the same way, the individual's point of view determines what facts and information will be noticed, the relative importance assigned to each bit of information, and even the acceptable solutions to the problem. You must take the time to recognize your own point of view and to affirm the right of others to have their own point of view.

Data, Information, and Evidence

Data and information are the basic material of reasoning. These are needed in order to define the prob-

lem under consideration and also find the solution. During the nursing education program you may often feel overwhelmed by the quantity of data and information that is presented to you. The result may be that you attempt to practice rote memorization. If data and information are seen as the evidence for reasoning and for problem-solving the process will be more than an exercise in memory. There is a logical relationship between the ideas and facts comprising the content of the nursing course. This logic can be discovered by reasoning. Once the logic is found, the use of the information for problem-solving will become possible. Be sure to also look for evidence against your position.

The nursing process steps related to the collection, analysis, and classification of data are assessment and evaluation. Your course in medical-surgical nursing will devote a considerable amount of time to the concepts required to identify appropriate data related to client care.

Concepts and Ideas

The evidence given in support of a conclusion consists of one or more statements relating the conclusion to the problem and to the supporting facts. Reasons must be logically related to the information; in other words, the conclusion cannot be based on something apart from the reasoning process. The concepts (such as pain, adaptation, and so on) that support the nursing process must be part of the evidence supporting a nursing judgment.

Inferences and Conclusions

Reasoning requires interpretation of facts and information. The interpretation must be justifiable in light of the relevant facts. It must be supported by logical connections to the problem and to appropriate data and information. Such interpretation can be called a judgment or inference. Too many times students state opinions as judgments or inferences. This occurs when interpretations are based on personal preferences, not on the information that is pertinent to the solution of the problem and the use of accepted authoritative information.

This way of reaching judgments or inferences is basic to thinking well. An inference results from this kind of thinking: "Because that is true, then this must be true." For example, you have learned that when the body's temperature goes above normal, the body's metabolic rate increases. You also know that increased metabolism requires more oxygen for the tissues. One way more oxygen can be delivered to the tissues is to increase the heart rate. From these facts you can infer that an elevated body temperature may result in an increased heart rate.

The product of reasoning is a conclusion in regard to the problem. The conclusion is the answer to the question that began the process. The conclusion must be logical and must answer the question. It must be based on the proper information and be logically related to the question.

Implications and Consequences

As an outcome of the reasoning process, more than one solution will usually be apparent. At this point, it will be necessary to examine the implications of each solution. This may include thinking about the ease with which a solution can be applied, the ability of a person to carry out the required actions, or the risks involved.

The outcomes of a particular approach to a problem under consideration are important. Consequences can result from action or inaction. Responsible problem-solving requires that all known consequences are acknowledged. Of course, it is not possible to predict all consequences, but the possible outcomes should be examined as completely as possible.

THE TRAITS OF A DISCIPLINED THINKER

The presentation in this chapter of some of the requirements of critical thinking will not make anyone think critically. By incorporating the idea that thinking about the quality of your own thinking in relation to universal intellectual standards is a desirable goal, you can improve your own thinking. Improved thinking is not something that can be acquired in a day or two. It is like any high level skill: it takes time, effort, and disciplined practice. The result is well worth it. Consistent efforts to improve your thinking can result in the acquisition of the traits of an educated person (Paul & Willsen, 1993). These traits or habitual characteristic ways of thinking can be recognized by others and make the person able to compete successfully in the high-tech world.

Reasonable

The educated person will be reasonable. This simply means that the person values reasoning in himself and in others. This person will not be interested in placing blame or dodging responsibility. There will be a commitment to problem-solving and to cooperative efforts aimed at logically solving the problems encountered in the workplace.

Humility

Another quality that results from consistent efforts to practice disciplined thinking is intellectual humility. To be intellectually humble means that an individual is aware of how much she does not know. There will be a willingness to examine conclusions and beliefs based on new evidence. There will be respect for the thoughts and ideas of others and a sense of continually learning and improving one's own thinking.

Courageous

The thinking person will be intellectually courageous. One of the characteristics of this trait is a willingness to take unpopular positions based upon reasoning. The conclusions and beliefs that direct activities will be the result of disciplined thinking, not the opinions of the group.

Integrity

Integrity refers to the constancy of one's actions based upon reasoning. The same standards are applied consistently; standards are not changed to suit circumstances or personal prejudices. The result is a person whose behavior is in harmony with his thinking.

Perseverance

Finally, this person will be capable of intellectual perseverance. This means that there is a willingness to undertake the challenge of completing hard intellectual tasks. Not giving up, pursuing a solution until its conclusion, and maintaining the quality of thinking are the qualities related to this trait.

CRITICAL THINKING AND THE NURSING PROCESS

The purpose of the nursing education program is to help you develop the logic of nursing. Another way to state this is to say that you will learn to think like a nurse. The method that nurses have adopted to implement the practice of nursing is called the nursing process. The nursing process is an application of the problem-solving process to the practice of nursing. A form of the problem-solving process is part of every scientific or human service discipline. The use of the nursing process requires critical thinking. If you can find the relationship between the content of the textbooks and the logic of nursing you will find the study of nursing to be an exciting and challenging process. Use of the nursing process will thus become the means by which the quality of your thinking is improved. The use of reasoning will enhance your use of the nursing process.

▶ *CASE STUDY*

At this point in subsequent chapters you will be given a client scenario or case study. This activity will be designed to give you an opportunity to apply the knowledge and skills you have gained. This will mean that you will be expected to use critical thinking skills to apply the nursing process as you explore selected nursing situations.

For this chapter the scenario is to be written by you and about you. In order to do this, you will use the nursing process to develop your plan for improving and utilizing your reasoning and thinking skills. This is a suggested way for you to approach this exercise.

1. Review the four basic skills for critical thinking: reading, writing, listening, and speaking.

2. Utilize the nursing process step of assessment to assess your skills in each area. Assessment implies that you will use the standards for skill in each of these areas to identify your own strengths and weaknesses.

3. Identify specifically the precise skills you want to improve. Write in your own words what you want to accomplish in terms of positive skills you will possess when you have implemented your plan and accomplished your goal. This means that you will identify specific performance measures for your reading, writing, speaking, and listening skills and time frames for points at which you will evaluate your performance. For example, if you set a goal of being able to identify the main points of assigned reading, how would you measure that? By comparison with others in your study group? By your test performance? Write down your evaluation criteria and the time for evaluation. This step corresponds to the nursing process steps of diagnosis and goal setting.

4. When you have clearly stated in writing which basic skills you will work on, you are ready to move to the next step of the nursing process, which is planning. Review the material in this chapter or from other resources to identify possible ways to work on your skills. Choose the most appropriate methods for you. Write down your plan. Be precise and specific.

5. Your next step, as in the nursing process, is to actually put your plan in action by doing what you have planned to do. This is the implementation step.

6. The final step of the nursing process is evaluation. This simply means look to see if your actions have resulted in the desired outcome. In order to perform a valid evaluation, you must have something with which to measure. In the case of the nursing process in client care, evaluation is based on the goals that were set during the problem identification and goal-setting steps. When the time for evaluation arrives, you make a judgment about how well your goal has been met. If the goal is met, reassess for the next area needing work and

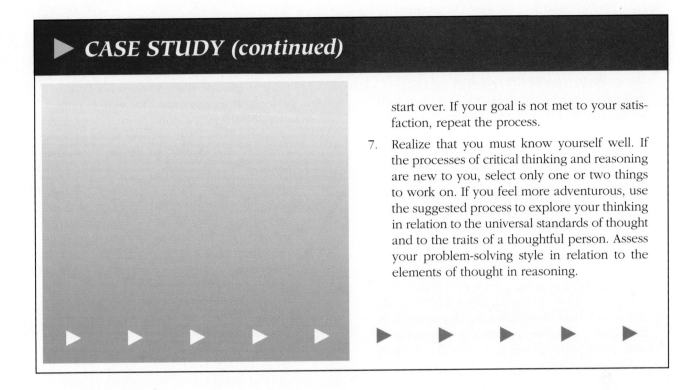

▶ **CASE STUDY (continued)**

start over. If your goal is not met to your satisfaction, repeat the process.

7. Realize that you must know yourself well. If the processes of critical thinking and reasoning are new to you, select only one or two things to work on. If you feel more adventurous, use the suggested process to explore your thinking in relation to the universal standards of thought and to the traits of a thoughtful person. Assess your problem-solving style in relation to the elements of thought in reasoning.

SUMMARY

- Critical thinking is a disciplined way of thinking that the nursing student can begin to develop. The effective use of the nursing process depends on the ability to think well.
- There are many ways to define critical thinking, but an exact definition does not lead anyone to become a good thinker. Essential components of any definition should emphasize that critical thinking is concerned with self-assessment of the quality of one's own thinking, according to standards of excellence and careful use of the elements of reasoning.
- There are four basic intellectual skills that are essential to quality thinking. These skills are critical reading, critical writing, critical listening, and critical speaking.
- The Spectrum of Universal Intellectual Standards can be the measure of competence in each of the basic skills.
- Reasoning is the process of applying critical thinking to some problem, to find an answer, to figure something out. Therefore, reasoning has a purpose. The process of reasoning requires that attention be paid to the elements of thought in reasoning and to the universal intellectual standards.
- When students begin to be aware of their own thinking and begin to assume responsibility for it, they will begin to use their own logic to discover the logic of nursing. The result will be better learning and the ability to use the nursing process to make high quality decisions related to client care.

- Consistent attention to improving the quality of thinking will produce the traits of an educated nurse. The student will become intellectually reasonable, humble, courageous, and possess intellectual integrity and perseverance.

Review Questions

This section in the following chapters will have a set of NCLEX style review questions. It will be important for you to understand that these questions provide an opportunity for you to practice your growing critical thinking skills. It is tempting to use review questions simply as a way to collect an isolated fact—the "correct" answer to this question. To improve your test-taking skills, look at each question as an opportunity to apply reasoning skills. To illustrate this, let's look at a possible thought pattern applied to a sample question.

Do not be concerned if you do not know the answer to this sample question. It has been selected deliberately to represent some knowledge you will probably be presented later in the course so that you will not guess or try to choose the answer intuitively. Focus on the thought processes illustrated.

Question: What is the most basic assessment to make about a client receiving IV potassium?

a. hourly urine output
b. vital signs
c. neuromuscular status
d. EKG recordings

This is an example of an approach to answering this question using the elements of thought in reasoning:

1. What is the purpose of this question? Why did the instructor choose this question?

    Possible answer: to test how well I understand the nursing implications for the IV administration of potassium.

2. State the problem to be solved. What is the question at issue?

    Possible answer: The question asks me to identify the most basic assessment to make when a client is receiving IV potassium. The key here is to identify the basic assessment that an LP/VN would be expected to make.

3. Read all of the possible answers in light of the question at issue. Apply the process of reasoning to each of them. Remember, it is as important to know why an answer is wrong for this question as to know why an answer is right. Let's look at each possible response.

    a. hourly urine output

        This may be a good choice because it is an assessment that you as an LP/VN will be prepared to make. Your knowledge base will also have provided the information that potassium is a vital electrolyte that is excreted by the kidney. You will also have learned that it can accumulate in the serum when urine output is decreased. This accumulation can lead to the adverse effects of too much potassium. At this point, you will consider this a good candidate for the right answer, but you will want to consider the other options as well.

    b. vital signs

        This looks good. Most students consider assessment of vital signs a good answer most of the time. Let's look at the evidence. Your knowledge base has included the information that a potassium deficit or excess can affect the blood pressure and the regularity of the heart beat. Before you select this answer, however, ask yourself when does this effect take place? When the levels are abnormal. What is the greatest danger of IV potassium? Too much potassium. But here is the key question: what is the most basic

assessment to make for IV potassium? What can cause the potassium level to be too high in this situation? Decreased excretion of potassium, which comes from decreased urine output. So this answer is not best for this question. Assessing vital signs is important and should be done for this client, but it is not the most basic because it is a later indication of change and not specific for potassium.

    c. neuromuscular status

        As usual, this answer also looks good. Your knowledge base will have given you the information that changes in potassium level can affect muscle tone and reflexes. Review the question one more time: which of the possible answers is the most basic assessment in relation to IV potassium. Again, changes in neuromuscular status are important to assess, but these changes are indicators of a problem resulting from changes in the potassium level. Urine output is an indicator of the ability of the body to handle potassium. So you conclude that this is not the best answer to this question. This does not mean that it is not an important assessment for this client. The question at issue is what is the most basic assessment.

    d. EKG recordings

        Here is another attractive answer. You will probably learn that changes in potassium can affect the EKG (ECG) tracing and cause cardiac dysrhythmias. There are two reasons why this is not the best answer for this question. First, these changes are late and do not match well with the potassium level, so this is not the most basic assessment. Second, most LP/VN students are not expected to make this kind of interpretation of EKGs. This does not mean that this is not an important assessment. It is not the most basic for an LP/VN.

So, this process, which takes much longer for me to write and for you to read than it does to do, leads us to the conclusion that response (a) is correct. You can see that preparing for and answering the review questions will be much more interesting than simply trying to memorize some fact or to identify the correct answer by memory.

CHAPTER
2

Legal Aspects of Nursing

Denise M. Jordan

► KEY TERMS

advance directives
assault
battery
confidential
durable power of attorney for health care
false imprisonment
felony
Good Samaritan Law
impaired nurse
incident report
informed consent
liability
libel
living will
malpractice
misdemeanor
negligence
nursing practice act
peer assistance programs
power of attorney
restraint
slander
standards of practice
tort

LEARNING OBJECTIVES

Upon completion of this chapter the learner should be able to:
- Define key terms.
- Describe the difference between criminal law and civil law.
- State the purpose of standards of practice and identify various sources.
- Discuss the difference between intentional and unintentional torts.
- Discuss the importance of accurate documentation.
- Discuss how informed consent relates to nursing practice.
- State the benefits of having one's own malpractice insurance policy.
- Discuss the concept of advance directives.
- List steps to take when suspecting a colleague is impaired by drugs or alcohol.
- State the purpose and correct utilization of an incident report.
- Discuss ways the nurse can reduce personal liability.

▶ *MAKING THE CONNECTION*

Refer to the topics in the following chapters to increase your understanding of nursing and the law.

INTRODUCTION

The uniqueness of nursing, which embodies a concern for the client in every aspect of life, encompasses a great responsibility, one that requires knowledge, skill, care, and commitment. As society advances and technology changes, the issues that affect nursing practice also change. We continue to recognize the importance of informed consent, of the right to decide what is best for one's self, and to believe in the client's bill of rights. However, difficult issues, such as living wills, advance directives, and Do Not Resuscitate (DNR) orders now face us. Nurses in the past did not have to contend with these controversial topics. Today's nurse needs to be informed on these and other issues. This chapter provides a general overview of many legal concepts that affect nursing.

KEY ABBREVIATIONS

The following abbreviations and acronyms are used in this chapter:

AMA	against medical advice
AMA	American Medical Association
ANA	American Nurses Association
DNR	do not resuscitate
DPAHC	durable power of attorney for health care
NCLEX	National Council Licensure Exam
NFLPN	National Federation of Licensed Practical Nurses

BASIC LEGAL CONCEPTS

It is useful to have a working definition of some basic legal concepts before applying them to a health care setting.

Definition of Law

Laws are rules of conduct that guide interactions among people. Laws are binding, enforceable, and necessary so that people can live and work together. If laws are broken, a penalty is incurred. Criminal law regulates the relationship between people and the government. Civil law, deals with the relationship between individuals.

Criminal law deals with those things that would affect all people or the state, an actual commission of a crime. Civil law deals with the interaction between private individuals and businesses, the protection of a person's civil rights.

Sources of Law

There are two primary sources of law, statutory law and common law. Statutory law is enacted by legislative bodies such as the state legislature, the Congress, or licensing boards such as state boards of nursing. Statutory laws are fixed and rarely change. However, there cannot be a law to regulate every single situation. Situations come up between people that have not been anticipated. Thus, we have what is known as common or case law. These are judicial decisions that can change on a case by case basis. Previous decisions may be used to help determine similar cases but they are not carved in stone.

Good Samaritan Law

The **Good Samaritan Law** may be a series of statutes enacted by a state, or common law, (case law precedent) to encourage off-duty health care professionals to render assistance in emergency situations. This law was necessary because physicians were sometimes reluctant to help at the scene of accidents, for example, because they were afraid of being sued by the families of accident victims. The Good Samaritan Law encourages their assistance and limits **liability**. This immunity from prosecution evolved to offer protection for other health care professionals as well, including nurses.

The Good Samaritan Law applies in emergency situations only, usually those outside the hospital setting. It stipulates that the health care worker must not be acting for an employer or receive compensation for care given.

In most states, health care professionals are not required to stop at the scene of accidents. However, if they do stop, they are held to higher standards than a lay person. Health care professionals are expected to use their specialized body of knowledge when providing care. They are expected to act as most other professionals with same background and education would. Liability would be incurred only in incidents of gross **negligence** or willful misconduct.

NURSING PRACTICE AND THE LAW

Nursing practice falls under both the criminal and civil sectors. Nurses are bound by rules and regulations stipulated by the **nursing practice act** as determined by the legislature in most states. Four states, Texas, California, Tennessee, and South Dakota have a title act for LP/VNs, instead of a practice act.

These laws are to protect the public. If these laws are broken, the nurse can be punished by paying a fine, losing her license, or being incarcerated. An example of this would be a nurse guilty of diverting drugs. This is a crime against the state. The nurse could lose his license and go to jail.

Civil laws deal with problems that occur between a nurse and the client. For example, if a nurse catheterizes a client and perforates the bladder, the client may bring a civil suit against the nurse. No law affecting the population as a whole has been broken, but the client has sustained injury. This is a problem between individuals—the nurse and the client or the nurse, the client, and the nurse's employer. The client may receive compensation for injuries, but no jail time is incurred for the nurse.

Standards of Practice

The state boards of nursing have been assigned the responsibility to determine and regulate nursing practice. The board indicates what is nursing and what is not, defines registered nursing and practical nursing, and sets educational guidelines for each program.

The state boards of nursing also stipulate who may practice nursing in that state (licensure). These criteria usually involve graduating from a state approved or accredited program, passing the National Council Licensure Exam (NCLEX), and meeting certain moral and legal standards. The boards have the authority to bring disciplinary action against a nurse for violation of its rules and regulations. Disciplinary action can include suspension or revocation of a nurse's license and/or a fine.

Under the auspices of the nursing practice act, guidelines have been developed to direct nursing care. These guidelines are called **standards of practice** or standards of care.

Standards of practice are derived from a variety of sources. As stated, they are usually defined by the board of nursing and described in the nursing practice act. However, professional organizations like the American Nurses Association (ANA) for the registered nurse and the National Federation of Licensed Practical Nurses (NFLPN) for the practical/vocational nurse also develop standards of practice. Books on nursing care planning, especially for specialized areas, are additional resources for developing standards of practice.

Policy and procedure manuals also represent standards of practice. Each facility, based on a rigorous review process, has identified specific ways of performing procedures such as passing medications, inserting catheters, and specimen collection. The nurse employed by that facility is expected to follow the guidelines as laid out by the policy and procedure manuals. For situations not covered in the policy and procedure manuals, the nurse is expected to exercise good judgment in the planning and providing of client care. In other words, the nurse is expected to act in a reasonable and prudent manner.

Liability

What defines a reasonable and prudent manner? This means that the nurse is expected to act as other nurses would at the same level, with the same amount of education or experience. If most nurses would respond to a particular situation in a certain way, and the nurse in question does also, then this nurse is acting in a reasonable and prudent manner. However, if most nurses would respond differently than this nurse, then this nurse is not behaving in a reasonable and prudent manner and can be held liable or responsible for damages. This liability is determined by whether or not the nurse adhered to the standards of practice. When a nurse is held liable for an action, it is either a criminal or civil offense. Criminal actions break the laws of the state. The nurse can be charged with a **felony**, which is a serious crime, resulting in loss of licensure and, in some states, imprisonment for a year or more. If charged with a **misdemeanor**, a less serious crime, the nurse may be fined, placed on probation, or spend up to a year in jail.

NURSE-CLIENT RELATIONSHIP

A variety of situations can develop between a nurse and a client that may require legal intervention. The following is a discussion of the types of legal circumstances that may arise.

Torts

Usually, when a case is brought against a nurse, it is a civil action that falls under the law of torts. A **tort** is a legal wrong committed against the person or property of another. Torts can be intentional or unintentional (see Table 2-1). The person committing an intentional tort knowingly and willfully violates the civil rights of another individual. Examples of intentional torts are **assault** and **battery**, defamation of character (**libel** and **slander**), **false imprisonment**, and invasion of privacy. Unintentional torts are those actions that cause harm to the client that result from a careless or negligent action of the nurse. If found liable, the nurse generally has to pay monetary damages. Prison terms are rare.

Intentional Torts

Assault and Battery   Assault and battery, though frequently used together, are actually two separate terms. Assault is the threat to do something that may cause harm or be unpleasant to another person. Battery is the unauthorized or unwanted touching of one person by another.

Fear and intimidation are the key elements in assault. The person assaulted must believe that the threat made can and will be carried out. For example, a client confined to a wheelchair is told, "If you do not finish your meal, you are going to sit there all night." The client complies because he believes the health care worker will leave him to sit for an uncomfortable period of time. The worker is in a position to carry out this threat and the client knows it.

The key factor regarding battery is consent. People have the right to be free of unwanted handling of their person. Striking a client is battery. Performing a procedure without the client's consent is battery. Forcing a person to take medication they do not want is battery. Any unwanted touching, regardless of outcome, can be construed as battery.

Table 2-1

SELECTED TORTS: DEFINITIONS AND EXAMPLES

Type of Tort	Definition	Example
Intentional		
Assault and Battery	Threaten or attempt to touch another person. Unconsented touching.	Nurse who unjustifiably forces a treatment against the client's will and in absence of consent.
False Imprisonment	Unwarranted restriction of the freedom of an individual.	Nurse who uses restraints on a client who is of sound mind and not in danger of self-injury or harm to another.
Quasi-Intentional		
Invasion of Privacy	All individuals have the right to privacy and may bring charges against any person who violates this right.	Nurse who discloses information about a client that is considered private knowledge, or photographs a client without consent.
Defamation (libel and slander)	Verbal (slander) or written (libel) remarks that may cause the loss of an individual's reputation.	Nurse who makes a statement that could ruin the client's reputation or cause the client to lose his or her job.
Unintentional		
Negligence	Failure to use such care as a reasonably prudent person would use under similar circumstances, which leads to harm.	Loss of client property. Medication error. Burns from improperly used equipment. Failure to observe and/or report a change in the client. Inaccurate sponge count in operating room.
Malpractice	Failure of a professional to use such care as a reasonably prudent member of the profession would use under similar circumstances, which leads to harm.	Nurse who makes an inaccurate nursing diagnosis and implements the wrong treatment. Nurse who does not follow physician's orders. Nurse who does not question physician's clearly erroneous order.

Libel and Slander Defamation is the use of words to harm or injure the personal or professional reputation of another person. If the words are written down, it constitutes libel. If the information is communicated verbally to a third party, it constitutes slander.

Nurses must be discreet as to how they characterize clients, peers, and other health care professionals. Negative or derogatory comments, which are untrue, leave the nurse no defense against charges of defamation. If comments are true, the relevancy of the information is important.

Cazalas (1978) relates a case where a nurse sued a hospital because of information released regarding her employment at that facility. A discrepancy in the narcotic count was noted on several occasions when this nurse worked. The director of nurses wrote a letter to the temporary agency that employed the nurse, declining further use of this nurse's services and listed the narcotic incidents. The nurse brought suit for libel.

The case was found in favor of the director. It was her legal duty, for the protection of the health care consumer, to communicate this information to the nurse's employer. She did not make the information public knowledge. There was no malicious intent. Therefore, the information was relevant. The interaction between the director and the temporary agency may be defined as privileged communication, in which information considered critical to the public's welfare superseded the nurse's individual right to privacy.

False Imprisonment False imprisonment is another example of an intentional tort. It is defined as the unlawful **restraint** of an individual's personal liberty or the unlawful detention of an individual (Cazalas, 1978). In other words, a person is prevented from moving about at will. Any mechanism used to confine a client or restrict movement can be considered a restraint. This includes threats, locked doors, physical restraints such as wrist or vest restraints, side rails, geriatric chairs, and psychotropic drugs.

Nurses find themselves in a quandary when a client chooses to leave the health care facility and no discharge order has been written. Possibly, the health care problem has not been resolved and the nurse feels that it is not in the best interest of the client to leave. If the client is of sound mind, he has the right to make this decision regardless of what others think best. Detaining the individual could result in charges of false imprisonment.

Documentation is very important in these situations. Document the client's reasons for leaving the facility and include any teaching or intervention related to the situation. Facilities have the client sign a form that indicates he or she is leaving against medical advice (AMA) and releases the facility of any liability. If the client is angry and refuses to sign the AMA form, document the client's refusal.

As indicated, any device used to restrict movement is called a restraint. To safeguard against possible charges of false imprisonment, the nurse should carefully assess the situation and include the client or significant other in the care planning process. If it is determined that a restraint is needed, explain the purpose and use of the restraint, how the restraint fits into the plan of care, how long the restraint may be necessary, and the expected outcome. Document the planning session in the client's medical record.

Assess the client in restraints frequently. Documentation must show:

- Restraints were checked hourly, released every two hours
- The client was toileted
- The client received food and water
- The client had position changes

In acute care settings, restraints can usually be applied temporarily as a nursing measure for client safety; however, a physician's order is needed within twenty-four hours. According to Fiesta (1994) "in the acute care setting, the nurse is more likely to be held liable for failing to restrain a client who should be restrained than for restraining one who should not be." In long-term care settings, a physician's order is required prior to utilizing any restraints.

Invasion of Privacy People are entitled to **confidential** (private) health care. This falls under the First Amendment, which guarantees every individual the right to privacy. Bandman & Bandman (1990) states that "The nurse safeguards the client's rights to privacy by judiciously protecting information of a confidential nature."

All information gleaned from working with a client or his medical records must be kept confidential. Therefore, a client's health status may not be discussed with a third party unless the client is present and has given verbal permission. Otherwise the permission should be in writing. This does not apply to discussing a client's health status with other health care workers involved in the care of the client.

Invasion of privacy occurs when a person's private affairs become public knowledge without their permission. From a legal perspective, invasion of privacy tends to concern physical acts related to exposure. Photographing a client without his consent is an invasion of privacy. Failing to pull curtains to shield clients while performing personal or intimate care is an invasion of privacy.

A common mistake made by health care personnel is discussing clients in public areas. It is difficult to gauge who overhears comments made while sitting in the cafeteria or waiting for the elevator (see Figure 2-1). The results can be detrimental to clients if they are embarrassed by this loss of privacy; jobs can be

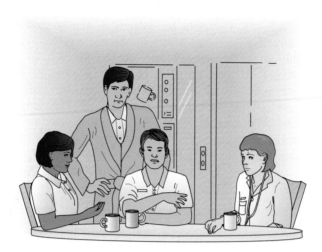

FIGURE 2-1   Do not discuss clients in public areas.

lost or family situations compromised depending on the nature of the information. For example, news of an abortion, positive HIV status, or venereal disease may be socially damaging to some clients. Do not discuss clients or their health care status in public areas or with those persons not directly involved in the care of the client.

All clients have the right to be free of unwanted public exposure. Obtain permission before going through a client's belongings. Keep doors closed and curtains pulled when providing personal care. People not involved in the performance of a procedure should not be invited to watch unless the client has given permission. Clients cannot be photographed or videotaped without their permission and a release form must be signed. Do not breach confidentiality by using a client's full name on care plans, case studies, or other assignments. Use initials only. Make sure these materials are not left laying around, making a client's private information public knowledge.

Public figures have less privacy in personal matters than the general public. For example, when a celebrity, such as the President of the United States, is hospitalized, details about diagnosis, treatment, and care become national news. However, there are guidelines for disclosure of information to fit these and other situations. The nurse must be familiar with the policies governing the release of information where she is employed. If things are not done according to protocol, confidentiality may not be maintained.

Nonintentional Torts

Nonintentional torts may include negligence and malpractice.

Negligence   All nurses, including student nurses, are expected to use good judgment when providing client care. This means that side rails should not be left down on confused clients' beds and sedated clients are not allowed to smoke unattended. Puddles and spills are cleaned up immediately to prevent falls, rather than waiting for housekeeping to take care of the matter. Any person, with or without the specialized knowledge required for nursing, could make these determinations. Should a nurse fail to protect a client in a situation such as these or one requiring similar judgments, the nurse could be found negligent.

Negligent or careless acts on the part of a nurse frequently come from not meeting the standards of care. In other words, from not doing what a reasonable and prudent nurse would do under similar circumstances. A nurse can be charged with negligence for acts committed or acts omitted. Failure to properly assess a client or to act upon assessment information are examples of omission. Giving a client the wrong medication because of improper identification procedures (not checking the armband) or improper setup (not using the medication administration record) are acts of commission.

Malpractice   Negligent acts on the part of a professional can be termed **malpractice** or professional negligence. More specifically, it relates to the conduct of a person while acting in a professional capacity. It can include attempting a procedure that the nurse is unfamiliar with or improperly performing a procedure resulting in client injury. Malpractice differs from negligence in that anyone can be accused of negligence; only professionals can be accused of malpractice.

Several factors must hold true for a nurse to be found guilty of malpractice.

- The nurse owed a special duty to the client; in other words, a nurse-client relationship existed.
- Criteria or standards of care guide the nurse-client interaction. For example, health care facilities have policies regarding medication administration or admission assessments.
- The nurse failed to meet the standards of care. Policy, procedure, or standards of care were not followed.
- Injury occurred as a result of the nurse's action or lack of action, a direct cause and effect.

The prudent nurse is protected by adhering to facility policy and procedure and attempting to meet the standards of care at all times. The case study discussed in Figure 2-2 illustrates some of the difficulties in distinguishing between malpractice and negligence.

Case Study: Standard of Care—Malpractice or Ordinary Negligence

Facts: A seventy-five-year-old patient fell and fractured a hip while in the hospital. The patient had been medicated with castor oil and a sleeping pill, and the nurse failed to raise the side rails on the bed. During the night the patient got out of bed to go to the bathroom and fell, fracturing a hip. The patient sued, alleging that the nurses had been negligent in failing to raise the side rails and in failing to tell the patient that a bedpan would be brought to the patient when needed.

Holding: The nurse's conduct constituted negligence. Unlike a malpractice action, no expert testimony was necessary to establish the applicable standard of care. The duty to raise side rails on a bed and to instruct the patient to use the call button beside the bed if assistance is needed did not involve the failure to render professional nursing or medical services requiring special skills. The jury, therefore, could evaluate the nurse's conduct under the standard of "the reasonably prudent person," rather than "the reasonably prudent nurse".

Norris v. Rowan Memorial Hospital, North Carolina Court of Appeals 1974.

Comment: This case points out the difficulties even courts have in drawing the line between ordinary negligence and malpractice. Cases involving a nurse's failure to raise bed rails are decided under the standard of ordinary negligence as often as they are decided under the standard of professional malpractice.

FIGURE 2-2 Case Study: Standard of Care—Malpractice or Ordinary Negligence? (*Courtesy Mitchell & Grippando,* Nursing Perspectives and Issues, 5th edition, *Delmar Publishers, 1993*)

Documentation

The best place to determine what takes place in a client's clinical history is the medical record, or the chart. The chart should be an accurate reflection of diagnosis, treatment, testing, clinical course, nursing assessment, and intervention. According to the law, "If it was not charted, it was not done." If a chart ever winds up in court, this is the standard the jury applies when trying to determine what happened and who is at fault.

Chart events as they happen. Do not wait until the end of the day. It is difficult to remember what takes place on an eight-hour shift, especially when caring for more than one client.

Do not chart medications before they are given or treatments before they are completed. It is a direct violation of the standards of practice for documentation and medication administration.

Use only accepted abbreviations. Each facility has its own list of approved abbreviations; be familiar with it. Do not assume abbreviations allowed at one facility are acceptable in another. If in doubt, write it out.

Documentation must be accurate and objective. The nurse should describe what he sees and does. Nurses' notes should reflect facts, not inferences or opinions about the client. Furthermore, it is not enough to chart nursing assessment or problems identified. The nurse needs to complete the task by documenting any actions taken—nursing interventions and physician orders received.

Entries must be neat, legible, spelled correctly, and written clearly. It is illegal to go back and change a chart. If an error in charting is made, simply draw a line through the incorrect entry and initial it. Do not scribble or use white correction fluid. Sloppy, mis-spelled charting might discredit excellent nursing care. Make the medical record work for you, not against you.

Figures 2-3 and 2-4 reflect situations where nurses identified client problems. In Figure 2-3, documentation was incomplete. In the situation presented in Figure 2-4, the nurses clearly identified the problem, the client's response, and the actions taken.

MALPRACTICE INSURANCE

Many nurses believe they do not need their own malpractice or liability insurance. They have been told the coverage provided by their employer is enough. This may be a misconception. There are several factors to consider when making this decision.

Nurses claim to be competent and knowledgeable health care providers. The health care consumer has heard the message and is holding the nurse accountable for his or her actions. As a result, nurses are named as defendants in malpractice suits. Under the doctrine of *Respondeat Superior,* employers are responsible for the actions of their employees. However, this responsibility stops when the employee leaves work. Also, if the nurse violates policy and the employer is forced to pay damages, the employer has the right to sue the nurse to recover losses.

Having a professional liability policy provides the nurse with an attorney, someone who will represent that nurse in court. An attorney representing the facility or a group of employees will be most concerned about the employer; the needs of an individual nurse will be secondary. The decision to settle a case or pursue a particular course of action may be based on the needs of the employer. The nurse, with private counsel, is better represented in court.

Incomplete Documentation : Mrs. Drew

Mrs. Drew, 85, was a resident on a transitional care unit. She lost 15 pounds over a three month period. When her chart was reviewed, the auditor targeted the weight loss as a problem. She examined the chart to discover what the nurses did to try to correct this situation.

The nurses had carefully documented the percentages Mrs. Drew had eaten at each meal, her lack of appetite, and the pattern of weight loss. They thought they had covered all bases. They were wrong.

The auditor referred to the standards of practice on weight loss in long-term care facilities. She questioned, "Did the nurses follow the guidelines?" No interventions were charted so it was presumed that nothing was done.

In fact, the nurses had called the dietitian to see this client several times to discuss her food preferences and a calorie count was initiated. Student nurses assigned to Mrs. Drew sat with her at meal times to encourage her to eat. The nurses had spoken with the doctor and her family about their concern over her lack of appetite and loss of weight. However, none of this was charted. There was no proof, other than the dietitian's entries, that any attempt had been made to intervene in this client's nutritional deficit.

FIGURE 2-3 Incomplete documentation: Mrs. Drew.

Complete Documentation: Roberta Wilson

Roberta Wilson is a 44 year old woman with a history of diabetes mellitus. Her diabetes is controlled by diet. She was admitted two days ago for abdominal pain. Ms. Wilson has been NPO since midnight for an ultrasound scheduled at 9:30 a.m. The doctor instructed she was to remain NPO until seen by a consultant. Her 11 a.m. accucheck revealed a blood sugar of 44. She was experiencing no symptoms of hypoglycemia.

What needed to be done and what needed to be documented to protect everyone involved? Hospital protocol stipulated giving 4 ounces of Coke for blood sugars less than 60, then repeating the accucheck in about 30 minutes. The nurses contacted the physician to cancel the NPO order, then administered the Coke. Roberta's blood sugar at 11:40 was 93. She was served an 1800 calorie ADA diet for lunch.

What was charted?

2/08/XX	11:10 a.m.	Accucheck 44. Client's skin is warm and dry, no complaints of nausea, tremors, or confusion. States she feels "fine." Physician notified of low blood sugar and client condition. Orders received to discontinue NPO status and resume previous orders.
2/08/XX	11:15 a.m.	4 ounces of Coke given.
2/08/XX	11:40 a.m.	Blood sugar 93. Served 1800 calorie ADA diet for lunch. Blood sugar to be repeated at 4 p.m.

FIGURE 2-4 Complete documentation: Roberta Wilson.

Frequently, family members and friends ask a nurse for advice or assistance on health care matters. This advice is sought because of the nurse's knowledge, experience, and role. Should the family member or friend later take issue with the results of the advice or treatment given by a nurse, they might bring a suit against the nurse.

Despite the fact that no money was exchanged for information or services, the nurse is still accountable for advice given. If the situation ends up in court, the nurse needs legal representation. Legal representation is costly. Judgments against the nurse can be costly. A professional liability insurance policy protects the nurse by providing legal representation and paying the judgments.

There are two basic types of liability protection, the claims made policy and the occurrence policy. The claims made policy protects the nurse against claims made during the time the policy is in effect. If a claim is made after the policy has been terminated, the nurse is not covered. Occurrence policies protect the nurse against events that took place during the period of time the policy was active even if a claim is filed after this policy is terminated. Occurrence policies seem to offer better protection for the nurse.

Opinions differ as to whether or not nurses should

carry individual liability insurance. Some attorneys and health care professionals believe this practice encourages lawsuits. Nurses must compare the cost and the benefits of having personal liability insurance against the cost of potential legal fees and loss of personal assets.

INFORMED CONSENT

Informed consent refers to the client's ability to make health care decisions based on full disclosure of the benefits, risks, potential consequences of a recommended treatment plan, and alternative treatments, including no treatment. This detailed explanation, provided by the physician, allows the client to make intelligent decisions about treatment options. The issue of informed consent deals with the right of the client to determine what happens to his or her person. Consent to treatment frees the health care worker from unwarranted charges of battery.

Whose Legal Responsibility to Obtain Consent?

Nurses must obtain consent for nursing procedures. Each client, on admission, signs a general care consent form. The nurse is obligated to explain what is to be done to the client and receive, at least implied consent when the client does not object. It is the physician's responsibility to obtain consent for medical or surgical treatment. The disclosure about the risks and benefits to treatment generally takes place at a time when the nurse is not present, often in the physician's office. It is usually on the basis of this discussion that the client decides whether or not to accept the treatment recommendation and sign the consent form. However, confusion arises because nurses are often delegated the duty of collecting the signature for invasive procedures such as surgery, cardiac catheterization, and other diagnostic procedures. Student nurses do not ask the client to sign a consent form, nor do they witness a consent form.

The Nurse's Role in Informed Consent

When a nurse has a client sign a consent form, the nurse is verifying three things:

1. The client's signature is authentic.
2. The client has the mental capacity to understand the things discussed with the physician.
3. The client was not coerced into signing the form.

If the nurse is unsure about the client's understanding or if the client still has questions, the client should not sign the form. Document the client's lack of under-

standing and contact the physician. Further clarification is needed and it must come from the physician. The responsibility for informed consent has been assigned, by law, to the physician. This duty cannot be delegated.

Clients over the age of 18 may give consent for their own health care. Parents or guardians give consent for minor children. However, minors who are married, live on their own, become pregnant, or require treatment for sexually transmitted diseases, mental illness, or substance abuse, may give consent for themselves.

A complicated area today is the question of minors refusing treatments to which parents have consented, or parents refusing consent or treatment for minors that has been deemed medically necessary. The court has had to intervene in these situations. At times like these, the child may be made a ward of the court and the decision-making capacity temporarily taken away from the parents. An example would be the child who needs a blood transfusion and the parents are Jehovah's Witnesses. While the parents have the right to refuse life-sustaining treatment for themselves on moral or religious beliefs, they may not refuse life-sustaining treatment for their child for religious or moral reasons.

Individuals declared incompetent have a guardian or someone who has **power of attorney** to make heath care decisions and give consent for treatment. In an emergency situation when immediate action is necessary to save a life or prevent the client from permanent physical harm, consent is implied. Written consent is waived. Once the emergency is over, consent must be obtained for any further care. Consent may be withdrawn, either verbally or in writing, at any time.

Invasive procedures or those that may have serious complications such as surgery, cardiac catheterization, or HIV testing, require written consent. Figure 2-5 illustrates a typical consent form used to obtain client permission for the performance of invasive procedures. Consent for procedures that are not invasive can either be given verbally or implied. The client implies consent when he cooperates with the procedure offered.

For example, the orderly says, "Mr. Jones, I am here to take you for your chest x-ray." Mr. Jones gets into the wheelchair. Consent is implied by Mr. Jones' cooperation.

In another situation, a nurse says to Mrs. Smith, "I have your medication, but I need to check your heart rate first." Mrs. Smith says, "Fine, I'll just lay this knitting aside until you're through." Consent has been given verbally.

IMPAIRED NURSE

One of the more sensitive issues we face within the nursing profession today is the subject of the **impaired nurse**. By definition, an impaired nurse is one under

CAYLOR-NICKEL
Bluffton, Indiana 46714

CONSENT AND PRE-OPERATIVE NOTE

☐ In-Patient   ☐ Out-Patient

I (we) hereby request and consent to the performance of the following operation or procedure on the patient by
_____ M.D. or members of the medical
staff and personnel of the CAYLOR-NICKEL HOSPITAL, the administration of anesthetics deemed advisable by the
physician performing the operation or procedure, the administration of blood or blood components or derivatives, and
extensions of the operation or procedure advisable by the physician performing the operation or procedure, and dis-
posal of any tissue, organ and body part, except as noted below:

Operation or procedure:_____

Exceptions, if any:_____

(If none, write "none")

DIAGNOSIS:
ALTERNATIVES:
BENEFITS:
RISKS:

_____
PHYSICIAN SIGNATURE   DATE

I acknowledge that I have discussed with a physician the operation or procedure, its purpose and nature, reasonable
alternatives possible consequences of remaining untreated, and risks and possible complications. I understand that
the practice of medicine is not an exact science, that it may involve the making of medical judgements based upon
the facts known to the physician at the time, that it is not reasonable to expect the physician to be able to anticipate
nor explain all the risks and complications, that an undesirable result does not necessarily indicate an error in
judgement, that no guarantee as to results has been made to nor relied upon by me, and I wish to rely on the
physician to exercise judgement during the course of the procedure or operation which he feels at the time, based
upon the facts then known, are in my best interest.

_____
(Patient or Person Authorized to Consent for Patient)   Date   Time

Witness Signature   Date   Time

SIGNATURES REQUIRED

1. If the patient is an adult (age 18 or over) —signature of patient, and if the patient is incompetent, the guardian's
   signature.
2. Minor patient (under age 18) —if emancipated (providing own support and living apart from the parents) patient's
   signature
   If married, signature of patient and spouse are required.
   Otherwise, signature of guardian is required.
3. In an emergency threatening the life or well being of the patient, and if signatures as required above are not
   available, there should be an entry in the chart documenting the emergency nature of the procedure and the
   need for prompt action, attested by the signatures of two physicians. Also, the signature of the closest adult
   relative should be obtained, if available.

FIGURE 2-5   Consent to operation. (*Courtesy Caylor Nickel Medical Center*)

the influence of alcohol or drugs. Job performance may not be immediately compromised, but eventually, the substance abuse does interfere with clinical judgment and performance. Because of the high levels of job-related stress and accessibility of drugs, the chem-ical dependency rate among nurses is greater than in the general public.

The primary concern is client care. In the role of client advocate, a nurse cannot let loyalties to co-workers interfere with duty to the client. Nurses suspected of being under the influence of drugs or alcohol must be reported to the proper authority at the place of employment. The second consideration is getting help for the impaired nurse. Do not be tempted to ignore the problem.

If you suspect a co-worker is diverting drugs or abusing alcohol:

1. Document the dates, times, and observed behavior. Be specific and descriptive about what you observed, not what you think. For example:

   > January 3, l996. P.P. working 3–11 shift. Client A and Client B complained of unrelieved postoperative pain. Documentation by P.P. stated both clients were comfortable after administration of Demerol 75 mg IM. Narcotic count at shift change satisfactory.

   > January 4, l996. Client C and Client D complained of unrelieved pain. Documentation by P.P. indicated both clients stated pain was relieved after administration of Demerol 100 mg IM. Narcotic count at shift change okay.

   > January 5, l996. Narcotic count showed 1 Demerol 100 mg syringe listed as broken and 1 Demerol 75 mg syringe listed as wasted, "client changed her mind." P.P. signed the narcotic sheet.

   or

   > March 1–2, l996. S.L. working the night shift. Strong odor of alcohol on his breath.

   > March 3, l996. S.L. observed walking with unsteady gait, speech is slurred, strong odor of alcohol on breath.

2. Go to your supervisor and report your concerns. Provide a copy of your documentation about the suspicious incidents. The supervisor will take responsibility for confronting the suspected employee. Intoxication requires immediate removal from the clinical area. In other situations, the supervisor will devise a plan before confronting the nurse.

3. Do not approach the co-worker yourself. He or she may become defensive and deny the problem or threaten you. Also, once the nurse is aware that you are suspicious, he or she will become more secretive, making detection less likely. Frequently, the nurse will quit one facility and go to another, repeating the same pattern.

Some employers offer an employee assistance program to rehabilitate the impaired nurse. In addition, most states have **peer assistance programs** (nurses helping nurses) under the auspices of the state nurses association in conjunction with the board of nursing.

The goals are to protect the public from impaired nurses, provide the needed assistance to the impaired nurse, assist the nurse to re-enter nursing, and monitor the nurse's compliance. With the help of the peer counselor, the impaired nurse develops a contract for treatment. Compliance is monitored, confidentiality is ensured. Successful completion of the program allows the nurse to return to the practice setting.

Participation in employer and peer assistance programs is optional. However, if the nurse chooses not to cooperate, employment may be terminated and sanctions by the board of nursing may follow.

INCIDENT REPORTS

An **incident report** is a risk management tool. It is used to help the facility identify or track problem areas and alert the legal department to possible lawsuits. An incident report is not meant to be a punitive device, although it is often perceived in that manner.

Incident reports are completed whenever any unusual event occurs to a client, visitor, or staff member. Unusual events include, but are not limited to falls, medication errors, forgotten treatment, injuries—anything that happens out of the ordinary. Another name for an incident report is a variance report or an occurrence report. The following three examples illustrate the types of occurrences that should be documented in an incident report.

1. Mrs. Jones had blood drawn for various laboratory tests. It was later discovered that the laboratory work had been ordered on Mrs. Smith, not Mrs. Jones. The requisition had been stamped with the wrong name.
2. Mrs. Barnes was given Lasix 20 mg p.o. at 9 A.M. When reviewing the physician's orders, the evening nurse discovered that Losec 20 mg had been ordered. Mrs. Barnes received the wrong medication.
3. Mrs. Gomez was visiting her daughter, who had just given birth to the family's first grandchild. While walking down the hall, Mrs. Gomez slipped and fell, injuring her right hip.

All of the above examples are incidents or variances that typically occur in health care settings. An incident report needs to be completed on each situation and channeled to the risk management department. They are not placed in the client's chart.

Under the auspices of risk management, a subgroup comprised of representatives from various departments such as nursing administration, dietary services, environmental safety, and others, reviews the incident report. This group tries to identify what factors, if any, contributed to the incident. Can the causal factors be eliminated or reduced? Does the possibility of a lawsuit exist as a result of the incident? What can be done to prevent this incident from occurring again?

Incident reports are filed by the person responsible for, witnessing, or discovering the incident. The report should state what was observed, not what was supposed. It should be factual and concise. "Mrs. Gomez found lying on floor outside room 222. Several puddles of liquid found under and around her; paper cup lying nearby." Incident reports should include a description of the care given to the client and the name of the physician who was notified.

Do not assign blame or accept responsibility. Just state the facts. Consider how inflammatory this statement could be: "Mrs. Gomez tripped and fell outside room 222. She slipped in a puddle of water."

Mrs. Gomez may have spilled the cup of water she was carrying during the fall. However, this note implies that Mrs. Gomez slipped in water that was already on the floor, thus implicating the facility. Just state the facts.

Chart the incident in the client's medical record but do not refer to the incident report in any way. The incident report is not a part of the medical record. However, the details described in the medical record and in the incident report should be the same.

When completing the incident report, be sure to include the date and time of incident, assessments, and interventions. Also include when family members and physicians are notified. Refer to nursing administration policy and procedure regarding follow-up documentation.

ADVANCE DIRECTIVES

Advance directives emphasize the right of the client to self-determination. They are instructions about health care preferences regarding life-sustaining measures. These instructions may indicate who may make health care decisions for the client, should he be unable to do so. In essence, they express the client's wishes about the kinds of medical treatment wanted and not wanted.

A client of sound mind retains the right to make all health care decisions and may even change his mind about previous decisions. However, should a situation arise when the person becomes incapable of making decisions, the information is there.

Advance directives serve as a guide to family members when discussing what kinds of treatment should or should not be allowed. They permit those involved in the decision-making process to know what "Mom" or "Dad" prefers. These instructions are best put in writing, but that is not always the case. Sometimes, health care preferences are shared verbally with family members or friends. There can be disagreement as to how verbal instructions are interpreted. This disagreement creates difficulty for all involved—the physician,

the health care facility, and the family. It is best to get this information in writing.

All health care facilities that receive Medicare or Medicaid monies are required to offer the opportunity to execute advance directives to all competent clients on admission. The client should be told about the purpose and availability of living wills and **durable power of attorney for health care** (DPAHC). If desired, the client should be offered assistance in completing these documents. In addition, the medical record must show that the client was afforded this opportunity. The documentation must indicate decisions made or not made at that time. Clients cannot be coerced into signing advance directives nor can they be discriminated against should they choose not to do so.

Facilities vary as to who provides the information on advance directives. Many health care facilities have the admissions office or social services take on this responsibility; others have the nurses do it. Regardless of which department is assigned this task, the nurse is frequently called upon to assist in the understanding of this information.

When discussing advance directives with a client, the nurse needs to be familiar with the Patient Self-Determination Act. Then, in the role of client advocate, the nurse explains the different types of advance directives to the client and family members. Terms such as "palliative care," "supportive care," "comfort measures," or "nutrition and hydration" may not be understood. The nurse can define those concepts more clearly and emphasize that the client has the right to choose what he believes is best for himself.

Point out that the client needs to discuss these preferences with the physician and family members. Emphasize that these advanced directives only go into effect should the individual become incompetent, have a terminal illness, or death is imminent. Care is not withheld in normal circumstances. The nurse should serve as a resource person, making needed referrals should the client wish to change his advance directives at a later date.

Meticulous documentation regarding all aspects of client contact and advance directives is required. The nurse must stay current on policies and procedures governing advance directives in the practice setting.

Durable Power of Attorney

A durable power of attorney for health care (DPAHC) is a legal document designating who may make health care decisions for a client when that client is no longer in a decision-making capacity. This health care representative is appointed by the client and is expected to act in the best interests of the client. This appointment can be revoked at any time the client chooses.

Part I. Durable Power of Attorney for Health Care

• If you do NOT wish to name an agent to make health care decisions for you, write your initials in the text ☐ Initials

This form has been prepared to comply with the "Durable Power of Attorney for Health Care Act" of Missouri.

1. Selection of agent. I appoint:
Name:_____
Address:_____

| It is suggested that only one Agent be named. However, if more than one Agent is named, anyone may act individually unless you specify otherwise. |

Telephone:_____
as my Agent.

2. Alternate Agents. Only an Agent named by me may act under this Durable Power of Attorney. If my Agent resigns or is not able or available to make health care decisions for me, or if an Agent named by me is divorced from me or is my spouse and legally separated from me, I appoint the person(s) named below (in the order named if more than one):

First Alternate Agent   Second Alternate Agent

Name_____   Name_____

Address:_____   Address:_____

_____   _____

Telephone:_____   Telephone:_____

| This is a Durable Power of Attorney, and the authority of my Agent shall not terminate if I become disabled or incapacitated. |

Part I. Durable Power of Attorney for Health Care (Continued)

3. Effective date and durability. This Durable Power of Attorney is effective when two physicians decide and certify that I am incapacitated and unable to make and communicate a health care decision.

• If you want ONE physician, nstead of TWO, to decide whether you are incapacitated, write your initials in the box to the right. ☐ Initials

4. Agent's powers. I grant to my Agent full authority to:

A. Give consent to, prohibit or withdraw any type of health care, medical care, treatment or procedure, even if my death may result;

• If you wish to AUTHORIZE your Agent to direct a health care provider to withhold or withdraw artificially supplied nutrition and hydration (including tube feeding of food and water), write your initials in the box to the right. ☐ Initials

• If you DO NOT WISH TO AUTHORIZE your Agent to direct a health care provider to withhold or withdraw artificially supplied nutrition and hydration (including tube feeding of food and water), write your initials in the box to the right. ☐ Initials

B. Make all necessary arrangements for health care services on my behalf, and to hire and fire medical personnel responsible for my care;

C. Move me into or out of any health care facility (even if against medical advice) to obtain compliance with the decisions of my Agent; and

D. Take any other action necessary to do what I authorize here, including (but not limited to) granting any waiver or release from liability required by any health care provider, and taking any legal action at the expense of my estate to enforce this Durable Power of Attorney.

5. Agent's Financial Liability and Compensation. My Agent acting under this Durable Power of Attorney will incur no personal financial liability. My Agent shall not be entitled to compensation for services performed under this Durable Power of Attorney, but my Agent shall be entitled to reimbursement for all reasonable expenses incurred as a result of carrying out any provision hereof.

Part II. Health Care Directive

• If you DO NOT WISH to make a health care directive, write your initials in the box to the right, and go to Part III. ☐ Initials

I make this HEALTH CARE DIRECTIVE ("Directive") to exercise my right to determine the course of my health care and to provide clear and convincing proof of my wishes and instructions about my treatment.

If I am persistently unconscious or there is no reasonable expectation of my recovery from a seriously incapacitating or terminal illness or condition, I direct that all of the life-prolonging procedures which I have initialed below be withheld or withdrawn.

I want the following life-prolonging procedures to be withheld or withdrawn:

| • artificially supplied nutrition and hydration (including tube feeding of food and water). . . . . | Initials |

• surgery or other invasive procedures. Initials
• heart-lung resuscitation (CPR) . . . . Initials
• antibiotic. . . . . Initials
• dialysis. . . . . Initials
• mechanical ventilator (respirator). . . . . Initials
• chemotherapy. . . . . Initials
• radiation therapy. . . . . Initials
• all other "life-prolonging" medical or surgical procedures that are merely intended to keep me alive without reasonable hope of improving my condition or curing my illness or injury. . . . . Initials

However, if my physician believes that any life-prolonging procedure may lead to significant recovery, I direct my physician to try the treatment for a reasonable period of time. If it does not improve my condition, I direct the treatment be withdrawn even if it shortens my life. I also direct that I be given medical treatment to relieve pain or to provide comfort, even if such treatment might shorten my life, suppress my appetite or my breathing, or be habit-forming.

IF I HAVE NOT DESIGNATED AN AGENT IN THE DURABLE POWER OF ATTORNEY, THIS DOCUMENT IS MEANT TO BE IN FULL FORCE AND EFFECT AS MY HEALTH CARE DIRECTIVE.

Part III. General Provisions Included in the Directive and Durable Power of Attorney

YOU MUST SIGN THIS DOCUMENT IN THE PRESENCE OF TWO WITNESSES. IN WITNESS WHEREOF, I have executed this document this_____day of _____, 19____.

_____
Signature

Print name _____
Address _____

The person who signed this document is of sound mind and voluntarily signed this document in our presence. Each of the undersigned witnesses is at least eighteen years of age.

Signature_____   Signature_____

Print name _____   Print name _____

Address _____   Address _____

| ONLY REQUIRED FOR PART I — DURABLE POWER OF ATTORNEY |

STATE OF MISSOURI   )
) as
_____OF_____   )

On this_____day of_____, 19_____, before me personally appeared to me known to be the person described in and who excuted the foregoing instrument and acknowledged that he/she executed the same as his/her free act and deed.

IN WITNESS WHEREOF, I have hereunto set my hand and affixed my official seal in the County of_____, State of Missouri, the day and year first above written.

_____
Notary Public

My Commision Expires:

FIGURE 2-6 Durable power of attorney for health care and health care directive. (*Developed and printed by the Missouri Bar*)

For example, if a client lapses into a coma and the prognosis is poor, the health care representative or the person appointed DPAHC can give consent for certain types of treatment or withhold treatment, even if the lack of treatment results in death. It is expected that the health care representative has discussed treatment preferences with the client and would know what the client desired. The DPAHC is activated only when the client is no longer competent to make health care decisions.

The person who has power of attorney or the authority to make decisions for a client in some areas does not necessarily have the same authority regarding health care issues. The granting of the right to make health care decisions has to be specified in the power of attorney agreement or a DPAHC must be signed (see Figure 2-6). Because of a possible conflict of interest, the health care representative may be different from the individual assigned the power of attorney.

A person who stands to benefit from the client's estate may not be appointed health care representative. A decision to terminate life support would benefit the designee financially; a conflict of interest exists. However, this person could have the right to make decisions about the client in matters not pertaining to health care.

Living Wills

Living wills are legal documents that allow a person to state her preferences about the use of life-sustaining measures should she be unable to make her wishes known. These preferences can be expressed with the use of the Living Will Declaration or the Life-Prolonging Procedure Declaration. These documents allow the client to specify in advance, what life-sustaining measures are to be done or not done.

The Living Will Declaration explains that certain life-prolonging treatments not be used. The individual prefers to die naturally. Food, fluids, and comfort measures are continued and the person is not abandoned. However, artificial means such as ventilators or feeding tubes may not be an option.

All states do not currently recognize living wills. However, consideration of the client's requests should be given due consideration when making health care decisions. The nurse needs to be knowledgeable about living will legislation in her state, and provide input through her professional organization. A sample living will is shown in Figure 2-7.

The Life-Prolonging Procedure Declaration indicates that the person wants all possible procedures done to delay the dying process (see Figure 2-8). This can include the use of ventilators and any other methods to keep the person alive by artificial means.

Where a form for a living will, durable power of attorney and/or health care representative is provided by statute, it should be utilized because health care providers are familiar with it. However, variations of the forms, if all the required elements are contained, may also be legal.

Sample Living Will

Declaration made this ____ day of __________, 19_____.
I, ______________________, willfully and voluntarily make known my desire that my dying not be artificially prolonged under the circumstances set forth below, and I do hereby declare:

If at any time I have a terminal condition and if my attending or treating physician and another consulting physician have determined that there is no medical probability of my recovery from such condition, I direct that life-prolonging procedures be withheld or withdrawn when the application of such procedures would serve only to prolong artificially the process of dying, and that I be permitted to die naturally with only the administration of medication or the performance of any medical procedure deemed necessary to provide me with comfort care or to alleviate pain.

It is my intention that this declaration be honored by my family and physician as the final expression of my legal right to refuse medical or surgical treatment and to accept the consequences for such refusal.

In the event that I have been determined to be unable to provide express and informed consent regarding the withholding, withdrawal, or continuaiton of life-prolonging procedures, I wish to designate, as my surrogate to carry out the provisions of this declaration:

Name: ____________________
Address: ____________________
____________________ Zip Code: __________
Phone: ____________________

I wish to designate the following person as my alternate surrogate, to carry out the provisions of this declaration should my surrogate be unwilling or unable to act on my behalf:

Name: ____________________
Address: ____________________
____________________ Zip Code: __________
Phone: ____________________

Additional instructions (optional):

I understand the full importance of this declaration, and I am emotionally and mentally competant to make this declaration.
Signed: ____________________

Witness 1:
Signed: ____________________
Address: ____________________

Witness 2:
Signed: ____________________
Address: ____________________

FIGURE 2-7 Sample living will. (*Courtesy of Choice in Dying, 200 Varick Street, New York, NY 10014*)

CAYLOR-NICKEL MEDICAL CENTER   Date of Birth   Clinic #

LIFE PROLONGING PROCEDURES
          DECLARATION

                                        Patient
                                        Name:

Declaration made this _____ day of _____ (month, year).

I ,_____ , being at least eighteen (18)
years old and of sound mind, willfully and voluntarily make known my desires that if at any time I have an incurable
injury, disease, or illness determined to be a terminal condition, I request the use of life-prolonging procedures
that would extend my life. This includes appropriate nutrition and hydration and the administration of medication
and the performance of all other medical procedures necessary to extend my life, to provide me with comfort care
or to alleviate pain.

Other instructions:

In the absence of my ability to give directions regarding the use of life-prolonging procedures, it is my intention that
this declaration be honored by my family and physician as the final expression of my legal right to request medical
or surgical treatment and accept the consequences of the request.

I understand the full impact of this declaration.

Signed _____

_____
City, County and State of Residence

The declarant has been personally known to me, and I believe (him/her) to be of sound mind. I did not sign the
declarant's signature above for or at the direction of the declarant. I am not a parent, spouse, or child of the
declarant. I am not entitled to any part of the declarant's estate and/or financially responsible for the declarant's
medical care. I am competent and at least eighteen (18) years old.

Witness _____ Date_____

Witness _____ Date_____

Forward to social service department

FIGURE 2-8   Life-prolonging procedures declaration. (*Courtesy Caylor-Nickel Medical Center*)

▶ *CASE STUDIES*

Case Study I: Helen Gee

Helen Gee is admitted for diabetes out of control. She is very nervous about this admission, despite the fact that she has been hospitalized several times before. Helen is unable to discuss advance directives with the social services representative at this time. "It makes me too nervous to think about that stuff," she explained to the social worker.

Later, Helen and two of her daughters were discussing a case they heard about on the news. A family had petitioned the court to disconnect a respirator on their daughter who had been in a persistent vegetative state for two years.

Helen said, "If I get bad, don't you kids pull the plug on me. I want you to do everything possible." Everyone laughed and the daughters made a couple of joking comments. The nurse joined in the discussion, asking pointed questions about Helen's beliefs regarding life-sustaining measures.

Case Study II: Mr. Jones

Mr. Jones is admitted for congestive heart failure. He is sixty-six years old, newly diagnosed, and acutely ill at this time. A student LP/VN is assisting the registered nurse (RN) with the admission. The student notes that Mr. Jones has a living will. Later she asks the RN, "Will you have to contact the doctor regarding a No Code status for Mr. Jones? He's got a living will so he doesn't want anything done."

The following questions are related to the case studies.

1. Was the nurse out of line to enter into a private discussion?
2. Does Helen's statement, "Don't pull the plug" qualify as an advance directive? List rationale.
3. List factors the nurse should emphasize when attempting to explain the concepts of advance directives.
4. Write a sample documentation of this interaction.

1. List factors the nurse should explain to assist the student in understanding the concept of the living will.
2. Describe how a cardiac arrest might impact this situation.

▶ CASE STUDIES (continued)

Mr. Jones' wife speaks privately with the nurse. She states, "I want everything possible done to save my husband. I don't care what it takes."

Mr. Jones is refusing a recommended treatment option. Mrs. Jones disagrees, and tells the doctor to go ahead with the recommended treatment plan.

Bob Smith came to the hospital for outpatient diagnostic testing. Passing an open door, he saw his high school principal, Mr. Jones, lying in a bed. A respiratory therapist was giving Mr. Jones a treatment and there seemed to be tubes and bags hanging everywhere. Alarmed, Bob went to the nurse's station seeking information. He pointed to Mr. Jones' name and room number listed on the board, and began asking questions.

3. Describe how this information may or may not affect the living will requests that Mr. Jones has made.
4. Write how the nurse might respond in this situation.
5. Identify a nursing diagnosis, two goals, and expected outcomes for Mrs. Jones.
6. How does the Patient Self-Determination Act affect Mr. Jones' refusal of treatment?
7. List the parameters allowing Mrs. Jones to consent or refuse treatment for her husband.
8. Discuss ways to calm Bob's fears without violating Mr. Jones' right to privacy.
9. Identify what situation(s) have already occurred to violate this client's privacy.

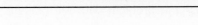

SUMMARY

- Laws are rules that guide personal interaction. They are derived from several sources and can be classified as civil or criminal.
- The nursing practice act indicates the scope of practice for nurses within most states. Standards have been developed to guide nursing practice.
- The nurse should be familiar with client rights. Care should be taken not to falsely imprison a client or violate the right to privacy.

- The client's chart is a legal document and should accurately reflect client status and care. Entries should be neat and timely.
- Informed consent is more than just signing a form. It includes an understanding of the risks, benefits, and alternatives to treatment.
- Whether or not to purchase malpractice insurance is a personal decision. However, having one's own policy provides coverage off the job and individual legal counsel.
- Impaired nurses are everyone's concern. Document

dates, times, and behaviors, and report to your immediate supervisor.

- Incident reports are a risk management tool. They are not meant to be used for punitive purposes.
- Advance directives are instructions about health care preferences. They protect the rights of the client and guide the family through difficult decisions.

Review Questions

1. Standards of practice are:
   a. different for each school of nursing.
   b. guidelines to direct nursing care.
   c. not legally binding.
   d. specific criteria on how to do procedures.

2. Immunity for nurses giving care in emergency situations is provided under the:
   a. Care and Good Faith Act of 1937.
   b. Good Samaritan Law.
   c. state nursing practice act.
   d. Patient Self-Determination act.

3. Select the situation that violates client privacy:
   a. copying information from the chart for a case study.
   b. discussing client status with clinical instructor.
   c. shutting the door and closing the curtain during a procedure.
   d. talking about an interesting client in the cafeteria.

4. To make the best use of time in the clinical area, the nurse should:
   a. chart events as they happen.
   b. chart in a block at the end of the shift.
   c. have a co-worker who is not busy chart for her.
   d. sign off all meds at the beginning of the shift.

5. The responsibility for informed consent rests with the:
   a. nurse.
   b. client.
   c. physician.
   d. unit clerk.

6. Informed consent occurs when the:
   a. nurse discusses the surgical procedure with the client.
   b. client gives consent verbally.
   c. client understands the risks, benefits, and alternatives to treatment.
   d. client signs the consent form.

7. If you suspect a co-worker is diverting drugs, you should:
   a. approach the co-worker and tell him what you think.
   b. document dates, times, observed behavior, and report to your supervisor.
   c. say nothing, it is none of your business.
   d. tell co-workers what you think so they can help you watch for suspicious behavior.

News Flash

The March, 1996 column of Legally Speaking in RN Magazine identified several issues placing nurses at risk for a variety of legal or ethical reasons. The issue that most affects the practical/vocational nurse is downsizing and the concurrent use of unlicensed assistive personnel. The current trend toward downsizing frequently places nurses in the position of having more work to do and less people to do it. In addition, reduced hospital stays have created a situation where client acuity is higher in both acute and long-term care settings. Higher acuity and less staff can pose a threat to the quality of client care.

Failure to assess or failure to intervene are major factors in litigation against nurses. An overburdened nurse may miss important assessment parameters or fail to intervene in a timely manner. Therefore, the nurse needs to carefully evaluate client assignments. If there is cause for concern, discuss the problem with the nursing supervisor before the assignment is accepted. In addition, use discretion when delegating to assistive personnel. Do not delegate or assign duties outside the person's scope or skill level. Follow up to see that assistive personnel are doing what is expected. Lack of knowledge is an inadequate defense.

(*Source: Infante, M. (1996). The legal risks of managed care.* RN (3), 57–59.)

8. Advance directives:
   a. are binding only if written.
   b. cannot be changed once they are notarized.
   c. guide family members through difficult decisions.
   d. prevent clients from determining the course of their health care.

9. The health care representative or durable power of attorney for health care:
   a. is appointed by hospital administrators to make medical decisions for the client.
   b. can give or withhold consent for treatment.
   c. is contacted to override the decisions the client makes for himself.
   d. is the client's physician or health care provider.

10. Which of the following situations reflects inappropriate use of an incident report?
    a. Mrs. Jones falls in the hall while visiting her daughter.
    b. A student nurse gives Losec instead of Lasix.
    c. The safety committee reviews incident reports regarding falls on the 3–11 shift on A-wing.
    d. An instructor, frustrated with a disorganized student nurse, fills out an incident report because the student gave a 9 A.M. medication at 9:25.

Critical Thinking Questions

1. How would you explain advance directives to your family?

2. How would you know if a client gave informed consent?

CHAPTER
3
Introduction to Ethics

Susan Halley

KEY TERMS

advocate
autonomy
beneficence
code of ethics
cultural values
deontological
ethical dilemma
ethical principles
ethical rights
ethics
fidelity
justice
legal rights
nonmaleficence
personal values
rights
teleological
values
value system
veracity

LEARNING OBJECTIVES

Upon completion of this chapter the learner should be able to:
- Define key terms.
- Discuss the relationship between ethics, rights, morals, and values.
- Identify how personal values and beliefs influence individual perspectives regarding ethical issues.
- Distinguish between the ethical principles of autonomy, beneficence, nonmaleficence, justice, fidelity, and veracity.
- Describe the cultural contexts that affect ethics in nursing.
- Discuss the role of the nurse and ethics in health care.
- Describe strategies for ethical decision making.

▶ *MAKING THE CONNECTION*

Refer to the topics in the following chapters to increase your understanding of ethics.

- **Chapter 1, Critical Thinking:** Reasoning and Problem-Solving, p. 12; Critical Thinking and the Nursing Process, p. 15.
- **Chapter 2, Legal Aspects of Nursing:** Informed Consent, p. 27.
- **Chapter 4, Biomedical Ethics:** Confidentiality, Privacy, p. 53; Clients' Rights Issues, p. 53; Organ Donation, Moral Views, p. 59; Reproductive Technology, Surrogate Motherhood, p. 62; Death and Dying Issues,

Euthanasia, p. 63, Assisted Suicide, p. 63; Genetics, p. 63; Abortion, Right to Life Issues, p. 64, Moral Issues, p. 65; Professional Gatekeeping, Impaired Colleague, p. 65.
- **Chapter 6, Cultural Aspects of Health and Illness:** Culturally Appropriate Nursing Care, Personal Cultural Assessment, p. 92, Client Cultural Assessment, p. 92, Nurse's Response, p. 94.
- **Chapter 7, Cultural Diversity in the Workplace:** Nursing Process and Spiritual Needs, p. 103; Nursing Implications, p. 113.

INTRODUCTION

As the health care industry continues to undergo dramatic changes, nurses are increasingly confronted by diverse ethical issues. Advances in medical technology and the limitation of health care resources create complex ethical client situations that challenge nurses daily. For example, a nurse may be challenged to meet the holistic needs of a new mother who, against her wishes, is required to be discharged from the hospital the day following the birth of her pre-term infant who must stay in the hospital for further treatment. The nurse's unique professional relationship with clients and families mandates that the nurse be responsibly aware of current health care issues and the ethical dimensions of nursing practice.

Ethics, personal rights, morals, duties, and a person's individual value system all affect the way a nurse delivers care and are addressed in this chapter. It is important for the nurse to understand the position of different moral views before trying to resolve ethical client situations. For nurses to make informed ethical decisions in client care, they must possess knowledge and skills acquired from the study of ethics. Nurses need to be aware of how their **personal values**, or beliefs they hold important, impact their decision making. Clarification of one's own value system, plus an understanding of ethical principles and theories, guide the nurse in making the best possible judgments in the care of clients.

The concepts discussed in this chapter are developed further in Chapter 4 which explores current topics in health care of ethical concern, such as life-prolonging technologies, surrogate motherhood, and abortion to name a few.

KEY ABBREVIATIONS

The following abbreviations and acronyms are used in this chapter:

AHA	American Hospital Association
DNR	do not resuscitate
NFLPN	National Federation of Licensed Practical Nurses

RIGHTS

It is especially important for nurses to consider the **rights** of others when planning ethical client care. The term rights is usually understood as a claim or entitlement. Rights infer that something is owed to someone. When rights are written as laws they are considered **legal rights** and are sanctioned by law. For example, the right to free speech is written in the Bill of Rights and guaranteed to all citizens of the United States. Rights define what a given society accepts as appropriate behavior and conduct from its citizens. A society's belief of what is acceptable behavior changes continually. Laws, too, continually change to reflect society's current beliefs. Chapter 2 provides additional information on nursing and the law.

While legal rights are guaranteed by laws, **ethical rights** are based on moral principle and are actually privileges. For example, a nurse is obligated to respect the uniqueness of all persons. This respect is an ethical right. People are awarded certain privileges because they are human. Ethical rights are applied equally to all persons, regardless of income, gender, race, or nationality. For example, the nurse may be among those on a committee that decides who should be granted a heart transplant. All heart transplant candidates have the ethical right to be considered for the heart transplant based on the degree of need and the chance for successful outcomes. Income, gender, race, or nationality should not enter into the decision of who is granted a heart transplant. The American Hospital Association (AHA) has developed A Patient's Bill of Rights that applies to every client in every health care institution (see Table 3-1). This document lists the rights of the client, how each client should be treated, and how care should be administered.

ETHICS

Ethics is a branch of philosophy that originated in Ancient Greece. Ethics involves the consideration of what is right and what is wrong, or what causes good and what causes harm. When formalized, ethics is gen-

erally organized as systems of appropriate behaviors. For example, the deontological theory of ethics (discussed later in this chapter), operates on the principle that actions are either right or wrong. On an individual level, ethics is based upon a person's **values**, or what a person believes to be true and right based upon his or her own unique experiences as a member of society. Organized groups, such as the National Federation of Licensed Practical Nurses (NFLPN), formalize agreed-upon ethical standards in a **code of ethics**. Unlike laws, adherence to a system of ethics is not enforced by legislation; however, membership in or affiliation with a professional organization is generally dependent on members following certain ethical standards.

Code of Ethics

A code of ethics assists members of a professional organization in choosing behaviors that are congruent

Table 3-1

A PATIENT'S BILL OF RIGHTS

PATIENT AND COMMUNITY RELATIONS

Introduction

Effective health care requires collaboration between patients and physicians and other health care professionals. Open and honest communication, respect for personal and professional values, and sensitivity to differences are integral to optimal patient care. As the setting for the provision of health services, hospitals must provide a foundation for understanding and respecting the rights and responsibilities of patients, their families, physicians, and other caregivers. Hospitals must ensure a health care ethic that respects the role of patients in decision making about treatment choices and other aspects of their care. Hospitals must be sensitive to cultural, racial, linguistic, religious, age, gender, and other differences as well as the needs of persons with disabilities.

The American Hospital Association presents *A Patient's Bill of Rights* with the expectation that it will contribute to more effective patient care and be supported by the hospital on behalf of the institution, its medical staff, employees, and patients. The American Hospital Association encourages health care institutions to tailor this bill of rights to their patient community by translating and/or simplifying the language of this bill of rights as may be necessary to ensure that patients and their families understand their rights and responsibilities.

Bill of Rights*

1. The patient has the right to considerate and respectful care.

2. The patient has the right to and is encouraged to obtain from physicians and other direct caregivers relevant, current, and understandable information concerning diagnosis, treatment, and prognosis.

Except in emergencies when the patient lacks decision-making capacity and the need for treatment is urgent, the patient is enti-

tled to the opportunity to discuss and request information related to the specific procedures and/or treatments, the risks involved, the possible length of recuperation, and the medically reasonable alternatives and their accompanying risks and benefits.

Patients have the right to know the identity of phsycians, nurses, and others involved in their care, as well as when those involved are students, residents, or other trainees. The patient also has the right to know the immediate and long term financial implications of treatment choices, insofar as they are known.

3. The patient has the right to make decisions about the plan of care prior to and during the course of treatment and to refuse a recommended treatment or plan of care to the extent permitted by law and hospital policy and to be informed of the medical consequences of this action. In case of such refusal, the patient is entitled to other appropriate care and services that the hospital provides or transfer to another hospital. The hospital should notify patients of any policy that might affect patient choice within the institution.

4. The patient has the right to have an advance directive (such as living will, health care proxy, or durable power of attorney for health care) concerning treatment or designating a surrogate decision maker with the expectation that the hospital will honor the intent of that directive to the extent permitted by law and hospital policy.

Health care institutions must advise patients of their rights under state law and hospital policy to make informed medical choices, ask if the patient has an advance directive, and include that information in patient records. The patient has the right to timely information about hospital policy that may limit its ability to implement fully a legally valid advance directive.

5. The patient has the right to every consideration of privacy. Case discussion, consultation, examination, and treatment should be conducted so as to protect each patient's privacy.

6. The patient has the right to expect that all communications and records pertaining to his/her care will be treated as confidential by the hospital, except in cases such as suspected abuse and public health hazards when reporting is permitted or

*These rights can be exercised on the patient's behalf by a designated surrogate or proxy decision maker if the patient lacks decision making capacity, is legally incompetent, or is a minor.

with the values of the profession. They are those general standards and ideals that members of a group strive to achieve. Codes of ethics do not provide members of an organization with answers to specific problems, but serve as a framework to assist members. Though not legally binding, the code of ethics of an organization can be used to guide others in determining whether someone acts as or like other individuals would have in any situation.

The NFLPN has developed a code of ethics that is commonly accepted as expectations of the licensed practical/vocational nurse (see Table 3-2). Each LP/VN, in accepting licensure, has a moral obligation to adhere to the standards of practice and conducts set forth in this code, which was originally developed in 1961 and revised in 1979 and 1991. Students of practical/vocational nursing should also familiarize themselves with the code and the standards of practice it outlines as they prepare themselves for licensure.

Ethical Principles

Ethics in health care is based on common **ethical principles** that are examined in ethical situations. **Autonomy**, **nonmaleficence**, **beneficence**, **justice**, **fidelity**, and **veracity** are key concepts in understanding health care ethics.

Autonomy

Autonomy is an individual's right of self-determination, independence, and freedom. To make an informed decision regarding their course of treatment, clients rely on health care providers to provide them with accurate, current, and understandable information regarding their conditions and the treatment options. Once health care workers provide the client with this information, the client then has the right to make independent choices about treatment plans. The

required by law. The patient has the right to expect that the hospital will emphasize the confidentiality of this information when it releases it to any other parties entitled to review information in these records.

7. The patient has the right to review the records pertaining to his/her medical care and to have the information explained or interpreted as necessary, except when restricted by law.

8. The patient has the right to expect that, within its capcity and policies, a hospital will make reasonable response to the request of a patient for appropriate and medically indicated care and services. The hospital must provide evaluation, service, and/or referral as indicated by the urgency of the case. When medically appropriate and legally permissible, or when a patient has so requested, a patient may be transferrred to another facility. The institution to which the patient is to be transferred must first have accepted the patient for transfer. The patient must also have the benefit of complete information and explanation concerning the need for, risks, benefits, and alternatives to such a transfer.

9. The patient has the right to ask and be informed of the existence of business relationships among the hospital, educational institutions, other health care providers, or payers that may influence the patient's treatment and care.

10. The patient has the right to consent to or decline to participate in proposed research studies or human experimentation affecting care and treatment or requiring direct patient involvement, and to have those studies fully explained prior to consent. A patient who declines to participate in research or experimentation is entitled to the most effective care that the hospital can otherwise provide.

11. The patient has the right to expect reasonable continuity of care when appropriate and to be informed by physicians and other caregivers of available and realistic patient care options when hospital care is no longer appropriate.

12. The patient has the right to be informed of hospital policies and practices that relate to patient care, treatment, and responsibilities. The patient has the right to be informed of available resources for resolving disputes, grievances, and conflicts, such as ethics committees, patient representatives, or other mechanisms available in the institution. The patient has the right

to be informed of the hospital's charges for services and available payment methods.

The collaborative nature of health care requires that patients, or their families/surrogates, participate in their care. The effectiveness of care and patient satisfaction with the course of treatment depend, in part, on the patient fulfilling certain responsibilities. Patients are responsible for providing information about past illnesses, hospitalizations, medications, and other matters related to health status. To participate effectively in decision making, patients must be encouraged to take responsibility for requesting additional information or clarification about their health status or treatment when they do not fully understand information and instructions. Patients are also responsible for ensuring that the health care institution has a copy of their written advance directive if they have one. Patients are responsible for informing their physicians and other caregivers if they anticipate problems in following prescribed treatment.

Patients should also be aware of the hospital's obligation to be reasonably efficient and equitable in providing care to other patients and the community. The hospital's rules and regulations are designed to help the hospital meet this obligation. Patients and their families are responsible for making reasonable accommodations to the needs of the hospital, other patients, medical staff, and hospital employees. Patients are responsible for providing necessary information for insurance claims and for working with the hospital to make payment arrangements, when necessary.

A person's health depends on much more than health care services. Patients are responsible for recognizing the impact of their life-style on their personal health.

Conclusion

Hospitals have many functions to perform, including the enhancement of health status, health promotion, and the prevention and treatment of injury and disease; the immediate and ongoing care and rehabilitation of patients; the education of health professionals, patients, and the community; and research. All these activities must be conducted with an overriding concern for the values and dignity of patients.

(Reprinted with permission of the American Hospital Association, copyright 1992)

Table 3-2

THE CODE FOR LICENSED PRACTICAL/VOCATIONAL NURSES

1. Know the scope of maximum utilization of the LP/VN as specified by the nursing practice act and function within this scope.
2. Safeguard the confidential information acquired from any source about the patient.
3. Provide health care to all regardless of race, creed, cultural background, disease, or lifestyle.
4. Refuse to give endorsement to the sale and promotion of commercial products or services.
5. Uphold the highest standards in personal appearance, language, dress, and demeanor.
6. Stay informed about issues affecting the practice of nursing and delivery of health care and, where appropriate, participate in government and policy decisions.
7. Accept the responsibility for safe nursing by keeping oneself mentally and physically fit and educationally prepared to practice.
8. Accept responsibility for membership in NFLPN and participate in its efforts to maintain the established standards of nursing practice and employment policies which lead to quality patient care.

(Reprinted with permission. Courtesy of National Federation of Licensed Practical Nurses, Inc., 1991 Revision).

client also has the right to refuse treatment. Informed consent is derived from the principle of autonomy, whereby the client's ability to make health care decisions is based on full disclosure of the benefits, risks, potential consequences of a recommended treatment plan, and alternative treatments, including no treatment. Refer to Chapter 2 for more information on informed consent.

Limits to client autonomy are only placed when the rights of others are infringed. For example, a client with a contagious disease may be placed in isolation or required by law to take medications to cure the disease to avoid endangering the wellness of others (Aiken & Catalano, 1994).

Nonmaleficence

"Do no harm" is key to the concept of nonmaleficence. Health care providers are required not to harm others intentionally or unintentionally. Furthermore, it is the responsibility of a nurse to be an **advocate** for those clients in their care who cannot protect themselves. Clients who may need extra protection might include the very young, the very old, those who are debilitated, the mentally incompetent or those under the influence of medications, and those who are uninformed.

Beneficence

Beneficence requires nurses to go beyond nonmaleficence and actively "do good" for clients. This is often viewed as the core of nursing practice. The nurse serves as a client advocate and promotes the rights of the client. The nurse is required to nurture the client and incorporate the desires of the client and the client's family into the plan of care. Sometimes, the nurse may have difficulty determining what is "good," especially when doing good for clients sometimes causes them discomfort. For example, a client who has been in a serious car accident may resist performing painful range of motion exercises and grow angry at the nurse for insisting. The nurse realizes the long-term value of the exercises, yet understands the client's physical and psychological pain.

Justice

Justice mandates that all persons be treated fairly. Nurses should treat people impartially without regard to race, gender, medical diagnosis, marital status, social standing, or religious beliefs. Access and allocation of health care resources are involved in this principle. The nurse may experience difficulty when deciding what is fair. For example, one client with a serious condition and no health insurance may not be able to remain in the hospital for the duration of treatment. Another client with the same condition and health insurance can remain until the condition stabilizes. Nurses may be challenged by such situations throughout their professional lives. Chapter 4 explores these issues in greater detail.

Fidelity

Fidelity is the duty to be faithful to commitments. A nurse has a duty to be faithful to the professional obligations assumed as a member of the nursing profession. As stated in the NFLPN code of ethics, the nurse must "know the scope of maximum utilization of the LP/VN as specified by the nursing practice act and function within this scope." Within the client-nurse relationship, nurses should be loyal to their responsibilities, keep promises, maintain privacy, and meet reasonable expectations of clients. This loyalty should extend beyond the client to include the client's family and co-workers. The nurse also has a duty to be faithful to him or herself. Conflict between commitments can complicate matters for the nurse who may also question who is owed fidelity. Remaining client-centered may help clarify this question, although it may not resolve the conflict. For example, the mother of a frightened teenage girl may try to pressure the nurse into revealing the results of her daughter's pregnancy test. While the nurse may believe the mother has the girl's best interests at heart, the nurse must protect the client's privacy.

Veracity

Veracity demands that nurses remain dedicated to telling the truth to clients and not deliberately misleading them. Deception can occur by giving false information or by omitting the truth. Telling the truth is sometimes uncomfortable for the nurse. However, discomfort is not a valid reason for avoiding the truth. Exceptions to truth telling are sometimes upheld by the principle of nonmaleficence, when the truth does greater harm than good. The act of giving placebo medications is an example of when telling the truth does greater harm than good.

Theories of Ethics

Theories of ethics, as mentioned earlier in this chapter, are formal organizations of basic ethical principles. Every nurse-client interaction creates an ethical situation. For example, the basic concepts of autonomy, nonmaleficence, beneficence, justice, fidelity, and veracity come into play: the nurse must respect the client's autonomy, endeavor not to harm the client, inform the client about the condition or treatment, and so on. Sometimes, during the course of care, the nurse may have a conflict with the client, the client's family, a physician, or another co-worker. When conflict occurs, the nurse may use one or more ethical theories to work through the problem. Clarification of the nurse's value system (discussed later in this chapter) also helps the nurse determine which ethical systems most closely reflect his or her own beliefs. **Deontological**, **teleological**, situational, and caring theories are commonly applied when ethical decisions are needed in the clinical setting and are summarized below.

Deontological Theory

Deontology is taken from the Greek word for duty or moral obligation. Deontological theory is also known as a "duty-oriented" theory because actions are viewed as inherently right or wrong, without regard to the end results. The duty or moral obligation is based on moral absolutes revealed by a higher power.

Those who follow the duty-oriented theory believe that the act of "promoting good" is not alone satisfactory when making ethical decisions. The "right" principle must guide a person's actions, not the consequences of those actions. This fundamental principle

at the foundation of the deontological theory is called the "categorical imperative." Examples of this include "life is worthy of respect, therefore, all persons should be treated the same"; "lying violates the obligation to tell the truth"; "human life has value."

The advantage of the deontological approach is that people have a clearer understanding of what actions are expected in a given situation. The disadvantage is that consequences of actions are not considered and, often, may do the client more harm than good.

Teleological Theory

Teleological is taken from the Greek word Telos which means "end." Teleological theory states that the "rightfulness" of an action is determined by the end result created from that action, i.e., the end justifies the means. Teleological theory is also known as utilitarianism. Behaviors that create the greatest good (or happiness) for the greatest number are considered the most moral. Concepts considered inherently good for all members of a society include health, strength, truth, freedom, security, and peace (Edge & Groves, 1994). In the health care setting, such goals as the prevention, elimination or control of disease, relief from unnecessary pain and suffering, amelioration of disabling conditions, and the prolongation of life are intrinsic goods (Beauchamp & McCullough, 1994).

On a smaller scale, the determination of what is good for the client (the end = client's happiness or well-being) versus what causes the client harm (means = pain, discomfort) may pose a challenge to the nurse. For example, a nurse caring for a client with cervical cancer may have difficulty watching the client undergo radium implant treatment, although the ultimate goal of the treatment is a return to wellness. In a more extreme example, a client suffering terribly from a terminal illness may seek an end to her suffering through assisted suicide. A strict believer of teleology would advocate the assisted suicide option. Chapter 4 explores such topics in greater detail.

The advantage of teleology is that the interest of the majority is protected. A major disadvantage is that minority and individual rights may be ignored. Also, determining what is meant by "good" or "happiness" is difficult in a health care setting.

Situational Theory

The situational theory holds that there are no set rules, norms or majority focused results. Each situation must be considered individually with emphasis on the uniqueness of the situation and respect for the person involved. Decisions made in one situation cannot be generalized to another situation (Pappas, 1994).

Caring-based Theory

Caring-based theory relies on relationships rather than principles for primary moral reflection. The theory is based on the premise that people do not make ethical decisions based on principles. Caring-based theory views decisions as being made with respect to relationships, caring, communication, a desire not to hurt others, and responsiveness. Caring focuses on emotions, feelings, and attitudes. The theory is sometimes referred to as the "voice of care" and contrasted with the "voice of justice." Justice and caring are not considered mutually exclusive, however (Beare & Myers, 1994).

VALUES

Values are perceptions or ideals that help shape a person's life and provide it with meaning. A person is not born with values; religion, family, societal norms and life experiences help forge a person's value system as he or she matures. A **value system** is an individual's collection of inner beliefs that guides the way the person acts and helps determine the choices made in life. For example, an individual who is strongly identified with family may choose to work part-time, if financially possible, in order to spend more time at home. Individual identity is reflected by a person's value system.

Values also influence client-nurse relationships since values determine both the client's and the nurse's behaviors. A client may misinterpret a nurse's behavior based on the client's personal value system. For example, a client with a value system of "grin and bear it" in the face of pain may be insulted by a nurse's attempts to offer pain medications. Nurses must be sensitive to the values expressed by the client, as well as clarifying their own belief systems so that effective client care can be given.

Acquisition of Values

The acquisition of values begins in childhood through socialization and role modeling of the adults in their environment. Values change as people grow intellectually and are influenced by varying life experiences. As adults, values give meaning to life and motivate them to understand their place in the universe (Hamilton, 1992).

People differ in the beliefs they consider important. A client's **cultural values**, or values determined by affiliation with a particular cultural group, may be extremely different from the nurse's values. For example, religious convictions may be deeply rooted and be a significant part of a person's life. A deeply religious Catholic nurse may be in a situation that creates con-

flict with values, such as working in a unit that performs abortions when abortions are in direct opposition to the nurse's value system. A nurse should make her values known to the employer before employment. Chapters 6 and 7 of this text discuss cultural values in greater detail.

Development Theories

As individuals grow from childhood to adulthood they develop a unique system of values, and their ability to perform moral reasoning matures. Much investigation has been done in this area of study by theorists such as John Dewey, Jean Piaget, and Lawrence Kohlberg. Piaget is often considered to have had the greatest influence in this area. Since ethics is based on the value of what is "good" in life, a review of moral development theories will assist the nurse to better understand the field of ethics.

Dewey

John Dewey outlined three levels of moral development: premoral, conventional, and autonomous. Individuals progress through these distinct stages as they mature. At the premoral stage, a person's behavior is triggered by biological or social impulses. This is considered the lowest level of moral development. For example, an infant is motivated by desires to eat, sleep, and excrete. A person matures to the second stage, called conventional, when a person's behavior mirrors the norms of society. Behavior based on critical thinking and deliberate analysis is reflective of the highest phase identified as the autonomy stage.

Piaget

Jean Piaget believed that a child's moral reasoning coincided with cognitive (intellectual) development and social experience. He believed that changes in children's thought processes result in a growing ability to acquire and use knowledge about their world (Piaget, 1969). As they mature and move through a series of cognitive development stages, children are better able to make judgments about right and wrong (see Table 3-3). As intellect is strengthened, moral reasoning is strengthened. For example, a child in the stage of concrete operational thought has the ability to understand cause and effect, or right and wrong (Oran, 1996). The child recognizes that if she does something understood as "wrong" (lying to her mother) consequences may result (she may be punished by her mother). In this stage, the child's focus is on the consequences of the act, rather than the nature of the act itself. As children move into the stage of formal operational thought, they begin to view right and wrong less as absolutes and more as the result of

Table 3-3

PIAGET'S STAGES OF COGNITIVE DEVELOPMENT		
Stage	**Age**	**Description**
Sensorimotor (amoral)	Birth–2 years	The child learns about the world through input from the senses and by motor activity. During this period, the child begins to link cause with effect and to recognize object permanence (i.e., that an object continues to exist even when it cannot be seen). Language provides the child with a tool for understanding the world.
Preoperational (amoral)	2–7 years	The child now thinks by using words as symbols, but logic is not well developed.
Concrete operational thought (moral realism)	7–11 years	The child develops a more accurate understanding of cause and effect, and reasons well if concrete objects are used.
Formal operational thought (autonomous morality)	11 years–adulthood	Mature intellectual thought is attained. The adolescent can reason abstractly and consider different alternatives or outcomes.

social agreement. For example, when the child lies to her mother, she will not only get in trouble, but might also influence her mother's opinion of her honesty, hurt her mother's feelings, feel badly herself, etc.

Kohlberg

Advancing Piaget's work, Lawrence Kohlberg expanded moral reasoning into three levels, with two stages each. Kohlberg believed that specific attainment of the stages is based on different degrees of maturity. Some persons never move beyond the lowest stages while others reach the highest stages. Lower stages reflect behaviors based on rigid, concrete principles. For example, young children accept authority since they have no comprehension of the concept of right and wrong. Higher stages are based upon abstract principles. For example, as children mature their concept of self strengthens and authority figures become less influential in the child's decision-making process. Concepts such as respect for the rights of others, justice, and following a person's conscience become the guide for ethical decision making (Edge & Groves, 1994). Table 3-4 outlines Kohlberg's stages of moral development.

Values Clarification

Values clarification is a method of identifying the priorities a person places in life. Beliefs about God, family, truth, love, sex, and pleasure are among those values that individuals clarify. Understanding one's own values helps decrease inner conflict. For example, a nurse who believes individuals have the right to determine their fate will have an easier time caring for

a client with a DNR order who ultimately dies, despite the sadness experienced over the client's death. Nurses who have clarified their values may also have an easier time making ethically sound decisions affect-

Table 3-4

KOHLBERG'S STAGES OF MORAL DEVELOPMENT
I. PRECONVENTIONAL MORALITY
Stage 1: Punishment and obedience orientation — Might makes right; obey authority to avoid punishment.
Stage 2: Individualism and relativist orientation — Look out for number one; be nice to others so they will be nice to you.
II. CONVENTIONAL MORALITY
Stage 3: Mutual interpersonal expectations — "Good girl, nice boy"; approval more important that reward.
Stage 4: Social system and conscience. — "Law and order"; contributing to society's good is important.
III. POSTCONVENTIONAL
Stage 5: Social contract — Rules are to benefit all, by mutual agreement; may be changed same way; the greatest good for the greatest number of people.
Stage 6: Universal ethical principles — Values established by individual reflection, may contradict other laws.

(*Adapted from* Beginnings and Beyond, 4e, *A. Miles Gordon & K. Williams-Browne: Delmar Publishers, 1995*)

ing client care, as long as they understand that personal values, preferences, and priorities do not take precedence over clients' values. Each person's value system is equally valid. For example, the nurse from the preceding example has spent time thinking through his personal beliefs regarding life-prolonging technologies and has come to the personal decision that he would not wish to be on life support, regardless of the situation. Familiar with his own deliberate process of values clarification, he should thus be able to understand the decision of a husband to prolong the life of his eighty-year-old comatose wife by means of life support, despite the fact that their values are in conflict.

Values clarification involves time and self-reflection. It may be useful to use a tool to help begin this process. Table 3-5 provides a systematic, seven step process designed to aid values clarification (Uustal, 1993).

Nurses also need to understand how their cultural values shape their perceptions about their environment and their personal beliefs about health care. Therefore, it is useful to perform a personal cultural assessment in conjunction with a values clarification exercise. Chapter 6 of this text discusses this activity in greater detail.

Table 3-5

EXAMINING VALUES

1. **Freedom to make own choices:**
   Who taught me my values? Have I given thought to my values? Are my values right?

2. **Choosing from alternatives:**
   What other values are possible? Have I thought about this alternative? Does it appeal to me?

3. **Choosing after considering the consequences:**
   What are the consequences from holding these values? What is the price to pay for my position? Is it worth it?

4. **Complement to other values:**
   Are my values consistent? Do they conflict with one another?

5. **Prize and cherish:**
   Do I feel good about my values? How important are my values?

6. **Public affirmation:**
   Am I willing to speak out for my values?

7. **Action:**
   Am I willing to put my values into action? Do my values guide my behaviors? Are my values ethical?

DUTIES AND OBLIGATIONS

Nurses as professionals have a duty and moral obligation to provide quality care to their clients. All clients are not compliant nor do they all speak pleasantly, but the nurse must still care for them all. A nurse who walks off the job could be sanctioned by the state board of nursing for abandoning her clients.

SOLVING ETHICAL DILEMMAS

Nurses are faced every day with rapid changes in technology that affect change in our social environment. Nurses are required to make judgments regarding client care in the midst of an evolving arena. Nurses solve problems by the nature of their work. Sometimes nurses are required to choose between equally undesirable alternatives and thus an **ethical dilemma** is a situation where right and wrong actions are not clear cut. When faced with ethical decision making, being systematic in reasoning brings clarity to the situation.

One systematic process is suggested by Aiken and Catalano (1994) and is as follows:

Step 1: Collect and analyze the data. Determine the facts and obtain enough to illustrate the issue.

Step 2: State the dilemma. Using the information collected, identify the ethical issue at hand.

Step 3: Consider choices of action. All possible choices without consideration of consequence should be listed.

Step 4: Analyze the advantages and disadvantages. Consider related outcomes to the possible choices. This reduces the list of realistic choices.

Step 5: Make the decision. Dilemmas by nature do not have a right or wrong answer. The best answer can be attained by using a systematic logical process and collaborating with others when appropriate. After the course of action has been acted upon, evaluate your decision to base future decisions regarding similar ethical clinical situations.

▶ CASE STUDIES

Case Study I

Janice is a forty-five-year-old woman who is pregnant with her fourth child. The pregnancy was unplanned and distressed Janice and her husband at first, but now they have accepted it and look forward to the delivery of their child. Janice has been receiving prenatal care from her family practice physician since her second month of pregnancy. She is now in her seventh month.

During her sixth month of pregnancy, the physician ordered laboratory tests and the results indicated a fetal abnormality. The physician requested to perform further invasive testing on the fetus during the seventh month. Janice and her husband refused further fetal testing. Although the physician explained the importance of the testing, the couple continued to refuse it.

After the couple leave the office the physician turns to the nurse and states, "Since they will not follow my suggestions, write them a letter and tell them I am terminating our relationship. Tell her to see a specialist." No arrangements for a referral have been made for Janice by the doctor. The doctor fears the high risk delivery predisposes him to a lawsuit.

The following questions are related to the case study.

1. Based on the information presented here, what are the primary moral/ethical issues?

2. What are your personal values in relation to the situation?

3. What course of action would you recommend for the nurse and why? What ethical/moral principles would guide you?

4. To what extent, in your opinion, is Janice non-compliant?

5. Was the medical intervention adequate? Is nursing to judge medical care?

6. What is the nurse's responsibility to ensure follow-up care?

▶ CASE STUDIES (continued)

Case Study II

Mr. Thomas is an eighty-nine-year-old resident in a long-term care facility. Mr. Thomas has a long history of diabetes with many complications. At present, he is losing his eyesight and has gangrene in his right foot. Mr. Thomas' family consists of two children, a son and a daughter, who visit for short periods every couple of weeks. Mr. Thomas says they are very busy running the business he started. Mr. Thomas' wife died four years ago and he misses her very much as he tells the nurse frequently. The pastor of Mr. Thomas' church visits at least weekly. The nurse has developed a special rapport with Mr. Thomas and he calls the nurse his "special nurse." Mr. Thomas has told the nurse he is ready to die and "does not want any of that stuff done to keep him alive." He asks the nurse to promise not to let them. When the nurse arrives for work, Mr. Thomas has been scheduled for surgery and is to be transferred. The nurse at report said Dr. Jones and Mr. Thomas' children made the decision and Mr. Thomas is not happy but no one is listening to him.

The following questions are related to the case study.

1. What are the moral/ethical issues?
2. Systematically collect and analyze all data and discuss their relevance to the ethical issues.
3. Are there emotional issues that are clouding the question?
4. What is the dilemma?
5. List all the choices of action.
6. Analyze the advantages and disadvantages of each choice.
7. What should you, Mr. Thomas' special nurse do, if anything?

SUMMARY

- Because nursing's primary concern is quality care of clients, nurses must possess a basic understanding of values, moral development, ethical principles, and ethical theories. A nurse's understanding of his or her values enhances the nurse-client relationship and helps the nurse make effective nursing decisions.
- Ethical rights are privileges based on moral principles and not guaranteed by laws. These rights apply equally to all persons, and are not determined by race, gender, income, or religion.
- A code of ethics helps members of a profession choose behaviors congruent with the values of that profession. The NFLPN has developed a code of ethics called "The Code for Licensed Practical/Vocational Nurses."
- Common principles examined in ethical situations include: autonomy, nonmaleficence, beneficence, justice, fidelity, and veracity.
- Ethical theories are formal organizations of basic ethical principles. Deontological, teleological, situational, and caring-based theories are commonly used ethical theories.
- Values are perceptions or ideals that help shape a person's life and provide it with meaning. A person's values develop as a result of family, religion, culture, and environment. Dewey, Piaget, and Kohlberg are theorists who have developed theories on the development of morality.
- Nurses should clarify their own values prior to working with clients because they will thus have an easier time making ethically sound decisions affecting client care. However, a nurse's personal values, preferences, and priorities do not take precedence over a client's values; each is equally valid.
- An ethical dilemma is a situation where right and wrong actions are not clear cut, and the choice is often between two equally undesirable alternatives. A nurse can use a system of reasoning to work through an ethical dilemma and come up with a choice.

Review Questions

1. An ethical right is a right that is:
   a. the same as a legal right.
   b. guaranteed by law.
   c. defined by a state nursing board.
   d. based on moral principle.

2. Nurses would use the Code for Licensed Practical/Vocational Nurses to:
   a. seek an answer to a client care problem.
   b. solve an ethical dilemma.
   c. understand the professional expectations required of them.
   d. develop a nursing care plan.

3. Values influence the nurse-client relationship because:
   a. the client's values take precedence over the nurse's values.
   b. every individual has a personal value system that helps determine his/her actions and reactions.
   c. the nurse cannot effectively care for a client with values that are different from her own.
   d. the nurse must help the client clarify his values to ensure effective nursing care.

4. By observing a client's body language, a nurse discovers his client is exceptionally modest about undressing for an examination. The nurse should:
   a. ignore the client's discomfort and get on with preparing the client for examination.
   b. respect the client's need for privacy, even if it seems excessive to him.
   c. explain to the client why he is being silly.
   d. call another nurse to intervene.

5. Values clarification is a useful exercise for the nurse to perform because it:
   a. helps the nurse make ethically sound decisions.
   b. establishes rules about right and wrong client care.
   c. helps the nurse avoid conflict with clients and co-workers.
   d. challenges the nurse to stay informed of new developments.

6. An ethical dilemma is:
   a. a choice between right and wrong.
   b. a series of problems the nurse encounters in each client care situation.
   c. a problem with two equally bad solutions.
   d. a problem the nurse cannot solve without the intervention of a physician.

News Flash

In 1995 a controversial survey was conducted to study the role of critical care nurses in circumstances involving euthanasia and assisted suicide in the United States. Of the 1,600 nurses surveyed, 1,139 responded. After certain exclusions were made, the results of the survey were based on 852 subjects. Of those, 141 nurses said they had received requests from clients or family members to perform euthanasia or assist in suicide; 129 nurses said they did participate in such acts; and thirty-five nurses said they hastened a client's death by pretending to provide life-sustaining treatment ordered by a physician. The most common method of euthanasia was administering high doses of an opiate to terminally ill clients. It was also reported that 342 nurses had wanted to perform euthanasia or assist in suicide, but did not for fear of getting caught and losing their nursing licenses because the practice is illegal, or because the client's wishes were not completely understood.

The survey focused predominately on critical care nurses because of the amount of time they spend with clients and the relationship they develop as compared to that of the client's physician, which is considerably lower. (Asch, 1996)

Critical Thinking Questions

1. A client who tests positive for HIV tells you he hopes his pregnant wife doesn't find out. His wife is waiting outside. How would you handle this situation?

2. The mother of a terminally ill child refuses treatment that could alleviate his pain. She says she "doesn't believe in the treatment." What do you do?

CHAPTER
4
Biomedical Ethics

Mary Jo Brock

KEY TERMS

▶ abortion
advance directives
allocation of funds
assisted suicide
bioethics
case management
competent
confidential
eugenics
euthanasia
gatekeeping
impaired colleague
incompetent
joint venturing
macroallocation
microallocation

LEARNING OBJECTIVES

Upon completion of this chapter the learner should be able to:
- Define key terms.
- List three situations that require breaching of confidentiality.
- Describe the purpose of an advance directive.
- Discuss nursing actions that protect the right to privacy.
- Compare and contrast active and passive euthanasia.
- List three sources of organ donation.
- Identify the nurse's role in relation to individual biomedical ethics presented in this chapter.

▶ *MAKING THE CONNECTION*

Refer to the topics in the following chapters to increase your understanding of biomedical ethics:

- **Chapter 1, Critical Thinking:** Reasoning and Problem-Solving, p. 12; Critical Thinking and the Nursing Process, p. 15.
- **Chapter 2, Legal Aspects of Nursing:** Good Samaritan Law, p. 20; Informed Consent, p. 27; The Nurse's Role in Informed Consent, p. 27, Impaired Nurse, p. 27, Incident Reports, p. 29; Advance Directives, p. 30.
- **Chapter 3, Introduction to Ethics:** Ethical Principles, p. 41; Values, p. 44; Solving Ethical Dilemmas, p. 46.
- **Chapter 6, Cultural Aspects of Health and Illness:** Influence of Culture on Beliefs and Practices About Health and Illness, p. 90; Culturally Appropriate Nursing Care, p. 92, Personal Cultural Assessment, p. 92, Client Cultural Assessment, p. 92.
- **Chapter 7, Cultural Diversity in the Workplace:** Nursing Implications, p. 113.

INTRODUCTION

As you read in Chapter 3, many ethical principles apply to health care. **Bioethics** involves ethical principles, case law, and philosophical ethics. In textbooks, ethical issues seem to be clearly stated. But in reality, when applying ethics to health care, other issues come to light. Nurses are not dealing with textbook cases, they are caring for human beings. Each human being is an individual who possesses religious or spiritual beliefs, cultural values, and social normative behavior along with an illness process that is leading the person to face an ethical dilemma. Each person experiences life and illness situations with an emotional bias. This bias influences the way the individual assesses and evaluates the ethical dilemma.

Health care has seen dramatic advances in technology, such as transplants, genetic screening and management, synthetic medications, laser treatments, implantable defibrillators, and computerized nerve tracking systems for paralyzed bodies. When first analyzed, these new technologies have a positive impact on people's lives, enabling them to return to an improved level of activity. However, there is another part to the world of technology, an ethical layer, that needs to be addressed. As we enter the twenty-first century, more ethical situations will be presented to health care professionals.

This chapter presents topics with ethical concerns. Each topic will discuss the pros and cons as they apply to the health care setting. A future nurse must analyze personal views regarding ethical concerns. To present an unbiased approach at the bedside is not easy. Critical thinking skills are used to gather all the information, analyze the situation, and select the appropriate action. The nurse's opinions, coupled with the knowledge of nursing and health care, will affect the nurse's approach. This discussion attempts to present information in an unbiased manner and a part of each section will contain practical information based on experience.

KEY ABBREVIATIONS

The following abbreviations and acronyms are used in this chapter:

HMO	health maintenance organization
UNOS	United Network of Organ Sharing

CONFIDENTIALITY

Handling situations in a **confidential** manner means that one person entrusts another with highly personal information. The entrusted person is to keep the information or situation secret between the two persons. Divulging the information would breach this confidential or trusted relationship.

Purpose

The client's right to privacy, the respect for autonomy, and the information shared by the client with the nurse, must be protected and is always handled in a confidential manner. The information is very personal and, as a part of the assessment process (data gathering), nurses need to reassure their clients that all the information will be kept confidential.

The strictest mode of confidentiality is between a Catholic priest and a person who is confessing sins. In no situation can the priest reveal what was shared in the confessional. How confidential is the handling of information within a multidisciplinary health care team? Think of all the persons who will have access to a client's chart: doctors, nurses, pharmacists, respiratory therapists, dietitians, discharge planners, therapists, pastoral ministers, consultants, medical records staff, and utilization reviewers. With all these people reading the chart, the potential exists for a breach in confidentiality.

There are two ways to breach confidentiality: (1) by failing to protect entrusted information and (2) by deliberately disclosing information. Failure to protect information can simply mean not monitoring who has access to the charts or to a computer screen displaying the client's data. Deliberately disclosing information means just that—telling information about the client that was disclosed in confidence. This is easy for nurses to do and is an occupational hazard. In a general conversation in an elevator or in the cafeteria a nurse may ask, "How's the guy in 411 doing tonight?" The other nurse may respond with a clinical report. The nurse does not consider the disclosure of information a breach of confidentiality; instead it is sharing information with a fellow worker who seems concerned about the client in 411 (Beauchamp & Childress, 1994). The nurse could have handled the situation better by simply saying, "He's doing better."

Privacy

Privacy means the condition of being secluded or isolated from the view of or from contact with others. Privacy is a right that protects the person's integrity; a right that limits physical or informational accessibility (Beauchamp & Childress, 1994). What is defined as a loss of privacy may differ depending on the societal norms and/or culture of the person. Every person cared for has the right to privacy. A person who cannot speak for himself has the right to privacy; the right not to be viewed or touched by others who are not involved in his care. This right is protected by common law, statutory law, and constitutional law. Review Chapters 2 and 3 of this text to learn more about privacy.

Communication

Information about people can be communicated by words between people, in writing, on a computer screen, by facsimile, the Internet, or telephone. All of these modes are used in the health care setting to obtain or share information concerning clients. Misuse

of these modes can lead to disclosure of information that was given in a private or confidential manner.

Required Reporting

There are times when a health care professional must break confidentiality and reveal information. The law requires health care professionals to report all gunshot wounds, whether self-inflicted, accidental, or intentional. The abuse or neglect of anyone must also be reported to authorities.

Health care professionals are required to break confidentiality to protect the welfare of the community or an individual, unless the law prohibits disclosure, such as AIDS cases. If someone tells of plans to harm another person, the information can protect the other person from harm and must be reported. An example of protecting the community would be the required reporting of a contagious disease.

Nurse's Role

Nurses protect information concerning the client. It is permissible to question someone reading a client's chart if the nurse does not recognize the person or the person does not wear proper identification. Nurses monitor the location of client information by ensuring charts are retained on the unit or accompany a client leaving the unit. Paper information is kept in file drawers that are locked at the end of each day. If another agency needs information from the records, the client must authorize an information release in writing. Care must be taken in disclosing information by telephone because it is difficult to verify whether or not the person requesting the information has been authorized to do so. The nurse's role is to protect client information.

CLIENTS' RIGHTS ISSUES

A right means that something is provided in accordance with the law, morality, and/or another standard. As stated earlier, clients' rights are listed in the Patient Bill of Rights (see Chapter 3).

Competence

A person is considered **competent** when she demonstrates the ability to make decisions based on sound judgment. The person must also meet other criteria set by law to be a decision maker, such as age eighteen years or older, or an emancipated teenager.

Incompetence

An **incompetent** person has either lost the ability to make decisions due to a medical condition, such as dementia, or the person never had competent decision-making ability because of mental retardation.

A third issue of competency comes into play in an acute care setting. A client receiving pain medication who is partially sedated may or may not be in a competent state. It may be necessary to wait until the medication level has diminished before asking the client to make a competent decision.

Informed Consent

Informed consent means more than the client signing the consent form. Informed consent means the client has been given an explanation of the illness and/or procedure at a level the client can understand. The physician tells the client what is likely to happen (prognosis), possible risks, benefits, and complications that could occur. Alternative treatments and the effects of no treatment must also be explained to the client. This information is given to the client by the physician allowing the client to make an informed decision (Dubler & Nimmons, 1992). Documentation of the conversation becomes a part of the client's record. With the emphasis on outpatient procedures, frequently the informed consent is obtained in the physicians' offices. The nurse verifies the client's information level before the procedure occurs by simply asking a few focused questions. If the client does not demonstrate informed consent, it is the nurse's role to inform the physician. The physician must explain the information again. Informed consent places the client in charge of health care treatment options. Based on the information, the client decides the course of action.

Informed consent does not always mean the person accepts the choices the physician has outlined. The person always has the right to decline all treatment options. The individual must be informed, in detail, of the consequences of that choice. This information must also be documented in the person's record.

Advance Directives

When a client decides to limit the amount of health care he receives, places his decision in writing, and shares his decision with family and/or physician, he has created an **advance directive**. In November 1991, the federal government authorized legislation on advance directives. The law stated that health care facilities needed to document three items:

1. Upon admission, the client must be asked if he has an advance directive.
2. The client's response must be documented as part of the record.
3. The client must receive information about advance directives.

Any adult eighteen years of age or older can complete an advance directive. Currently there are three types of directives: Living Will, Power of Attorney for Health Care, and Life-Prolonging Procedure. Each state has its own statutes for advance directives; not all states honor other states' directives. The forms can be obtained at a physician's office, pastoral care departments, attorney's office, or purchased at an office supply store. Legal counsel is not needed to complete an advance directive.

Living Will

A living will is a witnessed document that a person completes stating the level or amount of care he wishes to receive when he is diagnosed in a terminal state. The person completes the form, listing any specific treatments he wants to receive or not receive. The person should share the living will with the doctor, family or support system, and attorney.

Power of Attorney for Health Care

The Power of Attorney for Health Care is a document that a person completes naming the person who will be his decision maker when he no longer can make decisions. Again, the person can make his wishes about the amount of care he receives or does not receive known in this document. The document needs to be witnessed and notarized. It is imperative that the designated decision maker and the person completing the form discuss the contents of the form. Each person involved should retain a copy as a record.

Life-Prolonging Procedures

To ensure life-prolonging procedures, the client signs a form that simply states the person wants every treatment possible performed to keep him alive, no matter what his condition. This form also needs to be witnessed.

Many persons are uncomfortable discussing end-of-life decisions or putting them in writing. In light of life-prolonging technology, questions about how much individuals want done to keep them alive must be answered. When the organs wear out or are irreparably damaged from an accident, who will make the decision for the level of care received? Health care professionals assist people to make choices by explaining options in understandable language. The best time to complete the forms is when a person is not ill or facing a serious surgery.

Nurse's Role

Nurses can help educate the public about advance directives. Education can take place at health fairs, school PTA meetings, or meal sites for the elderly. It is also the nurse's role to ensure the advance directive is not only present on the chart, but is honored by the health care team.

ALLOCATION OF FUNDS

The **allocation of funds** involves the distribution of the scarce resources of health related services among various people.

Reimbursement Sources

In the United States, this distribution has been conducted by a variety of private businesses, such as insurance companies, Health Maintenance Organizations (HMOs) and government agencies. Prior ways of administering health care, the increase in population and length of life, combined with the dramatic increase in the cost of health care have led to reform of reimbursment sources.

Decisions about allocation of funds determine how much health care will be provided, thus opening the door for the concepts of limitation and selection. In other words, we cannot have it all. Questions and concerns are voiced when the subject is discussed. What kinds of services will be available and financed? Who will control the distribution? Will I see the same doctor as I have now?

Another aspect of allocation is a health budget. Health budgets are created at federal, state, and institutional levels. To those actually delivering care, the health care budget consists of giving acute, preventive, or curative care. That concept needs to be broadened. Health services also include programs provided by other community health professionals, such as pollution control, food and drug monitoring, sanitation, and occupational safety (Beauchamp & Childress, 1994).

Macroallocation and Microallocation

Health care allocations are commonly classified in terms of two levels of decision making: **macroallocation** and **microallocation**. Macroallocation determines the amount of resources available for particular kinds of services. Topics that represent macroalloca-

tion include hospital budgets, amount of national resources to be spent on preventive care, and high-technology or nonmedical interventions such as sanitation. Microallocation focuses on treatment decisions regarding particular persons. Topics representing microallocation include separation of conjoined twins, number of liver transplants for a certain child, or the amount of care given to a twenty-two week gestation newborn. Health care cannot be built focusing on one person at a time. When microallocation is discussed, a conflict with the health of society as a whole begins.

When one looks at health care resources, the question surfaces, "Is health care a right or a privilege?" To dissect the right/privilege discussion further, "Is it a moral right (owed on ethical grounds) or a legal right (entitled to by law)? An example of a legal right to health care is the Medicare program for the elderly. An example of a moral right to health care is the level of care given to a person in a terminal state. The moral right position receives heated debate. There are many views on the right to health care debate: market-based system, a system based on rights, and a system based on needs.

In the market-based system, persons believe that everyone is free to pursue his own life plan including economic and health aspects. Every person pays for his own health care, not sharing any part for another's care. No rights are violated in a market-based system. Persons are free to buy and sell as their resources allow. Critics of the market-based plan argue the plan does not ensure health care for those with insufficient economic resources. A market-based system stresses consumerism in health care. An educated consumer is able to understand cost and benefit analysis of medical options available. The poor, uneducated, and mentally challenged are discriminated against in this plan.

The right to health care holds that persons are entitled to receive some measure of health care. With this view, there are three possible ways the right to health care could be implemented. First, everyone would have access to the same level of health care. Second, to provide care to all, a marginal level of access would be given for the sake of equal treatment. A third aspect of the equal right is everyone receives every treatment that could possibly provide some benefit; this is difficult to imagine in a world of limited resources. One solution to the right to health care plan is to set an achievable standard of health care that could be guaranteed. Determining that standard presents a challenge, to say the least.

Another health care plan is based on the person's need rather than a right for care. A need is a condition or situation where something necessary or desirable is wanted or required. The "meeting the need plan" has several approaches. One approach is to meet the need until the person returns to optimal functioning.

Another is to meet the needs that provide significant health benefit. Defining "significant" could entail quality of life and length of life aspects. A third approach could assess need based on a priority status; need for acute care would receive attention over other needs.

Most people agree that a person should have access to basic goods such as food, shelter, clothing, and health care to carry out a life plan. Defining a standard of need could include three standards: (1) preventive; (2) acute care; and (3) tertiary care. When one looks at need, nonhealth care goods such as food, shelter, and education can have an impact on health and also need to be considered.

Rationing

Rationing means to restrict or limit a person's allotment of something. If rationing is used in the same sentence as health care, most people get very upset. In reality, there is and has been a rationing system in the United States called "the ability to pay system": those who are insured, receive Medicare or Medicaid or those who privately pay for their care receive health care. Those who do not have this financial ability do not receive health care (Lamm,1994). Because of advanced technology, people think that they should have it "all," but having it all does not work. It does not work fiscally. Disproportionate sums are spent on a few people for advanced technology, thus depleting financial resources available for others. Having it "all" also does not promote living a healthy lifestyle as some people believe that no matter how they treat their bodies, a medical miracle or a machine will reverse years of neglect and abuse.

Efficiency

Efficiency means without waste. Allocation of funds in an efficient manner involves evaluation of the cost/benefit ratio of health care delivered. Analyzing for efficiency can be performed by listing in one column all the preventive services that are or could be provided, in column two the number of persons impacted, and in column three the possible outcomes. This same evaluation format could be applied for acute care services, obstetrical services, and chronic illness services such as dialysis. It can be quickly understood how health care in the United States has expanded into an inefficient and expensive system.

Joint Venturing

Joint venturing means two or more agencies have joined together to provide a health care service. The agencies may be located in the same geographical area or across the country. Another form of joint venturing is the creation of hospital systems, when two or more hospitals join under one corporation. By joining a larger system, the buying power of the organization increases, there is a leaner management staff, and human resources can be shared. We will see more examples of creative management and budgeting as health care dollars shrink.

Case Management

Case management is a system designed by insurance companies in an attempt to limit the cost of health care. Physicians must call the company insuring the client and receive prior approval before the person can be admitted for acute care. The case manager, usually a nurse, must evaluate the case to verify that the person is sick enough for admission. The case manager would then monitor the amount of care given, the number of hospital days allowed, and set the discharge date for the client during the hospital stay. This has not been well received by physicians. The outcome, at least on the books, is a more efficient use of health care resources. The effects on the client are yet to be analyzed.

Some hospitals and home care agencies are adopting case management. A hospital may assign a primary nurse who as the manager of the case closely follows all treatments, lab tests, and client progress. The case manager works with all the team members to ensure the best care is given in the most efficient manner. Other hospitals may assign social workers to serve as case managers. No matter what organizational structure is chosen, the outcome to be expected is the use of health care resources in an efficient manner.

Care Mapping

Care mapping or clinical paths is a means of tracking and planning the client's care each hospitalized day. The maps are predesigned by a health care team and outline each day of care; for example, on day one, certain tests will be completed, the discharge plan is set, and certain medications are prescribed. Each day also has a set outcome goal to be achieved, signifying progress toward discharge. If the client does not meet the outcome for that day, a variance is reported which analyzes the change in plan. Figure 4-1 depicts a sample care map. Care maps can have a positive impact on health care by decreasing unnecessary tests or extended hospital stays, therefore saving money. The quality of care provided should not change. On the negative side, with a short hospital stay, the client may not feel strong enough to care for himself at home. Also, some clients are admitted with multiple illnesses and do not fit a simple care map plan. These clients receive care based on a plan that encompasses their multiple needs.

	DAY: 1 SURGERY DAY/POST-OP	DAY: 2 POD#1
Consults	* Notify consultants of room number. * Initiate or request a DIC consult if client is diabetic.	
Tests	AP/Lat of hip in PAC. O_2 Sat 4 h post-op. Call if O_2 < 90%.	Hemogram - call if Hgb < 8.0. Chem 8 (When indicated). O_2 Sat in AM on RA; call if O_2 Sat < 90%. Protime per Anticoag Orders.
Activity	Dangle - Progress to standing as tolerates PM of surgery.	Up in w/c. PT per protocol. Begin POD#1 in AM. OT per protocol. BRP on mabel prn.
Treatments	VS & CSM q 2 h X 8 q 4 h X 24 h then q shift. Voldyne q 1 h WA for all clients who had general anesthesia. Icebag X 48 h. O_2 2 L/NC. I&O X 72 h DC after 72 h & KOIV DC Reinforce drsg. X 24 h. Thigh High TEDS W/plexi pulse/int comp. stockings. Mt hemovac q 4 h X 4 then q shift Reinfuse autovac blood per protocal. Foley or straight cath X 2 if no foley anchored. Anchor on 3rd cath. Exercise sling, ankle pumps, quad sets and gluteal sets. Dressing to be changed on day of discharge by doctor or nurse for wound assessment.	May DC O_2 if Sat > 90%. After 1st 24 h change drsg prn saturated. Mt hemovac q shift.
Diet	Ice chips post nausea. Meds with sips of H_2O	Clear liquid diet. Advance diet as tolerated when good bowel sounds.
Meds	KO D5.45 N/S * Cefazolin 1 Gm q 8 h X 3 doses, if allergic Cleocin 600 mgm IV q 8 h X 3 doses. * Zantac 50 mgm IV BID X 48 h. May give 150 mgm po when tolerating diet to complete 48 h. * Home meds excluding ASA/NSAIDS. * Anticaog per protocal. * Colace 100 mgm po daily. * Administer Mantoux. PAIN MANAGEMENT: * PCA/IM/Epidural prn. PRN's:	KO IV til tol po fluids well and/or PCA DC'd then saline lock prn * Ferrous Sulfate 300 mgm 1 BID w/food.
Discharge Planning	Notify Social Service of Room #. Notify Case Manager.	Social Service assessment & discharge plan.
Teaching	* Reinforce teaching for post-op care. Exercise sling, ankle pumps, quad sets and gluteal sets.	* View hip video. * Pharmacy consult client teaching/Coumadin

(continued)

FIGURE 4-1 A sample care map. (*Courtesy of Lutheran Hospital, Fort Wayne, IN*)

	DAY: 3	POD#2 DAY: 4	POD#3 DAY: 5	POD#4
Consults				
Tests	Hemogram - call if Hgb < 8.0. Get UA when foley DC. Do C & S if indicated by dipstick. Protime per Anticoag orders.			
Activity	Up in w/c. PT per protocol. OT per protocol. BRP on mabel prn.			
Treatments	VS & CSM q 2 h X 8 q 4 h X 24 h then q shift. Voldyne q1h WA for all clients who had general anesthesia. DC ice bag 48 h post op use prn. I & O 72 h DC after 72 h and KO IV DC. After 1st 24 h change drsg prn saturated. Thigh high TEDS w/plexi pulse/int comp. stockings. DC hemovac 48 h post op. DC foley at 0600. Get UA and C&S if indicated by dipstick.	DC I & O after 72 h & KO IV DC'd.	* Report client's PT/OT progress to doctor for completing evaluation of appropriateness for discharge. Validate client has had BM since OR.	
Diet	* Evaluate if has had BM. If not, administer an appropriate plan. Clear Liquid diet. Advance diet as tolerated when good bowel sounds.			
Meds	KO IV til tol. po fluids well and/or PCA DC'd then saline lock prn. Zantac - DC 48 h post-op. Home meds excluding ASA/NSAIDS. Anticoag per protocol. Colace 100 mgm po daily. Ferrous Sulfate 300 mgm 1 BID w/food. Read Mantoux. PCA/IM/PO PRN. After physical therapy assess if client ready for conversion to po pain med. PRN's:	PO prn.		
Discharge Planning	Social service assessment & discharge plan.	SS finalize discharge plan.		
Teaching	* View hip video prn. * Pharmacy consult patient teaching/Coumadin.		* View hip video.prn. * Discharge to home or transfer to extended care facility	

FIGURE 4-1 (continued)

Nurse's Role

Until the 1990s, the role of the nurse did not encompass a working knowledge of health care funding or reimbursement issues. Nurses working with the budget of a specific unit counted supplies, figured salaries for staff, and practiced in a secure fee-for-service world. This meant that the unit was paid based on the charges submitted. There were very few questions asked.

Today, nurses need a working knowledge of reimbursement issues. Nurses must know how many days of service receive reimbursement, what is paid for as a skilled service, and how complications receive coverage. This knowledge base serves in any practice setting from acute care to home care. Nurses can help decrease the cost of care by wisely using supplies, demonstrating time management skills, and redesigning the work environment to promote efficiency.

Nurses cannot sit back and say, "Whatever they decide," as if nurses have no power in making the health care system more efficient. Nurses possess unique and valid information about how people become ill, live with illness, and what practices promote health. It is exactly that factual knowledge that must be shared with federal agencies, case managers, and the hospitals' managed care persons so the allocation of funds not only looks balanced on paper, but it also ethically promotes the use of health care resources.

ORGAN DONATION

Organ donation involves the removal and transplantation of a healthy organ from one person to benefit another. Major organs such as the heart, liver, kidney, and lung as well as skin, corneas, bone, and tendons can be transplanted. The person receiving the transplanted organ is returned to a higher level of wellness.

Ethical Principles

When discussing organ donation, ethical principles of autonomy, beneficence, and justice are applied. As stated in Chapter 3, autonomy means the client has the right to self-determination. The client or his surrogate has the right to decide without pressure, if organs are to be donated. Beneficence or "doing good" is the outcome of the donation process. The recipient is returned to a higher level of wellness without significantly harming the donor. All organ donations must be handled in a just manner; without partiality. Usually there are priority lists for those awaiting a donor from a nonfamily member. These lists rate the illness quotient of the person regardless of race, color, or creed. Each recipient is assigned a priority number and organs are distributed according to the list. The United Network of Organ Sharing (UNOS) is a computerized network that links all procurement organizations and maintains a list of potential organ recipients.

Religious Views

Organized religions have definite views on the subject of organ donation. The majority view donation as a positive act between human beings helping one another. There may be opposition to organ donation by some religious groups but it is not widely proclaimed. Some religions refer to donation as an individual choice.

Moral Views

Morality enters the donation process when the organs are incorrectly obtained, when autonomy is violated, or when organs are purchased. A gap exists between the demand for organs and the number of viable organs available. The gap has become wider, leading persons to solve the problem by importing organs from paid donors overseas. Persons with financial means have been known to advertise for donors and offer payment for the organ needed (Caplan, 1986).

Lastly, donors can sell their healthy organ to the highest bidder. This practice supports an unjust access to organs; only persons with financial means would receive an organ.

Source of Organs

Organ donors can be family members or other persons who match the tissue type of the client. These sources are labeled "live" donors. The person willingly donates the organ while alive. Examples of such donations would include a kidney, a part of a pancreas, or bone marrow. This type of donation benefits the client usually without causing significant harm to the donor.

A second type of donor source is labeled a "cadaver" donor. These donors have died and within a set number of hours the organs to be donated are surgically removed and implanted into the recipient. Almost any body part from the internal organs, bone, skin, and eyes can be donated. Some donors must meet certain criteria before the organ can be used, such as, most heart donors are under the age of 55. It is not necessary for nurses to remember all the criteria for donation. When or if a person or the person's family wish to donate organs, the nurse simply calls the state's donor line for direction.

With the shortage of organs for donation, scientists and society are investigating the use of other sources. This is when ethical issues arise. Why not obtain organs from prisoners, at least those on death row before they are executed? Why not use aborted fetal tissue?

The benefit and burden of these other sources need to be analyzed along with a question, "Does the means justify the end result?" If a piece of paper was divided into two columns, one marked benefit and one burden, what could be written to analyze the issue? In the benefit column, statements such as: the ill person could regain health; the prisoner would be helping society. Both statements are admirable and ethical. Now list some statements for the burden side: does the prisoner have the right to say no? If not, are we violating the prisoner's right to autonomy? Will these donations present a financial burden to society? Would a prisoner be considered to receive a donor organ? Who decides what organs are to be taken from which prisoner?

When analyzing the use of fetal tissue as a possible donor source, the question to be asked is, "does the end justify the means?" There are two sources of fetal tissue; one is the spontaneous abortion that naturally occurs. The other is an induced abortion to remove the fetus from the mother's womb. In the case of the spontaneous abortion, the tissue can be used if it is in a viable state depending on the gestational age of the fetus. The end, transplant of viable tissue, ethically justifies the means of obtaining the tissue from a dead fetus. It is viewed the same as a cadaver's donation.

The ethical debate intensifies when the source of the organ or tissue is from a deliberately aborted fetus. Does the end, transplant of viable tissue, justify the means, a purposely aborted fetus? Opponents state that killing a viable fetus never justifies the use of fetal tissue. Killing is not morally, legally, or ethically acceptable. Supporters of the issue state that it is permissible because the fetus is not considered alive and viable; it cannot live independently outside the mother's womb. The supporters also view the fetal tissue as a ball of cells, not a live infant, so it is not killing another human being to obtain the donation (Verklan, 1993).

The last source of organ donor is the person who is diagnosed as brain dead. Brain death literally means that the brain has permanently lost all function. When a person is brain dead, the MRI screen is totally black reflecting the absolute loss of all function. The brain dead person is literally dead; organs are being supported by equipment.

Nurse's Role

Nurses support the donor and/or family when they are making the decision to donate organs. The live donor receives most of the counseling and education from a transplant team. The preparation for donation includes physical, emotional, and psychological assessments.

Family members who are contemplating cadaver organ donation need to feel comfortable enough to ask questions. Examples include: "Are you sure he is dead?" This question is asked frequently by family members of a brain dead client simply because the person usually looks unharmed, like he is simply sleeping. It is hard for them to believe that their loved one is dead. "If I donate organs will he look different in the casket?" Now this may seem like a foolish question, but it is important to the person who is asking the question. The answer is no, this will not affect the viewing of the body. "Will this donation cost me any money?" At this time, the answer is no. There are no costs to the donor family or his estate."Will I know who receives the organs?" Yes, if the donor family and/or the transplant organization so wish, the transplant coordinator can inform the family.

Due to the short time frame from accident to brain death determination, the grief and stress the family is experiencing, and unfamiliarity with the health care environment, building a rapport with the family is a challenge for nurses. In situations where the donor is dead or dying, nurses need to quickly build rapport with the family. The nurse will be asking the family some difficult questions related to donation of organs. The nurse can rely on other team members to assist in family care, such as the chaplain, the family minister, other nurses, and physicians. Figure 4-2 is a sample consent form for organ donation.

REPRODUCTIVE TECHNOLOGY

In the United States, one in seven couples is involuntarily infertile (Beauchamp & Walters, 1994). When conceiving a child naturally is not physically possible, technology is now capable of assisting the couple. Like any other technological advancement, there are opinions, ethical and moral views, and financial issues to be discussed.

Artificial Insemination

Artificial insemination is one of the oldest forms of reproductive technology. A man's sperm is instilled into the woman's vagina. The sperm may be from the woman's spouse or an anonymous donor.

ALBANY MEDICAL CENTER &
CENTER FOR DONATION & TRANSPLANT

Consent for organ/tissue donation

I, _____ hereby make this anatomical gift from the body of _____ ,
who died on _____ , at _____ in _____ .

I am surviving:
1. ( ) Spouse
2. ( ) Son or daughter, 18 years of age or older
3. ( ) Parent
4. ( ) Brother or sister, 18 years of age or older
5. ( ) Guadian of the person of the decedent at the time of his/her death

I give, if medically acceptable for the purpose of:

1. ( ) Transplantation
2. ( ) Medical research/education

the following organs/tissues:

( ) Kidneys   ( ) Eyes
( ) Heart   ( ) Bone/connective tissue
( ) Lung   ( ) Heart valves
( ) Liver   ( ) Skin
( ) Pancreas   ( ) Saphenous/femoral vein
( ) Intestine   ( ) Other _____

I hereby authorize the center for donation & transplant and their designated physicians and agents, to perfom the necessary surgery to remove these organs and/or tissues consented to above, to obtain blood and tissue samples for the purpose of organ suitability, infectious disease and compatibility testing and to release post mortem examination results to the Center for Donation & Transplant at 218 Great Oaks Blvd. Albany, New York 12203, if applicable.

This donation is a gift for the benefit of mankind and is made in accordance with the anatomical gift act.

I acknowledge that I have read this document in its entirety and that I fully understand it.

_____   _____
Person obtaining consent   Signature of person consenting

_____   _____
Print name   Address

_____   _____
Witness signature   Address continued

_____   _____
Print name   Phone number

FIGURE 4-2 A sample consent form for organ donation. (*Courtesy of the Center for Donation & Transplant, Albany, NY*)

In Vitro Fertilization

In vitro fertilization and implantation literally means fertilization in glass. The first child conceived in a Petri dish, implanted into the mother's uterus and born alive in 1978 is Louise Brown. The simplest form of in vitro fertilization involves uniting the sperm and ova of the couple in the laboratory. The fertilized eggs then develop into embryos. All of the embryos are transplanted into the mother's uterus. There is no freezing or storing of these embryos. The technique can also involve donor sperm and ova. The resulting embryos can be donated for transplanting to a woman who has been unable to become pregnant, or the embryos can be used in research, genetic testing, stored, or allowed to die (Caplan, 1994).

Surrogate Motherhood

The last reproductive technology to be discussed is surrogate motherhood. This technique combines the old technology of artificial insemination with a new social arrangement (Beauchamp & Walters, 1994). A woman becomes pregnant with another couple's embryo implanted into her uterus and for a fee, carries and delivers the child. To clarify this further, if the surrogate mother is artificially inseminated (her ova and the father's sperm) she is the genetic mother of the infant. A gestational mother is implanted with a fertilized embryo from the genetic couple; she is the surrogate carrier.

Opposing Views

Opponents to reproductive technology are concerned with the effects of this technology on the family unit and on the resulting children. They see the laboratory production of human beings as no longer human procreation. Also in an overpopulated world, those with this view see it as wrong to actively take steps to create more human beings. Infertility is "God's will" for some couples. Opponents want these couples to accept their fate and go on with their lives. Lastly, the desire to have children is no more than a wish; it is not a human need like food or shelter. Money spent on reproductive technology takes away from the allocation of needed health care.

Supporters of reproductive technology view it as man controlling nature. Reproductive liberation is a major boom to the human species. The technology is morally justified because it is employed for good reasons. They believe that it is in a child's best interest to be reared by the biological parents. Through DNA testing, technology allows for implantation of the healthi-

est embryos. Genetically transmitted diseases could be eliminated.

There are some moral and ethical views on this subject. Three moral opinions exist for the treatment of the human embryo. First, the embryo is entitled to protection as a human being. Any research or manipulation that might damage the embryo or prevent its transfer to a uterus is ethically unacceptable, since it prevents the embryo from reaching its full potential of developing into a full-term fetus. Second, the embryo is not entitled to any moral status because it is not a human being. And third, is somewhere in the middle. The embryo meets some moral standard because it is a unique genotype and has potential (Beauchamp & Walters, 1994).

The treatment of the unused embryos is always an ethical concern. What is to be done with the unused embryos? If there are six embryos, who chooses the ones to be implanted? How many are implanted? How can a choice be made? If a person believes that life begins at conception and the unused embryos are discarded, is this killing?

Ethical views also center around the use of limited monetary resources for infertility research and treatment. The principle of justice comes into play when we discuss unequal access to infertility treatment. Currently, those who can pay for the care receive the care. It is not covered by federal or state monies. A large amount of money is spent to abort unwanted fetuses. Now, on the other hand, people are willing to go to extremes to become pregnant. It seems like these two sides could come together. If infertile couples could be paired with a woman contemplating abortion, the couple could support the pregnant woman and parent the fetus, creating a win-win situation.

DEATH AND DYING ISSUES

The care of clients who are dying can be a challenging nursing experience. It can be emotional for nurses, but to be able to give comfort to a client and his family is rewarding.

Natural

In the past, death was considered a natural part of life. Family members joined together caring for their dying loved one in the home, keeping the person comfortable with small amounts of food and fluid, clean linen, and love. To many people, care of the dying includes cultural and social rituals that are a part of their every day life. Death was not seen as a defeat but a part of the life cycle. In this era of acute care hospitals and advanced technology, United States culture tries to avoid death at all cost. Since 1976, case law and state statutes address end-of-life issues. The issue of death, dying, and limitation of treatment has left the private confines of the family and is now a part of the realm of health care.

Euthanasia

Euthanasia is a word with Greek roots that means "good or pleasant" death. There are two kinds of euthanasia: active and passive. Passive euthanasia means a person is allowed to die. It is ethically and legally permissible by stopping treatment and/or withholding treatment to the client even though the end will result in death. Active euthanasia means a person is helped to die by providing him with the materials to induce death.

Assisted Suicide

Assisted suicide means that someone assists or helps the person to end his life. In physician-assisted suicide the physician only provides the means of death, such as a medication, and the individual carries out the act. Supporters of physician-assisted suicide are proposing clinical guidelines for the process. First, the client must have an incurable condition associated with severe, unrelenting suffering. Second, the physician must ensure that the client does not suffer because of inadequate comfort care. Third, the client must repeat the request for assisted suicide several times of his own free will. Any ambivalence voiced by the client will abort the procedure. Fourth, the client must be capable of understanding the situation and the decision. Fifth, the physician-assisted suicide must be carried out in the context of a meaningful physician-client relationship. In other words, the physician must get to know the client personally. Sixth, consultation with another physician is required to ensure that the client is voluntarily requesting death (Quill, et al.,1994).

Palliative Care

Palliative care shifts the goal from cure and prolonging life to the alleviation of suffering and enhancing the quality of the person's remaining life (Latimer & McGregor, 1994). Palliative care supports the person's right to care and protection. In fact, supporters of palliative care are writing national standards, encouraging the topic be covered in the education of health care professionals, researching the effectiveness of palliative treatment and promoting public discussion (Erickson, et al., 1995). It is believed that good levels of palliative care would eliminate active euthanasia (Latimer & McGregor, 1994).

Ethical concerns about limitations of care include the freedom to self-determination, informed consent, benefits, and burdens. Before the person can make any decision about limitations of care, the person must give informed consent. As stated earlier, it means the person is given all the options, benefits, risks, and possible outcomes before being asked to make a decision. Many times the ill person sees himself as a burden on the family. Treatments are often seen as burdens, not benefits, by the ill person.

Concerns are also attached to euthanasia. Who will pay for the service? Religious sects and advance directives have begun to set guidelines for passive euthanasia. Who will set the guidelines for the practice of active euthanasia? If active euthanasia becomes a standard of care, will the poor, invalid, and elderly automatically receive active euthanasia when their level of care becomes too expensive or extensive?

Nurse's Role

Nurses provide care for the dying person and family. They have the opportunity to counsel the family, assist in the family's grieving process, and learn a great deal about the process of death and dying. It is the nurse's role to coordinate care for the dying person, thus preventing fragmentation or inconsistent completion of the person's wishes for limitation of care.

GENETICS

Ever since the family physician began reviewing a person's family history, health care has used genetic information. As early as the late 1800s, scientists were studying families who demonstrated musical talent, mapping the talent in a family tree format. In an attempt to improve society and eliminate "bad germs" (what early scientists called genes), proposals were written to curtail the entry of "aliens, lunatics, and idiots" into the United States. The prison system began mandating sterilization of male prisoners in the early 1900s, attempting to eliminate the "criminal germ." Today, we see the **eugenics** movement is continuing on a highly technological scale (Reilly, 1994).

Eugenics means the study of human improvement by genetic means. Genetic research involves the mapping and placing in proper sequence all of the human genes, numbering approximately three billion pairs.

In the United States, the research on human genes is called the Human Genome Project and is sponsored through the National Institutes of Health and the Department of Energy. In a laboratory, computers run constantly analyzing samples of human tissue and organs for genetic codes. In only three years, scientists have analyzed 83 million letters of the three billion total in the human genetic alphabet (Friend, 1995). Mapping the genetic codes will benefit mankind by discovering and deleting genes that cause disease, assisting in the development of treatments, and broadening the knowledge of basic human biology.

Genetic studies and analysis appear as an absolute wonder of science, but they are accompanied by numerous social and ethical concerns. Early in the twentieth century a search and destroy mission was started; search out the defective gene and destroy it. People believed that the poor, the indigent, and other vulnerable populations were inferior. Some states forced sterilization on the mentally handicapped resulting in the removal of their defective genes from the genetic pool.

In the 1960s, amniocentesis became available. Parents could now learn in the second trimester if a genetic defect was present in their fetus. The parents were given the choice of carrying the pregnancy to term or aborting the genetically defective fetus. The selective abortion choice was reasoned as positive and acceptable because it prevented a burden on the family and society, prevented suffering for the child, and did not add to the defective genetic pool.

Ethical concerns include confidentiality of genetic screening, requirement versus personal choice, and employment and insurance issues. All of the ethical concerns seem to link together around the principle of autonomy. If a person consents to genetic screening, who should know the results? Obviously, the person has a right to know. Now take the information to another level. If the insurance company the person has applied to requires genetic screening before it will cover the person or his family with insurance, who besides the insurance company has the right to know about this information? Can the company use the screening information to segregate who will be covered? Because the screen identified a person as prone to developing a certain disease, is this a preexisting condition? What are the ethical and moral ramifications of informing the person that he may or may not develop a disease? As you can see, this technology can have a great impact on a person's life.

The last comments on genetic management are made to stimulate thought. Readers of this chapter can list personal concerns. One that comes to mind is defining what is considered defective. Since no human being is perfect, how can a perfect genotype be created? Can people be mandated not to reproduce because they will pass on a defective gene? Who will write the definition of a deficit gene and who will determine characteristics that are detrimental? Discussion about deleting defective genes can evoke strong public response. Science and technology are moving at a rapid pace. It is imperative that the movement includes ethical components.

ABORTION

Abortion is the termination of a pregnancy before the fetus is viable. It may be spontaneous (miscarriage) or induced.

Induced Abortion

Induced abortion has been the subject of extensive debate on ethical and legal grounds. There are three views on abortion: conservative, liberal, and intermediate. The conservative approach states that induced abortion is never acceptable; conserving life at any cost is acceptable. The liberal approach holds that induced abortion is always permissible whatever the stage of fetal development. It supports freedom of choice and the right of the woman to decide what happens to her body. The intermediates believe that induced abortion is ethically acceptable up to a specified stage of fetal development or for some limited set of moral reasons, such as rape, that are sufficient to warrant an abortion (Beauchamp & Walters, 1994).

Right to Life Issues

The concept of human life, fetal life, and fetal rights play a role in the discussion. The beliefs attributed to the conservative approach and that of many religions is that life begins at conception. They attach a personhood to the fetus. Others argue that a fetus cannot be considered independent and alive. It cannot survive outside the uterus. They view the fetus as a ball of cells surrounded by a membrane.

A last approach is that a fetus is human at fertilization but not a person or a being. They agree that biological life, not a human life, is taken by abortion because the fetus is not a being. Obviously there are many other positions on when a fetus becomes a human being; the line is drawn somewhere between conception and birth.

Legal Issues

The legal side of abortion is based on the right to privacy and the control of the woman over her body. This was the basic framework for the Supreme Court ruling on *Roe* vs *Wade* which made abortion legal in the United States. The law also protects the person who is choosing the procedure from any harassment by opponents. Unfortunately, some of the extreme cases in this issue have involved the death of an abortion doctor by an anti-abortionist. Taking the law into one's own hands will not resolve this heated topic.

Moral Issues

Morality of the fetus also enters the debate. If the fetus has moral properties it means it qualifies under some moral protection. The conservative argument is that the fetus possesses full rights the same as anyone born. The liberal approach states that the fetus has absolutely no rights and the intermediate view is somewhere in between.

As pointed out in Chapter 3, an ethical principle applicable to this topic is nonmaleficence or do no harm. If one believes that a fetus is not a human being, then abortion is not morally wrong because another human being is not being harmed. On the other side, those who believe that a fetus is a human being attest that it is morally wrong to abort because a human being is harmed or killed (Beauchamp & Childress, 1994).

The intent of the abortion act is another part of this issue. The conservative approach states that the intent of an abortion is fetal death. The liberal view is that it gives the mother the opportunity to exercise her right of choice and autonomy regarding her body. If intent is an issue, then the abortion issue needs to broaden to include intrauterine surgery. If the intent of the action is to repair a fetal defect, but the procedure causes an abortion of the fetus, is the procedure morally wrong? Most ethicists argue that the procedure is not morally wrong because the intent was not fetal death, but fetal life. The principle of beneficence or do good was the deciding element in this ethical analysis.

Nurse's Role

Nurses who are opposed to abortion do not have to participate in the abortion procedure or work in an area where abortions are induced. A nurse may make it known, at the time of employment, that she wants no part in the care of clients who have had induced abortions. This is an area of health care where opinions are voiced very strongly. It is the nurse's role to gather health care information about the client in a nonjudgmental manner. The nurse's role in the area of abortion will be in counseling and educating the person. The nurse may not agree with the actions of the person but it is a license responsibility to care for the client.

PROFESSIONAL GATEKEEPING

Actions used to guard professional standards of practice and behavior is called **gatekeeping**. The nursing profession has a set of moral and ethical stan-dards based on the ethical principles outlined in Chapter 3. It is believed that nurses will act in an honest and trustworthy manner. When nurses violate that honesty in the classroom, it is called cheating. If a nursing student cheats on an exam, the cheating not only harms the student, but potentially harms future clients. If a fellow nursing student sees the student cheating, the responsible action is to report the offending student. When students take their licensure exam numerous interventions are employed to monitor cheating. If a nursing student is caught cheating during the exam, the student is dismissed from the exam.

Impaired Colleague

One of the hardest experiences in nursing is to report an **impaired colleague**. Impairment simply means the nurse is not in a state to deliver safe care. The colleague may be impaired due to the use of drugs or alcohol or due to an illness. According to state licensure laws, each nurse is responsible to report an impaired colleague. It should be reported to the immediate supervisor. In a case of substance impairment, many factors are evaluated, such as what substance is involved, the source of the substance, harm to the clients, and length of time used. Most institutions require on-site testing. Most state nursing boards have a rehabilitation program for nurses who are substance abusers. After rehabilitation, nurses can be returned to the practice area; some may have practice restrictions. Gatekeeping includes any impaired colleague. This person might be a surgeon who enters the operating room suite in a drunken condition. The nurse is responsible to protect the client from harm and must prevent the case from beginning.

Other Issues

Other professional issues include the breach of confidentiality by a peer, not reporting a medication error, or falsifying documentation. The nurse must report these incidents to the immediate supervisor.

A trusting relationship must exist between professionals. Without trust the team flounders and client care is compromised. Professionals demonstrate their value system, morals, and ethical behavior in everyday practice.

▶ CASE STUDY

Mrs. C. has been admitted to the hospital for treatment of a blood clot in her left leg. The following information was collected upon admission.

Mrs. C is a seventy-eight-year-old woman who has enjoyed fairly good health most of her life. She is a widow who never had children. There are no living relatives. She does not have an advance directive, nor has she discussed her wishes for health care with any friends, her physician, or clergy. Mrs. C. regularly attended the Methodist church but due to her declining health, has not attended routinely for the last six months.

On day two of her admission, Mrs. C. experiences a cerebral bleed which is exacerbated by the blood thinning medication she is receiving for her blood clot. Mrs. C. slips into a semicomatose state.

The following questions will guide your development of a Nursing Care Plan for the case study.

1. List subjective data a nurse would assess to verify the client's competency.
2. List two persons who could give consent for Mrs. C.
3. Write one nursing diagnosis and goal for Mrs. C.
4. List two ethical principles that apply in this case.
5. How can the nurse act as the client advocate for Mrs. C?

SUMMARY

- Every nurse needs to know who or where the resources are if there are ethical dilemmas to be resolved.
- Nurses serve as advocates for their clients.
- Nurses can have a positive impact on health care funding.
- Nurses use medical, nursing, legal, and ethical information when planning care for clients.

- Analyzing ethical issues involves critical thinking skills.
- Nurses must critically analyze health care technology.
- Nurses are educators of clients and families especially when options are presented.
- Nurses serve as gatekeepers to ensure safe delivery of care.

Review Questions

1. How can nurses protect the privacy of the client?

   a. Monitoring who has access to the chart.
   b. Keep computer covered.
   c. Discuss client only with other nurses.
   d. Keep the door to the clients room closed at all times.

2. Interventions that nurses can use to support efficiency in health care include:

   a. monitoring body systems.
   b. using a preventive approach to care.
   c. knowing signs of distress.
   d. keeping the client clean and dry.

3. Sources of organ donors are:

   a. comatose clients.
   b. family members.
   c. only nonrelated persons.
   d. only from a twin.

4. Active euthanasia means a person:

   a. helps a client to die.
   b. limits the amount of care.
   c. has an advance directive.
   d. chooses to stop pain therapy.

Critical Thinking Questions

1. How do you feel about euthanasia?

2. Discuss the ethics of organ donation.

News Flash

In Michigan, Dr. Kavorkian, a retired pathologist, has become known as "Dr. Death." He not only believes that people have a right to end their suffering, he assists them in ending their life. Dr. Kavorkian has been featured on television talk shows, in news magazines, and newspapers. He has appeared in court on possible murder charges but has never been convicted. Dr. Kavorkian has a group of physicians who have begun supporting his work. Dr. Kavorkian does visit with the client and family to assess their wishes for ending their life. He states that he does not assist all who ask for his service. There is also a group of physicians who do not agree with him. These physicians believe he is not honoring the Hippocratic oath. (Source, CNN, 1996).

CHAPTER
5

Communication

Lois White

KEY TERMS

active listening
aphasia
communication
congruent
dysarthria
dysphasia
empathy
feedback
hearing
listening
nonverbal
proxemics
rapport
therapeutic communication
verbal

LEARNING OBJECTIVES

Upon completion of this chapter the learner should be able to:
- Define key terms.
- Describe the process of communication and factors that influence it.
- Differentiate between verbal and nonverbal communication.
- Utilize therapeutic communication.
- Understand the psychosocial aspects of communication.
- Demonstrate proper telephone communication.
- Communicate effectively with clients and families.
- Demonstrate communicating with special clients who are visually impaired, hearing impaired, speech impaired, unconscious, and non-English speaking.
- Communicate effectively with terminally ill clients and their families.
- Communicate effectively with other members of the health care team.

▶ *MAKING THE CONNECTION*

Refer to the topics in the following chapters to increase your understanding of communication.

- **Chapter 1, Critical Thinking:** The Skills of Critical Thinking, p. 8; Critical Reading Skills p. 8; Critical Writing, p. 9; Critical Listening p. 9; Critical Speaking, p. 10; Reasoning and Problem-Solving, p. 12; Critical Thinking and the Nursing Process, p. 15
- **Chapter 2, Legal Aspects of Nursing:** Nurse-Client Relationship, p. 22; Informed Consent, p. 27
- **Chapter 6, Cultural Aspects of Health and Illness:** Culturally Appropriate Nursing Care, p. 92; Client Cultural Assessment, p. 92; Nurse's Response, p. 94

- **Chapter 7, Cultural Diversity in the Workplace:** Other Cultural Aspects Affecting Client Care, p. 103; Language, p. 103; Cultural Orientation, p. 105; Cultural Responses to Pain, p. 105; Cultural Responses to Grieving, p. 110; Cultural Response to Time and Space Orientation, p. 111; Nursing Implications, p. 113
- **Chapter 10, Nursing Assessment:** Techniques for Assessment, p. 167; Introduction of Nurse to Client/General Overview, p. 176
- **Chapter 18, The Dying Process/Hospice:** The Dying Person's Rights, p. 370; Grief, p. 370; The Dying Client's Family/Friends, p. 373; Nursing Assessments and Interventions, p. 374; Other Comfort Measures, p. 376

INTRODUCTION

Communication is a vital link between the client and the physician, nurses, and all other health care workers. Also, there must be accurate communication between health care workers. This chapter reviews the process of communication, the ways of communicating, and the importance of listening, observing, and having congruency of messages. Communicating with the client, family, and health care team is stressed. Self-communication is also discussed.

KEY ABBREVIATIONS

The following abbreviations and acronyms are used in this chapter:

CPR	computerized patient record
IOM	Institute of Medicine
WPM	words per minute

PROCESS OF COMMUNICATION

The simplest definition of **communication** is the sending and receiving of a message. The five aspects of communication are: sender, message, method for sending, receiver, and feedback.

Sender: The sender of a message is the person who has a thought, idea, or emotion to convey to another person.

Message: The message is the thought, idea, or emotion one person sends to another person.

Method for sending: The person sending the message must decide how to send the message. It might be sent verbally, nonverbally, or a combination of both.

Receiver: The person to whom the message is sent is called the receiver. The receiver must not only receive the message but also interpret that message in order to have meaning.

Feedback: **Feedback** is a response from the receiver so that the sender can verify that the message sent was the message received. If this is not the case, then more messages are sent and received until an understanding of the message is reached between the sender and receiver.

Both the sender and receiver are influenced by their education, culture, emotions, perceptions, and by the situation in which they find themselves. These are referred to as a person's frame of reference. Sometimes these influences help communication and sometimes they hinder communication. Figure 5-1 shows the process of communication and the influences on the sender and receiver.

METHODS OF COMMUNICATING

There are two methods of communicating: verbally and nonverbally. Which is better? Neither. It depends on what the sender is trying to communicate. Seldom is a spoken message sent without some nonverbal aspects. Some experts believe that nonverbal commu-

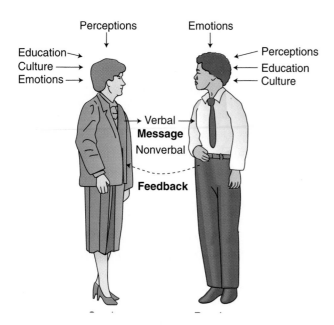

FIGURE 5-1 Process of communication.

nication is more honest than verbal communicatin because it usually is conveyed unconsciously by the sender. See Table 5-1 for methods of communicating.

Verbal Communication

Verbal communication is the use of words to send a message.

Speaking/Listening

Most commonly, speaking is thought of as verbal communication. The receiver of a spoken message must listen. Speaking and listening must both occur to have communication. Have you ever sent a spoken message to someone in the same room with you and received nonmeaningful, senseless feedback from that

Table 5-1

METHODS OF COMMUNICATING	
Verbal	**Nonverbal**
Reading	Eye contact
Writing	Tone of voice
Listening	Facial expressions
Speaking	Gestures
	Touch
	Gait
	Posture
	Body position
	Physical appearance

person or no feedback at all? More than likely, the other person was only hearing the message but not listening. **Hearing** is the act or power of perceiving sounds. **Listening** is more than hearing. It is interpreting those sounds and attaching meaning to them.

Communication experts say that people speak at a rate of 125–150 words per minute (WPM) but hear at a rate of 400–800 WPM. This extra time allows for distractions. Listeners are generally distracted because they are not concentrating on what is being said. Listening is one of the most difficult skills to learn.

Writing/Reading

The other mode of verbal communication is writing. The receiver of the written message must read the words. The reader must understand the words and attach meaning to them. With a written message there is generally no way for immediate feedback. Therefore, great care should be taken in the composition of a written message to ensure the message is clear.

Charting is a good example of written communication. The physician may read the chart when the caregivers who did the charting are off duty. There is little chance for immediate feedback. If, for instance, it is charted that a client was "uncooperative," the physician has no idea what the caregiver really means. Objective as well as subjective data should be written rather than drawing the conclusion "uncooperative." For example, chart "refused to eat lunch, refused to get out of bed and sit in chair."

Nonverbal Communication

Nonverbal communication, sometimes called body language, is the sending of a message without using words. There are many ways we communicate without words. Gestures, facial expressions, posture, tone of voice, touch, gait, eye contact, body position, and physical appearance are all ways of communicating nonverbally.

Nonverbal communication is generally unconscious—part learned behavior and part instinct. Feelings are most accurately expressed nonverbally since there is little conscious control.

Clients seem to believe and are particularly sensitive to nonverbal messages. Nurses must make an effort to be aware of their nonverbal messages. Some aspects of nursing care are not pleasant but must be done. Think how the client would feel if the nurse showed a facial expression of disgust or revulsion when changing a surgical dressing.

Nurses must also be sensitive to the client's nonverbal messages. Many clients do not want to bother the "busy" nurses, so they will say that they are fine or do not need anything. An astute nurse will observe the stiff posture, clenched fists, or frowning facial expression of a client. Further assessment must then be undertaken to determine why the client is sending these nonverbal clues. The verbal message may have been "no pain," but the nonverbal message seems to be saying "pain."

CONGRUENCY OF MESSAGES

It is important that verbal and nonverbal communications are **congruent**. That is, the same message is sent verbally and nonverbally. Saying "I really appreciate what you just did," with a smile and a happy tone of voice sends one message. Saying the same words with a frown and a disgusted tone of voice sends an entirely different message. These messages are not congruent. What does the message sender mean? Is the person pleased with what was done or is the person actually displeased and being sarcastic. Messages such as these are confusing to the receiver. Feedback is then necessary to clarify the message.

It is important for the nurse to watch for congruency in client messages. If they are not congruent, the nurse must ask for clarification.

LISTENING/OBSERVING

Listening and observing are two of the most valuable skills a nurse can have. These two skills are used to gather the subjective and objective data for the nursing assessment. Since the nursing diagnoses and nursing interventions are based on the assessment, it is imperative that the assessment be accurate.

The term **active listening** has been used to describe this behavior of listening and observing. It takes energy and concentration. The nurse who is at eye level with the client, who leans slightly forward toward the client, and who makes eye contact is showing undivided attention to the client and will be able to listen and observe more accurately. Responses from the nurse such as "go on," "tell me more," "yes," "what else," or "mmhm" encourages the client to continue and communicates that the nurse is really listening.

THERAPEUTIC COMMUNICATION

Therapeutic communication, sometimes called effective communication, is purposeful and goal directed. One person is the helper (nurse) and the other is being helped (client). The focus of the conversation is the client, the client's needs, or the client's problems, not the needs or problems of the nurse.

Goals of Therapeutic Communication

There are several goals or purposes of therapeutic communication. One or more of these goals guide every therapeutic communication in a nurse/client relationship. The goals are: obtain or provide information, develop trust, show caring, and explore feelings.

Obtain or Provide Information

It is important for the nurse to obtain information from the client about general health and specific health problems. It is with this information that the nurse can make an accurate assessment and plan of care.

The nurse provides information to the client from admission to discharge. It begins with the orientation of a new client to the hospital policies and routines. It continues throughout the hospital stay as the nurse explains procedures, treatments, and tests; teaches the client self-care; clarifies instruction from other health care workers; and answers client questions. The final aspect of providing information is the discharge instructions.

Develop Trust

Client and nurse are generally strangers at their first meeting. The nurse must work to establish trust with each client. Answering questions honestly, responding to call lights promptly, and following through are examples of ways that build trust. Trust develops faster when caring is shown.

Show Caring

Fluffing a pillow or offering a drink of water, without being asked, shows caring. Taking time to always greet the client by name, and knocking on the room door before entering are other ways to show caring.

When mutual trust is established between client and nurse it is termed **rapport**.

Explore Feelings

Once rapport is established, the nurse can encourage the client to explore feelings. Generally, most clients are anxious about their illness. Some fear the results of diagnostic tests and some are anxious about the hospital environment. Many clients do not want to admit they are anxious or fearful. By using therapeutic communication techniques the nurse is often able to help the client talk about feelings and reduce anxiety. Sometimes a clarifying statement is all that is needed to alleviate the fear or anxiety. Other times allowing the client to talk about the fear or anxiety reduces the fear or anxiety.

Behaviors/Attitudes to Enhance Communication

Some behaviors and attitudes enhance therapeutic communication. Included are: self-disclosure, caring, genuineness, warmth, active listening, empathy, and acceptance and respect.

Self-Disclosure

Self-disclosure means sharing something about yourself such as thoughts, expectations, feelings, or ideas. It does not mean sharing your personal problems. When the nurse shares something, such as future goals in nursing, it shows that the client is trusted with that knowledge. The more the client feels trusted, the more the client will trust the nurse and therapeutic communication is enhanced.

Caring

Caring is not only a goal of therapeutic communication but also an attitude that enhances communication. Caring is the foundation of a nurse/client relationship. A caring attitude is easily identified by the client. The client is made to feel important. Table 5-2 gives some examples of ways to show caring.

Genuineness

Effective communication must be genuine. The nurse must be himself. It means being honest about one's feelings. Sometimes it is "ok" to cry with a client.

It means being truthful and never attempting to answer a question when the answer is not known. The nurse should admit not knowing but offer to find the answer and then do so.

Being genuine builds trust. However, the nurse takes a risk when expressing negative thoughts or confronting a client, family member, or another health care worker.

Warmth

Warmth makes the client feel welcomed, relaxed, and unjudged. It is expressed predominantly by nonverbal communication. A smile helps the client feel relaxed.

Touch is an important method to show warmth, but it must be used appropriately. Society dictates the type of touching that is appropriate in different situations. Holding a client's hand or putting a hand on the shoulder can greatly enhance communication by providing a connection between the nurse and the client. Touch may not always be welcomed by the client.

Active Listening

As the words imply, listening is an active process requiring energy and concentration. It involves listening to the words spoken as well as being aware of nonverbal messages. The nurse listens to both the words spoken and the nonverbal messages.

Active listening requires responses from the listener. This indicates that the nurse is really listening to the client. It is important for the nurse to concentrate on the interaction at hand and not let other thoughts become a distraction. Refer to listening on previous page.

Empathy

Empathy is the capacity to understand another person's feelings. It is an objective awareness of, or a sensitivity to, another person's feelings and thoughts. Although the nurse does not share the thoughts and feelings of the client, with empathy the nurse is able to understand and accept the thoughts and feelings of the client.

Sympathy and empathy are not the same. In sympathy, the nurse becomes involved in the feelings and thoughts of the client which are generally related to a loss.

Table 5-2

WAYS TO SHOW CARING	
Activity	**Statements to Use with Activity**
Cover the client with a blanket.	"It feels chilly in here. Perhaps this blanket will help."
Assist the client to dress.	"I noticed you're having a little trouble getting your robe on. Perhaps I can help."
Serve a tray to the client.	"It's time to eat. I hope you're hungry because it really looks good."
Offer assistance.	"Here, let me help you. Perhaps together we can arrange these flowers."
When leaving the room.	"Is there anything more I can do for you before I go?" or "I'm leaving now, but I'll be back in twenty minutes."
Move the client up in bed.	"You look so uncomfortable. Let me move you up in bed."
Make the client's bed.	"Now you have a nice fresh bed."
Regulate environmental temperature.	"It seems very warm in here. Perhaps if I turn the air conditioner up, it will help."
Turn the client in bed.	"Changing position really makes a difference, doesn't it?"
Straighten a pillow.	"Let me straighten your pillow for you."

(Adapted from Kalman, N. & Waughfield, C. (1993). *Mental Health Concepts 3rd ed.* Albany, NY: Delmar Publishers.)

Acceptance and Respect

Accepting clients as individuals with beliefs and values of their own is an attitude that enhances communication. The nurse must be nonjudgmental, that is, accept the client at face value. The nurse may not agree with clients' values and beliefs but recognizes and accepts the fact that clients have different values and beliefs.

The nurse shows acceptance by not expressing differing values or beliefs but by simply accepting the statements or complaints of clients. Clients may then feel free to communicate and cooperate in their care.

Respect follows acceptance. Accepting clients in a nonjudgmental way leads to understanding them as unique individuals. Acceptance and respect by the nurse lets clients know that they can be themselves; and although the clients may have different values and beliefs than the nurse, the clients can feel they will still receive the best quality care. The nurse also shows respect by introducing himself and addressing the client by name (Mr., Mrs., or Ms.)

PSYCHOSOCIAL ASPECTS OF COMMUNICATION

The psychosocial aspects of communication include: style, gestures, meaning of time, meaning of space, cultural values, and political correctness. These aspects are based on individuality and culture. It is important to understand these aspects and how they vary in different persons and cultures.

Style

Each person has a style of communication that reflects the personality and self-concept of that person. According to Zerwekh and Claborn (1994), style can be divided into three common types: passive, aggressive, and assertive. It is important to remember that a person's style of communication is learned and reinforced over the years. The fact that communication style is learned indicates it can change.

When a person becomes a client in the health care system, fear and anxiety may change the person's style of communication. Fear and anxiety may cause the client's communication style to become passive or aggressive.

Passive

The person who uses the passive style of communication does not stand up for himself, is not able to share feelings or needs with others, has difficulty asking for help, and feels hurt and angry at others for taking advantage of him. This person uses apologetic words, has a weak soft voice, makes little eye contact, and is often fidgety. In other words, the person with a passive style of communication goes along with others. The client who has a passive style of communication is generally very compliant, asks for nothing, and gets little attention.

Aggressive

The person who uses the aggressive style of communication puts his own feelings, rights, and needs first and communicates them in a haughty or angry way. The voice is often demanding, and the eyes expressionless. This person also has an attitude of superiority, works to control or manipulate others, and shows no concern for anyone else's feelings.

Assertive

The person who uses the assertive style of communication stands up for himself without violating the basic rights of others. True feelings are expressed in an honest, direct manner and others are not allowed to take advantage of him. The voice is firm and confident and there is appropriate eye contact. This person also respects the rights, needs, and feelings of others; takes responsibility for the consequences of his actions; and behaves in a manner that enhances self-respect.

A person using the assertive style of communication effectively lets others know his thoughts, feelings, and needs. This style also allows the speaker to listen to and acknowledge another person's thoughts, feelings, and needs. If the thoughts, feelings, or needs of the persons communicating are in conflict, a compromise acceptable to both can usually be worked out by being assertive in their communication.

"I" messages—I think . . . , I expect . . . , I feel . . . , I need . . .—are excellent ways to begin assertive communication. It indicates ownership of the thought, feeling, or need—a fact with which no one can argue.

Gestures

Gestures are the movements of the hands and arms. Some gestures are known globally, such as: applause means approval, two fingers in a *V* means victory or peace, thumbs up means well done or good job. Some gestures have entirely different meanings in different countries. For example, a small circle made with the thumb and forefinger means "okay" in many places. However, in Japan it means "money" and in France it means "zero." In Brazil and Turkey that sign is an insult because it is considered a symbol for female genitalia.

Meaning of Time

In the United States, a great emphasis is placed on time and schedules. Being on time is very important. Time is precious. The clock tells us what we are to do and where we are to be every hour of the day and night. A person is considered dependable when scheduled appointments are kept. Time is often a noun, as reflected by our terms "save time," "waste time," and "spend time."

There are some cultures that know a day has passed because the sun has risen, set, and is rising again. In fact, some cultures do not even have an instrument for telling time. They have different ways of perceiving and dividing time. Scheduling in such cultures may mean "when they get around to doing it."

Meaning of Space

Gay (1993) discusses the work of anthropologist Edward T. Hall who for many years has studied proxemics. **Proxemics** is how people in diverse cultures use space. Hall says that humans like other animals are territorial. Some examples of human territoriality include: on a beach, people mark territory with a towel or blanket; in waiting rooms, people mark space with a jacket, hat, luggage, or newspaper; in a classroom, students generally sit in the same place and expect others to respect that space.

How close do you like to be to another person? Generally, this distance varies with the person and the situation. Age, sex of those interacting, and cultural values all influence the distance at which one person is comfortable with another person. Hall categorizes these comfort zones as intimate, personal, social, and public.

- Intimate—touch to 18 inches, usually limited to family and close friends. Necessary when performing most nursing procedures.
- Personal—18 inches to 4 feet, used with friends and co-workers. Probably most effective for many nurse/ client interactions.
- Social—4 to 12 feet, preferred distance with casual acquaintances.
- Public—12 feet or more, generally used with strangers in public places.

These distances will vary from person to person. Some people are quite comfortable being much closer to the person with whom they are interacting. Others prefer a greater distance. Nurses must always be aware of the client's space comfort. Much of nursing care involves touching the client. On admission, the nurse and client generally do not know each other. Thus, in a very short span of time, the nurse moves from the public space into the intimate space of the client when giving care. It may be more difficult when the client and nurse are friends or acquaintances. Care given competently and professionally will help the client feel comfortable when the nurse occupies the intimate space.

Cultural Values

It is important for the nurse to be familiar with the cultural values of the people in the region of employment. Smith (1992) discusses some cultural differences.

Optimal health for all is the focus of our culture. This is greatly different from some cultures where health is not the major concern and little financial or political effort is given to health.

Individualism is stressed in our culture. This contrasts with many cultures where the social group receives the primary consideration, not the individual.

A number of cultures have learned to enjoy what they have and do not feel the need to keep working for some goal or material object. In our culture persons are urged to work hard, to achieve, and to keep busy in order to be successful.

In our culture, cleanliness is closely related to optimal health, and it is a dominant value. There are few countries that emphasize cleanliness as we do. In fact many have no problem with being dirty, and may see it as a positive value.

Political Correctness

To be politically correct in communication means to use language that shows sensitivity to those who are different from oneself. It is intended to help eliminate prejudice by avoiding the use of language that offends. Politically correct language is designed to replace terms that suggest inferior status for members of minority groups and terms that exclude women, older people, and those with handicaps. Racist and bigoted language perpetuates prejudice, false ideas, and often leads to violence. Table 5-3 lists some politically correct terms.

Table 5-3

POLITICALLY CORRECT TERMS	
Politically Correct	**Meaning**
Person with disability	Disabled, handicapped
Hearing impaired	Deaf or hard of hearing
Visually impaired	Blind, unable to see well
Indigenous people	People native to a land
People of color	Non-Caucasian
Humankind	Mankind
Chairperson	Chairman
Manufactured	Man-made

Importance to Health Care System

It is important to understand these psychosocial aspects of communication and to be aware of them in individual clients. Communication will be more effective when these aspects are taken into consideration.

Effective communication has a positive influence on a client's well-being. Clients often judge nurses' competence by their communication skills. Good communication skills result in increased client satisfaction, and increased client satisfaction leads to increased compliance with the therapeutic regimen.

Communication is a key factor in the clients' perception of and the evaluation of the health care services provided.

NURSE/CLIENT COMMUNICATION

One of the most important aspects of nursing care is communication. Whether the nurse is gathering admission information, taking a health history, doing client teaching, or implementing care, good communication skills are essential.

Nurses have both an ethical and moral responsibility to use any information gathered from clients in the client's best interest. Information that affects the health status or care of the client should be shared with other members of the health care team. All information concerning a client is confidential and should never be discussed in elevators, the cafeteria, in hallways, or other public places outside the health care facility. Refer to Chapter 2 for the legal aspects of confidentiality.

Settings

Nurse/client communication takes place in different settings. Occasionally, a formal structured setting is most appropriate, but most of the time an informal setting works best.

Formal Setting

Formal interactions are used in a structured situation such as information gathering on admission or scheduled teaching sessions. Specific items are covered in a planned sequence. In this way, more information can be given or received in the shortest amount of time.

When gathering admission information or a health history, the nurse often uses closed questions. Even though this is considered a block to communication in other situations, it is the most efficient method to use when completing forms. Information relating to the current illness should be obtained using techniques for therapeutic communication. Encouraging the client to talk about the current illness provides information about the client's perception of the situation.

Informal Setting

While this occurs in an unstructured situation there is still a goal for the interaction. The majority of nurse/client interactions are informal. Information for nursing assessments and planning of care as well as implementing the care all make use of informal communication. Orienting a new client to the hospital is best accomplished with the informal approach.

Social Communication

Social communication is the everyday conversations held with family, friends, and acquaintances. Topics are generally those of interest to both parties and reflect their social relationship. Both parties share information, thoughts, and feelings. When getting acquainted with clients, social communication provides a way to learn about each other and begin a nurse/client relationship.

While social communication is not considered to be therapeutic communication, it is part of nurse/client communication. It puts the client at ease because it is nonthreatening, and allows the nurse to get to know the client and what is important to the client. Clients often interpret the social communication as expressions of caring on the part of the nurse. That is, the nurse cares enough about the client to spend some time communicating on a person-to-person level rather than on a nurse-to-client level.

Interactions

All nurse/client interactions should follow the same format whether formal or informal. Each interaction has three phases. The amount of time spent on each phase depends on the purpose of the interaction.

Introduction Phase

The beginning part of an interaction is usually fairly short. The client is greeted by name, the nurse introduces himself, and defines his role. Expectations of the interaction are clarified and mutual goals are set. A good format might be:

"Good morning, Mrs. Jones. My name is Paul Smith. I am a student practical (vocational) nurse and I will be caring for you today and tomorrow. I would like to teach you some breathing and coughing exercises that you will be asked to do after your surgery tomorrow."

Working Phase

Generally, this is the major portion of the interaction. It is used to accomplish the goal or objective defined in the introduction. The nurse should always ask for feedback to ensure understanding on the part of the client. In this situation, having the client demonstrate the breathing and coughing exercises and verbalize why the exercises are necessary would indicate understanding.

Termination Phase

The final phase of an interaction is the termination phase. There are several ways for the nurse to indicate the end of an interaction. Seldom do nurses have unlimited time to spend with one client. The nurse may ask if the client has any questions about the topic discussed. A summary by the nurse of the topic is also a good method to indicate closure.

Factors Affecting Nurse/ Client Communication

Factors influencing communication such as age, education, emotions, culture, language, proxemics, surroundings, and the congruency of messages affect both the nurse and the client in their communications.

Nurse

Many personal factors pertaining to the nurse can also influence nurse/client communication. Past experiences as a nurse, the nurse's state of health, home situation, work load, and staff relations can all impact the thinking, concentration, attitude, and emotions of the nurse. These in turn influence how the nurse sends messages and how messages are received by the nurse. Self-awareness is very important for the nurse when communicating.

Client

Special considerations for communicating with geriatric clients are provided in the box.

GERONTOLOGICAL CONSIDERATIONS

- Assess for sensory disturbances.
- Face the client when speaking.
- Have patience, response may be slow.
- Show respect and be considerate of the older client's personal dignity.

Some other factors related to the client that must be considered are: social, religious, family situation, visual impairment, hearing impairment, speech impairment, and level of consciousness.

Social Factors   Some illnesses are easy to discuss because they are socially acceptable. For example, having the gallbladder or appendix removed or having the flu. It may be more difficult to communicate with a woman having a breast removed. The symbolic meaning of the breast may make its removal hard for the client to accept and may influence how she relates to others. A person with a sexually transmitted disease or one who is HIV positive may be very reluctant to discuss any aspect of the illness.

Religion   Members of some religions seek healing through faith and not through conventional medical services. Others will not receive blood transfusion when an accident or disaster places these individuals in the health care system. These religious beliefs seem to be in conflict with those of the health care team and make communication difficult.

A client may have the priest, minister, or rabbi visit. Privacy for the visit should be provided if at all possible. The nurse must always be nonjudgmental.

Family Situation   Illness often brings family members together around the client. If the family has not been close to or supportive of the client before the illness, communication between the family and client may be strained. This stress may be noticed in the nurse/client interactions. The nurse must be careful not to discuss aspects of the client's condition or treatment in front of family members.

Generally, it is best to ask family members to step out of the room when any nursing care is being given. This should be followed whether assessing the client, providing physical care, or gathering information. The client's right to privacy and confidentiality is thus maintained.

Sometimes the client expresses a desire for a specific person to remain in the room. Unless contraindicated, this is usually allowed.

Visual Impairment   Communicating with the visually impaired does not seem to be a problem at first thought, since they can hear. However, the nonverbal part of a message is missed such as the facial expressions, gestures, and other body language. An important part of every message is lost to this client.

The visually impaired generally speak only when spoken to. Their speech may be loud if they are not sure where the other person is. Silence makes them uncomfortable if they are not sure of another person's presence in the room.

The nurse must include an explanation of "hospital sounds" when orienting a new client who cannot see. The room must be described in detail and the client guided around the room if possible. It is important for the nurses to always speak and identify themselves when entering the room. As with any client, all procedures should be explained. Each step of the procedure as well as any touching should be described before it is initiated. Always tell the visually impaired person before you touch so as not to startle them.

Hearing Impairment   Many hearing impaired persons can communicate by sign language, but few hearing persons can understand or use sign language. If the hearing impaired person is able to read, writing may be the easiest method of communication. Many hearing impaired persons have learned, at least to some degree, to speechread, formerly known as lip reading. Since many words look the same, speech-reading is not totally effective. Communicating with a hearing impaired patient requires time and patience.

The nurse should face the client and speak slowly and deliberately using slightly exaggerated word formation. Gesturing can also be very effective. Check to see if the client has a hearing aid and encourage its use while communicating.

The frustration of trying to communicate often makes the hearing impaired client stubborn or even hostile. The frustration is more from trying to understand others rather than from trying to make themselves understood. A touch on the arm, when the nurse enters the room, will let the client know someone is there and prevent feelings of paranoia.

Hearing impaired persons are usually able to speak. However, because they cannot hear themselves, their speech sounds hollow or monotonal and may be either soft or loud.

Speech Impairment   Dysphasia, the impairment of speech, and aphasia, the absence of speech, both can result from a brain lesion. They are most commonly seen as the result of a stroke. Other neurological diseases such as Parkinson's disease may also cause dysphasia. A dysfunction of the muscles used for speech is termed dysarthria. Dysphasia, aphasia, and dysarthria create communication problems.

A person with dysphasia has difficulty putting thoughts and feelings into words and sending a message. It should be remembered that seldom does this person have difficulty receiving and interpreting a message, so explanations should be given before doing anything. Inappropriate words, such as obscenities, may often be spoken clearly causing misunderstanding and frustration for the client and family. If the client can write, a magic slate or paper and pencil can be used for communication. A picture board, word board, or letter board may also be employed. If available and the client capable, a computer may be used as a means for the client to communicate.

Dysarthria makes a person's speech difficult, slow, and hard to understand. A person with these speech impairments may feel frustrated and helpless. Establishing some method of communication for the client provides hope and maintains self-esteem. At the same time feelings of depression, anger, and hostility are reduced or prevented.

Level of Consciousness   True communication cannot be accomplished with unconscious or comatose clients. However, it should be remembered that unconscious or comatose clients can hear even though they cannot respond. Caregivers should speak to these clients just as they would to alert clients. Always greet the client by name, identify yourself, and explain why you are in the room (what you are going to do). Then let the client know when you are leaving, and if possible when you will return. This is a one-sided interaction, yet so important to the client.

COMMUNICATING WITH FAMILIES

Hospital care deprives families of caring for their ill member. The family often feels helpless, cut off and isolated from their loved one. Therefore, client care should include the family so they can provide love, compassion, protection, and support. Communicating with the family helps them take an active part in the care and recovery of their loved one.

History of Family

Doherty (1992) discusses how the family has changed through the years. Until 1920 we had the "institutional family." The family was organized around economic production and the kinship network. Marriage was functional, not a romantic relationship. Family tradition and loyalty were more important than individual goals or romantic interests. The chief value was responsibility.

From 1920 to 1960 we had the "psychological family." Family affairs were more private and less tied to the extended kinship network. It was based on personal satisfaction and fulfillment of the individual members in a nuclear, two-parent arrangement. The chief value was satisfaction.

The social changes of the 1960s including gender equality and personal freedom caused changes in the family. Increase in the divorce rate may be attributed to the sexual revolution and the attitude that the individual deserves more and owes less to the family.

Today we have the "pluralistic family." No single family arrangement has a monopoly. Many types of families have emerged and are accepted. The chief value is flexibility.

Characteristics of Family

Family has come to be members of a shared household who have similar values and participate in shared goals. Fawcett (1993) discusses the characteristics of family. These characteristics are:

- Feeling love and affection
- Showing caring and compassion
- Feeling a sense of belonging and connectedness
- Having history and linkage to posterity
- Practicing rituals to rejoice
- Having a sense of place
- Accepting their members even with shortcomings
- Honoring their elders
- Having a system of earning and spending money
- Having competent manner of parenting or caretaking
- Dividing chores and labor

What is Family Today?

According to systems theory, families are considered to be interdependent, interacting individuals related by birth, marriage, or mutual consent (Sherman, 1994). This fits in with the pluralistic family described above. Examples of families today are: two-parent nuclear, single parent, blended, extended, cohabitating (never married), gay or lesbian, divorced families, adoptive, multi-adult household, and mixed marriage.

It is important to have the client identify family members. Then the nurse knows exactly who the client considers to be family.

Nurse's Objectivity

Each individual has a belief of what is family. This is shaped by personal experience and observation of other families. The nurse must remain objective and nonjudgmental when the client's family is different from the nurse's idea of family.

Family interaction patterns have an impact on the physical and mental health of the client. In some families the male makes all the decisions, in other families decisions are made jointly, and in others unrelated persons (godparents) are involved in decision making. It may help the nurse to remain objective when communicating with clients and families if the family health is assessed. This assessment can be used to guide communication. Table 5-4 illustrates family health assessment.

Table 5-4

FAMILY HEALTH ASSESSMENT	
Healthy	**Vulnerable**
Many social relationships	Few social relationships
Receive energy from outside	Receive little energy from outside
Strong structure	Weak structure
Access to resources	Limited resources
Receptive to change	Resistant to change
Good communication	Poor communication
Respect for family members	Lack of respect for family members

COMMUNICATING WITH NON-ENGLISH SPEAKING CLIENTS

Clients who do not speak English are generally from another culture. It is important to learn about the other culture especially the values and beliefs. This will help prevent the nurse from violating those values and beliefs.

If a family member speaks English, that person could be used as an interpreter. Sometimes another health care worker on the nursing unit may speak the same foreign language as the client. Consequently, as long as it does not interfere with their work, this person could be used as an interpreter.

A two-language dictionary or pictures are often helpful. If the other language is prevalent in the community, the nurse should learn some phrases in the other language that are useful in client assessment and in client care. Remember, gestures and other nonverbal communication send messages without the use of language.

COMMUNICATING WITH TERMINALLY ILL CLIENTS AND THEIR FAMILIES

Most terminally ill clients know they are dying. Yet they still have concern for those they love. Family and nurses often struggle for the proper response. No one knows for certain what happens after death, but many have beliefs concerning this matter. The unknown aspect after death is probably why some people fear death. No one can escape death, but many people do not want to discuss it. Death is often considered a defeat by health care workers and therefore is not a prime subject for discussion. It is important to remember that listening and silence are both part of communication.

Clients

Anytime a client initiates a conversation regarding death the nurse must be willing to participate. Too often nurses hesitate to communicate with the terminally ill for fear of saying the wrong thing. When the client wants to talk, a good listener is needed. Let the client guide the conversation. Try not to give advice, just listen and accept what the client says. This is very difficult to do.

Most dying people know that they are dying. They are usually afraid of what will happen before death and need information about what to expect. It is important for the client to have the company of those who will listen, those who understand the situation, and those who continue to offer love and friendship in the face of death.

Idle chatter about the news and weather keeps the terminally ill person from being able to talk. The client then feels lonely, isolated, and abandoned. Often they become resentful and angry.

Speaking should be done in normal, not hushed tones. Remember, the unconscious or comatose client can hear! The nurse is often a role model to the family. Communicating with the terminally ill client is one way the nurse shows caring.

Stages of Dying

Dr. E. Kubler-Ross (1969) described the stages of dying as denial, anger, bargaining, depression, and acceptance. There is usually no straight progression from denial to acceptance. The terminally ill client often moves back and forth from one stage to another as the situation changes. There is nothing right or wrong about the stages of dying. They are normal predictable responses to the dying process. Callanan & Kelly (1992) offer suggestions about communication during each of these stages.

Denial   When the client is in the denial stage, neither challenge nor encourage the denial. Acknowledge hopes or wishes but do not reinforce denial.

Anger   Anger is often caused by the frustration of helplessness. Sometimes there is also resentment or fear. Allow the client choices and control of the situation whenever possible. Respond to the frustration, resentment, or fear but not to the anger.

Bargaining   Most bargaining goes unnoticed and remains secret. It is done with anyone (God) thought to have the power to extend life a little longer. If the dying client does bring up the subject of bargaining, reflect what the client states and encourage verbaliza-

tion of those feelings. Do not encourage or promote the idea that death can be put off.

Depression   Depression grows out of grief. The terminally ill client grieves for what is lost (health, job, independence) and for what will be lost (personal relationships, life, future). Listen and try to understand.

Acceptance   Clients may have interludes of acceptance and then go to another stage. Permanent acceptance comes as death nears. With acceptance comes detachment or a drawing away. The presence of one or two important persons in the client's life is all that is needed.

Families

Communication with the families of terminally ill clients must be open and honest as all communication should be. This is a very emotional time. Often the family does not really listen to their loved one or understand what is being said. The nurse should help the family understand that a dying person often speaks in symbolic language because there are no words to describe what is being experienced.

The message of a dying person may be an attempt to describe what is being experienced while dying, or to request something that is needed for a peaceful death. The experiences being described may include being in the presence of someone not alive, preparing for travel to a place they alone can see, or knowing when death will occur. The requests may indicate a desire to reconcile personal, spiritual, or moral relationships or to remove some barrier to achieve peace.

Nearing Death Awareness

Assisting the family to understand nearing death awareness described by Callanan & Kelly (1992) is an important task for the nurse. Nearing death awareness develops in people dying slowly of progressive illnesses. They become aware of a dimension that lies beyond. The client may tell of talking to or seeing people no one else can see. Sometimes they see where they are going.

Often the client drifts between the present and this new dimension. They refer to the peace and beauty of a place invisible to us. Clients appear to be preoccupied or distracted. They seem to look through those around them and focus on something beyond. Family members may be upset, thinking that their loved one is confused or hallucinating. This can be very painful for those being left behind.

Clients experiencing nearing death awareness will assess their life and determine what remains to be finished before death. Often they know when they will die. Some need permission to die from the family they are leaving behind. They want to know that the remaining family have things under control and will be able to carry on.

The nurse and the family must work together to understand the strange ways in which the terminally ill client communicates. It takes persistence and insight to identify and decipher the messages. "Listening" to the client's gestures and facial expressions help to understand the message.

COMMUNICATING WITH THE HEALTH CARE TEAM

Providing care to clients is a team effort. For the team to work efficiently and effectively and to provide quality continuous care to clients, effective communication is necessary. This communication may be oral or written, individual or group, or even on a computer.

Oral Communication

Oral communication among the health care team is necessary for the appropriate planned care of the clients and for the efficient and effective functioning of the nursing unit. All persons who provide direct care to clients orally communicate with each other concerning client care to provide continuity of care.

Nurse/Nurse

This could be peer/peer or subordinate/superior communication. Peer/peer communication takes place many times every day. If each nurse uses effective communication with peers as well as clients, the unit will run more efficiently and client care will be more effective.

Superior/subordinate communication often directs the client care to be performed by the subordinate. The way in which this communication is handled will affect the attitude of the subordinate and the client care given. The situation can be stressful when performance of the subordinate is being evaluated, especially if the subordinate's performance has not been satisfactory. Evaluation should always be done face-to-face in a private place. Only statements of fact should be used. Judgmental statements will only hinder communication. It is very important for the superior to keep emotions under control.

Nurse/Nursing Assistant

The nurse is responsible for informing the nursing assistants of their duties. Taking time to answer questions and providing reasons for specific activities requested helps establish a relationship of trust and mutual respect.

An experienced nursing assistant can be of considerable assistance to the new graduate (RN or LP/VN). The nursing assistant is often much more comfortable and confident in providing bedside care. They should be included in planning care since they often have creative solutions to problems.

Nurse/Student Nurse

Student nurses must communicate not only with the clinical instructor but also with the staff nurses. How well the staff nurses interact with student nurses depends on how the staff nurses were treated as students and the experiences the staff nurses have had with other student nurses. Student nurses are involved in the clinical facility for specific learning experiences selected by the instructor and related to classroom topics. They must have time to review client records, observe others doing procedures, and communicate with and care for their clients. Students are limited in their nursing activities depending on how far they have progressed through the nursing curriculum. Since staff nurses retain responsibility for the care of clients even when clients are assigned to students, communication between student nurses and staff nurses is essential.

Generally, a complementary relationship develops between nursing students and staff nurses. Staff nurses often notify the student or instructor of potential learning experiences. Occasionally, a staff nurse will either view the student as an incapable invader or will try to protect the student from every stress. In these situations the instructor must intervene to ensure an adequate meaningful clinical experience.

Nurse/Physician

There have been much discussion and complaining about nurse/physician communication over the years. Some older physicians still think of nurses as handmaidens who must drop everything to meet any request and who are never to question an order.

Nursing education and expertise have evolved over the years to a professional level. Nurses are responsible for their own actions even if they follow a harmful physician order.

When the term *nursing diagnosis* was introduced, many physicians had difficulty understanding how nurses could make a diagnosis. Nursing diagnoses focus on human needs while medical diagnoses focus on disease conditions. Nurses must communicate openly and honestly with physicians showing their competence with accurate assessments and quality care.

Nurse/Other Departments

Communication with professionals in other departments should always be as peers. Clarification of goals for each client and ways to meet those goals should be the focus of communication. Listening to those in other departments and establishing mutual respect for each other's area of expertise provides the client with top quality care.

Group Communication

Client care conferences may be scheduled regularly or whenever there is a need. Some conferences may be solely for the staff of a particular nursing unit or, when necessary, members of other departments may be invited. Only persons directly involved with the care of the client should be invited.

The conference leader should establish the objectives for the conference and make all necessary arrangements. A conference room or other private place should be used as a meeting site. One person should be designated to record the discussion. If the conference is about a specific client, only facts should be documented on the client's chart. If the topic is general and not related to a specific client, then only a record of the discussion is needed.

Telephone

As a student, you will not be allowed to take telephone or verbal orders from the physicians. If you find yourself in such a situation, you must inform the physician that you cannot accept the order but that you will get the RN or LV/PN who will be able to take the order.

When the telephone rings and a student nurse is the only person available to answer, it should be answered with the name of the department or floor, personal name, and position (student nurse). Tell the caller the appropriate person will be right there. If a message must be taken, write it down, and read it back to the caller. Ask for the caller's name and have it spelled out. Do not give out any information about clients.

Written Communication

Most written communication is related to the client's chart. All aspects of client care are recorded on each client's chart.

Requisitions to x-ray, physical or respiratory therapy, or requests for laboratory services for a client are forms of written communication. The reports resulting from these requests become a part of the client's chart.

Other types of written communication, but not pertaining to a specific client are: interdepartmental memos requesting equipment, supplies, maintenance, or housekeeping. These are necessary to keep the nursing unit functioning efficiently and effectively.

Shift Report

Reports between shifts are vital to the continuity of client care. The most common method is an oral report. It may be that the charge nurse of the outgoing shift reports on all clients to the members of the incoming shift. Sometimes the charge nurse may give the report only to the incoming charge nurse who will in turn relay necessary information to primary nurses or to team members only about their individual clients.

Some nursing units have a taped report. That is, the charge nurse or each primary nurse records the information on each client for the next shift. These reports have a big disadvantage since there is no interaction between the nurses on the two shifts; there is no chance for feedback.

The other method of giving a shift report is called a "walking report." The charge nurse and/or primary nurses give the report to the oncoming nurses for each client as they walk from bed to bed. The client is included and is aware of what information is given to the oncoming shift. The nurses must be prepared to answer questions from the client.

Whatever method is used, the shift report about each client should be concise and complete. The report should begin with the client's name, room, and bed. This should be followed by age, physician, admitting diagnosis, and any surgery performed (see Table 5-5). Shift reports are to be focused on the clients and given in an orderly manner. It is not a time for social conversation.

Computers

Computers in health care agencies are being used extensively in the business office and have been for years. The introduction of computers into the departments of direct client care has been slower. In many

Table 5-5

INFORMATION FOR SHIFT REPORT

1. Client name, room and bed, age, sex.
2. Physician, admission date and diagnosis, and any surgery.
3. Diagnostic tests or treatments performed in the past 24 hours. Results if available.
4. General status, any significant change in condition.
5. New or changed physician's orders.
6. Nursing diagnoses and suggested nursing orders.
7. Evaluation of nursing interventions.
8. Intravenous fluid amounts, last PRN medication.
9. Concerns about the client.

places, computers are used by client care departments to send requisitions to other departments and to receive test results. There are programs used by the pharmacy that show safe dosages and drug interactions. There are programs for physicians to aid them in diagnosis and treatment of some conditions. Telemedicine uses videoconferencing integrated with medical devices so physician specialists in large medical centers can examine a client many miles away. The computerized patient record (CPR) as envisioned by the Institute of Medicine (IOM) is not yet available in the United States. Parts of the CPR have been implemented as described previously.

The IOM defines the CPR as an "electronic record that resides in a system specifically designed to support users through availability of complete and accurate data, practitioner reminders and alerts, clinical decision support systems, links to bodies of medical knowledge and other aids." This moves the client record from simply keeping track of client care to being a resource for health care delivery (Brandt, 1995).

Sigma Theta Tau International now publishes *The Online Journal of Knowledge Synthesis for Nursing.* It provides peer-reviewed electronic research that has been synthesized, analyzed, and translated into practice.

Before there is widespread use of the CPR, many questions have to be answered. Some of the questions are: How can changes in the data entered be prevented? How will charting errors be corrected? What happens when the computers are down? How will record security be maintained? What are the legal implications of electronic or digital signatures?

With the expanding use of computers in health care and the great potential for increased use, it is important for all health care workers to have some knowledge about computers.

COMMUNICATING WITH YOURSELF

Whether it is admitted or not, people talk to themselves every day. Many times it is in the form of thoughts, rather than speaking out loud. What people say to themselves influences their personality, and therefore how they interact with others. Sherman (1994) describes self-talk as positive or negative.

Positive Self-talk

Practicing positive self-talk is the key to positive self-esteem. Send positive thoughts to yourself about yourself. Better yet, say the thoughts out loud. Thinking, saying, and hearing positive statements about oneself adds reinforcement. Remind yourself about your good attributes and accomplishments. When you have had a difficult day, whether in the classroom or clinical area, pat yourself on the back for what you did accomplish. Each day verbally tell yourself what you learned or what good care you gave to your client(s).

Positive self-talk reinforces the desire to succeed. Memories of successes can be used as positive self-talk especially when things are not going well and frustration sets in.

Positive Affirmation

Positive affirmation is a positive thought or idea on which a person consciously focuses to produce a desired result. This can be used to change negative inner messages to positive messages. Instead of saying, "I don't know if I can pass this test," say "I know I can pass this test." Of course, positive affirmation is not a substitute for studying and preparing for the exam. Positive affirmation modifies the person's attitude about the situation.

Negative Self-talk

Whenever you say to yourself, "I can't do . . . ," you are decreasing your self-esteem with the negative self-talk. This negative self-talk may originate within you, or you may be replaying what others say about you. Negative self-talk is self-destructive. Your self-image is lowered by your own criticism and you begin to see yourself as a failure.

▶ CASE STUDY

Martha, a twenty-five-year-old Mexican-American female, is admitted for severe abdominal pain. Martha clung onto her mother's arm when the nurse asked the mother to leave the room during the admission procedure. The mother asked to stay in the room. The nurse looked at Martha who smiled but said nothing.

The following questions will guide your development of a Nursing Care Plan for the case study.

1. What subjective and objective data should the nurse gather?
2. What may be causing Martha to cling to her mother?
3. What can the nurse do to communicate with Martha?
4. Identify a nursing diagnosis for Martha.

SUMMARY

- Communication is influenced by education, age, culture, emotions, perception, and situations.
- Nonverbal messages are generally more accurate in communicating a person's feelings.
- Verbal and nonverbal messages must be congruent for clear communication.
- People have four comfort zones of closeness: intimate, personal, social, and public.
- Therapeutic communication is purposeful and goal directed.
- Almost every nurse/client interaction should involve therapeutic communication.
- Nurse/client communication is influenced by both the nurse and client.
- Psychosocial aspects of communication may aid or hinder communication.
- The nurse is often a role model for the family when communicating to the terminally ill client.
- Accurate communication among the health care team is needed for continuity of care.

Review Questions

1. Mr. George is looking out the window with his back to the door. A nurse opens the door and says, "You will not be able to eat or drink after supper because of tests tomorrow." Then the nurse leaves. Did communication take place?

   a. No, there was no feedback.
   b. No, there was no eye contact.
   c. Yes, Mr. George had to hear the message.
   d. Yes, there was a sender, receiver, and message.

2. What is the best way to communicate?

   a. verbally
   b. nonverbally
   c. it depends what the message is
   d. verbally and nonverbally together

3. Initial client assessment related to communication would include:

   a. vital signs.
   b. visual deficits.
   c. ambulatory ability.
   d. complete health history.

4. When performing a nursing procedure on a client the nurse should:

    a. only listen to what the client says.
    b. be aware of her own nonverbal messages.
    c. always have someone witness the procedure.
    d. tell the client how fortunate he is to be the nurse's client.

5. The nurse is aware that most nursing procedures are performed in which spatial comfort zone?

    a. public
    b. social
    c. personal
    d. intimate

6. Which of the following is the best way for a nurse to show caring?

    a. constantly stay with the client
    b. do everything for the client
    c. assist the client to learn self-care
    d. relay everything the client says to the physician

7. A terminally ill client denies that there is anything wrong and talks constantly about going back to work. The nurse should:

    a. listen but make no comments.
    b. acknowledge the hopes and wishes.
    c. advise the client that it will be impossible to return to work.
    d. assist the client to plan when to return to work.

8. The nurse uses therapeutic communication with the client to:

    a. cure the client of fear.
    b. discuss personal problems.
    c. obtain or provide information.
    d. relieve the client of all concerns.

9. The nurse is aware that communication among members of the health care team is necessary because it:

    a. provides for continuity of care.
    b. identifies who provides better care.
    c. allows team members to become friends.
    d. promotes competition between departments.

10. Mrs. Banc tells the nurse that she would rather die than have radiation. To whom should the nurse report this communication?

    a. the physician only
    b. everyone on the nursing unit
    c. the physician and charge nurse
    d. no one, the communication is confidential

Critical Thinking Questions

1. Discuss communicating with an unconscious adult.

2. Discuss communicating with a terminally ill client.

News Flash

In October, 1995 the Medical Records Confidentiality Act of 1995 (S1360) was introduced in the Senate. It provides: (1) federal safeguards for medical records whether they are in paper or electronic form; (2) clear rules governing the exchange and transfer of health information to ensure confidentiality of personally identifiable information; (3) strong and effective remedies for violations of this Act. As of this writing, the bill (S1360) is in the Labor Resources Committee. Currently, there are only thirty-four states that have medical privacy laws (Ravitch, 1996; Frawley & Asmonga, 1996).

UNIT
2

Cultural Aspects

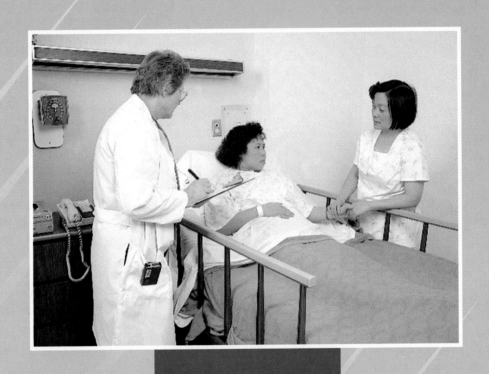

CHAPTER
6

Cultural Aspects
of Health and Illness

Susan Stranahan

LEARNING OBJECTIVES

Upon completion of this chapter the learner should be able to:
- Define key terms.
- Describe the impact of cultural beliefs on health and illness.
- Compare and contrast diverse health beliefs of major cultural groups in the United States.
- Analyze personal cultural beliefs and valves.
- Perform a cultural assessment.

► MAKING THE CONNECTION

Refer to topics in the following chapters to increase your understanding of cultural aspects of health and illness:

- **Chapter 3, Introduction to Ethics:** Rights, p. 39; Values, p. 44; Acquisition of Values, p. 44

- **Chapter 5, Communication:** Verbal Communication, p. 70, Nonverbal Communication, p. 70; Listening/Observing, p. 71; Psychosocial Aspects of Communication, p. 73, Gestures, p. 73, Meaning of Time, p. 74, Meaning of Space, p. 74, Cultural Values, p. 74; Factors Affecting Nurse/Client Communication, p. 76;

Communicating With Families, p. 77; Communicating with Non-English Speaking Clients, p. 78; Communicating with the Health Care Team, p. 80

- **Chapter 7, Cultural Diversity in the Workplace:** Aspects of Culture That Affect Client Care: Religion, p. 98; Other Cultural Aspects Affecting Client Care, p. 103, Language, p. 103, Cultural Orientation, p. 105, Cultural Responses to Pain, p. 105, Cultural Responses to Grieving, p. 110, Cultural Response to Time and Space Orientation, p. 111, Cultural Response to Nutrition, p. 112

INTRODUCTION

The social unrest of the 1960s and 1970s drew attention to the cultural and ethnic diversity that exists in the United States. America was once considered "the melting pot of the world" as waves of immigrants flooded the shores from Europe, Africa, and Asia during the nineteenth and twentieth centuries. Anthropologists are more inclined to describe the American experience in cultural diversity as a mosaic. Cultural groups who immigrated were not inclined to melt together to form one American culture. Rather, each group tried to preserve its identity through language, beliefs, values, and practices consistent with their country of origin. Native Americans were forced to retreat into pockets of isolation that inadvertently aided in preserving their cultural identity to some degree. While white European culture is considered to be the **dominant** American culture, **minority** or subcultures are not judged to be inferior even though they are different.

Medical anthropologists have observed that ethnic origin causes people to respond to illness and health events in different ways. The classic study conducted by Zola (1966) found that Irish and Italian Americans respond to pain very differently. The Italians were vocal and demonstrative about pain, whereas the Irish, experiencing the same type of pain, denied having any discomfort. The role that health and illness play in society depends on values, beliefs, and practices that are largely a function of culture. Illness behaviors stem from cultural beliefs and values and determine responses to illness.

The profession of nursing has recognized the need for nurses to acquire skill in cultural care because of the influence culture has on the human response to illness. Consequently, cultural diversity has become an integral curriculum component of nursing education since the National League for Nursing (NLN) mandated it in the 1980s. The aim of the NLN mandate is to develop culturally competent nurses who are able to appreciate the effects of culture on health and illness behavior and design culturally appropriate nursing interventions. Not only do nurses confront a culturally diverse clientele seeking health care, diversity based on ethnicity is found among students in nursing education programs, and subsequently in the health care workforce.

Diverse patterns of culture are likely to increase and play a prominent role in American life. Table 6-1 describes the distribution of population by the five major cultural groups in the United States according to the Bureau of the Census (*Statistical Abstract,* 1995). The white majority shows the smallest percent increase over the last decade while the four minority groups experienced the greatest percent increase. The proportion of the population contributed by minority groups will steadily increase over time until by the

Table 6-1

ETHNIC DISTRIBUTION OF POPULATION IN THE UNITED STATES IN THOUSANDS

Ethnic group	1980	1990	Percent increase
White	194,713	208,710	7.3
Black	26,683	30,486	14.3
Hispanic	14,609	22,354	53.0
Asian	3,729	7,458	100.0
Native American	1,420	2,065	45.4

Table 6-2

PERCENT DISTRIBUTION OF THE MAJOR ETHNIC GROUPS IN THE UNITED STATES (STATISTICAL ABSTRACT)

Year	White	Black	Hispanic	Asian/ American Indian
1990	83.9	12.3	9.0	3.8
1995	82.9	12.6	10.2	4.5
2000	81.9	12.8	11.3	5.3
2025	77.3	14.2	16.8	8.5

year 2025, approximately one person in four will not be white (Table 6-2).

Data suggest that disease is distributed along ethnic lines. Life expectancy in 1995 for white males and females was 73.4 and 80.2 respectively, but only 68.8 and 76.0 for black males and females. The United States Department of Health and Human Services (USDHHS) has attempted to narrow the gap in health status between whites and minority populations (1990). Various health objectives for the nation to achieve by the year 2000 have been established for ethnic groups who experience increased prevalence of certain health problems. For example, 44 percent of black women aged 20 and over are overweight as are 29 to 75 percent of Native Americans. The national objective is to reduce the overweight prevalence in these two groups to 30 percent by the year 2000. Only 18 percent of Hispanic women over age fifty have received mammograms. The goal is to increase this proportion to 60 percent by the year 2000. The highest rates for diabetes mellitus are found among Native Americans. The national objective is to reduce the prevalence of diabetes in this population group from 69 per thousand to 62 per thousand.

KEY ABBREVIATIONS

The following abbreviations and acronyms are used in this chapter:

AIDS	acquired immunodeficiency syndrome
HIV	human immunodeficiency virus
NLN	National League for Nursing
USDHHS	United States Department of Health and Human Services
WHO	World Health Organization

CONCEPT OF CULTURE

Definitions

Merriam Webster's Collegiate Dictionary (1995) defines **culture** as "the integrated pattern of human knowledge, belief and behavior that depends upon man's capacity for learning, and transmitting knowledge to succeeding generations" Patterns of behavior develop in universal areas such as language, social norms, political thought, supernatural beliefs, aesthetics, and beliefs about health and illness. These behavior patterns provide the unwritten and generally accepted rules for living within the homogeneous society. **Ethnic group** refers to individuals who share a unique cultural background, and subscribe to common patterns of behavior and beliefs. **Racial group** is a classification of people according to physical characteristics, such as skin pigmentation or facial features and is, therefore, not synonymous with ethnic group. Individuals may belong to the same racial group yet have very different patterns of behavior and, therefore, belong to different ethnic groups. For example, blacks from Africa and blacks from the Caribbean represent the Negroid race but do not necessarily share similar ethnicity. They may hold very different beliefs about rules for living and interpreting the universe.

Individuals who believe in the supremacy of their own ethnic group are described as **ethnocentric**. Until recently, the prevailing American attitude was that minority ethnic groups should absorb into the dominant culture and discard unique behavioral patterns and beliefs of subcultural groups. The "great American melting pot" analogy represents this view, and the process is called **acculturation**. Ethnocentricity prevents health care providers from examining their own cultural beliefs and those of their clients. It reveals an inability to understand the values and beliefs of another cultural group.

The increasing likelihood of a culturally diverse health care workforce and clientele underscore the need for each nurse to become aware of personal ethnocentric views. The demand is for flexibility and tolerance in attitudes toward individuals representing a different cultural heritage from one's own.

Components of Culture

Stewart has identified five components of culture that organize the way people think about life (in Lock, 1992).

1. Activity: identifies how people organize and value work.
2. Social relations: explain the importance and structure of friendships, gender roles, class.
3. Motivation: describes the value and methods of achievement.
4. Perception of the world: is the interpretation of life events and religious beliefs.
5. Perception of self and the individual: refers to personal identity, value, and respect for individuals.

This model is particularly helpful to nurses planning care for a client from another ethnic group. Work, social relationships, success, religion, and self-identity influence the definition cultural groups attribute to health and illness. The response to health events is determined by the role illness plays in a given society. If relationships are valued more than work, the sick role may permit an extended period of illness and sanction a lengthy time away from the employment site. However, where achievement is measured by output at work, illness may be interpreted in a negative manner. Individuals in this society may deny illness and delay seeking appropriate health care interventions.

Characteristics of Culture

Spradley and Allender (1996) have identified five characteristics shared by all cultures.

1. Culture is learned. Patterns of behavior are acquired as children imitate adults and develop actions and attitudes acceptable by others in society.
2. Culture is not inherited or innate. Culture is integrated throughout all the interrelated components. Activities, relationships, motivations, world views, and individuality are permeated with consistent patterns of behavior. They form a cohesive whole.
3. Culture is shared by everyone who belongs to the cultural group. Behavior patterns are not individually defined but are rather accepted and practiced by all.
4. Culture is tacit (unspoken), in that acceptable behavior is understood by everyone in the cultural group. Beliefs may not be written down nor spoken about but they are commonly known and espoused (adopted).

5. Finally, culture is dynamic; it is constantly changing. Each generation experiences new ideas that may generate different standards for behavior.

Relationship Between Culture and Religion

Anthropologists have identified the strength of the influence religion has on culture. In many cases, culture and tradition have been maintained and preserved through religious beliefs. Religion often includes the formal organizational structures for social behavior. The influence religion has on culture can be seen throughout the various components of culture. Attitudes toward activities, social relationships, motivations, interpretation of life events, and self-concept are closely tied to supernatural beliefs. Religion may determine dietary practices, interpretation and reaction to illness, therapeutic interventions, and choice of medical practitioner.

INFLUENCE OF CULTURE ON BELIEFS AND PRACTICES ABOUT HEALTH AND ILLNESS

It is common for diverse cultural groups to have a body of knowledge and beliefs about health and disease. Cultural practices can positively and negatively affect health and disease distribution. In cultures where raw foods are not consumed, the incidence of shigellosis may be lower. On the other hand, cultural taboos against eating protein during pregnancy have a deleterious (harmful or destructive) effect on fetal development. Human responses to illness are defined by cultural values. Whether an individual seeks professional care when ill and complies with prescribed treatment is related to cultural values.

Components of Health Subject to Cultural Influence

Beliefs and patterns of behavior affect attitudes about various aspects of health. Cause and origin of disease, practices for avoiding disease, definition of health, and types of medical or health practitioners vary by ethnic group.

Etiology

Peter Morley (1978), a noted medical anthropologist, presents four explanations for the origin of disease: supernatural, nonsupernatural, immediate, and ultimate causes. Supernatural causes for disease trace the origin of the disease to metaphysical forces such as witchcraft, sorcery, and voodoo. In this case, an individual might ascribe illness to evil spirits or a curse by a powerful spiritual person. Nonsupernatural causes are diseases that have an accepted cause-effect relationship even though that relationship may lack scientific rationale. For example, colic in an infant may be due to breast milk rendered impure when a nursing mother has sexual relations. For this reason, sexual relations in that culture are prohibited for nursing mothers. Immediate causes refer to diseases caused by known pathogenic agents. Ultimate causes describe determinates for diseases such as smoking in lung cancer. Most cultural groups will support a multietiologic origin, borrowing from three or all four explanations for how and why diseases occur.

Health Promotion and Protection

Strategies for achieving and maintaining good health varies by cultural group. Western culture has come to endorse a low-fat, high-fiber diet, regular exercise, and appropriate immunizations as means to promote and protect health. Other cultures may place greater value on meditation, prayer, and restored relationships, particularly where health protection and disease prevention are closely linked to beliefs about disease etiology. Preventing disease may require paying homage to ancestral spirits in order not to offend them and provoke their revenge through illness.

Definition of Health

The most popular definition of **health** was developed by the World Health Organization (WHO) and indicates that health is not the mere absence of disease but includes the concept of complete physical, mental, and social wellness. While the definition of health is broad enough to be global, what is understood by physical, mental, and social wellness is culturally defined. Any deviation from what is culturally understood as normal health is considered illness. A biological disease of immediate etiology might not be interpreted as an illness by some societies. Intestinal parasites are so common in some areas in Africa that the presence of ascaris in stools is considered normal. When the cultural group does not recognize certain behaviors or symptoms as illness, individuals are not likely to seek medical intervention when they appear. In this case, disease conditions may persist untreated to an irreversible state.

Practitioners and Remedies

Culturally diverse concepts of etiology and definitions for health and illness lead to variations in health/illness care providers. Alternative remedies and practitioners are characteristic of culturally diverse groups. When a scientific rationale for the etiology of disease is not accepted by a cultural group, standard western medicine may not be accepted for treatment either. Compliance with treatment regimes is unlikely when health care providers base therapy on principles of western medicine and prescribe treatments dissimilar to culturally traditional remedies. When disease etiology is traced to a supernatural cause, western medicine is not sought as a remedy. The individual is more likely to seek an intervention from a spiritual leader or traditional healer.

Health Beliefs of Selected Cultural Groups in the United States

While the population of the United States is represented by innumerable ethnic groups, four groups, African American, Hispanic, Asian, and Native American, emerge as the majority. They form the basis for the brief discussion of specific health beliefs affected by culture.

African American

In 1995, African Americans accounted for about 12.6 percent of the population in the United States. Their ancestors came to North America from various African countries, as either slaves or free immigrants, and also from the Caribbean. The different countries of origin as well as disparate educational levels, income, occupations, and religious beliefs explain the heterogeneous (different) cultural practices among African Americans today.

Some African American beliefs about health and illness are linked to either a supernatural or a nonsupernatural origin of disease. In traditional African societies, disease may be caused by disharmony in relationships. Discord may occur between a client and ancestral spirits, evil spirits, or living relatives. For example, following a wedding, a man may refuse to complete bride price payments to his in-laws. If he becomes ill, his illness may be attributed to the break in relations with his wife's family caused by his outstanding debt. Healing comes in restoration of harmony and may be achieved through prayer, mediation, or activities considered to be therapeutic such as offering a gift, wearing a charm, confessing of a wrong, and restitution. In this example, the man would have to pay his debt to his in-laws.

Disease may also be sent by God as a punishment for a serious infraction against Him or another person. Evil forces may account for illness in some cases. Treatments may be found in herbs and home remedies, consultation with a local healer, and certainly in prayer.

Hispanic

Hispanic Americans, 10 percent of the total population, comprise the second largest minority ethnic group in the United States. The majority originate in Mexico, Puerto Rico, and Cuba. Even though the Spanish language is common to most Hispanics, there is no single cultural pattern due to different countries of origin. In general, Hispanic Americans belong to a large extended family system where females are seen as subservient to males, but they also play a major role in family cohesiveness.

The influence of religion on culture is particularly evident in Hispanic populations. The majority have their roots in Catholicism, which has been blended with traditional Indian beliefs. Illness may have natural cause or be considered "an act of God" as punishment for sin, or the result of witchcraft or a curse by an enemy. Diseases may be traced to an imbalance between "wet" and "dry" or "hot" and "cold" forces. Treatment is determined by the cause. Western medicine is appropriate for some diseases while the native healer (curandera) may have to intervene for supernatural causes. Treatment may consist of herbal potions, diets based on "hot" and "cold" foods, or religious ceremonies.

Asian

Asian immigrants came from Pacific rim countries: Korea, Vietnam, Laos, the Philippines, Cambodia, China, and Japan. Generalization of a specific Asian culture is not possible from such a diversity of countries; however, certain similarities exist. Asian cultures are typically patrilineal, that is, family relations are traced through males. Males are heads of the households, and elders are respected.

Asians hold to a Yin (cold) and Yang (hot) etiology of disease. Yin and Yang are opposing forces and when in balance, there is health (see Figure 6-1). Illness occurs as a consequence of an imbalance in these forces. Foods are identified as either hot or cold and used as treatment. If Yang is overpowering Yin, then hot foods are avoided until balance is restored. Illness may also be caused by supernatural powers such as God, evil spirits, or ancestral spirits. In this situation, healing might be found through prayer or treatment from a traditional healer. Many Asian Americans rely on herbal remedies, acupuncture, and cupping and burning, a treatment that draws blood to the skin's surface when a warmed cup is placed on the skin. The inside and rim of the cup are heated with a candle flame. The rim of the cup is then applied directly to the client's skin and, as the cup cools, blood is drawn to the surface of the skin causing a bruised appearance.

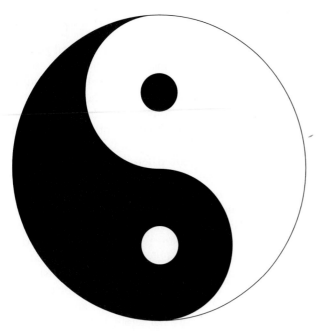

FIGURE 6-1   Yin and Yang.

Native Americans

The fourth major minority ethnic group in the United States is Native Americans. They form a very diverse group, stemming from over 200 different tribes across the United States. While many Native Americans have assumed Euro-American practices with regard to health, some still use traditional practices. Health is believed to result from a harmonious relationship with nature and the universe. Illness is frequently traced to a supernatural origin and precipitated by discord with the forces of nature. Use of witchcraft can cause illness and treatment may require exorcism of evil spirits. Prevention may be found in prayer, charms, and fetishes (objects having power to protect or aid the owner). Remedies often include herbal drinks. "Medicine men" are persons thought to hold supernatural powers of healing. Through prayers, rituals, ceremonies, and herbal drinks, health may be restored.

CULTURALLY APPROPRIATE NURSING CARE

Discussion has focused on the commonality of culture and certain concepts of culture that influence behaviors. All individuals, both clients and health care providers, come from a cultural background that, in some way, influences behavior and attitude about health and illness. Personal attitudes and behaviors determine not only how clients interpret health events and utilize health care but also how nurses interpret health events and provide health care. The central role that culture places in determining perception compels health care providers to evaluate their personal cultural views about health and illness before examining those of other ethnic groups. Nurses need to be able to recognize how culture affects the health care needs of clients and respond appropriately. Culturally sensitive nursing care begins with an examination of one's own culture and beliefs.

Personal Cultural Assessment

Spradley and Allender (1996) have identified five areas of examination in order to assess one's own culture and the influence it may have on personal beliefs about health care.

1. Influences from own ethnic/racial background
2. Own typical verbal and nonverbal communication patterns
3. Own cultural values and norms
4. Own religious beliefs and practices
5. Own health beliefs and practices

They suggest gathering as much information as possible on each issue then validating it with one or two other persons from the same cultural group.

Client Cultural Assessment

Having examined one's own culture and the influences it may have had in developing personal beliefs about sickness and health, the next step to providing culturally appropriate care is to assess the client's cultural background. Locate materials in the local library that describe the culture of interest. Through personal interviews, data may be collected from members of the culture to be studied or from others familiar with the culture.

Spradley and Allender (1996) have identified six categories of information necessary for a comprehensive cultural assessment of the client. These categories may be useful in organizing interviews with representatives from the culture.

1. *Ethnic or racial background.* Where did the client group originate and how does that influence their status and identity?
2. *Language and communication patterns.* What is the preferred language spoken and what are their culturally based communication patterns?
3. *Cultural values and norms.* What are their values, beliefs, and standards regarding such things as roles, education, family functions, childrearing, work and leisure, aging, death and dying, and rites of passage?
4. *Biocultural factors.* Are there physical or genetic traits unique to this cultural group that predispose them to certain conditions or illnesses?
5. *Religious beliefs and practices.* What are the group's religious beliefs and how do they influence life events, roles, health, and illness?

6. *Health beliefs and practices.* What are the group's beliefs and practices regarding prevention, causes, and treatment of illnesses?

The Cultural Assessment Guide presented in Table 6-3 provides topics of greater detail for conducting a cultural assessment.

Table 6-3

CULTURAL ASSESSMENT GUIDE

Category	Sample Data
Ethnic/racial background	Country(s) of origin Mostly native-born or U.S. born? Reasons for emigrating if applicable Racial/ethnic identity Experience with racism or racial discrimination?
Language and communication patterns	Language(s) of origin Language(s) spoken in the home Preferred language for communication How verbal communication patterns affected by age, sex, other? Preferences for use of interpreters Non-verbal communication patterns (eg: eye contact, touching, etc)
Cultural values and norms	Group beliefs and standards for male and female roles and functions Standards for modesty and sexuality Family/extended family structures and functions Values re work, leisure, success, time Values re education and occupation Norms for child-rearing and socialization Norms for social networks and supports Values re aging and treatment of elders Values re authority Norms for dress and appearance
Biocultural factors	Group genetic predisposition to health conditions (eg: hypertension, anemia) Socioculturally associated illnesses (eg: AIDS, alcoholism) Group attitudes toward body parts and functions Group vulnerability or resistance to health threats? Folk illnesses common to group? Group physical/genetic differences (eg: bone mass, height, weight, longevity)
Religious beliefs and practices	Religious beliefs affecting roles, childbearing and rearing, health and illness? Recognized religious healers? Religious beliefs and practices for promoting health, preventing illness, or treatment of illness Beliefs and rituals re conception and birth Beliefs and rituals re death, dying, grief
Health beliefs and practices	Beliefs re causes of illness Beliefs re treatment of illness Beliefs re use of healers (traditional and Western) Health promotion and illness prevention practices Folk medicine practices Beliefs re mental health and illness Dietary, herbal, and other folk cures Food beliefs, preparation, consumption Experience with Western medicine

(From Spradley, B. and Allender, J. (1996). Community health nursing: Concepts and practice (4th ed.). Philadelphia: J. B. Lippincott Company. Reprinted with permission.)

Nurse's Response

An understanding of personal cultural beliefs about health and illness as well as that of the client is the beginning of providing culturally appropriate care. Becoming aware of different beliefs based on culture is an important step. The next step is to apply cultural understanding to the nurse-client relationship. The following activities will help the nurse apply an understanding of cultural aspects of health and illness to an individual client.

- Be sensitive to behaviors and practices different from your own and respond accordingly.
- Listen for cues in the client's conversation that betray a unique ethnic belief about etiology, transmission, prevention, or some other aspect of disease. For example, a client might say, "I knew I would be sick today. I heard an owl last night."
- Respect clients for their different beliefs. Different is not bad nor wrong.
- Accommodate differences if they are not detrimental to health. A client may believe that eating onions may resolve his respiratory infection. While eating onions may not be therapeutic, it is also not likely to negatively impact health.
- Use the occasion to teach positive health habits if the client's practices are deleterious to good health. When asked about her diet, a pregnant woman may reply she never eats meat nor eggs while pregnant in the belief that gaining too much weight increases her risk of a difficult delivery. Such an event provides the nurse with an opportunity to provide nutritional instruction.

ILLNESSES ASSOCIATED WITH ETHNIC GROUPS

Patterns of frequencies of some diseases vary according to ethnicity. Explanations for the disparate (unequal) distribution focus on the biological differences between various ethnic groups. The degree to which environment, heredity, and cultural dietary practices account for the differences is not clearly understood. African Americans tend to be larger in size and weight than most whites, while Asians are smaller. African and Asian Americans mature sooner than whites. Hair texture, skin pigmentation, and food and drug metabolism differ among cultural groups (Clark, 1996).

Across the spectrum of major ethnic groups, diseases range from infectious to chronic. Many conditions, such as poor sanitation, tuberculosis, and infant mortality are associated with lower socioeconomic status. The impact of poverty on health cannot be ignored.

African Americans

African Americans have higher than average rates of hypertension, sickle cell anemia, cancer of the stomach and esophagus, coccidioidomycosis, and lactose intolerance (Stanhope & Knollmueller, 1996). African American populations experience higher incidences of cardiovascular disease, stroke, cancer, diabetes mellitus, cirrhosis, and homicide. Infant mortality rates are highest for this group. African Americans experience higher rates of AIDS.

Hispanic Americans

Hispanic populations experience elevated rates of diabetes mellitus, intestinal parasites, coccidioidomycosis, and lactose intolerance (Stanhope & Knollmueller, 1996). Hypertension, diabetes mellitus, obesity, AIDS, and alcohol are major health concerns for this population group.

Asian Americans

Rates of liver and stomach cancer are high in Asian populations. They also suffer from coccidioidomycosis, hypertension, and lactose intolerance (Stanhope & Knollmueller, 1996). Major health problems faced by Asian Americans are related to conditions under which they fled their countries of origin. They experience high rates of stress-related illnesses and suicides. Mental illnesses are common.

Native Americans

The incidence of accidents is elevated among Native Americans. Additionally, they experience higher rates of heart disease, cirrhosis of the liver, and diabetes mellitus (Stanhope & Knollmueller, 1996). They also have an increased incidence of arthritis and trachoma (Andrews & Boyle, 1995). Major health problems include diabetes, obesity, alcoholism and related fetal alcohol syndrome, and violence. Infectious diseases such as tuberculosis, influenza, impetigo, and dysentery occur at increased rates due to poverty, overcrowding, and poor sanitation. Lactose intolerance occurs among Native Americans at higher rates than in the general population.

Whites

Americans of European descent are a heterogenous group; consequently, it is more difficult to describe them in terms of common disease entities. In general, whites have higher rates of leukemia and breast cancer.

▶ CASE STUDY

Jose Santiago is a fifty-seven-year-old migrant worker who was brought to the evening screening clinic by his crew leader. The crew leader reported that Jose had collapsed in a cucumber field at 4:30 P.M. after ten hours of work and a midday sun temperature of 96°F.

Physical findings included:

B/P = 140/86; P = 120; R = 24;

T = 102° F

Height = 68″; Weight = 220 lbs.

Skin: Hot, red, dry

A diagnosis of heat stroke is made. A cold bath reduces the temperature to 100.8° F. Mr. Santiago refuses hospitalization and is sent home with a prescription for diazepam (Valium) 10 mg t.i.d., and instructions to monitor temperature and pulse q.i.d., and bed rest for two days. The community health nurse visited Mr. Santiago the next day and found him working in the cucumber field. In talking with him, she learns he visited the local healer during the night and did not get his prescription filled.

The following questions will guide your development of a Nursing Care Plan for the case study.

1. What are the most likely reasons Mr. Santiago returned to work the day after having a heat stroke?

2. Discuss the community health nurse's response to Mr. Santiago upon learning he visited the local healer and did not fill his prescription for diazepam.

3. Assess the health beliefs and practices of Mr. Santiago using the Cultural Assessment Guide (refer to Table 6-3, category 6).

4. Write three individualized nursing diagnoses and goals for Mr. Santiago. Include one culturally related nursing diagnosis.

5. List resources specific to location that could assist Mr. Santiago.

6. Describe the teaching that Mr. Santiago will need.

7. List at least three successful client outcomes for Mr. Santiago.

SUMMARY

- By the year 2025, one in four Americans will not be white.
- Response to health and illness is varied and determined by cultural origin.
- Culture is composed of beliefs about activity, relations, motivation, perception of the world, and perception about self.
- Culture is learned, integrated, shared, tacit, and dynamic.
- Culture is influenced by religion, which in turn affects beliefs and practices about health and illness.
- Beliefs about disease etiology, health promotion and protection, concepts of health, and treatment for disease are interrelated.
- Culturally appropriate care begins with an understanding of one's own cultural beliefs.
- Client cultural assessment is a prerequisite to providing appropriate nursing care.

Review Questions

1. The LP/VN who believes all clients should think about illness the way he/she does is:

    a. culturally appropriate.
    b. ethnocentric.
    c. culturally diverse.
    d. accommodating.

2. The LP/VN who believes all immigrants should assume an "American" outlook toward health is demonstrating:

    a. acculturation.
    b. ethnocentrism.
    c. cultural sensitivity.
    d. cultural awareness.

3. Which of the following is a characteristic of culture?

    a. culture is learned
    b. culture stays the same
    c. culture is biologically inherited
    d. culture is individually determined

4. Which of the following is descriptive of Hispanic Americans?

    a. they are culturally homogeneous
    b. their culture is not based on religion
    c. illness may be a punishment from God
    d. they always seek western medical intervention

5. When an African American says to the nurse, "I need to pray with my pastor in order to get well," the most appropriate response from the nurse is:

    a. "The medicine you take will make you well."
    b. "When you are released from the hospital, you can go to church and pray."
    c. "May I call your pastor for you and ask him to visit you?"
    d. "Why do you think prayer will make you well?"

6. It is important to be aware of cultural aspects of health and disease because:

    a. some cultural groups are represented in greater numbers than others.
    b. cultural groups respond differently to illness.
    c. differences in care should not be based on culture.
    d. reimbursement is related to ethnicity.

7. Which of the following statements is true about the distribution of ethnic groups in the United States?

    a. The proportion of whites is increasing while the proportion of Hispanics is decreasing.
    b. Blacks are increasing at a greater rate than Hispanics.
    c. Hispanics are increasing at a greater rate than whites.
    d. The proportion of Native Americans in the population is decreasing.

Critical Thinking Questions

1. What do you know about cultural or ethnic groups other than your own?

2. How does your culture influence your beliefs about health practices?

News Flash

Researchers have determined that pregnant black women have more than twice the rate of chronic hypertension than women of other races. Hypertension in this population may contribute to antepartum hemorrhage and other problems related to higher rates of low infant birth weight and infant mortality (AHCPR, June, 1996).

CHAPTER
7

Cultural Diversity in the Workplace

Joy E. Ache-Reed

▶ KEY TERMS

agnostics
atheists
cultural diversity
ethnocentrism
grieving
kosher
matrilineal society
novenas
prejudice
religious support system
shiva
spiritual care
spiritual needs
staple foods
therapeutic touch
yin and yang

LEARNING OBJECTIVES

Upon completion of this chapter the learner should be able to:
- Define key terms.
- Discuss the nurse's role in meeting the spiritual needs of the client and family.
- Discuss how the nurse's religious beliefs or lack of them can influence nursing care.
- Identify the general beliefs that account for the differences between Christian and non-Christian religions.
- Describe specific differences of cultural groups in relation to pain.
- Describe specific differences of cultural groups in relation to grieving.
- Describe specific differences of cultural groups in relation to time and space.
- Identify nutritional preferences held by various cultural groups.

▶ *MAKING THE CONNECTION*

Refer to the topics in the following chapters to increase your understanding of cultural diversity in the workplace:

- **Chapter 3, Introduction to Ethics:** Rights, p. 39; Values, p. 44, Acquisition of Values, p. 44
- **Chapter 5, Communication:** Methods of Communicating, p. xx, Verbal Communication, p. 70, Nonverbal Communication, p. 70; Listening/Observing, p. 71; Psychosocial Aspects of Communication, p. 73, Gestures, p. 73, Meaning of Time, p. 74, Meaning of Space, p. 74, Cultural Values, p. 74; Factors Affecting Nurse/Client Communication, p. 76; Communicating With Families, p. 77;

Communicating with Non-English Speaking Clients, p. 78; Communicating with the Health Care Team, p. 80

- **Chapter 6, Cultural Aspects of Health and Illness:** Concept of Culture, p. 89; Influence of Culture on Beliefs and Practices About Health and Illness, p. 90; Personal Cultural Assessment, p. 92
- **Chapter 8, Health Maintenance:** What Is Health?, p. 120; What Affects Health?, p. 124; Crucial Health Practices, p. 129; Prevention Works, p. 129
- **Chapter 12, Pain Management:** Definitions of Pain, p. 206; Assessment, p. 211; Alternative Delivery Systems, p. 218

INTRODUCTION

Both student nurses and licensed practicing nurses are confronted with people from different ethnic backgrounds on a daily basis. Some clients, their families, and co-workers belong to a different socioeconomic level and/or cultural group. Many will have values that appear different from the nurse's values. Undoubtedly, a nurse will be asked to provide holistic care to an individual who has a different religious philosophy than his or hers. The manner in which nurses provide nursing care to clients or the harmony in which nurses work alongside co-workers depend upon their understanding of **cultural diversity** (differences in beliefs, behaviors, and values), their educational background, and their personal maturity.

Nurses, like all humans, may be affected by the prejudices of others or even by prejudices of their own. It is imperative in nursing to accept people for who they are and recognize that all persons are created equal, regardless of their race or religious convictions. It is equally important that generalizations not be made and assume that since a person states he is Catholic, Protestant, Islamic, Jewish, or Native American, that the person practices every belief the religious group professes. Be careful not to generalize. Each person is unique and should be treated as such. It is the nurse's role to never assume knowledge, but to clarify information and respect the client's or co-worker's belief system.

Another important aspect of cultural diversity is that what differs between races and cultural groups is not so much the feelings or beliefs that they have, but the expression of those feelings. The nurse must take the time to acknowledge the expression of those feelings and beliefs and provide clients and co-workers with a sense of acceptance and acknowledgment of their rights.

ASPECTS OF CULTURE THAT AFFECT CLIENT CARE: RELIGION

Spiritual and religious beliefs are important in many individuals' lives. These beliefs can influence lifestyle, attitudes, and feelings about life, pain, and death. Some organized religions specify practices about diet, birth control, and appropriate medical care. Spiritual beliefs often assume greater significance at the time of illness than at any other time in a person's life. These beliefs help some people accept their own illness and explain illness for others. These spiritual beliefs often help people plan for the future. Religion can help people live a fuller spiritual life as well as strengthen or console them during suffering, and as they prepare for the inevitability of death. By providing a meaning to life and death, religion can supply the client, his family, and the nurse with a sense of strength, security, and faith during a time of need.

Spiritual needs are identified as an individual's need to find meaning and purpose in life, pain, and death. The spiritual realm is often identified as a very private area. However, in order to provide holistic care, the nurse must pay attention to the spiritual dimension of an individual, recognizing spiritual needs and assisting the client in meeting them.

The **religious support system** includes ministers, priests, rabbis, nuns, mullahs, shamans, and laypersons who are able to meet spiritual needs in the health care setting. The nurse has the responsibility of working with these individuals, including them in the client care team. A nursing intervention to provide spiritual care can involve contacting the religious support system members when necessary, and allowing them to have time and privacy with the client. Pastoral visits should be documented in the client care record and recognized as an alternative method of healing for the body and soul.

Another way a nurse can assist the client to meet spiritual needs is to understand his or her own spiritual beliefs and relationship to a higher being. It is important to acknowledge that while personal beliefs may have been effective for that individual, they may not be accepted by others. Once rapport has been established, the nurse may ask clients questions concerning their beliefs, concerns, and fears. The nurse can use therapeutic communication skills to show interest and caring. Becoming involved with clients' rituals and practices is a good way to show commitment. If clients request that the nurse read them scripture or pray with them, do so. In so doing, the nurse will be assisting the client to meet spiritual needs.

Many clients belong to a specific denominational group. A denominational group is a select group of individuals who share a belief system about a particular concept of God. Each group may have different rituals or practices that set them apart from other groups. They may also have symbols or objects such as jewelry, rosaries, statues, pictures, and scripture books that make them feel closer to God. Nurses must be aware of the general religious philosophies of their clients' denominations. The nursing diagnosis, spiritual distress, can be apparent in a client who is unable to practice religious rituals due to illness or confinement in a health care institution. Be aware that there are individuals who do not have a belief in a higher being. **Agnostics** believe that the existence of God cannot be proved or disproved. **Atheists** do not believe in God or any other deity.

Christian religions believe in Jesus Christ and the truth as taught by Him. Some religions identify with prophets who lived in ancient times as their link to God, or they may believe in other deities. It is important to identify particular beliefs from these various religions that can influence client care activities. Some of these beliefs concern: baptism, communion, Sabbath day practices, dietary concerns, rules for daily living, prayer times, religious books or symbols, and religious support systems.

Since there are over two thousand identifiable religious groups in the United States, it is impossible to include them all in this discussion. The following information is not intended to be an exhaustive treatment of the beliefs of various religious faiths, but to indicate some practices that nurses may encounter in the course of their duties.

Religions

Christian religions encompass a broad spectrum and include: Protestant, Roman Catholic, Orthodox, Jehovah's Witness, Mormon, Christian Science, and Amish. The majority of the Christian religions worship on Sunday, and their primary written reference is the Holy Bible. Do not place other items on top of the Bible and never place it on the floor or out of the reach of the client.

Protestant

Many separate denominations (over 1,200) constitute the group known as Protestant. Protestant groups include such denominations as Baptist, Episcopal, Lutheran, Methodist, Presbyterian, and Seventh Day Adventist.

Baptist   Baptists do not practice infant baptism. For them, baptism is a rite to be performed only after a believer reaches an age of understanding and confesses his acceptance of the saving work of Jesus Christ. Baptism is performed by full immersion in water and not by sprinkling. Communion is a spiritual act and symbolizes the suffering, death, and resurrection of the Lord.

Episcopal   Episcopalians have a number of similarities with Catholics, including confession, anointing of the sick (Holy Unction), communion, and baptism. Holy Unction is most often given as a healing sacrament. Episcopalians believe that a dying infant should be baptized, and the nurse may perform the rite. The usual administration of these sacraments is by an Episcopal priest. The Book of Common Prayer is of great use to members of the Episcopal Church and may be found at the bedside along with the Bible.

Lutheran   Traditionally Lutherans practice baptism of infants and adults by sprinkling. Emergency baptisms may be performed by any baptized Christian. When performing a baptism, pour water over the client's forehead and, at the same time, say aloud, "I baptize you in the name of the Father, and of the Son, and of the Holy Spirit." The Lutheran churches have a more restrictive definition of sacrament than the Roman Catholic and Orthodox churches do, and only recognize baptism and Holy Communion (Eucharist) as meeting that definition. Holy Communion is understood as the body and the blood of the Lord and is often administered to those who are ill or awaiting surgery. Central to their belief is the doctrine of "justification by faith." People are redeemed by God solely on the basis of God's grace, which they receive through faith or acceptance of what God has done for them.

Methodist   Methodists acknowledge the baptismal rites of other Trinitarian Christian religions and practice both infant and adult baptism. They believe that religion is a matter of personal belief, and they use the conscience as a guide for living.

Presbyterian   Presbyterians also practice communion (remembering the death of Jesus Christ for them) and baptism. Salvation is believed to be a gift from God.

Seventh Day Adventist   Seventh Day Adventists do not believe in infant baptism, but baptize individuals when they reach an age of accountability. They practice both public and private worship. They generally are vegetarians, using soybean products as a protein source. Some individuals may eat meats that are specified in the Bible, but never consume pork. Adventists generally do not smoke or drink alcohol products and some members may avoid the use of over-the-counter medications and beverages containing caffeine. Their Sabbath worship is observed from sunset on Friday to sunset on Saturday. They do not pursue their jobs or worldly pleasures during this time.

Roman Catholic

Various rites known as Sacraments (sacred) are performed by the priest at appropriate times in the life of the Catholic. Sacraments that might be encountered in the health care setting are: anointing of the sick, baptism, the Eucharist, and confession.

Baptism   Baptism is administered only once in the life of a Catholic. Catholics believe that baptism is absolutely necessary for salvation. If a Catholic priest is unavailable, any baptized Christian may perform an emergency baptism. It is performed as in the Lutheran church. If unsure if the client has already been baptized, then prefix the baptismal words with, "if you are capable of being baptized, I baptize you in the name of the Father. . . ." Inform the hospital chaplain, the client's family, and the client's priest that you administered an emergency baptism and record the fact in the client record.

Eucharist   Eucharist is also called communion. The Catholic believes that he receives by way of bread and wine, the body and blood, soul, and divinity of Jesus Christ. A client preparing to take communion is normally asked to abstain from food or drink for an hour before the rite, although water and medications are allowed at any time.

Confession   Confession is a rite for the forgiveness of sins. The Catholic client's confession must be heard

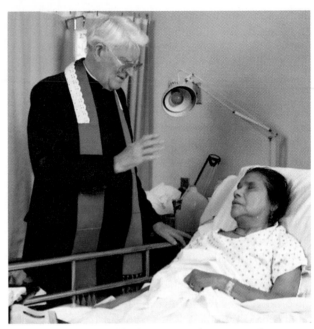

FIGURE 7-1   A Catholic priest administers the Sacrament of the Sick to a gravely ill client.

by a priest, who then pronounces absolution (forgiveness). It is a very private matter and should be respected. To a Catholic client this sacrament may be a form of therapy as valuable as medication and treatment.

Sacrament of the Sick   The Sacrament of the Sick, in which the client is anointed with holy oil, was formerly known as the "last rites" given to someone near death (see Figure 7-1). It is intended to confer a special grace on those who are gravely ill or who are experiencing physical limitations sometimes inherent in old age.

Sabbath Day Rituals   Mass is the central prayer of the Catholic religion and is a responsibility for practicing Catholics. Catholics are excused from Mass if ill; these clients may wish to read prayer books, recite prayers in the hospital room, or watch televised Mass on Sunday mornings to fulfill this obligation. It is important for the nurse to give adequate privacy during these times.

Dietary Practices   Ash Wednesday and Good Friday are the only days that require complete fasting and abstinence from meat. When sick, a Catholic is excused from fasting (giving up food for a specified period of time) and abstaining (giving up meat for a specified time).

Religious Books or Symbols   Catholic clients may request that religious pictures and objects (crucifix, rosary beads, prayer book, religious medals) be kept at the bedside or on their person. These are reminders of God's presence in their lives and are sources of consolation. Respect these objects and take care not to misplace them.

Orthodox

The Orthodox churches express their love of God through worship liturgies. It is important to the church that they remain faithful to the teachings of the ancient church. Holy Unction is practiced using oil to anoint the body for healing of bodily and spiritual infirmities. Baptism is also important; in life-threatening situations involving an unbaptized child an emergency baptism is performed.

Jehovah's Witness

Jehovah's Witnesses are prohibited from receiving any blood or blood products, including plasma. They also will not eat anything containing blood. To receive such products is viewed as a violation of the law of God and condemnation will result. Blood volume expanders are permissible if they are not derivatives of blood. In some cases, children have been made wards of the court so that they could receive blood when a medical condition requiring blood transfusion was life-threatening. Jehovah's Witnesses do not celebrate Christmas, Easter, or other traditional Christian holidays, but they do have a special observance of the Lord's Supper. Faith healing is not sought, but an elder of the church will pray with the sick client and read scriptures to comfort the individual, which can lead to healing of the mind and body. Autopsies are acceptable only if it is required by law. However, no parts are removed from the body. Man's spirit and body are never to be separated.

Mormon (Church of Jesus Christ of the Latter Day Saints)

Mormons do not believe in baptizing infants, but will baptize at the age of eight years. If necessary, baptism of the dead will be performed for adults. Mormons refrain from using caffeine-containing beverages (tea, coffee, cola drinks), alcohol and tobacco. Mormons fast (no food or water is permitted for twenty-four hours) on the first Sunday of each month. Mormons wear a special undergarment that has special significance symbolizing dedication to God. This garment may be worn under the hospital gown.

Christian Science

Christian Scientists generally believe that illness can be eliminated through prayer and spiritual understanding. Healing is considered an awakening to this belief. When a critically ill Christian Scientist client is admitted to a health care facility they may wish to have a Chris-

tian Science practitioner contacted to give treatment through prayer. Christian Scientists ordinarily do not use medicine, agree to surgical procedures, or accept blood transfusions. Immunizations/vaccines and autopsies are acceptable only when required by law.

Amish

Amish do not believe in health insurance or social security and rely on mutual aid from other Amish in the community during a time of need. Amish prefer that children not have childhood immunizations. They believe that sudden fright or blood loss may cause loss of the soul. Females do not approve of cutting their hair and married men do not shave their faces. Amish can be recognized by their characteristic plain clothing similar to that worn in the pioneer days. Modesty in covering the body by wearing undergarments under the hospital gown should be permitted. Amish do not have recognized pastoral leaders, but take turns leading worship in their own homes.

Judaism

Judaism is both a religious faith and an ethnic identity. It is based on the five books of Moses called the Torah. Culture and religion are deeply interwoven in the Jewish faith. As a result, ritual, tradition, ceremony, religious and social laws, and the observance of holy days are major influences in the Jewish daily life.

There are three groups in Judaism: Orthodox, Conservative, and Reformed. All share the fundamental teachings of Judaism but vary in how strictly they follow the traditions. Orthodox Jews strictly observe all traditional practices. The Conservative group observes many of the traditional practices, and the Reformed group interprets traditions loosely.

The rabbi is the spiritual leader of the Jewish congregation and is the representative to be informed when a client of the Jewish faith requests it.

The Jewish Sabbath, a day devoted to prayer, study, and rest begins at sunset on Friday and ends at sunset on Saturday. The Sabbath meal is an important ritual that includes family members and special foods. Traditional observance of the Sabbath requires a self-imposed restriction to do no work on the Sabbath. This, for the most observant, would keep the client from turning on or off electrical appliances. It is, however, acceptable for the nurse to perform these actions for the client. In addition, many Jewish clients may not desire surgical procedures or diagnostic exams to be performed on them during the Sabbath. Just as the cross is recognized as the symbol of Christianity, the Star of David is identified with Judaism and may be found on many of their religious books or symbols.

Circumcision is a religious custom in Judaism that is performed on the male infant eight days after birth. It may be done by the pediatrician or by the Mohel who may be a rabbi. Jewish boys receive their names at this ceremony. Jewish girls receive their names at their parents' synagogue (house of worship).

Dietary practices vary among the three Jewish groups. These practices date from early Jewish history. **Kosher,** meaning clean or fit to be eaten, are restrictions that apply to meats, fish, and dairy products and to the utensils in which they are prepared and served. Make arrangements with the dietary department for separate utensils for preparing and serving meat. These foods can be served in the original containers or on paper plates. Meat may be consumed a few minutes after drinking milk, but six hours must pass after eating meat before drinking milk again. Meats that are not permitted on a kosher diet include: pork products, eel, oysters, crab, lobster, shrimp, or eggs with blood spots. Today, many food products are manufactured in accordance with kosher dietary standards. These foods are marked with the symbol ⓤ; packaged products that are marked with the term *pareve* may be served with meat or dairy products.

The Jewish culture dictates that an individual should never die alone. A family member, rabbi, or other members of the community should be permitted to remain in the room if requested to do so. When a life-threatening situation occurs, life may be preserved by the use of standard medical protocol. CPR, surgery, and blood transfusions, along with medication, are permitted. Life support measures should be discussed with the client, the family, the rabbi, and the physician. Autopsy is permitted only when required by state law. Many branches of Judaism will bury the dead before sundown of the day of death.

Islam

The religion of Muslims is Islam. Islam believes that Allah is the supreme deity and that Mohammed, the founder of Islam, is the chief prophet. The Muslim's holy day of worship extends from sunset on Thursday to sunset on Friday. Some Muslims may desire to pray to their god Allah five times a day (after dawn, at noon, at mid-afternoon, after sunset, and at night). If the client requests that he face Mecca, the holy city of Islam, a bed or chair may be positioned facing the southeast direction (if you are in the continental United States). If a Muslim brings the Koran, the holy book of Islam, to the health care institution, do not touch it or place anything on top of it. The Muslim client may be wearing an article of writing from the Koran on a piece of string around his neck, arm, or waist. This should not be allowed to get wet or to be

removed. Rules of cleanliness include eating with the right hand and cleansing self with the left hand after urinating or defecating. Hand medication or other materials to the Muslim client with your right hand so as not to offend them as they consider the left hand dirty. Some Islamic females prefer to be clothed from head to ankle. During the physical examination, they may prefer to undress one body part at a time. Islamics are forbidden to eat pork in any form or to drink alcoholic beverages. In addition, Muslims refrain from eating or drinking during the daytime hours for the month of Ramadan (the ninth month of the Muslim lunar year), but are permitted to eat after sunset.

Buddhism

Buddhism is a general term that indicates a belief in Buddha, "the enlightened one." Buddha's teachings include the Four Noble Truths and the Noble eightfold way. Nirvana, a state of greater inner freedom and spontaneity, is the goal of existence. When one achieves Nirvana, the mind has supreme peace, purity, and strength. Buddhism does not dictate any specific practices or sacraments. There are no religious restrictions for therapy or special holy days. Buddhists do not believe in healing through faith. The religious support system for the sick is the priest. The Buddhist believes in reincarnation. The body is considered a shell; therefore, autopsy and cremation are permitted.

Hindu

Hinduism has no common creeds or doctrines that bind Hindus together. The major distinguishing characteristic is the social caste system. The religion of Hinduism is founded on the Scripture called the Vedas. Brahma is the principal source of the universe and the center from which all things proceed and to which all things return. Reincarnation is a central belief in Hindu thought. The goal of existence is freedom from the cycle of rebirth and death and entrance into what the Hindus, like the Buddhists, call Nirvana. Hindu temples are dwelling places for deities to which people bring offerings. Some Hindus believe in faith healing; others believe that illness is God's way of punishing a person for sins. The eating of meat is forbidden because it involves harming a living creature.

Implications of Religious Aspects

After examining the basic beliefs of these religious groups it is important not to make generalizations or assumptions about a client's lifestyle, attitudes, or feelings about life, pain, or death based on religious affiliation. It is important to determine what an individual of a specific religious belief personally believes to be important. The only way to do this is to ask the client, or, if the client is unable to communicate this information personally, ask a close family member. Making assumptions about a client's religious belief system on the basis of their cultural or religious affiliation may lead to wrong conclusions. Acknowledgment of individual variation is as important as appreciation of religious diversity. Individuals share some part of the religious heritage of their group, but not necessarily all of it. It is critical that the nurse take the time to validate an assumption with each client before planning a nursing intervention. Clarify with the Jewish client if a kosher diet is desired. Do not assume that all clients from a Jehovah Witness background will refuse blood products. Furthermore, it should be noted that not all clients will desire to have their religious support system notified of their hospital admission. Refer back to Chapter 6 to review cultural assessment.

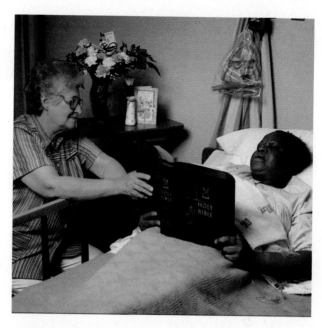

FIGURE 7-2 Spiritual needs often increase when individuals are sick.

Nursing Process and Spiritual Needs

Although spiritual needs are recognized by many nurses, **spiritual care** (to recognize and meet spiritual needs) is often neglected. Spirituality is characterized by an individual's search to find meaning and purpose in life. The goal of spiritual nursing care is to enable clients to identify and utilize their spiritual beliefs when faced with a health crisis as coping mechanisms. Among the reasons that nurses fail to provide spiritual care are the following:

• They feel that spirituality is a private matter.
• They are uninformed about the religious beliefs of others.
• They have not identified their own spiritual beliefs.
• They view meeting the spiritual needs of the client as a family or pastoral responsibility, not a nursing responsibility.

Spiritual nursing care is appropriate if the nurse cares about the client's well-being as it affects the client's emotional, physical, and psychosocial health. The spiritual dimension must be balanced with these other needs for overall good health (see Figure 7-2).

The focus of the nursing diagnosis, spiritual distress, is to help the client maintain his spiritual health (see Table 7-1). When religious beliefs are contributing to the client's overall health problems (i.e., malnutrition due to inappropriate use of a vegetarian diet) the nurse should ask questions to identify the problem and nonjudgmentally encourage the client's problem solving.

OTHER CULTURAL ASPECTS AFFECTING CLIENT CARE

Unlike changeable opinions, preferences, or attitudes, cultural and ethnic behaviors are strongly integrated and are difficult to alter. Clients reveal their cultural differences each time they interact with the world around them. In an unfamiliar situation, such as admission to a health care setting, these differences may seem even greater because in times of stress, most people will hold tightly to what is familiar in order to protect themselves from the unknown. A way that a nurse can show caring is to acknowledge the expression of these differences and to let the client retain what is familiar.

Language

Language is common to all human beings, but not everyone shares the same language. This cultural difference can lead to misunderstanding and frustration. When the client speaks with a different language or accent, it does not make his needs any different, only his means of expressing them. When communication is restricted because of language differences, find alternative methods of communication. Often when people think someone does not understand English, they tend to speak louder; instead, remember to speak slowly, distinctly, and at a normal volume. Also remember that the client's family may be able to assist you when there

Table 7-1

SPIRITUAL DISTRESS

DEFINITION

Spiritual Distress   The state in which an individual or group experiences or is at risk of experiencing a disturbance in the belief or value system that provides strength, hope, and meaning to one's life.

DEFINING CHARACTERISTICS

Major (Must Be Present)

Experiences a disturbance in belief system

Minor (May Be Present)

Questions meaning of life, death, and suffering
Questions credibility of belief system
Demonstrates discouragement or despair
Chooses not to practice usual religious rituals
Has ambivalent feelings (doubts) about beliefs
Expresses that he or she has no reason for living
Feels a sense of spiritual emptiness
Expresses concern—anger, resentment, fear—over the meaning of life, suffering, death
Requests spiritual assistance for a disturbance in belief system

RELATED FACTORS

Pathophysiological

Related to challenges to belief system or separation from spiritual ties secondary to

Loss of body part or function
Terminal illness
Debilitating disease
Pain
Trauma
Miscarriage, stillbirth

Treatment-Related

Related to conflict between (specify prescribed regimen) and beliefs

Abortion
Surgery
Blood transfusion
Dietary restrictions
Isolation
Amputation
Medications
Medical procedures

Situational (Personal Environmental)

Related to death or illness of signifcant other

Related to embarrassment at practicing spiritual rituals

Related to barriers to practicing spiritual rituals

Intensive care restrictions
Confinement to bed or room
Lack of privacy
Lack of availability of special foods/diet

Related to beliefs opposed by family, peers, health care professional

OUTCOME CRITERIA

The person will

1. Continue spiritual practices not detrimental to health
2. Express decreasing feelings of guilt and anxiety
3. Express satisfaction with spiritual condition

INTERVENTIONS

1. Communicate acceptance of various spiritual beliefs and practices
2. Convey nonjudgmental attitude
3. Acknowledge importance of spiritual needs
4. Express willingness of health care team to help in meeting spiritual needs
5. Provide privacy and quiet as needed for daily prayer, for visit of spiritual leader, and for spiritual reading and contemplation
6. Contact spiritual leader to clarify practices and perform religious rites or services if desired.
7. Maintain diet with spiritual restrictions when not detrimental to health.
8. Encourage spiritual rituals not detrimental to health
9. Provide opportunity for individual to pray with others or be read to by members of own religious group or a member of the health care team who feels comfortable with these activities
10. For parent conflict over treatment of child.
    a. If parents refuse treatment of child, encourage consideration of alternative methods of therapy (e.g., utilization of Christian Science nurses and practitioners; special surgeons and techniques for surgery without blood transfusions); support individual making information decision—even if decision conflicts with own values.
    b. If treatment is still refused, physician or hospital administrator may obtain court order appointing temporary guardian to consent to treatment
    c. Call spiritual leader to support parents (and possibly child)
    d. Encourage expression of negative feelings
11. Give "permission" to discuss spiritual matters with nurse by bringing up subject of spiritual welfare if necessary
12. Use questions about past beliefs and spiritual experiences to assist person in putting this life event into wider perspective
13. Offer to pray/meditate/read with client, if you are comfortable with this, or arrange for another member of health care team if more appropriate
14. Be available and willing to listen when client expresses self-doubt, guilt or other negative feelings.
15. Offer to contact other spiritual support person (such as pastoral care, hospital chaplain, etc.) if person cannot share feelings with usual spiritual leader.

(*From Carpenito, L.J. (1996). Handbook of nursing diagnoses (6th ed.). Philadelphia: J. B. Lippincott Company. Reprinted with permission*) is a block in communication. Family members can interpret procedures and instructions to the client and communicate the client's thoughts and questions to the nurse (see Figure 7-3). If no family members are available, ask the hospital social worker to find an interpreter. When family members or interpreters are not present at the bedside, flash cards can be used to facilitate communication. One side can contain the word or phrase in the client's language, and the other side can include the English equivalent. Involve family members to help create individualized flashcards and include their use on the client's care plan. Loneliness and fear are difficult to handle, and health care workers only increase the client's isolation when they do not seek alternative methods to assist the client to understand and to be understood.

Cultural Orientation

People's reactions to situations will vary according to their cultural orientation. Customs and habits are learned behaviors that are considered appropriate within a cultural group. Behaviors that are appropriate or correct in one culture may cause controversy within another. When conflict occurs, it is important that an interpreter explains the cultural differences so that the client can adjust to the requirements of the health care setting. It will also help the nurse adapt the nursing care routine to the client's cultural beliefs. For example, do not expect that a client will willingly carry out your instructions to bathe every morning after breakfast if his belief or custom is to bathe several times a week before going to bed at night.

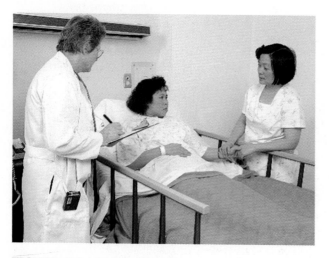

FIGURE 7-3 Family members can often serve as interpreters to help clients who do not speak English understand procedures and instructions and to communicate the client's thoughts and questions to the nurse.

Ethnocentrism is the belief that one's own cultural beliefs are the most desirable or best. This is demonstrated by a superior attitude to another's cultural lifestyle and a refusal to understand the beliefs of another culture. Ethnocentrism cannot be tolerated in the health care setting. Ethnocentrism may result from a lack of exposure or knowledge about another culture. A first step in becoming culturally sensitive is to assess the beliefs and attitudes of one's own culture and to acknowledge that different viewpoints are possible. **Prejudice**, the strongly held opinion formed about some topic or group of people, can be corrected by education when it occurs due to ignorance or misinformation. All people have some prejudice. Problems occur when people in authority allow prejudice to affect their relationships with culturally different clients. It is important for the nurse to examine personal ideology and prejudice.

Cultural heritage plays an important role in a client's perception of health and illness. Some people believe that illness is caused by an evil spell, by improper food, or by actions of family members. Some view illness as an imbalance between the yin and yang (this will be explained later). These different beliefs directly affect a person's behavior and health practices. Cultural practices will influence the way an individual and his family react to pain, grieving, time and space concepts, and nutritional preferences. Having knowledge of these cultural behaviors will assist the nurse to provide culturally sensitive care. Table 7-2 presents some nursing diagnoses with cultural implications.

CULTURAL RESPONSES TO PAIN

A client's response to pain is culturally determined. In many cultures, pain may be considered a punishment for sin or bad deeds. Therefore, the individual is to tolerate the pain silently in order to atone for sins. Some cultural groups believe that there is a lesson to be learned from pain—that it can make them become a stronger individual because of it. Many Asians believe that life is suffering, or enduring the pain, so if they are experiencing pain it is part of life and they must accept it. Yet they long for others to notice their pain. In Japan, displaying pain in a public place brings disgrace. For clients from the Middle East or African cultures, self-inflicted pain is often used as a sign of mourning or grief. For still other groups, such as Native Americans, pain is to be anticipated as part of ritualistic rights of passage and, therefore, tolerance of pain signifies strength and power. During painful

Table 7-2

NURSING DIAGNOSES WITH CULTURAL IMPLICATIONS

- Anxiety
- Body image disturbance
- Breast feeding
- Communication, impaired, verbal
- Coping, individual, ineffective
- Decisional conflict
- Family coping, ineffective
- Fear
- Grieving
- Health maintenance, altered
- Health seeking behaviors
- Nutrition, altered
- Pain
- Role performance, altered
- Sleep pattern disturbance
- Social interaction, impaired
- Spiritual distress

experiences, periods of silence are observed among many tribes; one who interrupts the silence is seen as immature and unknowing.

There are many ways to express pain: stoic denial, objective reporting, social withdrawal, crying, screaming, writhing, or complaining. Individuals of some cultural groups desire to tolerate their pain privately, whereas others want the sympathy and support of family members, loved ones, and caretakers.

It is important that the nurse consider the methods of pain relief used by different cultural groups. Chinese use acupuncture, and the Hindus often use yoga and meditation. Today, various groups control pain by combining herbal remedies used in ancient Egyptian and Chinese cultures with Western medicine. **Therapeutic touch**, or healing touch, is practiced today in modern cultures. This "laying on of hands" produces a transfer of energy from the "healer" to the client that improves the client's own healing potential. Cultural healers that may be useful for certain clients in the relief of pain include shamans, curanderos, espiritos, spiritualists, and herbalists.

Nurses need to identify their own attitude toward pain and not transfer their beliefs about pain and pain expression to their clients. Studies have been done that show that the majority of nurses in America are white, middle-class women of European descent who value self-control in response to pain. Client expression of pain such as crying or screaming should be viewed within each culture's context. Nursing awareness and acceptance of various cultural behaviors related to pain can ease discomfort as the client gains feelings of acceptance from the nurse.

Sample Nursing Care Plan: The Family With Ineffective Coping

Mrs. Chang, a seventy-four-year-old housewife, was admitted to the hospital with complaints of nausea and difficulty keeping food down related to recurrent breast cancer with bone metastasis. For the past few weeks her appetite has been decreasing. She is able to drink some fluids.

Mrs. Chang's husband of fifty-three years remains at her bedside along with their two grown daughters. She insists that they remain at her bedside so that she does not have to bother the nurses for her basic care. Mr. Chang remains at her bedside leaving only to go home and shower; when he does so, both daughters remain with Mrs. Chang.

The nurses notice that Mr. Chang is looking exhausted and appears to have lost weight. The daughters have tried to relieve their father at night so he can go home and rest, but he insists on remaining at the hospital. Mrs. Chang insists that the oldest daughter bathe her and walk her to the bathroom.

Even though Mrs. Chang never voices discomfort, she has her husband and daughters constantly massaging her back and legs. She changes position slowly and grimaces with each movement. She does not verbalize to the nursing staff, but lets her family do the talking for her. She denies pain when questioned by the nurse, but she complains of pain to her family. She does not sleep well.

Mrs. Chang's treatment plan is supportive. The hospital staff has mentioned the idea of hospice care to the family. Mrs. Chang has stated that she wants to go home.

Nursing Diagnosis Ineffective family coping, high risk for, related to deteriorating course of disease of a family member.

Goals	Nursing Interventions	Rationale	Evaluation
Family will plan a specific rotation schedule to meet each other's need for rest and support while caring for their mother.	Provide empathy and support for the husband and daughters who need to be at the bedside. Permit them to have unlimited visitation, adequate space for members who stay overnight, and privacy.

Assess family members for signs of fatigue or overexertion.

Explore with husband and daughters other possible extended family members who would be willing and be accepted by Mrs. Chang to keep her company and give her support. | The family is one of the most important factors in the life of the Japanese American. A sense of obligation to intervene and assist is highly valued. Casual help from strangers is avoided.

Japanese Americans value self-control and self-sufficiency. To ask for help would mean loss of face and dignity.

This family will not be able to keep up this vigil for an unknown period of time. Family obligations take precedence over individual desires. | Family sharing bedside care responsibilities. Husband remains at bedside during daytime hours with eldest daughter. Youngest daughter rests at home during the day and exchanges places with father and sister at night. Mrs. Chang is agreeable and does not put guilt on family members as they leave for rest at home. |

(continued)

Goals	Nursing Interventions	Rationale	Evaluation
Open communication will be maintained between family members.	Develop trusting and respectful relationships with Mrs. Chang and family members.	Japanese Americans tend to be reserved with those viewed to be in authority. The nurse should remember that this family needs to establish a caring, trusting relationship before they participate in self-disclosure.	Mr. Chang meets with both daughters to discuss their mother's plan of care. He includes the primary care nurse in the discussion and asks for her input on how to get Mrs. Chang to take more nourishment.
	Encourage Mr. Chang to have family meetings as necessary to discuss realistic plans and expectations of other family members, using health care providers as needed.	Japanese traditionally value authoritarian styles of leadership where the father makes unilateral family decisions. Authority and communication come from the top down. Discouragement of verbal communication, avoidance of discussion of personal problems, and limited expression of emotion have been noted as common patterns in the traditional Japanese family. However, cultural change in family norms occurs with tendency to adopt more Western family norms and behaviors.	
	Encourage and assist family to explore outside resources to assist them in dealing with the crisis.	This family structure cannot maintain bedside attendance without help. The outside resource might be extended family, sisters, brothers, nieces, or nephews of Mrs. Chang who live in the neighborhood.	

Goals	Nursing Interventions	Rationales	Evaluation
Family members will perform client care without compromising their own physical and emotional health.	Assess if basic physical and emotional needs of Mrs. Chang and family members are being met.	The ideal pattern of communication in Japanese society is silent communication. Stoic reactions to pain and other uncertain situations is common. Direct expression of negative feelings is unusual. The nurse will need to assess for nonverbal clues indicating the status of needs.	Mr. Chang and his daughters continue to provide the physical care for their wife/mother. Mr. Chang appears more rested and has put on some weight. The daughters express gratefulness that their father is stronger and has taken on the leadership role.
	Monitor ability of family members to carry out treatment plan and provide safe care.	When care is provided by family members who are exhausted safety will always be an issue. The nurse is ultimately responsible for the well-being of the client.	
	Discuss management of personality changes and mood swings with those who are providing Mrs. Chang's care.	The family may not expect changes in personality to occur if they have never been in a chronic life-threatening situation before. Communication styles may be threatened when emotional outbursts occur from normally stoic personalities and shame may be felt from losing "face."	
	Teach coping strategies to manage tension and strain if previous techniques are no longer effective.	Coping strategies to maintain healthy emotional and psychological health may be necessary. This is especially true for a society who has been taught not to put individual needs or emotions ahead of the family.	

CULTURAL RESPONSES TO GRIEVING

Grieving has been identified as the normal subjective response to loss. It is essential for good mental and physical health and helps in coping with the loss, gradually accepting it as part of life. How grief is expressed is often determined by the customs of the culture. There are many rituals that people use from their cultural group to help them cope with death. Grief, like pain, is universal. What differs between the races and cultural groups is not so much the feelings of grief, but their forms of expression of that grief. By understanding some of the cultural differences related to death, dying, and bereavement, the nurse can individualize the care given to clients and their families.

In the United States, the Protestant ethic of individualism, self-sufficiency, autonomy, and hard work lead to the sharing of grief with only significant others, and not the community. Unless extended family are present, grief is handled by the nuclear family (husband, wife, and children).

Although nurses frequently encourage clients and their families to express their grief openly, many are reluctant to do so in the health care setting. The nurse often sees the family at a time when they are still in shock over the death, and trying to comprehend what has just happened, rather than expressing their grief.

Many Americans have the belief that grief is a private matter that is kept internal and not shared. Emotions are to be repressed and not discussed. Men have especially been socialized to be strong and not show tears.

In the non-Western world, the family is often more important than the individual. The family members are expected to spend time with the ill client. They show their love and respect to the ill family member by the amount of time they spend at the bedside. A nurse may find it difficult to perform nursing duties when the client's room is full of visitors who stay for hours. Recognizing this as the family's cultural way of caring may ease a difficult situation. Family should be looked upon as the best resource for meeting the needs of the client.

Some cultural groups value social support and expression of loss from individuals outside of their family group. In African American congregations, grief is expressed with much emotion. For them, religion has functioned as an escape from the harsh reality of daily life. The African American church has produced respect in spite of poverty and has promoted a high degree of self-respect among the African American community. The church family plays an important role in the grieving process for the family who has experienced a loss.

In Mexican American groups where strong family ties are maintained, support is provided by family members and open, unrestrained expression of grief is encouraged. Many view wellness and illness, including death, as the will of God. Because Roman Catholicism is the dominant religion, religious rituals such as masses, rosaries, and **novenas** (nine consecutive days during which family and friends gather to pray for the deceased) are practiced to benefit both the deceased and the surviving family members. During dying and death, Mexican Americans utilize their church, families, and friends as their support system. Some Spanish-speaking groups believe the human spirit will not be able to enter into the next life if that person has not been able to finalize relationships with significant others before death. To complete relationships with the dying person, it is important that friends and family can say their good-byes.

Grief is communicated by some people as a seizure-like behavior, a display of hostility, or sometimes lethargy. These behaviors are socially accepted as a way of venting grief and anger over a death. Males in the United States generally are raised to retain feelings of suffering inside; bereaved Mexican American men often refuse grief counseling and may resent being told that it is acceptable to cry.

Jewish people believe in sitting **shiva**. This is a formal mourning period of seven days during which friends visit and comfort the bereaved in the home of the deceased.

The attitudes toward death and dying in ancient Chinese society have continued in the immigrants who have made their home in the United States. In general, Chinese Americans tend to be unemotional and fatalistic when experiencing terminal illness and death. In the Asian world, the Chinese traditionally follow the practice of double burial. In the first burial, the body is buried in a coffin for seven years, then the remains are exhumed and placed in an ornate urn. Reburial in an elaborate family tomb represents the second burial. It is believed that after this second burial, the deceased has a beneficial effect (good luck) on descendants.

Some Southeast Asian refugees have been greatly exposed to the stress of bereavement. They have already suffered the loss of many family members as a result of the Vietnam War. In the United States, their traditional mourning practices must be altered. Traditional Vietnamese practices include preparation of the body by family members, placement of a coin in the mouth of the deceased to assist the spirit in the next life, and the use of divination when selecting the burial site.

When questioned who would be utilized for comfort and support in times of grief, many people frequently name a family member or a member of the clergy. A nurse who has worked with a client and the family throughout the dying process may feel rejected at the time of death when the grieving family turns to other family members, and the nurse is left out.

Another important point regarding cultural expression of grief is that the expression of grief may differ depending on the lines of emotional attachment and control. In **matrilineal societies**, where the female is considered the head of the family, it is socially acceptable for a woman to mourn over the death of male members of her maternal family, such as her father and brothers. It is not acceptable behavior for her to mourn over the loss of her own husband.

Finally, a perceptive nurse is aware of cultural desires regarding body preparation. As was mentioned earlier, many non-Anglo cultural groups believe body preparation is very important. While many cultural groups have assumed the practice of letting the mortician prepare the body, there are still some who want to retain their native customs. For example, certain groups such as the Vietnamese and Jews believe that family and friends of the same sex as the deceased should wash and prepare the body for burial. Depending upon the cultural practices of the family, they may view nursing staff "preparing" the body as an invasion of their cultural ways and an intrusion on a duty that belongs to them alone. The nurse should question the family members concerning their preference of body preparation.

CULTURAL RESPONSE TO TIME AND SPACE ORIENTATION

Time and space orientation is another variable among cultural groups that needs to be understood by nurses. Generally, society in the United States tends to be future oriented. People plan for the future, establish long-term goals, and are increasingly concerned with prevention of future illnesses. In daily life, people are oriented to time of day constantly referring to clock time; meals are taken at a specified time, and clients have appointments with health care professionals as well as other time obligations. The nurse must also be very attentive to time. Medications are given at assigned times and work begins and ends at specified times. Other groups that are often future oriented are Japanese, Jews, and Arabs. They view time as a commodity to achieve future goals.

However, not all cultural groups are future oriented. People of other cultures (e.g., Asians), may be oriented to the past. For Asians, this orientation is demonstrated by how ancestor worship and the influence of Confucianism affect the present. Other cultures, such as Native Americans are said to be present oriented. Many Native Americans do not own clocks,

and they live one day at a time showing little concern for the future. Mexican Americans and African Americans often value relationships with people in the present more than the future. African Americans are present oriented in health care behaviors. They often express the fatalistic belief "it's going to happen anyway, so why bother" and fail to seek medical attention until a disabling condition occurs. The African American culture often teaches flexible attention to schedules; what is happening now is what is most important. The nurse needs to consult with the black client about when he may want to have his physical therapy treatment or about rescheduling his bath time if the hospital's schedule conflicts with his normal bathing time preference. At the same time, strict schedules for medication requiring therapeutic blood level maintenance may have to be maintained. In these instances explanations about the necessity of time scheduling must be given to the client. In essence, a compromise approach between the nurse and the client must occur.

How does time orientation affect health care? An individual's orientation to time may affect promptness or attendance for health care appointments, compliance with self-medication schedules, and reporting the onset of illness or other health concerns. Clients might not see the necessity for preventive health care measures if they experience no difference in their health today when they follow a special diet or exercise programs. The nurse teaches clients when timing is critical in health care situations and practices patience when working with people who are not future- or clock-time oriented.

Territoriality or personal space is also influenced by the individual's culture. Territoriality is a pattern of behavior resulting from an individual's belief that certain spaces and objects belong to that person. Personal space is the distance a person prefers to maintain from another during communication. In general, people of Arabic, South European, and African origin frequently sit or stand relatively close to each other when talking, whereas people from Asian, North European, and North American countries are more comfortable when talking further apart. Refer to Chapter 5 for additional information on communicating with clients from other cultures.

Asian cultures believe in harmony in social relationships and the need to maintain dignity and "save face." Asian adults do not touch one another very often. Communication using body language is very important. The head is believed to be sacred; nurses should not touch it without the client's permission to do so. Affection and caring behavior are not communicated by touch in their culture. Do not to take it personally if an Asian client moves away from your touch. When you are working with clients from cultures that react negatively to touch use the universal sign of caring, the smile. Take time to fluff the pillow, fill the water pitcher, and do other thoughtful things that demonstrate caring behaviors to the client and his family. Inquire about any needs that are not being met.

Politeness and respect toward adults and the elderly are emphasized and practiced in some cultural groups more than others. The elderly are highly respected in the Mexican American, Native American, and Far Eastern cultures. Some Mexican Americans may kiss the hand of the elders while greeting them as a form of respect. Although calling people by their first name in the Anglo society is acceptable, nurses should remember to call their adult Mexican American, Native American, African American, and Asian clients by their last names. The people of these cultures also emphasize modesty and privacy. Many clients feel embarrassed when wearing a hospital gown or when they must undress for an examination. The nurse must respect the client's attitudes about modesty and prevent exposure of them at all times. Many female clients from these cultures may refuse to be treated by male physicians or male nurses.

CULTURAL RESPONSE TO NUTRITION

The foods people eat and the customs associated with food vary widely among cultures, subcultures, and ethnic groups. For example, the **staple food** (chief food consumed in the diet) of Asians is rice; of Italians, pasta; and of Eastern Europeans, wheat bread. Even families who have been in the United States for several generations often continue to prepare and eat the staple food from their country of origin.

Hospitalized clients often have very little choice about the food they are served. Menus are often restrictive in choice and may not contain the ethnic food or staple food desired by a client. Many cultural groups view their foods as comforting. Unfamiliar foods can be alienating, reminding them that they are away from home with little control over their food practices. The nurse can encourage family members to bring in special meals from home if the client's health status permits. These foods from home can be comforting and contribute to their recovery. In case the client does not understand English, instructions regarding meal planning for special diets at home may have to be explained to younger members of the family who are fluent in English or they may be given to a health worker of the same culture who can act as an interpreter. When clients are taught about a special diet, nurses must be sensitive to the cultural significance of food and to the staple foods that the client traditionally eats. For example, it may be inappropriate to arrange for "Meals On Wheels" if the service is unable to provide the foods the client prefers, i.e.,

bean sprouts and vegetables for the Japanese client or fish and rice for the Chinese client.

Each culture may assign specific meaning to foods. For example, Native American tribes assign symbolic meaning to foods. Their practice of food restrictions vary from tribe to tribe and are cultural or religious in origin. After healing ceremonies are performed for the Navajo people, they are not to eat certain foods such as organ meats, chicken, or eggs for the rest of their lives. This food restriction enables them to regain and maintain their health. Delaware Indians do not permit a person with a fever to eat meat. It is believed that meat will elevate the temperature of an already ill individual. Many food restrictions are frequently used during pregnancy and for one year following childbirth while the mother is still breast-feeding. In certain Native American tribes, custom dictates that women are denied salt while others are denied fish and berries. It is believed that these foods are unhealthy for the mother and her infant. These tribal food restrictions are reinforced by the oral traditions in each tribe that are passed down from generation to generation. Most Indian tribal groups believe corn has healing properties.

African Americans often believe that health is maintained by a proper diet that includes a hot breakfast. The term *soul food* used by the African American represents a feeling of kinship among Blacks. Salt pork and bacon seasoning are the key to many soul food vegetable preparations. An African American superstition is that the black-eyed pea, a soul food, must be eaten on New Year's Day for good luck the entire year. Whenever a meal is prepared there is always enough food for friends and relatives who may drop in because sharing food is a way to extend hospitality and friendliness. Pork is the main meat source (fried, barbecued, roasted, smoked, pickled, spicy, and hot). Client assessment should include the identification of potentially harmful dietary practices or those that vary from traditional African American eating patterns (Black Muslims). For example, some African Americans with hypertension may refer to their condition as "high blood" and drink brine from pickles or olives or take epsom salts to help the blood "go down." Include ethnic foods, whenever possible, in the diet plan to promote individualism of the diet and to increase the African American's compliance to the dietary plan. Arrange for alternative choices to maintain a low-fat, low-cholesterol, and low-sodium diet.

Asians practice the concept of **yin and yang** to balance a meal. Yin is cold and includes fruits, vegetables, cold drinks, and hot melon soup. Yang is hot and includes soups containing ginger and scrambled eggs. The concept of hot and cold has nothing to do with the temperature of the food. A Chinese client who is believed to be ill with a "hot disease," such as an eye infection, may wish to eat cold foods rather than hot foods in order to get well. When a "cold disease" is suspected, the client will be treated by serving him foods that are considered hot. This will return balance to his being and the illness will be cured.

Traditional foods for Mexican Americans are beans and tortillas. Traditional foods can present a problem when a special diet is required. Mexican Americans generally prefer rice to potatoes and the manner of preparing the rice is important. Mexican Americans also use the concept of hot and cold to balance their meals and to treat diseases. They take great pride in their ethnic food and music and use them to celebrate important social gatherings for the family and the community.

Food also plays an important role in Arab culture. When family members gather, it is often around elaborate meals. Affection and care are communicated by using food. Christian Arabs consume pork and alcohol, whereas Muslim Arabs do not. Muslims are forbidden by doctrine to eat any pork products. Some Arab Americans find hospital food too bland, preferring a more spicy menu. The nurse can encourage food to be brought to the client from home.

NURSING IMPLICATIONS

The nurse is responsible for the client's well-being regardless of his race, nationality, or religion. Clients have the right to receive holistic care that is individualized to their cultural orientation. The nurse must understand and incorporate these cultural differences into the plan of care. Mutual respect and tolerance can be the bridge to give adequate nursing care. There is no need to change cultural traits or habits unless they are destructive to the well-being of the client. Client rights are protected and respected regardless of the nurse's feelings about the client's cultural ways.

People of various cultural and religious beliefs are part of the health care environment. These differences must be respected in the workplace, and all co-workers must be treated with respect. It is a nurse's legal responsibility and ethical duty to report to the appropriate individual any discrimination occurring in the workplace.

▶ *CASE STUDY*

Maria Garcia brings her Catholic, eighteen-year-old sister, Rosa, to the hospital emergency room with a high temperature, chills, vomiting, and complaint of right lower quadrant pain. She brings her three children, ages 3, 2, and 1 year old, with her. Maria understands and speaks broken English, but Rosa is fluent in Spanish only. The nurse directs Maria to the waiting room with her children, then takes Rosa to the examination room. Rosa is examined by a male nurse who promptly complains at the nurses' station about how uncooperative Rosa was during the physical examination. Rosa is admitted for inpatient care with a diagnosis of appendicitis requiring emergency surgery. Maria is left in the waiting room unaware of the difficulty the nursing staff has had communicating with Rosa. Rosa is taken upstairs to her room to await her surgical preparation. Maria is notified that she can go upstairs for a few minutes but must then leave because her children do not meet the age requirement for visitor privileges. Maria finds Rosa weeping nearly hysterical. The physician walks in and asks Maria why she waited so long to bring Rosa in for treatment. He informs her that Rosa's appendix was close to rupturing and that treatment should have been started three days ago when her symptoms first began. Maria informs him that she had taken Rosa to the curandero, who had given her some herbal tea to drink, but that when it did not help she had brought Rosa to the hospital.

The following questions will guide your development of a Nursing Care Plan for the case study.

1. Why was communication between Maria, Rosa, and the health care professionals a problem?
2. What Mexican American cultural diversities were not addressed by the health care professionals?
3. What needs of Maria and Rosa are being ignored by the health care professionals?
4. What questions do you feel need to be asked by the health care professionals to give them a better understanding of this situation?
5. Write three individualized culturally sensitive nursing diagnoses and goals for Rosa.
6. Recalling the diagnoses and goals identified in question 5, list pertinent nursing interventions for Rosa.
7. List resources that the nurses could use to assist Rosa in her recovery.
8. List at least three successful client outcomes for Rosa.

SUMMARY

- Spiritual and religious beliefs are important in many people's lives. They can influence lifestyle, attitudes, and feelings about illness and death.
- The nurse should not make assumptions about clients based on the client's religious and cultural affiliations. Individuality will exist among all peoples. A nurse's information must be accurate.
- The focus of nursing care is to help the client maintain his own beliefs in the midst of a health care crisis and to use those personal beliefs to strengthen coping patterns.
- Differences between races and cultural groups is not so much feelings, but the expression of those feelings.
- Unlike opinions, preferences, and attitudes which change, cultural characteristics are deeply rooted and difficult to change. Clients reflect their cultural and ethnic heritage every time they interact with the world around them.
- Understanding and encouraging client differences are important aspects of being a nurse.

Review Questions

1. Select the trait to avoid when studying about persons of different cultures.

   a. diversity
   b. acculturation
   c. stereotyping
   d. unbiased attitude

2. A mother is observed breast-feeding her four-year-old son who is a client in the pediatrics wing of the hospital. A nurse is overheard talking in the nursing station about the weird ways the mother has continuing to breast-feed a four-year-old. She comments that the American way is the best. The nurse is guilty of:

   a. ethnocentrism.
   b. stereotyping.
   c. unusual break behavior.
   d. not insisting that the mother stop breast-feeding .

3. Which religious group teaches that physical healing exclusively comes through prayers and readings?

   a. Roman Catholic
   b. Jewish
   c. Christian Science
   d. Seventh Day Adventist

News Flash

Is there a relationship between ethnicity and health care wishes? A group of researchers examined the preferences of a group of 1,193 older adults, all of whom were enrolled in the Program for All Inclusive Care of the Elderly (PACE) in ten national sites. Researchers examined whether individuals in the group, comprised of non-Hispanic whites, blacks, Hispanics, and Asians, were more or less likely to use advance directives, living wills, durable powers of attorney, and health care proxies.

Findings revealed that the different groups differed widely in their choices and there may be some correlation to ethnicity. Blacks were less likely to choose living wills and durable powers of attorney, compared to whites and Asians, but more likely to choose "full code" (aggressive life-prolonging measures, such as CPR or ventilator support) than whites, Asians, or Hispanics. The team speculated that fear of exploitation on the part of some of the black participants, many of whom grew up in the segregated "Deep South," may have created a reluctance to "sign anything." A high level of religiosity was attributed to the desire of this group to choose full code. Similar to blacks, Hispanics were also unlikely to choose advance directives, and the team speculated that language barriers and the low utilization rate of health services by this population may be the cause. Hispanics were also likely to choose full code measures, and again, the team attributed high religiosity as well as the daughter's role as the primary caregiver to this finding. Of the group, non-Hispanic whites were the most likely to have written advance directives and the least likely to select health care surrogates. Whites were more likely than Hispanics and blacks to choose "no code, " or reject aggressive, life-prolonging procedures. Finally, the Asians studied (79 percent being Chinese) were unlikely to select advance directives or choose aggressive life-saving procedures. Language barriers, the cultural value of the spoken word over written documents, and religious belief in a natural time for death were some of the factors attributed to these findings (Eleazer, et al., *JAGS,* 1996).

4. Which religious group observes the Sabbath from sunset Friday until sunset Saturday?
   a. Mormons
   b. Jews
   c. Presbyterian
   d. Islam

5. A client of this religious denomination would most likely refuse a blood transfusion even if his life was in jeopardy.
   a. Hindu
   b. Jehovah's Witness
   c. Jew
   d. Mormon

6. The nursing diagnosis that might be used for a client who is hospitalized and has religious practices that are difficult to maintain is:
   a. emotional depression.
   b. guilt and misery.
   c. spiritual distress.
   d. spiritual manipulation.

7. It is important for the nurse to know the client's religion in order to:
   a. chart it on his record.
   b. give holistic care.
   c. meet his physical needs.
   d. know how to pray for him.

8. The kosher practice refers to:
   a. the religious worship services of the Jewish faith.
   b. the Jewish calendar.
   c. Bar Mitzvah ceremonies in the Jewish faith.
   d. Jewish dietary laws.

Critical Thinking Questions

1. Describe your religious support system.

2. How do you express grief?

UNIT
3

Physical and Mental Integrity

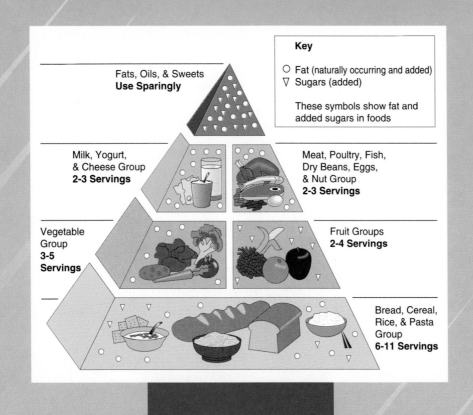

Key

○ Fat (naturally occurring and added)
▽ Sugars (added)

These symbols show fat and added sugars in foods

Fats, Oils, & Sweets
Use Sparingly

Milk, Yogurt,
& Cheese Group
2-3 Servings

Meat, Poultry, Fish,
Dry Beans, Eggs,
& Nut Group
2-3 Servings

Vegetable
Group
**3-5
Servings**

Fruit Groups
2-4 Servings

Bread, Cereal,
Rice, & Pasta
Group
6-11 Servings

CHAPTER
8

Health Maintenance

Lois White

LEARNING OBJECTIVES

Upon completion of this chapter the learner should be able to:
* Define key terms.
* Discuss guidelines for healthy living.
* Describe the scope of prevention.
* Explain the importance of *Healthy People 2000*.
* Discuss the use and benefits of a genogram.
* Make a teaching plan for ways to maintain health.

▶ MAKING THE CONNECTION

Refer to the topics in the following chapters to increase your understanding of health maintenance.

* **Chapter 6, Cultural Aspects of Health and Illness:** Influence of Culture on Beliefs and Practices About Health and Illness, p. 90 (Components of Health Subject to Cultural Influence, p. 90, Health Beliefs of Selected Cultural Groups in the United States, p. 91); Culturally Appropriate Nursing Care, p. 92; Illnesses Associated with Ethnic Groups, p. 94 (African Americans, p. 94, Hispanic American, p. 94, Asian American, p. 94, Native American, p. 94);

* **Chapter 9, Substance Abuse:** Factors Related to Substance Abuse, p. 138; Prevention, p. 139; CNS Depressants, p. 141
* **Chapter 16, Care for the Older Adult:** Health Promotion and Maintenance, p. 333, (Personal Hygiene, p. 333, Exercise, p. 335, Nutrition, p. 335, Psychosocial Considerations, p. 336, Health Care, p. 336);
* **Chapter 31, Female Reproductive System:** Breast Self-Examination, p. 866
* **Chapter 32, Male Reproductive Disorders:** Testicular Self-Examination, p. 927

INTRODUCTION

The responsibility for maintaining health rests squarely on the shoulders of each individual adult. Parents are responsible for maintaining their children's health and teaching them a healthy lifestyle. Health maintenance deals with the whole person and the person's whole life. It includes prevention of disease and the early detection and treatment of disease. Maintaining health requires constant effort by focusing on all aspects of a person's life.

Simon (1992) quotes Dr. Wood Hutchinson who wrote in the *Journal of the American Medical Association* "our system's philosophy might be condensed in the motto 'millions for health care and not a penny for prevention'." This was written in 1896. One hundred years have passed and we still spend less than three cents of each health dollar on prevention and education.

The United States is the world leader in medical science and education, yet is only 16th among nations in life expectancy. We spend more for health care than any other country, yet we are 24th in infant mortality. In 1991, there were 82,902 positions for residents in specialty areas and only 202 in preventive medicine. Many doctors have not incorporated preventive medicine into their practices (Simon, 1992).

There is no profit in prevention. Insurance premiums buy illness insurance, not health insurance, since insurance companies often will not pay for preventive testing and treatment. Compensation for clinical care makes illness the priority, not health. Diagnosis and treatment of illnesses are what insurance pays for, not maintaining health.

Corporate America is always focused on the bottom line. Their advertising glamorizes overeating, overdrinking, smoking, promiscuity, and fast cars when the key to health is prudent living. It is unrealistic to think that all diseases and illnesses can be avoided, but diseases causing the majority of disabilities and death in the United States are not inevitable. Many of these diseases are related to body abuse or disuse or exposure to environmental hazards such as smoking, lack of regular exercise, and not wearing seat belts (Simon, 1992).

KEY ABBREVIATIONS

The following abbreviations and acronyms are used in this chapter:

EPA	Environmental Protection Agency
Td	Tetanus/diphtheria
USDHHS	United States Department of Health and Human Services
WHO	World Health Organization

WHAT IS HEALTH?

A widely accepted definition of **health** comes from the World Health Organization (WHO). They define health as a state of complete physical, mental, and social well-being, not merely the absence of disease or infirmity.

Other concepts of health focus on motivation. A eudaemonistic approach to health (from the Greek, meaning fortunate or happy) views the individual as motivated by joy and self-fulfillment. Health is when full potential is realized. Illness is viewed as an impediment.

Those who hold the adaptive view of health are motivated by altering the risks in self or the environment such as dietary or exercise programs or reducing exposure to environmental hazards. Illness is when the individual is unable to cope with the risks and stresses.

When the health focus is role performance, the individual is motivated by being able to meet responsibilities at home, work, play, and in the community. Health is when the individual fulfills the obligations and responsibilities to family, job, and community.

In the clinical health focus, the individual is motivated by the absence of disease. As long as no disease is diagnosed the individual considers himself healthy. One's personal definition of health influences life choices and personal health decisions.

Wellness is often equated with optimal health; with the individual moving toward integration of human functioning, maximizing human potential, taking responsibility for one's own health, and having greater self-awareness and self-satisfaction. Floyd, et al. (1995), Hafen & Hoeger (1994), and Seiger, et al. (1995) describe the behaviors exhibited by individuals in a state of wellness. There is some overlapping in the various areas of wellness.

Emotional Wellness

Emotions bridge the gap between mind and body. The person who is emotionally well understands his own feelings and knows when to express them appropriately. This individual accepts his limitations, has the ability to adjust to change, copes with stress in healthy ways, enjoys life, is optimistic and happy, and shows respect and affection to others.

Mental Wellness

Mental wellness is exhibited by the individual who is alert, creative, logical, curious, open-minded, clear thinking, and accepting of others. This person also has common sense, a good memory, and a desire for continual learning.

Intellectual Wellness

The ability to think, process information, and solve problems is evident in the person with intellectual wellness. This person questions and evaluates information and situations, learns from life experiences, is flexible, creative, and open to new ideas.

Vocational Wellness

The individual who has school and/or job satisfaction and works in harmony with others has vocational wellness.

Social Wellness

Social wellness is evident when a person shows concern, fairness, affection, and respect for others; communicates effectively; has satisfying relationships; and interacts well with others. This person has a network of family and friends, is a member of various organizations, and works with a spirit of teamwork. Other behaviors exhibited are honesty, loyalty, confidence, and tolerance.

Spiritual Wellness

Spiritual wellness gives meaning, direction, and purpose to life by way of values, ethics, and morals. This person has faith, optimism, and high self-esteem.

Physical Wellness

Physical wellness is noted in the person who avoids risky sexual behavior; tries to limit exposure to environmental contaminants; and restricts the intake of alcohol, tobacco, caffeine, and drugs. Regular exercise, eating a well-balanced diet, and regular physical examinations also assist in physical wellness.

HEALTH PROMOTION

Health promotion means more than preventing illness. It means assisting individuals to enhance their health, well-being and functioning and to maximize their potential. Health promotion focuses on healthy behaviors rather than avoiding illness. The goal is for individuals to control and improve their health. Health promotion is appropriate for the individual and the population as a whole.

Healthy People 2000

In 1980 and again in 1990, the United States Department of Health and Human Services released a list of objectives for disease prevention and health promotion (USDHHS, 1990). In 1990, more than 10,000 individuals representing 300 national organizations were involved in developing the health objectives for the year 2000. More than 300 health objectives for the nation to achieve by the year 2000 evolved. These objectives were published in a document titled *Healthy People 2000: National Health Promotion and Disease Prevention Objectives*.

This document address three important issues:

- Personal responsibility—each individual must be health-conscious and practice responsible, informed health behaviors.
- Health benefits for all people—everyone must have health benefits for the nation to be healthy.
- Health promotion and disease prevention—health care must change from a treatment focus to a prevention focus to cut costs and to increase the quality of life.

A sample of the objectives is found in Table 8-1. The entire document may be ordered from the United States Department of Health and Human Services, Washington, DC, DHHS Publication No. (PHS) 91–50212.

Smith & Lancashire (1995) report on the progress made in meeting the more than 300 objectives of *Healthy People 2000*. Eight percent of the goals have been met and progress has been made in another 41 percent. The other 51 percent of the goals either had mixed results, no change, no data yet available, or actually moved away from the goal. Highlights of the report are:

- There has been a slight increase in the number of adults who exercise regularly. Yet almost one in four adults report having a sedentary lifestyle.
- Smoking continues to decline among adults.
- The death rate for alcohol-related motor vehicle crashes has declined markedly, and has surpassed the year 2000 goal.
- The suicide death rate among teenagers, ages fifteen to nineteen, has remained stable over the past few years, but the suicide attempts have increased.
- Mortality due to heart disease and stroke is down.
- There has been a decline in cholesterol levels, smoking, and intake of dietary fat—all risk factors of heart disease and stroke. However, the number of overweight adults and teenagers has increased.
- Colorectal cancer death rate decreased to the year 2000 goal by 1992.
- Breast cancer death rate is down. More women are receiving mammograms.
- Births to teenagers are down and births to unmarried mothers may have stabilized.

Table 8-1

SAMPLE OF HEALTH OBJECTIVES FOR THE YEAR 2000

I. Physical Activity and Fitness	• Increase the proportion of people who engage regularly, preferably daily, in light to moderate physical activity for at least 30 minutes per day. • Reduce the proportion of people who engage in no leisuretime physical activity. • Reduce overweight to a prevalence of no more than 20 percent among people aged 20 and older and no more than 15 percent among adolescents aged 12 through 19.
II. Nutrition	• Reduce dietary fat intake to an average of 30 percent of calories or less and average saturated fat intake to less than 10 percent of calories among people aged 2 and older. • Increase complex carbohydrate and fiber-containing foods in the diets of adults to five or more daily servings for vegetables and fruits, and to six or more daily servings for grain products. • Increase calcium consumption in the diet. • Decrease salt and sodium intake in the diet.
III. Chronic Diseases	• Increase the proportion of adults with high blood cholesterol who are aware of their condition and are taking action to reduce their blood cholesterol to recommended levels. • Increase the proportion of people with high blood pressure who are taking action to help control their blood pressure. • Reverse the rise in cancer deaths. • Reduce coronary heart disease deaths. • Reduce hip fractures among older adults.
IV. Mental Health and Disorders	• Reduce the prevalence of mental disorders. • Reduce the suicide rate. • Reduce the proportion of people who experience adverse health effects from stress.
V. Tobacco	• Reduce the incidence of cigarette smoking • Reduce the initiation of cigarette smoking by children and youth. • Increase the proportion of worksites with a formal smoking policy that prohibits or severely restricts smoking at the workplace.
VI. Alcohol and Other Drugs	• Reduce the proportion of young people who have used alcohol, marijuana, and cocaine. • Reduce deaths caused by alcohol-related motor vehicle crashes. • Reduce drug-related deaths.
VII. AIDS, HIV Infection, and Sexually Transmitted Diseases	• Confine annual incidence of diagnosed AIDS cases to no more than 98,000 cases. • Confine the prevalence of HIV infection to no more than 800 per 100,000 people. • Increase the proportion of sexually active, unmarried people who used a condom at last sexual intercourse.
VIII. Family Planning	• Reduce the number of pregnancies that are unintended. • Reduce the proportion of adolescents who have engaged in sexual intercourse. • Increase the proportion of sexually active, unmarried people aged 19 and younger who use contraception, especially combined-method contraception that both effectively prevents pregnancy and provides barrier protection against disease.
IX. Unintentional Injuries	• Increase use of occupant protection systems, such as safety belts, inflatable safety restraints, and child safety seats among motor vehicle occupants. • Increase use of helmets among motorcyclists and bicyclists.

(Adapted from U.S. Department of Health and Human Services, Public Health Service. Healthy People 2000: National Health Promotion and Disease Prevention Objectives)

SCOPE OF PREVENTION

Prevention, hindering, obstructing, or thwarting a disease or illness from occurring, incorporates both old and new ideas. The taboos, dietary laws, and traditions of various cultural, ethnic, and religious groups were begun for a reason. If scientific research has not proved these incorrect or harmful, there is no reason not to practice the old ways.

All stages of life should embody the tenets of preventive health. It must begin before conception with healthy parents and prenatal care, and continue through the life span. Scientific advice based on firmly established medical data and reasonable probability should be heeded. Interventions for health maintenance may be lifestyle changes, costing little or nothing, or high tech procedures that are very expensive.

Before the full impact of disease prevention can be discovered, there must be major changes in health care delivery, funding, and insurance coverage. The health care system must insist on more research relating to prevention and then use the results of the research. More prevention practices must be implemented by the health care system and the individual. The rewards will be: enhanced health, longer life expectancy, and a population who feels better, looks better, and functions better.

Types of Prevention

Prevention extends to all stages of health. There are three types of prevention: primary, secondary, and tertiary.

Primary Prevention

Primary prevention takes place before disease begins. It includes all practices to prevent health problems from developing. Not smoking to prevent lung cancer, and eating calcium-rich foods to prevent osteoporosis are both examples of primary prevention. Primary prevention should be the focus for every individual and the health care providers. It is usually the least expensive and provides the greatest benefits.

Secondary Prevention

Secondary prevention is early detection and intervention to reduce the consequences of a health problem. That is, disease or illness is identified before the individual has any symptoms or functional impairment. Performing monthly breast self-exam is an example of secondary prevention. When there are no known methods of primary prevention for a specific disease or illness, the focus should be on having a regular physical exam and testing.

Tertiary Prevention

Tertiary prevention is caring for a person who already has a health problem. The disease or illness is treated after symptoms have appeared so as to prevent further progression of the disease or illness. For example, taking antibiotics for an ear infection should eliminate the infection. Potential complications and the disability of hearing impairment are prevented. Rehabilitation is an important aspect of tertiary prevention focusing on preventing deterioration of a person's condition and minimizing the loss of function. One example is providing range of motion exercises for a client who had a stroke.

Secondary and tertiary prevention have been, and still are, the main focus of our health care system. They are also the most expensive.

PREVENTION HEALTH CARE TEAM

The prevention health care team consists of the individual assisted by nurses and the primary physician.

Individual

The individual is the center of the prevention health care team. It is the individual who must incorporate the knowledge related to preventive health care and make the behavioral changes necessary to live a more healthy life.

Individuals should tell their physician what they want and expect in health care. Honesty with self, the nurses, and physician is necessary. Be assertive and ask questions of the physicians and nurses. Ask for and keep a copy of all test results. Be an active, informed health care consumer. The ultimate responsibility for health care belongs to the individual.

Nurses

Nurses, especially nurse practitioners, often do the initial health screening in clinics and physician offices. This gives them a great opportunity to inquire about lifestyle and the preventive health habits of the client. Nurses are often excellent listeners. This gives the clients time to discuss health care habits and ask questions. Nurses are also great teachers of preventive health habits. Simon (1992) states that most physicians know that their nurses are their greatest asset.

Primary Physicians

Primary physicians generally are family practitioners, pediatricians, or internists. These are the family doctors, the physicians seen on a regular basis. They have the opportunity and obligation to inquire about, advise, and discuss preventive health habits. When necessary, they refer clients to specialists for specific problems. After the problem has been resolved, the client returns to the primary physician for further care.

WHAT AFFECTS HEALTH?

A great many things affect health. They can be categorized into four topics:

- Genetics and human biology
- Personal behavior
- Environmental influences—biological agents that cause disease, exposure to chemicals, radiation, physical and climatic trauma
- Health care—immunizations, regular exams and screening tests, preventive medications

Genetics and Human Biology

Inherited traits and the way the human body functions are included in this category. For several decades now, genetic counseling has been available to prospective parents. This counseling discusses the genetic disease or problem in question and gives an educated estimate of the probability of the prospective parents' children showing the disease or problem. Rather recently, technology has produced the ability to perform genetic engineering. While this is still experimental, it has raised many ethical and moral questions.

Ince (1995) describes how good news from a genetic test frees people from the terrible uncertainty and enables them to make plans for their future. Yet, with the rapid discovery of many gene-related diseases, geneticists and consumers are having second thoughts about how the findings are used. Insurance companies have used the results of genetic testing to justify coverage cancellation and to deny coverage.

Human biology affects health because normal body functioning prevents some illnesses and makes us more susceptible to others. The female and male hormones, estrogen and testosterone, respectively, are responsible for many of these effects (see Table 8-2, [Hoffman, 1995]).

Table 8-2

FEMALE AND MALE HORMONE EFFECTS		
	Hormone	
Tissue	**Female: Estrogen**	**Male: Testosterone**
Cardiovascular	Increases arterial dilation Causes vascular spasms. Improves cardiac function.	Increases size of heart.
Liver	Inhibits production of triglycerides, LDL (bad) cholesterol, and free glucose. Decreases drug metabolism prolonging action.	Produces triglycerides, LDL (bad) cholesterol., and free glucose. Increases drug metabolism shortening action.
Fat	Encourages fat deposits in breasts, hips, and thighs and suppresses the movement of fat from these areas.	Less body fat with deposits in the abdomen.
Gastrointestinal	Slows down motility and favors formation of gallstones.	
Respiratory	Increases respiratory rate and basal body temperature.	
Musculoskeletal	Enhances bone density (postmenopausal at risk for osteoporosis).	Ensures bond density and strength.
Immune	Enhances antibody production and suppresses T cell-mediated processes (prevents rejection of sperm and fetus).	
Blood	Suppresses RBC development, lowers Hgb levels, increases coagulation.	Increases RBC development, increases Hgb levels.
Integumentary	Increases skin vitality, collagen, and water content.	Promotes body hair.

(*Adapted from Hoffman, E. (1995). Our health, our lives. New York: Pocket Books.*)

Personal Behavior

This is the area having the most factors affecting health, and it is controlled entirely by the individual. It is the individual's decision whether these factors will promote health or lead to illness and disease.

Diet

Use the Food Guide Pyramid (Figure 8-1) and Dietary Guidelines for Americans (Table 8-3) to plan the daily diet. Eat a wide variety of foods; eat less rather than more. Use fresh foods, skim milk, and low-fat or nonfat dairy products. Prepare foods simply without butter and sauces. Cut back on junk foods. Snack on raw fruits and vegetables or unbuttered popcorn. Use nonstick cooking utensils. Eat slowly and share mealtime with family and friends. Read the nutrition label on foods. Drink plenty of water.

Exercise

Integrate physical activity into daily life by walking and climbing stairs. Exercising 30 minutes three times a week is minimal, but exercising 30 minutes five times a week is better. Try swimming, walking, bicycling, ballroom dancing, water aerobics, or low-impact aerobics. Be sure to warm up before exercising and cool down after exercising. Do not overdo it; exercise should not be painful.

Exercise improves circulation, muscle strength, and emotional well-being. It lowers blood pressure, increases endurance, and reduces the chances of heart

Table 8-3

DIETARY GUIDELINES FOR AMERICANS

- Eat a variety of foods.
- Balance the food you eat with physical activity—maintain or improve your weight.
- Choose a diet with plenty of grain products, vegetables, and fruits.
- Choose a diet low in fat, saturated fat, and cholesterol.
- Choose a diet moderate in sugars.
- Choose a diet moderate in salt and sodium.
- If you drink alcoholic beverages, do so in moderation.

(*Source: U.S. Department of Agriculture, U.S. Department of Health and Human Services. 1995. Home and Garden Bulletin No. 232, Fourth edition*)

attack, stroke, and osteoporosis. The individual who exercises regularly looks healthier and feels better.

Many people have joined health clubs in an effort to meet their need for exercise. Health clubs can be a source of disease as reported in *Industry Week* (Nov. 6, 1995). For example, perspiration on exercise machines is a prime source of impetigo. As a safety precaution, wear thigh-length shorts and always keep a towel between the body and the exercise equipment.

Personal Care

Maintain normal weight for body height by combining a nutritionally sound diet plan, emphasizing low

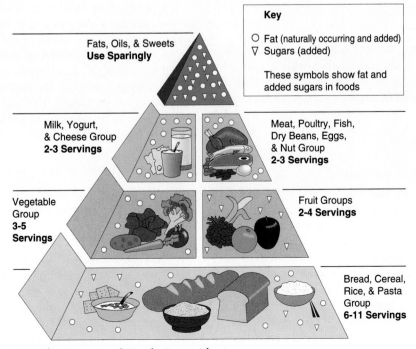

FIGURE 8-1 Food Guide Pyramid.

fat and high fiber foods and daily exercise. Keep weight within 10 percent of the ideal weight for body frame and height. This will decrease the chance of heart disease, stroke, and postoperative complications.

The skin protects the body from outside elements. It works with the immune system to defend the body against harmful bacteria, fungi, viruses, and allergens. The skin must be kept clean and supple. Shower or take a bath daily, use a moisturizer afterward. Liberally apply sunscreen before spending time in the sun. Clean all scrapes and cuts with water and allow to air dry. The hair must be kept clean. Wear a hat in the sun. Keep nails clean and trimmed. Wash hands after toileting, before preparing food, and frequently as needed at other times.

Schedule regular eye exams with tonometry for glaucoma. Wear sunglasses. Avoid loud noises, especially continuous loud noises. Schedule regular dental exams. Floss and brush teeth daily. Use a soft toothbrush and fluoridated toothpaste. Schedule regular physical exams.

Avoid constipation and sitting on the toilet and reading for any length of time. This encourages the formation of hemorrhoids. Avoid the use of laxatives.

Always use proper posture. When standing or walking keep the back straight, shoulders back, and head up. Sit with the back straight and both feet on the floor. Practice proper body mechanics. Squat down to pick up objects so leg muscles, which are stronger, are utilized. Hold objects being carried close to the body.

Get a good night's sleep to feel refreshed, alert, and in good spirits. Most adults require between seven and nine hours of sleep each night. A short nap in the afternoon may be helpful for some people.

Safe Sex

Abstinence, no sex, is the safest. The next safest is to have a monogamous relationship with a partner who is also monogamous. If neither of the first two suggestions is available or acceptable, use a latex condom but never reuse the condom.

Control Stress

Not all stress is harmful. Limited stress makes one more alert and raises the energy level. How one responds or copes with stress determines whether stress is relieved or made worse. Controlling stress involves some of the topics already discussed: eat well-balanced meals regularly, exercise regularly, and get adequate sleep. Take time to relax during the day. One of the best relaxation techniques is to consciously focus on breathing; increase the length of expiration; and breathe slowly, deeply, quietly, and regularly. Participate in meaningful activities (work and play). Take time to enjoy the pleasures of life (defined by the indi-

vidual). Take time from work and regular activities for oneself. Stay connected with nature and the earth. Slow down and observe plants and flowers whether in a garden, city park, or wilderness. Own a pet if feasible. Pets give unconditional love and are always good listeners. Talk things over with a spouse, parent, sibling, or a friend. Be involved in the community, serve as a volunteer. Associate with family members including extended family. Connect to a higher power. Love yourself. Think positively.

Avoid Tobacco and Drug Abuse

Do not smoke or use tobacco in any form. When a smoker gives up the habit, the health risks decrease at once; but it takes 10 to 15 years to eliminate all the effects from smoking on the lungs. The person who smokes provides the second-hand smoke that is a health risk to those who do not smoke.

Addiction to both illegal and prescribed drugs is one of the most serious medical and social problems of our time. Drugs prescribed by a physician are abused if they are not taken as directed, or by passing them along to another person. Many prescribed drugs can be addicting when not taken as directed. For every prescribed drug, find out what effect should occur, any side effects, any food or beverage to avoid, and the maximum amount of the drug that can be safely taken in one day. Taking a tranquilizer or sedative makes driving a motor vehicle unsafe; mixing either of them with alcohol can be deadly. Refer to Chapter 9, Substance Abuse, for more information.

Limit Alcohol

If a person uses alcohol, it should be limited to one or two drinks a day. *Industry Week* (Feb. 5, 1996) reports that up to two drinks of red wine daily reduces the blood's tendency to clot and raises the blood level of HDL, which is good cholesterol. More alcohol intake does not increase the health benefits, but may lead to health problems. The use of alcohol plays a significant role in drownings, adult fire deaths, traffic fatalities, falling fatalities, and suicides.

Safety

Practice safety in all aspects of life. All homes should have functioning smoke detectors that are tested at least every six months. Keep a fire extinguisher in the kitchen. Have an escape plan that all members of the household know. Practice several times a year. Check heating equipment yearly. Keep matches and lighters out of children's reach.

House plants can improve air quality. They use carbon dioxide and give off small amounts of oxygen. Make sure there is good ventilation in the home and workplace.

Use of protective gates keeps small children and others who may wander safe. Wipe up spills immediately so no one slips or falls. Use a step stool or ladder, not a chair, to reach items on high shelves. Install a safety rail in the tub and shower.

Keep medicines and cleaning materials in locked cabinets. Watch small children who may be fascinated by visitors' purses that may contain medicines. Firearms should be empty of ammunition and kept in locked cabinets.

Safety practices are important in various methods of transportation. As a passenger in an airplane, keep the seat belt fastened and count the rows to the nearest exit. Boaters should have and use all Coast Guard required safety equipment. Wear a life jacket. Passengers in a motor vehicle should use seat belts properly. Infants and small children should always be put in approved car seats and the belts fastened properly. This reduces injuries, prevents unrestrained adults from landing on a child, and prevents death from ejection. Infants have been killed in accidents when the car was going only five miles an hour. As the driver of a motor vehicle, wear a seat belt and drive safely; never drive after drinking alcohol or taking drugs; obey traffic laws and take a safe driving course.

Know what to do in case of poisoning, choking, strangling, or suffocation. Keep the poison control telephone number in a prominent place. Become certified in CPR and encourage others to do the same. Learn the Heimlich maneuver.

Environmental Influences

Be aware of health risks such as carbon monoxide, lead, mercury, and chemicals used at work or in the home. Try not to live in heavily industrialized areas or where air pollution reaches dangerous levels frequently. Air pollution contributes to the occurrence of lung cancer and emphysema. Avoid having unnecessary x-rays. Avoid exposure to the sun especially between 10 A.M. and 3 P.M.. Always use sunscreen.

Is the water safe? Use bottled water if uncertain. To find the telephone number of the regional water management office, call the Environmental Protection Agency (EPA) at 1-800-424-9065. If there is a water softener in the home, consider using potassium chloride crystals instead of sodium chloride crystals in the softener; both crystals soften water. According to experts, potassium is something many Americans need more of to lower the risk of high blood pressure and stroke (Quench strokes, 1995).

Safety proof the home against falls and accidents. Always use tools and equipment for the task for which they were intended.

Follow safe practices in food preparation, serving, and storage to avoid food-borne illnesses. Always wash hands before preparing food. Use separate utensils for each food and for raw foods and cooked foods.

Health Care

Most people use the health care system when they are ill for the treatment of their disease or condition. That is as it should be. However, a more effective use of the health care system is health promotion and disease prevention. Routine physical exams with minimal testing are invaluable for maintaining health and preventing disease. Healthy adults should consider health care services based on factors in the individual's family health history, personal health history, personal habits, or the presence of symptoms that may alter the time frame for suggested health care services.

Physical Exam

The physical examination should begin with a review of family health history, personal health history, personal habits (tobacco, alcohol, drugs), and concerns or questions the client may have. Before visiting the physician, the client should write down questions and concerns so none will be forgotten. Individuals between the ages of twenty and thirty-nine should have a complete physical exam every one to three years; those forty to forty-nine years of age, a complete physical exam every one to two years; and those over fifty years of age, a complete physical exam every year. Women should have a breast exam with every physical exam before age forty and yearly thereafter. Men should have a testicular exam with every physical exam and a rectal exam to check the prostate with every physical exam after age forty.

Immunizations

Those adults who have not had the recommended schedule of immunizations as children should discuss it with their primary physician. Depending on the client's risk factors, the physician may recommend having the immunizations as an adult. See the childhood immunization schedule in Figure 8-2.

Each adult should have a tetanus booster immunization every ten years for life. Those at high risk of exposure, such as health care workers and college students; those who have chronic pulmonary, heart, or kidney disease, or diabetes; and those sixty-five years of age and older should have an influenza immunization every year and a pneumococcal pneumonia immunization every six years.

Tests

The following tests should be done with every physical exam: complete blood count, blood sugar,

Recommended childhood immunization schedule — United States, January-June 1996

Vaccines are listed under the routinely recommended ages. Bars indicate range of acceptable ages for vaccination. Shaded bars indicate catch-up vaccination: at 11-12 years of age, hepatitis B vaccine should be administered to children not previously vaccinated, and Varicella Zoster Virus vaccine should be administered to children not previously vaccinated who lack a reliable history of chickenpox.

Vaccine▼ Age▶	Birth	1 mo	2 mos	4 mos	6 mos	12 mos	15 mos	18 mos	4-6 yrs	11-12 yrs	14-16 yrs
Hepatitis B[1,2]		Hep B-1								Hep B[2]	
			Hep B-2			Hep B-3					
Diphtheria, Tetanus Pertussis[3]			DTP	DTP	DTP	DTP[3] (DTaP at 15+ mos)			DTP or DTaP	Td	
H. influenzae type b[4]			Hib	Hib	Hib[4]	Hib[4]					
Polio[5]			OPV[5]	OPV	OPV				OPV		
Measles, Mumps, Rubella[6]						MMR			MMR[6] or MMR[6]		
Varicella Zoster Virus Vaccine[7]						Var				Var[7]	

Approved by the Advisory Committee on Immunization Practices (ACIP), the American Academy of Pediatrics (AAP), and the American Academy of Family Physicians (AAFP)

[1] **Infants born to HBsAg-negative mothers** should receive 2.5 g of Merck vaccine (Recombivax HB) or 10 g of Smithkline Beecham (SB) vaccine (Engerix-B). The 2nd dose should be administered ≥ 1 mo after the 1st dose. **Infants born to HBsAg-positive mothers** should receive 0.5 mL hepatitis B immune globulin (HBIG) within 12 hrs of birth, and either 5 g of Merck vaccine (Recombivax HB) or 10 g of SB vaccine (Engerix-B) at a separate site. The 2nd dose is recommended at 1-2 mos of age and the 3rd dose at 6 mos of age. **Infants born to mothers whose HBsAg status is unknown** should receive either 5 g of Merck vaccine (Recombivax HB) or 10 g of SB vaccine (Engerix-B) within 12 hrs of birth. The 2nd dose of vaccine is recommended at 1 mo of age and the 3rd dose at 6 mos of age.

[2] Adolescents who have not previously received 3 doses of hepatits B vaccine should initiate or complete the series at the 11-12 year-old visit. The 2nd dose should be administered at least 1 mo after the 1st dose, and the 3rd dose should be administered at least 4 mos after the 1st dose and at least 2 mos after the 2nd dose.

[3] DTP4 may be administered at 12 mos of age, if at least 6 mos have elapsed since DTP3. DTaP (diphtheria and tetanus toxoids and acellular pertussis vaccine) is licensed for the 4th and/or 5th vaccine dose(s) for children aged ≥ 15 mos and may be preferred for these doses in this age group. Td (tetanus and diphtheria toxoids, adsorbed, for adult use) is recommended at 11-12 years of age if at least 5 years have elapsed since the last dose of DTP, DTaP, or DT.

[4] Three H. influenzae type b (Hib) conjugate vaccines are licensed for infant use. If PRP-OMP (PedvaxHIB [Merck]) is administered at 2 and 4 mos of age, a dose at 6 mos is not required. After completing the primary series, any Hib conjugate vaccine may be used as a booster.

[5] Oral poliovirus vaccine (OPV) is recommended for routine infant vaccination. Inactivated poliovirus vaccine (IPV) is recommended for persons with a congenital or acquired immune deficiency disease or an altered immune status as a result of disease or immunosuppressive therapy, as well as their household contacts, and is an acceptable alternative for other persons. The primary 3-dose series for IPV should be given with a minimum interval of 4 wks between the 1st and 2nd doses and 6 mos between the 2nd and 3rd doses.

[6] The 2nd dose of MMR is routinely recommended at 4-6 yrs of age or at 11-12 yrs of age, but may be administered at any visit, provided at least 1 mo has elapsed since receipt of the 1st dose.

[7] Varicella zoster virus vaccine (Var) can be administered to susceptible children any time after 12 months of age. Unvaccinated children who lack a reliable history of chickenpox should be vaccinated at the 11-12 year-old visit.

FIGURE 8-2   Childhood immunization schedule.

cholesterol, urinalysis, stool for blood, and for women a Pap smear. An electrocardiogram (EKG or ECG) should be done at ages twenty and forty and every five years thereafter (yearly if at high risk). Women should have a baseline mammogram between ages thirty-five and forty and yearly after age fifty. Men should have a testicular exam and rectal exam of the prostate with each physical exam. Each woman should perform a breast self-exam after every menstrual period. Each male should perform a testicular self-exam on a monthly basis. Refer to Chapter 31 for the breast self-exam and Chapter 32 for the testicular self-exam.

Dental

A dental exam, prophylaxis, and needed treatment should be performed every six to twelve months throughout life.

Eye Exam

An eye exam including tonometry for glaucoma should be performed every two to three years from age forty to forty-nine and every one to two years after the age of fifty.

CRUCIAL HEALTH PRACTICES

Simon (1992) states that in the United States, all the medical progress from 1900–1990 has increased the life span of an average adult four years; but simple lifestyle changes increased the life span of an average adult eleven years. He describes ten crucial health practices that seem to sum up everything discussed in this chapter.

- Tobacco and drugs—do not use at all.
- Alcohol—no more than two ounces per day.
- Eat a diet low in fat, cholesterol, and salt; but high in fiber, fruits, vegetables, and fish.
- Exercise regularly—one hour each week is helpful, three is ideal.
- Stay lean.
- Drive cars with air bags and wear the seatbelts; drive prudently, and never drink before you drive.
- Avoid excessive stress.
- Minimize your exposure to radiation, ultraviolet rays, chemical pollutants, and other environmental hazards.
- Protect yourself from sexually transmitted diseases.
- Obtain regular medical care including immunizations and screening tests.

PREVENTION WORKS

If one examines the controllable factors for the leading causes of death, the crucial health practices identified by Simon (1992) can be found. The controllable factors overlap, that is they affect more than one cause of death. Therefore, following the crucial health practices will work to eliminate the leading causes of death. The uncontrollable factors of family history, advancing age, and gender will always be present. Table 8-4 identifies the controllable factors for the leading causes of death.

MAKE A GENOGRAM

A **genogram** is a method of visualizing family members, their birth and death dates or ages, and specific health problems. It should include at least four generations: the individual, the children, the parents, and the grandparents. Then it is easy to follow the health problems in the family through the generations. The individual can identify the health problems that may be encountered, take steps to prevent them, and have the appropriate screening tests performed. Figure 8-3 shows a sample genogram.

Table 8-4

CONTROLLABLE FACTORS FOR LEADING CAUSES OF DEATH	
Cause of Death	**Controllable Factors**
Heart Disease	Smoking, high blood pressure, high cholesterol, lack of exercise, excessive stress, diabetes, obesity
Cancer	Tobacco, radiation, alcohol abuse, improper diet, environmental exposures
Stroke	Tobacco, high blood pressure, high cholesterol, lack of exercise
Accidents	Alcohol, drug, and tobacco use, not using seat belts, fatigue, stress, recklessness
Chronic lung disease	Tobacco, environmental exposures
Pneumonia and influenza	Chronic lung disease, environmental exposures, tobacco, alcohol abuse, lack of immunization
Diabetes	Obesity, improper diet, lack of exercise, excessive stress
Suicide	Excessive stress, alcohol, drugs
Liver disease	Alcohol, exposure to toxins (ingested and environmental) lack of immunizations
Atherosclerosis	Tobacco, high cholesterol, high blood pressure, lack of exercise

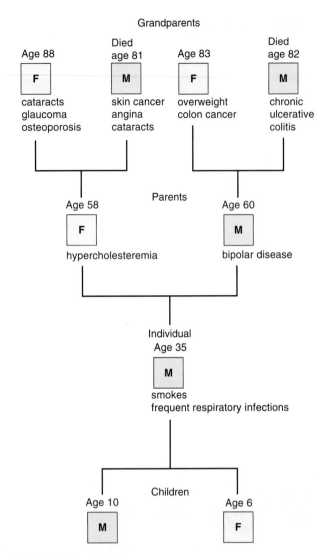

FIGURE 8-3   Sample genogram.

PREVENT COMMON HEALTH PROBLEMS

Lifestyle factors are identified that may help prevent selected health problems. Most are primary prevention, those with asterisks are secondary prevention.

Heart Disease

- Eat a diet low in fat and cholesterol, and high in fiber.
- Exercise regularly, 30 minutes three to five times a week—walking, swimming, cycling.
- Quit smoking or do not start to smoke.
- Handle stress appropriately, use relaxation or meditation.
- No excessive use of caffeine or alcohol.
- Maintain appropriate weight for height.
- *Maintain normal blood pressure.
- *Have a regular physical exam.

Osteoporosis

- Throughout life eat calcium-rich foods (milk and milk products) and a balanced diet.
- Get plenty of exercise.
- Discuss the need of a calcium supplement and estrogen replacement therapy (females) with the primary care physician.
- Do not smoke.

Cancer

- Do not smoke.
- Avoid exposure to unnecessary radiation.
- Protect skin from ultraviolet rays—use sunscreen.
- Avoid exposure to harmful chemicals.
- Minimize exposure to pesticides, herbicides, and poisons.
- Limit alcohol intake.
- Eat a well-balanced diet with adequate fiber.
- Exercise.
- Practice safe sex.
- *Have cancer screening tests—mammogram, Pap smear, fecal occult blood test and rectal exam—with each physical exam.

Low Back Pain

- Regular exercise.
- Good posture.
- Use proper body mechanics.

Colds and Flu

- Wash hands frequently.
- Use paper tissues and dispose of properly.
- Have flu shots yearly.
- Follow Food Guide Pyramid for balanced diet.
- Drink plenty of fluids.
- Do not smoke.

Breast Cancer

- Low fat diet.
- Regular exercise.
- Limit alcohol and caffeine intake.
- *Breast self-exam.
- *Mammogram.

Sexually Transmitted Diseases

- Abstinence.
- Monogamous sex between noninfected individuals.
- Use latex condom.

Tuberculosis (especially for health care workers)

- *Mantoux test.
- *Isoniazid preventive therapy—any newly exposed and infected individual taking a full course of therapy (Reichman & Mangura, 1996).

Urinary Tract Infections

- Drink plenty of water.
- Empty bladder frequently, especially before and after sexual intercourse.
- Wear underwear with a cotton crotch.
- Wipe from front to back.
- Drink cranberry juice.
- Avoid bubble bath, douches, and scented or colored toilet paper.

Sickle Cell Anemia and Thalassemia

- *Genetic screening and counseling.

Cataracts

- Wear sunglasses and a hat with a brim.
- Eat well-balanced diet.
- Do not smoke.

Glaucoma

- *Tonometry.
- *Optic nerve exam.

Sunburn

- Always wear suncreen, with SPF 15, when out in the sun.

Dental Caries and Periodontal Disease

- Brush after each meal, floss daily.
- Use fluoride toothpaste.
- Professional cleaning twice a year.
- *Dental exam yearly.

Environmental Hazards

There are many hazards to health in our environment. Some can be eliminated or reduced and some cannot.

Home

- Lock cupboards with medicines and cleaning materials.
- Maintain working smoke alarms and fire extinguishers.
- Use carbon monoxide alarm with gas appliances and heaters.
- Plan escape routes in case of fire and have fire drills.
- Safety proof home against falls.
- Know water safety rules.

Work

- Follow workplace safety regulations.
- Report unsafe equipment or practices.

Travel

- Wear seat belt.
- Do not drink and drive.
- Drive safely and defensively.
- Use infant and child seats and restraints.
- Wear a helmet when riding a bicycle or motorcycle.
- Never swim alone.

Overweight - Underweight

- Follow Food Guide Pyramid for a balanced diet.
- Exercise thirty minutes daily.
- If overweight, eat the least number of servings recommended.
- If needed, use raw fruits or vegetables as snacks between meals.
- If underweight, eat the largest number of servings recommended.
- Eat a nutritious snack between meals.

Stress

- Identify source of stress.
- Establish realistic goals and expectations.
- Be flexible.
- Express your thoughts and feelings.
- Do not depend on alcohol or drugs for relaxation.
- Exercise.
- Practice deep breathing and muscle relaxation.
- Get enough sleep.
- Have a sense of humor—laugh.
- *Use professional help when needed.

▶ *CASE STUDY*

Use the genogram in Figure 8-4. The individual has a high level administrative position at a large university. He must attend many luncheon and dinner meetings. Free time is spent reading novels or watching television.

1. Identify the possible health problems for the individual.
2. List the lifestyle changes the individual must make to lower his risk of health problems.
3. Identify secondary preventive measures the individual should take.
4. Identify the possible health problems for the children.
5. List ways the children can lower their risk for the health problems identified in statement 4.
6. Identify the secondary preventive measures the children should be taking.

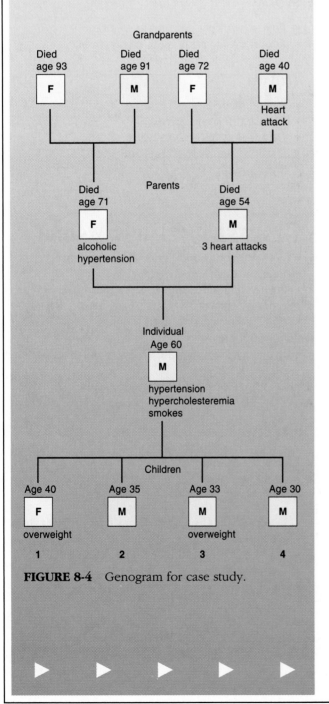

FIGURE 8-4 Genogram for case study.

SUMMARY

- Health maintenance includes prevention, early detection, and treatment of health problems.
- The best way to maintain health is to follow the Food Guide Pyramid and the Dietary Guidelines for Americans, exercise regularly, reduce stress, prevent accidents, and receive routine health exams.
- The leading causes of death can be significantly reduced by lifestyle changes.
- Physical, mental, emotional, social, and spiritual aspects play a key role in the development of disease; and also, in the ability to resist disease and maintain health.

Review Questions

1. The person responsible for health maintenance and disease prevention is the:
   a. nurse.
   b. physician.
   c. individual.
   d. nurse practitioner.

2. The *Healthy People 2000* objectives:
   a. are related only to physical fitness.
   b. are related to only disease conditions.
   c. address the treatment of disease conditions.
   d. address the issue of personal responsibility for health behaviors.

3. Primary prevention:
   a. begins with the physician.
   b. is curing a disease in a week.
   c. takes place before disease begins.
   d. includes all diseases or conditions.

4. The prevention health care team is composed of the:
   a. dietitian, nurses, and pharmacist.
   b. individual, physician, and nurses.
   c. physician, pharmacist, and laboratory.
   d. radiology, laboratory, and individual.

5. Health is improved by:
   a. not smoking.
   b. not drinking alcohol.
   c. eating more sweet foods.
   d. sleeping nine to ten hours each night.

6. How often should an individual have a physical exam?
   a. every year
   b. every two years
   c. every three years
   d. it depends on the person's age

7. A genogram is used for:
   a. building a family tree.
   b. identifying potential health problems.
   c. preventing most diseases and illnesses.
   d. identifying the genes a person inherits.

8. Colds and flu can best be prevented by:
   a. smoking.
   b. staying warm and dry.
   c. washing hands frequently.
   d. having a flu shot every three years.

9. Cataracts can be prevented by:
   a. wearing prescription glasses.
   b. wearing sunglasses and a hat.
   c. washing the eyes with saline.
   d. having plenty of light when reading.

10. What is the secondary prevention for stress?
    a. use professional help
    b. have a sense of humor
    c. do not depend on drugs or alcohol
    d. establish realistic goals and expectations

Critical Thinking Questions

1. What lifestyle changes would benefit you and your family?
2. How can you assist a client to identify potential health problems?
3. What is the relationship between stress and health?
4. What kind of preventive health care should be received by a person 20 years old, 42 years old, and 65 years old?
5. How does the nurse's state of health affect client care?

News Flash

Coprocytobiology is being developed by scientists at the United States Department of Agriculture and Johns Hopkins University as an alternative to colonoscopy. It is a painless and less costly procedure for detecting colon disease. The client collects a fresh stool (a grape-size piece), places it in a screw-capped tube containing a special medium, and shakes to disperse the stool. The tube is packed in ice to maintain the stability of the cells shed by the lining of the colon into the feces, and taken to the laboratory. Simple laboratory procedures yields millions of cells that can then be studied (Brown, 1995).

CHAPTER
9
Substance Abuse

Lois White

KEY TERMS

abuse
addiction
behavioral tolerance
co-dependent
confabulation
cross-tolerance
dependence
detoxification
hallucinations
intoxication
Johnsonian intervention
misuse
opisthotonos
relapse
reverse tolerance
substance
synthesiasis
teratogenic
tolerance
withdrawal

LIST OF TOPICS

► Alcohol
► Benzodiazepines and other sedative-hypnotics
► Cannabis
► Cocaine
► Amphetamines
► Caffeine
► Nicotine
► Methylphenidate HCl (Ritalin)
► Phencyclidine - PCP
► Opioids
► Inhalants
► Anabolic Steroids
► Nursing Process
► Co-dependency
► Impaired Nurse

LEARNING OBJECTIVES

Upon completion of this chapter the learner should be able to:
• Define key terms.
• Differentiate between dependence, abuse, and intoxication.
• Describe issues related to drug testing.
• Discuss substances frequently abused.
• Use assessment skills to identify possible substance abuse.
• Describe nursing interventions in working with substance abusers.
• Describe stages of alcoholism and the impact on the individual, family, and society.

- Discuss medications frequently used in the treatment of substance abuse.

- Describe an impaired nurse.
- Identify goals of programs for impaired nurses.

▶ *MAKING THE CONNECTION*

Refer to the topics in the following chapters to increase your understanding of substance abuse.

- **Chapter 2, Legal Aspects of Nursing:** Impaired Nurse, p. 27
- **Chapter 4, Biomedical Ethics:** Confidentiality, p. 52; Privacy, p. 53; Required Reporting, p. 53; Nurse's Role, p. 53; Professional Gatekeeping, p. 65; (Impaired Colleague, p. 65)
- **Chapter 8, Health Maintenance:** What Is Health?, p. 120; Emotional Wellness, p. 120; Mental Wellness, p. 120; Intellectual Wellness, p. 121; Social Wellness, p. 121; Spiritual Wellness, p. 121; Scope of Prevention, p. 123; Prevention Health Care Team, p. 123; What

Affects Health?, p. 124 (Genetics & Human Biology, p. 124; Personal Behavior, p. 125; Environmental Influences, p. 127); Crucial Health Practices, p. 129; Prevention Works, p. 129
- **Chapter 10, Nursing Assessment:** Inspection, p. 167; Vital Signs, p. 176
- **Chapter 16, Caring for the Older Adult:** Special Consideration, p. 332 (Losses, p. 332); Health Promotion and Maintenance, p. 333
- **Chapter 19, Respiratory Disorders:** Pneumonia, p. 399; Asthma, p. 423; Emphysema, p. 428
- **Chapter 34, Digestive Disorders:** Esophagael Varices, p. 974; Cirrhosis, p. 996

INTRODUCTION

Substance use has taken place for many centuries. It is not a new problem for society. A **substance** is a drug, legal or illegal, that may cause physical or mental impairment. With the great increase in world population there are more people involved in substance abuse. Today's speed of travel and communication has made it easier for the distribution of substances.

Many street drugs are "cut" (mixed) with substances that should not be consumed such as talcum powder, rodent exterminating powder, or even strychnine. The purity (strength) of the drug is then not known and overdose easily occurs. Fatalities can occur from the substance with which the drug is cut.

In the United States, substance disorders affect male and female, all ethnic groups, and persons of all levels of education and income. From the newborn to the elderly, all ages can be affected.

Substance disorders may be classified as intoxication, abuse, or dependence (addiction). The reversible effect on the central nervous system (CNS) soon after the use of a substance is termed **intoxication**. **Abuse** is the recurrent use of a substance, but abstinence does not cause withdrawal symptoms. **Dependence (addiction)** is reliance on a substance to such a degree that abstinence causes physical withdrawal symptoms and/or a psychological craving for the substance. The person has no control over use of the substance and only feels pleasure when using the substance. Table

9-1 shows diagnostic criteria for abuse and dependence.

KEY ABBREVIATIONS

The following abbreviations and acronyms are used in this chapter:

AA	Alcoholics Anonymous
ADDH	attention deficit disorder with hyperactivity
AWS	alcohol withdrawal syndrome
DEA	Drug Enforcement Administration
DETOX	detoxification
DSM-IV	*Diagnostic and Statistical Manual of Mental Disorders,* fourth edition
DTs	delirium tremens
FAE	fetal alcohol effects
FAS	fetal alcohol syndrome
FDA	Federal Drug Administration
LSD	lysergic acid diethylamide
MADD	Mothers Against Drunk Driving
MAOI	monoamine oxidase inhibitors
NA	Narcotics Anonymous
OTC	over the counter
PCP	phencyclidine
SADD	Students Against Driving Drunk

Table 9-1

DIAGNOSTIC CRITERIA FOR SUBSTANCE ABUSE AND DEPENDENCE

Abuse	In a 12-month period, the person is involved in one or more of the following situations when impaired by a substance.	• Failure to fulfill role obligations at home, work, or school • Performs physically hazardous activity (driving a car) • Legal problems—arrests • Social or interpersonal problems caused or worsened by effects of substance • Has never met criteria for substance dependence
Dependence	In a 12-month period, three or more of the following occur at any time.	• Tolerance—need increasing amount of substance to have desired effect. Same amount produces less effect • Withdrawal—characteristic symptoms when substance is no longer used • Larger amounts used or used longer than intended • Persistent desire or unsuccessful attempts to control use • Much time spent obtaining substance, using substance, or recovering from its effects • Occupational, social, or recreational activities given up or reduced because of substance use • Continued use despite knowledge that physical or psychological problems are caused by substance use

(Adapted from American Psychiatric Association. (1994). Diagnostic and statistical manual of mental disorders (4th ed.). Washington DC: American Psychiatric Association.)

HISTORICAL PERSPECTIVES

Nearly 6,500 years ago, ancient Egyptians used opium for pain relief. Later they used it for recreation when they discovered it provided anxiety relief, a pleasurable experience, and an escape from reality. China's attempt to control drug abuse led to the Opium War of 1839. China lost the war and became the main source of opium for the world.

Drug problems began in the United States with the Civil War in 1861. Wounded soldiers were given their own supply of morphine. Its use was uncontrolled. The drug problem was as great in 1900 as it is today. Dependence-producing drugs such as cocaine, heroin, and morphine were given freely to clients by the doctors. Patent medicines, many containing alcohol, cocaine, and heroin, were said to cure almost any ailment a person might have.

The Pure Food and Drug Act of 1906, requiring accurate labeling of drugs, was the first to control drugs in the United States. In 1914, The Harrison Act, made the use of certain narcotics illegal. Physicians then became unwilling to give individuals these drugs. Drug use actually increased as those persons already using drugs turned to an illegal market for a supply. In 1919 Congress passed the 19th Amendment to the Constitution declaring the making and selling of alcohol illegal. Prohibition lasted until 1933 when the 19th

Amendment was finally repealed. It had not controlled drunkenness or alcoholism as was intended.

Many medical, law enforcement, and legislative efforts in the 1930s slowed narcotic addiction. Then marijuana flooded the market. The Marijuana Tax Act of 1937 was to raise revenue, identify the persons involved in its use, and discourage the recreational use of marijuana. Marijuana was removed in 1941 from the official list of drugs United States physicians could prescribe. World War II disrupted supply routes of drugs from Asia and Europe, and large-scale drug use disappeared in the United States.

The 1960s saw drug use move into the mainstream of life in the United States. Drugs were used as a form of relaxation. It is estimated that during the 1970s, 50 million United States citizens in every occupation and every socioeconomic level used marijuana. The Comprehensive Drug Abuse Prevention and Control Act was passed in 1970. It is commonly referred to as the Controlled Substance Act. This act regulates the manufacturing, distributing, and dispensing of controlled substances. To enforce the provisions of this act, the Drug Enforcement Administration (DEA) was organized. There are five classifications or schedules of these substances. The schedules indicate the degree of control. Table 9-2 identifies and explains the five schedules.

In the 1980s, marijuana and other drug use declined,

Table 9-2

SCHEDULES OF CONTROLLED SUBSTANCES	
Schedule I (C-I)	High abuse and dependence potential. No accepted medical use in the United States. Includes heroin, mescaline, LSD, and psilocybin. Can be obtained legally for limited research programs.
Schedule II (C-II)	High abuse and dependence potential. Have currently accepted medical use. Includes narcotics, barbiturates, and amphetamines. Obtained only with physician's prescription, nonrefillable.
Schedule III (C-III)	Less abuse potential, moderate dependence likely. Includes nonbarbiturate sedatives and some narcotics in limited doses. Prescription refills good for six months. Fewer controls than for Schedule II.
Schedule IV (C-IV)	Even less abuse potential, limited dependence likely. Includes some sedatives and antianxiety agents and nonnarcotic analgesics.
Schedule V (C-V)	Limited abuse potential. Includes cough medicines containing codeine and antidiarrheals. May be sold over-the-counter in pharmacies to persons over 18 years old. A record is kept of the buyer's name.

especially with high school students. Cocaine and its derivative, crack, were the new drugs of choice. The lure of making huge amounts of money attracted new drug dealers. The increased supply hooked many people into heavy drug use. The 1990s have seen an increase in the use of all substances. Our society is antidiscomfort and impatient for relief.

DSM-IV CRITERIA

The American Psychiatric Association has identified specific criteria for mental disorders, including substance intoxication, substance abuse, and substance dependence. These criteria can be found in the *Diagnostic and Statistical Manual of Mental Disorders,* fourth edition. Most definitions for intoxication, abuse, and dependence are based on these criteria.

FACTORS RELATED TO SUBSTANCE ABUSE

The use of substances is a defense mechanism that blurs reality but does not alter the situation. There are many factors that interact to influence a person's substance abuse. Many people who have stopped substance abuse **relapse** (go back to substance abuse) because of these same factors. These factors may be categorized as individual, family, lifestyle, environmental, and developmental.

Individual Factors

Genetic factors are being researched as a possible reason for a person's susceptibility to substance abuse. According to Santomier & Hogan (1991), research has produced some evidence to suggest the presence of an abnormal chromosome in addicted individuals. This does not guarantee addiction, but may predispose the person to addiction.

Other research suggests that variations in the intensity of the flow of neurotransmitters may cause certain individuals to be more susceptible to addiction. The personality traits of sensation seeking and being impulsive may make it easier for the person to experiment with substances.

Family Patterns

Substance abuse, especially in the adolescent, seems to be related to family relationships. Close family relationships, with the parents involved in their children's activities, appears to discourage substance abuse. Families with positive relationships between parents and children generally have less use of illicit drugs.

Parental attitudes about substance abuse and their own drug-using behaviors contribute to drug use by the children. Parents who use alcohol, often have children who also use alcohol. Parent-child interactions that show a lack of closeness, lack of maternal involvement in the children's activities, lack of or inconsistent discipline, and low aspirations for the children's education contribute to the prediction of substance abuse by the children.

Families of adolescent substance abusers generally have negative communication patterns. That is, there is a lack of praise and a great deal of blaming and criticism. Often there are unreal expectations of the children by the parents, inconsistent or unclear behavioral limits, and a pattern of self-medication by family members.

Lifestyle

All dimensions of a person's life that influence how that person lives is termed lifestyle. First is the physical dimension which includes food, clothing, shelter, and health care. The second is the social dimension that includes friends, organizations, and activities with others. Third is the intellectual/emotional dimension including education, parental support of education, self-esteem, and how the individual is treated by others. The fourth dimension is spiritual and includes a belief in a "higher being," caring and compassion for others, and being in touch with the inner self. A lack of any of these aspects of a person's lifestyle may have a negative effect on the person. Substance use, abuse, or dependence may be the coping mechanism used by an individual who has problems in any dimension of lifestyle.

Environmental Factors

There are many environmental factors that may encourage or predispose an individual to substance abuse. The social environment in which persons find themselves, the groups, clubs, gangs, sororities, fraternities, and other organizations influence the acceptance or rejection of substance abuse. The stresses in a person's life, including accidents, disabilities, illnesses, stressful family relations, frequent job changes, divorce, death, or precarious financial conditions may be too much for that person to handle. The maladaptive coping of substance abuse offers temporary relief. Because the symptoms of the stressors are reduced, substance abuse is reinforced.

Advertising can influence people in subtle ways to become involved in substance use and abuse. Landau (1995) describes how Camel cigarette consumption by the eighteen- to twenty-four-year-old age group soared when the character Joe Camel was introduced in advertising promotions in 1988. It was "cool" to be associated with Joe Camel. Pictures of happy couples drinking beer or liquor implies that drinking makes or keeps the couple happy. Other advertising connects caffeine, nicotine, or alcohol with success, sexuality, and power.

The accessibility of substances in the urban areas encourages abuse. In general, there is more anonymity and less social responsibility in the big cities. People are more alone and must cope individually. Rural areas and small town populations tend to know each other, give each other emotional support, and take responsibility for the community as a whole.

Social traditions, especially in the use of alcohol, may open the door for abuse in certain individuals. Some examples of these social traditions include having wine with meals, making toasts at weddings and other celebrations, serving "holiday cheer," and going to "happy hour." For some individuals, these situations may predispose them to alcohol abuse or dependence.

Peer activities, especially during adolescence, may result in substance abuse. Even adults often feel they must go along with certain activities to get ahead in their career. Career advancement is allowed to guide their behaviors instead of their own personal values and beliefs.

Some occupations, like health care, seem to be more associated with substance problems than others. Physicians and nurses, particularly, have access to many substances of abuse. Refer to section on Impaired Nurse discussed in this chapter and in Chapter 2.

Developmental Factors

Many individuals have not had good role models in their life. They have not learned to identify with others and do not understand that their behavior affects others. Not learning the skills and attitudes of problem-solving leaves the individual unable to apply personal resources to situations and escape seems the only answer. Substances provide that escape.

Learning the intrapersonal skills of self-discipline, self-control, and self-assessment helps the individual to cope with tension and stress. These skills also work to prevent dishonesty with self, inability to defer gratification, and low self-esteem. A lack of interpersonal skills results in dishonesty with others, resistance to feedback, inability to share feelings, and give or accept help. Not learning to take responsibility or adapt one's behavior to a situation results in irresponsibility, not accepting the consequences of behavior, and seeing oneself as a victim of circumstances.

PREVENTION

Prevention of substance abuse must be a proactive process to empower people to constructively confront stressful situations in their lives in adaptive ways. Marlatt (1992) describes three levels of prevention. Primary prevention focuses on preventing the initial use or preventing further uses that may lead to abuse or dependence. This is usually aimed at school-age children. Children need to hear the message that drugs are not good for them. Education about substances and their effects must also emphasize personal, social, and health risks. Children need role models to teach them how to cope with life without drugs, to resist social and peer pressure, and to make effective decisions. They need to feel good about themselves (positive self-concept) and to know how to have fun. A safe place to ask questions about drugs is also needed. When parents cannot provide their children with these requirements, then prevention programs must offer them.

Secondary prevention focuses on preventing ongoing use from becoming a situation of abuse or dependence. If abuse is already evident, the focus is to return the client to a state of abstinence or at least reduced use.

Tertiary prevention focuses on returning the client to a drug-free state. If this is not possible, at least physical and psychosocial problems are kept from getting worse.

COMMON DIAGNOSTIC TESTS

Clients who have a problem with substance abuse or dependence often have abnormal liver function tests and electrolyte levels. Diagnostic criteria for specific substance-related disorders can be found in DSM-IV.

Drug Screening

Tests may be done with either a blood or urine specimen. A positive test only indicates that the person has been exposed to the substance. It does not indicate abuse, addiction, or intoxication (except alcohol). Positive screening tests should be confirmed by a more specific test using a different process. Drugs for which tests can be done include alcohol, benzodiazepines, barbiturates, cocaine, crack, amphetamines, opiates, synthetic narcotic analgesics, cannabis, and PCP.

Urine is usually the body fluid tested because it is easily obtained and tested. Most substances are detectable for less than seven days. Chronic marijuana use, however, may be detected for up to thirty days. When obtaining a urine specimen for drug screening, the client should be observed so as to prevent adulteration of the specimen by the client such as substituting another person's drug free urine. A "chain of custody" is maintained by having each person who handles the specimen sign an attached paper until the specimen has been tested.

Detection of a substance depends on the amount used and the time since last used. Cocaine, barbiturates, amphetamines, and opiates are detectable for less than two days and alcohol less than one day. A false negative may result if the client's drug level falls below the threshold of sensitivity for the test.

Positive results for reasons other than substance abuse can occur. This is called a false positive. Poppy seeds may give a positive result for opiates for up to sixty hours after ingestion. Using a Vicks® Inhaler or over-the-counter diet aids may give a positive result for amphetamines. The client should be asked about the use of these items.

Other Specimens

Breath specimens can be used to determine alcohol levels. Law enforcement officials do this with the breathalyzer tests. If hair is not cut, hair analysis can detect substance use for up to a year after the person has used a drug for only two or three days. Testing meconium (first stools) from a newborn can detect illicit drug use by the mother during pregnancy.

TREATMENT/RECOVERY

Treatment depends on many factors including the amount and frequency of substance use, age, health, diet, and overall lifestyle of the individual. Infection from the use of unsterile needles and/or tissue or organ damage caused by the substance used, such as lung damage from smoking crack or marijuana or using inhalants, will also require treatment.

Recovery requires abstinence along with intrapersonal and interpersonal changes. Most individuals need professional treatment and participation in a self-help program. Daley, et al. (1993) describe four areas of recovery: physical recovery, psychological and behavioral recovery, social and family recovery, and spiritual recovery.

Physical recovery means eliminating the substance from the body. This is termed **detoxification**. If the client cannot stop using the substance or if withdrawal symptoms are present, admission to a detoxification unit is usually necessary. After detoxification, treatment must focus on restoring the client's physical health and dealing with the cravings for the substance now removed from the client's body. It helps if environmental cues such as drug paraphernalia and alcohol bottles or cans are removed.

Psychological and behavioral recovery become evident when the client no longer denies the problem and accepts the inability to consistently control the substance abuse. The client will have developed a desire for abstinence and accepted the need for long-term recovery and support. Emotional stability will be restored when the client learns to cope with uncomfortable emotional states.

Social and family recovery occurs when the client no longer denies the impact on the family and makes amends to family members and significant others who have been negatively affected by the substance abuse. The client works to improve family relationships and develops a recovery support system. Also, the client learns to resist social pressures to use alcohol or other drugs, and participates in healthy leisure-time activities. The client's family should also attend a program for recovery. If a client returns to a dysfunctional family, it may be difficult for the client to maintain recovery.

Spiritual recovery is when the client has resolved the feelings of guilt and shame and developed a meaning for life and a relationship with a higher power.

SUBSTANCE USE PATTERNS

Patterns of substance use have changed throughout the years. Coffee (caffeine) and cigarettes (nicotine) are legal in our society and have been widely used in the past. While many people still drink coffee, more and more are using decaffeinated coffee. Cigarette use has decreased in the older population as the addictive nature and negative effects of nicotine have become more evident. However, cigarette use has increased in the adolescent population.

The substance of choice is alcohol. It is legal and easily obtained. Many high school seniors have been drunk and some are already regular drinkers. There are still more alcoholic men than women, but the number of identified women alcoholics is increasing.

Elderly persons are more commonly addicted to prescription medications, especially minor tranquilizers and sleeping pills. Alcohol may be used by the elderly to soothe feelings of isolation and loneliness. Depression and paranoia may be identified as senility rather than a problem with alcohol.

Moderate consumption of alcohol may have been influenced by Mothers Against Drunk Driving (MADD) and Students Against Driving Drunk (SADD). Laws that make bars and individuals liable if they let guests leave and drive while drunk and famous people like Betty Ford and Liza Minelli sharing with the public their illness and recovery are other influences.

CNS DEPRESSANTS

Central nervous system depressants usually decrease the heart and respiratory rates as well as voluntary muscle responses.

ALCOHOL

Alcohol is a CNS depressant. Low doses of alcohol first depress areas of the brain that are inhibitory causing diminished self-control and judgment. Continued alcohol ingestion may cause unconsciousness and even death.

The active ingredient in alcoholic beverages is ethanol. Depending on the alcoholic beverage consumed, varying amounts of ethanol are ingested. It is metabolized at an average rate of 10 mL/hr. Table 9-3 shows the alcohol content in some beverages.

One ounce of alcohol provides 200 Kcal but no other nutrients. It is not converted to glycogen. The blood alcohol level depends on the size of the person, the amount ingested, and the time since ingestion. Most states have set the legal limit for blood alcohol while driving a motor vehicle at 100 mg/dL (0.1%).

Incidence

Anthenelli and Schucket (1991) report that in Western countries most men and women drink alcoholic beverages. Several national surveys have found that

Table 9-3

ALCOHOL CONTENT IN BEVERAGES

Beverage	Percent Alcohol	Equivalent amounts
Beer	4	12 ounces
Wine cooler	4	12 ounces
Wine	14	4 ounces
Hard liquor	40	1½ ounces

(Adapted from Woolf, D. (1991). CNS depressants: alcohol. In Bennett, E. & Woolf, D. Substance abuse, 2nd ed. Albany NY: Delmar Publishers.)

approximately two-thirds of the population have more than an occasional drink. Men are likely to drink more frequently and in greater quantity than women. The heaviest drinking occurs in men under the age of thirty, and there is a higher proportion of abstainers in adults over the age of fifty.

The vast majority of individuals with an alcohol problem are blue- or white-collar men and women—not the "skid-row bum." Some alcoholics drink little or none in public or with friends. They are "at home" or "hidden" alcoholics and are more likely to be women. It often takes a family quite a while to realize there is a problem with alcohol by one of the family members.

The individual with an alcohol problem often learns **behavioral tolerance**. Hollandsworth (1990) describes behavioral tolerance as a compensatory adjustment made by an individual under the influence of a particular substance. The person under the influence of alcohol learns how to compensate for the deterioration of motor performance and speech.

Signs and Symptoms

The ingestion of alcohol causes a feeling of euphoria, relaxation of skeletal muscles, changes in mental activity such as altered judgment, and reduced self-control. It has a diuretic effect which, in heavy drinkers, may cause increased loss of electrolytes, especially potassium, magnesium, and zinc. Increased levels of alcohol depress the cardiovascular and respiratory systems and produce a toxic effect on the intestinal mucosa resulting in decreased absorption of thiamine, folic acid, and vitamin B_{12}. Excess consumption of alcohol often results in a severe lack of nutrient intake. Finally, coma and death can result.

Psychosocial aspects include memory blackouts, secretive drinking, rationalization of drinking behavior, trouble with family and employer, loss of outside interests, neglect of food intake, impaired thinking, and moral deterioration. **Confabulation,** making up information to fill in memory gaps, is used by individuals abusing or depending on alcohol.

Potential for Addiction

The potential for addiction is high.

Associated Problems/ Disorders

Liver

Chronic alcohol abuse causes three distinct diseases of the liver. They are fatty liver, an accumulation of triglycerides in the liver caused by obesity, excessive alcohol consumption, and certain drugs; alcoholic hepatitis, an acute toxic liver injury from excess alcohol consumption; and cirrhosis, a chronic degenerative liver disease that can be caused by alcohol consumption. Fatty liver is reversible but alcoholic hepatitis and cirrhosis are not reversible situations. Liver cells will not function once the scar tissue of cirrhosis develops. Esophageal varices are associated with cirrhosis and could cause death if they bleed. See Chapter 34, Digestive Disorders.

Gastrointestinal Disturbances

Alcohol damages the lining of the stomach and esophagus by irritating the mucosa and causing inflammation or ulcer formation. Aspirin with alcohol can result in greater irritation and bleeding in the gastrointestinal (GI) tract. Gastric pain, vomiting, and diarrhea are common in alcohol abuse and are often what brings the individual to the health care system.

Pancreatitis

An alcoholic has a higher risk of developing pancreatitis than an abstainer. Severe pancreatitis can result in death.

Wernicke's Encephalopathy

This inflammatory hemorrhagic and degenerative condition of the brain is caused by a thiamine deficiency. It is characterized by delirium, memory loss, unsteady gait, a sense of apprehension, and an altered level of consciousness. Thiamine intake improves the situation.

Korsakoff's Psychosis

Disorientation, amnesia, insomnia, hallucinations, and peripheral neuropathologies characterize this psy-

chosis. Both thiamine and B$_{12}$ deficiencies contribute to the degeneration of the brain and peripheral nervous system. Frequently, there is bilateral foot drop and pain over the long nerves. Thiamine and B$_{12}$ intake may improve the situation.

Cardiovascular Disturbances

Moderate amounts of alcohol cause cutaneous vasodilation (flushed skin). This causes rapid heat loss and the core temperature may drop to a dangerous level. Blood pressure decreases with intoxicating doses of alcohol. There may be irregularities in cardiac rhythm. Hematologic alterations such as bone marrow depression, anemia, leukopenia, or thrombocytopenia may also occur.

Fetal Alcohol Syndrome (FAS)

The **teratogenic** (causing abnormal development of the embryo) effects of alcohol are related to the amount of alcohol ingested and the stage of pregnancy when the alcohol is ingested. Even a small amount of alcohol can be detrimental. For a diagnosis of FAS, the infant must meet certain criteria. Table 9-4 gives these criteria.

If only some of the FAS criteria are met, it is called fetal alcohol effects (FAE). The only treatment for FAS or FAE is prevention. Women who are pregnant or are trying to get pregnant should abstain from alcohol consumption.

Withdrawal

Withdrawal is the symptoms produced when a substance on which an individual has dependence is no longer used by that individual. Alcohol withdrawal syndrome (AWS) appears when the blood alcohol concentration of the alcoholic decreases. The onset of symptoms usually occurs six to twelve hours after drinking stops and may last up to five days. If physical

Table 9-4

INFANT CRITERIA FOR FETAL ALCOHOL SYNDROME

Prenatal and/or postnatal growth retardation (weight, length, or head circumference below the 10th percentile)

CNS involvement (signs of neurologic abnormality, developmental delay, or intellectual impairment)

Craniofacial anomalies, at least two of the following (microcephaly or head circumference below 3rd percentile, microopthalmia or short palpebral fissure, poorly developed philtrum, thin upper lip, or flattening of maxillary area)

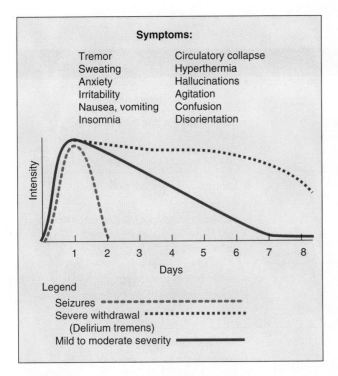

Symptoms:

Tremor	Circulatory collapse
Sweating	Hyperthermia
Anxiety	Hallucinations
Irritability	Agitation
Nausea, vomiting	Confusion
Insomnia	Disorientation

Legend

Seizures `-------------------`
Severe withdrawal `··················`
(Delirium tremens)
Mild to moderate severity `━━━━━━━`

FIGURE 9-1   Alcohol withdrawal patterns.

dependence is low, the withdrawal symptoms of nausea, tremulousness, weakness, anxiety, and insomnia usually last only a few hours. Chronologically, how long the drinking has occurred and the amount of alcohol consistently consumed are factors in the severity of the withdrawal symptoms.

Greater physical dependence will cause more severe withdrawal symptoms that will last longer. Symptoms may include anxiety, agitation, irritability, diaphoresis, tachycardia, systolic hypertension, temperature elevation (less than 101°F), nausea, vomiting, diarrhea, anorexia, insomnia or vivid dreams, seizures within the first forty-eight hours of abstinence, disorientation, hallucinations, or delusions. Figure 9-1 shows alcohol withdrawal patterns.

Delirium Tremens

Delirium tremens (DTs) is the most advanced stage of alcohol withdrawal. It develops two to three days after alcohol drinking has stopped. Symptoms may include disorientation, delirium, agitation, diaphoresis, tachycardia, fever, and cardiovascular collapse. If alcohol abuse continues, symptoms of subsequent withdrawals are generally more severe. Up to 15 percent mortality is estimated for untreated DTs. Early recognition and treatment lowers the mortality to approximately one percent (Woolf, 1991). It is recommended that withdrawal be medically monitored to decrease the chance of fatality.

Treatment/Rehabilitation

Many treatment programs are based in hospital or residential treatment centers. These are generally called inpatient programs and last thirty days. Many insurance companies are encouraging clients to participate in lower cost outpatient programs. Currently, there is no evidence that inpatient programs are more effective than outpatient programs.

Many outpatient programs have both day and evening sessions so clients can maintain their usual occupations. The programs usually consist of a four-week intensive session with follow-up sessions for six to twenty-four months. The first part of either type of treatment program is detoxification.

Detoxification

The goal of detoxification (DETOX) is to halt or control the neuronal overactivity that occurs when the alcohol level is reduced or alcohol is no longer present in the client's body. This is done by substituting a pharmacologically similar drug and gradually reducing the dose given. The benzodiazepine drugs, chlordiazepoxide (Librium), diazepam (Valium), lorazepam (Ativan) and clorazepate dipotassium (Tranxene) are the most commonly used.

During DETOX, other problems such as malnutrition, vitamin deficiencies (B vitamins, especially thiamine), dehydration, and potassium and magnesium deficiencies must also be treated. A client with hypoglycemia should be given thiamine before administering dextrose to prevent Wernicke's encephalopathy. Ignoring these problems complicates the management of detoxification.

Psychologic Intervention

The classic psychologic intervention technique was originally described by Johnson (1973). Although several modifications have been published and used since then, the technique is still used and is known as **Johnsonian intervention**.

This early intervention technique compresses into one dramatic confrontation all the past crises caused by the person's alcohol abuse. Instead of waiting until the client "hits bottom," this intervention is designed to help the client immediately. The confrontation helps eliminate denial so the client will agree to treatment.

The client's significant others (spouse, teenage or older children, one or two close friends, possibly employer) meet with a professional addiction counselor. This group rehearses in order that they may present a united front when confronting the client. They present specific examples of painful or embarrassing behaviors by the client while intoxicated that caused problems and concerns. It is difficult for the client to

Table 9-5

ALCOHOL WITH OTHER DRUGS

Drug Classifications with examples		Interaction
Narcotic Analgesics	meperidine hydrochloride (Demerol) proproxyphene HCl (Darvon) hydromorphone HCl (Dilaudid)	• Loss of effective breathing (respiratory arrest) • Can be fatal
Nonnarcotic Analgesics	aspirin (Bayer Aspirin)	• Stomach and intestinal bleeding
Anticoagulants	warfarin sodium (Coumadin, Panwarfin) dicumarol	• Increases drugs ability to stop blood clotting • May cause life-threatening or fatal hemorrhage
Antidepressants	imipramine HCl (Tofranil) desipramine HCl (Pertofrane) perphenazine and amitriptyline HCl (Triavil)	• Reduces CNS functioning • Chianti wine may cause hypertensive crisis
Antihistamines	Most cold remedies pseudoephedrine HCl and triprolidine HCl (Actifed) chlorpheniramine maleate and acetominophen (Coricidin)	• Increased calming effect • Person becomes very drowsy • Driving is hazardous
Antihypertensives	reserpine (Serpasil) methyldopa (Aldomet)	• Orthostatic hypotension
Antimicrobials	metronidazole (Flagyl) cefotetan disodium (Cefotan) rifampin (Rifadin)	• Possible disulfiram-like reaction, nausea, cramps, vomiting, headache, flushing or hepatotoxicity
CNS Stimulants	Most diet pills dextroamphetamine sulfate (Dexedrine) caffeine (No Doz) methylphenidate HCl (Ritalin)	• May reverse depressant effect of alcohol and give a false sense of security
Diuretics	chlorothiazide (Diuril) furosemide (Lasix)	• May reduce blood pressure and cause dizziness
Antipsychotics	thioridazine HCl (Mellaril) chlorpromazine HCl (Thorazine)	• Added CNS depression and impairs voluntary movements • Causes respiratory depression • Can be fatal
Sedative-hypnotics	glutethimine (Doriden) pentobarbital (Nembutal)	• Reduces CNS functioning • Sometimes causes coma and respiratory arrest • Can be fatal
Antianxiety Agents	diazepam (Valium) chlordiazepoxide (Librium)	• Reduces CNS functioning • Decreased alertness and judgement • Can lead to household and driving accidents

maintain denial in this situation. Then the group encourages the client to accept professional help. If the client refuses help, each individual of the group must plan to minimize co-dependent behavior in the future. This technique can also be used for substances other than alcohol. Examples of confrontations may be found in Johnson's books (1973, 1988). Co-dependency is discussed later in the chapter.

Education

The abuse of or dependence on alcohol is a maladaptive way to cope with life stressors. Learning basic life skills to improve personal competence and provide adaptive coping mechanisms help the individual resist the use of alcohol.

One adaptive coping mechanism is exercise. Assist clients to become active in an exercise program and encourage them to participate. Exercise helps relieve feelings of stress and promotes feelings of well-being.

Teach clients about the Food Guide Pyramid for an adequate, balanced diet. Most clients have, in the past, received the majority of their calories from alcohol. They must now learn how to maintain health by eating nutritious foods.

The interaction of alcohol with other drugs should also be taught. Some effects can be life threatening. Table 9-5 shows the interaction of alcohol with some classifications of drugs.

Self-help Groups

Alcoholics Anonymous (AA), begun in 1935, is the model for other self-help groups such as AL-ANON for adults, AL-ATEEN for teenage children and AL-ATOT for younger children in the family of an alcoholic. The holistic approach of AA to the individual with alcohol problems is described in the Twelve Steps, and the Twelve Traditions of Alcoholics Anonymous speak to the functioning of the group (Table 9-6).

Table 9-6

THE TWELVE STEPS OF ALCOHOLICS ANONYMOUS	THE TWELVE TRADITIONS OF ALCOHOLICS ANONYMOUS
1. We admitted we were powerless over alcohol—that our lives had become unmanageable.	1. Our common welfare should come first; personal recovery depends upon A. A. unity.
2. Came to believe that a Power greater than ourselves could restore us to sanity.	2. For our group purpose, there is but one ultimate authority—a loving God as He may express Himself in our group conscience. Our leaders are but trusted servants; they do not govern.
3. Made a decision to turn our will and our lives over the care of God *as we understood Him.*	3. The only requirement for A. A. membership is a desire to stop drinking.
4. Made a searching and fearless moral inventory of ourselves.	4. Each group should be autonomous except in matters affecting other groups or A. A. as a whole.
5. Admitted to God, to ourselves and to another human being the exact nature of our wrongs.	5. Each group has but one primary purpose—to carry its message to the alcoholic who still suffers.
6. Were entirely ready to have God remove all these defects of character.	6. An A. A. group ought never endorse, finance, or lend the A. A. name to any related facility or outside enterprise, lest problems of money, property, and prestige divert us from our primary purpose.
7. Humbly asked Him to remove our shortcomings.	7. Every A. A. group ought to be fully self-supporting, declining outside contributions.
8. Made a list of all persons we had harmed, and became willing to make amends to them all.	8. Alcoholics Anonymous should remain forever non-professional, but our service centers may employ special workers.
9. Made direct amends to such people wherever possible, except when to do so would injure them or others.	9. A. A., as such, ought never be organized; but we may create service boards or committees directly responsible to those they serve.
10. Continued to take personal inventory and when we were wrong promptly admitted it.	10. Alcoholics Anonymous has no opinion on outside issues; hence the A. A. name ought never be drawn into public controversy.
11. Sought through prayer and meditation to improve our conscious contact with God, *as we understood Him,* praying only for knowledge of His will for us and the power to carry that out.	11. Our public relations policy is based on attraction rather than promotion; we need always maintain personal anonymity at the level of press, radio, and films.
12. Having had a spiritual awakening as the result of these steps, we tried to carry this message to alcoholics, and to practice these principles in all our affairs.	12. Anonymity is the spiritual foundation of all our traditions, ever reminding us to place principles before personalities.

The Twelve Steps and Twelve Traditions are reprinted with permission of Alcoholics Anonymous World Services, Inc. Permission to reprint the Twelve Steps and Twelve Traditions does not mean that A. A. has reviewed or approved the contents of this publication, nor that A. A. agrees with the views expressed herein. A. A. is a program of recovery from alcoholism only—use of the Twelve Steps and Twelve Traditions in connection with programs and activities which are patterned after A. A., but which address other problems, or in any other non-A. A. context, does not imply otherwise.

Disulfiram

Disulfiram (Antabuse) may be given to some alcohol abusers as a deterrent to drinking. It inhibits the enzyme needed to metabolize alcohol. Drinking alcohol with disulfiram in the body causes flushing of the neck and face, blurred vision, nausea, vertigo, anxiety, palpitations, tachycardia, and hypotension. Clients must be instructed not to use cologne, mouthwash, aftershave, over-the-counter cold preparations, cough syrups, vitamin-mineral tonics, as well as candies, sauces, and foods made with alcohol. These items will cause the same reaction as if the person took a drink of alcohol.

Therapy should not be started until at least 12 hours after the last drink of alcohol. The effects of disulfiram with alcohol can occur for six to twelve days after taking the disulfiram. As with any drug, there are side effects such as drowsiness, fatigue, and impotence. Garlic-like breath occurs frequently and is sometimes used as an indicator of compliance in taking the disulfiram. Disulfiram is contraindicated in clients with cardiovascular disease, hypothyroidism, suicide ideation, and in clients receiving antihypertensives or monoamine oxidase inhibitors (MAOI).

BENZODIAZEPINES AND OTHER SEDATIVE-HYPNOTICS

With the introduction in 1961 of chlordiazepoxide (Librium), the benzodiazepines have replaced most of the short-acting barbiturates and other nonbarbiturate sedative-hypnotics that were in use prior to that time. Table 9-7 lists drugs in these categories.

Incidence

Benzodiazepines are not commonly used as recreational drugs but are widely prescribed and are thus available for abuse. Statistics are not available because some clinicians are still denying that addiction to these drugs occurs. Withdrawal symptoms are subtle and delayed, and the symptoms are not always connected to the benzodiazepines.

Barbiturates and other sedative-hypnotics are more abused but less prescribed. These are available on the illegal market.

Signs and Symptoms

Benzodiazepines in low doses produce drowsiness or sedation. Larger doses produce sleep but surgical anesthesia cannot be induced. Respirations are not depressed and there is little effect on the cardiovascu-

Table 9-7

BENZODIAZEPINES, BARBITURATES, AND OTHER SEDATIVE-HYPNOTICS

Generic Name	Trade Name	Routes of Abuse
Benzodiazepines		
chlordiazepoxide	Librium	PO, IM, IV
diazepam	Valium	PO, IM, IV
lorazepam	Ativan	PO, IM, IV
oxazepam	Serax	PO
prazepam	Centrax	PO
flurazepam hydrochloride	Dalmane	PO
chlorazepate dipotassium	Tranxene	PO
temazepam	Restoril	PO
clonazepam	Klonopin	PO
alprazolam	Xanax	PO
halazepam	Paxipam	PO
triazolam	Halcion	PO
Barbiturates		
amobarbital	Amytal	PO, IM, IV
secobarbital	Seconal	PO, IM, IV
pentobarbital	Nembutal	PO, IM, IV
phenobarbital	Luminal	PO, IM, IV
butabarbital	Butisol	PO
secobarbital/ amobarbital	Tuinal	PO, IM, IV
Others		
ethchlorvynol	Placidyl	PO, IV
chloral hydrate	Noctec	PO
meprobamate	Equanil, Miltown	PO
methaqualone	only on illicit market	PO
paraldehyde	Paral	PO

(Adapted from Bennett, E. & Woolf, D. (1991) *Substance abuse.* 2nd ed. Albany, NY: Delmar Publishers.)

lar system unless extremely large doses are taken. Then a decrease in systolic blood pressure and an increase in heart rate may result. Side effects may include motor incoordination, ataxia, increased hostility or rage, confusion, metalic-like aftertaste, headache, and blurred vision. **Tolerance** (a decreased sensitivity to subsequent doses of the same substance) to other benzodiazepines and **cross-tolerance** (tolerance to other substances in the same category) to other CNS depressants occur with chronic use.

Barbiturates depress all areas of the CNS, some selectively according to the dosage. They do not reduce pain. Respirations are depressed but not significantly when therapeutic doses are taken. When a barbiturate is given to a client in pain, excitement rather than sedation may occur. Side effects may include drowsiness, residual effects on motor skills, and especially in the elderly, excitement, irritability, or delirium. An overdose of barbiturates causes decreased respirations, rapid and weak pulse, cyanosis, coma, and sometimes respiratory paralysis. Tolerance results from chronic use or abuse.

Other sedative-hypnotics that are often abused include:

- chloral hydrate (Noctec)—which when mixed with alcohol is called a "Mickey Finn," has an offensive taste, and is a gastric irritant. Toxic doses cause cardiac arrhythmias. Chronic abuse results in gastritis, hepatic and renal damage, and tolerance.
- paraldehyde (Paral)—has a putrid odor and taste. Large doses cause respiratory depression and hypotension. It is chemically unstable, and open bottles must be discarded after 24 hours. Must be kept in glass container and administered in a glass container.
- ethchlorvynol (Placidyl)—gives mint-like taste. Large doses produce pulmonary edema.
- meprobamate (Miltown, Equanil)—main effects are drowsiness and ataxia.
- methaqualone (Quaalude)—withdrawn from United States market but widely abused from illegal sources. Fatigue and dizziness are frequent side effects. Others may include nausea, abdominal cramps transient paresthesia, or feelings of depersonalization.

Potential for Addiction

The potential for addiction is high for all of these substances.

Withdrawal

Symptoms of withdrawal for benzodiazepines include cramping, sweating, disorientation, confusion, tremors, depression, hallucinations, and paranoia. Barbiturate withdrawal symptoms include anxiety, weakness, anorexia, insomnia, tremors, convulsion, and delirium. Withdrawal reactions related to other sedative-hypnotics include nausea, headache, cramping, toxic psychosis, insomnia, and convulsions.

Treatment/Rehabilitation

Ideally, treatment for benzodiazepines is a gradual reduction in the amount taken until the client is no longer taking any. Sometimes phenobarbital is given to control symptoms and then its dosage is reduced.

Treatment for barbiturate and other sedative-hypnotics overdose or withdrawal is symptomatic.

Rehabilitation that focuses on teaching clients alternative methods of coping with the anxiety and stressors in their lives is necessary. Supportive individual psychotherapy or a self-help recovery group is almost always advisable. The goal is to assist the client to abstain from the drug use.

CANNABIS

Marijuana was used in China as early as 2737 B.C. (Bennett & Woolf, 1991). Marijuana is the most common type of cannabis used. It is composed of dried leaves, stems, and flowers of the plant *Cannabis sativa* and can be smoked or added to food. Hash or hashish is a potent concentrate of the resin from the flowers. Hash oil is extremely concentrated, made by boiling hashish in a solvent and filtering out the solid matter.

Incidence

Use in the United States began in the early 1900s, peaked in the period 1978 to 1980, and has steadily decreased since. According to Johnston, et al. (1991), the prevalence of marijuana use in high school increased from 20 percent in the class of 1969 to 60.4 percent in the class of 1979 and fell to 50.2 percent in the class of 1987 and fell again to 40.7 percent in the class of 1990. The use among college students declined from a peak of 51 percent in 1980 to 29 percent in 1990. Males are more likely to use marijuana than females.

Signs and Symptoms

The general effects of marijuana use include a sense of relaxation and well-being, euphoria, altered sensory perception, decreased attention span, impaired psychomotor function, compromised driving ability, disorganized thought processes, and disorientation. Prolonged use causes pulmonary toxicity, impaired immune response, and personality and behavioral changes. A **reverse tolerance** can develop whereby a smaller amount of marijuana will elicit the desired psychic effects.

Potential for Addiction

The potential for psychologic addiction is moderate. Physiologic dependence does not usually develop even with long-term heavy use.

Associated Problems/Disorders

There is still controversy as to whether the use of marijuana leads to the use of stronger drugs. Marijuana is generally used before the individual uses depressants, hallucinogens, cocaine, or heroin. Positive experiences with marijuana may encourage experimentation with other drugs. The acquisition and use of marijuana often facilitate meeting individuals who use and have access to other drugs.

Withdrawal

Nausea, myalgia, restlessness, irritability, nervousness, insomnia, and depression may appear after ceasing to use marijuana. Symptoms may not appear for up to a week after the last use.

Treatment/Rehabilitation

Treatment focuses on relapse prevention and the development of new coping mechanisms, ways of living, and how to have fun without drugs. Weekly group therapy sessions to maintain a commitment to abstinence and enhance interpersonal skills is often used. Participation in a self-help group is encouraged.

CNS STIMULANTS

Drugs that stimulate the CNS include cocaine, amphetamines, caffeine, and nicotine. They increase cortical alertness and electrical activity in the brain and spinal cord. There is tachycardia and an increase in blood pressure.

COCAINE

Cocaine is extracted from the leaves of the coca plant, *Erythroxylum coca*. It may be heated and the fumes inhaled. This is termed *free-basing*. As a white powder, cocaine may be snorted by inhaling it through the nose. It may also be heated to a liquid state and injected intravenously. Crack is a crystallized form of cocaine that is melted in a water pipe and smoked. New forms of cocaine appear frequently.

Incidence

Cocaine abuse and dependence was the major illicit drug problem for the United States in the 1980s. The introduction of crack dramatically increased cocaine abuse among the poor. Crack is low cost and gives an intense "high."

Signs and Symptoms

The immediate reaction, less than ten seconds, is an intense euphoria that lasts ten to fifteen minutes. This short response time leads people to binge on cocaine. That is, they repeatedly use cocaine to maintain the euphoria.

The heart rate increases and blood pressure goes up. Normal pleasures are magnified, anxiety decreases, self-confidence increases, social inhibitions are reduced, communication is facilitated, and sexual feelings are enhanced. Other psychological effects are inability to concentrate, insomnia, reduced sense of humor, antisocial behavior, hallucinations, and compulsive behavior.

An overdose may occur with the first use since there is little quality control of drug strength in the street drug culture. A client with an overdose may have arrhythmias, tremors, convulsions, respiratory failure, cardiovascular collapse, and death.

Potential for Addiction

The potential for addiction is high.

Withdrawal

The crash, a period of exhaustion, occurs in the client; there are symptoms of depression, anxiety, and a great need for sleep. The depression may be to the point of suicidal behavior. The client has no energy, shows little interest in the surroundings and seems to have little ability to experience pleasure. These symptoms are the most intense during the first three days, but continue for one to four months. An intense craving for cocaine is felt, including dreaming about cocaine. Then there is a period of less intense craving for cocaine called extinction and may last months or even years. Withdrawal does not result in a medical emergency as seen with alcohol.

Treatment/Rehabilitation

Treatment is aimed at reducing the craving and managing the severe depression. Careful monitoring of the client is necessary to identify and prevent actions aimed at carrying out the idea of suicide. The intense craving for cocaine and strong denial that cocaine is addicting creates a problem in engaging an individual, with a history of cocaine usage, in treatment. Inpatient programs for some clients with cocaine dependence should therefore be recommended, while other clients can be effectively treated in outpatient programs.

Medications

Bromocriptine mesylate (Parlodel) in small doses seems to reduce the withdrawal symptoms. Amantadine hydrochloride (Symmetrel) also has some success in treating cocaine withdrawal. Desipramine hydrochloride (Pertofrane) seems to reduce the craving for cocaine.

Education

Individual or group therapy should focus on helping the client feel pleasure again, improve energy level, and reduce cocaine craving. Peer support groups and self-help groups, such as Cocaine Anonymous, may be very effective. Random and regular urine testing is an external support to promote abstinence.

AMPHETAMINES

Amphetamines (also called uppers, speed, bennies) include dextroamphetamine sulfate (Dexedrine), amphetamine sulfate (Amphetamine), and methamphetamine hydrochloride (Desoxyn). These are all controlled substances, Schedule II.

Incidence

Amphetamines have been abused since the early 1930s. World War II greatly increased use and abuse when military personnel used amphetamines to decrease fatigue and increase alertness. Today, abuse ranges from truck drivers and college students who want to ward off sleep and increase alertness to the heavy abuser who injects methamphetamine.

Signs and Symptoms

Besides suppressing fatigue and increasing alertness, amphetamines enhance psychomotor performance, induce a temporary state of well-being and give an instantaneous euphoria. Like cocaine, after several days the person becomes exhausted and lapses into a long period of sleep and depression (crash). Amphetamines' action lasts much longer than cocaine and there is a greater potential for adverse reactions and severe toxicity.

High abuse doses may cause insomnia, tachycardia, headache, arrhythmias, hypertension followed by hypotension, nausea, vomiting, cramping, diarrhea, hyperreflexia, convulsions, and death. The psychologic effect is termed amphetamine psychosis and closely resembles paranoid schizophrenia. Symptoms include paranoid ideation, confusion, compulsive behaviors, and visual and auditory hallucinations. Tolerance does develop.

Potential for Addiction

The potential for addiction is high.

Withdrawal

Physical symptoms of withdrawal are fatigue and muscle pain. Psychological changes include apathy, irritability, depression, and disorientation.

Treatment/Rehabilitation

Urinary acidifiers, such as ascorbic acid (vitamin C), increase the excretion of amphetamines. Diazepam (Valium) is given for sedation to ease the withdrawal crash. Bromocriptine mesylate (Parlodel) or levodopa (Dopar) may help decrease the craving. A quiet environment is also helpful.

Behavioral therapy is used to help the client recognize and accept the need to stop using amphetamines. Supportive individual or group therapy, and especially self-help groups aid the client to stay abstinent and in treatment.

CAFFEINE

Caffeine is found in coffee, tea, cola beverages, cocoa, chocolate, and some nonprescription drugs.

Incidence

Caffeine is probably the best known and most frequently used and abused CNS stimulant.

Signs and Symptoms

Caffeine causes relaxation of smooth muscles in blood vessels and bronchi, diuresis, an increased gastric acid secretion, suppression of appetite, increased feeling of energy, and constriction of cerebral blood vessels. Increased levels of caffeine intake causes jitteriness, restlessness, nervousness, excitement, flushed face, palpitations, and nausea.

Potential for Addiction

The potential for addiction is moderate.

Withdrawal

Withdrawal produces headache, irritability, and tremulousness.

Treatment/Rehabilitation

A gradual reduction of caffeine intake can reduce or eliminate the withdrawal symptoms. The client can then drink decaffeinated coffee and tea and caffeine-free soft drinks. The intake of cocoa and chocolate should be greatly reduced or eliminated. Caffeine can be avoided by reading labels and not using nonprescription products that contain caffeine.

NICOTINE

Nicotine is found in tobacco in a one to two percent concentration. There is no therapeutic use for nicotine. Smoking and other uses of tobacco have been in and out of favor several times during the past five centuries. This century has seen the greatest degree of abuse. Reasons for this increase are related to the mass production of tobacco products, mass advertising campaigns, and the psychologic dependence produced by the nicotine. Tobacco, even when used in moderation, will likely produce disease and death.

Incidence

About 28 percent of the adult population uses tobacco. However, persons with less education and some ethnic minorities (Native Americans, Hispanics, and African Americans) have a rate of 20 percent to 60 percent higher (Naegle, 1991).

Signs and Symptoms

Nicotine causes decreased skeletal muscle tone, decreased sensitivity of some receptor sites (pain, heat, taste buds), reduced appetite, vasoconstriction, decreased body temperature, and increased blood pressure. Tolerance develops so the daily intake must increase to continue the desired effect.

Potential for Addiction

The potential for addiction is moderate to high. Even first time users can become dependent within weeks of their initial use.

Associated Problems/ Disorders

Tobacco causes more morbidity and mortality than all other psychoactive drugs combined. Other ingredients in the smoke (tar, carbon monoxide, and incompletely burned waste products) are largely responsible for the negative health consequences.

Respiratory

Chronic obstructive pulmonary disease is caused by the many changes tobacco use makes in the respiratory system. Smokers are more prone to develop pneumonia, and asthma is exacerbated by smoking. Chronic exposure to smoke inhalation gives children higher rates of otitis media and respiratory illnesses.

Cardiovascular

Ischemic heart disease is twice as likely to develop in a smoker than in a nonsmoker. Cerebrovascular accidents and peripheral vascular disease are strongly associated with smoking. Cessation of smoking, about ten years, reduces the risks for these three vascular diseases to the nonsmoker's level.

Cancer

Many cancers, oral, pharyngeal, laryngeal, esophageal, lung, pancreatic, kidney, and bladder are strongly associated with tobacco. Janerick, et al. (1990) estimate that 17 percent of lung cancer cases in nonsmokers could be the result of exposure to passive smoke during their childhood and adolescent years. The Surgeon General's report in 1982 stated that cigarette smoking is the major single cause of cancer mortality in the United States.

Pregnancy

Smoking by a pregnant female is associated with low birth weight of the infant, miscarriage, stillbirth, and bleeding problems during pregnancy.

Withdrawal

Short-term effects of nicotine withdrawal include nausea, diarrhea, headache, drowsiness, insomnia, irritability, and poor concentration. Increased appetite along with an intense craving for tobacco may persist for months.

Treatment/Rehabilitation

Most people who quit using tobacco do so unassisted by any formal program or medication. Encouragement and counseling by the physician or nurse may be helpful. Nicotine replacement therapy by patch or gum may help some individuals break the habit. It is important that the client not smoke while using the patch. Serious adverse effects may be experienced with a high serum nicotine level. It can be toxic. Later, a gradual withdrawal of the nicotine patch can be accomplished.

An exercise program will help with stress management and minimize possible weight gain. Relaxation techniques will also reduce stress. Support by family and significant others for the person quitting tobacco use may help the process. A lack of support may greatly increase the difficulty of quitting for the individual.

METHYLPHENIDATE HYDROCHLORIDE (RITALIN)

Currently, there is an increase in the use (misuse and overuse) of Ritalin that is becoming a growing problem. Ritalin is an accepted treatment for children with attention deficit disorder with hyperactivity (ADDH). Although Ritalin is a CNS stimulant, there is a paradoxical calming effect on children with ADDH. Too many children are being given Ritalin without thorough testing to eliminate other causes of attention deficit. These children have the potential for dependence.

HALLUCINOGENS

Hallucinogens refers to a group of naturally occurring and synthetic agents that produce essentially the same mind altering effects.

Lysergic acid diethylamide (LSD), a manufactured chemical compound, is perhaps the most widely known and used of these drugs. In the past, LSD has been used as a legitimate medication and in research. In the 1960s when its abuse became so widespread, the manufacturer refused to supply it for research. It had already been discontinued as a useful medication. It is generally taken orally but can be injected intravenously.

Psilocybin and psilocin are naturally occurring organic compounds found in some mushrooms that grow in the United States and Mexico. These mush-

rooms have been used for centuries in southern Mexico primarily in religious ceremonies. Fresh or dried mushrooms, sometimes mixed with food, are ingested orally.

Dimethyltryptamine (DMT) and diethyltryptamine (DET) are found in tropical plant leaves and seeds. For centuries they have been dried and powdered and used as snuff. They are not orally active. Sometimes the powder is added to tobacco or marijuana.

Mescaline is the active ingredient in peyote cactus found growing in the southwestern United States and Mexico. It is the only legally used hallucinogen. Members of the Native American Church of the United States may use it for religious purposes. It is ingested orally. A cross-tolerance to LSD and psilocybin occurs. There are several amphetamine-like hallucinogens. Probably the two best known are 2,5 dimethyl-4-ethylamphetamine (DOM) and methylenedioxyamphetamine (MDMA, ecstasy) which are chemically manufactured compounds. These are usually taken orally but may be injected intravenously or inhaled.

Incidence

The use of hallucinogens declined throughout the 1980s. The early 1990s indicated that LSD was making a comeback. The 1990 and 1991 annual survey of high school seniors found that for the first time since 1976, more seniors had used LSD than cocaine in the previous twelve months (Nagy, 1992; Seligmann, et al., 1992).

Signs and Symptoms

The functioning of both the peripheral nervous system and the central nervous system is altered by hallucinogens. They increase blood pressure and body temperature, produce mydriasis (dilated pupils), distort time and distance, impair rational judgment, and cause visual **hallucinations** (seeing things that are not really there) and delusions. **Synthesiasis**, hearing colors and seeing sounds, occurs. A state of either euphoria or depression is experienced. The depression with feelings of anxiety, panic, or suicidal tendencies is termed a "bad trip." Flashbacks may occur years after taking the drug. Their occurrence and frequency are unpredictable but seem to happen in times of high stress.

Potential for Addiction

There is no physical dependence but possible psychological dependence.

Associated Problems/Disorders

Personality changes occur with LSD use and may happen after a single LSD experience. Acceptable social behaviors seem to diminish with the use of hallucinogens.

Withdrawal

There is no withdrawal seen.

Treatment/Rehabilitation

A person on a "bad trip" should be carefully watched to prevent self-injury. Reassurance, support and "talking down" should be done in a quiet, pleasant manner. Keep the person sitting up or walking. Closing the eyes intensifies the "bad trip." Remind the person that the drug is doing this and the effects will soon go away.

After cessation of chronic hallucinogen use, long-term psychotherapy is usually required to determine what needs were fulfilled by the use of these drugs. A twelve-step program and family assistance are usually necessary to reinforce the decision to remain abstinent. If the client is upset by flashbacks or the fear of flashbacks, an anxiolytic drug such as diazepam (Valium) may be ordered.

PHENCYCLIDINE (PCP)

PCP was made for use as an anesthetic agent but it produced such adverse reactions that it was withdrawn from clinical trials. Abuse was so great that legal manufacture was stopped in 1978. However, it can easily be manufactured in an unsophisticated laboratory from simple materials. The degree of purity varies widely. It is often found as a contaminant in other street drugs.

Incidence

PCP is primarily used by adolescents and young adults with the first use between the ages of thirteen and fifteen years. About three percent of those between the ages of twelve and seventeen years have used PCP (Nagy, 1992).

Signs and Symptoms

There are usually four phases with the symptoms dose related. Acute toxicity is characterized by visual disturbances, auditory hallucinations, combativeness, catatonia, convulsions, and coma, and lasts about three days. The toxic psychosis phase has visual and auditory hallucinations, agitation, paranoid delusions, and disturbed judgment, and lasts about seven days. The third phase has psychotic episodes including thought disorders, paranoid ideation, and effect disorders much like schizophrenia and lasts a month or more. Depression is the fourth phase that may include suicide. The use of other street drugs may alleviate the depression. Behavior is highly unpredictable. Death can occur from respiratory depression.

Potential for Addiction

Even chronic use does not produce physical dependence. Psychological dependence does develop as evidenced by a craving for PCP.

Associated Problems/Disorders

Seizures are a common occurrence with PCP. Hypertension and hyperthermia must be treated before they become a crisis situation. **Opisthotonos**, a complete arching of the body, usually is relieved as the blood level of PCP decrease. Cardiac arrhythmias may need interventions by a cardiologist. Acute renal failure may result from the use of PCP. Strokes also have been reported.

Withdrawal

PCP is fat soluble and its effects are felt weeks after the last use as it is gradually released from the fatty tissue into the circulation.

Treatment/Rehabilitation

Treatment should begin in an inpatient setting because of the high risk of suicide. The goal is to keep the client from resuming drug use. Sedatives may be used and urinary acidifiers such as ascorbic acid may be given to increase excretion of PCP. Minimal confrontation should be used. Provide a nonthreatening, supportive environment. Decrease stimulation and do not try to "talk down" as with the hallucinogens. This may precipitate an acute psychotic reaction.

Expect minimal involvement initially in group or individual therapy. Vocational counseling and training may enhance self-esteem. Body awareness, yoga, and progressive relaxation help the client focus and improve attention span and concentration. Encourage participation in a self-help group such as Narcotics Anonymous (NA).

Table 9-8

OPIOIDS

Natural Opiates:

    morphine sulfate

    codeine sulfate

Semisynthetic opiates:

    heroin

    hydromorphone hydrochloride (Dilaudid)

    oxymorphone hydrochloride (Numorphan)

    oxycodone (in Percodan)

    hydrocodone (in Hycodan)

Synthetic opiates:

    meperidine hydrochloride (Demerol)

    methadone hydrochloride (Dolophine)

    propoxyphene (Darvon)

Agonist-antagonists:

    pentazocine (Talwin)

    nalbuphine hydrochloride (Nubain)

    butorphanol tartrate (Stadol)

OPIOIDS

Opioids is a term used to include the naturally occurring opiates, the semisynthetic opiates, the synthetic opiates, and the agonist-antagonists. Table 9-8 provides examples of these opioids.

Incidence

Kleber (1994) describes the 1990s as the decade of heroin. Cocaine addicts are switching to heroin. Heroin is easily available, the purity is higher than in decades, and the cost continues to drop.

Signs and Symptoms

All of these drugs affect the central nervous system causing mental changes, euphoria, drowsiness, analgesia, constricted pupils, and depressed respirations. These changes become more pronounced as the dose is increased.

Opioids increase stomach tone, decrease intestinal peristalsis, and increase the tone of the anal sphincter. This all adds up to constipation. Prolonged drug use may result in a fecal impaction.

Peripheral blood vessels are dilated by opioids and orthostatic hypotension frequently occurs. The work of the heart is not changed by opioids so they are frequently used to treat the severe pain of a myocardial infarction.

Tolerance may develop to one or more of the effects of opioids but not to others. For example, morphine addicts will always have pinpoint pupils even when the euphoric effects are not experienced. Tolerance to one opioid usually means tolerance to other opioids as well. Withdrawal symptoms from one opioid can be suppressed by using another opioid.

Potential for Addiction

The potential for addiction is high.

Associated Problems/ Disorders

Abuse of opioids is not associated with the induction of physical diseases. However, the intravenous route of drug abuse is considered a factor in contracting acquired immune deficiency syndrome (AIDS).

Withdrawal

Withdrawal symptoms are dependent on drug purity, dose, and route of administration. It is characterized by a rebound excitability of those functions that had been depressed. Symptoms include stomach cramps, nausea, vomiting, diarrhea, diaphoresis, hypertension, aching of bones and muscles, lacrimation, rhinorrhea, gooseflesh, yawning, mydriasis, anxiety, irritability, restlessness, and sometimes paranoia, violence, fear, or depersonalization.

Morphine withdrawal symptoms begin within eight to twelve hours after the last dose and the acute phase is over in about ten to fourteen days. Figure 9-2 illustrates the signs and symptoms of morphine withdrawal. This is the basic pattern of withdrawal for all opioids.

Codeine withdrawal symptoms may be a little less severe than morphine withdrawal. Dilaudid and heroin withdrawal may begin slightly earlier than morphine withdrawal. Meperidine (Demerol) withdrawal begins within three hours and peaks in eight to twelve hours. Propoxyphene (Darvon) withdrawal is considerably milder.

Methadone withdrawal is slower to develop and lasts longer. Symptoms may not occur for one to two days with acute symptoms lasting two to three weeks but not disappearing until six weeks after abstinence begins. Symptoms of fatigue, sluggishness, and irritability may last up to six months.

Withdrawal from the agonist-antagonists begins in

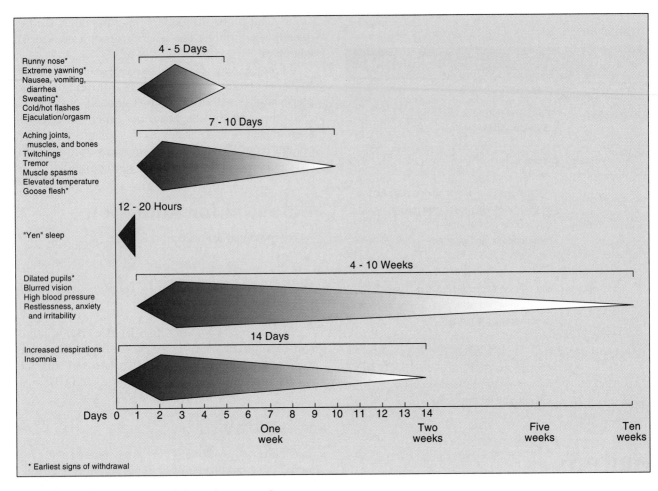

FIGURE 9-2 Morphine withdrawal signs and symptoms.

six to eight hours and is usually over in eight days. The symptoms are the same as morphine only in a milder form.

Treatment/Rehabilitation

Initial treatment is symptomatic and supportive of vital functions until the acute phase is over.

Detoxification

Several methods currently used for opioid detoxification are: methadone, clonidine, and clonidine/naltrexone.

Methadone   Methadone is given and the dose adjusted to keep withdrawal symptoms under control. The dose is gradually reduced over a period of three to six months. Routine and random urine testing is usually done to ensure no other drug use.

Clonidine   Clonidine hydrochloride (Catapres), an antihypertensive, has not yet been given Federal Drug Administration (FDA) approval for use in controlling withdrawal. However, clonidine has been so widely used to suppress opioid withdrawal symptoms both in the United States and abroad, that it has become an accepted alternative to gradual methadone reduction. Clonidine should not be used on clients who have taken tricyclic antidepressants within three weeks, on pregnant clients, those with a history of psychosis, cardiac arrhythmias, hypotension, or those on antihypertensive medications. The time frame for methadone and clonidine detoxification is approximately the same.

Clonidine/naltrexone   Naltrexone hydrochloride (Trexan) produces immediate severe withdrawal from opioids by replacing the opioid at the receptor site. By giving clonidine an hour or two before the naltrexone, the withdrawal symptoms are substantially relieved. Also, oxazepam (Serax) is often given to relieve muscle spasms and prochlorperazine (Compazine) to prevent vomiting. Detoxification is completed in five days. Naltrexone alone may be continued to prevent a relapse.

Counseling/Self-help Groups

Individual and/or group counseling must go hand in hand with the detoxification to help the client learn new methods of coping with life's stresses. Participation in Narcotics Anonymous (NA) helps the client maintain abstinence from drugs.

INHALANTS

Inhalants are inexpensive and easy to obtain. Examples are toluene (glues), gasoline, kerosene, isopropyl alcohol, lacquer thinner, acetone, benzene, naptha, carbon tetrachloride, fluorocarbons (aerosols), correction fluid, and nitrous oxide. They are rapidly absorbed into the brain and stored in body fat.

Incidence

Male junior high students are the most common users.

Signs and Symptoms

The desired effect of euphoria is followed by nausea, headache, and amnesia. Other effects of using inhalants include dizziness, unsteady gait, slurred speech, auditory and visual hallucinations, drowsiness, hypotension, heightened sexual response due to profound vasodilation, stupor, unconsciousness, and coma. Heavy use can lead to hypoxia, multiple organ damage, and death. Airway freezing and/or laryngospasm can be caused by nitrous oxide.

Behaviors that may indicate inhalant abuse include decreased school performance; loss of interest in extracurricular, family, and social activities; and the onset of legal problems.

Potential for Addiction

The potential for addiction is high for psychological dependence only.

Associated Problems/ Disorders

Chronic pulmonary irritation and/or chemical pneumonitis may be caused by the use of inhalants. Toluene may cause renal tubular acidosis. Fluorocarbons sensitize the myocardium to catacholemines and may cause arrhythmias.

Withdrawal

There are no withdrawal symptoms.

Treatment/Rehabilitation

Initial treatment is to provide oxygen and respiratory support. Participation in a traditional chemical dependency program is often needed. An adolescent twelve-step group is very helpful. Individual and family counseling are essential.

ANABOLIC STEROIDS

Anabolic steroids are compounds made from testosterone or made synthetically. They cause both androgenic (masculinizing) and anabolic (tissue building) effects. Most people use anabolic steroids for their anabolic effects. Medically, they are used in the treatment of some anemias and in some cancer therapies. The use of anabolic steroids is banned by the International Olympic Committee and the National Collegiate Athletic Association.

Incidence

Primarily, athletes and young males abuse anabolic steroids for the effect on muscle mass.

Signs and Symptoms

The commonly perceived effects of anabolic steroids are an increase in skeletal muscle mass, enhanced physical performance of the skeletal muscles, increased body weight, and improved athletic ability. However, there is no conclusive evidence that these perceived effects are medically accurate.

Other effects found when anabolic steroids are used include hepatocellular damage, cholestasis, hepatoadenoma, hepatocarcinoma, acne, hirsutism, male-pattern baldness, a deepening of the voice, increased cholesterol level, increased blood pressure, decreased glucose tolerance, mood swings, aggressiveness, depression, psychosis, and hepatitis or HIV infection if needles are shared. In males, there is testicular atrophy, oligospermia, impotence, prostatic hypertrophy, prostatic carcinoma, and gynecomastia. In females, there is amenorrhea, clitoromegaly, uterine atrophy, breast atrophy, and teratogenicity.

These effects seem to be reversible when the anabolic steroids are no longer taken except for the male-pattern baldness, liver tumors, and gynecomastia in males; clitoral enlargement, virilization, and male-pattern baldness in females. The increased aggressiveness and euphoria are probably beneficial during athletic competitions but otherwise may cause severe social problems.

Potential for Addiction

The potential for addiction is moderate.

Withdrawal

Symptoms of withdrawal include lethargy, abdominal muscle cramps, constipation, headache, and depression.

Treatment/Rehabilitation

Treatment of withdrawal focuses on providing symptom relief for the client and counseling to build self-esteem and self-confidence in abilities without the use of anabolic steroids.

NURSING PROCESS

Assessment

The subjective and objective data given are related to substance abuse and dependence in general. Data specific to a specific substance have already been given throughout the chapter.

Subjective Data

The client will often describe being very relaxed, feeling wonderful, having a headache, fatigue, depression, sleep disturbance, suppression of appetite, dizziness, hallucinations, paranoia, anxiety, emotional lability, memory loss, heightened sexual desire (with early use), or loss of sexual desire (with continued use). Problems in various areas of life are common, such as frequent job changes; marital conflict, separation and/or divorce; work related accidents, lateness, absenteeism; and legal problems including arrest for driving while intoxicated. The client may describe having falls or fights and financial problems. Assess normal diet pattern and the presence of any disease conditions.

Ask the client, "How often do you use drugs/alcohol? How much do you usually use? Have you ever used drugs/alcohol more than you use them now? When? Under what circumstances? What substance did you last use?" The information received from the client may not always be accurate. Validation with the family or significant other is helpful.

Objective Data

Neglect of health and personal care is often evident. The client may have dental caries, bad breath, gingivitis, unkempt appearance, and be undernourished or malnourished. If substances have been inhaled, there may be irritation and bleeding of the nasal mucosa, destruction of the nasal mucosa and cartilaginous structures, or depression of respirations. If substances have been injected intravenously, there will be scarring of veins (needle marks, track marks), possibly skin infections, enlarged lymph nodes, and hematomas.

The client may appear older than the stated age, have chronic cough producing brown to black sputum, dilated or pinpoint pupils, tremors, slurred speech, lack of coordination, frequent episodes of sexually transmitted diseases, jaundice, or vomiting. There may be tachycardia, hypertension, ascites, or petichiae.

Nursing Diagnoses

Possible nursing diagnoses for a client with substance abuse or dependence may include:

1. Nutrition, altered, less than body requirements.
2. Self-care deficit.
3. Injury, high risk for.
4. Sleep pattern disturbance.
5. Activity intolerance.
6. Physical mobility, impaired.
7. Sensory-perceptual alterations.
8. Communication, impaired, verbal.
9. Infection, high risk for.
10. Fluid volume excess.
11. Thought processes, altered.
12. Coping, individual, ineffective.
13. Self-esteem disturbance.
14. Violence, high risk for.
15. Anxiety.
16. Social interaction, impaired.
17. Hopelessness.
18. Powerlessness.
19. Family coping, compromised, ineffective.

Goals

There are several overall goals for the care of a client with a substance abuse problem.

1. The client will abstain from using psychoactive substances.
2. The client will adhere to the treatment plan.
3. The client will make lifestyle changes to maintain abstinence.
4. The client will engage in behaviors that foster good health.

Other goals specific to nursing diagnoses must be formulated on an individual basis.

Nursing Interventions

Nursing interventions include active listening, providing care in a nonjudgmental manner, teaching health promotion, and referral to self-help groups or individual counseling. Other nursing interventions must be specific for the goals and nursing diagnoses identified for the individual client.

1. Provide well-balanced diet. Monitor intake and lab tests results. Assess for GI bleeding.
2. Assist with personal hygiene. Encourage self-care.
3. Administer medications as ordered to decrease or prevent symptoms of withdrawal. Keep call light in client's reach. Keep side rails up.
4. Provide warm milk at bedtime. Plan with client a time for bed. Encourage use of relaxation techniques. Reassure client that insomnia will improve.
5. Encourage client to do active ROM exercises. Encourage adequate diet intake.
6. Assist client to turn in bed. Assist client to ambulate as able. Answer call light promptly.
7. Do not argue with client if having hallucinations. Remind client of day, time, and place.
8. Watch client's nonverbal communication. Ask "yes-no" questions.
9. Encourage good personal hygiene. Inspect skin for integrity. Administer antibiotics as ordered. Monitor vital signs.
10. Monitor I & O. Monitor lab tests results.
11. Administer vitamins as ordered. Provide cues as needed. Encourage adequate diet intake.
12. Assess coping patterns to identify strengths and weaknesses. Actively listen to client. Refer to appropriate community agencies.
13. Assist client to identify areas of low self-esteem. Encourage client participation in group therapy. Refer to individual counseling as needed. Actively listen to client.
14. Administer medications as ordered. Monitor client closely. Use restraints as ordered. Keep bed in low position and side rails up.
15. Encourage use of relaxation exercises. Refer client for counseling as needed. Encourage participation in physical exercise.
16. Introduce client to other recovering persons. Encourage client to participate in self-help group.
17. Provide spiritual support if asked. Encourage client to verbalize loss of hope. Encourage client to have hope.
18. Involve client in decision making when possible. Give positive reinforcement for abstinence.
19. Encourage family to participate in treatment program. Refer to counseling as needed.

Evaluation

Each goal must be evaluated to determine how it has been met by the client.

GERONTOLOGICAL CONSIDERATIONS

- The older smoker is less motivated to quit—has survived this long.
- Misuse, using drug for something other than intended or exceeding the dose of prescription and over-the-counter drugs, is more common than abuse or dependence.
- Alcohol impairs cardiac function and decreases cardiac output and efficiency.
- Substances that decrease respirations can increase the frequency of mental confusion.
- Decreased coordination from alcohol or other substances is associated with more falls leading to fractures of the wrist, back, and hips.
- Chronic medical conditions can be made worse from even minimal use of alcohol or other drugs as they can change the effect of prescribed medications.
- Unrealistic expectations of retirement may lead to use of mood altering substances to relieve depression and boredom.

CO-DEPENDENCY

Co-dependency was first recognized by those working with families of alcoholics. It is a learned pattern of feeling and behaving, a problem with relationships. In healthy relationships, people share love, concern, and respect for each other. There is equal give-and-take. This is termed interdependence. In unhealthy relationships, people are often out of touch with their own needs and feelings. They may be unwilling or unable to take care of themselves and have little self-esteem. Only by fulfilling the expectations of others do they feel good about themselves. This is termed co-dependence. Co-dependent persons live based on what others think of them. They always try to meet the needs of others, demand love from others, and manipulate and control the lives of others.

Serious family problems like addictions, abuse, family secrets, or other major stresses cause confusion and put a family at risk. Co-dependent behavior thrives when fear, guilt, blame, and low self-esteem become evident. When family members do not relate to each other in positive ways or when their interactions do not provide a healthy environment, the family is called dysfunctional. Many children grow up in dysfunctional families and learn to be co-dependent.

Co-dependency tends to run in families. Parents cannot teach their children how to cope in healthy ways if they do not know how themselves. Without intervention or a conscious change by the individual, a pattern of co-dependent behavior will continue in other relationships.

Characteristics

Persons who are co-dependent have specific characteristics or traits. They have low self-esteem, never feel they are good enough, and often feel shame. Emotions are denied. They are out of touch with their own feelings and deny their own needs. Their smile is phony much of the time. Problems with communication become evident as they have trouble expressing their needs and feelings. Often they say the opposite to hide their true feelings. They expect others to read their mind. Relationship problems occur because they are afraid of being hurt or that others might learn of their secret feelings and reject them. They cannot risk loving and losing. Relationships are desired but walls are always put up.

Co-dependent persons live through others. They are people pleasers who would rather give than take. The approval of others means they are "OK." They think they can fix others. The feeling of powerlessness occurs because they give power to others by looking to them for approval. They go to extremes. For a while they will try very hard for approval and then they will not try at all or they will keep negative feelings inside

---

Table 9-9

CHARACTERISTICS OF THE CO-DEPENDENT PERSON	
Caretaking	"I always give to others. No one gives to me."
Obsession	"I can't stop worrying about ____ problems."
Denial	"I pretend I don't have problems."
Poor communication	"No one understands me."
Lack of trust	"I don't trust myself."
Anger	"I resent feeling controlled and manipulated."

(Adapted from Kalman, N. and Waughfield, C. (1993). Mental Health Concepts *3rd ed. Albany, NY: Delmar Publishers, Inc.)*

---

with a smile on their face and then blow up over some little thing. Table 9-9 lists some characteristics of the co-dependent person.

Treatment

Professional help is usually necessary to change co-dependent behavior. The goal of treatment is to help the co-dependent person feel happy and good about himself or herself. Therapy sessions focus on identifying and reconnecting with the true self, dealing with feelings, learning how to communicate feelings, learning to trust, setting boundaries for relationships, and taking charge of their own life.

THE IMPAIRED NURSE

Most states now have peer assistance programs to help nurses impaired by either alcohol or other substances. Substance abuse and dependence are greater problems among nurses than among the general public. Nurses have access to many controlled substances. The impaired nurse often requests to give medications, makes medication errors, and "wastes" drugs frequently. This nurse may wear long sleeves and spend an extraordinary amount of time in the bathroom.

Peer assistance programs first appeared in 1980. They have been formed through the state nursing association, the state board of nursing, or through joint effort of both the state nursing association and the state board of nursing. The goals of the peer assistance programs are to assist the impaired nurse to receive treatment; protect the public from impaired nurses; help the recovering nurse reenter the nursing workforce in a planned, safe manner; and monitor the nurse's recovery for a time. The state board of nursing may restrict access to controlled substances for the recovering nurse for some period of time.

Prior to the peer assistance programs, impaired nurses were generally just dismissed from employment. Then they would find employment at another health care agency where substance abuse or dependence would continue. This often went on for years.

As the name implies, peer assistance programs are staffed with nurses to help nurses. Many of the staff are volunteers who work in psychiatric nursing or substance abuse centers or who are themselves recovering from substance abuse. According to Lippman (1992), it is best not to cover up for a colleague with a substance abuse problem. Report the situation to a supervisor who can arrange for the nurse to receive help.

► CASE STUDY

Joe, age nineteen, quit school three years ago. He has a part-time job at a fast food place but has been tardy or absent quite often lately. Sometimes he is easy to get along with, and sometimes he is aggressive and difficult. His mother, with whom he lives, says he is a good boy and does not give her any trouble. Joe was brought to the emergency room by a friend after he passed out. His temperature is 99°F, respirations 10, and pupils are pinpoint. There are track marks on both arms.

The following questions will guide your development of a Nursing Care Plan for the case study.

1. List signs and symptoms, other than Joe's, that a client may experience as a heroin addict.

2. List diagnostic tests that may be ordered.

3. List subjective and objective data the nurse should obtain.

4. Write three individualized nursing diagnoses and goals for Joe.

5. List resources within the medical center and local area that could assist Joe.

6. Describe the use of methadone in heroin addiction.

7. List teaching that Joe will need as a part of his rehabilitation.

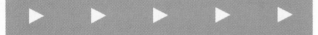 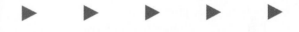

SUMMARY

- Substance abuse and dependence have been problems for centuries.
- Factors related to substance abuse include individual, family patterns, lifestyle, environmental, and developmental.
- A false positive result on a drug screening test may be caused by ingestion of poppy seeds or use of a Vicks® inhaler.
- Detoxification is the first step in the treatment and rehabilitation of a substance abuser or dependent.
- Street drugs vary in strength and purity. Cheaper or easier to obtain drugs are often mixed with a higher priced drug.
- Neglect of health and personal care are often evident in substance abuse and dependence.
- Nurses have a higher incidence of substance abuse and dependence than the general public.
- Most states have peer assistance programs for impaired nurses.

Review Questions

1. Schedule II substances:
   a. can be sold as over-the-counter drugs.
   b. have high abuse and dependence potential.
   c. can have prescription refilled for six months.
   d. have no accepted medical use in the United States.

2. Substance use and abuse are:
   a. influenced by advertising.
   b. caused by a lack of education.
   c. rejected by all religious groups.
   d. caused by a chromosomal abnormality.

3. Prevention of substance abuse must be focused on:
   a. parents.
   b. children.
   c. teenagers.
   d. young adults.

4. Drug screening tests:
    a. are very accurate.
    b. indicate the level of abuse.
    c. indicate exposure to a substance.
    d. can test for all substances of abuse.

5. The substance most often chosen for abuse or dependence is:
    a. heroin.
    b. cocaine.
    c. alcohol.
    d. marijuana.

6. Alcoholics Anonymous is:
    a. the newest self-help group.
    b. a short-term temporary help group.
    c. a government agency to help those with an alcohol problem.
    d. a self-help group providing a holistic approach to abstinence.

7. Urinary acidifiers are used in the treatment of:
    a. opioids and LSD.
    b. amphetamines and PCP.
    c. alcohol and CNS stimulants.
    d. inhalants and benzodiazepines.

8. The use of inhalants:
    a. can be fatal.
    b. includes only glue and paints.
    c. has severe withdrawal symptoms.
    d. is a harmless activity of young male teenagers.

Critical Thinking Questions

1. What is your attitude toward substance abusers?

2. Should drug testing of all health care workers be required?

News Flash

Touted as a potent "date-rape" drug, Rohypnol, a sleeping pill, is sold by prescription in sixty countries but not in the United States. It is used to "doctor drinks" causing the recipient to black out for twelve to fourteen hours. Rohypnol enhances the effects of alcohol. Using them together raises the possibility of an overdose.

Rohypnol is not approved for use in the United States, but until March 11, 1996 travelers could bring in a three-month supply for personal use. Most of the drug was entering from Mexico through Texas. In a recent three-week period, an estimated 100,000 doses came into the country. Many authorities know little about this drug and only find it when they make a "bust" for other drugs. Classified as a Schedule IV drug, Rohypnol possession is a very minor offense. The United States Customs Service has now banned Rohypnol from being brought into the country. The Drug Enforcement Administration (DEA) wants to make it a Schedule I drug like heroin and LSD. This would make possession a greater offense and allow more severe penalties.

"Rohypnol has become one of the fastest-growing problem drugs among teens, gang members, and 20-something clubcrawlers. . . ." The little white pills have many street names such as roofies, la rocha, ropies, rips, roachies, and rope (Rodriguez, P., 1996).

SECTION II

UNIT
4

Concepts of
Medical-Surgical Care

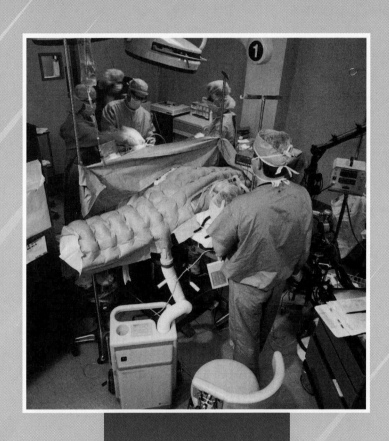

CHAPTER
10

Nursing Assessment

Susan L. Bredemeyer
with Cheryl Erickson

▶ KEY TERMS

adventitious
affect
amplitude
aneroid
ascites
auscultation
borborygmi
crackles
cyanosis
dullness
flatness
inspection
orthostatic hypotension
palpation
percussion
pleural friction rub
rate
rhythm
sibilant wheezes
sonorous wheezes
tympany

LEARNING OBJECTIVES

Upon completion of this chapter the learner should be able to:
- Define key terms.
- Identify the components of functional health patterns.
- Utilize the framework of functional health to facilitate a holistic assessment process.
- Analyze the components of the head-to-toe assessment.
- Incorporate the four assessment techniques within the head-to-toe assessment.
- Utilize the head-to-toe assessment in clinical situations.

▶ *MAKING THE CONNECTION*

INTRODUCTION

Within the scope of the nursing profession, a complete health history and physical assessment are necessary tools used to analyze each client's needs in a holistic manner. Nursing assessment includes both physical and psychosocial aspects to evaluate a client's condition. A nurse demonstrates caring, respect, and concern for each client when doing a nursing assessment.

A thorough nursing assessment must include the use of both a health history and a physical assessment. To perform a health history, the nurse interviews a client and identifies how she adjusts to or lives within her environment. This data is subjective data or what a client says about oneself or aspects of one's life during the history-taking interview. During the physical examination the nurse collects objective data, which includes observations made by the nurse while utilizing the assessment techniques of inspection, palpation, percussion and auscultation. Other sources of objective data are laboratory tests, x-rays, and measurements of the client's vital signs, height and weight.

The health history and the physical examination assist the nurse in focusing on the client as a whole. Nursing assessment, therefore, delves into the art and science of nursing to bring forth the most complete history and physical examination possible.

KEY ABBREVIATIONS

The following abbreviations and acronyms are used in this chapter:

AP	apical pulse
BP	blood pressure
LOC	level of consciousness
P	pulse
PERRLA	pupils equal, round, react to light and accommodation
R	respirations
RLQ	right lower quadrant
T	temperature

FUNCTIONAL HEALTH PATTERNS

The health history format provides a guideline for the interview. The nursing health history is different from the medical history in that it focuses on the client's response to the illness. A physician takes a medical history to assist in diagnosis and treatment of an illness. A nurse utilizes a health history to provide individualized care, to determine the impact the illness has on the client and the family, to determine health teaching needs, and to begin discharge planning.

Margory Gordon identified functional health patterns to guide data collection and aid in client problem identification. The functional assessment focuses on the psychosocial, physical, and environmental needs and abilities of clients. It determines the abilities of clients to care for themselves. It includes assessment of Activities of Daily Living (ADLs), such as dressing, toileting, and eating. Other aspects of functional assessment include the determination of ability to cook, manage finances, maintain social relationships, along with assessment of self-concept and coping abilities.

Gordon's Eleven Functional Health Patterns are as follows:

- Health perception/Health management
- Nutritional/Metabolic
- Elimination
- Activity/Exercise
- Sleep/Rest
- Cognitive/Perceptual
- Self-perception/Self-concept
- Role relationship
- Sexuality/Reproductive
- Coping/Stress tolerance
- Value/Belief

According to Bowers et al. (1992), functional assessment explores how individuals adapt and adjust to the environment in which they exist. Throughout the performance of a functional assessment, the interviewer's questions focus more on the norms and usual environment of the client. These questions assist in establishing what is ordinary or purposeful to each individual person. This establishes the holistic identification of the client's life and lifestyle.

Topics for questions the nurse can ask within each of these eleven functional health patterns are described and clarified in Table 10-1. Both a health history as well as a physical examination can be performed by the nurse through the use of topics shared in Table 10-1.

To perform the physical examination or assessment, the nurse may use either a systems format or head-to-toe format. When utilizing a systems approach the nurse assesses all pertinent information related to a particular body system; for example, the neurological, cardiovascular, or respiratory system. The systems format can be difficult to remember, whereas the client's body provides a reminder of what should be systematically assessed in the head-to-toe format. This chapter will focus on head-to-toe assessment. The physical exam column in Table 10-1 does not follow a head-to-toe appraoch. The data acquired in the head-to-toe assessment are grouped under specific health patterns to aid in the identification of client problems and nursing diagnoses.

The initial nursing assessment generally occurs within twenty-four hours of a client's admission to a health care facility, and continues throughout the stay. In a physician's office or health care clinic, the nursing assessment would be completed immediately. Usually a health history is completed prior to the physical examination. However, in emergency situations or when performing care in a health care facility after the initial admitting assessment, it will be necessary to incorporate history-taking within the physical examination. When incorporating a health history within the head-to-toe assessment, the nurse must remember to incorporate questions about the client's habits or usual patterns along with the physical data collected in the head-to-toe assessment. Functional assessment is best done within the framework of the physical assessment since the environment in which each client resides and participates becomes a part of the physical assessment. The functional assessment brings the environment in which the client lives and the physical needs of that client together to establish a holistic picture.

TECHNIQUES FOR ASSESSMENT

The nurse performs the physical or the head-to-toe assessment by using specific assessment techniques. These techniques include: **inspection**, **palpation**, **percussion**, and **auscultation**.

Inspection

Inspection consists of a thorough visual assessment of the client. This visual assessment gives the nurse a description of the body's outward response to its internal functioning. Inspection of the skin, for example, can assist the nurse in identifying signs of a fever through the client's flushed facial cheeks. The skin can also be an indicator of a decreased oxygen supply when **cyanosis**, a bluish or dark purple coloration, is noted in the client's lips or nail beds. Sharing observations with the client during inspection enhances the holistic data collected. For example, when the nurse mentions the observation of visible scars, the client may discuss previous surgeries or hospitalizations.

Table 10-1

GUIDE SHEET FOR NURSING ASSESSMENT

HEALTH HISTORY	PHYSICAL EXAM

HEALTH PERCEPTION/HEALTH MANAGEMENT

HEALTH HISTORY		PHYSICAL EXAM
• *Health Perception*	(1) Statement from patient about how patient views overall health (2) Statement from patient about why patient is hospitalized	• *General Appearance:* *Race:* Caucasian, black, Hispanic, Chinese, other *Gender:* male, female *Age group:* child, teenager, young adult age, middle aged, elderly
• *Lifestyle*—lives:	Alone or specify with whom Type of home Nursing home No known residence	*Body build:* small, average, large *Stature*: (comparison of height and weight): emaciated, obese, stout, stocky, robust, cachectic, rotund) *Grooming*
• *Health Maintenance*		• *Signs of Distress:*
Habits:	*Use of alcohol:* none, type and amount per day, week, month	Any grossly abnormal signs In acute distress = describe In no acute distress
	Use of tobacco: none, quit date, pipe, cigar, cigarettes < 1 pack per day, 1–2 packs per day, > 2 packs per day	• *Mental Status*
	Other Recreational or OTC Drugs: No, yes, Type, Usage	
Preventive Health Behaviors:	*Breast or testicular self-examination:* yes or no *Date of last physical examination* *Date of last dental examination*	
• *Problems that could contribute to falls or accidents*	Age 65 or over Confused and disoriented, hallucinating History of falls Recent history of loss of consciousness, seizure disorder Unsteady on feet/physical limitations Poor eyesight Poor hearing Drug or alcohol problem Postop condition/sedated Language barrier Attitude (resistant, belligerent, combative, fearful) Postural hypotension	
• *Family History—Risk Factors*		

NUTRITIONAL/METABOLIC

HEALTH HISTORY		PHYSICAL EXAM		
• *Previous Dietary Intake:*		• *Height and Weight:*		
Diet:	Regular, no added salt, ADA, soft, low cholesterol, high fiber, low residue, clear liquids, NPO, list other	• *Body Temperature:*		
		• *Skin:*	Color:	Light pink to dark pink or light brown to dark brown.
Vitamins or supplements:	Name			Pallor, flushed, cyanotic, ashen, glossy, jaundiced
Food Preferences:	List		Color Variations:	Erythema, ecchymosis/contusion, petechiae, vitiligo, pigmented
Appetite:	Normal, increased, decreased, presence of nausea or vomiting, decreased taste sensation		Lesions:	Macule, patch
• *Nutritional Impairment:*				Papule, plaque, nodule, tumor, wheal, verruca, nevus
	Inability to swallow (dysphagia): none, to solids or liquids			Vesicle, bulla, pustule, furuncle
	Inability to chew			Erosion, ulcer, fissure
	Inability to feed self			Crust, scab
				Excoriation, abrasion, laceration, incisions

HEALTH HISTORY	PHYSICAL EXAM

NUTRITIONAL/METABOLIC (continued)

HEALTH HISTORY	PHYSICAL EXAM
• **Weight Fluctuations Last 6 months:** None, lbs.Gained/Lost	*Texture:* Smooth, soft, rough, thick, scaling
	Turgor: Return Immediate/return greater than 30 seconds
• **Dentures:** Upper (partial/full), lower (partial/full) Usage—describe	*Temperature and Moisture:* Warm, dry, extremely cool, extremely warm, wet, oily
• **Allergies:** List, NKDA	*Edema:* Absent/0, or 1+, 2+, 3+, 4+
	• **Hair:** *Color:* describe
• **Skin:**	*Length:* describe
History of Skin/ *Healing Problems:* none, abnormal healing, rash, dryness, pruritus, excess perspiration/diaphoresis	*Texture:* Fine, coarse, pliant, brittle, dull, shiny, lustrous, glossy
	Amount: thick, thin, normal
Usual Hygiene *Practices:* Bath/shower, give frequency	*Distribution:* Even, alopecia, hirsutism, sparse
Skin Care Aids: List	• **Nails:** *Color:* Pink, pale, cyanotic splinter hemorrhages, poor capillary return
	Shape: Beau's lines, clubbing, spooned
	Texture: Smooth, hard, jagged, soft
	Nailbed: Smooth, firm, pink, inflamed
	• **Decubitus Risk Factor:** Calculate and give score
	• **Mouth:**
	Mucous Membranes: *Color:* Pink, pale, cyanotic, reddened
	Consistency: Smooth, moist, dry, bleeding, ulcers, presence of white patches, describe lesions
	Teeth: *Number:* Within Normal Limits, edentulous
	Position/condition: Stable fixation, smooth surfaces and edges, loose or broken teeth, jagged edges, dental caries, sordes, crooked, protruding, crowded, irregular, broken
	Color: Pearly white and shiny, darkened, brown discoloration
	Gums: Pink, pale, reddened, moist, clearly defined margins, dry, firm, edematous, tenderness, bleeding, ulcers, white patches, receding, shrunken
	Tongue: *Symmetry/texture:* Moist, papillae present, symmetrical appearance, midline fissures, dry, nodules/ulcers present, papillae or fissures absent, asymmetrical, coated, swollen
	• **Dietary Intake:** regular, no added salt, ADA, soft, low cholesterol, high fiber, low residue, clear liquids, NPO, list other

	Amount eaten: 50% or less = poor
	    50–75% = fair
	    75–100% = good

	• **Fluid Intake during care:**
	Oral: give in cc's *IV:* give in cc's

(continued)

HEALTH HISTORY	PHYSICAL EXAM

ELIMINATION

HEALTH HISTORY	PHYSICAL EXAM
• *Previous Urinary Pattern:*	• *Urinary* Mode: indwelling catheter, external catheter, incontinence
Frequency of voiding: every _____ hours or _____ times/day	Color: pale to dark yellow, straw colored, amber
Problems: Presence of incontinence, dysuria, hematuria, nocturia, urgency, hesitancy	Characteristics: clear, cloudy, hazy, sediment, aromatic
• *Previous Bowel Pattern:*	• *Bowel/Stool:*
Number of BMs/day, constipation, diarrhea, incontinence, presence of ostomy	Bowel Sounds: audible, hyperactive, hypoactive, inaudible, present, active, not present equally in all quadrants
Use of laxatives, enemas, suppositories	Abdominal appearance: *Contour:* rounded, flat, distended, rotund, scaphoid, enlarged, protruding, hard, rigid, relaxed, taut, pendulous, tympanites
Last bowel movement	*Symmetry:* symmetrical, asymmetrical
• *Presence of heavy perspiration/diaphoresis*	*Surface motion:* no movement, bounding peristalsis, bounding pulsations
	Feces: *Color:* dark brown, med. brown, mustard yellow, green, dark red/bright red, black, tarry, clay-colored
	Amount: small, med., large
	Consistency: soft, semisolid, formed, hard, loose
	Characteristics: mucoid, foul-smelling, aromatic, pencil-like, bulky, pasty
	• *Drainage:*
	Amount: give in cc's, describe size on dressing
	Color: pink, red, green, brown, white, yellow
	Odor: aromatic, unique, strong
	Consistency: thick, mucoid, watery, thin, frothy, tenacious
	Characteristics: purulent, suppurative, mucopurulent, sanguineous, blood tinged, serosanguineous, serous
	• *Emesis:* hematemesis, bile-colored, amount, contents
	• *Fluid output during care:*
	Categorize each type in cc's, then total

ACTIVITY/EXERCISE

HEALTH HISTORY	PHYSICAL EXAM
• *Previous pattern of activity:*	• *Present pattern of activity:*
eating/drinking, bathing, dressing/grooming, toileting, bed mobility, transferring, ambulating, stair climbing, shopping, cooking, home maintenance. Rate as independent, use of assistive device, assistance from others, assistance from person and equipment, dependent/unable	eating/drinking, bathing, dressing/grooming, toileting, bed mobility, transferring, ambulating, stair climbing, shopping, cooking, home maintenance. Rate as independent, use of assistive device, assistance from others, assistance from person and equipment, dependent/unable
• *History of tolerance limitations:*	• *Musculoskeletal:*
pain, stiffness, dyspnea, fatigue, frequent pauses in activity to rest, dizziness	*Posture:* relaxed, shoulders back, tense, rigid, slumped, asymmetrical posture, kyphosis, lordosis

HEALTH HISTORY	PHYSICAL EXAM

ACTIVITY/EXERCISE (continued)

HEALTH HISTORY	PHYSICAL EXAM
• **Mobility aids:** crutches, bedside commode, walker, cane, splint/brace, wheelchair, other.	*Muscle tone:* slight resistance, spasticity, rigidity, flaccidity
• **Exercise pattern/wellness activities:** Type, frequency, length	*Muscle strength:* Rate all major muscle groups according to the following scale—
• **Limitations in ability:** missing limbs, paralysis, deformities, casts	0 = No muscular contraction
• **Vital sign ranges:** either since hospitalization or verbal from patient	1 = Barely flicker of contraction
• **Use of diversional activities**	2 = Active movement with gravity removed
	3 = Active movement against gravity
	4 = Active movement against gravity and some resistance
	5 = Active movement against full resistance with no fatigue
	Gait: Spastic hemiparesis, scissors, steppage, sensory ataxia, cerebellar ataxia, Parkinsonism
	Balance: Steady, unsteady
	Range of motion: unlimited, full, limited with crepitation or pain, immobile, decreased, restricted
	Weight bearing: Give in percentages, ability to stand on left/right heels/toes, weakness, inability to use either extremity
	• **Cardiorespiratory:**
	Lungs:
	Breath sounds: clear, crackles, rhonchi, wheezes
	Rate: apneic, eupneic, tachypneic, bradypneic
	Rhythm: Regular, irregular
	Depth: deep, shallow
	Cough: continuous, persistent, frequent, productive, nonproductive, spasmodic, paroxysmal, tight, loose, deep, dry, hacking, harsh, painful, rasping, exhaustive
	Use of O_2: flow rate and method of delivery—mask, nasal cannula
	Heart:
	Rate: give in numerical value, tachycardic, bradycardic
	Rhythm: regular, irregular, regularly irregular, irregularly irregular
	Peripheral Vascular:
	BP
	Peripheral Pulses: strong, equal, bounding, thready, imperceptible, weak asymmetrical, absent, 1+, 2+, 3+, 4+
	Sensation: nontender, can identify light and deep touch, paresthesia, tenderness, pain, tingling, burning, stinging, prickling, numb
	Motor: Hand grasps and foot movement: equal, strong, weakness, paralysis
	• **Present tolerance for activity:** pain, stiffness, dyspnea, fatigue, frequent pauses in activity to rest, dizziness

(continued)

HEALTH HISTORY	PHYSICAL EXAM

SLEEP/REST

HEALTH HISTORY	PHYSICAL EXAM
• *Sleep patterns:*	• *Observe appearance:*
Bedtime, hours slept. Routine: AM nap, PM nap, work night shifts, variable work *+-shift	pale, puffy eyes, dark circles
• *Sleep aids used:* medication, food, rituals.	• *Observe behavior:* yawning, dozing, irritability, short attention span
• *Position of comfort*	
• *Problems:* none, early waking, insomnia, nightmares	

COGNITIVE/PERCEPTUAL

HEALTH HISTORY	PHYSICAL EXAM
• *Knowledge level*	• *Memory:*
• *Educational level achieved*	*Long term:* intact, impaired; give example
• *Primary language spoken*	*Short term:* intact, impaired; give example
• *Developmental level*	• *Speech:*
• *Past history of cognitive/perceptual illness*	*Paralanguage:* qualities of speech—pitch, intonation, rate of speaking, voice volume, words that are stressed or accented
• *Past history of sensory perception:*	*Articulation:* articulate, not articulate: describe
Heat, Cold, Taste, Smell, Touch, Vertigo, Hearing, Sight	*Sequencing:* logical, illogical: describe
• *Pain Assessment:* location, intensity, duration, quality, predisposing factors, grade on 1–10 scale	*Appropriateness of content:* appropriate, inappropriate
	Ability to express self verbally: words or types of expression used
	Ability to follow verbal/ written instructions: yes; if no, explain
	• *Neurological:*
	Orientation: person, place, time
	Pupil reaction: sluggish, brisk, PERRLA
	Grasp Strength:
	Level of consciousness: comatose, unresponsive to verbal or painful stimuli, semiconscious, stuporous, drowsy, lethargic, alert, responsive
	• *Perceptual—Cognitive:*
	Hallucination: absent, present
	Delusions: Absent, present
	Attention span: intact, not intact: describe
	• *Sensory:*
	Visual Impairment: absent, present: describe
	Visual Aids: absent, present, glasses, contacts, prosthesis
	Auditory Impairment:: Absent, present: describe—impaired, deaf, tinnitus
	Auditory aide: absent, present
	Other sensory impairments: absent, present: describe

HEALTH HISTORY	PHYSICAL EXAM

SELF-PERCEPTION/SELF-CONCEPT

• *Developmental stage of Life:*	• *Posture*
Give supporting data	• *Eye contact:* present, absent, describe
• *Ability to accomplish age level tasks:*	• *Facial expression (affect):*
Describe	animated, sad, fixed, describe
• *Present health goals:*	• *Grooming:* Hair groomed: yes, no
Ask the patient: How would you describe yourself?	Hygiene: good, poor: describe
What do you consider to be your strengths?	Makeup: present, absent
Are the goals and responses age related?	Shaven: yes, no
• *Body Image*	Dress: neat, not neat: describe
	• *Attitude:* describe
	• *Appropriateness of behavior:*
	appropriate, inappropriate, describe
	• *Mood:* describe
	• *Self-derogatory comments:*
	present, absent, describe
	• *Self-affirmative comments:*
	present, absent, describe
	• *Powerlessness:*
	present, absent, describe
	• *Hopelessness:*
	present, absent, describe
	• *Low self-esteem:*
	present, absent, describe

ROLE RELATIONSHIP

• *Patterns of relating to others*	*Observe patient's interaction with others*
• *Identification of own role*	• Verbal, nonverbal communication: describe
• *Response to authority, peers, subordinates*	• Does patient have visitors?
• *Age, marital status, occupation*	
• *Perceptions of responsibilities in life:*	
situation at home, work, and in the community	

SEXUALITY/REPRODUCTIVE

• *Number of living children, abortions, miscarriages, stillbirths*	• *Breasts:* round, pendulous, sagging, equal, pink with/without presence of striae
• *Sexual self-feelings toward sex, role self-concept*	*Areola:* pink to dark brown, round oval, everted presence of discharge
• *Effect of illness or impairment to sexuality*	• *Genitalia:* presence and distribution of pubic hair, sexually mature, visible lesions, odor, drainage
• *Present sexual activity*	
• *Use of birth control*	
• *Age of onset of menses, menopause*	
• *Last Pap, mammogram*	

(continued)

HEALTH HISTORY	PHYSICAL EXAM
COPING/STRESS TOLERANCE	

• *Coping patterns:* Use of counseling, usual methods of problem solving
• *Support system*
• *Recent loss or change in life situation*
• *Presence of stress-related disorders*
	• *Behavior patterns:* Abusive to self or others
	
	   Nervous, relaxed, controlled, agitated, mood swings: describe
	• *Appearance*
	• *Affect*
	• *Ability to reason and make sound decisions:*
	   able, unable: describe

VALUE/BELIEF	

• *Health/Illness beliefs*
• *Spiritual, cultural, ethnic heritage and pattern of participation in*
• *Concern with meaning of life/death:*
   present, absent, describe
• *Concern with meaning of suffering:*
   present, absent, describe
• *Anger toward God/religion:*
   present, absent, describe
	• *Symbols of Faith:* present, absent, describe
	• *Current religious/cultural ties:*
	   present, absent, describe (Praying, meditation, reading religious materials, clutching religious artifacts, wearing religious jewelry)
	• *Visits from clergy*

(*Courtesy: Lutheran College, Ft. Wayne, IN*)
Barkauskas, V, Stoltenberg-Allen, K., Baumann, L. & Darling-Fiisher, C. (1994) *Health and physical assessment.* St. Louis: Mosby.
Bates, B. (1995) *A guide to physical examination and history taking.* (Sixth ed). Philadelphia: J. B. Lippincott.
Carpenito, L. (1993) *Nursing diagnosis: Application to clinical practice.* (Fifth ed). Philadelphia: J. B. Lippincott.
Cox, H., Hinz, M., Lubno, M., Newfield, S., Ridenour, N., Slater, M., & Sridaromont, K. (1993) *Clinical applications of nursing diagnosis: Adult, child, women's, mental health, gerontic, and home health considerations.* (Second ed). Philadelphia: F. A. Davis.
Taylor, C., Lillis, C., & LeMone, P. (1993) *Fundamentals of nursing: The art and science of nursing care.* (Second ed). Philadelphia: J. B. Lippincott.
Weber, J. (1993) *Health assessment.* (Second ed). Philadelphia: J. B. Lippincott.

Palpation

In palpation, the nurse uses her hands and sense of touch to gather data about the client. The nurse's fingertips touch and put pressure on the client's skin. The purpose of palpation is to detect temperature, texture, pulsations, masses, or tenderness. The nurse's finger pads are placed flat against the client's skin, exerting slight pressure as seen in Figure 10-1. Assessment of the kidneys, liver, spleen, bowel, and fundal height may be accomplished through deep palpation. Pulses are also palpated. The abdomen is palpated for distention, softness, firmness, rigidity, or tenderness.

Percussion

Percussion is used to assess underlying organs and tissues for their location and size and to determine if an organ is solid or filled with fluid or gas. The nurse uses her fingertips to tap the client's body to produce

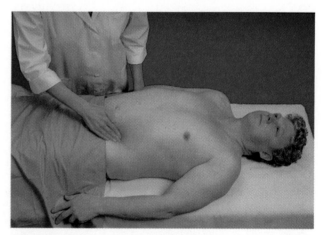

FIGURE 10-1 Palpation, a technique used in physical assessment.

sounds and vibrations. The sounds indicate the density of tissue. The nurse places the middle finger of her nondominant hand on the client's skin in the area to be percussed, then taps lightly with the middle finger of her dominant hand on the distal phalanx of the middle finger positioned on the body surface (Figure 10-2). The nurse taps twice in one place before moving to a new area. Percussion should not be painful to the client. If it is painful, discontinue the percussion and document what happened. Percussion is a skill that requires much practice to master and it is important to be familiar with the sounds produced when percussion is used. A hollow organ, such as the stomach, produces a high-pitched, drumlike sound called **tympany**. The liver, a dense organ, will produce a low-pitched, thud-like sound termed **dullness**. Dullness would also be produced when a client presented with **ascites**, which occurs when the abdomen is filled with fluid. Muscle produces a soft, high-pitched, flat sound called **flatness**. Table 10-2 describes the various percussion tones.

Auscultation

Auscultation is listening to body functions through a stethoscope. It is used whenever the physical assessment requires identification of specific sounds within the body. For example, auscultation of breath sounds enhances the knowledge of lung function. The respiratory, cardiovascular, and gastrointestinal systems also produce sounds that may be auscultated. The apical pulse and bowel sounds are also assessed by auscultation. Identification of fluid in the lungs can be ascertained when abnormal sounds such as crackles or wheezes are heard. Figure 10-3 identifies auscultation.

Utilization of these assessment techniques helps to facilitate a complete and thorough head-to-toe assessment.

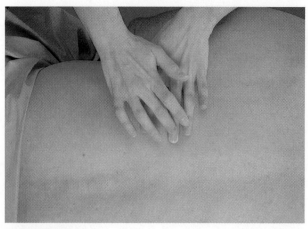

FIGURE 10-2 Percussion, a technique used in physical assessment.

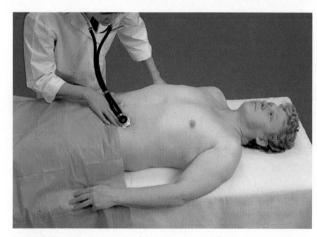

FIGURE 10-3 Auscultation, a technique used in physical assessment.

Table 10-2

DESCRIPTION OF PERCUSSION TONES

Tone	Intensity	Pitch	Duration	Quality	Normal Location
Dullness	Medium	High	Medium	Thudlike	Liver
Flatness	Soft	High	Short	Extreme dullness	Muscle
Hyperresonance	Very Loud	Very Low	Long	Booming	Child's lung
Resonance	Loud	Low	Long	Hollow	Peripheral lung
Tympany	Loud	High	Medium	Drumlike	Stomach

HEAD-TO-TOE ASSESSMENT

Prior to beginning the examination, keep in mind some important concepts to be utilized throughout the examination. Provide for the client's privacy by pulling the curtain, closing the door, and providing appropriate draping of the client. When possible, try to stop distracting noises such as radio or television and people talking. Remember to utilize standard precautions when in contact with any body fluids by using gloves, gowns, or masks when appropriate. Be sure to explain all procedures to the client and maintain confidentiality of data acquired during the examination.

Introduction of Nurse to Client/ General Overview

The nurse's introduction to the client is an important first step at the start of a complete head-to-toe assessment. It is important for the nurse to identify herself and to express her intent for the care of the client and the time frame involved. During this introductory time, it is appropriate for the nurse to utilize inspection to make a general assessment of the client. This overview is the first impression the nurse will have of the client. It is the beginning point of the assessment of the client from head to toe. It includes such aspects as the general state of health, notation of any signs of distress, such as pain or breathing difficulties. It also includes observations regarding the client's awareness of his or her surroundings, body type and posture, facial expressions, and mood. These aspects are assessed throughout the physical assessment as well as initially.

Vital Signs

Once the nurse has established rapport with the client through introductions, measurement of vital signs is the next step in a head-to-toe assessment. Vital signs are the "signs of life" of an individual. They provide a way of connecting the external inspection of each client with the internal functioning of the client's organs. When checking vital signs, the nurse obtains the temperature, pulse, respirations, and blood pressure of the client. See Table 10-3 for normal values and variations.

Temperature

When assessing the client's temperature (T), the nurse can either use an electronic or mercury thermometer. Body temperature can be taken by four routes: oral, rectal, axillary, or tympanic membrane. The route is chosen depending upon the client's age and physical condition. Factors such as age, sex, physical activity, and environment can affect a person's temperature.

Pulse

Assessment of the client's pulse (P) includes the **rate**, **rhythm**, and **amplitude**. The rate is the number of heartbeats counted during a sixty second time frame. The regularity or irregularity of each heartbeat is described as the rhythm, while the amplitude of each heartbeat denotes the fullness of the pulse. If the radial pulse is irregular when palpated, the nurse should check the apical pulse (AP). The other major pulses, temporal, facial, carotid, brachial, femoral, popliteal, posterior tibial, and dorsalis pedis should be assessed when disease or injury are present in those areas.

Usual assessment of the radial pulse occurs for thirty seconds and the number of beats is doubled for documentation. If the pulse rhythm is irregular, assessment must occur for sixty seconds. During the pulse assessment, the nurse should integrate questions about

Table 10-3

VITAL SIGNS AND NORMAL VARIATIONS		
Vital Signs	**Normal Ranges**	
Temperature	Axillary	36.5°C or 97.6°F
	Tympanic	37°C or 98.6°F
	Oral	37°C or 98.6°F
	Rectal	37.5°C or 99.6°F
Pulse	60–100 beats/min.	
Respirations	16–20 resp./min.	
Blood Pressure	90/60–140/90	

Vital Signs	**Variations**	
Temperature	< 36°C or 96.8°F Hypothemia	
	> 38°C or 100.4°F Pyrexia	
Pulse	< 60 Bradycardia	
	> 100 Tachycardia	
Respirations	< 16 Bradypnea	
	> 20 Tachypnea	
Blood Pressure	< 90/60 Hypotension	
	> 140/90 Hypertension	

AGE VARIATION AND PULSE RATE	
Age	**Pulse Rate**
At Birth	70–170
Neonate	120–140
1 year	80–140
Toddler	80–130
Adult	60–100

endurance, fatigue, and any possible episodes of palpitations, "feeling the heart beating," over the chest area. Through verbal communication, palpation, and auscultation, a complete assessment of the pulse is obtained.

Respiration

The assessment of respirations may be accomplished while taking the radial pulse. Place the client's wrist from which the radial pulse is being assessed over the abdomen. The respiratory rate can more readily be assessed with the client in this position.

Assessment of external respirations (R) should include specific characteristics of respirations as well as the use of any type of oxygen equipment. Each respiration includes one complete inhalation (breathing in) and exhalation (breathing out) by the client. When identifying the characteristics of respirations, determine the rate, depth, and rhythm of each breath. Terms used to describe respirations are even, easy, regular, irregular, quiet, noisy, labored, or unlabored. Respirations should be even, quiet and easy, or unlabored. It is also important to observe for nasal flaring and the use of accessory muscles for breathing as evidenced by sternal, costal, and subclavicular retractions. Observation of the use of thoracic or abdominal muscles for respirations is indicated. Children and males typically utilize abdominal muscles to breathe and women use thoracic muscles (Fuller & Shaller-Ayers, 1994). If a client is receiving oxygen, determine if it is it by mask or nasal cannula and assess the flow of oxygen in L/min.

During the assessment of respirations, the nurse may determine functional ability by asking about any periods of shortness of breath, any difficulty in breathing with increased exercise, or problems following through with activities of daily living.

Blood Pressure

After checking a client's respirations, assessment of the client's blood pressure (BP) is the next task. Blood pressure is measured utilizing either an **aneroid** or a mercury sphygmomanometer. An aneroid sphygmomanometer is connected to a round calibrated dial with a needle that indicates pressure. A mercury sphygmomanometer consists of a mercury filled cylinder or tube calibrated in millimeters of mercury (mm/Hg) (Taylor et al., 1993). When assessing a client's blood pressure, incorporate the use of auscultation as well as palpation assessment techniques.

A person's blood pressure is the result of the interaction of cardiac output and peripheral resistance, and will be dependent on the speed with which the arterial blood flows, the volume of blood supplied, and the elasticity of the walls of the artery. The force exerted by the blood against the wall of the artery as the heart contracts and relaxes is called the arterial pressure. When the ventricles contract and blood is forced into the aorta and pulmonary arteries, the systolic arterial pressure is measured. This is the first sound heard. When the heart is in the filling or relaxed stage, the force is described as the diastolic blood pressure. This is when the last sound is heard. Refer to Table 10-3 for norms and variations of blood pressure. The difference between the systolic and diastolic blood pressures is called the pulse pressure. A pulse pressure is usually between 30–40 mmHg.

This is an appropriate time to ask if the client ever becomes lightheaded or dizzy when moving from a reclining position to a sitting or standing position. This may occur as a result of an abnormally low blood pressure caused by the inability of the peripheral blood vessels to compensate quickly for the change in position and is referred to as **orthostatic hypotension**.

Head Assessment

Assessment of the head follows checking the client's vital signs. The nurse will assess the head and neck and determine the client's mental and neurological status, and the client's overall **affect** or mood.

The hair and scalp of a client should be inspected. When assessing the hair, note the hair distribution, quantity, texture, and color. The scalp should be smooth and free of any debris or infestations.

The eyes should be examined to determine if they are symmetrical. Look at the eyebrows and eyelids to determine if there is any drooping, which may be a sign of muscle weakness or neurological impairment. Determine the color of the sclera, conjunctiva, and if there is any drainage present.

The pupils should be assessed to determine their size, shape, and reaction to light. This is accomplished by darkening the room and asking the client to gaze into the distance. Move a light in from the side and notice if the pupil constricts. This is called the direct light reflex. Determine the pupil size in millimeters both before and after the light response (Figure 10-4).

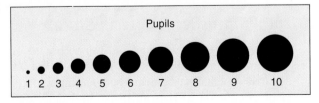

FIGURE 10-4 Scale used to measure pupil size, in millimeters.

Test for accommodation by asking the client to focus on an object in the distance. This will dilate the pupils. Next, have the client move his gaze to a near object such as a pen or finger held approximately three inches from the nose. The pupils should constrict as they focus on the near object and the eyes will converge or move in toward midline. This normal response is documented as PERRLA or Pupils Equal, Round, React to Light and Accommodation.

Determine if the client utilizes glasses and for what reason. Ask the client if they are experiencing any eye problems such as blurry vision, diplopia (double vision), or difficulty seeing at night.

The nose should be symmetrical, midline, and in proportion to other features. Determine if there is any deformity or inflammation or if the client has experienced any trauma to the nose. Test the patency of the nostrils by asking the client to sniff inward while closing off each nostril. Ask the client if the following are ever experienced: nosebleeds, dryness, history of surgery, or decrease in sense of smell.

The lips and mucous membranes of the mouth are observed for color, symmetry, moisture, or lesions. Note if the client has dentures or partial plates and ask them to remove them for a more thorough inspection of the mouth. Note any unusual breath odors. Inspect the oral mucosa by inserting a tongue depressor between the teeth and the cheek. The mucous membranes and gums should be pink, moist, smooth, and free of lesions. Inspection of the tongue assists in determining the client's hydration. The tongue should be pink with a slightly rough texture. Determine during the examination if the client is able to enunciate words appropriately and if there have been any voice changes such as hoarseness. Discuss usual dental hygiene practices and obtain the client's history of tobacco usage.

The neck should be assessed to determine if there is full range of motion. The accessory neck muscles should be symmetrical. As the client moves the head note any enlargement of the lymph nodes or enlargement of the thyroid gland. Normally none is present. Observe for any pulsations in the neck. The carotid pulsation is seen just below the angle of the jaw. Normally there are no other visible pulsations while the client is in the sitting position.

Mental Status/Neurological Status

All head-to-toe assessments must incorporate an assessment of the client's mental and neurological status. A client's mental status includes identification of the level of orientation to person, place, and time. Also included within the mental status is the client's responsiveness to the environment. When assessing for responsiveness, observe for the client's ability to follow directions, respond appropriately to comments and to their name when called. Refer to mental status in Chapter 27.

Neurological assessment of the client focuses on the following: level of consciousness (LOC), pupil response, hand grasps, and foot pushes. Each of these assessments will be discussed in the area of the head-to-toe assessment in which it will be observed. The level of consciousness is the client's degree of wakefulness. For example, a client who is alert is fully awake with eyes open and responds to environmental stimuli. The client who is less awake will be drowsy and slow in response to environmental stimuli. Refer to the Glasgow Coma Scale in Chapter 27.

Affect

Incorporated within each head-to-toe assessment is the description of the client's affect (mood or emotional expression). When documenting the client's affect, utilize terms that are descriptive and expressive of the client's overall mood. Use of words such as pleasant, happy, cooperative, nice, good, unco-operative, angry, depressed, hostile, or judgmental statements may lead to legal consequences. The description of affect should focus specifically upon the behaviors exhibited by the client, or specific quotations of the client shared with the nurse. In doing this, the nurse not only maintains the accuracy of the conversation or the behaviors observed, but also maintains the legal appropriateness of the assessment.

Skin Assessment

Assessment of the skin should be performed as each area of the body is assessed. The color of the skin as well as its moisture or dryness should be noted. Inspect and palpate the condition of the client's skin, assess the turgor, integrity, color, moisture, sensation, and vascularity. Palpation of the skin with the dorsal aspect of the hand on the right and left sides of the body provides a comparison of the client's skin temperature. The client should also be asked if any pain or discomfort in relation to the skin and/or mucous membranes has occurred. Identification of the skin's turgor is best accomplished by pinching the skin of the forearm and observing for the return of the skin to its previous position. Terms to describe skin turgor include: supple, fair, and loose. If the skin stays pinched during assessment, it may indicate dehydration, and further assessment should occur.

The location, size, distribution, and appearance of

skin lesions throughout the body should be determined. Documentation of any breaks in or changes in the skin integrity is an important aspect of nursing assessment. Scratches, bruises, skin tears, cuts and scars from previous injuries or surgeries are examples of skin characteristics that should be noted. A survey of the general hygiene of the skin is indicated and the client's usual skin care routines need to be assessed.

Thoracic Assessment

Within the head-to-toe progression, thoracic assessment follows head and neck assessment. During thoracic assessment, the nurse will determine the condition of the client's cardiovascular and respiratory systems along with assessment of the breasts. Pay attention to the client's skin, observing the condition of any wounds, drains, or tubes.

Cardiovascular Status

Assessment of the client's cardiovascular status focuses specifically on listening to the apical pulse, identifying heart tones, and checking the nailbeds and mucous membranes. The apical pulse is determined by using auscultation and palpation. To assess the apical pulse, palpate over the apex of the heart at the fourth or fifth left intercostal space at the midclavicular line. A slight, short duration tap against the fingers will be felt, and this is where the apical pulse will be auscultated (Figure 10-5). Listening to the apical pulse is the most accurate assessment of the heart rate, and should occur for sixty seconds. The apical pulse is assessed first with the diaphragm of the stethoscope for the regularity or irregularity of its rhythm. Second, the bell of the stethoscope is used to differentiate the loudness or tones of the heart. Along with the apical pulse, other pulse points to assess when focusing on a client's cardiovascular status are: temporal, carotid, brachial, radial, femoral, popliteal, posterior tibial, and dorsalis pedis (Figure 10-6). Along with palpation of these other pulse points, assess the color and vascularity of all extremities.

The focus of the history includes personal habits contributing to, or preventing disease, such as chest pain, shortness of breath, fatigue, syncope, and edema. Determine the client's personal exercise habits. Also ask questions that elicit responses regarding past chest pain or shortness of breath. Have the client describe any pain, its location, duration, precipitating factors, and what is done to alleviate the pain. Ask if the client has ever fainted or felt dizzy, noticed any swelling or what causes the swelling.

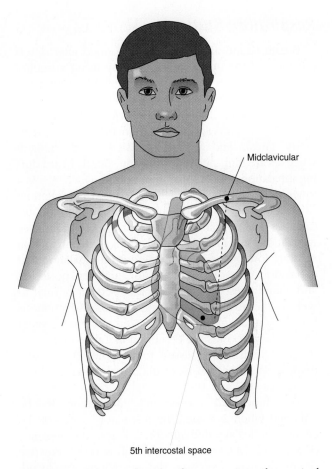

FIGURE 10-5 Landmarks for assessing the apical pulse.

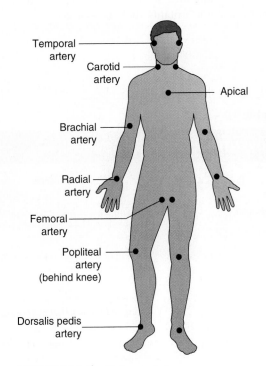

FIGURE 10-6 Pulse points.

Respiratory Status

Breath sound assessment is performed after determination of the apical pulse rate. By using auscultation, assess breath sounds in all lung fields, noting any **adventitious** sounds. Adventitious sounds are abnormal sounds including **sibilant wheezes** (formerly wheezes), **sonorous wheezes** (formerly rhonchi), **crackles** (formerly rales), and **pleural friction rubs**. Sibilant wheezes are high-pitched, whistling sounds heard during inhalation and exhalation. A sonorous wheeze is a low-pitched snoring sound that is louder on exhalation. Coughing may alter the sound if caused by mucous. Crackles are popping sounds heard on inhalation or exhalation, not cleared by coughing. Pleural friction rubs are low-pitched grating sounds on inhalation and exhalation. Breath sounds of the anterior, posterior, and lateral chest wall must be assessed for normal as well as the adventitious breath sounds. Adventitious breath sounds must be monitored on a consistent basis. These sounds are described in Table 10-4.

Lung fields are assessed for clearness. The lung fields auscultated consist of the areas shown in detail in Figures 10-7 and 10-8.

The functional assessment information to be obtained when assessing the respiratory status of the client includes any difficulty breathing or the presence of a cough. Determine if the cough is nonproductive or productive. Describe the secretions produced. Terms used to describe secretions expectorated would be thick, thin, yellow, green. The client's occupational or home environment may affect breathing patterns. Determine exposure to dust, chemicals, vapors or paint fumes, and irritants such as asbestos.

Wounds, Drains, Tubes, Dressings

When assessing the thorax, the nurse should note any type of wounds, drains, tubes, or dressings the client may have. Assessment of these must include the location, size, and amount of drainage or discharge, and if present, signs of inflammation. Use of appropriate medical terminology to describe these terms assists in facilitating a more complete documentation of the wound, drain, tube, or dressing.

Breasts

Assessment of the breast tissue should be done for both males and females. Begin by inspecting the breast for size and symmetry. It is common to have a slight difference in size in breasts. Look for any obvious masses, dimpling (a depression in the surface skin), or inflammation. The skin normally is smooth and even in color. Determine if the nipples and areolae are symmetrical in size, shape, and color, and note any discharge from the nipples.

Palpate any abnormal area for size, consistency, mobility, tenderness, and location of the lesion. Another area to include in breast assessment is the axillary lymph nodes which drain the breasts. Palpate the axilla for enlarged or inflamed lymph nodes and ask if there is any tenderness. Determine if and when the client performs self-breast exams. Ask if the client has had mammography and when the last x-ray was taken. Refer to Chapters 15 (Oncology) and 31 (Female Reproductive Disorders) for further information.

Table 10-4

ADVENTITIOUS BREATH SOUNDS		
Type	**Definition**	
Crackles	Popping sounds heard on inspiration or expiration. Not cleared by coughing	
Sonorous wheezes	Snoring or gurgling sound, will someimes clear after coughing. Louder on exhalation	
Sibilant wheezes	High pitched whistling sound, possibly heard on both inspiration and expiration.	
Pleural friction rub	Low-pitched grating sound on inspiration and expiration	

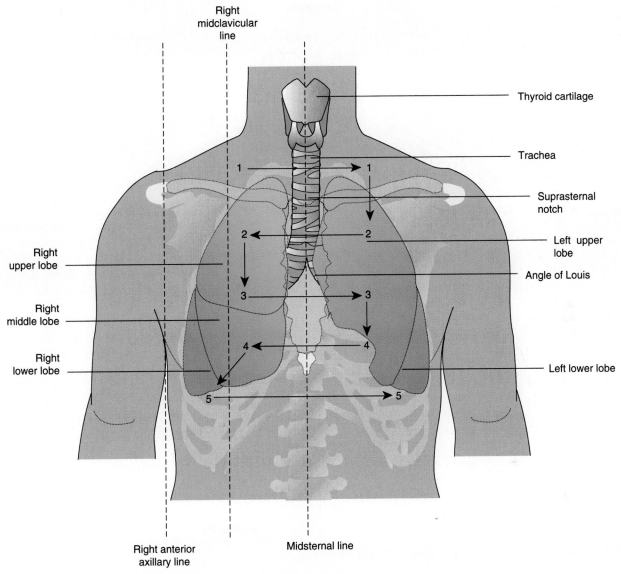

Right
midclavicular
line

Thyroid cartilage

Trachea

Suprasternal
notch

Right
upper lobe

Left upper
lobe

Right
middle lobe

Angle of Louis

Right
lower lobe

Left lower lobe

Right anterior
axillary line

Midsternal line

FIGURE 10-7 Symmetrical assessment of breath sounds (anterior).

Abdominal Assessment

During abdominal assessment the nurse determines the status of the client's gastrointestinal, urinary, and reproductive systems. The nurse should assess the client's skin as well for the presence and condition of wounds, drains, tubes, or ostomies.

Gastrointestinal Status

To determine a client's bowel status, the nurse uses the assessment techniques of inspection, auscultation, percussion, and palpation, in that order. Inspect, then auscultate, the abdomen, since palpation of the abdomen is likely to initiate peristalsis, which could potentially affect the bowel sounds. Inspect the abdomen for rashes and scars and inquire about their occurence. Determine if the abdomen is flat, rounded,

or distended. Observe the abdomen for symmetry and visible signs of peristalsis or pulsations. If the abdomen is distended, ask questions pertaining to the client's bowel movements and urinary status. See the discussion of urinary status assessment that follows.

Auscultation is the second component of the abdominal assessment of a client's bowel status. Listen for the "bubbly-gurgly" sound, caused by peristalsis and movement of the intestinal contents, by placing the stethoscope on each quadrant of the abdomen and listening for approximately one minute. These sounds should be present in all four quadrants of the abdomen. Begin in the right lower quadrant (RLQ) and move clockwise around the four quadrants as shown in Figure 10-9. When approximately 5 to 20 bowel sounds are heard per minute, or one at least every 5 to 15 seconds, the bowel sounds are considered active.

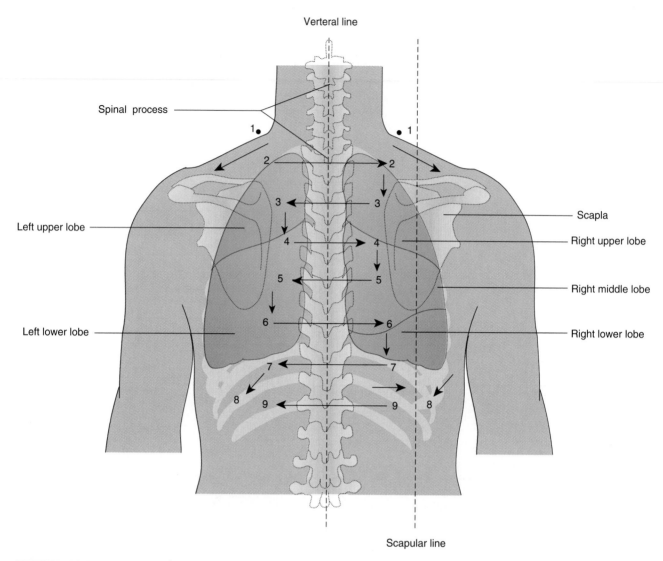

FIGURE 10-8 Symmetrical assessment of breath sounds (posterior).

The absence of bowel sounds during one minute of auscultation in each quadrant is documented as absent bowel sounds. Bowel sounds of less than five "bubbly-gurgly" sounds per minute are described as hypoactive, while an excess of 20 or more bowel sounds per minute is defined as hyperactive. High pitched, loud rushing sounds heard with or without a stethoscope are termed **borborygmi**. This is caused by the passage of gas through the liquid contents of the intestine.

Percussion of the abdomen should occur in all four quadrants. The predominant abdominal percussion sound is tympany caused by percussing over the air-filled stomach and intestines.

Palpation of the abdomen is done to assess for muscle tone, masses, pulsations, or any signs of tenderness or discomfort. Abdominal muscles may be palpated and should feel relaxed on light palpation, not tightly contracted or spastic. If the client is anxious, muscle contraction may be evident. Palpation of a separation of the rectus abdominous muscle may be felt, especially in clients who are obese or pregnant. The rectus abdominous muscle includes two large, midline muscles that extend from the xiphoid process to the symphysis pubis, and can be palpated midline as the client raises his or her head. Rebound tenderness, indicating possible inflammation of the appendix, may be elicited by depressing the abdomen and quickly withdrawing your fingers. This examination is done at the end of the abdominal assessment because of the possibility of increasing the client's level of pain. After assessment of bowel sounds, the nurse should question the client about diet, usual bowel patterns, appetite, weight changes, indigestion, heartburn, nausea, pain, and use of enemas or laxatives.

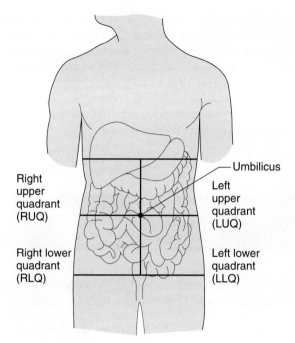

FIGURE 10-9 The four quadrants of the abdomen.

Genitourinary Status

Assessment of the client's urinary and reproductive status is accomplished mainly by inspection and use of interview skills. Genitourinary assessment includes examination of the abdomen, urinary meatus and genitalia, and assessment of the client's urine.

Inspect the abdomen for any enlargement or fullness. In the normal adult, the abdomen is smooth, flat, and symmetrical. Inspect the urinary meatus for any abnormalities such as inflammation and discharge, which may signal a urethral infection.

In females, observe the appearance of the genitalia (labia, clitoris, vaginal opening). Questions to ask the client which focus on the reproductive history include: pregnancies, use of birth control, menstrual cycle history, present sexual activity, use of protection during intercourse, the date of the last Pap test and determination of how any present illness has or will affect sexual activity.

In males, assessment of the genitalia includes inspection of the penis, urethral meatus, foreskin (if uncircumcised), and scrotum. Questions to ask the client which focus on the reproductive history include: present sexual activity, use of protection during intercourse, and also how the present illness has or will affect sexual activity. Determine if the client performs testicular self-examinations.

Note any lesions or ulcerations that may indicate sexually transmitted diseases. Determine if the client has had any history of urinary tract infections, kidney

stones, if there is any change in the urinary stream, or if there is painful urination or nocturia. Refer to Chapters 31, 32 , 33, and 35 for further information.

Wounds, Drains, Tubes, Dressings, Ostomies

The nurse should note any type of wounds, drains, tubes, dressings, or ostomies the client may have. Assessment of these must include the location, size, and amount of drainage or discharge, and if present, any signs of inflammation. Chapter 36 describes ostomies in more detail. Use of appropriate medical terminology to describe these items assists in facilitating a more complete documentation of the wound, drain, tube, dressing, or ostomy.

Musculoskeletal and Extremity Assessment

Symmetry and strength of major muscle groups can be assessed throughout the head-to-toe assessment. Any time during the assessment when the client is repositioned, observe the range of movement the client utilizes to make that position change. Every joint in the body has a normal range of motion, or greatest range of movement. Asking the client to walk across the room, or noting the client's movements and stance when sitting up in bed are observations made to assess gross motor movement and posture. Assessment of the client's handshake gives an estimate of muscle strength. Palpating muscles lightly determines swelling, tone, or any specific changes in shape of the muscles.

Hand grasps and foot pushes assess the strength and equality of the client's extremities. Upper extremity strength is assessed by having the client grasp the nurse's index and middle fingers of each hand. The grasp should be equal in both hands. Foot pushes assess the lower extremities. The nurse's hands should be placed on the soles of the client's feet. The client is asked to push both feet against the nurse's hands. The push should be equal in both feet. Asking the client to touch the tip of her nose with a finger and then the tip of the nurse's finger as it is moved to different locations, tests the client's coordination skills.

Strength and symmetry of some of the major muscle groups can be assessed by watching gait and postural movements. Ask the client if any aids to ambulation are utilized. Symmetrical examination of muscles should occur in pairs, first one extremity and then the other; observe for equality of size, contour, tone, and strength.

The skin of the lower extremities should be carefully assessed to determine color changes, loss of feeling or hair, change in temperature within the extremity and from one extremity to the other, presence of varicose veins, ulcers, and edema. Determine if the client experiences any leg pain or cramps.

Assessment of the client's nails can provide information regarding the client's health status and self-care practices. The nails should be observed for color, consistency, symmetry, cleanliness, and smoothness.

Ask the client if she experiences muscle weakness or has difficulty or pain when walking or performing routine daily activities. The functional assessment should also include asking the client about routine activities such as cooking, shopping, exercise, yard work, or hobbies. Tolerance limitations can also be observed by assessing for stiffness, crepitus, or fatigue during ambulation. Safe and appropriate performance of function essential for home life and activities of daily living need to be determined.

▶ CASE STUDY

Tom Turner, age forty, was admitted to the hospital with pneumonia. He had never been hospitalized before. His wife and three children are all at home. Because his wife has just given birth to their third child, Tom's wife cannot drive the other two children to school. Tom provides the sole income for his family, and he only has three more sick days to use at work before he will be off without pay.

Tom's vital signs are BP 120/72, P 100, R 34, T 100.6° F. His breath sounds show sonorous wheezes throughout, cleared by coughing. His cough is frequent and productive of foamy, cloudy, yellow secretions. His AP is 102 and regular, but distant heart tones were noted. The abdomen is firm and distended with hypoactive bowel sounds noted in all four quadrants. He moves all extremities slowly but per self and with purpose.

Tom is oriented to person, place, and time. His pupils are PERRLA. Hand grips are strong and equal bilaterally, as are foot pushes. He speaks only when spoken to, and his eye contact with staff is minimal. Whenever his wife visits, his voice raises and his heart rate increases about

The following questions will guide your development of a Nursing Care Plan for the case study.

1. List the functional assessment data collected from Mr. Turner that identify psychosocial concerns.

2. List the data supporting Mr. Turner's diagnosis of pneumonia.

3. What are two possible reasons for identifying the added information about Mr. Turner in the last paragraph?

4. Write 2 or 3 nursing diagnoses that are supported by the health history and physical assessments documented about Mr. Turner.

5. Write goals and nursing interventions for each nursing diagnosis.

6. The priority actions to be taken for Mr. Turner while he is in the hospital focus specifically on which functional patterns?

7. List at least two ways the nurse could evaluate Mr. Turner's physical recovery from pneumonia.

▶ **CASE STUDY (continued)**

2–5 beats. At one point, Tom stated, "How much more of this can we take?" Tom's wife mentions that their church would love to help, but Tom refuses to take charity. Tom states, "Any income for this family has to come from me."

Other added information acquired during the assessment included the fact that Tom has a history of drinking 1 to 2 beers daily, and has not performed testicular self-exams. He eats and drinks what he likes, and he states he really "hates seafood." Usually he bathes daily in the early morning and helps to bathe two of their children each evening. His job is 9-5:30 P.M., five days per week, and also some Saturday mornings. Tom pays all of the household bills, and is the sole decision maker of the family.

▶ ▶ ▶ ▶ ▶ ▶ ▶ ▶ ▶ ▶

SUMMARY

- Psychosocial needs of clients are identified within the scope of a functional assessment.
- The health history and the physical head-to-toe assessment used together present a holistic view of client needs.
- Margory Gordon's eleven functional health patterns provide a systematic means by which to obtain a complete functional assessment.
- The four assessment techniques used in a head-to-toe assessment include: inspection, palpation, percussion, and auscultation.
- Introduction of the nurse at the beginning of a physical assessment enhances the ability to accomplish the complete assessment necessary.
- Collection of vital signs is the foundation to each

head-to-toe assessment and includes: temperature, pulse, respirations, and blood pressure.
- Assessment of a client's mental status and neurological status is performed when the nurse obtains information about the client's level of consciousness, pupil response, as well as hand grip and foot push capabilities.
- When describing a client's affect, the nurse must utilize terms that are descriptive of the specific behavior observed, not the nurse's judgment about the behavior.
- Assessing the cardiovascular status of each client includes inspection of specific pulse points.
- Auscultation of lung fields assists in collection of data regarding the breath sounds of the client.
- An abdominal assessment includes use of inspection, auscultation, percussion, and palpation within

the four quadrants of the abdomen to establish bowel status and function.

- Through observation of client gait and overall range of movement, the nurse is able to obtain some knowledge of the symmetry and strength of muscles.

- During the assessment of wounds, drains, dressings, and other external devices, the nurse must maintain accurate documentation of the amount of drainage, color, or other changes noted.

Review Questions

1. Jim's apical pulse is 102. He states to the nurse that he can feel his heart pounding. Which of the following charting terms would accurately describe Jim's statement of concern regarding his heart rate?

   a. bradycardia
   b. changing of rhythm
   c. palpitation
   d. tachycardia

2. Mrs. Jones is fifty-four years old. While performing your assessment overview, Mrs. Jones states, "I just get so lightheaded when I first get up in the morning." Mrs. Jones most likely has:

   a. cyanosis.
   b. hypertension.
   c. orthostatic hypertension.
   d. orthostatic hypotension.

3. According to Gordon's Eleven Functional Health Patterns, which pattern focuses on: the health and wellness of the person, performance of self-exams, lifestyle, and habits that could influence a person's state of wellness?

   a. coping-stress tolerance
   b. health perception-health management
   c. role relationship
   d. self-perception/self-concept

4. During the physical head-to-toe assessment of the client, the nurse checks his pulse and blood pressure. Which of the four assessment techniques did the nurse utilize?

   a. auscultation, palpation, and inspection
   b. auscultation, percussion, and inspection
   c. auscultation and palpation
   d. palpation and inspection

5. The client and the nurse were discussing the following data. In which of the eleven functional health patterns would you place the majority of this data?

   - abdomen firm, distended, hypoactive bowel sounds
   - eats and drinks what he likes
   - states he really hates seafood
   - Temperature 100.6° F
   - bathes daily in early AM

   a. activity-exercise
   b. elimination
   c. health perception-health management
   d. nutritional-metabolic

6. The nurse is collecting health history and physical assessment data about a newly admitted twelve-year-old girl experiencing difficulty breathing. Of the data listed below, which would be of lowest priority?

   a. dietary intake
   b. skin color
   c. vital signs
   d. weight and height

7. Upon admission to your unit, the client verbalizes an increased pain in her left leg. What would be the pertinent assessment information to collect about this client?

   a. listen to the client's bowel sounds
   b. check circulation in the right leg
   c. assess both of the client's legs
   d. ask the client about her current diet

8. Which of the pulses should be assessed when trying to identify good circulation to the lower extremities?

   a. dorsalis pedis
   b. femoral
   c. temporal
   d. popliteal

9. How often a nurse assesses a client's vital signs depends upon:

   a. availability of personnel.
   b. doctor orders.
   c. nurse's discretion.
   d. client's condition.

10. The nurse checks the radial pulse for 30 seconds and multiplies by 2. She notices an irregularity in the beat. What is the next action the nurse should take?

    a. Check the radial pulse for 60 seconds.
    b. Listen to the apical pulse for 60 seconds.
    c. Listen to the apical for 30 seconds and multiply by 2.
    d. Continue on with the rest of the assessment.

Critical Thinking Questions

1. How do you feel about performing a complete physical assessment on a client?

2. How do you feel when you receive a complete physical assessment?

MEDICAL TERMINOLOGY

The following word parts are associated with physical assessment.

Auscult/a-	listen
Auscultation	listening to sounds from within the body
Dia-	across; through
Diagnos/o-	knowledge of current status of a disease
Diagnosis	a statement of the nature of a disease a client is currently experiencing or going "through"
Endo-	inner; within
Endoscopy	the process of examining the interior of the body
Eti/o-	cause
Etiology	the study of disease causes
-gram	record of
-graph	instrument for recording
-metry-	process of measuring
Palpa-	touch
Palpation	the process of touching
Percuss/o-	to beat; tap
Percussion	the process of tapping
Scop/o-	examine
Son/o-	sound
Sonography	the process of recording sound waves
Steth/o-	chest
Stethoscope	an instrument used to examine the chest (steth = chest)
Therm/o-	heat
Ultra-	beyond; excess

News Flash

What will happen to nursing physical assessment in the future? Imagine the possibilities, and how you will play an integral role. From the knowledge we have available, computers will be leading and directing the way into the next century. Bedside computers, in some hospital settings, are maintaining complete and up-to-date assessment data on each client. The data entered may travel halfway around the world to aid in diagnosis of some rare disease. In the future the nurse may enter data via a voice-activated headset. As the nurse assesses the client all the data may be transmitted directly to the physician's office or other pertinent departments. Use of bedside computers by respiratory therapists at Lutheran Hospital in Fort Wayne, Indiana has enhanced the accuracy of assessment of respiratory status and assists in maintaining up-to-date data on the care of all clients. Incorporation of similar bedside computer systems for the nursing staff is on the horizon. Nursing care plans are developed, updated, and evaluated through computer technology. Where will computers take nursing in the future? The possibilities are limitless. The potential of computers has just begun to be tapped. Perhaps nurses will be acquiring vital signs through completely electronic means. Perhaps auscultation of breath sounds and bowel sounds will happen without the use of a stethoscope. . . . Advances in computer and electronic technology will continue to propel all nurses into a new and perhaps unimaginable future. Ready, set, computerize!

CHAPTER
11
Anesthesia

Michael A. Fiedler

LEARNING OBJECTIVES

Upon completion of this chapter the learner should be able to:
- Define key terms.
- Describe the difference between regional and general anesthesia.
- List the purposes of sedation and when it might be useful.
- Describe the effects of sedation or general anesthesia on memory and cognitive function.
- Describe the types of monitoring necessary to ensure client safety during sedation.
- Describe the risks of oversedation.
- Describe some of the tasks an anesthetist must perform during an anesthetic in addition to administering anesthetic drugs.
- List the purposes of an endotracheal tube used during general anesthesia.
- Describe the dangers involved in aspiration of gastric contents and how gastric aspiration is prevented during anesthesia.
- List, in general, the medications that are usually given on the day of surgery.
- List and describe briefly the different types of regional anesthesia.
- Describe the risks involved with regional and general anesthesia.
- Describe the residual effects of anesthesia and how they affect the client.
- Recall why oxygen should be administered to clients receiving sedation or recovering from general anesthesia.
- Describe the dangers to the client and clinical appearance of residual muscle paralysis following general anesthesia.
- Recall how long after a general anesthetic may be necessary for complete elimination of anesthetic agents.
- List two reasons why clients shiver after general anesthesia and what nursing interventions can reduce or eliminate the shivering.
- Describe the reason why clients may have a greatly increased urine output postoperatively.
- List several different methods of postoperative pain management and explain briefly how each is administered.

▶ *MAKING THE CONNECTION*

Refer to the topics in the following chapters to increase your understanding of anesthesia.

- **Chapter 2, Legal Aspects of Nursing:** Informed Consent, p. 27
- **Chapter 12, Pain Management:** Pharmacological Treatments, p. 214; Invasive Techniques, p. 223

- **Chapter 13, Perioperative Nursing:** The Nursing Process in the Postanesthesia Care Unit, p. 247
- **Chapter 14: Fluid Electrolyte, and Acid-Base Balances:** Basic Physiology of Body Fluids and Electrolytes, p. 268

INTRODUCTION

The delivery of general **anesthesia** for the purpose of preventing pain during surgery began in the United States in the 1800s. When surgeons began using anesthesia routinely, they soon realized the need for someone trained in its administration and turned to the nurses with whom they worked daily. Early nurse **anesthetists** were trained on the job by the surgeons with whom they worked. Anesthesia is now a specialty of both nursing and medicine. Nurse anesthetists work not only in the United States, but in many other countries around the world. Experienced Registered Nurses with a baccalaureate degree can become Certified Registered Nurse Anesthetists (CRNAs) after completing two or more years of graduate education in Nurse Anesthesia at one of approximately ninety nurse anesthesia programs throughout the country. There are currently about 25,000 CRNAs in the United States. CRNAs administer the majority of all anesthetics given in the United States every year, often working in groups with, or under the supervision of physician **anesthesiologists**.

Prior to an anesthetic, the anesthetist will assess a client's health status, discuss anesthesia with the client, and plan an anesthetic appropriate for the client and the surgical procedure. The surgical nurse can help prepare clients to talk with their anesthetist by encouraging them to ask any questions they have about anesthesia and the care they will receive. Some clients are reluctant to ask questions even when they have significant fears and concerns. Oftentimes by answering their questions a client's anxiety can be significantly reduced.

The delivery of an anesthetic is essential to the health and well-being of clients undergoing surgery. Yet, while anesthesia prevents the sensation of what would be extreme pain, anesthesia also temporarily eliminates or diminishes the client's ability to control many essential physiologic functions such as respiration, heart rate, and temperature regulation. In addition to ensuring adequate levels of anesthesia throughout a surgical procedure, the anesthetist monitors and, when necessary, controls physiologic functions. Prior to the end of the surgery and anesthetic, the anesthetist administers appropriate medications to ensure that the client is comfortable while emerging from the anesthetic. Pain relief may be accomplished with local anesthetic infiltration, opioid analgesics, or nonopioid analgesics. In addition to the provision of anesthetics, nurse anesthetists are often involved in emergency airway management throughout the hospital, obtaining circulatory access (arterial and intravenous lines), and providing postoperative pain management.

KEY ABBREVIATIONS

The following abbreviations and acronyms are used in this chapter:

BP	blood pressure
CNS	central nervous system
CRNA	Certified Registered Nurse Anesthetist
CSF	cerebrospinal fluid
EKG	electrocardiogram
ETT	endotracheal tube
HR	heart rate
IVPCA	intravenous patient controlled analgesia
NPO	nothing by mouth
NSAID	nonsteroidal anti-inflammatory drug
PCA	patient-controlled analgesia
PDPH	postdural puncture headache

PREANESTHETIC PREPARATION

Preparing a client for anesthesia and surgery is a cooperative effort involving the surgeon, the anesthetist, and the nursing staff who will care for the client both before and after surgery.

Oral Intake

Normally, only air should enter into the trachea and lungs. The body prevents foreign material from entering the trachea by coughing forcefully when something other than air enters or by tightly closing the vocal cords to prevent entry of the foreign substance. Anyone who has ever been drinking something and had it go down the wrong way knows how uncomfortable it is and how hard the body works to cough up the foreign substance.

General anesthesia removes a person's ability to guard the airway by coughing or closing the vocal cords. Passive regurgitation of stomach contents into the back of the throat can occur at any time during a general anesthetic. Aspiration of gastric contents into the lungs can cause significant illness or death. An important step in preventing aspiration of gastric contents is ensuring that the stomach is as empty as possible. In the past, adults have been instructed not to eat or drink anything for at least eight hours prior to surgery, usually nothing past 12:00 midnight. Infants and children have a higher metabolic demand and are subject to shorter periods of fasting. More recent information, however, strongly indicates that adults need not go without water for eight or more hours prior to surgery (Phillips, Hutchinson, & Davidson, 1993; Soreide, Holst-Larsen, Reite, Mikkelsen, Sorejde, & Steen, 1993). In fact, the amount of liquid in a person's stomach at the time of surgery may actually be decreased if water is taken a couple of hours before surgery. Some anesthesia providers still prefer that their clients not have anything to eat or drink for at least eight hours prior to surgery. Others may allow water up to two hours before leaving for the operating room.

Instructions for oral intake prior to surgery in adults may vary from the traditional "NPO past midnight" to no food after midnight but allowing clear fluids up to two hours prior to surgery. Any instructions about oral intake prior to surgery should be followed, and the nurse should be aware that the length of time for which water is denied prior to surgery may vary. The variability in length of time that food or water is withheld is due to differences in client age and the preference of the anesthesia providers.

Preoperative Medication

Most scheduled medications that a person receives while in the hospital or takes at home every day will be continued up until the time of surgery. Most oral medications should be given with just enough water to swallow them, even when a client is going to have surgery first thing in the morning. The anesthetist will usually write orders to specify how the morning medication should be handled. Cardiovascular medications such as antihypertensives and heart medications are especially important for the client to receive.

Exceptions to the rule include drugs such as insulin and oral antihyperglycemics, nonsteroidal anti-inflammatory drugs (NSAIDs) like aspirin, and anticoagulants like heparin or coumadin. Since food is being withheld, giving insulin or oral antihyperglycemic drugs is likely to result in a dangerously low blood sugar level. How insulin and glucose administration is handled will depend on the severity of the client's disease and the preference of the physician and anesthesia provider. NSAIDs and anticoagulants affect bleeding. Naturally, the surgeon wants as little bleeding as possible during surgery. Some types of surgery are more prone to the bleeding caused by aspirin like drugs or low dose heparin than others. In some cases, no NSAIDs are allowed for ten days to two weeks prior to surgery. In other circumstances they may be given right up until surgery. Low dose heparin or heparinoids may be given preoperatively to prevent postoperative thromboembolism but higher doses of heparin and any dose of coumadin will almost certainly be stopped prior to surgery to allow the return of normal coagulation.

Additional medications may be ordered to prepare the client for surgery or anesthesia. Surgeons often order prophylactic antibiotics. The anesthetist may order a sedative to help the client sleep the night before surgery or to ease the client's anxiety while waiting for surgery. Opioids like morphine or meperidine (Demerol) may also be used for pain relief or to ease the induction of anesthesia. Some anesthetists, however, do not order any preoperative medication. They may not be sure when the client's case will start or they may prefer to give preoperative medications in the operating room to precisely control the medication's effect on the client. This is especially true for very sick clients.

Consent

Consent for anesthesia is usually obtained on the same form with the surgical consent. The anesthesia department may have a separate consent form that they use instead of or in addition to the combined consent. In either case, for an informed consent to be obtained the anesthetic must be discussed with the client by someone with expert knowledge of anesthesia. Discussion of anesthesia should be undertaken by either an anesthesia provider or the surgeon (see Table 11-1). It is unwise for the surgical nurse to discuss anesthesia with the client. Even seemingly trivial aspects, like the type of anesthesia a client will have, can result in client anxiety or worse, legal consequences. For example, a case may be posted for a general anesthetic only to have new information become available that indicates that a regional anesthetic would be safer for the client. After discussion with the surgeon the anesthetist begins to talk to the client about a regional anesthetic. The client may become concerned about the change because the surgical nurse had already told him that he would have a general anesthetic. For more information about the legal aspects of consent see Chapter 2, Legal Aspects of Nursing.

SEDATION

Sedation always involves some degree of central nervous system (CNS) depression. Sedation is used to decrease awareness of events, relieve anxiety, control the physiologic changes that often accompanies anxiety, and ease the induction of general anesthesia. This is welcome news to many clients who fear local or regional anesthesia because they do not want to be awake and see and hear everything during a surgery or diagnostic procedure.

Table 11-1

KEY CONSIDERATIONS FOR PREANESTHETIC CARE

- Make sure all preoperative orders are executed, especially blood tests, preoperative medications, and orders for blood from the blood bank.
- Check, verify, and document the presence or absence of drug allergies in each client.
- Administer regular daily PO medications with a small sip of water as ordered.
- Remind the client of the importance of refraining from eating or drinking anything before anesthesia.
- Administer preoperative medications as close to the ordered time as possible. Timing can be crucial to achieve the desired effect at the correct time.
- If the client responds abnormally to the preoperative medication notify the anesthesia department immediately.
- Make sure the client's chart is complete when it goes to the operating room with the client. Recent diagnostic test results are especially important to include; otherwise surgery may be delayed while these results are sought.
- Make sure the client's consent is in order and included in the chart when it leaves for surgery.

Some drugs are better sedatives than others although many drugs have sedative properties. Oftentimes different sedatives, given in combination, have a greater effect on the client than the sum of their individual effects. This phenomenon is called **synergism**. (An analogy to illustrate the concept of synergism would be 1 + 1 = 3. The two "1s," given in combination, have a greater effect "3" than the sum of their individual parts, which is "2.") The synergistic effect that occurs when different sedative drugs are administered together makes respiratory depression and unconsciousness more likely when combinations of sedative drugs are used. In general, the benzodiazepines (diazepam [Valium] and midazolam hydrochloride [Versed]) are better sedatives than the opioids (morphine and fentanyl [Sublimaze]). Even so, if a client's anxiety is due to pain an opioid is going to be a better sedative than a benzodiazepine because it will relieve the pain that caused the anxiety. There is a great deal of variability in the dose of drugs needed to sedate different clients. While many drugs given for specific effects are administered by a set "mg per kg" dose alone, this is not possible when drugs are used for sedation. Sedation should be given based on the client's physical condition, weight, mental state, the procedure being performed, and in concert with close observation of the effect of the drugs on the client.

The amount of sedation a client requires to be comfortable is always in balance against the amount of stimulation they are experiencing due to pain or anxiety. A client who is only mildly stimulated (little anxiety) will be well sedated with a relatively small dose of sedative medication. A client who is greatly stimulated (undergoing a painful procedure or terribly frightened) will require a much larger dose of sedative to be comfortable. Because sedation involves CNS depression, as does the induction of general anesthesia, sedation and anesthesia exist on a continuum. As sedation becomes deeper and deeper it eventually becomes general anesthesia. Sometimes the line between sedation and general anesthesia is very difficult to distinguish. When sedation becomes general anesthesia all the risks of general anesthesia are present, including airway obstruction and the possibility for aspiration of gastric contents. For this reason, all but the lightest sedation should be administered by an anesthetist or another provider skilled and experienced in airway assessment, protection, and management as well as assessment of oxygenation and ventilation.

Sedation and Monitoring

Sedation is often used during procedures performed under local anesthesia to alleviate client anxiety and discomfort. Properly performed, local anesthetic injection blocks the painful stimulus of small incisions and minor surgical procedures. However, the needlesticks necessary for local anesthetic injection can be significantly uncomfortable to some people. Injection of local anesthetic may be uncomfortable due to tissue irritation caused by the acidity of the local anesthetic solution. Additionally, most clients are uncomfortable knowing that they are being operated on and prefer to be less alert during the procedure. Sedation decreases the client's perception of these physical and mental discomforts.

During local anesthesia and sedation, the client must remain conscious and in control of his own airway and breathing reflexes. Oversedation is likely to result in airway obstruction and places the client at risk for aspiration of gastric contents. Since sedatives are CNS depressants, and therefore respiratory depressants, supplemental oxygen should be given to almost all clients during sedation. Monitoring during sedation should begin with an individual knowledgeable and experienced in the assessment of respiratory volume and airway patency by observing the client. Monitoring should also include an electrocardiogram (EKG), blood pressure, pulse rate, respiratory rate, and continuous oxygen saturation monitoring (pulse oximetry). In all but the most healthy, lightly sedated clients undergoing very short procedures, the individual monitoring the client's breathing and vital signs should be devoted to that task to the exclusion of any other duties.

Residual Effects of Sedation

Sedation usually persists beyond the duration of the surgical procedure itself. The length of time it takes to recover from sedation depends on the health of the client, the properties of the drugs used, other drugs the client may be taking, and the amount of sedative drugs administered.

Amnesia produced by sedatives commonly lasts longer than the procedure itself even in a client who appears to be completely recovered. This is important knowledge since these clients will probably not remember any instructions given them during or soon after the procedure. Since minor procedures and surgery are commonly performed on an outpatient basis, the client may actually be discharged at a time when he or she is still unable to remember verbal instructions. All instructions should be given in writing and explained to the person responsible for taking the client home.

If heavy sedation has been used or an uncomfortable procedure ends suddenly, the client may remain significantly sedated after the procedure is over. This results because the CNS stimulation has ended while the CNS depressant effect of the sedative remains. When this occurs the client should be closely monitored until the effects of the sedative medications have worn off enough that the client is awake and oriented.

REGIONAL ANESTHESIA

What Is It and How Does It Work?

Regional anesthesia is a method of temporarily rendering a region of the body insensible to pain by injecting a local anesthetic. Local anesthetics are a class of drugs that temporarily block the transmission of small electrical impulses through nerves. The duration of anesthesia produced by a local anesthetic depends on what drug is used, how much is injected, and into what part of the body it is injected. In general, nerves carry either sensory information to the brain or instructions from the brain to muscles telling them how and when to contract. Both types of nerves can be blocked by local anesthetics. Sensory nerves are highly subspecialized to carry specific types of information to the brain. One type carries the pain we experience when stuck with a needle and another carries the sense of joint position that tells us, without looking, whether our arm is down by our side or elevated over our head. There are many different types of nerves and not all of them are blocked to the same degree or at the same time when a local anesthetic is injected. The amount of insulation surrounding a nerve fiber, the anatomical location of different fibers, and the diameter of the nerve fiber itself all modify the ease with which nerve impulses are blocked by local anesthetics.

Types of Regional Anesthesia

There are several types of regional anesthesia: local, nerve blocks, and spinal and epidural blocks.

Local Anesthesia

Clinically the use of local anesthetics to block nerves is identified by different names depending on the amount of local anesthetic used and where it is injected. When a small amount of local anesthetic drug is injected into the skin and subcutaneous tissues around a cut, or at the site of a needle puncture for a central line placement, it is called *local anesthesia*. When a local anesthetic is injected in this way, it is not aimed at a specific nerve but is more of a "shotgun" approach to anesthetize whatever small superficial nerves are in the area. Local anesthesia is most commonly performed with lidocaine (Xylocaine) and lasts about an hour. Occasionally, this type of anesthesia may be used over a large area of the body for some types of plastic surgery. When this is the case, longer acting local anesthetics may be used. Local anesthesia is technically easy to perform and involves little risk of bleeding or nerve damage. Since very small amounts of local anesthetics are generally used the risk of local anesthetic toxicity is also small.

Nerve Blocks

When a local anesthetic is injected more deeply into the body and/or is directed at a specific nerve or nerves it is called a *nerve block*. Often nerve blocks are called by the name of the specific nerve or nerves they block. Examples would include an ulnar nerve block in the arm or a brachial plexus block of all the nerves in the arm. Nerve blocks are technically more difficult to perform and involve a variable risk of bleeding or nerve damage since the needle is usually directed into deeper structures that are often close to major veins or arteries (Selander, Dhuner, & Lundborg, 1977). Nerve blocks are often performed with lidocaine (Xylocaine), mepivacaine (Carbocaine), or bupivacaine (Marcaine) and may last from one to twelve hours. Larger volumes of drug are needed than what are used for local anesthesia and local anesthetic toxicity is a rare but known complication of these types of blocks.

Spinal and Epidural Blocks

Blocks may also be identified by where the local anesthetic is injected. An example of this is an *epidural block* in which local anesthetic is injected into the epidural space near the spinal cord to anesthetize a number of spinal nerves at once. With *spinal blocks* (also called subarachnoid blocks) the local anesthetic is injected into the cerebrospinal fluid where it can bathe uninsulated spinal nerves as they exit the spinal cord to the periphery of the body (see Figure 11-1). Opioids (morphine, fentanyl citrate [Sublimaze]) may be added to the local anesthetic in either of these blocks to intensify the analgesic or anesthetic effect or provide postoperative pain relief after the block has worn off (Abouleish, Rawal, & Rashad, 1991; Cousins & Mather, 1984; Liu et al., 1995; Robertson, Douglas, & McMorland, 1985; Rosen, Dailey, & Hughes, 1988; Wells & Davies, 1987).

Spinal and epidural blocks are generally used to anesthetize a significant area of the body. They are capable of safely producing anesthesia sufficient for surgery in the abdomen, pelvis, perineum, or lower extremities. When an epidural block is performed a catheter is usually inserted into the epidural space making it possible to inject additional doses of drug. Epidural blocks have an added advantage in that the density of the block can be varied to produce **analgesia** (pain relief without producing anesthesia), complete anesthesia, and even profound muscular relaxation (needed for some types of surgery) by varying the way the local anesthetic is used. This allows epidural anesthesia to be used not only for surgical procedures but for labor analgesia and postoperative

pain relief as well. Spinal anesthetics are most often performed with lidocaine (Xylocaine) or bupivacaine (Marcaine) and last from one to three hours. Epidural anesthetics are most commonly performed with bupivacaine (Marcaine) and the block can be continued as long as local anesthetic is injected through the catheter into the epidural space (Figure 11-2).

One type of complication is peculiar to spinal and epidural regional anesthetics. When CSF leaks out through a hole made in the dural membrane during performance of a subarachnoid block or an accidental dural puncture during the attempted performance of an epidural block, a postdural puncture headache (PDPH) may result. The headache is caused by the loss of CSF from around the brain. The hallmark of a PDPH is its postural nature. The headache is relieved by lying down and returns when the individual sits up or stands. Commonly, it is in both the front and the back of the head, sometimes with neck and shoulder stiffness. Photophobia or double vision may be present with severe headache. The onset of the headache is usually not immediate but may take one to two days to become bothersome. Postdural puncture headaches may be mild and shortlived or severe and last for a week or more. In general the headache is worse when the dural puncture is made with a larger needle (17 gauge epidural needle) because more CSF can leak out. Treatment involves adequate hydration to allow the normal production of CSF, analgesics, and bed rest in a supine position. Oral caffeine (Camann, Murray, Mushlin, & Lambert, 1990) and sumatriptan succinate (Imitrex) (Carp, Singh, Vadhera, & Jayaram, 1994) are effective in preventing and treating PDPH in some people. The definitive treatment for significant or persistent PDPH is a procedure called an epidural blood patch that involves injecting 15 to 20 mL of the client's own blood into the epidural space. Once the blood clots, it plugs the hole in the dural membrane.

Local anesthetic drugs always block the sympathetic nerves that control the dilation or constriction of blood vessels before they block sensory or motor nerves. This results in vascular dilation. With most blocks the blood vessels that dilate as a result of sympathetic block are not sufficient to result in a change in blood pressure. With widespread spinal or epidural blocks, blood pressure may decrease due to sympathetic nerve block. To prevent this the anesthetist will often infuse an extra volume of IV fluid or administer a vasoconstrictor such as ephedrine before the sympathetic block sets up. Client harm from hypotension is rare.

Spinal and epidural blocks are techniques at which many anesthetists are very skilled. Like other nerve blocks they carry some risk of bleeding (Dickman, Shedd, Spetzler, Shetter, & Sonntag, 1990; Horlocker, Wedel, & Offord, 1990; Horlocker, Wedel, Schroeder, et al., 1995; Onishchuk & Carlsson, 1992) and nerve

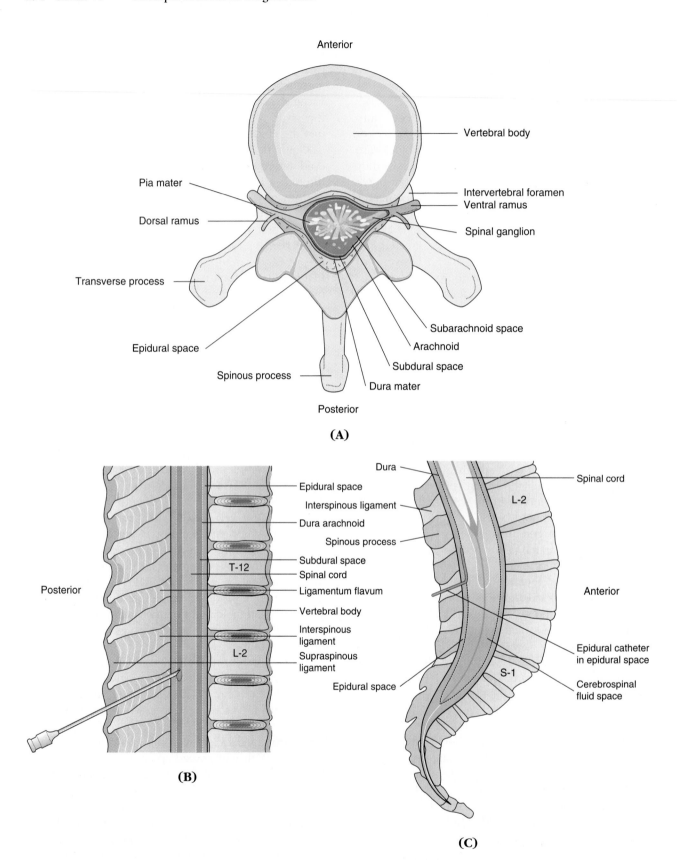

FIGURE 11-1 **(A)** Cross sectional anatomy of the spine where spinal and epidural blocks are injected. **(B)** Side view of the anatomy of the spine with the tip of an epidural needle placed in the epidural space. **(C)** Side view of the anatomy of the spine with the tip of an epidural catheter placed in the epidural space.

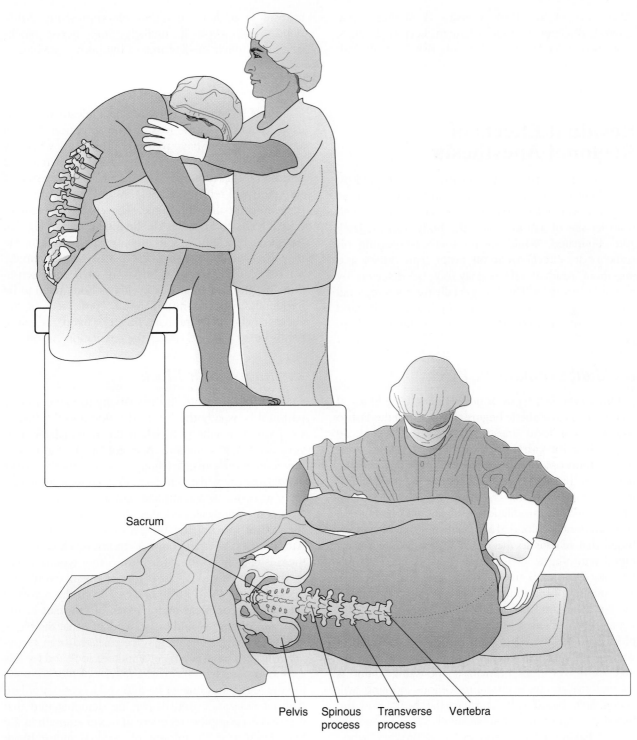

FIGURE 11-2   Correct positions for performing a spinal block or inserting an epidural catheter in the lumbar area. The assistant is crucial to the proper positioning, reassurance, and safety of the client.

damage (Ben-David, Vaida, Collins, Naum, & Gaitini, 1994; Bromage, 1993; Kane, 1981; Kroll, Caplan, Posner, Ward, & Cheney, 1990), but the high degree of expertise that many anesthesia providers have in these blocks minimizes the risk. Only a small dose of local anesthetic is needed for a spinal block so local anesthetic toxicity is very unlikely. Variable amounts of local anesthetic are used for an epidural block and some doses can approach the upper limits of safety. Anesthetists are careful to avoid overdoses of local anesthetics with this block and toxicity is exceedingly rare. If opioids like morphine are added to the local anesthetic solution there is a risk of the drug migrating to the brain and causing respiratory depression

(Abouleish, et al., 1991; Cousins & Mather, 1984; Renaud, Brichant, Clergue, Chauvin, Levron, & Viars, 1988; Rosen, et al., 1988) but this risk is small with careful dosing and is easily detected in time to prevent client harm.

Residual Effects of Regional Anesthesia

No anesthetic currently available can be turned off like a light switch. All anesthetics must wear off as the drug responsible for causing the anesthesia is removed from its site of action within the body, metabolized, and eliminated. While an anesthetic is wearing off some of its effects wear off faster than others and important residual effects may not be detected by casual observation. This is especially true of a regional anesthetic since the client may be wide awake and able to carry on a conversation as if nothing has happened.

Residual Sympathetic Block

One of the first types of nerve fibers to be blocked when a local anesthetic begins to work and the last to recover as a local anesthetic wears off are those responsible for carrying instructions to the muscles that surround blood vessels. When these sympathetic nerves are blocked, veins and arteries dilate decreasing the blood pressure. The venous system has a large capacity and venous dilation results in the pooling of a large amount of blood. This decreases the amount of blood that returns to the heart. When the amount of blood returning to the heart decreases, the heart has less blood to pump and the blood pressure decreases. The amount of blood that pools is greatest in parts of the body that are furthest below the level of the heart. Even so, in a client who has had a spinal or epidural block and is lying supine a significant amount of venous pooling still occurs and the blood pressure may be lower than normal. If the same client is allowed to sit up even more venous pooling will occur, little blood will return to the heart, and the blood pressure will fall substantially. This phenomenon of having a large drop in blood pressure when sitting up or standing is called **orthostatic hypotension**. Orthostatic signifies that it involves body position and hypotension means low blood pressure. Clients who have had a spinal or epidural block are more likely to have orthostatic hypotension the higher the level of their block. Someone who has a block up to their midchest is more likely to have low blood pressure when sitting up than someone who has a block that only comes up to their waist. If someone with a high block has low blood pressure when they are sitting up, lowering the head of their bed is likely to result in an increase in their blood pressure. Orthostatic hypotension is unlikely after nerve blocks because a much smaller area of the body is involved.

Residual Sensory Block

One of the effects of any regional anesthetic that is used for surgery is the loss of pain sensation. Normal sensation may not have returned completely when the client is discharged from the recovery area and returned to his room. As the regional block wears off sensation will return gradually. Not all types of sensation return at the same time. The client may experience a "pins and needles" feeling in an arm or leg that has been blocked as sensation begins to return. He may feel touch or pressure before recovering complete sensation. Until complete recovery of normal sensation any blocked areas of the client's body need to be frequently checked and carefully protected as the client may be unaware that a finger or hand, for example, is being pinched or has the circulation cut off.

Residual Motor Block

Motor block results in the inability to move a body part and is usually the last to develop and the first to wear off. It results only when the regional block is very dense and complete. A motor block is a temporary condition caused when local anesthetic blocks nerves that carry instructions to skeletal muscles telling them to contract. A complete motor block results in a temporary paralysis and the client is not physically capable of moving the blocked part no matter how hard he tries. When a complete motor block is present there is usually no function in any other type of nerve in the same area. Because this is true it would be unusual for a client to be released from the recovery area with a complete motor block of any part of the body since there would be no evidence that the block was wearing off. Clients may be released from recovery with residual (incomplete) motor block and for this reason anyone who has had any type of block involving the legs should never be allowed to get out of bed without assistance until it can be demonstrated that they have a complete recovery of motor strength in the legs. Even a small amount of residual motor block greatly increases the possibility that a client will fall.

As a regional block begins to wear off, motor function begins to return. Sensation begins to return next. Sympathetic nervous function returns last. Motor function and sensation can be detected easily by asking the client to move the blocked part or by touching the skin and asking the client if it feels normal. The return of sympathetic function is more difficult to detect. Because sympathetic nervous function returns last, orthostatic hypotension may still occur even after motor and sensory function have completely returned and the regional block appears to have worn off. To prevent fainting, clients should not be allowed to get out of bed without the presence of a nurse until after they have been able to do so without any dizziness or a significant decrease in blood pressure.

GENERAL ANESTHESIA

What is General Anesthesia?

General anesthesia produces unconsciousness, complete insensibility to pain, amnesia, motionlessness, and surgical muscle relaxation with powerful drugs. General anesthesia also takes away the body's ability to control many important functions. These functions include, for example, the ability to maintain an airway to breathe through, the ability to control vital functions like breathing and heart rate, and the ability to regulate temperature. These functions are controlled by the anesthetist during a general anesthetic.

Overview of a General Anesthetic

A general anesthetic is divided into four overlapping periods: induction of anesthesia (going to sleep), maintenance of anesthesia, emergence from anesthesia (waking up), and recovery from the effects of anesthesia.

Induction and Airway Management

The induction of general anesthesia is a short, but critical, period of time during which the client is rendered unconscious, his vital functions are controlled, and enough anesthetic drug is introduced into the body to keep the client asleep during surgery. In adults, drugs are usually injected into an intravenous line to quickly produce unconsciousness and then additional anesthetic is inhaled through a breathing circuit. In small children, an anesthetic vapor is inhaled which produces unconsciousness a little more slowly and then an intravenous line is started and additional intravenous drugs are administered.

Immediately after the induction of general anesthesia the anesthetist will usually secure the airway with a cuffed endotracheal tube (ETT). The ETT is usually inserted under direct vision with the aid of a laryngoscope, an instrument designed to provide visualization and illumination of the trachea as shown in Figure 11-3. An endotracheal tube provides a breathing passage from outside the client to within the client's trachea. The endotracheal tube cuff seals the space between the ETT and the trachea making it difficult, though not impossible, for air to escape from or gastric contents to

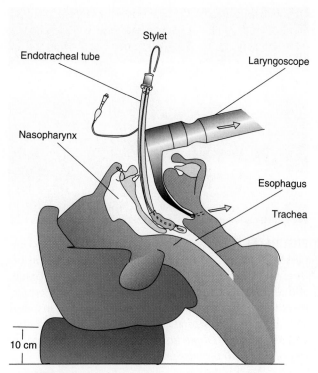

FIGURE 11-3 Performance of a laryngoscopy to place an endotracheal tube in the trachea under direct vision.

enter into the lungs. The ETT cuff decreases the possibility that stomach acid or food particles will enter the client's trachea. An ETT also provides a dependable way to provide oxygen and ventilation to the client. Breaths given through a properly positioned cuffed ETT go directly into the lungs and prevent any gas from entering the stomach.

Maintenance

General anesthesia is maintained with some combination of intravenous and inhaled drugs. Some of these drugs are only used as general anesthetics and others are used for other purposes but are also useful as anesthetics. Isoflurane (Forane) is an example of a drug used only for anesthesia. It produces all the components of a general anesthetic by itself. Figure 11-4 shows a client connected to an anesthesia machine by a breathing circuit. Benzodiazepines and opioids (sometimes called narcotics) are used for many other purposes but are also used as part of a general anesthetic. Neither produces all the components of a general anesthetic by itself. In healthy clients undergoing simple surgeries anesthetic drugs may be all that are needed. In critically ill clients and those undergoing complicated types of surgery other drugs may be needed to strengthen the heart, control the blood pressure, or produce complete paralysis of skeletal muscles.

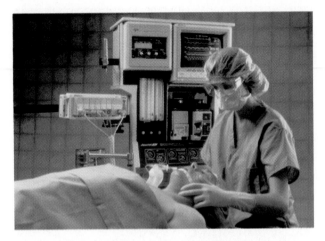

FIGURE 11-4 A typical anesthesia machine is a complex equipment set. This machine has anesthetic vaporizers and flowmeters to deliver oxygen, nitrous oxide, and air and also contains a small ventilator and equipment to monitor ventilation, oxygen content of inspired gas, client oxygen saturation, blood pressure, heart rate, and respiration. *(Ohmeda Excel 210 SE. Reprinted courtesy of and with permission of Ohmeda, Inc.)*

Skeletal Muscle Relaxation Some types of surgery require complete relaxation of skeletal muscles. In these cases the anesthetist administers a skeletal muscle relaxant like pancuronium bromide (Pavulon) or vecuronium bromide (Norcuron) to completely paralyze the client. These types of drugs prevent clients from breathing on their own but anesthetists are very skilled at ventilating clients during surgery. Usually a mechanical ventilator is used. Paralysis must be eliminated prior to emergence from anesthesia in order for the client to be able to breathe independently again. Once the skeletal muscle relaxant has begun to wear off, an anticholinesterase drug (neostigmine methylsulfate [Prostigmin], pyridostigmine bromide [Regonol]) is used to antagonize the remaining paralysis. The antagonism of residual paralysis is commonly called reversal. Once the paralyzing effect of an anesthetic muscle relaxant has begun to wear off on its own, the anesthetist can administer an anticholinesterase drug to reverse the remaining paralysis. This normally results in a quick return of muscle strength and the ability to breathe.

Inadequate reversal of paralysis may present as anything from total skeletal muscle paralysis to the inability of the client to cough and clear his airway. Typically, a client with partial paralysis has uncoordinated large muscle movements and is weak. If only small levels of paralysis remain the client may complain of difficulty swallowing or difficulty breathing deeply. Any detectable paralysis in a postoperative client should immediately be brought to the attention of someone from the anesthesia service for evaluation. If the client is having difficulty breathing basic life support should be provided until the arrival of an anesthetist.

Emergence

Emergence from general anesthesia occurs when anesthetic drugs are allowed to wear off. The anesthetist must carefully control when and how much anesthetic drug is given in order for the client to emerge from general anesthesia at, not before, the desired time. This takes experience and a detailed understanding of the drugs used and the client's response to those drugs. The initial phase of emergence is usually quite quick, allowing the client to awaken enough to obey commands and maintain his own airway. After this time, the client's breathing tube can usually be removed and the client taken to the post anesthesia care unit (recovery room). If, for some reason, the client must be left on a ventilator with a breathing tube in place the anesthetist may take the client to an intensive care unit asleep instead of waking the client up from the anesthetic.

Recovery

Recovery from general anesthesia is not complete simply because the client has regained consciousness. The client may not remember what has happened for minutes or even hours after the anesthetic. The ability to think clearly often takes longer to return, with some residual thinking difficulty persisting for several days or even weeks. Inhalation anesthetics are eliminated from the body through the lungs and very small amounts of anesthetic are still being exhaled during this time (Yasuda, Lockhart, & Eger, 1991). Many anesthetic drugs are stored in body fat and released back into the bloodstream very slowly after the anesthetic has ended. How long depends on the amount of anesthetic given during the surgery, the length of the surgery, and how deeply the client is breathing.

Oxygenation and Ventilation Almost all anesthetics are respiratory depressants. Benzodiazepines, opioids, and inhalation anesthetic agents have significant respiratory depressant effects. Any one of these drugs may be used during a general anesthetic in a dose that causes apnea. When used in combination their effect on respiration is at least additive. When the rate or depth of respirations decrease, the elimination of carbon dioxide is retarded and carbon dioxide builds up in the blood and in the lungs. The buildup of carbon dioxide actually blocks the entry of oxygen into the bloodstream and makes it harder to keep the client adequately oxygenated. Even small amounts of supplemental oxygen given to a client whose rate or depth of breathing is decreased adds significantly to the amount of oxygen in the bloodstream. This is the most important reason why oxygen is given to even healthy clients while they are recovering from general anesthesia.

Heart Rate and Blood Pressure General anesthesia has few direct effects on heart rate (HR) and blood pressure (BP) regulation during recovery. Some anesthetic techniques that are heavily based on opioids like fentanyl (Sublimaze) or sufentanil citrate (Sufenta) can cause a slow heart rate but as long as the blood pressure is maintained no specific treatment is necessary. Although most general anesthetics are myocardial depressants, these effects are mild with modern agents and have little effect once anesthetic administration is ended. Some individuals will become sympathetically activated during the initial period after regaining consciousness. This occurs most commonly in clients with cardiac or vascular disease (hypertension, coronary artery disease, peripheral vascular occlusive disease). If the increase in HR or BP is a danger to the client it can usually be successfully treated with a combined alpha and beta blocker like labetalol hydrochloride (Normodyne) or a calcium channel blocker such as nifedipine (Procardia).

Most HR and BP changes during recovery are due to factors related indirectly to the anesthetic. Both HR and BP increase due to sympathetic stimulation. Pain, hypoxia, and fear can all result in sympathetic stimulation with an increase in HR and BP. Pain results when inadequate analgesia has been provided as the client emerges from anesthesia. Administering an opioid such as morphine or meperidine (Demerol) will relieve the pain. The residual effects of anesthesia on respiratory centers or airway muscles in the throat may result in hypoventilation or airway obstruction. Providing supplemental oxygen, proper airway management, and mechanical ventilation if necessary, will ensure adequate oxygenation. Discovering the source of client's fear and addressing it often reduces the anxiety. When the causes of sympathetic stimulation are addressed HR and BP should become normal as well.

Temperature Regulation and Shivering General anesthesia defeats the body's natural ability to regulate temperature. General anesthetic agents dilate the blood vessels close to the surface of the body exposing the client's warm blood to the cool exterior. During the time the client is anesthetized he is in a cold operating room, mostly uncovered, and the area of the body to be operated on is cleaned with cold solutions. Once this is done, the client's insulating covering (skin and subcutaneous fat) is cut open to expose the warm interior of the body and allow its heat to escape, room temperature intravenous fluids are infused into his veins, and the client breathes cool gases. Surgical clients lose a lot of heat while the body is least able to

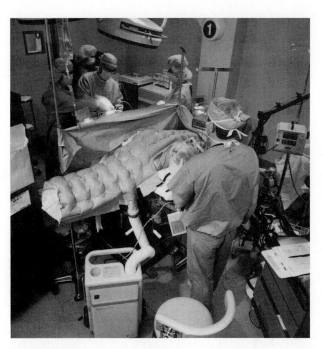

FIGURE 11-5 A forced air warming blanket applied to the upper abdomen, chest, and arms of a patient during surgery. The unit on the floor to the left of the anesthetist (standing in the foreground) is the heating unit and contains a fan that pushes warm air through the hose into the blanket much like a furnace pushes warm air through the heating ducts in a house. Warm air exits hundreds of pinholes on the surface of the blanket next to the patient. (*Courtesy of Mallinckrodt Medical, Inc.*)

do anything about it. Hypothermia adds to the central nervous system depression present from any residual anesthetics. Surface warming with a forced air warming blanket is a much more effective way to increase the temperature of a client recovering from general anesthesia than cloth blankets or heating lamps. Forced air warming blankets are also used to prevent or limit the development of hypothermia intraoperatively. Figure 11-5 shows a forced air warming blanket.

All potent inhalation agents are associated with shivering during emergence from general anesthesia when the blood level of the anesthetic agent is very low. This was first associated with halothane and called the "halothane shakes," but it can occur following any inhalation anesthetic. The cause of the shivering is not clear but it does not appear to be related to the client's body temperature. (Of course, postoperative clients also shiver if they are cold.) The key to eliminating shivering postoperatively is to make sure the client is warm and encourage deep breathing so that the anesthetic is eliminated as quickly as possible.

Fluid Balance Surgical procedures and the injuries that necessitate them have major effects on the body's distribution of fluid. Appropriate care during anesthesia sometimes necessitates the delivery of a large volume of intravenous fluid. This IV fluid does not stay in the vascular system long. It moves out of the vascular space to replace losses from the interstitial and intracellular spaces.

Trauma, whether due to an accidental injury or a surgical incision, results in fluid losses or shifts in three general areas as follows: direct blood loss, evaporation through the surgical wound, and fluid shifts. The surgical wound can lose large volumes of fluid into the air, especially during abdominal procedures. A major abdominal procedure, for example, can result in the loss of up to 10 cc/kg/hour of fluid by evaporation. Following an acute tissue injury, due to trauma or surgery, a shift of body fluid to a so called *third space* occurs. This *third space* is not really a different place at all but rather a concept. The fluid is actually in the interstitial space between cells in a tissue. Anesthetists like to think of the fluid separately from other body fluids because it is unavailable for the body to use (therefore, we conceptualize it as being in a totally different place, a third space). It does not transfer nutrients or metabolites. It is not available to move into the vascular space to replace blood loss. This shift in fluid is a physiologic response to trauma and is unrelated to the volume of blood lost or the volume of intravenous fluid replaced. A major abdominal surgery can result in the shifting of 10 cc/kg/hour or more fluid to this third space in addition to what is lost due to evaporation. In healthy clients, a third space fluid shift persists for one to three days postoperatively and is then mobilized and eliminated as urine.

POSTOPERATIVE PAIN MANAGEMENT

Pain has many causes. Postoperative pain is due to tissue injury, release of local and hormonal substances, inflammation, mental outlook, and perhaps also neural hyperexcitability from excessive noxious input. As such, baseline postoperative pain, pain from pressure on an incision, and pain from client movement may each respond best to different pain relieving strategies. Enough is now known about postoperative pain management that there is seldom an excuse for inadequate pain relief.

The amount of medication needed to relieve pain depends on the intensity and type of pain, the size of the client, and client age. The dose requirement for most opioids decreases dramatically in the elderly. An eighty-nine-year-old needs 50 percent less opioid analgesic than a twenty-year-old (Scott & Stanski, 1987).

Intravenous Patient-Controlled Analgesia

Patient-controlled analgesia (PCA) allows clients to self-administer pain medicine by pushing a button when they experience pain. When an intravenous catheter is in place a client controlled analgesia pump is connected "piggyback" into the IV line. The pump is programmed to deliver a predetermined dose of morphine or meperidine (Demerol) when the client pushes a button. It will not, however, deliver unlimited amounts. A set time must pass between each successive dose and once the total dose of opioid given in any hour reaches a preset limit, the pump will not deliver any more medicine until the next hour. Properly programmed, PCA allows the client a great deal of control over when pain medicine is received which is likely to help decrease anxiety. PCA also results in a shorter interval between the need for pain medicine and its administration, better pain relief than intermittent IM injections, and a reduction in nursing time necessary for the delivery of pain medicine. It does not, however, decrease the need for client assessment while the PCA machine is in use. An important safety feature of PCA is that if the client's level of consciousness becomes depressed from excessive medicine the client will not be able to push the button to administer more drug. For this reason only the client should push the button to administer another dose. Nursing personnel and visitors should be instructed not to push the button.

Regional Analgesia

Regional analgesia and anesthesia have many applications in the relief of postoperative pain. Regional anesthetics do not end when the surgery ends and provide pain relief for a variable period of time afterwards. The duration of postoperative pain relief can be extended by continuing the infusion of pain medicine into the epidural space or by adding opioids to either epidural or spinal anesthetics.

Local Anesthetics

Local anesthetics, either alone or in combination with opioids, can be administered into the epidural space at low concentrations that do not cause complete anesthesia. This type of pain relief is most commonly used for women in labor who receive labor epidural analgesia. Low concentrations of local anesthetic are powerful analgesics. If they are administered in a way to include the lower extremities in the area of pain relief, clients will usually be confined to bed. Even dilute concentrations of local anesthetic may affect the strength of leg muscles enough to increase the risk of falling. Clients receiving epidural analgesia should be watched carefully to make sure they do not develop pressure necrosis in the blocked areas. Local anesthetic pain relief can occasionally do such a good job at relieving pain that the client may be unaware that pressure necrosis is occurring (Cohen, Van Duker, Siegel, & Keon, 1993).

Opioids

The spinal cord has receptors for opioids and when opioids are added to a spinal or epidural anesthetic, they provide pain relief even after the anesthetic block has worn off. When morphine is added to a spinal or epidural anesthetic it can provide hours of postoperative pain relief, often enough that no other pain medicine is needed (Abouleish, et al., 1991). It may even provide better pain relief than IM injections or intravenous PCA (Kilbride, Senagore, Mazier, Ferguson, & Ufkes, 1992). Opioids may be added to spinal or epidural anesthetics as a single dose or infused into the epidural space postoperatively. Although spinal and epidural morphine provides excellent pain relief, it may also produce significant respiratory depression. Respiratory depression with properly dosed epidural or spinal fentanyl (Sublimaze) is exceedingly rare (Renaud, et al., 1988; Brockway, Noble, Sharwood-Smith, & McClure, 1990; Wells & Davies, 1987). Fortunately, the respiratory depression following spinal or epidural morphine administration is rarely quick in onset. With modern client selection and dosing protocols, life-threatening respiratory depression is a rare event. When it does occur, it can be detected long before it causes harm by observing the client frequently, noting respiratory rate and depth, and periodically measuring oxygen saturation by pulse oximetry. Table 11-2 lists the key considerations in postanesthetic care.

Table 11-2

KEY CONSIDERATIONS IN POSTANESTHETIC CARE

- Report any difficulty breathing to the anesthetist or surgeon immediately.
- Report a falling blood pressure or a rising heart rate to the surgeon or to the anesthesia department immediately.
- Verify that clients are able to stand or walk with normal motor strength and coordination and without any dizziness while in your direct care before allowing them to get up without assistance.
- Do not allow clients to rub their eyes. Clients who are still drowsy may try to rub out protective eye moisturizer and in the process cause painful corneal abrasions.
- Observe clients immediately for bladder distention. Both regional and general anesthesia can sometimes cause temporary urinary retention.
- If clients are using Intravenous Patient Controlled Analgesia (IVPCA), do not allow anyone other than the client to push the activating button. If nursing staff or visitors push the button, an overdose may result.
- If clients have an epidural catheter for postoperative pain management ensure that they change positions from time to time to prevent pressure necrosis. Do not allow the lateral aspect of the leg to rest on the side rails.
- Report a headache that gets worse when sitting up or standing to the anesthesia department as soon as possible.
- Verify that client's ability to remember instructions has returned before giving discharge instructions. Always share discharge instructions with the individual responsible for taking the client home and provide the client with a written copy of the instructions.

▶ CASE STUDY

Mrs. Jones is in the recovery room follow-ing outpatient surgery. She had a general anesthetic and is now awake, breathing deeply, and talking to the staff. She has received meperidine (Demerol) intrave-nously and is quite comfortable. Before being discharged home from the day surgery center Mrs. Jones rests in an easy chair in the transitional recovery area. The nurse taking care of her notices that she asks questions about things that have already been discussed and has even asked one question three times.

The following questions will guide your develop-ment of a Nursing Care Plan for the case study.

1. After making these observations what nursing diagnoses and goals might the nurse identify for Mrs. Jones?

2. List the nursing interventions to be performed in caring for Mrs. Jones.

3. Identify how teaching should be done.

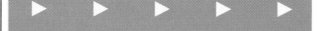
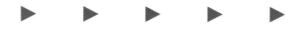

SUMMARY

- In addition to ensuring adequate levels of anesthe-sia throughout a surgical procedure the anesthetist monitors and controls physiologic functions.
- Some anesthetists prefer that clients not have any-thing to eat or drink for at least eight hours prior to surgery. Others allow water up to two hours before leaving for the operating room.
- Most scheduled medications that a client takes every day will be continued up to and including the morning of surgery.
- Sedation depresses the brain, decreasing aware-ness, reducing anxiety, and easing the induction of general anesthesia.
- Oversedation results in airway obstruction and places the client at risk for aspiration of gastric contents.
- Regional anesthesia temporarily renders a "region" of the body insensible to pain by the injection of a local anesthetic.
- General anesthesia produces unconsciousness, com-plete insensibility to pain, amnesia, motionlessness, and muscle relaxation.

- Emergence from general anesthesia occurs when anesthetic drugs are allowed to wear off.
- A person is unlikely to remember what has hap-pened for minutes or hours after sedation or a gen-eral anesthetic.
- Everyone needs supplemental oxygen following a general anesthetic.
- Intravenous patient controlled analgesia (PCA) allows clients to self-administer pain medication by pushing a button on the PCA machine. Limits are programmed into the machine to prevent overdose.
- Local anesthetics, alone or in combination with opi-oids, can be injected into the epidural space at low concentrations to provide postoperative analgesia.
- Spinal and epidural morphine can produce danger-ous respiratory depression that can be detected long before it causes client harm by frequent obser-vations of the client's respiratory rate and depth and periodic measurement of oxygen saturation by pulse oximetry.

Review Questions

1. Who is qualified to explain anesthesia and its risks and benefits in a manner sufficient to secure an informed consent from a client or their legal guardian?
   a. a medical/surgical staff nurse
   b. an anesthetist or surgeon
   c. an operating room nurse
   d. a nursing supervisor

2. Why are clients at risk for aspiration of gastric contents into the lungs when they have a general anesthetic?
   a. General anesthesia causes stomach distention.
   b. General anesthesia eliminates protective airway reflexes.
   c. Gastric peristalsis is reversed during general anesthesia.
   d. Vomiting normally occurs during general anesthesia.

3. What is the most important result of oversedation?
   a. client will not obey commands
   b. longer recovery time delays discharge
   c. prolonged amnesia
   d. inability to breathe adequately

4. What is the most convincing sign that a client has a post dural puncture headache following a spinal or epidural regional anesthetic?
   a. It gets better after drinking plenty of liquids.
   b. It began after the surgical procedure.
   c. It gets worse when the client sits up or stands.
   d. The client is confused in addition to having a headache.

5. In addition to keeping the client unconscious, preventing the sensation of pain, and relaxing muscles to hold the client still and allow for surgical exposure, what does an anesthetist do to ensure a safe anesthetic?
   a. control vital functions like breathing and heart rate
   b. record how much anesthesia is used
   c. monitor how long the surgery is taking
   d. administer prophylactic antibiotics

6. How long after a general anesthetic might it be before a client can think as clearly as before the client had an anesthetic?
   a. before being discharged from the recovery room
   b. within two hours
   c. six hours
   d. several days

7. What effect might a spinal or epidural anesthetic still have after normal sensation and motor function have returned?
   a. decrease in pulse rate while client is lying in bed
   b. decrease in blood pressure when the client stands up
   c. inhibition of protective airway reflexes
   d. sore muscles

Critical Thinking Questions

1. Why is physical assessment important relative to anesthesia?

2. What is the best kind of anesthesia?

News Flash

For many years clients scheduled for elective surgery have been instructed not to eat or drink anything after midnight (NPO past midnight). This practice was meant to allow the stomach to empty completely and thus decrease the risk that stomach contents might regurgitate into the back of the throat where they could be aspirated into the lungs. Aspiration of gastric contents holds two different types of danger. First, stomach acid has a very low pH and the acidity of gastric liquid can cause extensive damage to the air passages and alveolar sacs in the lungs. This damage causes fluid to leak into the lungs. Inflammation and swelling of lung tissue also occurs after acid aspiration. Second, food particles obstruct breathing tubes limiting the movement of air into the lungs. Both of these problems result in a decreased ability to absorb oxygen and causes hypoxia.

Although clients are still instructed not to eat for at least eight hours before elective surgery, many anesthesia professionals now question the need to withhold water, and perhaps other clear liquids, from adults for so long. (Infants and small children have always been permitted sugar water up until two to four hours before surgery.) After all, not hav-

ing anything to drink is uncomfortable, especially if surgery is scheduled for later in the day. Research over the last few years has shown that allowing adults to drink reasonable amounts of water, and perhaps other clear liquids such as apple juice (Vincent, McNeil, Spaid, MacMahon, Maxwell, Brenner, et al., 1991), up until two hours prior to surgery does not result in an increase in the volume of stomach contents (Phillips, et al., 1993; Read & Vaughan, 1991; Soreide, et al., 1993). In fact, some studies have shown that the volume and acidity of gastric contents are less at the beginning of surgery in clients who have had several ounces of water to drink two hours before surgery.

While most anesthesia providers still require clients to be NPO for eight hours there is growing evidence that liquids can safely be permitted up until two hours before elective surgery. As more anesthetists and surgeons become aware of the current research in this area surgical nurses should expect to see more liberal orders for oral intake prior to surgery. Of course preoperative instructions should be respected in this area even if a particular provider or department chooses not to allow more liberal fluid intake.

CHAPTER
12
Pain Management

Mary E. A. Laskin

KEY TERMS

acupuncture
acute pain
addiction
adjuvant
analgesia
analgesic
ceiling effect
chronic pain
cordotomy
endorphin
epidural analgesia
gate control theory
intrathecal analgesia
modulation
nociceptor
noxious stimulus
opioid
pain
perception
referred pain
rhizotomy
somatic pain
tolerance
transduction
transmission

LEARNING OBJECTIVES

Upon completion of this chapter the learner should be able to:
- Define key terms.
- Identify the four components of pain conduction.
- List three guidelines that should be included in a thorough pain assessment.
- Identify three general principles of pain management.
- List the nurse's responsibilities in administration of analgesics.
- Identify site of action of both nonopioid and opioid analgesics.
- Describe three examples of nonpharmacological measures for pain relief.

▶ *MAKING THE CONNECTION*

Refer to the topics in the following chapters to increase your understanding of pain management.

- **Chapter 7, Cultural Diversity in the Workplace:** Cultural Responses to Pain, p. 105
- **Chapter 13, Perioperative Nursing:** The Nursing Process in the Postanesthesia Care Unit,

p. 247; Ambulatory Surgery, p. 258; Elderly Clients Undergong Surgery, p. 259
- **Chapter 15, Oncology Nursing:** Symptom Management, Pain, p. 315

INTRODUCTION

Pain is a phenomenon that crosses all specialties of nursing. No matter the setting a nurse practices in, including neonatal intensive care, intraoperative, home care, or clinics, the nurse will be exposed to challenges in pain management. While other health care team members address pain management with clients, it is the nurse who spends the most time with the client experiencing pain. For example, in an acute care setting, the physician orders the **analgesics** (substances that relieve pain) for the client, but may only spend ten to fifteen minutes each day with that client. The nurses are the ones who are present twenty-four hours a day, administer the medications, assess the client's response, and report the response to the physician. It is for this reason the nurse is often called the "backbone" or "cornerstone" of pain management. The nurse's role can be pivotal in relieving the client's pain.

Pain management in health care settings has been shown to be inadequate. Studies document undertreatment of pain of all types and in all age groups for the past two decades (Liebeskind & Melzack, 1987). In one such study, the researchers interviewed medical and surgical clients, finding that 58 percent had experienced excruciating pain in the previous seventy-two hours. Fifty-five percent of these clients could not recall a nurse asking about their pain (Donovan, et al., 1987). A more recent study examined pain management in metastatic cancer clients in an outpatient setting. Forty-two percent of the clients with pain were not given adequate analgesic therapy (Cleeland, et al., 1994).

It is generally thought that this undertreatment of pain is partially due to the lack of knowledge in both physicians and nurses. It is, therefore, important for the nurse to understand not only the psychological and physiological components that add up to the pain experience, but also the wide range of interventions available to provide relief. Another reason for undertreatment may be the health care worker's own biases regarding pain. Consequently, nurses should also rec-

ognize their own responses to pain and how they respond to others' expressions of pain. This chapter provides an overview of the complex phenomenon of pain, including: pain definitions, pain physiology, and pain assessment. Strategies to control pain will also be discussed, including pharmacological, noninvasive, and invasive techniques. The nurse who is equipped with this knowledge-base in pain management will be able to function as the strong backbone the client deserves.

KEY ABBREVIATIONS

The following abbreviations and acronyms are used in this chapter:

APS	American Pain Society
AHCPR	Agency for Health Care Policy and Research
ATC	around the clock
IASP	International Association for the Study of Pain
IVP	intravenous push
NSAID	nonsteroidal anti-inflammatory drug
PCA	patient controlled analgesia
PRN	*pro re nata,* Latin for "as required"
OTFC	oral transmucosal fentanyl citrate
ORIF	open reduction internal fixation
SBP	systolic blood pressure
TENS	transcutaneous electrical nerve stimulation
TMJ	temporomandibular joint

DEFINITIONS OF PAIN

The phenomenon of **pain** is evidenced in ancient history with references being made as far back as the Babylonian clay tablets. Aristotle (fourth century B.C.) described pain as an emotion, being the opposite of pleasure. While emotions certainly play an important role in pain perception, we now know there is much more to the experience than the feelings involved.

In the Middle Ages, pain was viewed with religious connotations. Pain was seen as God's punishment for sins, or as evidence that an individual was possessed by demons. This definition of pain is still embraced by some clients, who might tell the nurse that the suffering is their "cross to bear." Pain relief may not be the goal for those individuals who believe in this definition of pain. Spiritual counseling may need to be implemented before this person is willing to work toward relief.

Currently, the most widely accepted definition of pain was developed by the International Association for the Study of Pain (IASP). This organization defines pain as "an unpleasant sensory and emotional experience associated with actual or potential tissue damage or described in terms of such damage" (Merskey, 1979). This definition incorporates both the sensory, or nerve stimulation, component along with the emotional component of pain. It also acknowledges that evidence of actual tissue damage is not required in order for the pain to be considered real. For example, in the case of low back pain where no damage is seen on the x-rays or a magnetic resonance image (MRI), the client may be treated as if the pain was psychosomatic. According to this definition, however, the pain in this client would be considered actual pain.

Many pain experts emphasize the subjective nature of pain. Unlike a blood pressure or a blood glucose measurement, the intensity of discomfort the client is feeling cannot be measured with an instrument. Margo McCaffery (1979) says it best by defining pain as "whatever the patient says it is, existing whenever the patient says it does." When a nurse states that the client does not "look like she's in that much pain," it must be remembered that the pain is a subjective experience. The nurse must believe the client. This philosophy is emphasized in professional pain management guidelines. For example, the Agency for Health Care Policy and Research (AHCPR) guideline for cancer pain states, "Health professionals should ask about pain, and the patient's self-report should be the primary source of assessment." The (APS) American Pain Society also stresses the importance of self-report, "Pain is always subjective . . . The clinician must accept the patient's report of pain" (1992).

Though pain has had many definitions throughout humankind's history, research in pain physiology has shown that pain is a complex phenomenon. In defining pain in clinical practice, the nurse should keep in mind that pain has both sensory and emotional components, plus it may be described in terms of actual or potential tissue as defined by IASP. The nurse also needs to make the client's report of pain a priority, due to the subjective nature of pain, as defined by McCaffery (1979).

ACUTE VS. CHRONIC PAIN

Pain is usually divided into two categories: acute and chronic. It is important to understand the difference between the two, as they each present a different clinical picture. Unfortunately, most health professionals learn about pain in the acute model. Therefore, if the client's signs and symptoms do not fit that model, it may be difficult to believe in the client's pain.

Acute Pain

Acute pain is considered pain that has lasted less than six months (see Table 12-1). It can usually be associated with a specific injury or disease that has caused tissue damage. Acute pain should diminish as healing occurs. Everyone has experienced acute pain, for example: headaches, toothaches, skinned knees, muscle pain, childbirth, postoperative pain, a sprained ankle. The client will describe the pain as highly localized and is usually able to pinpoint where the hurt is. Characteristics of acute pain are often described as sharp, although if the pain is deep, **somatic pain**, it may be described as dull and aching. Accompanying signs will be those of the activation of the sympathetic nervous system, that is, the fight or flight response. Therefore, the client will exhibit elevated heart rate, respiratory rate, and blood pressure. The client may become diaphoretic and have dilated pupils. These signs resemble those of anxiety, which often accompanies acute pain. Behaviors may include crying and moaning, rubbing the site of pain, guarding, frowning, and grimacing. The client will usually complain of the discomfort.

Chronic Pain

Chronic pain is considered pain that lasts longer than the expected healing time (refer to Table 12-1). The usual time frame is pain lasting longer than six months. This time frame was initially chosen arbitrarily, but has since become the most widely accepted measure. The client may have difficulty pinpointing the location of the pain. Characteristics of chronic pain are often described as dull and aching. The signs and symptoms of chronic pain can look very different from acute pain. The body could not tolerate the sympathetic nervous system signs for such a long period of time and, therefore, adapts. The vital signs will often be normal, with no accompanying pupil dilatation or perspiration. Lack of these signs may prompt some health care workers to question the client's description of pain. The signs and symptoms of chronic pain, such as hopelessness, listlessness, loss of libido and weight, are often similar to depression. The client will often complain of exhaustion and fatigue. Behaviors include

Table 12-1

ACUTE PAIN VERSUS CHRONIC PAIN		
	Acute	**Chronic**
Time span	Less than six months	More than six months
Location	Localized, associated with a specific injury	Difficult to pinpoint
Characteristics	Often described as sharp, diminishes as healing occurs	Often described as dull, diffuse, and aching
Physiologic signs	• Elevated heart rate • Elevated BP • Elevated respirations • May be diaphoretic • Dilated pupils	• Normal vital signs • Normal pupils • No diaphoresis • May have loss of weight
Behavioral signs	• Crying & moaning • Rubbing site • Guarding • Frowning • Grimacing • Complains of pain	• Physical immobility • Hopelessness • Listlessness • Loss of libido • Exhaustion & fatigue • Only complains of pain when asked

no complaints of pain unless asked and physical inactivity or immobility that can lead to functional disability. The crying, moaning, guarding, and grimacing that most clinicians associate with pain are absent. Treatment of chronic pain is more complex than acute pain. It is viewed by pain experts as a disease state, rather than a symptom (Bonica, 1990). Management includes identifying the cause of pain, recognizing emotional and environmental factors that may be contributing to the pain, and rehabilitation to improve the client's functional abilities. Successful chronic pain programs often use a multidisciplinary team approach.

PURPOSE OF PAIN

Pain serves an important purpose as a protective mechanism. It tells us to withdraw from the **noxious stimulus** that is causing the tissue damage. For example, if a person touches a hot stove, the pain signal will cause them to pull their hand away immediately. The skin would be seriously burned if this did not happen. So pain has an important purpose. Not only does it protect us, but it prompts clients to seek out medical care. Pain is usually the chief complaint of people accessing health care.

Pain is also useful as a diagnostic tool. Characteristics of the pain, such as the quality and duration, can give important clues in determining a client's medical diagnosis. For example, in acute appendicitis, the clin-

ician looks for rebound tenderness (the pain increases when pressure is released) when palpating the abdomen. This particular type of pain helps to determine the diagnosis of appendicitis rather than other gastrointestinal disorders. Once pain has served its purpose, there is no reason to let it continue. Pain control needs to be a therapeutic goal for all clients, and is a basic client right.

PHYSIOLOGY OF PAIN

The Gate Control Theory

The most widely accepted theory of pain processes is the **gate control theory** of pain, proposed by Melzack & Wall (1965). This theory proposes that sensory, motivational-affective, and cognitive processes all combine to determine how a person perceives pain. The theory suggests that nerve fibers that contribute to pain transmission converge at a site in the dorsal horn of the spinal cord. This site is thought to act as a gating mechanism that determines which impulses will be blocked and which will be transmitted to the thalamus. The image of a gate can be useful in teaching clients and their families about pain relief measures. If the "gate" is closed, the signal is stopped before it reaches the brain, where **perception** (being aware of) of pain occurs. If the gate is open, the signal will continue on through the spinothalamic tract to the cortex, and the client will feel the pain. Whether the gate is opened or closed is influenced by the impulses from peripheral nerves (the sensory components), and nerve signals that descend from the brain (motivational-affective and cognitive components). For example, stimulation of some types of peripheral nerves by cutaneous stimulation such as massage can close the gate, whereas stimulation of the **nociceptors** (nerves that receive and transmit the pain signal) will open the gate.

If a person is anxious, the gate can be opened by signals sent from the brain down to the mechanism in the dorsal horn of the spinal cord. On the other hand, if the person has had positive experiences with pain control in the past, the cognitive influence can send signals down to the gating mechanism and close it. The gate theory offered a great benefit by suggesting new approaches to relieving both acute and chronic pain. Pain could be relieved by blocking the transmission of pain impulses to the brain by both physical modalities and by altering the individual's thought processes, emotions, or other behaviors.

Conduction of Pain Impulses

Conduction of pain impulses refers to the physiologic processes that occur from the initiation of the pain signal to the realization of pain by the individual. There are four processes involved in the conduction of this signal. The first of these, **transduction**, is the step where a noxious stimulus triggers electrical activity in the endings of afferent nerve fibers (nociceptors). Once the signal is triggered, **transmission** occurs. The impulse travels from the receiving nociceptors to the spinal cord. Projection neurons then carry the message to the thalamus, and the message continues to the somatosensory cortex. This is where the third step, perception of pain occurs. It is here that neural messages are converted into the subjective experience. The fourth process, **modulation**, is a central nervous system pathway that selectively inhibits pain transmission by sending blocking signals back down to the dorsal horn of the spinal cord.

Each of the four steps has implications for treating pain. Understanding the neurophysiology of conduction and pain explains the rationale for pain relieving interventions.

Transduction

Transduction is the step where an action potential is generated in the nociceptors that will be transmitting the pain signal. This is the peripheral pain system. Chemical energy (biochemical mediators) is changed to electrical energy (the action potential in the neuron).

There are two types of primary afferent pain fibers

or nociceptors: the A-delta fibers (acute pain), are myelinated and, therefore, transmit the signal rapidly. The slower conducting chronic pain or C-fibers, are smaller and unmyelinated (see Figure 12-1). The two types of neurons explain the two types of pain felt with an injury. For example, if you bump your elbow, you feel the first sharp pain immediately (A-delta fibers), followed by a throbbing, aching pain (C-fibers). The C-fibers are those that are associated with chronic pain.

A noxious stimulus (either mechanical, thermal, or chemical) causes the release of biochemical mediators, which activate the afferent neurons. These mediators lead to the generation of an action potential in the neuron. Biochemical mediators that activate or sensitize the nociceptive response include: potassium, hist-

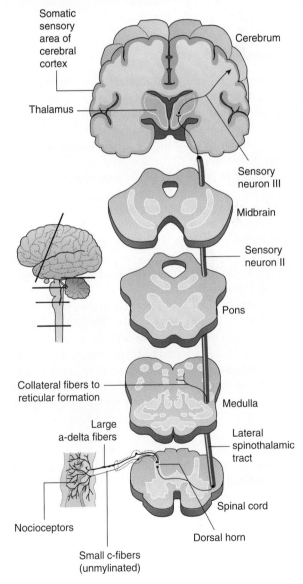

FIGURE 12-1 Nociceptors: primary afferent nerve fibers. The A-delta fibers are myelinated, the small C-fibers are unmyelinated.

amine, neurotransmitters (e.g., substance P), prostaglandins, leukotrienes, bradykinin.

Clinical implications at this step of pain conduction include inhibition of prostaglandins. Prostaglandins formed from precursors that are released by damaged cells contribute to the pain by activating the nociceptive response. Some of the nonopioid analgesics are potent prostaglandin-blockers (referred to as nonsteroidal anti-inflammatory drugs, or NSAIDs). Another implication is the use of anticonvulsant or anesthetic drugs (referred to as membrane stabilizers) which prevent the generation of an action potential in a neuron. An example of an anticonvulsant is carbamazepine (Tegretol), and examples of anesthetics are mexiletine HCl (Mexitil HCl). and lidocaine (Xylocaine). By preventing transduction, the pain signal is stopped at the peripheral level before new impulses responsible for the experience of pain reach the cortex and the client feels the pain.

Transmission

Transmission is the term that refers to the traveling of the nociceptive signal. The first leg of the journey is along the afferent fibers, terminating in the dorsal horn of the spinal cord. Neuropeptides and other substances, primarily substance P, are released from the neuron. Substance P diffuses across the synaptic gap to secondary neurons and binds with receptor sites. It is this synapse which is the proposed "gate" in the gate control theory. This triggers an action potential in those nerve cells. These neurons are called spinothalamic tract neurons, which carry the signal to the other side of the spinal cord and terminate in the thalamus, although some terminate in the midbrain. The signal then continues to the cortex.

The primary clinical implication at this stage of the process is the action of **opioids**. These drugs bind to opiate receptor sites on the afferent neuron in the dorsal horn of the spinal cord (see Figure 12-2). This prevents release of the neurotransmitters, such as substance P and stops the signal at the spinal cord level. This explains why opioids work so well intraspinally or epidurally. They are delivered close to the site of action.

Another clinical implication of this step in conduction is the **cordotomy** procedure, or the surgical ablation of the pain-conducting tracts in the dorsal horn of the spinal cord. Because these transmission fibers occur in a well-defined region in the spinal cord, neurosurgeons can inhibit the pain message by ablating (severing) the tract surgically.

Perception

As previously discussed, perception is the process where sensory messages become the subjective feel-

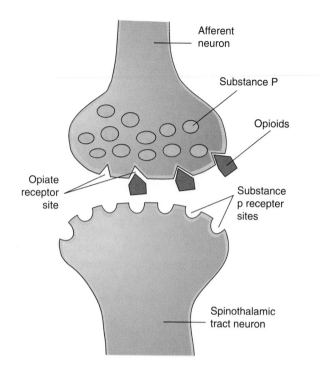

FIGURE 12-2 Mechanism of opioids. The opioids bind to the afferent neuron in the dorsal horn of the spinal cord. This prevents the neurotransmitter, substance P, from being released from the afferent neuron. Thus, the pain signal is not continued in the spinothalamic tract neuron, but blocked at the spinal cord level.

ings of pain. This step occurs when the signal reaches the brain. Neurons from the thalamus transmit the nociceptive message to several areas in the cortex. The signal terminates in two areas in the parietal lobe: the somatosensory cortex (associated with the intensity and quality of pain) and the association cortex (associated with affective types of pain). The signal also terminates in the limbic system (associated with anxiety). This is the stage where a person realizes pain. It is the least understood of all the stages in pain conduction.

Modulation

Modulation is the body's own ability to change the pain signal. The neurons that terminate in the midbrain stimulate regions that send descending signals to the dorsal horn of the spinal cord (see Figure 12-3). These neurons inhibit the transmission of nociception by releasing substances such as serotonin, norepinephrine, and endogenous opiates (**endorphins**). They bind to the afferent neuron and prevent the release of substance P as do the opioid medications.

Clinical implications of modulation include activities that may increase the release of endorphins, for example, TENS and hypnosis. Due to the presence of norepinephrine, a neurotransmitter in the descending

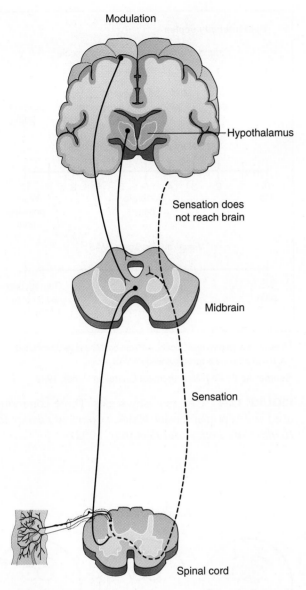

FIGURE 12-3 Modulation. Neurons that terminate in the midbrain stimulate regions that send signals to the dorsal horn of the spinal cord, blocking the transmission of pain.

fibers, clonidine HCl (Catapres) (a medication similar to norepinephrine), has been administered epidurally and intraspinally to relieve pain. However, the hypotensive effects are significant. Another implication of modulation is the use of tricyclic antidepressants. Antidepressants inhibit the reuptake of serotonin back into the descending neuron, which allows more serotonin to remain available in the synaptic cleft. This inhibits the pain transmission by "closing" the gate.

The combination of the gate control theory and the four processes involved in the conduction of the pain signal describe the physiology of pain. Knowledge of these processes gives the nurse rationales for the pain control measures utilized in pain management practices.

ASSESSMENT

Assessment of the client's pain is a crucial function of the nurse. Failure to assess pain correctly may lead to its undertreatment. During the assessment process, the nurse needs to be aware of his or her own values and expectations about pain behaviors. Just as the client's experience and cultural background help determine how pain is demonstrated, the nurse's culture and experience will determine which pain behaviors are viewed as acceptable. The nurse needs to be aware of these values and avoid letting them create biases when assessing client pain and planning client care. Once a self-assessment about pain has been conducted, the nurse is ready to assess the client. A systematic method of organizing the initial pain assessment will help to identify the cause and develop a plan for managing the pain.

Subjective

Due to the subjective nature of pain, the subjective data takes priority in the pain assessment. Whenever subjective and objective data conflict, the subjective reports of pain are to be considered the primary source.

Location

Have the client point to the location of the pain on their own body or locate it on a body diagram on a pain assessment tool. Ask if there is more than one site of pain. Have the client indicate if the pain radiates, and if so to where. Ask if the pain is deep or superficial.

Case Example During intershift report on a postoperative client recovering from abdominal surgery, the nurse reported that the client had stated she had pain and had been medicated with IM Demerol. When greeting her client, the nurse asked the client about the pain she had experienced during the night. The client replied, "Oh, it is fine now, I only had a headache." The night nurse had assumed the client's pain was in her surgical site and chose the medication accordingly. The headache probably could have been relieved with a milder medication.

Onset and Duration

Ask how long the client has had the pain. Other questions that the nurse might ask include, "Is there anything that triggers its onset?" "Are there any patterns to the pain, for example is it worse at certain times of the day or night?" It is common for the client's pain to be worse at night when there are less distractions. Teaching the client that this is normal can be reassuring as the client may attribute the increased pain to complications of her illness.

Quality

Ask the client what the pain feels like, and record the words used to describe the pain. Clients may use sensory-type words, such as "pricking," "burning," or "throbbing." However, some clients use words that have an affective connotation, such as, "fearful," "sickening," or "punishing." Other words used may be evaluative, such as "miserable" or "unbearable." The quality of pain provides information that may be useful in diagnosing the cause of the pain. For example, pain described as "burning" or "freezing" is usually neuropathic in origin.

Intensity

The client may have difficulty in judging the intensity of pain. However, it is important to obtain an estimate of the severity of the pain. This information allows the clinician to evaluate the effectiveness of pain relief measures tried by comparing intensity before and after the interventions.

There are several tools available to measure intensity (see Figures 12-4 and 12-5). A tool that is easy to use in almost any setting is a numeric rating scale. Ask the client to rate the pain on a scale of "0" to "10," where 0 is no pain, and 10 is the worst pain imaginable. Some clients may respond with answers off the scale, such as "50." However, the tool will still provide the clinician with important information, especially if the client rates it as "30" after medication. There are some individuals who have difficulty in relating numbers to their pain. In these cases, a verbal scale, such as using progressively more severe words, can be used.

There are several intensity tools developed for use with children, the one most commonly used is the "Faces Pain Rating Scale," developed by Whaley & Wong (1987), shown in Figure 12-5. This scale is a drawing of a series of faces ranging from smiling to crying. The client is told that each face is for a person who is happy or sad because of the pain ("hurt" or "owee") that she has. Choose the words for pain that are appropriate for the individual child. The Faces Pain Rating Scale is recommended for children over three. It can also be used in clients where a language barrier exists, as long as a translator is used initially to explain what the faces represent.

On initial assessment, assess the intensity of the pain: pain at present, pain at its least, pain at its worst.

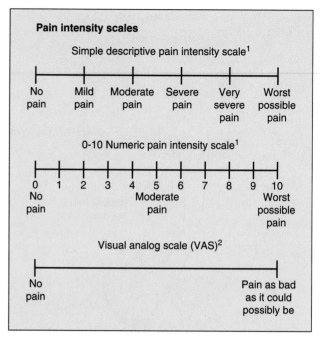

¹ If used as a graphic rating scale, a 10-cm baseline is recommended.
² A 10-cm baseline is recommended for VAS scales.

Source: Acute Pain Management Guideline Panel, 1992.

FIGURE 12-4 Pain intensity scales. Three commonly used self-report intensity scales. (*Courtesy Agency for Health Care Policy and Research, 1992*)

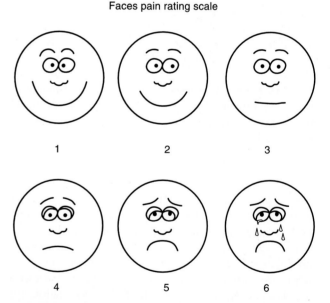

FIGURE 12-5 Faces Pain Rating Scale. (Face 1 is the happiest because she has no pain, Face 2 hurts a little bit, and so on until Face 6 who is very sad because she hurts as much as you can imagine.) (*From Wong, D.L.: Whaley & Wong's Nursing Care of Infants and Children, 5th ed., 1995. Used with permission*)

Subsequent assessments of intensity are used to assess the effectiveness of interventions.

Aggravating and Relieving Factors

Question the client about what makes the pain worse and what makes the pain better. Are there behaviors or activities that influence the pain? This information provides input into developing the plan of care for the client in pain. If there are specific activities that relieve the pain, the nurse can incorporate them into the care plan. Being aware of activities that increase the pain can allow for interventions that may prevent the pain. For example, if physical therapy exercises trigger an increase in pain, the nurse can administer an analgesic as ordered prior to treatment.

Effects of Pain

The initial pain assessment should include the impact of pain on the activities of daily living. Pain may cause changes in sleep patterns or the ability to work and carry out the many roles in a client's life. Pain may affect appetite, mood, sexual functioning, or the ability to participate in recreational activities. If pain is interfering with daily life, the client's quality of life can be greatly affected.

Meaning of Pain

Due to the motivational-affective components of the pain experience, the meaning of pain can have a great impact on how the client perceives the pain. A frequently cited classic study on this phenomenon was conducted by Beecher (1956), who compared the pain perceived by soldiers wounded in battle to pain perceived by civilians with similar surgical wounds. He found that only 32 percent of the soldiers required narcotics for pain relief, whereas 85 percent of the civilians needed the narcotics. This was interpreted that for the soldiers, the wound represented a ticket away from the battlefield, while for the civilians, the surgical wound was a depressing event.

The nurse should explore with the client what implications the pain may have for the individual. Does it mean that the client's cancer is metastasizing? Or that the client's condition is worsening? All of these interpretations may influence the pain experience for the client.

Cultural Considerations

Culture determines the way persons derive meaning from their lives and determine appropriate behaviors. One's cultural upbringing will teach behaviors, including those that are exhibited when in pain. People from different cultures use different types of words to describe pain (for example, in sensory or emotional terms). These differences should not be ignored, but the nurse also needs to be careful not to prejudge a client based on cultural background or ethnicity. Due to the unique experience of pain, the person will exhibit individualized behaviors even though they are influenced by cultural upbringing.

Objective

As discussed when addressing acute versus chronic pain, the objective data often will present a different picture depending on the type of pain the client has.

Physiologic

Acute pain will activate the sympathetic nervous system and the client may exhibit the following: elevated heart rate, elevated respiratory rate, elevated blood pressure, diaphoresis, and dilated pupils. These signs resemble those of anxiety, which often accompanies acute pain. The signs and symptoms of chronic pain show adaption, and, therefore, are different from acute pain with vital signs being normal and no accompanying pupil dilation or perspiration.

Behavioral

Acute pain behaviors may include crying and moaning, rubbing the site of pain, a distorted posture, guarding the painful area, frowning, and grimacing. The client usually states discomfort and may be restless or afraid to move. The client will usually complain of the discomfort. The client in chronic pain may demonstrate behaviors similar to depression such as hopelessness, listlessness, and loss of libido and weight. Often there will be no complaint of pain unless specifically asked. Chronic pain also often leads to physical inactivity or immobility, which can lead to functional disability.

Pain Assessment Is Ongoing

The initial assessment obtains a baseline of information regarding the client's pain. Subsequent assessments provide information regarding the effectiveness of the interventions. Physiologic and behavioral signs, and most important, the client's subjective pain ratings of the intensity will all help the health care team determine whether the interventions should be continued or changed. Perform the pain assessments when the intervention should be providing the most relief. For example, the onset of intravenous morphine is rapid, peaking at approximately twenty minutes after administration. If the client has not obtained relief by twenty minutes, the intravenous morphine was ineffective, and the plan of care would need to be changed.

NURSING DIAGNOSES

The current NANDA-approved nursing diagnoses for the phenomena of pain are:

- Pain, acute
- Pain, chronic

The time frame for chronic pain is any pain that lasts longer than six months. Pain may be used as an etiology for other problems, for example: Physical mobility, impaired, related to arthritic hip pain. Whether the pain is addressed in the problem statement or the etiology will be determined by the client's primary problem. There are many diagnoses that can be related to the client in pain depending on the effects of the pain:

- Activity intolerance
- Anxiety
- Body image disturbance
- Breathing pattern, ineffective
- Constipation
- Coping, ineffective individual
- Fatigue
- Fear
- Hopelessness
- Knowledge deficit
- Physical mobility, impaired
- Powerlessness
- Role performance, altered
- Sleep pattern disturbance
- Social interaction, impaired
- Therapeutic regimen (individual), ineffective management of
- Thought processes, altered

THERAPEUTIC APPROACHES TO PAIN

Planning the care for the client in pain can be difficult due to the individual nature of pain. The nurse often needs to combine several approaches until adequate relief is obtained. No matter which type of intervention is being utilized, there are general principles that apply.

General Principles

The general principles to keep in mind when planning for pain relief are: individualization, prevention, and utilization of a multidisciplinary approach.

Individualize the Approach

A variety of pain relief measures can be tried in many combinations until the goal of pain relief is reached. This often means some trial-and-error of interventions until the right combination is found. It is important to include measures that the client believes will be effective. The cognitive component of pain perception can have a powerful influence on the effectiveness of interventions. This may mean including folk remedies or nonscientific relief measures. It is important to keep an open mind. This comes with the caution that the nurse needs to avoid those remedies that may harm the client.

Use a Preventive Approach

Pain is much easier to control if it is treated before it gets severe. Interventions should be implemented when pain is mild, or when it is anticipated. For example, medicate a client prior to a painful dressing change or treatment rather than waiting for the pain to occur.

Use a Multidisciplinary Approach

Pain relief is a complex phenomenon requiring input from various members of the health care team. The nurse's role is pivotal in managing a client's pain. The physician also plays a key role, diagnosing and treating the medical cause of the pain, which includes prescribing appropriate medications. In complex cases, other professionals, such as physical therapists, psychologists, social workers, or chaplains may be needed. The multidisciplinary team approach is the most successful way to manage chronic pain and improve the quality of a client's life.

Categories of Therapeutic Approaches

There are three main categories of pain control measures: 1) Pharmacological, 2) Invasive, and 3) Noninvasive. Each category will be discussed separately. The nurse needs to be aware that the client may need a combination of measures from any or all of the categories.

PHARMACOLOGICAL TREATMENTS

Medications are the interventions most frequently used for pain control. United States society emphasizes this in many ways, such as television, magazine, and radio advertisements. Clients expect medication for pain management. There are many effective analgesics and **adjuvants** (drugs that have an additive effect to analgesia) available to manage pain. Drug therapy is the mainstay of treatment for pain control.

It is speculated that one of the primary reasons for the undertreatment of pain is the lack of knowledge about the use of analgesics. The American Pain Society (1992) and AHCPR (1992, 1994) have published guidelines that give specific recommendations for the use of drug therapy in pain control. These guidelines were developed by panels of experts who analyzed current research available on pain control and represent concise information that can help nurses, physicians, and other health care workers to effectively administer medications for pain relief. As more clinicians become aware of these guidelines and start to implement their use, it is hoped that the undertreatment of pain will begin to decrease.

Nurses' Role in Administration of Analgesics

As discussed earlier, the nurse is the backbone of controlling the client's pain. The nurse is the health care professional who spends the most time with the client in pain and is the team member who is most often able to assess the effectiveness of pain control interventions. When analgesics are prescribed, the nurse is often given choices of drug, route, and interval. For example, the postop client may have the following orders:

- Morphine 10-15 mg IM or IV q 2-4 hours prn severe pain
- Vicodin i-ii tabs q 3-4 hours prn moderate pain

When this client complains of pain, which analgesic should the nurse choose to administer? Which route? Which dose? How frequently? The nurse in this situation carries a large responsibility in making these decisions. The nurse also has autonomy in making these decisions. The client may not be aware of all the available choices. Each nurse may make a different decision, often based on the nurse's own biases.

These choices and autonomy require responsibility on the part of the nurse. The following are the responsibilities of the nurse in administering analgesics (McCaffery & Beebe, 1989). (See Table 12-2 for a summary.) The nurse must determine whether or not to give the analgesic, and if more than one is ordered, which one. The nurse must assess the client's response to the analgesic, including assessing the effectiveness in pain relief and occurrence of any side effects. The nurse must also report to the physician when a change is needed, including making suggestions for changes based on her knowledge of the client and pharmacol-

Table 12-2

NURSES' RESPONSIBILITIES IN ADMINISTERING ANALGESICS

1. Determine whether or not to give the analgesic.
2. Determine which one to give, if more than one is ordered.
3. Assess client's response to the analgesic.
4. Report to physician when a change is needed.
5. Teach the client and family regarding analgesic use.

(Adapted from McCaffery & Beebe, 1989)

ogy. The last responsibility is to teach the client and family regarding the use of analgesics. This can include the general principles, dispelling misconceptions, and guidelines for taking medications. The nurse who takes these responsibilities seriously can play a vital role and has a positive influence on the client's pain experience.

Principles of Administering Analgesics

"How an analgesic is used is probably more important than which one is used" (McCaffery & Beebe, 1989). There are principles that should be applied in the administration of analgesics, no matter which one is given. These principles discussed in the next section will help ensure that the analgesic(s) will provide the most effective means of pain relief.

Preventive Approach

Pain is much easier to control if treated when it is anticipated or at a mild intensity. Once pain becomes severe, the analgesics ordered may not be effective enough to relieve it. Many clinicians still teach their clients to wait to take medication until they are sure they really need it. This practice leads to uncontrolled pain. There are two ways the preventive approach may be implemented:

- ATC (Around the clock)—when pain is predictable, for example, the first few days following surgery or with chronic cancer pain, the medication is administered on a scheduled basis. This prevents the peaks and valleys of serum drug levels that can lead to oversedation or toxicity and recurrence of pain, respectively. If the analgesics are ordered by the physician to be given PRN, it can still be a nursing measure to administer the drugs ATC, as long as they are given within the time constraints of the order.

- PRN (Latin for *pro re nata,* which means "as required")—pain cannot always be predictable, therefore PRN dosing may be required. For some clients this may be used in addition to scheduled dosing for "breakthrough" pain (pain that surpasses the level of **analgesia**, or pain relief, that the steady level of analgesics is providing). Examples of this include a cancer client on prolonged-release morphine who needs extra analgesics to participate in activities such as shopping or receiving visitors. Another example would be the orthopedic client who is receiving regularly scheduled analgesics for postop pain who needs additional pain relief for therapy sessions. In order to implement the preventive approach with PRN dosing, the medications should be given as soon as the pain appears, or when it is anticipated to begin.

Titrate to Effect

Due to the unique nature of the pain experience, the analgesic regimen needs to be titrated until the desired effect is achieved. This involves adjusting the following:

- *Dosage*—some clients may require more or less than the standard dose. There are many factors that may influence the pharmacokinetics in an individual client. The individual's response is assessed and the dosage of the analgesic is regulated accordingly. In clients with chronic cancer pain, opioid analgesics are recommended to be increased until pain relief is obtained or unacceptable side effects occur. This may be done due to the lack of a **ceiling effect** (the dosage beyond which no analgesia occurs) in pure opioids. The lack of a ceiling effect means there is no limit to the dose that can be given. For example, cancer clients have been known to receive over one gram per hour intravenously. Because the dosage is gradually increased, the client develops a **tolerance** (progressive decrease in drug effectiveness) to the side effects of the opioid.
- *Interval*—some clients may metabolize the analgesics faster than others. For example, young adults tend to metabolize opioids faster, therefore they may need more frequent doses. Elderly clients tend to metabolize them slower, therefore they will require a longer interval between doses.
- *Route*—the appropriate route is chosen depending on how rapidly pain relief is required, the client's ability to take medications orally, the client's diagnosis, and assessment of the client's response to the current route. Intravenous administration provides the most rapid onset of pain relief. All other routes

require a lag time for absorption of the analgesic into the circulation. In postoperative pain, IV is the preferred route for opioids when the oral route is not appropriate. If IV access is not available, sublingual and rectal routes should be considered over IM or subcutaneous (AHCPR, 1992).

With cancer pain, the oral route is preferred. If these clients are unable to take oral medications, rectal and transdermal routes are preferred since they are relatively less invasive than other routes (AHCPR, 1994). In addition, tolerance develops at a slower rate with the oral route compared to the more invasive routes.

- *Choice of drug*—if one drug is not providing relief or has unacceptable side effects, another analgesic may be tried.

The key to administering an analgesic is to monitor the client's response to it. This includes assessing the effectiveness of pain relief and the occurrence of side effects.

Classes of Analgesics

There are three classes of drugs used for pain relief: (1) nonopioid analgesics, which includes salicylates, acetaminophen, and nonsteroidal anti-inflammatory drugs (NSAIDs), (2) opioid analgesics; and (3) analgesic adjuvants (World Health Organization, 1986). Each class of drugs will be addressed separately, as indications and side effects are different for each one.

Nonopioids

The medications in this category are useful for a variety of painful conditions, including surgery, trauma, and cancer (American Pain Society, 1992). The indications include mild to moderate pain, and used in conjunction with opioids. These drugs differ from opioids in several ways:

- there is a ceiling effect to analgesia, that is, there is a limit to attaining an increased pain relief with an increased dose
- they do not produce the effect of tolerance or physical dependence
- they are antipyretic, and should not be given in cases where they may mask an infection

Action Action of these drugs is thought to inhibit prostaglandin formation. As discussed earlier, prostaglandins sensitize the nociceptors in the afferent neuron that receives the signal of pain (transmission step of pain conduction). If prostaglandins are inhibited, the sensory neurons are less likely to receive the pain signal. Thus, this class of analgesics work in the peripheral nervous system.

There are several types of nonopioid drugs:

- *Salicylates*—these include aspirin and other salicylate salts. Common side effects of aspirin include gastric disturbances and bleeding due to the antiplatelet effect. Some of the salicylate salts, such as choline magnesium trisalicylate (Trilisate) and salsalate (Salgesic) have fewer gastrointestinal and bleeding effects than aspirin.
- *Acetaminophen*—this is a nonsalicylate which is similar to aspirin in its analgesic action, but has no anti-inflammatory effect. Its mechanism of action for pain relief is not known.
- *NSAIDs*—the effectiveness of these drugs vary, with some being close to the effectiveness of aspirin and acetaminophen, while others are much stronger. Clients tend to vary in response, so once the maximum recommended dose has been tried with ineffective results, it would be worth trying another NSAID. The drugs in this group inhibit platelet aggregation, and are contraindicated in clients with coagulation disorders or on anticoagulation therapy.

Opioids

This class of analgesics are the foundation of treatment for severe acute pain (such as postoperative pain or trauma pain) and chronic cancer pain. Their use for chronic nonmalignant pain is currently controversial among pain experts. The pure opiates produce no ceiling effect, therefore their dose can be continually increased to gain increased pain relief, although their dose is limited by the side effects.

Action Opioids act in the central nervous system by binding to opiate receptor sites on afferent neurons. This prevents substance P from being released into the synaptic junction; therefore a new action potential is prevented from being triggered in the spinothalamic tract neurons. The pain signal is stopped at the spinal cord level, and does not reach the cortex where pain is perceived.

Examples There are several opioids available in the United States. Some are weak, appropriate for moderate pain, such as codeine or hydrocodone bitartrate (found in Lortab and Vicodin). Others are strong narcotics, appropriate for severe pain, such as morphine or hydromorphone hydrochloride (Dilaudid).

Side Effects Opiates have several side effects, the most serious of which is respiratory depression. Reassuringly, if respiratory depression does occur, it can be reversed with the antagonist, naloxone hydrochloride (Narcan). Clients who receive chronic opiate therapy tend to develop tolerance to the side effect of respiratory depression. Other side effects include sedation, nausea and vomiting, and constipation. Sedation can be treated by decreasing the dose, or supplementing the medication with an adjuvant stimulant, such as caffeine. Due to this side effect, it is important to teach the client to avoid driving or using hazardous equipment while taking the opioids, unless they have been taking them long enough to develop a tolerance to this response. Nausea and vomiting can be managed with antiemetic medications. Any client taking opiates is susceptible to constipation and should increase fiber consumption and take a mild laxative. It is important to discuss this side effect with the client in order to prevent the potentially uncomfortable problem of constipation. Side effects of opiate therapy include: respiratory depression, sedation, nausea and vomiting, constipation, hypotension (usually transient), and miosis (abnormal constriction of the pupil).

Fears About Opioid Use It is proposed that one of the main reasons for the undertreatment of pain is the fear surrounding opioid use. Clients and their families, physicians, and nurses hesitate to use opiates due to fears of **addiction** and tolerance.

In our "just say no" society, many people have concerns of addiction developing from taking drugs from the opioid family. The evidence, however, shows that when opiates are taken for pain relief, addiction is a rare phenomenon. When the pain stops, most people stop taking the medication. Addiction is defined as an overwhelming preoccupation with obtaining and using a drug for its psychic effects. This is quite different from the occurrence of withdrawal symptoms if the opioid is abruptly discontinued. Withdrawal symptoms are treated by tapering the dosage of the opioid gradually down instead of abruptly stopping it. The incidence of addiction is less than 1 percent.

In a study that examined almost 12,000 clients who had received at least one opioid in the course of being hospitalized, only four clients became addicted (Porter & Jick, 1980). Simply, addiction is exaggerated by clients and health professionals. Failing to treat pain because of these fears will most likely lead to clients suffering rather than protecting clients from becoming addicted.

Tolerance is the phenomenon where an increased dose of an analgesic is required to obtain the same amount of pain relief. Fears of tolerance are reflected in statements such as, "I can't take the morphine now, because I might need it later when the pain gets worse." This is a common fear in clients with prolonged pain or terminal illness. The reassurance for those with these fears is that when tolerance does occur, the dose of opioid may be increased safely. This is because while tolerance occurs with the analgesic effect, it also occurs with the side effects such as respiratory depression. This, plus the lack of ceiling effect in the pure opioids, allows the dose to be increased as high as the client needs it.

> **Case Example** A nineteen-year-old client was admitted to the orthopedic ward for uncontrolled pain due to metastasis of Ewing sarcoma. Despite attempts of multiple treatments for her pain, including an unsuccessful cordotomy and an implantable intrathecal catheter for intermittent injections of morphine, her pain remained out of control. The intrathecal catheter became infected and had to be removed. The client was finally treated with continuously increasing doses of a continuous IV morphine infusion. This brought the pain to a tolerable, but never comfortable level. When she died, she was receiving 550 mg of morphine per hour. She had been alert and oriented to person, place, and time on this dose.

A Word About Meperidine Meperidine (Demerol) has several disadvantages when compared to similar opioids. It is relatively short-acting. Its duration only lasts two to three hours. It has poor oral potency, requiring 300 mg po to obtain the same dose as 75 mg IM. This high dose is not recommended due to problems with toxicity. The potential of toxicity, caused by its metabolite normeperidine, can be serious. Signs of toxicity range from irritability to grand mal seizures. Clients at risk for developing toxicity are those with repetitive dosing or high doses. Those with impaired renal function are particularly at risk. It is for this reason that Demerol is rarely the drug of choice when the client requires opioid analgesia for a period longer that six days, requires high doses, or has evidence of renal dysfunction. The AHCPR Guideline for Management of Cancer Pain states, "Meperidine should not be used if continued use is anticipated" (1994).

Alternative Delivery Systems

Opioids are administered in more than just the traditional routes of oral, subcutaneous, intramuscular, intravenous, and rectal.

Patient-Controlled Analgesia (PCA)

PCA is a system that allows the client to self-administer the drug, usually by a programmable

pump. This system helps to eliminate the time required for the nurse to draw up the medication, and allows the client to feel some control over the pain. The pump has the safety feature of locking out once a maximum dose has been reached. This prevents the client from overdosing. The PCA has been successfully used with many types of pain and in many settings, including pediatrics and home health.

Epidural/Intrathecal Analgesia

Epidural analgesia refers to administering the opioid via a catheter that terminates in the epidural space, the space outside the dura mater that protects the spinal cord (Figure 12-6). **Intrathecal analgesia** refers to administering the drug directly into the cerebrospinal fluid. These may be administered as a one time injection by the anesthesiologist, or via a catheter that has been placed there. Both of these routes are occasionally referred to as intraspinal anesthesia. Because the opioid is delivered close to the site of action, these routes require much lower doses of opioid (usually morphine [Duamorph] or fentanyl [Sublimaze] are used) for pain relief. The incidence of systemic side effects are also much lower with these routes. Duration is longer than systemic routes, for example, the

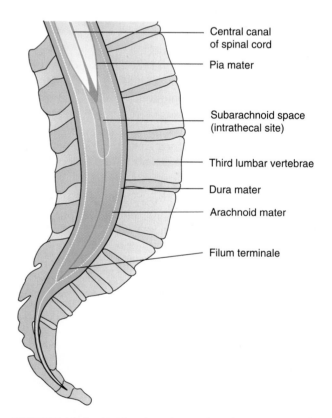

Central canal
of spinal cord

Pia mater

Subarachnoid space
(intrathecal site)

Third lumbar vertebrae

Dura mater

Arachnoid mater

Filum terminale

FIGURE 12-6 Epidural and intrathecal sites. Opioids may be administered through a catheter that terminates in the epidural space or the subarachnoid space (referred to as "intrathecal" site)

duration of one dose of intrathecal morphine can last twenty-four hours.

Transdermal

Another route of opioid administration is the transdermal patch. The only opioid drug currently available via this route is fentanyl (Duragesic). This medication is on an adhesive patch that attaches to the skin. It is available in 25, 50, 75, and 100 mcg/hour dosages. The fentanyl transdermal patch is the source of the drug that infuses slowly through the skin. The fentanyl patch is indicated for continuous pain with high dosage requirements. The advantage of this route is that it is simple to apply and it is effective for seventy-two hours. The disadvantages are that dosage adjustments are difficult to make due to the slow infusion rate. In addition, side effects may not be reversed as rapidly as administering opiates via the oral route. During initial application, a short-acting analgesic should be used for the first twenty-four hours, as it may take this long to reach its full effect. If the patch is removed, it can take up to seventeen hours for the fentanyl serum level concentration to fall by 50 percent. Therefore, if converting to another route of analgesic, initiate treatment twelve to eighteen hours after removing the patch. This avoids the risk of overdosing the client. Due to its ease of application and the frequency of use (every three days), the fentanyl patch offers a route that sufficiently serves clients with steady, continuous pain.

Adjuvants

Adjuvants are not a primary analgesic drug, but have been shown in research studies to have analgesic properties. These are often used in conjunction with opioid or the nonopioid classes of drugs. They may be used to enhance the pain relieving effect of the analgesic, or to counteract the side effects of the analgesics. Examples of adjuvant drugs include corticosteroids such as dexamethasone (Decadron) to elevate the mood and to increase the appetite. Membrane stabilizers, including anticonvulsants such as carbamazepine (Tegretol) and anesthetics such as mexiletine hydrochloride (Mexitil) are especially helpful in treating neuropathic pain. Tricyclic antidepressants are also useful in treating neuropathic pain. The action of the antidepressants is thought to be due to their effect on mood, potentiation of opioid analgesia, and direct analgesic effects (AHCPR, 1994).

WHO Analgesic Ladder

The World Health Organization (WHO) has made worldwide relief of cancer pain one of their primary goals (1990). In order to help meet this goal, it devel-

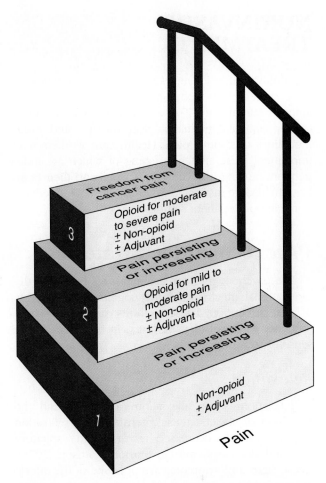

FIGURE 12-7 WHO Analgesic Ladder. Gives guidelines for choosing analgesic therapy for cancer pain, based on the level of pain the patient is experiencing. (*Courtesy World Health Organization, 1990. Used with permission.*)

oped an analgesic ladder to help the clinician determine which analgesic to prescribe (see Figure 12-7). The ladder recommends that the analgesic, plus or minus an adjuvant is chosen based on the level of pain the client is experiencing. For mild pain, the ladder recommends a nonopioid. If the pain persists or if the client has moderate pain to begin with, WHO recommends a weak opioid, plus or minus the nonopioid, plus or minus an adjuvant. If pain persists, a strong opioid is used. This ladder gives health care workers guidelines in determining if the drug regimen is appropriate for the client with cancer pain.

With the many choices of drugs available for pain relief, most painful conditions can be controlled adequately with medications. The nurse plays a key role in administering analgesics to clients. With a strong knowledge base in the pharmacology of pain relief, the nurse is able to fulfill his or her expected responsibilities in a manner that best benefits the client. Administering analgesics in the appropriate manner can maximize their effectiveness in managing pain.

NONINVASIVE TREATMENTS

Noninvasive relief measures consist of psychocognitve strategies and physical modalities that use cutaneous stimulation. These treatments can be used to supplement pharmacological therapy and other modalities to control pain. Health care workers may implement these strategies, some of which are independent nursing interventions. Clients and their families can also be instructed to utilize these treatments at home and in inpatient settings.

Psychocognitive Strategies

The psychocognitive relief measures influence the motivational-affective and the cognitive components of pain perception. These methods can not only help influence the level of pain, but help the client gain a sense of self-control.

Relaxation

Relaxation is the alleviation of anxiety and the reduction of skeletal muscle tension. The relaxation response includes decreased heart rate and respiratory rate and decreased muscle tension (Benson, 1974). These signs and symptoms are opposite of the effects of sympathetic nervous system activation that occurs with acute pain. The body's response to pain is almost "tricked" into reversing itself when relaxation exercises are implemented.

Relaxation exercises help reduce pain by decreasing anxiety and decreasing reflex muscular contraction. There are a wide variety of relaxation techniques, including focused breathing, progressive muscle relaxation, and meditation. Simple techniques should be used during episodes of brief pain (for example, during procedures) or when pain is so severe that the client is unable to concentrate on complicated instructions.

To teach simple relaxation techniques, instruct the client to: (1) take a deep breath and hold it; (2) exhale slowly and concentrate on going limp; and (3) start yawning (McCaffery & Beebe, 1989). The yawning triggers a conditioned response in the client, that is, the body associates yawning with relaxation, and will relax when the client yawns. The technique can be enhanced if the nurse starts yawning . . . it is so contagious that even the client compromised by severe pain will usually start yawning with the nurse.

A more complex technique is progressive muscle relaxation. This involves contracting a series of muscle groups and subsequently relaxing them. This type of technique is especially useful for clients who do not know what muscle relaxation feels like. By purposely contracting and releasing the muscle groups, the client is able to compare the difference and identify feelings of relaxation. Meditative relaxation techniques are also available, including audiotapes sold in most bookstores.

Relaxation is a learned response. The more frequently the client practices these techniques, the more skilled the body will be in learning to relax. Ideally the best time to teach the client these methods is when pain is controlled, or before the pain occurs (for example, in the preoperative period). The client can learn more effectively than when distracted by pain.

Distraction

Distraction focuses one's attention on something other than the pain, therefore placing pain on the periphery of awareness (McCaffery & Beebe, 1989). Successful use of distraction does not eliminate the pain, it makes it less troublesome to the client. The main disadvantage of distraction is that as soon as the distractive stimuli stop, the pain returns in full force. For this reason, the most appropriate use of distraction techniques is for the relief of brief, episodic pain. For example, it can be effective for procedural pain or the period of time between administration of an analgesic and the onset of the drug. Examples of distraction include:

- Active listening to recorded music (have the client tap their fingers in rhythm to the beat)
- Reciting a poem or rhyme (children do this well)
- Describe a plot of a novel or movie
- Describe a series of pictures

The key to distraction techniques is that they must involve the client enough to truly take the mind off the painful experience. Often watching television or listening to music without the physical involvement of tapping the rhythm is not enough to distract the client.

Guided Imagery

Guided imagery is using one's imagination to provide a pleasant substitute for the pain. This modality incorporates features of both relaxation and distraction. The client imagines a pleasant experience, such as going to the beach or the mountains. The experience should include use of all five senses in order to fully involve the client in the image. For example, when describing a beach scene, the nurse may include descriptions of:

- The *feel* of the hot sand crunching beneath the client's feet and the cool water washing over the ankles as each wave comes in.
- The *sight* of the sunlight glinting off each breaker as it peaks.

- The *sound* of the waves crashing rhythmically on the shore, the sea gulls crying out overhead, and the children laughing as they run in and out of the water.
- The *taste* of the salt in the air with each deep breath.
- The *smell* of the suntan lotion on the skin.

The images chosen need to be ones that are pleasant for the client. Describing an ocean cruise would not be appropriate for a person who becomes seasick.

The nurse can help lead the client through the experience by reading a script or describing a situation for the client to imagine. This is a passive form of guided imagery. The nurse may also ask the client questions to let the client create the scenario with help of the nurse's guidance. For example, the nurse can prompt the client with questions such as, "Look around, what do you see?" and "Tell me what do you hear?" The positive images that guided imagery provides can help restore feelings of self-control and hope in the client. These skills do not require a physician's order, and therefore can be included in the care plan independently.

Humor

The old saying, "Laughter is the best medicine," carries some truth to it. While there is nothing very funny about pain, laughing has been shown to provide pain relief. The act of laughing can cause distraction from the pain, induce relaxation by taking deep breaths and releasing tension, release endorphins, and provide a pleasant substitute for pain. Norman Cousins (1979) relates obtaining two hours of pain relief from watching episodes of the *Candid Camera* television show and Marx Brothers films. The nurse can implement this technique by encouraging the client to watch humorous movies, read funny books, or listen to comedy routines. One San Diego oncology unit has taken this to heart and established a library of humorous materials (including books, videos, and audiotapes). Because different people see humor in different types of situations, the nurse needs to be sensitive to what the client views as funny. The nurse should use caution to avoid using humor at the expense of the client.

Client Teaching

Client teaching can play a vital role in the overall pain management plan. This is due to the cognitive influence of pain perception. The education needs to involve the client and the family/significant others. If the family has misconceptions and fears about pain control, it will be difficult for the client to adhere to the pain management plan. The teaching plan should include pain relief measures and the rationale for them (including brief explanations of the physiology of pain). The general principles of pain management need to be reviewed, with special emphasis on using the preventive approach. Details about the analgesic regimen and how to manage side effects are key concepts to incorporate into the teaching plan. Taking the medications properly can determine their effectiveness. Use of the noninvasive relief measures are also key concepts in client education. Client teaching can play a vital role in the overall pain management plan.

Cutaneous Stimulation

The technique of cutaneous stimulation involves stimulating the skin to control pain. It is theorized that these techniques provide relief by stimulating nerve fibers that send signals to the dorsal horn of the spinal cord to "close the gate." The main advantage of this therapy is that many techniques are easy for the nurse to implement, and easy to teach the client and family to perform. They are not usually meant to replace analgesic therapy, but to complement it.

Methods of Skin Stimulation

There are a variety of techniques used to stimulate the skin. Due to the unique nature of the pain experience, the client may need to try several different methods or combinations of methods before finding what will provide the best relief.

Heat and Cold Application In addition to stimulating nerves that can block pain transmission, superficial heat application serves to increase the circulation to the area, which can promote oxygenation and nutrient delivery to the injured tissues. It can also decrease joint and muscle stiffness. Heat is contraindicated in cases of acute injury because it can increase the initial response of edema. It is also contraindicated in rheumatoid arthritis flare-ups, and over topical applications of mentholated ointments. Heat treatments should be limited to twenty to thirty-minute intervals because maximum vasodilatation occurs in that time.

Cold therapy induces local vasoconstriction and numbness, therefore altering the pain sensations. It is contraindicated in any condition where vasoconstriction might increase symptoms, for example, peripheral vascular disease. For best results, limit cold therapy to twenty to thirty-minute intervals. In deciding whether to use heat or cold, either modality can be used as cutaneous stimulation unless one is specifically contraindicated. Cold often provides faster relief (McCaffery & Beebe, 1989). If the client has used heat or cold before, the nurse should incorporate the modality that the client believes will be the most effective. Combining the two might provide better relief. An example of this would be to apply a hot pack for four minutes, followed by an ice pack for two minutes, repeated four times. In a hospital setting, a physician order is required for this therapy. If the order is worded, "Apply cold and/or heat packs as needed for pain relief," it will provide the nurse flexibility in finding the combination and the site that is most effective for the client.

Massage and Acupressure One of the first responses to pain is to rub the painful part. Instinctively people seem to understand the pain relieving aspects of this intervention. In addition to blocking the pain transmission through nerve stimulation, massage can also promote relaxation. Acupressure is a type of massage that consists of continuous pressure on or rubbing acupuncture points. It is based on the same principles of acupuncture, but needles are not used. Massage also provides a form of nonverbal communication that can be therapeutic on its own. The painful area can be rubbed, or other areas such as the back, feet, and hands. It is recommended to use oil, lotion, or powder to reduce friction on the skin. When massaging a client, instruct the client to keep talk to a minimum, but inform the nurse if the strokes are too hard. This helps to emphasize the nonverbal communication taking place and lets the client focus on the soothing feelings experienced. The client should also be instructed to not "help;" let the nurse lift the arm or turn the head. This promotes further skeletal muscle relaxation.

> **Case Example** A client was recovering from an ORIF of multiple comminuted tibia-fibula fractures. In the immediate postoperative period he received morphine 10 mg IVP every 4 hours. It provided some relief initially, but the duration did not last the four hours. The nurse administered a back rub lasting fifteen minutes. The client stated that not only was the pain relief more effective than the morphine, but it lasted for an hour.

Mentholated Rubs Ointments or lotions containing menthol are thought to provide relief by providing a counter-irritation to the skin. The menthol gives the client the perception that the temperature of the skin has changed (becoming either warmer or cooler). This alters the sensation of pain or provides a distraction from the pain. Client response varies to mentholated rubs; some gain effective relief, others have poor results. Their use is contraindicated on broken skin, mucous membranes, or if pain increases.

Transcutaneous Electronic Nerve Stimulation (TENS) Transcutaneous electronic nerve stimulation is the process of applying a low-voltage electrical current to the skin through cutaneous electrodes (see Figure 12-8). This modality modulates the pain trans-

mission as do other cutaneous stimulation methods but also distracts the client from pain. Research supports the effectiveness of using TENS for the relief of postoperative pain (AHCPR, 1992). It has also been used successfully in many pain syndromes, for example: chronic low back pain, menstrual cramps, temporomandibular joint (TMJ) syndrome, phantom limb pain, and others. It is administered by health professionals especially trained in its use, usually a physical therapist.

Sites

The site chosen on which to apply the skin stimulation will depend on the client's diagnosis, treatments or procedures being performed, and client preference. There are several options to choose from:

- *Site of pain*—apply stimulation directly to the site
- *Around the pain*—apply stimulation in circular motion around the site
- *Proximal*—apply between site of pain and the center of the body (McCaffery & Beebe refers to this as "between pain and the brain.")
- *Contralateral*—apply stimulation to the opposite side of the body (This is effective due to the crossing over of the nerves in the spinal cord.)
- *Acupuncture points*—stimulation is applied to specific sites defined by Oriental medicine that is based on a system of meridians
- *Trigger points*—apply stimulation to areas that cause **referred pain**, or pain felt in a point other than the point of origin, when compressed.

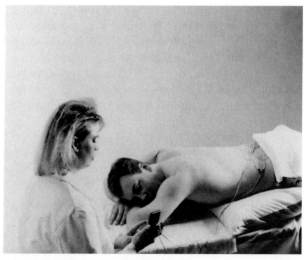

FIGURE 12-8 Patient using TENS unit for pain relief (EPIX XL Transcutaneous Electrical Stimulator [TENS]. (*Photo courtesy of Empi, Inc., Minneapolis, MN. All rights reserved.*)

Positioning

The final noninvasive technique is proper positioning and body alignment. Moving the client with the least possible stress on joints and skin will minimize exposure to painful stimuli. This includes supporting joints appropriately and maintaining wrinkle-free sheets.

Noninvasive techniques include the psychosocial therapies and the physical modalities that stimulate the skin. They provide options for pain relieving measures that can be incorporated into the client's plan of care. They are meant to complement the pharmacologic interventions in order to find the individualized care plan that will provide the best pain relief.

INVASIVE TECHNIQUES

Invasive interventions are meant to complement behavioral, physical, and pharmacological therapies in those clients who do not obtain relief from those measures alone (AHCPR, 1994). Invasive measures are indicated primarily for chronic cancer pain and in some cases of chronic benign pain. These procedures are usually only tried when noninvasive measures have been attempted first with poor results.

Nerve Block

Neural blockade is the process of injecting a local anesthetic or neurolytic agent into the nerve. An anesthetic agent may be injected to act as a diagnostic tool in order to identify the nerves involved in a pain syndrome. A neurolytic agent is a chemical agent that causes destruction of the nerve, and, therefore, creates an interruption in the pain signal.

Neurosurgery

Neurosurgical measures for pain control include neurostimulation procedures and destructive or ablative procedures. Neurostimulation procedures involve the implantation of electrical stimulation devices that send impulses to different parts of the nervous system. Some of these devices stimulate areas of the brain, others stimulate the spinal cord. Relief is thought to be provided by blocking the afferent fiber input at the spinal cord level, or by stimulating release of endorphins using the body's ability to modulate pain.

Destructive or ablative procedures are used to destroy part of the nervous system that conducts pain. By interrupting the pain signal, it is prevented from reaching the cortex where realization of pain occurs. These procedures are reserved for clients with terminal illness, as the pain usually returns either from regeneration of nerve fibers or the development of collateral pain pathways. One such procedure is cordotomy, which is the division of a portion of the spinal cord. The targeted area is the dorsal horn of the spinal cord, where the afferent nerve fibers synapse with the spinothalamic tract neurons. Another procedure is a **rhizotomy**, which is the sectioning of the spinal nerve root just before it enters the spinal cord.

Radiation Therapy

Radiation can be used as a palliative measure for pain relief in clients with cancer pain. It can relieve both metastatic pain and pain caused by tumors at the primary cancer site. It enhances other pain management strategies such as analgesic therapy because it is aimed specifically at the cause of the client's pain. When administered for pain relief, the smallest dose of radiation is utilized to minimize the side effects that accompany radiation therapy.

Acupuncture

Acupuncture is the insertion of small needles into the skin at selected (or hoku) sites. The specific sites will be chosen after the practitioner takes a detailed history and uses traditional Oriental diagnostic techniques. The needles used for acupuncture have rounded ends that enter the skin without cutting the tissue. The practitioner may twirl or vibrate the needles manually or electrically. The advantages of this therapy is that it can complement other pain management techniques and has few side effects. The disadvantages are that it requires a skilled practitioner. Some insurance plans may not cover the costs. It is important that the nurse keep an open mind when the client chooses this therapy, or the client may be reluctant to discuss its use with the nurse.

▶ CASE STUDY

Johnny Prince, a twenty-seven-year-old male, is admitted to the medical unit diagnosed with hemophilia and septic arthritis in his left ankle. He has a history of epilepsy, arthritis, artificial knee joints (bilateral), and two hip surgeries. Medications taken at home include: factor VIII, phenobarbital 100 mg hs, and Naprosyn 5 mg tid. His chief complaint is swelling and severe pain in his left ankle.

Current RX: *Colace, MOM, ceftriaxone sodium (Rocephin) IV piggy-back, phenobarbital 100 mg q hs, FeSO₄, multivitamins, vitamin C, oxacillin (Bactocill), factor VIII 20,000 IVP q 12 hrs, hydromorphone HCl (Dilaudid) 8 mg po q 8 hrs (hold SBP < 90, resp. < 12), MS 4 mg IVP q 4 hrs prn, flurazepam HCl (Dalmane) 30 mg po q hs prn*

The following questions will guide your development of a Nursing Care Plan for the case study.

1. What will you include in assessing Mr. Prince's pain?
2. What factors in his history will influence his pain perception?

Your pain assessment gives you the following information:

- Location—through center of ankle
- Intensity—pain at time of assessment is 5 (medicated thirty minutes prior to interview) on scale of 0–10, at its worse = 25, at its best = 3.
- Quality—describes pain as throbbing at times, a jabbing pain. It hurts worse between 9 and 10 A.M., and 9 and 12 at night. Mainly worse when medicine wears off.
- Effects of pain—only gets two or three hrs of sleep, often dreaming about it. Pain makes him avoid activity, get grumpy and snappy. Concentration turns totally to pain.
- Behaviors—he yells at times, but doesn't like to. He'd prefer to "sweat it out." Also grimaces, grips hands and tries repositioning.

3. Why did the physician order the analgesics on that schedule?
4. Mr. Prince requests a dose of morphine. The narcotic drawer has the following available in prefilled syringe cartridges: 2 mg per cc, and 8 mg per cc. Which cartridge(s) should the nurse select?
5. Why is the morphine ordered IVP, not IM?
6. Why did the physician order colace and MOM?
7. What are some noninvasive relief measures that might be tried with Mr. Prince?
8. What can the nurse do, using medications from current orders, to promote better sleeping patterns for Mr. Prince?
9. Write three individualized nursing diagnoses and goals for Mr. Prince.
10. What teaching will Mr. Prince need before discharge?

SUMMARY

- Pain may be defined as "an unpleasant sensory and emotional experience associated with actual or potential tissue damage," and "whatever the client says it is, existing whenever the client says it does."
- The gate control theory proposes that several processes (sensory, motivational-affective, and cognitive) combine to determine how a person perceives pain.
- There are four processes in the conduction of pain signals: transduction, transmission, perception, and modulation.
- Assessment of pain helps establish a baseline of data, and helps to evaluate the effectiveness of interventions.
- The subjective data to gather includes: location of pain, onset and duration, quality, intensity (on a scale of 0 to 10), aggravating and relieving factors, and how pain affects the activities of daily living.
- The three general principles to follow with pain relief measures are: (1) Individualize the approach; (2) Use a preventive approach; and (3) Use a multidisciplinary approach.
- The nurse carries a great deal of autonomy in administering analgesics, which leads to specific responsibilities for which the nurse is accountable.
- Undertreatment of pain has been related to fears of opioid use. Incidence of addiction is actually very rare, far less than one percent.
- Noninvasive treatments for pain relief are measures that can supplement pharmacological and invasive treatments for pain relief.
- Invasive techniques are interventions used when the noninvasive and pharmacologic measures do not provide adequate relief. Methods include nerve blocks, neurosurgery, radiation therapy, and acupuncture.

Review Questions

1. According to McCaffery, pain may be defined as:
   a. discomfort resulting from identifiable physiologic or iatrogenic sources.
   b. a syndrome of behavioral and physical manifestations that can be objectively identified by the nurse.
   c. whatever the patient says it is, whenever and wherever the patient says it does.
   d. a sensory response to noxious stimuli.

2. Which of the following is a useful tool for assessing the intensity of pain that is easy to use?
   a. the gate control scale.
   b. acute pain monitor.
   c. numeric pain scale.
   d. pressure pain monitor.

3. Mr. Levy, forty-five, has experienced chronic low back pain since a fall eight years ago. He describes his pain as "a gnawing, constant dull pain" that makes him feel tired. The nurse caring for him recognizes that one of the differences between acute and chronic pain characteristics is:
   a. acute pain is more severe.
   b. chronic pain is often described as dull and is difficult to localize.
   c. chronic back pain is often not real.
   d. acute pain is more diffuse and difficult to describe.

4. Mrs. Nancy Johnson, eighty-four years old, is recuperating from a total hip replacement. Morphine, 8 mg IV q 4 hours prn, is prescribed for Mrs. Johnson. Her respiratory rate is 18, her pulse rate is 96 beats per minute, and her blood pressure is elevated slightly above her normal level. She is complaining of severe pain, 8 on a scale of 0–10. The most appropriate initial nursing intervention is:
   a. question the physician regarding the dosage amount for a client this age.
   b. turn her and then reevaluate her need for opioid analgesia.
   c. administer the medication as ordered.
   d. advise Mrs. Johnson to cough and breathe deeply since you are unable to give her anything for pain until her respiratory rate is 20.

5. Ms. Redgrave, fifty-five years old, is hospitalized with an exacerbation of rheumatoid arthritis. She has a favorite television show she watches every afternoon. She reports feeling comfortable during this show and seldom requests pain medication when she is watching it. The nurse's assessment of this phenomenon is that:
   a. the assessment of pain that prompted hospitalization is inaccurate.
   b. Ms. Redgrave is bored and the boredom usually makes her pain seem worse.
   c. inactivity is the best approach to Ms. Redgrave's pain.
   d. distraction is an effective modifier of the pain experience for Ms. Redgrave.

6. At what anatomical site does perception of the pain occur?

    a. dorsal horn of the spinal cord.
    b. nociceptors.
    c. thalamus.
    d. cortex.

7. One of the general principles of pain management is:

    a. anticipated or mild pain is easier to relieve than severe pain.
    b. the more experience a person has with pain, the better able he will be able to tolerate it.
    c. no pain, no gain.
    d. the cause of pain must be identified in order to relieve it.

Critical Thinking Questions

1. What are your responses to pain?

2. Would you use methods, other than medications, for pain relief? If yes, which ones and why?

News Flash

Lollipops for pain relief? A new innovation in administering opioids for pain relief is the development of oral transmucosal fentanyl citrate (OTFC). This is a fentanyl-impregnated sweet lozenge that is attached to a plastic handle. As the client sucks on the lozenge, most of the short-acting opioid fentanyl diffuses across the oral mucosa, while the remaining is swallowed and is absorbed in the gastrointestinal tract. The "suckers" were recently approved by the FDA for use as a premedicant before surgery and for use in monitored anesthesia care. The lozenges are available in 200 mcg, 300 mcg, and 400 mcg dosages. The side effects are similar to other opioids, along with mild pruritus (usually limited to the face), nausea and vomiting, and decreases in O_2 saturation below 90 percent (although it usually returns with verbal stimulation). The primary advantage is that OTFC provides a less painful and less frightening route of opioid administration for children (no needles are required). Other advantages are it provides a rapid onset (ten minutes) and a noninvasive route for clients who are not able to swallow analgesics. Nursing considerations are to administer supplemental oxygen, carefully monitor respiratory status, and know possible side effects. Though its use is currently limited to preop and anesthesia care, possible future applications include breakthrough cancer pain, painful procedures in emergency departments and dental clinics. With the advantages OTFC has to offer, this "lollipop" has important implications for relieving clients' pain (Streisand, 1994).

CHAPTER
13

Perioperative Nursing

Cathy Greer
Diana L. Case

► **KEY TERMS**

Aldrete Score
anesthesiologist
anesthetist
asepsis
aseptic technique
circulating nurse
dehiscence
evisceration
first assistant
informed consent
intraoperative
nosocomial
perioperative
postoperative
preoperative
scrub nurse
sterile
sterile conscience
sterile field
surgeon

LEARNING OBJECTIVES

Upon completion of this chapter the learner should be able to:
- Define key terms.
- List risk factors to be identified in a preoperative nursing assessment.
- List information to include in a general teaching plan for a preoperative client.
- Identify common nursing diagnoses and nursing interventions for the preoperative, intraoperative, and postoperative phases of surgery.
- Identify members of the surgical team and their functions.
- Describe the principles of asepsis and their application to nursing practice.
- Identify nursing interventions to prevent or treat postoperative complications.
- Identify information needed by the postoperative client prior to discharge.

▶ *MAKING THE CONNECTION*

Refer to the topics in the following chapters to increase your understanding of perioperative nursing:

INTRODUCTION

Surgery is a unique experience with no two persons responding alike to similar operations. The same person may not even respond in a like manner to the same or different surgeries. As for the typical surgical client, there is no such being. Each client is a unique individual with varying socioeconomic backgrounds, and filling different family and community roles. Regardless of these differences, surgery is a major stressor for all clients. To a client about to undergo surgery, there is no such thing as minor surgery; anxiety and fear are normal. Surgery, even when planned well in advance, is a stressor that produces both psychologic (anxiety, fear) and physiologic (neuroendocrine responses) stress reactions. Surgery is a stressful experience because it involves entry into the human body and is sometimes a threat to life itself.

Surgeries are classified as minor (prevents little risk to life) or major (may involve risk to life), and may be performed for a variety of reasons. Table 13-1 lists indications for surgery.

Table 13-1

INDICATIONS FOR SURGERY		
Type	**Purpose**	**Example**
Diagnostic	• Determine cause of symptoms	• Biopsy • Exploratory laparotomy
Curative	• Removal of diseased part or replacement of body part or replacement of body part to restore function	• Cholecystectomy • Total knee arthroplasty
Palliative	• Relieve symptoms without curing disease	• Tumor resection associated with cancer
Restorative	• Strengthen a weakened area	• Herniorrhaphy
Cosmetic	• Improve appearance • Change shape	• Face lift • Mammoplasty

The term **perioperative** encompasses the **preoperative** (before surgery), **intraoperative** (during surgery), and **postoperative** (after surgery) phases of surgery. Each phase identifies a particular time during the surgical experience, and each requires a wide range of specific nursing behaviors and functions. Perioperative nursing has one continuous goal: to provide a standard of excellence in the care of the client before, during, and after surgery. Perioperative nursing is client-oriented. Therefore, the nursing activities must be geared to meet the client's psychosocial needs as well as immediate physical needs.

Surgical intervention is a distinctive event for clients. Individuals face this particular event with their own values. Every client not only has specific expectations of the surgical experience but also has distinct hopes for the outcome of the surgery. The perioperative nurse must take an active part in this process in order to ensure quality and continuity of client care.

KEY ABBREVIATIONS

The following abbreviations and acronyms are used in this chapter:

AIDS	acquired immunodeficiency syndrome
ALT	alanine aminotransferase
AORN	American Operating Room Nurses
AST	aspartate aminotransferase
BUN	blood urea nitrogen
CRNA	Certified Registered Nurse Anesthetist
DO	doctor of osteopathy
EENT	eyes, ears, nose, and throat
EKG	electrocardiogram
ESU	electrical surgical unit
ET	endotracheal
Hct	hematocrit
Hgb	hemaglobin
IV	intravenous
JCAHO	Joint Commission on Accreditation of Healthcare Organizations
MD	doctor of medicine
NPO	nothing by mouth
OR	operating room
PACU	postanesthesia care unit
PCA	patient controlled analgesia
PT	prothrombin time
PTT	partial thromboplastin time
RNFA	registered nurse first assistant

PREOPERATIVE

The preoperative phase is a particular time during the surgical experience beginning with the client's decision to have surgery, and ending with the transfer of the client to the operating table.

The outcome of surgical treatment is tremendously enhanced by accurate preoperative nursing assessment and careful preoperative preparation. The client must be assessed by the nurse both physiologically and psychologically. Assessment of the client involves the integration of factors relating to the client's illness, physical condition, related medical conditions, and the current surgical diagnosis. Regardless of how minor the surgical procedure, a thorough health history is essential and should be available to the perioperative team throughout the client's surgical experience.

In addition to the client's health information, the psychological well-being of the client may have an impact on the surgical outcome. The surgical client is at high risk for anxiety related to the surgical experience and the outcome of surgery. Fear and anxiety can affect the client's ability to cooperate with the proposed plan of care. Anxiety is a normal adaptive response to the stress of surgery. Individuals differ in their perception of the meaning of surgery and will respond in various ways. However, if fear and anxiety become excessive, these emotions can interfere with recovery by magnifying the normal physiologic stress response. Objective signs and symptoms of anxiety include decreased attention span, lack of eye contact, increased heart rate, lack of self-confidence, decreased concentration, rapid speech patterns, diaphoresis, dry mouth, clammy skin, nausea, urinary frequency, hyperventilation, and precordial chest pain. Subjective signs and symptoms of anxiety include the client's statements of nervousness. The nurse, by assessing and being aware of the fears and anxieties of the surgical client can provide support and information so that stress does not become overwhelming. The most common fears related to surgery are:

- Fear of the unknown
- Fear of pain and discomfort
- Fear of mutilation and disfigurement
- Fear of anesthesia
- Fear of disruption of life patterns
  - Separation from family/significant others
  - Sexuality
  - Financial
  - Permanent/temporary limitations
- Fear of death/not waking up
- Fear of not being in control

Fear of the unknown is the most prevalent fear prior to surgery and the fear in which the nurse can most easily intervene.

Preoperative Physiologic Assessment

Physiologic assessment should include the physical examination and review of the client's laboratory values and diagnostic studies. Laboratory and diagnostic studies may be divided into those that are routine and those that are done for specific reasons to evaluate the client's primary disease process or coexisting condition. The following summarizes common preoperative laboratory tests:

- Hemoglobin and hematocrit (Hgb and Hct)
- White blood cell count (WBC)
- Blood typing and cross matching (screening)
- Serum electrolytes
- Prothrombin time (PT) and partial thromboplastin time (PTT)
- Bilirubin
- Liver enzymes: alanine aminotransferase (ALT) and aspartate aminotransferase (AST)
- Urinalysis
- Blood urea nitrogen (BUN) and creatinine

It is common practice to obtain a chest film for many clients admitted to the hospital, but this study is increasingly omitted on healthy children and healthy adults under the age of forty in whom the physical examination is normal and there is no reason to suspect pulmonary or cardiac disease. Additional radiographic or fluoroscopic examinations, sonograms, radioisotopic scans, magnetic resonance imaging, and computerized tomography scans give useful information as to the nature of the disease process, its anatomic location, and extent. Any organ that is undergoing major surgery should be adequately evaluated prior to the operation.

Electrocardiograms are routinely performed in middle-aged and elderly clients undergoing surgery because of the prevalence of ischemic heart disease in these age groups. It is also of value to have a baseline study for comparison should subsequent electrocardiograms be needed.

Preoperative testing may be done several days before the date of surgery. The type and amount of routine preoperative screening will depend on the age and condition of the client, the nature of the surgery, and the surgeon's preference. **Surgeons** (doctors who perform surgery) are coming under increasing economic pressure to minimize routine testing procedures. Presently, the trend is based on cost versus benefits, moving away from extensive testing in the absence of indicative/warranting data from the health history and physical examination.

The nurse's role is to ensure that the tests are ordered, performed, and the results are placed in the client's chart. Abnormal results are reported to the physician immediately in case surgery may need to be delayed or canceled. The management of diagnostic tests is considered a portion of the preoperative physiological assessment.

The physiologic nursing assessment is completed prior to surgery. Preoperative assessment can take place in the surgeon's office, during hospitalization, or the day of surgery in the hospital or ambulatory surgery unit. The nurse collects client health data by interviewing the client, the family, significant others, and health care providers. Data collection can also be accomplished through review of the client records, assessment, and/or consultation. Assessment is essential to establishing nursing diagnoses and predicting outcomes (AORN, 1995). When performing the nursing assessment, the nurse screens the client for risks that may contribute to complications in the perioperative period. Table 13-2 lists risk factors and possible complications of each. The nurse's role in the preoperative phase assures client safety, understanding, and compliance with health care treatment.

Age

Surgery can be performed on individuals of any age, although persons at both extremes of age (infants, elderly) may be less able to tolerate the stress of surgery. Infants can easily become dehydrated or fluid overloaded with resultant electrolyte imbalances. Their metabolic rate is two to three times that of an adult. Therefore, infants can have formula up to six hours before surgery and breast-fed infants may be nursed up to four hours before surgery. Infants may then have clear liquids for up to two hours before surgery.

Infant renal, body temperature regulatory, immune, and respiratory systems are different than the adult. Renal function in the infant is decreased due to a lower glomerular filtration rate and less efficient renal tubular function than an adult (Atkinson & Fortunato, 1996). This may lead to retention of anesthesia and medications and also to fluid overload. Due to the larger ratio of body surface area to body mass, infants are also more prone to hypothermia when placed in a cool environment or have large areas of exposed body surface. Infants are more susceptible to infections due to an immature immune system. Because of their smaller and weaker anatomic structure with enlarged tongues and lymphoid tissue, infants are also more prone to respiratory obstruction. Infants have very special needs and the nursing process must be tailored to meet the unique needs of each client.

Elderly clients have many physiologic changes associated with aging and are more likely to have multiple organ degenerative disease, including many of the risks described in Table 13-2. The elderly are more likely to be dehydrated and thus have less reserve adaptation to fluid loss during surgery. The elderly are

Table 13-2

RISK FACTORS AND RELATED COMPLICATIONS

Variable	Related Risk Factors	Possible Complications	
Age	**Infants**	• Dehydration • Fluid overload • Hypothermia	• Infection • Respiratory obstruction
	Elderly	• Decreased metabolism and elimination of anesthetics and medications • Hypothermia • Hypervolemia • Hypovolemia and shock • Deep vein thrombosis, thrombophlebitis, pulmonary embolus • Decreased urinary output/renal failure • Urinary incontinence/retention	• Urinary tract infections • Poor wound healing • Pressure sores • Atelectasis/pneumonia • Constipation/fecal impaction • Infection • Physical injury (falls or joint overextension)
Nutritional Status	**Malnourishment**	• Fluid and electrolyte imbalance • Delayed wound healing • Wound infection	• Poor tolerance to anesthetics • Bleeding/hemorrhage
	Obesity	• Retention of anesthetics and medications • Wound infection • Delayed wound healing	• Deep vein thrombosis, thrombophlebitis, pulmonary embolus • Atelectasis • Pneumonia
Fluid and Electrolyte Status	**Deficits and Excesses of Fluids and Electrolytes**	• Anorexia, nausea, vomiting • Diarrhea and cramps • Constipation • Paralytic Ileus • Hypotension • Hypertension • Edema (including pulmonary edema) • Confusion • Lethargy • Tetany • Weakness	• Parathesias • Paralysis • Restlessness • Delusions and hallucinations • Seizures • Laryngospasm • Respiratory arrest • Tachycardia • Dysrhythmias • Cardiac arrest • Renal failure
Respiratory Status	**Acute Respiratory Infections**	• Bronchospasm • Laryngospasm • Hypoxemia	• Atelectasis • Pneumonia
	History of Chronic Respiratory Diseases/Smoking	• Atelectasis • Pneumonia	
Cardio-Vascular Status	**History of Preexisting Cardiac Disease**	• Dysrhythmias • Hypotension/syncope • Myocardial infarction • Congestive heart failure	• Cardiac arrest • Stroke • Shock • Deep vein thrombosis, thrombophlebitis, or pulmonary embolism

(continued)

Variable	Related Risk Factors	Possible Complications	
Renal or Hepatic Status	History of Pre-existing Renal or Hepatic Diseases	• Fluid and electrolyte imbalances • Bleeding/hemorrhage • Infection	• Impaired wound healing • Hyperglycemia/hypoglycemia • Decreased metabolism and elimination of anesthetics and medications
Neurological Musculo-skeletal and Integumentary Status	Surgical Positioning or Prolonged Immobility	• Pressure alopecia • Pressure point compression • Pressure sores • Nerve injury to axillary neurovascular bundle, subclavian neurovascular bundle, brachial plexus, facial, peroneal, radial, and ulnar nerve • Neck pain, lower back pain, joint damage	• Postural hypotension • Pressure alopecia • Eye abrasion • Ear compression • Atelectasis on dependent side • Air embolism • Facial and airway edema
Endocrine and Immune Status	Diabetes	• Fluid and electrolyte imbalances • Deep vein thrombosis, thrombophlebitis, and pulmonary embolism • Infection including respiratory and urinary tract	• Neurogenic bladder • Impaired wound healing • Hyperglycemia/hypoglycemia • Ketoacidosis
	Immuno-compromised	• Infection • Respiratory infections	• Pressure sores • Impaired wound healing
Medications	Chemical Dependency	• Increased or decreased effectiveness of anesthetic agents, narcotics, and/or sedatives	• Drug interactions • Symptoms of withdrawal—hallucinations, disorientation, convulsions

also more sensitive to central nervous system depressants used during the perioperative period. However, even the elderly can favorably tolerate extensive surgery when carefully assessed and managed.

Nutritional Status

Nutritional assessment includes recognition of individual deficiencies or excesses that can increase the surgical risk. Surgery increases the body's need for nutrients necessary in normal tissue healing and resistance to infection. The malnourished individual may have diminished stores of carbohydrates and fats, and thus the proteins would be utilized for energy instead of tissue building and restoration. Nutritional deficiencies of vitamins B complex and C are also significant, since these substances are essential to healing. This predisposes the client to a higher risk for alteration in fluid and electrolyte balance, delayed wound healing, and incidence of wound infections. When liver and kidney functioning is affected, anesthetic agents are poorly tolerated and the client becomes prone to bleeding. If time allows, the nurse should encourage malnourished clients to increase the intake of carbohydrates, proteins, and vitamins. Total parenteral nutrition or enteral nutrition may be given to the malnourished client for several days to weeks prior to surgery as ordered by the surgeon.

Nutritional excesses or obesity increases the risk for respiratory, cardiovascular, and gastrointestinal complications. Obesity makes access to the surgical site more difficult which prolongs surgical time. Thus, the client requires more anesthesia. Since inhalation anesthesia is absorbed and stored by adipose tissue and released postoperatively, anesthesia recovery time is slower. Adipose tissue is less vascular and more difficult to suture, which predisposes the client to wound infection, delayed wound healing, and increased incidences of wound complications including postoperative incisional hernias. Failure to exercise and ambulate increases the chances of decreased respiratory function with atelectasis and pneumonia, and also may lead to decreased wound healing, and an increased risk of thrombus formation. Often, obese clients also have other chronic conditions such as hypertension or diabetes mellitus which increase the likelihood of developing complications. Nursing care of the obese client involves encouraging activity, encouraging a weight reduction diet, and assisting in the control of chronic conditions. In some situations, such as joint replacement, surgery may be delayed until nutritional status improves when the client loses weight.

Fluid and Electrolyte Balance

Dehydration and hypovolemia, with correlating electrolyte disturbances, predisposes a client to complications during and after surgery. Both may be caused by diarrhea, excessive nasogastric suctioning, inadequate oral intake, vomiting, and/or bleeding. The complications of fluid and electrolyte imbalances are numerous and varied as demonstrated in Table 13-2, and range from minor (but may prolong recovery) to major (resulting in death). "Changes in fluid and electrolyte balance affect renal function, cellular metabolism, and oxygen concentration in the circulation" (Atkinson & Fortunato, 1996). Nursing care focuses on the administration of parenteral fluids or blood products as prescribed, keeping a detailed intake and output record, and the surveillance of correlating laboratory studies.

Respiratory Status

Respiratory assessment should include detection of acute and chronic problems. Because acute respiratory infections may lead to bronchospasms or laryngospasms, surgery may be delayed or contraindicated. Chronic respiratory problems, such as asthma and chronic obstructive pulmonary disease impairs the client's gas exchange and increases the risk associated with inhalation anesthesia. Clients with chronic respiratory problems are more likely to develop atelectasis and pneumonia.

Respiratory assessment by the nurse includes assessing the client's breath sounds and color of the skin, and mucous membranes. It also involves assessing the client for presence of shortness of breath (dyspnea), clubbed fingers, and coughing. In addition to a chest x-ray, arterial blood gases or an oxygen saturation baseline may be ordered. Restriction of smoking should be encouraged at least four to six weeks before a scheduled surgery, when possible. All clients, and especially those clients who smoke and have a chronic lung disease, should be taught deep breathing, use of incentive spirometry, coughing, and turning preoperatively (Table 13-3).

Cardiovascular Status

Cardiovascular assessment focuses on diseases that would require close observation by the nurse and make necessary the avoidance of sudden changes of position, overhydration with intravenous fluids, and prolonged immobilization. Examples of such diseases include angina, recent myocardial infarction or cardiac surgery, hemophilia, hypertension, and congestive heart failure. Clients with a history of cardiac disease are prone to develop complications such as dysrhythmias, hypotension, myocardial infarction, congestive heart failure, cardiac arrest, stroke, shock, deep vein throm-

bosis, thrombophlebitis, or pulmonary embolism. It should be noted that the client "who fears dying while under anesthesia runs a greater risk of cardiac arrest on the operating table than clients with known cardiac disease" (Atkinson & Fortunato, 1996, p. 389). The psychological condition of the client can have a stronger influence than the physiologic condition.

The nursing assessment also includes assessment for anxiety and for the presence of an elevated blood pressure, slow, rapid, or irregular pulse, chest pain, edema, coolness or cyanosis/discoloration of extremities, weakness, and shortness of breath (dyspnea). All clients must be taught postoperative leg exercises (Table 13-4). The goal of nursing care is to improve the client's cardiovascular condition to the highest extent possible by promoting rest alternating with activity; a low-sodium and low-cholesterol diet; administering heart medications; and judiciously administering parenteral fluids while recording a detailed intake and output record.

Renal and Hepatic Status

Renal and hepatic insufficiency are a major concern since many medications and anesthetic agents are detoxified by the liver and excreted by the kidneys. Renal disease affects fluid and electrolyte balance and protein equilibrium. Liver disease may be accompanied by bleeding tendencies or carbohydrate, fat, and amino acid imbalances which impair wound healing and increase the incidence of infection. The nurse assesses for symptoms of urinary frequency, dysuria, and anuria, and notes the color and amount of the urine. The nurse also assesses for a history of bleeding tendencies, easy bruising, nosebleeds, and use of anticoagulants. The most commonly ordered preoperative tests to assess renal function are urinalysis, blood urea nitrogen (BUN), and creatinine. The most common liver tests are prothrombin time (PT), partial thromboplastin time (PTT), bilirubin, and the liver enzymes alanine aminotransferase (ALT) and aspartate aminotransferase (AST). Nursing care focuses on administering fluids and adequate nutrition, monitoring fluid intake and output, and surveillance of laboratory tests.

Neurological, Musculoskeletal, and Integumentary Status

The nurse assesses the client's overall mental status including the level of consciousness; orientation to person, place and time, and the ability to follow commands. The nurse assesses the condition of the skin and notes any rashes, bruises, lesions, previous incisions, and turgor. Client mobility and sensation are also assessed through observation of range of motion, ability to ambulate, gait, and through client statements. The nurse notes any abnormalities, injuries, previous

Table 13-3

PREOPERATIVE INSTRUCTION FOR POSTOPERATIVE DEEP BREATHING, INCENTIVE SPIROMETRY, COUGHING, AND TURNING

Activity	Description	Instruction
Deep Breathing	• Mode of breathing during which the diaphragm expands fully allowing expansion of the thorax, upper abdomen, and alveoli as air enters; followed by abdominal and diaphragmatic contraction during expansion	• Sit in semi-Fowler's position with hands placed over lower ribs and upper abdomen • Inhale deeply through the mouth and nose • Hold the breath for five seconds • Exhale fully through mouth and nose • Repeat 15 times with short rest periods as needed • Perform twice daily
Incentive Spirometry	• Method of using a commercial cylinder which measures deep breaths during inhalation with a float that rises	• Sit as upright as possible • Seal lips around mouthpiece • Inhale and watch float rise • Hold deep breath for five seconds • Remove mouthpiece and exhale slowly • Repeat 10–12 times per hour • Cough after the last breath
Coughing	• Cough moves secretions from smaller airways to larger airways to promote the removal of lung secretions	• Sit as upright as possible • Splint incision with hands or pillow • Inhale deeply using deep breathing technique • Cough several times until it feels as if no air left in lungs • May continue with another deep inhalation followed by one or two strong coughs • Repeat one time per hour
Turning	• Method of alternating position from back to either side to promote circulation, lung expansion and drainage, and relief from pressure areas	• Change position every one to two hours (assistance and support pillows may be required)

surgery, and assesses the risk for falls. Since the presence of a prosthesis or implant may require preoperative antibiotics, the presence of internal or external prostheses or implants such as pacemakers, heart valves, or joint prosthesis is noted.

Thin clients, clients undergoing long surgical procedures or vascular procedures, and the elderly are the most vulnerable to neurological, musculoskeletal, or integumentary injuries. Some underlying disease processes also contribute to a higher risk of injury such as clients with edema, infection, cancer, osteoporosis, arthritic joints, neck or back problems. Clients who are malnourished, anemic, obese, hypovolemic, paralyzed, or diabetic are also prone to skin breakdown. Information gathered about the neurologic, musculoskeletal, and integumentary systems is used for preparation of the surgical site, surgical positioning,

and as a comparative basis for postoperative assessments, activity, and screening for complications. Table 13-2 lists complications from surgical positioning and prolonged immobility after surgery.

Endocrine and Immunological Status

Diabetics require special consideration while undergoing surgery. Diabetics should be scheduled as early in the morning as possible. and a fasting glucose drawn immediately prior to surgery. Surgery is a stress and stress raises the serum glucose level in the diabetic client. The serum glucose may vary significantly so the morning dose of insulin may be eliminated or only one half of the normal amount given. While anesthetized during surgery, the client exhibits very few symptoms of hypoglycemia. Therefore, the serum glu-

Table 13-4

POSTOPERATIVE LEG EXERCISES

Activity	Instructions
• Leg lifts	• While lying on back or in a semi-sitting position, bend the leg and raise it. • Hold for count of five. • Lower leg to the bed. • Repeat five times then proceed with other leg. • Perform every hour.
• Dorsiflexion of feet	• Flex ankle and raise toes. toward head, stretching posterior calf. • Hold for count of two. • Relax. • Repeat five times then proceed with other foot. • Perform every hour.
• Foot circles	• Point the toe and raise the leg slightly off the bed. • Trace a circle in the air with the great toe. • Repeat five times then proceed with other foot. • Perform every hour.

cose needs to be checked frequently during surgery, usually by the anesthesiologist. Stability is attained by the administration of insulin or glucose or both. Besides hyperglycemia and hypoglycemia, a diabetic client is more prone to fluid and electrolyte imbalances, infection including respiratory and urinary tract infections, neurogenic bladder, impaired wound healing, ketoacidosis, deep vein thrombosis, thrombophlebitis, and pulmonary embolism.

Since the immunological system protects the client from infections, the immunocompromised surgical client is very prone to infection. Clients taking steroids or chemotherapy, or clients with systemic lupus erythematosus, Addison's disease, or Acquired Immunodeficiency Syndrome (AIDS) are considered to be immunocompromised. The immune response in these clients is weakened or deficient resulting in an increased incidence of infection. The role of the nurse is to communicate the presence of potential immunosuppression to other health care team members. Since surgery breaks the integrity of the skin, the normal inflammatory response is suppressed and wound healing may be impaired. Strict adherence to aseptic technique, covered later in this chapter, is even more imperative. Prevention of infection becomes crucial to these clients.

Medications

Knowledge of the client's use of drugs for recreational or therapeutic purposes is essential to preoperative assessment. The history of medication usage by the client should include type and frequency of use for both over-the-counter and prescription drugs. The use of certain drugs (Table 13-5) can affect the client's reaction to anesthetic agents and surgery. Surgical risks are increased by certain drugs and these medications usually are temporarily discontinued when a client goes to surgery. Some medications such as heart or hypoglycemic medications may still be given even though the client is going to surgery. The surgeon or anesthesiologist will write specific orders for this. Dosages of medications may also be adjusted during the perioperative period.

Chronic alcohol use increases the surgical risk as it is often accompanied by impaired nutrition and liver disease. Postoperatively, the client may exhibit delir-

Table 13-5

CLASSIFICATION OF MEDICATIONS AND POSSIBLE EFFECTS WITH ANESTHETIC AGENTS AND SURGERY

Classification	Possible Effects
• Antibiotics	• Respiratory paralysis when combined with certain muscle relaxants
• Anticoagulants	• Hemorrhage
• Anti-Parkinsonian drugs	• Increase hypotensive effects of anesthetic agents
• Diuretics	• Electrolyte imbalances
• Hypoglycemics	• Hypoglycemia or hyperglycemia
• MAO inhibitors (Monoamine)	• Hypertensive crisis when combined with certain anesthetics
• Steroids	• Cardiovascular collapse if abruptly withdrawn • Impairs physiologic response to stress • Delayed wound healing • Increase risk of infection
• Street drugs and alcohol abuse	• Tolerance to narcotics
• Tranquilizers	• Potentiates narcotics and barbiturates

ium tremens or acute withdrawal syndrome. Pain medication may have decreased effectiveness.

Psychosocial Health Assessment

The psychosocial health status of the client is also assessed. The nurse elicits the client's perceptions of surgery, expectations of care, and determines coping mechanisms used by the client. The nurse determines the client's knowledge level and ability to understand. The nurse identifies religious and cultural beliefs and practices that may affect care. The data collected is incorporated into nursing care throughout the perioperative experience.

Surgical Consent

An **informed consent** is a form signed by the client and witnessed by another person, granting permission to have the procedure described by the client's physician. An informed consent is needed for any procedure when:

- anesthesia is used
- the procedure is considered invasive
- the procedure is nonsurgical but has more than a slight risk of complications (such as an arteriogram)
- radiation or cobalt therapy is used

All clients must consent to any treatment. Figure 13-1 shows a typical surgical consent form. Four conditions must be met for the informed consent to be valid. First, the client has a right to know what is to be done and why it should be done along with the risks and possible complications, disfigurement, and removal of body parts. The client also needs to be informed of alternative means of treatment available and have a general idea of the time frame and what to expect during recovery. The second condition for a valid consent is that the client must demonstrate understanding of the information. The third condition is that the client must be competent. In order to meet the fourth condition for valid consent, the client must always sign the consent voluntarily. The physician writes a note in the medical record to document that detailed explanation about the procedure, risks, and alternatives took place to the satisfaction of the client.

Informed consent protects not only the client against unauthorized procedures but the physician, the health care institution and its employees from claims that an unauthorized procedure was performed. The ultimate responsibility for obtaining the informed consent lies with the physician, although it is often the nurse who obtains and witnesses the client's signature, ensuring the client signed the consent form voluntarily, and was alert and comprehending of the action. If

a client is confused, unconscious, sedated, mentally incompetent, or considered a minor, consent may be given by a parent, spouse, next of kin, legal guardian, or the person named in a durable power of attorney for health care. In an emergency, oral consent may be obtained by phone with two witnesses hearing the consent simultaneously or the physician can obtain a court order.

Most hospitals use a standard preprinted form so the information written by the health care personnel must be specific to the individual client. The client's signature on the consent form indicates the information has been read and is correct. The client has the right to refuse treatment even after the consent has been signed. When this occurs, the nurse must inform the physician immediately of the client's decision.

Preoperative Teaching

The client about to undergo surgery is at high risk for a knowledge deficit related to preoperative procedures, protocols, and postoperative expectations. Preoperative teaching is the giving of information to the client prior to a surgical procedure. The potential benefits of preoperative teaching include more rapid recovery with fewer complications and shorter hospitalization. Due to the reduction of anxiety, the client also usually requires less medication for pain. The purpose of preoperative teaching is to (1) answer questions and concerns about surgery; (2) determine the client's present knowledge of the intended surgery; (3) determine the need or desire for additional information; and (4) provide the information in the most conducive manner for learning to take place.

One-to-one sessions provide the most personal method of instruction. The nurse should always try to include the family or significant other. The level of learning increases when using more than one teaching medium. For example, using verbal and visual material such as video tapes, charts, tours, anatomic models, pictures, and brochures appeals to modes of learning other than auditory. Demonstration with return demonstration are helpful. Written instructions provide a reference for later use. Instructions should be simple with minimal medical jargon. Any unfamiliar words or concepts should be thoroughly explained. Clients are most interested in any sensory information that describes the sights, sounds, tastes, feelings, odors, and temperature of what they are about to experience. For example, the feeling of relaxation from preoperative medications, the sounds of instruments or equipment in the operating room (OR), the pressure from the automatic blood pressure cuff, the warmth or coolness of skin preparation solutions, or the brightness of the operating room lights are all sensations the client may experience. Analogies or stories of real or fictitious situations of sensory experiences help the client

LUTHERAN HOSPITAL OF INDIANA

Name of Patient _____ Date ___/___/___ Time _____ A.M. P.M.

Proposed Operations or Procedures _____

(Name of Patient)

_____

I authorize the performance upon _____

of the operation/procedure as described above, by _____

and associates and assistants of his choice.

The nature and purpose of the operation, possible alternative methods of treatment, the risks involved, and the possibility of

complications have been discussed with me by my physician/surgeon and any questions answered by him. No guarantee or

assurance has been given by anyone as to the results that may be obtained.

I consent to the administration of such anesthetics as may be considered necessary or advisable by the physician responsible

for this service.

Any tissue or members severed in any operation or procedure may be disposed of at the discretion of the pathologist, except

_____

_____

My signature below constitutes my acknowledgment that I have read and agreed to the foregoing paragraphs; that the proposed

operations or procedures have been satisfactorily explained to me by my doctors and that I have all the information that I desire,

and that I hereby give my authorization and consent.

_____   _____

Signature of Patient   Signature of Witness

Date ___/___/___ Time _____ A.M/P.M.   Date ___/___/___ Time _____ A.M./P.M.

AUTHORIZATION FOR AND CONSENT TO SURGERY, SPECIAL

DIAGNOSTIC OR THERAPEUTIC PROCEDURES

ADDRESSOGRAPH

FIGURE 13-1 Sample surgical consent form. (*Courtesy IOM Health System, L.P. d/b/a Lutheran Hospital*)

understand concepts being presented and remain interested. The teaching methods used by the nurse strongly influences the degree of learning and the retention of information.

Preoperative teaching needs to begin as soon as the client has decided to have surgery, and can occur in the surgeon's office. With so many clients being admitted the day of surgery or having ambulatory surgery, time does not always allow adequate instruction. In these situations, over-the-phone and/or mailed instructions are beneficial. Just prior to surgery, a brief review with additional information tailored to the needs of the client may be given. The client should be given an opportunity to ask questions. All applicable instructions need to be reinforced in the postoperative period. Preoperative teaching should include the content areas listed in the teaching tips.

Teaching Tips

- Introduce self
    Identify purpose
- Determine knowledge level and need or desire for additional information
- Explain the routine for the day of surgery
    Absence of food or fluid
    Intravenous fluids
    Premedication
    Time of surgery
    Anticipated length of surgery
    Transportation to the operating room
    Special skin preparations
- Familiarize the person with the operating room environment
    Operating room lights and table
    Accessory equipment
    Monitoring equipment
    Anesthesia induction
- Include significant others
    Time to arrive at the hospital
    Location of surgical waiting area
    What to expect when person returns to the unit
- Explain postanesthesia care unit
    Location of recovery room
    Purpose of recovery room
    Routine of postanesthesia care
- Identify anticipated dressings, drains, catheters, casts, etc.
- Demonstrate and evaluate client's performance of:
    Cough and deep breathing exercises
    Turning
    Incentive spirometry
    Extremity exercises
    Any special transfer procedures or aids required after surgery

Information should always be tailored to the client's needs. Teaching plans should be tailored according to the client's level of anxiety. Mild to moderate anxiety actually heightens a person's alertness and motivates learning. Mildly anxious clients should receive the most complete instructions. Moderately anxious clients should receive less information but more attention to specific areas of concern. Severely anxious clients should receive only basic information but should be encouraged to verbalize their concerns. Clients in a state of panic are unable to learn, so no instruction is given and the surgeon should be notified.

Physical Preparation

Extreme care must be given to identifying the proper client verbally and reading the identification name band. Then the nurse begins the important task of verifying the operative procedure. This needs to be completed through client statements, surgeon verification, and the signed surgical consent form. Pay particular attention to differentiating between right and left operative sites.

In order to reduce the chance of infection, special care is given to the preparation of the operative site. To reduce the number of microorganisms on the skin, the operative site is cleansed the night before surgery either in the hospital or at home with an antiseptic soap such as povidone-iodine. Typically, the operative site is no longer shaved; but if it is shaved, the shave takes place immediately prior to surgery in the operating room. To reduce the number of bacteria in the gastrointestinal tract for gastrointestinal, peritoneal, perianal, and pelvic surgery, enemas are ordered. Enemas prevent contamination of the peritoneal cavity by fecal content. The reduction in colon size from the loss of bulk also helps prevent colon injury and increases visualization of the operative site. Enemas are usually given the night before surgery. If the enemas are done at home, the client must be given detailed instructions. Many types of surgery require special preparations. The specific protocol for each surgical procedure is usually available at the health care facility.

The nurse checks the vital signs, including blood pressure, temperature, pulse and respirations. Due to anxiety, some increase in vital signs is normal. If marked differences exist from the baseline data, the surgeon must be notified.

The nurse assists the client in putting on a hospital gown, hair cap, and if ordered, antiembolic hose. According to institutional policy, jewelry is removed, but wedding rings may be taped on and left in place. If removed, the nurse records the disposition of the jewelry. Hairpins, wigs, and prostheses must also be removed. If policy requires, nail polish (at least one nail if dark polish) is removed so oxygen saturation may be read by pulse oximeter. Some pulse oximeters may be able to read oxygen saturation through nail polish. Make-up is also removed so skin color can be observed.

Medication, food and chemical allergies (including contrast agents), and previous blood reactions are verified. The nurse needs to differentiate between a medication intolerance and a true allergic reaction. With a medication intolerance, the client may suffer side effects that are unpleasant. For example, many clients state allergies to meperidine (Demerol) when nausea is experienced. A true allergy produces a skin reaction or anaphylactic reaction where the client experiences cardiorespiratory reactions that may be life threatening, such as hypotension and pulmonary edema. A client with multiple food allergies is more prone to have additional hypersensitivities to medications. When allergies are identified, the client's chart is marked accordingly and an allergy wrist band is applied. By being aware of and making other team members aware of the client's allergies, safety and comfort of the client is maintained.

The nurse verifies the NPO status of the client for the amount of time specified by the surgeon's order (see Chapter 11 for additional information on NPO). Restricting oral intake reduces the possibility of aspiration pneumonia. Typically, the client is placed NPO after midnight. If surgery takes place in the afternoon, the client may have a clear liquid breakfast if ordered by the surgeon. Careful client instruction is required since if the client consumes food or fluid, the surgery may be postponed. The following are nursing actions to implement NPO status for a client:

- Explain reasons for NPO status to the client
- Remove any food and water from client's over bed table and night stand
- Mark client door and bed with NPO sign
- Mark the client Kardex or other nursing information sources
- Notify dietary department

In addition to the above preparations, dentures and bridgework are removed to prevent loss or damage and to prevent possible dislodgement and airway obstruction during the surgery. The nurse also ensures the client has an empty bladder by allowing time for the client to void prior to transfer to surgery.

The nurse should identify any sensory deficits in clients and communicate this information to other health care team members. Glasses and hearing aids are usually removed to prevent loss or damage. But if policy allows, it is better to leave these items in place so the client is able to see and hear better and then to communicate their presence to other health care team members.

Following is a list of geriatric considerations:

GERONTOLOGICAL CONSIDERATIONS

- Increased risk of complications including infection
- Increased incidence of coexisting conditions
- Unpredictable response to medications and anesthetics
- Greater need for family and significant other support
- Increased skin and bone fragility
- Possible nutritional and financial deficiencies
- Impaired visual and auditory senses
- Impaired or slowed thought processes and cognitive abilities
- Fear of death, loss of independence, and change in lifestyle

The surgeon or **anesthesiologist** (a doctor trained in providing anesthesia) may order preoperative medication. Table 13-6 lists medications that may be given alone or in combination to reach the desired effects for the individual client. The nurse gives the medication in the ordered route (usually intramuscular, but may be given intravenously or orally) at the specified time (typically one hour prior to surgery). Often preoperative medications are ordered "on-call" and the nurse is notified from a member of the surgical team when the preoperative medication needs to be given. Ask the client to void prior to receiving the medication. After administering the preoperative medication, raise the side rails of the cart or bed and instruct the client not to get up without assistance.

When the surgical team is ready, the client is transported on a cart by a member of the surgical team. The client is always transported feet first with side rails up to reduce the incidence of dizziness and nausea. If the client is on a clinical nursing unit, the client may be taken to a preoperative holding area first where additional verifications of client identification, preparation, diagnostic tests, and surgery to be performed are made. According to institutional procedure, the nurse attentively instructs the family or significant others where to wait.

Much of the information collected in the preoperative preparation is documented in the client record, usually on a preoperative checklist. Figure 13-2 illustrates a typical preoperative checklist. This checklist is completed prior to the client leaving the clinical unit or upon admission to ambulatory surgery. The nurse needs to also communicate verbally with other health care members the necessary information collected.

Table 13-6

COMMON CLASSIFICATIONS, EXAMPLES, AND DESIRED EFFECTS OF PREOPERATIVE MEDICATIONS		
Classification	**Example**	**Desired Effects**
• Tranquilizers	• diazepam (Valium) • lorazepam (Ativan)	• Reduce anxiety • Decrease motor activity • Promote rapid induction of anesthesia
* Sedatives	• phenobarbitol sodium (Luminal Sodium) • secobarbital (Seconal) • midazolam hydrochloride (Versed)	• Promote sleep • Decrease anxiety • Reduce amount of anesthesia required
• Narcotics	• morphine sulfate • meperidine (Demerol)	• Reduce pain • Relax the client • Reduce anxiety
• Vagolytic Agents (anticholinergics)	• atropine sulfate • scopolamine hydrobromide • glycopyrrolate (Robinul)	• Reduce tracheobronchial secretions • Dry mucous membranes • Interrupt vagal stimulation • Produce sedative and amnesia effects
• Antinausea Agents	• droperidol (Inapsine) • promethazine hydrochloride (Phenergan)	• Reduce nausea • Prevent vomiting • Provide mild relaxation
• H$_2$ Receptor Antagonists	• cimetidine (Tagamet) • ranitidine hydrochloride (Zantac) • famotidine (Pepcid)	• Decrease gastric secretions

INTRAOPERATIVE

The intraoperative phase is a particular time during the surgical experience beginning when the client is transferred to the operating room table and ending upon admission to the postanesthesia care unit (PACU).

Physical Description of the Operating Room Environment

For the purposes of preventing wound infections, the surgical suite is an environmentally controlled area of the hospital or clinic. Personnel restriction and geographic isolation provide part of this control. Constant filtered airflow and positive air pressure in the operating rooms also aid in environmental control. Clean and contaminated areas are separated within the suite as well. The surgical suite centralizes equipment and supplies needed for each client so that members of the surgical team do not have to leave the area. The design of the surgical suite is to prevent surgical wound infections.

Operating rooms vary in size, depending on the amount of equipment needed for each particular type of operation. For example, open-heart surgery rooms are usually the largest; minor procedure rooms are usually the smallest. Supplies and furniture are limited to prevent dust collection. The plain furniture is usually made of stainless steel to withstand corrosive disinfectants, yet easily movable on wheels. Besides general illumination with ceiling lights, overhead operating lights illuminate the operative site. Figure 13-3 shows the appearance of an average operating room. The temperature of the room can be adjusted but usually remains a cool 66°F to 68°F. This provides comfort for the surgical team (wearing gowns, gloves, and masks under hot lights is sometimes overbearing), comfort for the client underneath layers of sterile drapes, and an unfavorable environment for bacterial incubation and growth. Although the modern operating room is designed to prevent wound infections, the surgical client views it differently, attributing impersonal and uncaring characteristics to this strange environment.

LUTHERAN HOSPITAL OF INDIANA   DATE _____

	Yes	No	N/A	To be completed in holding area	Pending to be sent to OR		Yes	No	N/A	To be completed in holding area	Pending to be sent to OR
Operative consent(s) signed?						Only cap and gown on patient?					
Operative area prepped?				By:		Hairpins, hairpieces, make-up, nail polish removed if appropriate?					
ID band on patient?						Sensory/motor disabilities? e.g. HOH, deaf, visually impaired, blind, contractures (circle disabilities)				Specify others:	
Allergies:						Language barrier? e.g. aphasia, foreign language				Specify:	
Allergy band applied?											
Lab results on chart?						Do you use recreational drugs?					
Blood/blood products ordered?						OR notified of weight over 300 pounds?					
Blood band # _____						PAR notified of bed transfer?					
Indicate number of units ready____						Voided/catheterized? Time					
X-ray report(s) on chart?						Patient made NPO at:					
EKG report on chart?						Pre-op teaching done and documented?					
Filter removed from IV?											
MD notified of abnormal results?				Comment:		Family/significant other informed to wait in:					
History & physical ☐ on chart ☐ dictated											
Meds be sent to OR?											

Removal or disposition of:	Yes	No	Disposition
Jewelry			
Contact lenses/glasses			
Dentures/partial plates			
Hearing aids			
Prosthesis			

Time_____ Temperature _____ Pulse _____ Respirations_____ Blood pressure_____

FOR HOLDING AREA ONLY

Time_____ Temperature _____ Pulse _____ Respirations_____ Blood pressure_____
☐ Shallow ☐ Dyspneic
☐ Regular ☐ Unlabored

Skin: ☐ Dry ☐ Pale ☐ Pink ☐ Dusky ☐ Warm ☐ Cool ☐ Moist ☐ Jaundice
Level of consciousness: ☐ Alert/oriented ☐ Arouses to verbal ☐ Confused ☐ Not responding
☐ Calm ☐ Anxious ☐ Other _____

CATHETERS/DRAINS

(Specify)	☐ None	Clamped	Unclamped

IV THERAPY

Location	Site condition	Solution	Rate	Initials

Nurse notes:_____

ADDRESSOGRAPH

Unit nurse signature_____ Initials _____
Holding area nurse signature_____ Initials _____
10708
1/95
PREOPERATIVE CHECKLIST

FIGURE 13-2 Sample preoperative checklist. (*Courtesy IOM Health System, L.P. d/b/a Lutheran Hospital*)

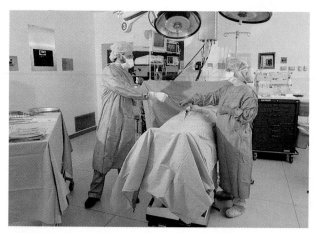

FIGURE 13-3 A typical operating room demonstrating proper surgical attire. (*Photo courtesy of the U.S. Army*)

The client entering the operating room sees an environment that does not look friendly and inviting. The operating room is cold. The people caring for the client dress in characteristic surgical scrubs with hair covered in a cap and faces covered by surgical masks as demonstrated in Figure 13-3. This attire makes the operating room personnel look impersonal and distant. The clanging hollow sounds of the equipment being prepared are sometimes alarming to the client. The terminology used in conversations is foreign. All of these experiences combined with the sight of a barren room and ominous overhead lights while lying on a hard operating room table, add to the client's fear, anxiety, and feelings of powerlessness.

Members of the Surgical Team

The client has many unknown friends in the operating room to act as his advocate. These friends are collectively called the surgical team. At no other time during hospitalization will the ratio of personnel to client be higher than when the client is undergoing surgery. The surgical team includes **sterile** (without microorganisms) team members who are: the surgeon, **first assistant** (assists the surgeon), and **scrub nurse** (passes the instruments to the surgeon). Sterile team members scrub their arms and hands, don sterile gowns and gloves, then perform their duties in the sterile field. The **sterile field** is an area surrounding the client and the surgical site, which is free from all microorganisms. It is created through a process of draping the work area and the client with sterile drapes. Nonsterile team members include the Anesthesia Care Provider (an **anesthesiologist** or **anesthetist** [provides anesthesia under direction of the anesthesi-

ologist]) and **circulating nurse** (RN responsible for all activities during surgery). The nonsterile team members perform their duties outside of the sterile field and do not enter it. Each team member has a clear definition of their role and duties. Clear communication between team members and coordination of their activities improve the chances of the most favorable outcome for the client. Table 13-7 describes members of the surgical team and their duties.

Asepsis

The prevention of infections is the responsibility of the entire surgical team. The environment of the surgical client contains both pathogenic (disease producing) and nonpathogenic microorganisms. When the skin, a prime barrier to infection, is accidentally or purposefully broken, as during surgery, the susceptibility of the client to a bacterial invasion is increased. Bacteria do not "fly," but bacteria carried by dust or nose and throat droplets are easily transported by air currents. When unnecessary activity occurs in the room, or when a team member pulls off his mask while assisting in the transfer of a client to the cart, the environment of the operating room is affected and a wound can easily be invaded by undesirable microorganisms. **Asepsis** is the absence of pathogenic microorganisms. **Aseptic technique** is a collection of principles used to control and/or prevent the transfer of microorganisms from sources within (endogenous) and outside (exogenous) of the client. For example, scrubbed persons wear sterile gowns and gloves; sterile drapes are used to create a sterile field; items used in a sterile field must be sterile; and those working within a sterile field must maintain the integrity of the sterile field. In other clinical nursing units, dressing changes require the application of some of the principles of aseptic technique as does inserting a foley catheter or preparing for an obstetrical delivery. Thus, the practice of aseptic technique applies to other clinical nursing units and other procedures as well.

Practicing aseptic technique requires the development of the sterile conscience. The **sterile conscience** does not allow the surgical team to vary in their adherence to the principles of aseptic technique. Aseptic technique must be strictly followed. This requires constant assessment and monitoring of self and others. It also requires honesty. Sometimes it is easier or less expensive for surgical team members to overlook an infraction of aseptic technique rather than correct the infraction. This must never be allowed to happen. Compromising the principles of aseptic technique may increase the likelihood of an infection, thus harming the client.

Table 13-7

MEMBERS OF THE SURGICAL TEAM: QUALIFICATIONS AND RESPONSIBILITIES

Type of Team Member	Name of Team Member	Typical Qualifications and Responsibilities
Sterile Team Members	Surgeon	• Completed a residency program approved by the American Board of Surgery and may or may not be Board Certified • May be a doctor of medicine (MD) or osteopathy (DO), oral surgeon, or podiatrist specially trained and qualified • Identifies need for surgery • Determines and plans appropriate treatment • Discusses surgical risks, benefits, possible complications, and treatment alternatives with the client • Obtains informed consent • Performs the surgery
	First Assistant	• Assists the surgeon • May be an associate physician in practice, referring physician, or surgical resident • May be a Registered Nurse First Assistant (RNFA) who has been approved by the American Operating Room Nurses (AORN) and endorsed by the American College of Surgeons • Retracts tissue and aids in the removal of blood and fluids at the operative site • Assists with hemostasis and wound closure
	Second or Third Assistants	• May be a qualified Registered Nurse, Licensed Vocational Nurse, or Surgical Technologist who is qualified by training or experience • Usually holds retractors
	Scrub Nurse	• May be a Registered Nurse, Licensed Vocational Nurse, or Surgical Technologist who is qualified by training or experience • More than one scrub nurse may be needed for complicated operations • Provides services under the direction of the circulating nurse • Opens sterile supplies • Scrubs, dons sterile gown and gloves • Assist in gowning and gloving other sterile team members • Prepares instrument tables • Maintains integrity, safety, and efficiency of sterile field • Assists with sterile draping of client's operative site • Passes instruments, sutures, etc. to the surgeon • Assists with instrument, sponge, and sharp counts • Aids in cleaning room after procedure
Nonsterile Team Members	Anesthesiologist or Anesthetist	• An anesthesiologist may be a doctor of medicine (MD) who has completed a two-year residency in anesthesia and is preferably board certified by the American Board of Anesthesiology • An anesthesiologist may also be a doctor of osteopathy (DO) who specializes in anesthesia • An anesthetist may be a qualified Registered Nurse, dentist, or an MD who administers anesthetics • A Certified Registered Nurse Anesthetist (CRNA) is a Registered Nurse with critical care nursing experience who has completed an accredited program of nurse anesthesia and has passed a certifying examination • Anesthetists work under the direct supervision of an anesthesiologist or a surgeon • Assesses client during a preoperative visit • Chooses, induces, and maintains anesthesia • Monitors oxygenation and gas exchange • Manages untoward effects of anesthesia during surgery and postoperatively • Monitors and replenishes fluid and electrolyte balance

(continued)

Type of Team Member	Name of Team Member	Typical Qualifications and Responsibilities
	Circulating Nurse	• Always a Registered Nurse
		• Responsible and accountable for all activities during a surgical procedure
		• Manages personnel, equipment, supplies, the environment, and communication throughout the operation
		• Arranges furniture and equipment in room
		• Opens sterile supplies
		• Ties gowns of sterile team members
		• Attends to needs and supplies of sterile team members
		• Identifies and assesses client
		• Brings client to operating room and transfers to operating room table
		• Applies and assists in insertion of monitoring devices
		• Assists anesthesiologist with induction of anesthesia
		• Positions client for surgery
		• Performs designated surgical skin preparation
		• Assists with sterile draping and setup of sterile field around operative site
		• Monitors sterile technique of surgical team
		• Collects, labels, and distributes specimens
		• Completes intraoperative record
		• Monitors blood and fluid loss
		• Counts sponges, instruments, and sharps with scrub nurse—reports results to surgeon
		• Communicates with surgical team members and others such as client family, pathologist
		• Applies dressing
		• Assists in transferring client to cart—may assist in transporting to postanesthesia care unit
		• Aids in cleaning room after procedure

The Surgical Hand Scrub

An item is sterile when all microorganisms are removed, but the skin cannot be sterilized. Thus, the sterile team members wear gloves as a barrier between the sterile field and the skin. Since accidental tearing or puncturing of the surgical glove is possible, microorganisms may be introduced into the surgical wound. Therefore, the sterile team members must perform the surgical hand scrub before gowning and gloving to lower the number of microorganisms on their hands and arms. The surgical hand scrub removes soil and transient (not always present and easily removed) microorganisms from the hands and forearms. The antimicrobial soap lowers the count of resident (almost always present and not easily removed) microorganisms and continues to prevent sudden bacterial rebound or regrowth after the scrub is completed. The purpose of the surgical scrub is to reduce the possibility of transmission of microorganisms from the surgical team to the client.

During the surgical hand scrub, watches, rings, and bracelets are not worn. Fingernails must be short, clean, and healthy. Artificial nails may not be worn,

but freshly applied, unchipped fingernail polish that has been applied within the last four days may be worn (AORN, 1995). The hands and forearms should have no breaks in skin integrity. Jewelry, artificial nails, polished nails chipped or worn longer than four days, and skin breaks harbor greater numbers of microorganisms.

To perform the surgical scrub, an antimicrobial soap, usually iodophor or chlorhexidine, is applied to moistened hands and arms, making lather. The subungual (under the nails) areas are cleaned. Then a sterile brush with the same antimicrobial soap is used on all four sides of each finger, the hands, and the forearms for a minimum of five minutes or until the time stated in the institutional policy has been completed. Hands are always held higher than the elbows, allowing the fluid to run from the cleanest area (the fingers and hands) to the dirtiest area (the forearms and elbows).

Two Minute Hand Scrub

The surgical hand scrub reflects practices used by all nurses in all clinical areas when washing their hands. A shorter version of the surgical hand scrub, usually two minutes, is practiced at the beginning of the day and between clients to reduce **nosocomial** infections. Nosocomial infections are those infections acquired from the hospitalization. Frequent and thorough handwashing prevents the cross-contamination of microorganisms from client to client and personnel to the client.

For the two minute hand scrub, jewelry is kept to a minimum. Nails are short with no artificial nails. Polish may be worn but should be freshly applied and not chipped. An antimicrobial soap approved by the hospital is applied to moistened hands and forearms. All surfaces are exposed to soap. Rather than using a brush, friction occurs from vigorous handwashing. The hands and forearms are well-rinsed and dried with a paper towel. Then the same paper towel is used to turn off the faucet before discarding. By following the two-minute scrub procedure between clients, clients are less likely to acquire a nosocomial infection from the hands of hospital personnel.

Surgical Skin Preparation

Another skin surface that cannot be sterilized is the client's incision site. Like the surgical hand scrub, the goal of surgical skin preparation of clients is to lower the number of microorganisms on and near the incision site. The surgical skin preparation also removes soil and transient (not always present and easily removed) microorganisms from the incision site. The antimicrobial soap lowers the count of resident (almost always present and not easily removed) microorganisms and continues to prevent sudden bacterial rebound after the scrub is completed. The purpose of the surgical skin preparation is to reduce the possibility of postoperative wound infections from microorganisms on the client's own skin.

Typically, the client is asked to shower or wash the operative site before arrival at the surgical facility or immediately prior to surgery. The client is then transferred to the operating room. After general anesthesia induction, regional block completion, or before local infiltration of the operative site, the circulating nurse performs the surgical skin preparation. Using aseptic technique, the circulating nurse scrubs the area with an antimicrobial soap. Typically this soap is povidone iodine (containing iodine) or chlorhexidine. Potential allergies to iodine must be verified. The circulating nurse scrubs a generous area around the operative site to allow for extension of the surgical incision if the need arises. The scrub is completed in an ever-widening circular motion from the incision site which is considered clean, to the periphery which is considered dirty. Once the periphery is reached, the same sponge is never brought back toward the center of the area. The concept of cleansing from the center (incision site) to the periphery applies for skin preparation of other

procedures in other clinical nursing units such as IV (intravenous) insertion, chest tube insertion, thoracentesis, or subclavian catheter placement. The surgical skin preparation lasts five to ten minutes. After the scrub is completed, the area is blotted dry with sterile towels. An antiseptic solution that is often also iodine-based is applied in the same manner.

Safety and Protection of the Client

The success of nursing process in the operating room is measured by client outcomes. The AORN has established client outcome standards for perioperative clients to be evaluated upon completion of surgery. These outcomes state the client is to be free from infection and injury related to positioning, foreign objects, or chemical, physical, and electrical hazards. In addition, skin integrity and fluid and electrolyte balance are to be maintained. Consequently, nursing care in the operating room strives to provide these standards to all clients undergoing surgery.

Although the responsibilities of the circulating nurse and scrub nurse seem to be a series of tasks or duties, these same tasks and duties are providing nursing interventions to provide quality nursing care to the client. Nursing care in the operating room focuses on the safety and protection of the client. The planning phase of the nursing process for the circulating and scrub nurse involves selecting equipment and supplies, room preparation, and formation of the sterile field prior to the delivery of actual nursing care. The nursing process focuses on preventive nursing actions rather than restorative nursing actions.

Clients undergoing surgery are at high risk for infection related to the invasive procedure undertaken and the exposure to pathogens from the environment, personnel, and client. Some clients are at a higher risk for developing nosocomial infections. Clients undergoing surgery longer than two hours or surgeries of the abdomen or thorax are more prone to infection. Poor nutritional status, the presence of an underlying disease process, obesity, and smoking or substance abuse also place a client at high risk for infection. In addition, the very young (less than one year old) and the elderly (older than sixty-five years of age) are at risk. Regardless of risk factors, nursing care for all clients requires strict aseptic technique to prevent nosocomial surgical wound infections.

Clients undergoing surgery are at high risk for injury related to positioning during surgery. Injuries may include postural hypotension, pressure alopecia, lower back or neck pain, facial and airway edema, eye abrasion, ear compression, joint damage, and nerve injury to brachial plexus, suprascapular nerve, subclavian neurovascular bundle, axillary neurovascular bundle and peroneal, radial, or ulnar nerve. The choice of the client's position during surgery is usually determined by the surgical approach, the surgeon's preference, and individual considerations. The ideal surgical position does not interfere with respiration and circulation, and it should not cause pressure on any nerve. Proper positioning provides access to the operative site and allows easy access for the administration of anesthesia. Proper body alignment is maintained as much as possible to prevent postoperative discomfort. The goal of nursing care is for the client to be free from injury related to surgical positioning.

Some clients are at a higher risk for developing injuries related to positioning. Thin clients, clients undergoing long surgical procedures or vascular procedures, and the elderly are the most vulnerable to injuries related to positioning. Some underlying disease processes also contribute to a higher risk of injury such as clients with edema, infection, cancer, osteoporosis, arthritic joints, neck, or back problems. Clients who are malnourished, anemic, obese, hypovolemic, paralyzed, or diabetic are also prone to skin breakdown due to pressure from positioning. Refer back to Table 13-2 which lists potential complications from surgical positioning. During assessment of the surgical client, the circulating nurse recognizes potential client problems that may put a client at a greater risk for injury due to positioning, but care is taken in positioning all clients.

Since the client is usually positioned after being anesthetized, the client is never moved without the anesthetist's guidance. The circulating nurse ensures availability of positioning devices and adequate personnel for lifting or turning. Proper body alignment is maintained. Client exposure during positioning is minimized to preserve client dignity. After proper positioning, the client is secured with a safety strap.

The client is at high risk for injury related to retained foreign objects left in the wound. The placement of some foreign objects is deliberate and recorded. For example, vascular replacement grafts or orthopedic implants are designed to be left in the surgical wound as part of the surgical procedure. Occasionally, a wound may be packed with gauze or sponges for a physiological purpose such as hemostasis. Inadvertent retention of a foreign object is not desired. Nursing interventions to prevent this type of injury include using only x-ray detectable sponges on the operative field, and the circulating nurse and scrub nurse count sponges, instruments, and sharps according to institutional policy. The circulating nurse reports the results of the various counts to the surgeon and documents counts on the operative record. The goal of nursing care is for the client to be free from injury related to inadvertent retained foreign objects.

The client undergoing surgery is at high risk for injury related to chemical, physical, and electrical hazards. Clients are exposed to numerous chemicals used to clean the environment, prepare the skin, and sterilize instruments. Since anesthetized clients are not able to protect themselves, bodily injury is more likely to occur during positioning, transfers, or falling. Physical hazards may also include the use of both ionizing (x-ray) and nonionizing (laser) radiation when the surgical procedure warrants their use. The majority of equipment used during surgery requires electricity thus exposing the client to electrical hazards. A frequently used piece of equipment is the Electrical Surgical Unit (ESU) or cautery which stops bleeding through electrical coagulation of blood vessels. The goal of nursing care is for the client undergoing surgery to be free from injury related to chemical, physical, and electrical hazards.

Nursing care focuses on minimizing and documenting the exposure to these hazards. Skin integrity is assessed prior to and after completion of the surgical procedure. Allergies to antimicrobial soap are verified. Pooling of preparation solutions beneath the client is prevented. Institutional protocols are followed for radiation and laser safety. In addition, after surgery the area around the dressing site is cleansed to remove any residual antibacterial soap and antiseptic paint solution. Equipment is set up, checked prior to use, and operated according to the manufacturers' recommendations. Care of the surgical client includes multiple interventions from the surgical team. The circulating nurse remains with the client at all times, acting as the client advocate during a time when the clients cannot act for themselves.

The client undergoing surgery is at high risk for altered tissue integrity related to positioning, electrical hazards, and chemical hazards. Nursing actions ensure no bruising, areas of skin breakdown, reddened areas, discolored skin, open skin lesions, excoriation, or itching after surgery. Nursing care to prevent skin breakdown is similar to those actions to prevent injury related to positioning and chemical, physical, or electrical hazards. The goal of nursing care is to maintain the client's skin integrity.

The client undergoing surgery is at high risk for alteration in fluid and electrolyte balance related to abnormal blood loss and NPO status. The goal of nursing care is to maintain fluid and electrolyte balance. Application of hemodynamic monitoring devices by the circulating nurses and anesthesiologist allows the physiologic monitoring of fluid and electrolyte parameters. Intravenous patency is protected and maintained. Nursing care is aimed at monitoring and replacing fluid loss. The circulating nurse accomplishes this by assisting the anesthesiologist in estimating blood loss in sponges and suctioning and monitoring urine output. Intravenous fluids and blood products are administered according to the anesthesiologist's instructions. Fluid and electrolyte values and vital signs should be consistent with preoperative measurements.

After completion of surgery, the circulating nurse applies and secures the dressing. When the anesthesiologist is ready, the client is transferred to a cart. The unconscious or semiconscious client is placed in a side-lying or semiprone position unless contraindicated by the surgical procedure. If the client is supine, the client's head is turned to the side. The client is then taken to the postanesthesia care unit (PACU) accompanied by the anesthesiologist and another surgical team member.

POSTOPERATIVE

The postoperative phase is a particular time during the surgical experience beginning from the end of the surgical procedure until the client is discharged from medical care by the surgeon, not just from the hospital or institution. Upon transfer from the operating room, the client usually goes to the PACU. All clients who receive general anesthesia, spinal anesthesia, or regional anesthesia are admitted to the PACU. Occasionally, clients who have undergone surgery with local anesthesia or no anesthesia or have received intravenous sedation only are placed in postanesthesia care for a short period to be monitored closely until their conditions stabilize. The PACU is usually located next to the operating room. Typically, it is one large room with individual units for clients along the perimeter of the room. Within reach at the head of the client's cart, each of these units has an oxygen delivery system, suction, various other supplies, and cardiac, respiratory, and blood pressure monitoring devices. Curtains can be pulled to provide privacy if needed, but an open view allows continual assessment of all clients.

The postanesthesia care nurse is a registered nurse specially trained in caring for immediate postoperative clients. The goal of the postanesthesia nurse is to promote recovery from anesthesia and the immediate effects of surgery. The immediate postoperative period is a period of physiologic transition for the client, from the intraoperative phase to the postoperative phase. The postanesthesia nurse has knowledge and skill in recognizing and treating anesthetic and surgical complications very quickly. The postanesthesia nurse is empathetic and is able to assess and manage pain for the client who may not be able to express himself. The client is constantly monitored and assessed.

The Nursing Process in the Postanesthesia Care Unit

Upon arrival to the PACU, the anesthesiologist verbally reviews the client's anesthesia and the operative procedure with the postanesthesia nurse. The postanesthesia nurse begins the following nursing assessment in the immediate postoperative period:

- Time of arrival in recovery room
- Patency of airway
- Respirations
- Presence of artificial airway devices
  - Oral airway
  - Nasopharyngeal airway
  - Endotracheal airway
- Oxygen saturation
- Need for supplemental oxygen
  - Mode of administration
  - Flow rate
- Color of skin, nail beds, and lips
- Presence of cardiac dysrhythmias
- Other vital signs
  - Blood pressure, pulse
- Skin condition (moist or dry, warm or cool) and skin temperature
- Initiate Aldrete Score
- Level of consciousness
- Activity level
- Intravenous infusion
  - Type of solution
  - Amount in bottle or bag
  - Flow rate
  - Appearance and location of IV site
- Dressings
  - Amount and character of drainage
- Drains and tubes
  - Intactness and function
  - Connection to drainage and/or suction
  - Amount and character of drainage
- Other assessments according to surgical procedure
- Pain

The postanesthesia nurse notes the client's arrival time to the unit and immediately begins to assess the patency of the airway by placing a hand above the client's nose and mouth to feel exhalation. The quality and quantity of respirations are then immediately observed along with observing for the presence of artificial airways. The client is attached to a pulse oximeter and breath sounds are auscultated. Noting the color of the client and the skin condition is completed as part of the respiratory assessment. Peripheral cyanosis may be an indication of hypothermia and not necessarily respiratory distress. Thus, correlating with the

"A-B-Cs" of airway, breathing, and circulation, the respiratory system is assessed first.

Since the vast majority of clients admitted are in an unconscious state and have received muscle relaxants during surgery, respiratory exchange is often affected. Snoring, stridor, labored chest movement, sternal retractions, cyanosis, and apnea are all signs of respiratory distress. Respiratory distress is the most grave of all complications since respiratory crisis and subsequent death can occur in a matter of minutes if distress is not observed and treated quickly. In the event of any signs of respiratory distress, the postanesthesia nurse must be alert to the possibility of respiratory arrest and ready to initiate cardiopulmonary resuscitation.

Respiratory complications can occur with any anesthetized client. The postoperative client is at high risk for ineffective airway clearance. Often airway obstruction occurs from the tongue falling backward over the pharynx. Nursing interventions include manually lifting the jaw forward to raise the tongue from the pharynx and open the airway (see Figure 13-4). Because of airway obstruction, clients will often arrive in PACU

with an artificial airway inserted. Figure 13-5 shows three common airways: a nasal trumpet, oral airway, and endotracheal tubes (ET tube).

Laryngospasm is the spastic contraction of the lar-

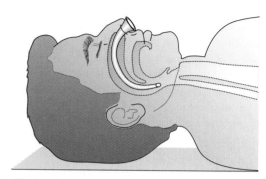

(A) Nasal trumpet

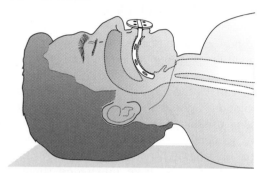

(B) Oral airway

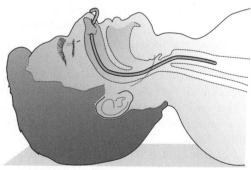

(C) Nasal endotracheal tube

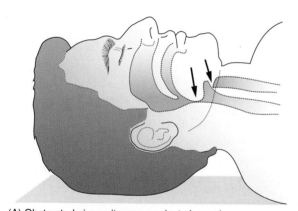

(A) Obstructed airway (tongue against pharynx)

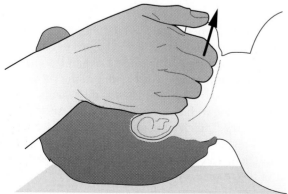

(B) Jaw thrust (anterior displacement)

FIGURE 13-4 An obstructed airway with manual jaw lift.

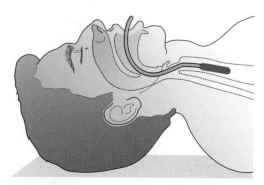

(D) Oral endotracheal tube with cuff inflated

FIGURE 13-5 Three types of artificial airways: nasal trumpet, oral airway, and endotracheal tubes.

ynx that effectively causes airway obstruction. It is often caused by irritation of the larynx from the endotracheal tube or is a possible side effect of some of the anesthetic gases. Laryngospasm is most likely to occur after removal of the ET tube. The client develops an acute inspiratory stridor with sternal retractions. The postanesthesia nurse starts oxygen via a mask, reassures the client, and notifies the anesthesiologist immediately for medication orders of intravenous atropine.

The surgical client in PACU is at high risk for ineffective breathing pattern. Hypoventilation is most likely due to the depressant effects of anesthesia. In hypoventilation, oxygen and carbon dioxide are not exchanging adequately in the alveoli of the lung. Additional oxygen is provided to the client, as needed, through the oral airway or nasal catheter or mask if indicated. The client's oxygen saturation is monitored via a pulse oximeter. It is desirable to maintain the oxygen saturation above 90 percent with the aid of additional oxygen if needed. Pallor, hypotension, tachycardia, and respiratory distress are other indications for oxygen administration. Oxygen may be provided prophylactically to clients who have undergone prolonged or traumatic surgery.

The postoperative client is also at high risk for aspiration. Aspiration of stomach contents, oral secretions, bloody secretions, and foreign bodies into the lungs is another form of airway obstruction. The client temporarily loses the gag and cough reflexes necessary to protect the lungs. Aspiration later causes pneumonia and atelectasis. The postanesthesia nurse intervenes by having suction ready and using it frequently to prevent aspiration. Antiemetics are given as needed to prevent nausea and vomiting. Coughing and deep breathing are initiated as soon as the client is able to follow directions.

The cardiovascular system is assessed next according to the A-B-Cs of airway, breathing, and circulation. The client is attached to an EKG monitor. Then the blood pressure and pulse are taken and along with respirations, are reported to the anesthesiologist if still present in the PACU. If a client does not already have a skin thermometer or another means to obtain temperature, one is applied and the temperature noted. Skin condition is observed for temperature and the presence of diaphoresis. The **Aldrete Score** is initiated.

The Aldrete Score, also known as the Postanesthetic Recovery Score, was developed by J. Antonio Aldrete, MD, MS (see Table 13-8). For approximately 25 years, the Aldrete Score has been used in postanesthesia care units to objectively assess the physical status of clients recovering from anesthesia and has served as a basis for dismissal from the PACU. The Aldrete Score has recently been adapted to assess the readiness for clients to be dismissed from ambulatory surgery. The first five indexes are used for dismissal from PACU. Clients are assessed at the time of admission to PACU

Table 13-8

ALDRETE SCORE/POSTANESTHETIC RECOVERY SCORE

Aldrete/Postanesthetic Recovery Score

Activity	Able to move 4 extremities voluntarily or on command	2
	Able to move 2 extremities voluntarily or on command	1
	Able to move 0 extremities voluntarily or on command	0
Respiration	Able to breathe deeply and cough freely	2
	Dyspnea or limited breathing	1
	Apneic	0
Consciousness	Fully awake	2
	Arousable on calling	1
	Not responding	0
Circulation	B/P ± 20% of preanesthetic level	2
	B/P ± 20% to 50% of preanesthetic level	1
	B/P ± 50% of preanesthetic level	0
Color	Pink	2
	Pale, dusky, blotchy, jaundiced, other	1
	Cyanotic	0

Additional Assessments: Aldrete Score/ Postanesthetic Recovery Score for Clients Having Anesthesia on an Ambulatory Basis

Dressing	Dry and clean	2
	Wet but stationary or marked	1
	Growing area of wetness	0
Pain	Pain free	2
	Mild pain handled by oral medication	1
	Severe pain requiring parenteral medication	0
Ambulation	Able to stand up and walk straight	2
	Vertigo when erect	1
	Dizziness when supine	0
Fasting/feeding	Able to drink fluids	2
	Nauseated	1
	Nausea and vomiting	0
Urine output	Has voided	2
	Unable to void but comfortable	1
	Unable to void and uncomfortable	0

and every fifteen minutes until dismissal. The first five indexes include assessing activity, respiration, circulation, consciousness, and oxygen saturation. Each of the five indexes is scored from 0 to 2, according to the degree of functional disturbance. The score is expressed as a total score with 10 being the maximum. Typically, a minimum score of 8 is required for dismissal from the PACU. As complete as the Aldrete Score may seem, it does not consider some problems that may warrant continued stay in the PACU or admission to a critical care unit. Cardiac dysrhythmias that do not affect blood pressure, bleeding at the incision site, uncontrollable severe pain, and persistent nausea and vomiting may be present even if the client has an Aldrete Score of 10, indicating a need to stay in PACU or be transferred to a critical care unit until the problem is resolved. Regardless, the Aldrete Score has proven effective, reliable, and safe in clients evaluated with this method in the United States and many Latin American countries. It has been adopted as suggested criteria by the Joint Commission on Accreditation of Healthcare Organizations (JCAHO) and corresponding agencies in other countries (Aldrete, 1995). As indicated, the Aldrete Score has been modified to include additional assessments for dismissal from ambulatory surgery.

The postoperative client is at high risk for decreased cardiac output. Hypotension is frequently encountered during the immediate postoperative period. Hypotension can be caused by blood loss, residual effects of anesthesia, narcotics or tranquilizers, position changes, and even pain.

The cardiovascular assessment includes comparing the present blood pressure to the preoperative blood pressure and the blood pressures during surgery. Besides a lowered blood pressure, the postanesthesia nurse assesses symptoms of hypotension such as pallor, clammy skin, diaphoresis, rapid weak pulse, rapid shallow respirations, and restlessness. An imperceptible blood pressure and weak pulse are reported to the surgeon and anesthetist immediately. Oxygen is begun; the intravenous rate is increased; and the client is placed in the Trendelenburg position while evidence of bleeding is sought. If the blood pressure is low but all other signs are normal, the client is watched closely until the client has a chance to awaken; he may be merely depressed from anesthesia. If the pulse is slow (below 50 and not comparable to the preoperative range) or irregular but other signs are normal, the anesthesiologist should be notified. Again, in the event of cardiac arrest, the postanesthesia nurse is ready to initiate cardiopulmonary resuscitation.

The surgical client in the PACU is also at high risk for fluid volume deficit. Blood loss usually ranges from 100 mL to 500 mL in an average surgery. Usually blood transfusions are not given unless more than one unit of blood is needed and the blood loss is greater than 500

mL. Hypovolemic shock usually does not occur until the client has lost more than 1.5 L to 2.0 L of blood or 20 percent to 25 percent of the blood volume (Lewis, Collier, & Heitkemper 1996). If hypotension is due to the residual effects of anesthesia, the effects are usually mild and the client's blood pressure gradually returns to the preoperative level. Giving narcotics may potentiate the effects of residual anesthesia and may contribute to hypotension. Blockages of sympathetic nerves in the spinal cord during spinal and epidural blocks may result in arterial dilation and decreased venous return, producing hypotension. Whereas mild to moderate pain may cause an increase in blood pressure, severe pain may cause hypotension as a result of the release of norepinephrine which then decreases the heart rate and reduces cardiac output. Hypotension may even have existed preoperatively.

Hypertension may also be assessed in the postoperative period. The client may have preexisting hypertension so the blood pressure is compared to the client's normal and admitting blood pressure. Hypertension can be due to pain, the response to anesthesia or medication used, and restlessness or apprehension. Increased intracranial pressure, increased or rapid fluid intake, hypoxia, and fighting the artificial airway may also increase blood pressure. The postanesthesia nurse uses judgment and then proceeds to treat the probable cause by medicating for pain, slowing the intravenous rate, removing an artificial airway, administering oxygen, or raising the head of the bed. If these measures fail, or if the blood pressure is dangerously high, the surgeon or anesthesiologist is notified and orders are followed.

The next system to be assessed is the neurological system. In the Aldrete Score, the level of consciousness and activity level are assessed. The level of consciousness is typically labeled as able to answer questions clearly; arousal only when called; or unresponsive to verbal stimulation. The neurological assessment does not include orientation to person, place, and time. A surgical client is usually oriented to person. Due to the amnesic effects of some medications, the client may be oriented to the facility, and may not be oriented to the specific area of the facility even after being told. Because the postoperative client loses the ability to track time while undergoing some types of anesthesia and has no way of knowing how long the surgical procedure has taken, the client may be oriented to year and month but is rarely oriented to the specific time of the day. Therefore, assessing orientation to person, place, and time is not included as part of the neurological assessment. The level of consciousness affects the ability to breathe, maintain oxygen saturation without assistance, and the ability to move upon command. The assessment of the level of consciousness as described in the Aldrete Score is significant during recovery from anesthesia.

Part of the neurological assessment involves assessing the activity level or the ability to move extremities voluntarily. Voluntary movement is assessed by the ability to move extremities upon command. Hearing is the first sensation to return after being anesthetized. Clients in PACU are asked to squeeze the postanesthesia nurse's hands and to plantarflex and dorsiflex the feet. Due to a regional block or previous condition, the client may not be able to move more than two extremities. Thus, the postoperative client is at high risk for sensory/perceptual alterations.

The surgical client in PACU is also at high risk for injury and high risk for altered thought processes. Some clients are in a state of delirium, in which bizarre and uncontrollable physical movements occur. All clients are restrained with the side rails up, and the cart safety strap applied across the torso and the cart wheel brakes are locked. Some clients showing signs of restlessness may need additional physical restraints. Safety is the utmost concern but when placing restraints, the postanesthesia nurse must first differentiate that the restlessness is due to the state of anesthesia and not pain or anoxia.

Following the neurological assessment, the fluid intake and output is assessed. The intravenous solutions and amount hanging are identified as well as any medications added. The intravenous fluids are infused according to the surgeon's order and run at a specified rate. The intravenous site is assessed for patency, redness, and swelling. The client is restrained as necessary to maintain patency of the intravenous site. In addition, all other infusions and irrigations are also assessed.

The postanesthesia nurse checks dressings and/or peripads for any evidence of bloody drainage and notes the amount so that any subsequent appearance of blood may be accurately evaluated. All drainage tubes are then connected and recorded according to physicians' orders. Table 13-9 lists common types of drains placed in surgery. The amount and kind of drainage are recorded. Nursing care includes making sure tubes are not kinked. Urinary output is also monitored. Scanty urinary drainage is noted (less than 50 cc/hour or as ordered) and reported to the surgeon.

Surgical drains are placed so the wound can drain freely of blood clots, body fluids, pus, and necrotic material that otherwise would collect in the wound and provide a rich medium for bacterial growth. All drains are inserted at the operative site and exit through the incision or a separate stab wound adjacent to the incision. The type of drain is chosen according to the location of wound, size of wound, and type of drainage anticipated. The use of drains decreases pain and infection while increasing wound healing. However, if the wound is draining the skin is not closed so a pathway exists for microorganisms to enter. Drains can then be a source of infection. Complications of drains include hemorrhage, sepsis, loss of the drain, and bowel herniation. Therefore, nursing care of all drains includes assessing the color, character, and odor of drainage, assuring the patency of the drain (making sure there are no kinks in the tubing) and assuring the drain does not accidentally become dislodged. Table 13-10 lists additional assessments according to surgical procedure.

After the client has been admitted and assessed in PACU, the postanesthesia nurse checks the surgeon's and the anesthesiologist's orders and initiates any therapy designated for PACU. All stat IV or IM medications are given; inhalation therapy and specific equipment are initiated as ordered. The clinical unit is notified of any unusual equipment.

Narcotics are given in PACU in reduced amounts according to the client's state of consciousness and the type of anesthesia administered during surgery. A usual dosage is one-half or less of an ordered dose, which may be repeated in one-half hour if the client continues to have pain. Some anesthesiologists write specific orders for narcotics while in PACU. Clients who are medicated typically stay one-half hour after the first medication and fifteen minutes after the second medication. The postanesthesia nurse considers the client's need for medication and dosage based on the length of time it takes to arouse the client, type of anesthetic agent used during surgery, type of surgery performed, and the client's general condition and age.

The postanesthesia nurse charts on a separate nursing record for PACU. Notations are kept to a minimum but anything unusual must be documented adequately. The postanesthesia nurse checks vital signs every fifteen minutes if in the normal range. If unstable, the vital signs are taken every five minutes or as often as necessary until stable. If vital signs fail to stabilize, the surgeon and anesthesiologist are notified. The surgical site is checked at least every thirty minutes. If any initial bleeding has not subsided, the surgeon is notified. The routine checks are continued until dismissal from PACU.

The Aldrete Score is assessed every fifteen minutes along with the skin temperature. The temperature may be checked with a thermometer if there is a question. If the temperature is abnormal, the surgeon and/or anesthesiologist is notified. A significantly elevated temperature can be indicative of malignant hyperthermia, a potentially fatal complication of some anesthetics in sensitive individuals, characterized by a hypermetabolic crisis.

The postanesthesia nurse determines if the client meets the criteria for discharge from PACU. Typically, the client's vital signs must be stable and within the client's normal limits. The Aldrete Score must be 8 to 10. If 7 or less, a surgeon's or anesthesiologist's order is required for dismissal. The dressing must be checked, changed, or reinforced according to orders.

Table 13-9

DESCRIPTION, USES, AND NURSING CARE OF COMMON DRAINS PLACED IN SURGERY

Type	Example	Description	Uses	Nursing Care
Passive	Penrose	A single lumen, soft latex tube that works with gravity directly from the surgical incision	To remove drainage when more than a minimal amount of drainage is expected	• Inspect dressing • Check underneath client to assure drainage has not leaked from the side of the dressing • A dressing must always be in place
	T-tube	A single lumen tube shaped like a T, made of latex	Used after Common Bile Duct Exploration to keep bile drained from the duct as suture lines heal and swelling decreases	• May be attached to a drainage bottle or to a T-tube bag
Active	Hemovac Jackson Pratt J-Vac Relia Vac Surgivac	Closed wound drainage system with drain and reservoir having self-suction when reservoir is compressed	Used after multiple types of procedures to provide continuous gentle suction of the operative site to increase drainage of serosanguinous fluid and to collapse tissue for increased healing	• Assess the drainage system as appropriate to client's condition for 1. Continued drainage 2. Maintained decompression 3. Air-tight tubings 4. Need for emptying • To reactivate suction wash hands, wear gloves, and eye/face protection • Reservoirs are emptied every 8 hours, when drainage nears the full line, or as ordered by the physician
Passive or Active	Davol Sump Axiom Sump	Large, multilumen tube with larger main port for drainage and/or suction; and smaller side port(s) for irrigation and/or air venting to help prevent tissue from being suctioned against catheter and damaged	Used to drain intra-abdominal fluids from abscesses, cysts, or hematomas	• If using continuous irrigation, use one of the smaller or sump ports • Calculate intake and output carefully with irrigations • Place impervious pads underneath client • Change dressings frequently when saturated • If not attached to suction, may be attached to catheter drainage bag • Do not plug sump ports
	Chest Tube ThoraKlex Pleure Vac	Large single lumen drain attached to closed water-seal drainage system	Used to drain fluid or air from pleural cavity	• Assess breath sounds and respirations including depth, rate, symmetry of chest expansion, color of mucous membranes, and presence of crepitus with suction off or tubing clamped • If present, assess amount and type of suction • Assure connections are tight and sealed with tape • Keep chest tube drainage reservoir lower than client's chest • Observe for air leaks in air leak indicator or drainage chamber of drainage reservoir • Place petroleum jelly gauze nearby for quick access should the tube become dislodged • Measure drainage at least every 8 hours (more frequently if in a critical care unit or client condition warrants it) • Clamp or milk the chest tube only with a surgeon's order • Notify surgeon if drainage is greater than 100 cc/hour • Change drainage system when ⅔ full

Table 13-10

ADDITIONAL ASSESSMENTS ACCORDING TO CLASSIFICATION OR TYPE OF SURGICAL PROCEDURE

Classification or Type of Surgical Procedure		Nursing Care
Orthopedics		• Expose wet casts to the air • Check surgeon's orders for positioning of client. Most operated extremities are elevated • Check for digital warmth, color, mobility, circulation (pulses) and sensation of affected extremity
Urologic		• Attach all catheters to drainage • Monitor continuous irrigations closely to assure flow in and out are equal; if obstructed, the bladder could rupture • Increase or decrease irrigation flow rate according to amount of bleeding • Assess for chills or elevated pulse indicating possible hemolysis or bacterial infection • Assess abdomen for signs of distension and rigidity and report especially if client complains
Oral		• Suction frequently and carefully around sutures • Watch breathing; make sure dranage or packing does not obstruct • Apply ice bag when ordered • Remove dental packs as ordered and assess every 15 minutes for further bleeding
Eye, Ears, Nose, & Throat (EENT)	• Ear Surgery • Eye Surgery • Nose Surgery • Tonsillectomies	• Assess edema and tracheal patency (listen for stridor and observe for restlessness) • Assess for facial paralysis • Minimize head movements, coughing, vomiting, and restlessness • Maintain open airway, suction orally, and apply ice • Place on side to facilitate drainage. Elevate head of bed. Keep suction available. Observe closely for bleeding, vomiting, and obstruction
Neurologic	 • Laminectomy or Discectomy • Craniotomy	• Assess level of consciosness; be aware of drowsiness, slurring of speech, disorientation, or irritability that may differ from preoperative state • Observe for pupil changes: inequality, constriction, and nonreactivity to light • Assess for respiratory changes such as snoring, retraction of cheeks and trachea, shallowness, and slowing of rate • Monitor blood pressure and pulse; an elevated blood pressure with lower pulse leads to shock • Observe extremity movement for weakness, paralysis, rigidity, and unilateral drooping of facial features • Use caution when medicating • May move as ordered • Assess sensation, circulation, and motion of extremities distal to incision site • Position as ordered • Complete a neurological check • Do not use Trendelenburg position without permission of surgeon
Vascular (all grafts, carotid endarterectomy, femoral-popliteal bypass)		• Assess color, sensation, warmth, and mobility of extremity • Observe presence and strength of pedal pulse and post tibial pulse • Complete a neurological check for carotid endarterectomy • Check all dressings and area beneath client frequently

(continued)

Classification or Type of Surgical Procedure	Nursing Care
Thoracic	• Observe chest tube closely for patency, amount of bleeding, and presence of air leaks. Tape all connections. Mark drainage container on admission and discharge. Assess fluctuation of drainage in tubing. Attach suction as ordered
	• Observe respirations closely for color change, restlessness, apprehension, dyspnea, or mediastinal shift
	• Elevate head of bed 30 degrees unless contraindicated
	• Encourage coughing and deep breathing
	• Use caution in giving narcotics, especially morphine sulfate, as client cannot afford respiratory depression
* Pneumonectomy	• Do not turn on nonoperative side. Turn from back to operated side alternately
• Lobectomy and resection	• May be turned to either side
Gynecologic	• Assess vaginal drainage

All other parameters are reassessed and charted. All adults are kept in PACU for a minimum of one hour except outpatients, who go to ambulatory surgery when awake and postmedication time has been fulfilled. Children stay only until awake, stable, and have an Aldrete score of 8 to 10. When criteria for dismissal are met, the postanesthesia nurse calls the clinical unit or ambulatory surgery unit and reports the client's name, vitals, surgery, and all pertinent information. The client is then transferred to the appropriate unit.

Later Postoperative

Prior to the client's arrival to the clinical unit, the nurse has prepared for the client. The linen has been changed, the bed clothing folded down, and the room is free from clutter. Special required equipment, as notified by the postanesthesia nurse, has been gathered. An emesis basin and tissue are available. The nurse is ready to assess the client in an organized manner, focusing on the body system affected by surgery.

Upon the client's arrival to the clinical unit, the nurse assists in the transfer of the client to the bed. The nursing assessment of the client upon admission to the clinical unit includes:

• Time of arrival to unit
• Transfer from cart to bed
  Place bed in lowest, locked position with side rails up
  Place in position of comfort
• Vital signs including airway assessment and breath sounds
• Color of skin, nail beds, and lips
• Skin condition (moist or dry, warm or cool)
• Level of consciousness
• Activity level

• Intravenous infusion
  Type of solution
  Amount in bottle or bag
  Flow rate
  Appearance and location of IV site
• Dressings
  Amount and character of drainage
• Drains and tubes
  Intactness and function
  Connection to drainage and/or suction
  Amount and character of drainage
• Urinary output
  Need to void or time of voiding
  Presence of catheter, patency, and output/hour
• Pain
  Last dose of analgesia
  Current pain location, intensity, quality
• Compare assessment with PACU report
• Call light within reach
  Reorient client to usage
• Location of family or significant others
• Postoperative orders

A brief assessment including vital signs is completed every fifteen minutes for an hour; every one-half hour for two hours; and every hour for four hours. The possibilities of postanesthetic complications continue, but as time proceeds different postsurgical complications may develop.

Respiratory complications can still occur with any anesthetized client. The postoperative client is at high risk for ineffective airway clearance, ineffective breathing patterns, and aspiration as in PACU. Now nursing measures begin toward preventing ineffective airway clearance caused by atelectasis and hypostatic pneumonia, both of which usually occur within the first forty-eight hours postoperatively. In postoperative atelectasis, the bronchioles of the lungs become plugged with mucous so air cannot reach the alveoli. The alveoli then collapse. The client develops dyspnea, fever, tachypnea, tachycardia, and cyanosis. In postoperative hypostatic pneumonia, the stagnant mucous promotes the growth of bacteria and atelectasis then develops into a secondary infection. To prevent these complications, the client is actively encouraged by the nurse to cough, deep breathe (with and without incentive spirometry), and turn as instructed preoperatively. In addition, the client is encouraged to sit up and ambulate as soon and often as possible. The nurse needs to ensure adequate pain relief measures so mobility is tolerated well.

Within the cardiovascular system, the client continues to be at high risk for decreased cardiac output and fluid volume deficit, but as the postoperative period progresses the client then becomes at high risk for peripheral neurovascular dysfunction, fluid volume excess/deficit, and activity intolerance. The nurse implements measures to prevent deep vein thrombosis, thrombophlebitis, pulmonary embolism, complications of fluid overload, fluid deficit, hypokalemia, and syncope.

The stress response to surgery, inactivity, pressure from body position, obesity, and injury to pelvic veins during surgery may contribute to the formation of a deep vein thrombosis, thrombophlebitis, and pulmonary embolism. These complications may appear immediately postoperatively or one to two weeks later. The nurse assesses routinely for a positive Homan's sign and for warm, tender, reddened, hardened areas in the calves. To assess for Homan's sign, the client is asked to forcefully dorsiflex the foot. If pain is felt in the calf of the leg, it is considered positive; if no pain is felt, it is considered negative. A positive Homan's sign may be indicative of thrombophlebitis and should be reported to the surgeon. Deep vein thrombosis and thrombophlebitis may lead to a pulmonary embolus. However, there may be no warning of the client developing a pulmonary embolus. When a pulmonary embolism occurs, the client may experience dyspnea, chest pain, cyanosis, cough, hemoptysis, tachycardia, and fever with an elevated white blood cell count. If the embolism is large enough, shock may develop rapidly. Pulmonary embolism may be fatal.

To prevent the formation of a deep vein thrombosis, thrombophlebitis, and pulmonary embolism, the nurse should encourage the client to ambulate to the extent possible. When in bed, the client should perform postoperative leg exercises each hour. Antiembolism stockings are usually ordered as well as a sequential compression device. A sequential compression device has two components, two sleeves and a pump. The sleeves are plastic, inflatable foot wraps held around the feet, calves, and/or thighs by Velcro. They are connected by small tubes to a pump placed at the foot of the bed. The pump is programmed to

inflate the sleeves regularly in a sequential manner from the most distal portion of the foot to the more proximal. This action mimics walking by pumping the venous plexus in the arch of the foot. This action causes blood to move from the extremities toward the heart and thus helps to prevent pooling of the blood preventing deep vein thrombosis, thrombophlebitis, and pulmonary embolism. The sleeves and antiembolism stockings should be removed every day for bath and skin care. It is very important to note that antiembolism stockings and the sequential compression device are not substitutes for leg exercises. Leg exercises must still be performed.

When ordered, the nurse also administers low dose heparin therapy to hemostatically stable clients more than forty years of age having undergone pelvic, abdominal, or thoracic surgery. Usually, heparin is given subcutaneously every twelve hours until discharge. At low dosages, no laboratory test is necessary during therapy to determine the drug's effect if preoperative prothrombin time, partial thromboplastin time, and platelet count were within the normal range. This regimen is followed and ordered at the discretion of the surgeon.

The nurse measures intake and output and monitors laboratory findings (e.g., electrolytes, hematocrit, hemoglobin, and serum osmolality) and signs and symptoms of hemorrhage by assessing vital signs, skin color and condition, dressings, drains and tubes as performed in PACU.

Often, the client may experience syncope when changing from a lying position to a sitting or standing position. The nurse can prevent this by assisting the client to change positions slowly, proceeding in steps, allowing time for the client's internal equilibrium to adjust. The nurse checks the radial pulse frequently and asks the client for subjective statements of dizziness or nausea. If syncope occurs while ambulating, the nurse can ask for assistance with a wheelchair for the client, use a nearby chair, or lower the client to the floor until the client recovers. This is frightening for the client, but not physiologically threatening except if the client is injured while falling.

Gastrointestinal complications become more prevalent after the immediate postoperative recovery. The client may be at high risk for altered nutrition—less than body requirements related to nausea and vomiting and NPO status. The client also may experience pain related to hiccoughs and slowed GI function.

Nausea and vomiting are caused by anesthetic agents, narcotics, hypotension, and the manipulation of the bowel during surgery. Handling of the bowel during pelvic and abdominal surgery causes peristalsis to stop or slow severely. Bowel function normally returns between two to five days postoperatively. If bowel inactivity persists, a paralytic ileus may develop. As bowel function resumes, the nurse continues to assess the client for bowel sounds and if a nasogastric tube is present, a reduction in drainage. As peristalsis returns in a discontinuous fashion, the client may experience distention with flatulence and gas pains. Once bowel sounds resume in all quadrants, the client may be removed from NPO status according to the surgeon's orders. A transitional diet is now available instead of progressing from clear liquids to diet as tolerated (see News Flash). The nurse may suggest this new diet to the surgeon or may move the client as quickly as tolerated from a clear liquid diet to a regular diet. The nurse also provides good oral hygiene while the client is NPO and administers antiemetics as needed for nausea and vomiting.

Hiccoughs are caused by irritation of the phrenic nerve. Impulses then cause the diaphragm to contract rhythmically and violently. Abdominal distention, gastric distention, and the presence of a nasogastric tube are common causes, but electrolyte and acid-base disturbances, intestinal obstruction, and intra-abdominal bleeding may also initiate hiccoughs. The nurse may need to notify the surgeon when hiccoughs are prolonged.

Signs and symptoms of abdominal distention and gas pains may be minimized with early and frequent ambulation and resumption of an oral intake. Gas pains might also be helped by frequently repositioning the client to encourage movement of air through the intestines. As air rises and peristalsis moves from right to left, the client can be moved from lying on the left side (where air will rise on the right), to supine, to the right side (where air will rise on the left). If the client can tolerate it and there are no contraindications, lying prone with the head turned to the side places pressure on the abdomen, forcing air to rise and move out through the rectum. Other nursing care measures to relieve abdominal distention might include irrigation of the nasogastric tube. Irrigating the nasogastric tube may also relieve hiccoughs.

Constipation is a major source of discomfort for the client. Analgesics combined with decreased activity and NPO status are very constipating. Oral fluids and activity should be encouraged. If ordered, the medical regimen of stool softeners and suppositories may be indicated.

The client is at high risk for developing urinary retention related to anesthesia, immobility, and pain. The client is also at high risk for infection related to foley catheter placement. The quantity and quality of urine are more directly related to cardiac output and the perfusion of the kidneys, although a stress response following surgery causes the body to retain fluids for 24 to 48 hours postoperatively. Urine output should be at least 30 cc per hour if a catheter is in place. The catheter must be assessed for patency. If not catheterized, the client should void at least 200 cc

at the first voiding. Most clients void within six to eight hours after surgery. If the client has not voided, the nurse should palpate, inspect, and percuss the bladder. Often the surgeon orders a foley catheter to be placed if the client has not voided after eight to ten hours. Since a foley catheter offers a direct route into the bladder, the risk for developing a nosocomial infection is greater. Strict aseptic technique is required for catheter insertion and clean technique is required for catheter care and handling of the catheter.

Urinary retention occurs frequently in the postoperative period especially in abdominal or pelvic surgery. Anesthesia depresses the urge to void. Narcotics, vagolytic agents (anticholinergics), and spinal anesthesia also interfere with the ability to initiate voiding. The nurse can facilitate voiding by encouraging fluid intake and assisting the client to void in an anatomically correct position as the client's condition warrants. Privacy, running water, indirect bladder pressure (placing a firm hand over the bladder), and warm water over the perineum may encourage voiding.

Alterations in neurological function vary and may be expressed as pain, fever, or delirium. The client may become at high risk for sensory perceptual alterations related to anesthesia, narcotics, change of environment, fluid and electrolyte imbalances, sleep deprivation, hypoxia, and sensory deprivation or overload. The client may also experience pain related to the surgical incision; hypothermia related to anesthesia and surgical environment; and hyperthermia related to infection. Assessing the level of consciousness is a priority. A change in the level of consciousness may be the first indication of a stroke and/or increased intracranial pressure. Determining the level of consciousness may be difficult, especially in the elderly or at night. Often thoughts will clear if the client is given the opportunity to become thoroughly awake. Encouraging the presence of loved ones, offering explanations, and listening to the client may decrease sensory perceptual alterations. Encouraging previous sleep patterns, providing uninterrupted sleep, and alternating rest and activities may also be beneficial.

Pain assessment is essential. Subjective data regarding the location, intensity on a scale of 0 to 10, quality, duration, and factors contributing to pain are assessed and recorded. Objective data such as grimacing and crying are also recorded. Analgesics are usually ordered to be administered via Patient Controlled Analgesia (PCA), epidural analgesia, directly intravenous or intramuscular by the nurse, or orally, all on a PRN (as needed) basis. The client needs to be encouraged to ask for the medication before the pain becomes severe. The nurse should offer medication before activity or painful procedures such as wound irrigation. The nurse needs to attend to analgesic requests promptly. Ensuring comfort allows full participation in coughing, deep breathing, turning, and ambulation by the client.

Hypothermia is common postoperatively for the first few hours. The nurse can offer blankets as needed. From the normal inflammatory response, the temperature may later elevate to a low-grade fever. If the temperature becomes higher than 101°F, the surgeon needs to be notified. Atelectasis and dehydration may cause an elevated temperature (more than 101°F) in the first twenty-four to forty-eight hours postoperatively. After forty-eight hours, an elevated temperature (more than 101°F) may be indicative of a wound, respiratory, or urinary tract infection and can even be indicative of thrombophlebitis or pulmonary embolism.

The nurse's primary role is to prevent infection using aseptic technique. Once a fever has occurred, the nurse follows orders to determine the cause of the elevation such as urine, wound, blood, or sputum cultures. The nurse also administers antipyretics as ordered. Providing light covers and clothing, frequent linen changes, cool washcloths, and a cool environment are nursing measures that may increase comfort.

The nurse automatically forms two nursing diagnoses for any surgical client: Impaired skin integrity related to surgical incision and high risk for infection related to surgical incision. Generally, the nurse does not remove the primary dressing without an order. Bleeding may be monitored by circling the drainage on the dressing and then reassessing later to see if the drainage parameter has increased in size. The dressing may also be reinforced with additional absorbent dressings as needed. In some institutions, the nurse may change the dressing as necessary after the first dressing change. Dressings may not be necessary if there are no drainage or drains, but this is usually the surgeon's preference.

Drainage on dressings and in drains typically changes from sanguinous to serosanguinous to serous over several hours to several days, depending on the type of surgery. The amount should also decrease over the same time period. Purulent, odorous drainage may be a sign of an infection. A sudden increase in drainage may be a sign of impending wound separation. The surgeon should always be notified of any excessive or abnormal drainage.

All wounds heal by primary, secondary, or tertiary intention. In primary intention, the wound layers are sutured together with no gaping edges. The wound generally heals in eight to ten days, but may take up to three months. There is minimal scar formation. Most surgical wounds are of this type.

In secondary intention, the wound heals by filling in the wound with granulation tissue. This wound heals by contraction where the skin edges are not approximated. This method is used in ulcers where there is not enough tissue to approximate the edges or when dealing with an infected wound where drainage is desirable. Wounds healing by secondary intentions are assessed by the presence of granulation tissue with a red granular appearance. Wound healing is slow and can take many months, up to two years. Thus, wound healing by primary intention is preferable.

In tertiary intention, the approximation of tissue edges is delayed. This allows an infection to drain or an area of extensive tissue removal to begin healing. The edges of the wound are closed four to six days later. Since areas of granulation tissue are brought together at this time, the scar is usually much wider.

Wound **dehiscence** and **evisceration** are serious complications of wound healing. Dehiscence occurs when the wound edges separate. Evisceration occurs when there is complete wound separation and the viscera protrude from the wound. Both of these are more likely to occur seven to ten days postoperatively and are preceded by a sudden spillage of serosanguinous drainage. Dehiscence and evisceration are more likely to occur in the very elderly, the malnourished, those with an infection, or clients with abdominal distention who are straining severely. If evisceration occurs, the viscera should be immediately covered with sterile saline dressings and the surgeon notified of the wound disruption.

During dressing changes and after the dressing has been removed, the surgical wound is assessed for the approximation of skin edges, edema, and bleeding. The skin edges may be slightly reddened and swollen from the normal inflammatory response. Signs of a wound infection might include increased suture tension, warmth, erythema, drainage, odor, pain, and induration around the incision site. The nurse can enhance wound healing by promoting nutrition, discouraging smoking, and cleaning the wound properly. The practice of aseptic technique cannot be emphasized enough in preventing nosocomial infections in a surgical incision.

Many clients undergo a psychological adjustment to surgery. Clients are at high risk for anxiety or ineffective individual coping related to disturbance in body image, change in lifestyle, financial strain, or a poor prognosis. Taking time to talk and listen to the client combined with simple explanations and reassurances may be all the support the client needs to combat anxiety.

As the client recovers and is dismissed from the hospital, the client is at high risk for knowledge deficit related to home care. Hopefully, the client has been instructed routinely since admission about home care. Adequate teaching about home care results in a quicker recovery, fewer complications, and greater independence.

Teaching Tips

Topics of information the client and family must know for proper home care:

- Medication instructions
- Diet
- Activity restrictions
- Follow-up appointments
- Wound care
- Special instructions

AMBULATORY SURGERY

Ambulatory surgery is defined as surgical care performed under general, regional, or local anesthesia with less than twenty-four hours of hospitalization. Other names for ambulatory surgery include Same-Day, One-day, Outpatient, In and Out, or Short-stay Surgery. Whatever the term, the goal of ambulatory surgery remains the same: "to give high quality care to the patient requiring surgery and to decrease patient complications with the most efficient use of time and money" (Beare, 1994).

A trend in health care is for promoting a philosophy of wellness. Clients are encouraged to accept more personal responsibility for their state of health. In the past, the message given to clients was that the client is sick and the medical community will provide all care. Now ambulatory surgery clients are asked to believe a totally different concept and that is the postoperative client is not sick and except for a few minor limitations, can often resume normal daily activities soon after anesthesia and surgery are completed.

Ambulatory surgery has grown dramatically. The competitive health care environment emphasizes cost containment. Short-stay surgery has the longest period of time, usually twenty-three hours, for the client to obtain skilled postoperative care or monitoring without being formally admitted to the hospital. This attempts to overcome the risk of premature dismissal while meeting fiscal requirements. The emphasis on cost containment coupled with government changes in Medicare-Medicaid provisions, has further promoted the concept of ambulatory surgery.

To further reduce health care costs, few clients are admitted to the hospital prior to the day of surgery. Most surgical clients are processed through the ambulatory surgery unit. These clients are called Day of Surgery or AM Admit Clients. Necessary laboratory work, radiology tests, or other examinations are completed on an outpatient basis prior to the day of surgery. Even clients undergoing extensive surgeries such as open-heart surgery (a coronary artery bypass), craniotomy, or total joint replacement, can be admitted the day of surgery for an elective procedure. Then,

after dismissal from the perioperative suite, the client may either be admitted to the hospital as an inpatient or may be dismissed from the ambulatory surgery unit.

Besides fiscal reasons, ambulatory surgery has grown through technological advances. Clients experience a shorter recovery due to new procedural technology, such as laporoscopic cholecystectomy. The introduction of shorter-acting anesthetic agents also decreases the immediate postoperative recovery time so clients are more able to function independently upon dismissal from ambulatory surgery settings.

Ambulatory surgery encompasses many different types of surgeries. There is no predetermined list as to what types of procedures are to be performed as ambulatory surgery. The physician or a third party payer selects the surgical setting. The selection must account for the client's unique medical, social, and psychological needs. As a client advocate, the nurse is able to influence the surgical setting decisions either in a preoperative office setting, or on the actual day of surgery or the postoperative decisions in the ambulatory surgery setting based on the nursing assessment.

The benefits of ambulatory surgery are many. Ambulatory surgery decreases cost to the client, institution, insurance carriers, and government agencies. Since clients are hospitalized for such a short period of time, the risk of acquiring a nosocomial infection during the perioperative period is decreased. The client experiences less personal life disruption and also experiences decreased psychological distress from hospitalization. With ambulatory surgery, the client especially benefits from early postoperative ambulation.

Ambulatory surgery is performed in several different settings. Hospital-based integrated facilities are formal ambulatory surgery programs incorporated into existing inpatient surgery programs. The clients are cared for preoperatively and postoperatively in the ambulatory surgery unit but are mixed with inpatients in the operating room schedule. This type of facility also allows preoperative processing of Day of Surgery clients. Hospital-affiliated facilities encompass a separate department with designated preoperative, intraoperative, and postoperative areas. This facility may be located within the hospital, adjacent to the hospital, or at a satellite location. Free-standing facilities are independently owned and operated and are not affiliated with a hospital or medical center. Physicians have generally owned these in the past, but the trend is for health care corporations to own these. Some doctors' offices also have facilities to complete minor ambulatory surgery. The multiple types of facilities provide safe, convenient, and cost-effective surgery administered to basically stable, healthy individuals who will assume responsibility for postoperative self-care at home.

Nursing care in ambulatory surgery is similar to care

given to clients in the hospital-based surgical suite. The client still possesses basic pathology that requires surgical intervention. The surgical techniques and technology used to implement these techniques are similar. The surgical team must be skilled and knowledgeable in surgical techniques. The surgical team must consciously practice strict aseptic technique. Unexpected anesthetic and surgical emergencies may occur. Since there is no such thing as minor surgery to the client, clients have the same fears whether they are undergoing ambulatory surgery or inpatient surgery. The client remains dependent on the surgical team during surgery and anesthesia.

The Aldrete Score has been modified for use with clients having anesthesia on an ambulatory basis. The popularity of ambulatory surgery has not only required dismissal criteria from PACU but also criteria when clients can be discharged home. Five other assessments were added to the Aldrete Score and similarly graded 0, 1, or 2 according to the criteria described in Table 13-8. Attainment of these criteria indicates clients should be able to care for themselves at home and accomplish activities of daily living independently and safely. The points are totaled at regular intervals (usually every one-half hour) and clients may be discharged to home when their total score is 18 or higher.

Differences do exist between ambulatory and inpatient surgery. In ambulatory surgery, the emphasis is on wellness with increased client and family responsibility in the home setting. The surgical team loses control in assuring the clients' compliance with preoperative instructions. Elective procedures generally are performed on healthier clients. Typical procedures are shorter, often using local infiltration of the surgical site as the method of anesthesia. The relatively short stay compresses time for assessment, planning, and intervening with the nursing process. The differences between ambulatory and inpatient surgery are a challenge to the surgical team to ensure quality care while remaining economical.

ELDERLY CLIENTS UNDERGOING SURGERY

Elderly clients (more than sixty-five years of age) are at high risk for developing complications from surgery or anesthesia. Unfortunately, because an increase incidence of disease correlates with increasing age, more elderly require surgery than any other age group. As the percentage of elderly persons in the whole population rises, the number of surgeries on the elderly will also rise. Because of the complex needs of the elderly client undergoing surgery, the nurse must be knowledgeable in promoting health and rehabilitation in the elderly.

Surgery is a stressor. The elderly may not have sufficient resilience to react defensively to this stressor because of insufficient energy sources. The risk of complications from surgery becomes even greater with elderly clients who have one or more chronic diseases. Surgery then can become the source of a downward spiraling effect toward debilitation or possibly death.

The elderly vary in the ability to respond to the stress of surgery. Physiologic changes have occurred due to the aging process that inhibit the elderly from readily coping with surgery. The physiologic changes in the very elderly (more than eighty years of age) are markedly greater than the number of changes in those in their sixties and seventies. The breathing capacity, renal blood flow, cardiac output, and conduction velocity of the nervous system diminish. Table 13-11 lists physiologic changes in the elderly and correlating nursing interventions. Aging affects all body systems, and the nurse needs to be familiar with these changes and the interventions geared toward each to prevent and detect complications of surgery.

In the cardiovascular system, the elderly experience decreased elasticity of the blood vessels and decreased pumping action of the heart resulting in less blood reaching the peripheral circulation. Ultimately, the blood flow is slower and less blood reaches vital organs such as the brain, heart, lungs, liver, and kidneys. Decreased blood flow to vital organs inhibits the older adult client from eliminating anesthetics and medications through the lungs, liver, and kidneys as readily as younger adults. Decreased elasticity of the blood vessels does not allow vasoconstriction and vasodilation to compensate for hypovolemia and hypervolemia so the elderly are more prone to hypotension and shock or conversely, fluid overload or hypervolemia. Slower blood flow in addition to an increased incidence of atherosclerosis, the presence of other cardiovascular diseases, combined with decreased mobility increases the likelihood that elderly surgical clients are at high risk for developing deep vein thrombosis, thrombophlebitis, and accompanying pulmonary emboli. Decreased blood flow to vital organs may cause confusion, decreased urinary output, and drug retention or overdose. Decreased peripheral circulation may also contribute to poor or delayed wound healing as well. The effects of aging on the cardiovascular system increase the likelihood of multiple complications from surgery for the elderly client.

As with the cardiovascular system, the respiratory system in elderly clients demonstrates less elasticity also, and expansion of the chest wall and lungs are affected. As a result, elderly clients are unable to exhale fully, causing increased air retention in the lung (residual lung volume) and decreased ability to forcefully exhale air (forced expiratory volume). The amount of air inhaled and exhaled (vital capacity) is decreased. Less air reaches the alveoli causing

Table 13-11

PHYSIOLOGIC CHANGES OF AGING		
	Change	**Nursing Intervention**
Cardiovascular System	• Decreased elasticity of the vascular system • Decreased cardiac output • Decreased peripheral circulation	• Closely monitor vital signs and peripheral pulses • Encourage early ambulation • Use antiembolism stockings • Monitor intake and output including blood loss • Monitor preoperative response to activity and compare tolerance to activity postoperatively
Respiratory System	• Decreased vital capacity • Decreased alveolar volume • Decreased movement of cilia	• Closely monitor respirations • Auscultate breath sounds frequently • Encourage coughing and deep breathing • Turn frequently • Monitor oxygen saturation
Urinary System	• Decreased glomerular filtration rate • Decreased bladder muscle tone • Weakened perineal muscles	• Monitor intake and output q 1 to 2 hours • Assist frequently with toileting • Monitor fluid and electrolyte status
Gastrointestinal System	• Loss of gastric and intestinal motility • Altered digestion and absorption • Decreased food consumption	• Assess for obesity and malnutrition • Encourage fluids and activity • Encourage high protein foods and supplements • Assist with meals as needed • Provide companionship during mealtime
Immunological System	• Decreased levels of gamma globulin • Decreased plasma proteins	• Follow strict aseptic technique • Monitor temperature • Assess incision site
Nervous System	• Decreased conduction velocity • Poor vision • Loss of hearing • Decreased sensation	• Allow use of glasses and hearing aids • Orient to environment • Provide for safe environment • Repeat information as needed • Use medications sparingly • Provide written instructions • Allow extra education time
Integumentary System	• Lack of elasticity • Loss of collagen • Decreased subcutaneous fat	• Lift to position to prevent shearing forces on skin • Pad bony prominence • Use paper tape • Use warm prepping solutions, irrigating solutions, and intravenous solutions intraoperatively • Give extra blankets • Provide warm room temperature • Turn frequently • Encourage early ambulation

decreased alveolar volume. Decreased vital capacity and alveolar volume results in lower carbon dioxide and oxygen exchange in the lungs. The cilia, lining the passageways of the lung, do not move as efficiently thereby decreasing the cough reflex of the elderly. All of these changes may lead to atelectasis, pneumonia, and postoperative confusion.

The urinary system is affected by age as well. Kidney function decreases as blood flow to the kidneys is decreased. Waste products are not excreted as quickly and urine output is less. The decreased blood flow decreases the glomerular filtration rate. Decreased bladder muscle tone causes urinary retention and weakened perineal muscles can cause urinary incontinence. The effects of aging increases the likelihood of renal failure, urinary incontinence, and urinary retention.

A combination of age-related changes in renal and liver function, related to decreased perfusion rate, results in a slower drug metabolism. The elderly client may need a reduced dosage, given less frequently, or smaller more frequent doses to avoid side effects of postoperative analgesics. Decreased peripheral circulation may reduce or delay the absorption of intramuscular analgesics. Oral analgesics may also not be well absorbed due to decreased gastrointestinal motility and decreased mesenteric blood flow. Intravenous analgesia may be preferred for the elderly to provide careful dosing according to the individual response and need.

In the gastrointestinal system, loss of gastric and intestinal motility in aging results in constipation and fecal impaction. Loss of muscle strength and limited range of motion causes decreased activity, thereby contributing to constipation. As elderly clients are often less mobile after surgery, constipation and fecal impaction become very common.

The nutritional status of the elderly client prior to surgery may also have a profound effect on wound healing, susceptibility to infection, degree of postoperative recovery, and length of hospital stay (Talabiska, 1995). Factors that influence nutritional status include the presence of a chronic illness. With a chronic illness, the client requires more energy or may expend more energy to maintain metabolism and activities of daily living. Dementia, depression, and altered mental status may also affect nutritional status. Because the elderly take multiple medications, drug-food interactions are more common. Food consumption, gastric motility, and digestion and absorption are decreased. The financial situation and social status of the elderly client may also contribute to poor nutritional status. Poorly fitting dentures can negatively affect the nutritional status of the elderly. The nutritional status of the elderly client needs to be carefully assessed both preoperatively and postoperatively to enable optimum recovery from surgery. Nutrition is one area where nursing can directly intervene.

Elderly clients are more prone to infections such as wound infections, pneumonia, and urinary tract infections. Delayed wound healing, including wound dehiscence or evisceration, are also more frequent in the elderly. Changes in the metabolism and the immune system of the elderly may contribute to these

effects. The levels of gamma globulin and plasma proteins fall causing inadequate inflammatory responses. The body has a decreased ability to protect itself from pathogenic microorganisms when there are fewer killer T-cells and decreased response to foreign proteins. Normally, an increased production of leukocytes and temperature for forty-eight hours postoperatively is a normal inflammatory response. If the temperature is markedly elevated and continues longer than this, an infectious process may be occurring. In the elderly, a reduction in the basal metabolic rate causes a reduced normal temperature. Thus, fever in the elderly is even more significant.

The conduction velocity of the nervous system diminishes in the elderly, slowing movements and impairing equilibrium. Other sensory changes also increase the risk of injury for the elderly surgical client. Poor vision, loss of hearing, and decreased sensation contribute to falls, burns, and other injuries. Overstimulation and the lack of a familiar environment often cause confusion, another factor in injury. Chronic conditions limiting mobility such as arthritis or previous strokes may also contribute to the incidence of injury. The physiologic changes in the nervous system may lead to integumentary complications as mobility and sensation are decreased.

Due to the lack of elasticity and loss of collagen, the skin of the elderly is dry, flaky, and itchy. The skin becomes thin and easily bruised and abraded. The lack of subcutaneous fat and decreased circulation makes the older adult more prone to hypothermia and pressure sores.

The elderly have a lifetime of individual experiences affecting their response to surgery. A lifetime of watching family and friends experience surgery, illness, and dying influences personal reactions to impending surgery. Regardless of whether the impressions from experiences are correct or incorrect, the client perceives the experiences as fact. Due to the variation in these experiences, each client reacts differently to similar situations. Simply talking with the client to correct misconceptions or listening to realistic fears helps in preparing for the future.

Often, the effects of third party reimbursement policies require elderly clients to undergo surgical procedures on an outpatient basis. Since many elderly clients have neurological deficits and other chronic disease processes, the elderly outpatient poses a particular challenge for the nurse. Additional self-care deficits may be added postoperatively as a result of the surgical procedure and the effects of anesthesia. Often the elderly live alone and lack support systems needed for care at home. In order to provide realistic discharge planning, the nurse needs to assess the ability of the client, family, and friends to provide care at home.

▶ CASE STUDY

Mr. Glen Stone, a seventy-four-year-old retired schoolteacher who is married and the father of four and grandfather of sixteen, weighs 275 lbs, has undergone a right hemicolectomy in which the right side of his colon has been removed because of cancer. He has a history of smoking, but has no other health problems. The surgery was uncomplicated and he is in the PACU. He has a midline incision with a Penrose drain and a stab wound with a Jackson Pratt drain adjacent to the incision. He has a nasogastric tube attached to low intermittent suction. He is alert and oriented and moves all four extremities. His blood pressure is normal for him in comparison to preoperative levels. He is breathing regularly and easily at a rate of 16 breaths per minute, has pink mucous membranes, but his oxygen saturation is 86 percent with additional oxygen given via mask.

The following questions will guide your development of a Nursing Care Plan for the case study.

1. What will you include in assessing risk factors for developing postoperative complications for Mr. Stone?

2. What is his Aldrete Score at this point?

3. What nursing measures can you institute to promote oxygenation?

4. What type of drainage is expected from his incision and drains for the first 1 to 2 days?

5. What nursing observations can be made and reported to indicate to the surgeon that nasogastric tube can be removed?

6. What nursing measures can be implemented to prevent deep vein thrombosis, thrombophlebitis, or pulmonary emboli?

7. Write three individualized nursing diagnoses and goals for Mr. Stone.

8. What information will Mr. Stone need prior to discharge?

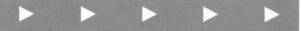

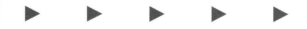

SUMMARY

- Surgery is a major stress for all clients. Anxiety and fear are normal. Fear of the unknown is the most prevalent fear prior to surgery and the easiest for the nurse to intervene.

- The outcome of surgical treatment is tremendously enhanced by accurate preoperative nursing assessment and careful preoperative preparation, thus ensuring client safety, understanding, and compliance with health care. Information gathered through preoperative assessment and risk screening is later used for preparation of the surgical site, surgical positioning, and as a comparative basis for postoperative assessments, activity, and screening for complications.

- The teaching methods used by the nurse strongly influences the degree of learning and the retention of information.

- Aseptic technique is a collection of principles used to control and/or prevent the transfer of microorganisms from sources within (endogenous) and outside (exogenous) of the client. These principles are practiced within all clinical nursing units. The sterile conscience governs personal behavior in adhering to aseptic technique.

- Nursing care in the operating room focuses on the safety and protection of the client so the nursing interventions are primarily preventive rather than restorative.

- Postoperative nursing assessments are completed in

an organized manner, focusing on the priorities of airway, breathing and circulation, then the body system affected by surgery.

- The nurse can prevent the formation of deep vein thrombosis, thrombophlebitis, and pulmonary embolism through early ambulation, postoperative leg exercises, and providing antiembolism stockings and sequential stockings if ordered.
- The client must be encouraged to ask for the medication before the pain becomes severe, and the nurse should attend to analgesic requests promptly to allow full participation in coughing, deep breathing, turning, and ambulation by the client. The nurse should offer medication before activity or painful procedures such as wound irrigation.
- Ambulatory surgery is defined as surgical care performed under general, regional, or local anesthesia with less than 24 hours of hospitalization. Cost containment, government changes, and technological advances have all promoted the concept of ambulatory surgery.
- Because of the physiologic changes and complex needs of the elderly client undergoing surgery, the nurse must be knowledgeable in promoting health and rehabilitation in the elderly surgical client.

Review Questions

1. The nurse, while doing client teaching, implements which one of the following?

    a. assesses barriers to learning
    b. completes teaching in a single time frame
    c. provides information in one mode of learning
    d. allows little time for questions

2. Client education is:

    a. completed when time allows.
    b. started when discharge is scheduled.
    c. always more beneficial when completed in a structured group setting.
    d. directed toward the client's family when the client is unable to learn.

3. The role of the nurse in obtaining consent includes which of the following?

    a. judging the quality of the explanation and ascertaining the client's understanding of the consent form
    b. acting as a witness to the signature of the client
    c. administering the preoperative medication before the client signs the consent
    d. ensuring coercion was used to obtain the client's signature on the consent

4. The use of drains will:

    a. increase postoperative pain.
    b. prevent tissue healing.
    c. increase scarring.
    d. eliminate fluid accumulation.

5. Upon admission to the PACU, the nurse first:

    a. takes the client's blood pressure.
    b. assesses the airway.
    c. assesses the level of consciousness.
    d. checks the incision site.

6. The nurse is making a preoperative assessment on a client. Which of these assessments is the most important to know for a client who is having general anesthesia?

    a. hearing impaired
    b. a right leg amputee
    c. color-blind
    d. a smoker

7. Which of the following persons is responsible and accountable for all activities during a surgical procedure?

    a. surgeon
    b. anesthesiologist
    c. circulating nurse
    d. scrub nurse

8. The surgical skin preparation will:

    a. sterilize the skin.
    b. cleanse and inhibit bacterial growth.
    c. prevent fingernails from growing.
    d. remove the dermis.

9. The single nursing intervention that reduces almost all surgical risks is:

    a. encouraging activity and early ambulation.
    b. assessing the blood pressure.
    c. assuring adequate nutrition.
    d. monitoring intake and output.

10. Surgical risk increases in the elderly due to:

    a. type of surgery.
    b. physiologic aging changes.
    c. exposure to infectious processes.
    d. number of children.

Critical Thinking Questions

1. Could you develop a "sterile conscience" and have the integrity to acknowledge a break in aseptic technique?

2. How can you explain to a client what it is like having surgery?

News Flash: The Transitional Diet

Traditionally, the clear liquid diet has been the initial feeding on return to an oral intake despite its poor nutritional quality and unacceptable palatability. Theoretically, clear liquids cause fewer symptoms of intolerance such as nausea, vomiting, diarrhea, and/or abdominal distention. Health care workers have continued the use of clear liquid diets without a scientific basis for doing so. But clients find the clear liquid diet choices unacceptable. Perhaps the limitation of solid foods plants seeds of doubt in the clients' minds about their ability to take in and tolerate other foods which may lengthen the clients' progression to an adequate diet even farther. The transition from clear to full liquids is also problematic for clients with a lactose intolerance or milk allergy. They find little on a full liquid tray that they can safely eat and are limited to clear liquids with hot cereal at a time when they had hoped to put broth and flavored gelatin behind them.

A new diet available as an alternative is the Transitional Diet. It is an option for clients to aid in returning to oral intake after surgery, extended parenteral nutrition, or a period of nausea and vomiting. It contains items such as chicken noodle soup, toast, crackers, and mashed potatoes. This diet more readily optimizes nutrient intake and supplies more calories and higher protein content with food choices that are more readily accepted and easily tolerated. With the Transitional Diet, clients are more satisfied with few signs of intolerance. This could potentially decrease length of hospital stays.

Sample Menu of the Transitional Diet

Breakfast
- peach nectar
- cream of wheat
- two slices of toast
- margarine/jelly
- decaffeinated tea

Lunch
- chicken noodle soup/saltines
- mashed potatoes/margarine
- fruit gelatin
- custard
- 7-up

Dinner
- beef noodle soup/saltines
- rice
- cottage cheese
- canned fruit cup
- sherbet
- apple juice

HS snack
- applesauce
- graham crackers

Other allowed foods
- eggs
- cold cereal
- milk
- juices
- broth-based soups
- lean meats
- vanilla wafers

(Adapted from "Transitional diet" by K. Goodman 1995. Current Topics in Nutrition Support. Fort Wayne, IN: Lutheran Hospital.)

CHAPTER
14

Fluid, Electrolyte, and Acid-Base Balances

Diane R. Behrens

▶ **KEY TERMS**

acidosis
active transport
alkalosis
buffer systems
diffusion
edema
electrolytes
filtration
fluid volume deficit
fluid volume excess
homeostasis
osmolality
osmosis
pH
solute
solvent

LIST OF DISORDERS

Fluid Balance
▶ Fluid Volume Deficit
▶ Fluid Volume Excess
Electrolyte Balance
▶ Hyponatremia
▶ Hypernatremia
▶ Hypokalemia
▶ Hyperkalemia
▶ Hypocalcemia
▶ Hypercalcemia
▶ Hypomagnesemia
▶ Hypermagnesemia
▶ Hypochloremia
▶ Hyperchloremia
▶ Hypophosphatemia
▶ Hyperphosphatemia
Acidosis
▶ Metabolic Acidosis
▶ Respiratory Acidosis
Alkalosis
▶ Metabolic Alkalosis
▶ Respiratory Alkalosis

LEARNING OBJECTIVES

Upon completion of this chapter the learner should be able to:

- Define key terms.
- Discuss the basic physiology of fluid, electrolyte, and acid-base balances within the human body.
- Describe causes, assessment data, nursing interventions, and criteria for evaluating effectiveness of care for clients with a nursing diagnosis of fluid volume deficit or fluid volume excess.
- Describe causes, assessment data, nursing diagnoses, nursing interventions, and criteria for evaluating the effectiveness of nursing care for clients with sodium, potassium, calcium, and magnesium imbalances.
- Relate principles of nursing management for clients receiving fluids and electrolytes via oral supplements, intravenous solutions, enteral feedings, and total parenteral nutrition.
- Differentiate between the causes, assessment data, and nursing management of metabolic and respiratory acidosis and alkalosis.

▶ *MAKING THE CONNECTION*

Refer to the topics in the following chapters to increase your understanding of fluid, electrolyte and acid-base balance.

- **Chapter 13, Perioperative Nursing:** Postoperative, The Nursing Process in the Postoperative Care Unit, p. 247; Later Postoperative, p. 254.
- **Chapter 15, Oncology Nursing:** Oncological Emergencies, Hypercalcemia, p. 317.
- **Chapter 19, Respiratory Disorders:** Anatomy and Physiology Review, p. 388; Adult Respiratory Distress Syndrome (ARDS), p. 421; Acute Respiratory Failure, p. 423.
- **Chapter 20, Cardiac Disorders:** Congestive Heart Failure p. 455; Dysrthythmias, p. 456
- **Chapter 21, Vascular Disorders:** Anatomy and Physiology Review, p. 491.

- **Chapter 22, Blood and Lymph Disorders:** Anatomy and Physiology Review, Blood, p. 518.
- **Chapter 29, Endocrine Disorders:** Anatomy and Physiology Review, p. 780; Diabetes Insipidis, p. 800; Parathyroidism, p. 813; Adrenal Glands, p. 817; Addison's Disease, p. 819
- **Chapter 30, Diabetes:** Acute Complications of Diabetes, p. 840.
- **Chapter 34, Digestive Disorders:** Peritonitis, p. 992; Cirrhosis, p. 996: Pancreatitis, p. 1002.
- **Chapter 35, Urinary Disorders:** Anatomy and Physiology Review, p. 1015; Acute Renal Failure, p. 1039: Dialysis, p. 1048; Hemodialysis, p. 1048; Peritoneal Dialysis, p. 1049.
- **Chapter 36, Ostomies:** Pathophysiology of Bowel and Bladder, p. 1061.

INTRODUCTION

Fluid, electrolyte, and acid-base balances are essential to maintain **homeostasis**, a state of balance between the supply and demand of essential substances within the body. Environmental factors, personal behaviors, psychological influences, therapeutic modalities, and diseases all can create situations that can alter internal stability. Fundamental to all nursing care is an understanding of the homeostatic mechanisms involved in the maintenance of internal stability. Early detection of imbalances in fluids, electrolytes or acid-base and the application of effective nursing interventions promote restoration of vital substances to a state of equilibrium.

COMMON DIAGNOSTIC TESTS

The following is a table of the commonly used diagnostic tests for clients who present electrolyte imbalances.

Test	Explanation/Normal Values	Nursing Responsibilities
Sodium (Na⁺)	Measure level of serum sodium 135–145 mEq/L Function in the body: Major electrolyte in extracellular fluid Regulates fluid balance Stimulates conduction of nerve impulses Helps maintain neuromuscular activity	Explain to the client that blood will be drawn for this laboratory test. No food or fluid restrictions are required.
Potassium (K⁺)	Measure level of serum potassium 3.5–5.0 mEq/L Function in the body: Major electrolyte in intracellular fluid Maintains normal nerve and muscle activity Assists in cellular metabolism of carbohydrates and proteins Regulates acid-base balance	Explain to the client that blood will be drawn for this laboratory test. No food or fluid restrictions are required. If the client has hypokalemia or hyperkalemia, evaluate the client for cardiac dysrhythmias.
Calcium (Ca⁺⁺)	Measure level of serum calcium Total serum calcium 9.0–10.5 mg/dl Ionized serum calcium 4.5–5.6-mEq/L Function in the body: Essential role in bone and teeth integrity, clotting smooth, skeletal and cardiac muscle functioning and nerve impulse transmission Vitamin D is needed for absorption of calcium from gastrointestinal tract	Explain to the client that blood will be drawn for this laboratory test. No food or fluid restrictions are required.
Magnesium (Mg⁺⁺)	Measure level of serum magnesium 1.5–2.5 mEq/L Function in the body: Combines with calcium and phosphorous in intracellular bone tissue Essential for neuromuscular contraction, synthesis of protein and body temperature regulation	Explain to the client that blood will be drawn for this laboratory test. No food or fluid restrictions are required.
Chloride (Cl⁻)	Measure level of serum chloride 100–110 mEq/L Function in the body: Major electrolyte in extracellular fluids Functions in combination with sodium to maintain osmotic pressure Assists in maintaining acid-base balance	Explain to the client that blood will be drawn for this laboratory test. No food or fluid restrictions are required.

(continued)

Test	Explanation/Normal Values	Nursing Responsibilities
Phosphate (PO4⁻⁻)	Measure level of serum phosphate 1.8–2.6 mEq/L Function in the body: An essential intracellular electrolyte Exists in an inverse relationship with calcium	Explain to the client that blood will be drawn for this laboratory test. The client is NPO after midnight. Sometimes IV fluids containing glucose are discontinued several hours before the test is done.

KEY ABBREVIATIONS

The following abbreviations and acronyms are used in this chapter:

ABGs	arterial blood gases
ADH	antidiuretic hormone
Ca⁺	calcium ion
Cl⁻	chloride ion
CO₂⁻⁻	carbon dioxide ion
ECF	extracellular fluid
H⁺	hydrogen ion
H₂CO₃	carbonic acid
H₂0	water
HCO₃⁻	bicarbonate ion
ICF	intracellular fluid
K⁺	potassium ion
Na⁺	sodium ion
Mg⁺⁺	magnesium ion
PCO₂ (PaCO₂)	partial pressure of carbon dioxide
pH	potential hydrogen, a scale that measures the acidity of a solution
PO₂ (PaO₂)	partial pressure of oxygen
PO₄⁻⁻	phosphate ion
PPN	peripheral parenteral nutrition
PTH	parathyroid hormone
TPN	total parenteral nutrition

BASIC PHYSIOLOGY OF BODY FLUIDS AND ELECTROLYTES

Fluids (water) and electrolytes are vital to the proper functioning of the body. An understanding of how and why they move in the body is basic to quality nursing care.

Fluid Compartments

Approximately 60 percent of total human body weight is water, which is found in either intracellular compartments or extracellular compartments as shown in Figure 14-1. The majority of body fluid, or 65 percent, is located within cells and is known as intracellular fluid (ICF). The remaining body fluid, or 35 percent, is found outside the cell membranes and is called extracellular fluid (ECF).

ECF is divided into two subclassifications: interstitial fluids and intravascular fluids. Interstitial fluids are found in the spaces around cells. About three-fourths of all ECF is located in these interstitial compartments. Intravascular fluids are composed primarily of blood, plasma, and lymph located in blood and lymph vessels throughout the body. Tears, saliva, sweat, cerebrospinal fluid, digestive secretions, synovial fluid, aqueous humor, perilymph, endolymph, and serous fluid are sometimes classified as specialized extracellular fluids. A constant exchange of water occurs between the intracellular and extracellular compartments to maintain fluid balance.

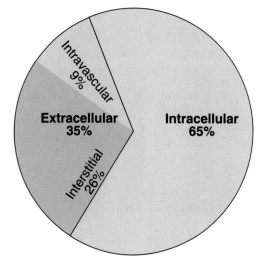

FIGURE 14-1 Body fluid compartments.

Third Spacing

As a result of certain pathological disorders, such as portal hypertension, pancreatitis, complete bowel obstruction, or major abdominal surgery, additional fluid may move into the interstitial space. This is known as third spacing or third space syndrome. The tissue injury increases capillary membrane permeability and allows fluid and protein (albumin) to leave the capillaries and enter the interstitial space. The resulting change in osmotic pressure pulls more fluid from the intravascular space (plasma) into the interstitial space. This causes abdominal distention, sacral edema and a high I&O ratio. With adequate fluid intake, there is a decrease in urine output. This is the objective data that fluid is trapped in the interstitial space.

Treatment for third spacing focuses on infusing adequate isotonic fluids to prevent persistent hypovolemia. The nurse must constantly observe for signs of hypervolemia (jugular vein distention, hypertension, dyspnea, pulmonary edema, and increased urinary output) as the fluid shifts back to the vascular system.

Electrolytes

Electrolytes, or electrically charged elements (ions), are present in both intracellular and extracellular fluids. When dissolved in water, they are either positively charged (cations) or negatively charged (anions). Common cations include hydrogen (H^+), sodium (Na^+), potassium (K^+), calcium (Ca^{++}), and magnesium (Mg^{++}). Common anions are chloride (Cl^-), phosphate (PO_4^{--}) and bicarbonate (HCO_3^-). The number of positive and negative charges must be equal in all fluid compartments for electrolyte balance to be maintained. This is accomplished by the constant movement of ions between the two compartments.

Fluid and Electrolyte Movement

Maintaining a state of homeostasis within the body necessitates the movement of fluids and electrolytes between extracellular and intracellular compartments. Membranes separate the compartments. A **solute** is a substance dissolved in a **solvent**. A solvent is any solution capable of dissolving solutes. Water is the most common solvent within the body. Small molecule solutes pass easily across membranes. Larger molecule solutes, on their own, have a harder time. The four major methods of electrolyte movement are **osmosis**, **diffusion**, **filtration**, and **active transport**.

Osmosis

Osmosis is the movement of water from an area of low solute concentration through a semipermeable or selectively permeable membrane to an area of high solute concentration to equalize the concentrations of salt or other solutes. The number of molecules in water, not their weight, determines the **osmolality** of a solution. Normal blood plasma osmolality, the osmotic pressure of a solution expressed in osmols or milliosmols per kilogram of water, is 275–295 mOsm/kg H_2O. Any solution put into the body with the same osmolality as blood plasma is isotonic. Those with more molecules in solutions are hypertonic. Those with less molecules in solution are hypotonic.

Diffusion

Diffusion is the movement of a solute, such as potassium, from an area of higher concentration to an area of lower concentration until equilibrium is reached. As a result, the concentration of the solute on both sides of the membrane are equal.

Filtration

Filtration occurs when both water and substances move together as a result of hydrostatic pressure (water pressure). This commonly occurs in the body when the pressure in the capillary beds is higher than that in interstitial fluids. Therefore, water, electrolytes, and dissolved substances within the capillaries move out and become interstitial fluids. The reverse also occurs when the pressure in the interstitial spaces is higher than that in capillary beds.

Active Transport

Active transport is the movement of substances across cell membranes with the help of chemical energy and specific carrier molecules. It allows larger molecules to pass through cell membranes. An example of active transport is the binding of insulin to glucose, which facilitates the movement of glucose from blood plasma into cells. Active transport also promotes the movement of molecules from an area of lower concentration to one of higher concentration.

Hormonal Control

The kidneys are the primary organs responsible for controlling fluid and electrolyte balance. They function under the direct influence of a number of hormones and physical processes. The kidneys reabsorb or secrete water and electrolytes based upon hormonal influences. Refer to Chapter 35 for more information on the urinary system.

Antidiuretic hormone (ADH), aldosterone, glucocorticoids, parathyroid hormone, and thyrocalcitonin are hormones that directly influence fluid and/or electrolyte balance.

Antidiuretic Hormone

ADH is secreted by the posterior pituitary gland in response to high blood osmolality. The higher the concentration, the more ADH is released. It signals the renal tubules to increase reabsorption of water. Consequently, urinary output decreases and additional water is added to circulating blood, lowering the osmolality.

Aldosterone

Aldosterone, a mineralocorticoid secreted by the adrenal cortex, plays a role in regulating sodium, potassium, and water balance. It promotes reabsorption of sodium and water and excretion of potassium in the renal tubules.

Glucocorticoids

Glucocorticoids, also secreted by the adrenal cortex, affect water and electrolyte balance. When levels are elevated, as seen in clients with Cushing's disease or those taking corticosteroids, sodium and water retention occurs. Potassium loss also develops.

Parathyroid and Thyroid

Calcium balance is regulated by hormones secreted from the parathyroid and thyroid glands. When the serum level of calcium becomes low, parathyroid hormone (PTH) is released. It increases calcium reabsorption by the renal tubules and increases absorption in the gastrointestinal tract. Calcium is also released from bone cells and put into circulating blood. Thyrocalcitonin, one of the hormones secreted by the thyroid gland, inhibits the release of calcium from bone.

Normal Intake and Output of Body Fluids

In the average adult, approximately 2500 mL of fluid is lost on a daily basis through respiration, perspiration, urination, and defecation. The majority occurs through urination, but about 1000 mL of daily fluid loss is a result of the combined excretory functions of the lungs, skin, and GI tract. About 300 mL is replaced through water taken in when breathing and from metabolic water. To maintain a balance, the rest must be made up by liquids and foods consumed (see Table 14-1). Multiple factors can lead to imbalances (see Table 14-2).

Essential to basic nursing care is the evaluation of client fluid intake and output. This involves recording, or having the client record, fluids consumed and lost. Liquids taken into the body orally, via tube feedings or intravenously, including IV solutions and blood products, are recorded as intake. Urine, emesis, NG suctioning, chest tube drainage, wound drainage and/or

Table 14-1

NORMAL ADULT 24 HOUR FLUID LOSS AND REPLACEMENT			
Fluid Loss (Output)		**Fluid Replacement (Intake)**	
Respiration	300–400 mL	Respiration and Metabolism	200–300 mL
Perspiration	400–500 mL		
Defecation	150–250 mL	Liquids consumed	1000–1600 mL
Urination	1400–1600 mL	Water in foods eaten	700–1200 mL
Total Fluid Loss (Output) and Fluid Replacement (Intake) Should Be Equal			

watery discharge from the lower gastrointestinal tract, i.e., diarrhea or ileostomy drainage, are all calculated when determining output. Accurately recording intake and output is an essential nursing intervention for any client with a potential or real fluid imbalance (see Figure 14-2) Ideally, intake should equal output. A significant difference indicates either a deficit or an excess.

Effects of Age

The very young and the elderly are especially prone to fluid and electrolyte imbalances. Approximately 75 percent of a newborn infant's weight is water. Since the total percentage is so high, even small fluid losses can dramatically affect the balance, causing major complications. As one ages, this percentage decreases. In the elderly, less than 50 percent of their body weight is water. Fat cells contain very little water. Therefore, obese individuals have an even smaller percentage of body weight from water. If a fluid loss occurs, little is available in reserve to make up for the deficit. Renal function deteriorates in the elderly, making regulation of imbalances even more difficult. Consequently, infants and obese elderly clients are especially prone to fluid and electrolyte imbalance.

Effects of Atmospheric Conditions

High atmospheric temperatures affect fluid and electrolyte imbalance. In an effort to stay cool, the body eliminates water and sodium through perspiration. When the humidity is high, the rate of perspiration is greater, yet the cooling effect is less. This is because the air is already saturated, thereby slowing down evaporation of the perspiration. If lost water and sodium are not replaced, imbalances develop.

Table 14-2

FACTORS WHICH LEAD TO FLUID IMBALANCES		
	Fluid Deficit	**Fluid Excess**
Environmental Factors	Exposure to sun or high atmospheric temperatures	
Personal Behaviors	Fasting Fad diets Exercise without adequate fluid replacement	Excessive sodium/water intake Venous compression due to pregnancy

Psychological Influences	Decreased motivation to drink due to
	    Fatigue
	    Depression
	Excessive use of
	    Laxatives
	    Enemas
	    Alcohol
	    Caffeine
		Low protein intake due to anorexia

Therapeutic Modalities	Diarrhea due to infusion of high osmolar tube feedings	Corticosteroid medications Compromised lymphatic drainage secondary to mastectomy

Consequences of Diseases	Fluid losses due to
	    Fever
	    Wound drainage
	    Vomiting
	    Diarrhea
	    Heavy menstrual flow
	    Burns
	Difficulty swallowing due to
	    Oral pain
	    Fatigue
	    Neuromuscular weakness
	Excessive urinary output due to
	    Uncontrolled
	        Diabetes mellitus
	        Diabetes insipidus
		Fluid retention due to
		    Renal failure
		    Cardiac conditions
		    Congestive heart failure
		    Valvular diseases
		    Left ventricular failure
		    Cirrhosis
		    Cancer
		    Impaired venous return

Effects of Exercise

Exercise raises body temperature. When undertaken during periods of high atmospheric temperature and humidity, individuals are even more prone to fluid and electrolyte imbalances.

► FLUID BALANCE

Two conditions may develop as a result of internal changes in fluid balance: **fluid volume deficit** (dehydration) or **fluid volume excess** (overhydration). Each condition is discussed in this section.

► FLUID VOLUME DEFICIT

Fluid volume deficit occurs when an individual has less water than normal in the intracellular, intravascular, or interstitial spaces as a result of either inadequate fluid intake or excessive fluid losses or both.

Environmental factors, personal behaviors, psychological influences, therapeutic modalities, and consequences of diseases can all contribute to the development of fluid volume deficit (see Table 14-2).

3 - 11 Intake					
Hour	Type of fluid	Oral	I.V.	Tube feedings	Other *IVPB*
1800	Coffee	240			
2030	Juice	200			
2230	H₂O	300			
8 Hour Total		740	760	0	100

Total intake= *1600*

3 - 11 Output				
Hour	Urine	Suction	Drains *JP #1*	Other *JP #2*
1630	360			
1945	440			
2230	550			
8 Hour Total	1350		85	120

Total output= *1555*

FIGURE 14-2 Sample I & O sheet.

▶ Medical/Surgical Management

▶ Medical

Medical management is aimed at replacing lost fluids. In mild cases, oral intake may be all that is required for replacement. In more severe cases, intravenous fluid replacement is needed. The type of solution given will depend upon the client's lab results and the cause. Generally, isotonic solutions, such as lactated Ringer's solution, are used. Additional electrolytes may be added based upon individual client need.

▶ Nursing Process

Assessment

Subjective Data Client history often reveals a negative balance between fluid intake and output. Further questioning may elicit information indicating complaints of thirst, nausea, and/or anorexia.

Objective Data Physical symptoms include elevated temperature, pulse and respiratory rates, low blood pressure, dry skin and mucous membranes, decreased skin turgor, slowed capillary refill, sunken eyeballs, and a drawn facial expression. Urinary output is usually decreased, unless excessive urination is the cause of the fluid deficit. Diarrhea may be a contributing cause. Constipation may develop as a consequence of other contributing factors. Weight loss may also occur.

Serum hematocrit, electrolyte and blood urea nitrogen levels elevate due to decreased amounts of intravascular fluid. Urine specific gravity is increased as the kidneys compensate for the deficit by retaining water.

▼ ▼

Possible nursing diagnoses for a client with fluid volume deficit may include:

Nursing Diagnoses	Goals	Nursing Interventions
▶ *Fluid volume deficit related to decreased oral intake.*	The client will increase fluid intake to at least 2000 mL/day. The client will maintain a normal urine specific gravity.	Monitor intake and output. Intake should be at least 2000 mL over a twenty-four hour period. Urine output should be between 1000 and 1500 mL over the twenty-four hour period. Sometimes, urine output is measured each hour. In this case, the client would have a catheter with a drainage bag containing a urometer (Figure 14-3). Teach the client to drink something every hour and teach family members to encourage the client to do so. Provide large glasses or containers of water and liquids within reach to promote cooperation. Use a refractometer to measure the urine specific gravity. Notify the physician immediately when hourly recordings fall below 30 cc/hr for two consecutive hours.
	The client will demonstrate no signs or symptoms of dehydration.	Weigh clients on the same scale, with the same clothes, at the same time of each day since daily weight provides an excellent measure of the effectiveness of fluid replacement. A 5 to 9 percent weight loss indicates a moderate level of dehydration. If a client's weight remains the same or decreases despite fluid replacement, additional fluid is needed. If a client's weight increases dramatically i.e., 5 to 9 percent weight gain, the client may be getting too much fluid and developing fluid volume excess.
▶ *Fluid volume deficit related to abnormal fluid loss.*	The client will verbalize understanding of the cause of abnormal fluid loss and methods to decrease the loss and replace fluids.	Avoid caffeine-containing drinks (coffee, colas, and tea) or other beverages, such as grapefruit juice, since they act as diuretics.
	The client will demonstrate a balance between intake and output.	Monitor intake and output.
	The client will maintain a normal urine specific gravity.	Notify the physician immediately when hourly recordings fall below 30 cc/hr for two consecutive hours.

▶ *Evaluation*

Each goal must be evaluated to determine how it has been met by the client.

▲ ▲

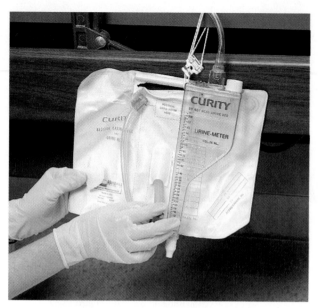

FIGURE 14-3 Hourly urometer.

▶ FLUID VOLUME EXCESS

Fluid volume excess occurs when an individual develops intracellular or interstitial fluid overload as a result of excessive fluid intake or inadequate fluid excretion. Personal behaviors, psychological influences, therapeutic modalities, and consequences of diseases can all contribute to the development of fluid volume excess (see Table 14-2). Usually it is related to the effect of a condition which interferes with the body's ability to remove excess fluid, such as compromised regulatory mechanisms secondary to renal failure. Another example is decreased cardiac output

secondary to congestive heart failure. Occasionally, excessive intake of sodium and/or fluids is the causative factor. Interstitial fluid becomes hypotonic to the cells and the cells increase in size. This could occur if an IV solution were infused at a very rapid rate.

▶ Medical/Surgical Management

▶ Medical

Medical management involves the use of diuretics, such as furosemide (Lasix) or spironolactone (Aldactone) to remove excess fluid along with the treatment of the contributory condition.

▶ Nursing Process

Assessment

Subjective Data Client interview may reveal a previous history of cardiac, renal, or liver disease or a recent consumption of large amounts of water.

Objective Data Physical symptoms include elevated blood pressure, bounding pulse, rapid, labored respirations, crackles, distended neck veins, moist, shiny skin, weight gain and **edema**, an abnormal accumulation of fluid in the interstitial spaces of the body. Confusion and/or coordination problems may be present.

Serum hemoglobin, hematocrit, electrolyte, and blood urea nitrogen levels show a decrease due to dilution of blood plasma. Urinary specific gravity is decreased.

▼ ▼

Possible nursing diagnosis for a client with fluid volume excess may include:

Nursing Diagnoses	Goals	Nursing Interventions
▶ *Fluid volume excess related to a decreased ability to excrete fluids, or to excess intake of sodium and/or water.*	The client will relate causative and contributing factors of fluid volume excess.	Help the client identify the causative and contributing factors of the fluid volume excess.
	The client will demonstrate methods to prevent fluid volume excess.	Teach the client to eat a diet low in sodium and maintain an adequate protein intake. For example, lemon, vinegar, or spices can be used in place of salt and canned or frozen foods should be avoided since they are often high in sodium.
	The client will exhibit a decrease in signs and symptoms of fluid volume excess.	

Nursing Diagnoses	Goals	Nursing Interventions
		Elevate edematous extremities above the level of the heart. If this is not possible, have client place legs on a stool or ottoman when sitting. Discourage client from crossing the legs or ankles.
		Teach client to avoid clothing that constricts blood vessels, such as girdles, garters, and knee-high stockings. Recommend antiembolic stockings.
		If immobility is a problem, instruct client to perform range of motion exercises every four hours to promote fluid return.
		Inspect edematous skin, which is especially prone to injury, on a daily basis for signs of breakdown.

▶ Evaluation

Each goal must be evaluated to determine how it has been met by the client.

▲ ▲

▶ ELECTROLYTE BALANCE

Electrolyte balance is the state of equilibrium between the electrically charged ions within and around cells. It is essential for normal body functioning. Alterations can lead to life-threatening conditions.

SODIUM

Sodium (Na^+) is the major electrolyte in extracellular fluid. It regulates fluid balance through osmotic pressure because water follows sodium in the body. Sodium stimulates conduction of nerve impulses and helps maintain neuromuscular activity. The major source is diet. Excretion occurs primarily via the kidneys. The normal adult serum sodium concentration is between 136 and 145 mEq/L.

▶ HYPONATREMIA

A person with below normal serum sodium level, < 136 mEq/L, has hyponatremia. Possible critical level = < 120 mEq/L. Causes of hyponatremia are a decreased sodium intake, increased sodium loss or increased amounts of body water. A diet low in sodium or the administration of nonelectrolyte IV solutions limits sodium intake. Sodium losses develop as a result of vomiting, nasogastric suctioning, diarrhea, diaphoresis, large open wounds, burns, fistula drainage, massive edema, ascites, kidney and adrenal insufficiency. Increased body water develops when excessive amounts of water are consumed and in clients with diabetes insipidus. Consequently, the serum sodium concentra-

tion is decreased. As serum sodium level decreases, water moves into the cells causing them to swell. When this occurs, potassium moves out of the cells; it is likely that the client will also have a potassium imbalance.

▶ Medical/Surgical Management

▶ Medical

As with all electrolyte deficiencies, treatment is focused on replacement of the abnormally low ion. In mild cases, eating foods and/or drinking fluids high in sodium may be all that is required. In more severe cases, IV administration of fluids containing sodium, such as normal saline (0.9 percent sodium chloride) or lactated Ringer's may be required to restore a normal level.

▶ Nursing Process

Assessment

Subjective Data   Client history may reveal complaints of headache, nausea, abdominal cramps, fatigue, and lack of appetite.

Objective Data   Physical symptoms include elevated body temperature, postural hypotension, muscle weakness, vomiting, confusion, and personality changes. In severe cases or prolonged deficit situations, convulsions and/or coma can develop. Laboratory tests often reveal a serum osmolality between 285 and 295 mOsm/kg and urine specific gravity below 1.010.

▼ ▼

Possible nursing diagnoses for a client with hyponatremia may include:

Nursing Diagnoses	Goals	Nursing Interventions:
▶ Therapeutic regimen, ineffective management of, related to insufficient knowledge of methods to maintain a normal sodium level.	The client will describe methods to increase sodium level.	Teach clients to increase their intake of foods high in sodium, such as corn or potato chips, cheeses, ham, bacon, hot dogs, sausage, and canned soups.
		Limit water intake to no more than 1000 mL per day.
		Give client liquids containing sodium to replace lost fluids.
▶ Fluid volume excess related to excessive intake of hypotonic fluids.	The client will have a serum sodium level within normal limits.	Monitor I&O and lab reports for serum sodium level.

▶ Evaluation

Each goal must be evaluated to determine how it has been met by the client.

▲ ▲

▶ HYPERNATREMIA

A person with an above normal serum sodium level, > 145 mEq/L, has hypernatremia. Possible critical level = > 160 mEq/L. Hypernatremia develops due to increased sodium intake, decreased sodium loss, or excessive water loss. Excessive intake of sodium may be either oral or intravenous. This can occur through eating excessive amounts of foods high in salt or rapidly infusing hypertonic IV solutions.

▶ Medical/Surgical Management

▶ Medical

In mild cases, limiting sodium intake until the serum level returns to normal may be all that is required. In more severe cases, oral intake of pure water or intra-venous administration of a hypotonic solution may be needed. Identification of the causative factors leading to the development of hypernatremia is necessary to prevent further episodes.

▶ Nursing Process

Assessment

Subjective Data   Client history may reveal a recent period of extreme thirst, fatigue, and a diminished urge to urinate.

Objective Data   Physical symptoms include flushed skin, decreased urinary output, dry mouth, fatigue, and increased heart rate. If untreated it can progress to convulsions and coma.

Laboratory tests may reveal the serum osmolality above 295 mOsm/kg and specific gravity above 1.030.

▼ ▼

Possible nursing diagnoses for a client with hypernatremia may include:

Nursing Diagnoses	Goals	Nursing Interventions
▶ *Therapeutic regimen, ineffective management of, related to insufficient knowledge of methods to maintain normal sodium level.*	The client will identify factors that cause hypernatremia.	Teach client to avoid salt, foods high in sodium and processed or canned foods. Preferred foods include fresh fruits, vegetables, chicken, meats, and unsalted grains.
	The client will describe methods to reduce sodium intake and relate an intent to practice health behaviors necessary to maintain a normal sodium level.	Encourage client to drink water. Salt substitutes may be used, unless potassium restriction is advised.
▶ *Fluid volume deficit related to low intake of fluid or high intake of sodium.*	The client willhave a serum sodium level within the normal range.	Monitor I&O and lab reports for serum sodium level.

▶ *Evaluation.*

Each goal must be evaluated to determine how it has been met by the client.

▲ ▲

POTASSIUM

Potassium (K⁺) is the major electrolyte in intracellular fluid. Its concentration inside cells is about 150 mEq/L, while its concentration in the blood serum is less than 5 mEq/L. Consequently, slight changes can dramatically affect body functioning. Potassium maintains normal nerve and muscle activity, especially the heart, and osmotic pressure within body cells. Potassium is mainly excreted by the kidneys. The kidneys prefer to retain sodium and excrete potassium even when both electrolytes are depleted. Potassium assists in the cellular metabolism of carbohydrates and proteins. Sodium and hydrogen ions move into the cells when potassium moves out. This aids in regulating acid-base balance. The normal adult serum potassium level is between 3.5 to 5.0 mEq/L.

HYPOKALEMIA

A person with a below normal serum potassium level, less than 3.5 mEq/L, has hypokalemia. Possible critical level = < 2.5 mEq/L. Causes of hypokalemia are decreased potassium intake, increased potassium loss or a shift into the cells. A diet low in potassium and the administration of nonpotassium containing IV solutions leads to decreased intake. Excessive loss develops as a consequence of diarrhea, vomiting, fistula drainage, NG suctioning, cellular loss from trauma or burns, use of potassium-losing diuretics (such as furosemide [Lasix] or chlorothiazide [Diuril]), Cushing's syndrome, or large doses of corticosteroids. Clients who are taking digitalis for cardiac arrhythmias must be carefully monitored since hypokalemia can potentiate digitalis toxicity. A potassium shift to the intracellular compartment may be a consequence of IV administration of insulin, glucose, and calcium.

▶ Medical/Surgical Management

▶ Medical

Mild cases are treated with a diet high in potassium rich foods and/or oral potassium supplements, such as potassium chloride (Micro-K, K-Dur or Slow-K). More severe cases require intravenous administration of potassium.

▶ Nursing Process

Assessment

Subjective Data   Client history may reveal feelings of being tired all the time and a lack of appetite.

Objective Data   Objective data includes muscle weakness, cardiac arrhythmias, leg cramps, nausea, and vomiting. Physical symptoms may develop when potassium level falls below 3.0 mEq/L. As the level continues to fall, blood pressure drops, flaccid paralysis develops, and cardiac and respiratory arrest are eminent.

An electrocardiogram (ECG) may show a U wave and/or ventricular dysrhythmias. (Refer to Chapter 20, Cardiac Disorders).

▼ ▼

Possible nursing diagnoses for a client with hypokalemia may include:

Nursing Diagnoses	Goals	Nursing Interventions
▶ Therapeutic regimen, ineffective management of, related to insufficient knowledge of methods to maintain normal potassium levels.	The client will describe methods to promote potassium intake.	Encourage clients to eat more foods high in potassium (fruits, especially bananas and oranges, and vegetables). If a potassium supplement is prescribed, it should be taken with a full glass of water or juice and sipped slowly to avoid GI irritation.
	The client will have a serum potassium level within the normal range.	Monitor lab reports for serum potassium level.
▶ Activity, intolerance, related to muscle weakness.	The client will increase activity as potassium level increases.	Assist client with ROM exercises. Assist client to ambulate as strength returns.
▶ Injury, high risk for, related to use of IV potassium.	The client will not be injured by use of IV potassium.	If potassium is added to IV solutions, administer it no faster than 20 mEq/hour. In some severe incidences, it may be ordered at a faster rate for a short period. When this is the case, the largest possible vein should be used to facilitate adequate dilution and prevent damage to the lumen of the vessel.
		Carefully monitor the client's heart rate for the development of tachycardia and abnormal rhythms.
		Since potassium is caustic to tissues, the IV site needs to be carefully monitored for early signs of infiltration.

▶ Evaluation

Each goal must be evaluated to determine how it has been met by the client.

▲ ▲

▶ HYPERKALEMIA

A person with a higher than normal serum potassium level, above 5.0 mEq/L, has hyperkalemia. Possible critical level is > 6.5 mEq/L. Causes of a high level are the results of metabolic disease states or excessive potassium intake. Clients with renal disease develop hyperkalemia because potassium cannot be excreted adequately by the kidney. Extensive trauma also leads to hyperkalemia, as the potassium is released from the cells and enters the bloodstream. An elevated level also occurs in clients with decreased adrenal function, i.e., Addison's disease. Ingestion of large amounts of potassium-rich foods or salt substitutes, overuse of potassium supplements, or rapid administration of IV solutions containing potassium all lead to hyperkalemia. Hyperkalemia is a much more critical situation than hypokalemia.

▶ Medical/Surgical Management

▶ Medical

In mild cases, oral supplements are discontinued and potassium-rich foods are eliminated from the diet until the level returns to normal. In severe cases, IV calcium may be prescribed to block cardiac effects. IV insulin and glucose or sodium bicarbonate may be given to force potassium back into cells. Sodium polystyrene sulfonate (Kayexalate) may be prescribed to force excretion of potassium. It is administered orally or in the form of an enema.

▶ Nursing Process

Assessment

Subjective Data   Client history reveals a diminished urge to urinate and feelings of anxiety, nausea, abdominal cramps, numbness, and tingling.

Objective Data   Physical symptoms include irregular pulse rate, muscle weakness and irritability, vomiting, decreased urinary output, and cardiac arrhythmias.

An ECG may reveal a widening of the QRS complex, peaked T wave and lower than normal P wave, usually after the potassium level exceeds 7.0 mEq/L and cardiac and respiratory arrest are eminent if the condition is not quickly corrected.

▼ ▼

Possible nursing diagnoses for a client with hyperkalemia may include:

Nursing Diagnoses	Goals	Nursing Interventions
▶ *Therapeutic regimen, ineffective management of, related to insufficient knowledge of methods to maintain a normal serum potassium level.*	The client will describe methods to reduce potassium intake. The client will have a normal serum potassium level.	Teach clients to avoid foods high in potassium, potassium supplements, and salt substitutes containing potassium. Encourage range of motion exercises to improve muscle tone and reduce cramps. Monitor intake and output and lab reports for serum potassium level.
▶ *Injury, high risk for, related to muscle weakness (heart).*	The client will not be injured by a weak heart muscle.	Give medications as ordered. Monitor vital signs frequently.

▶ Evaluation

Each goal must be evaluated to determine how it has been met by the client.

▲ ▲

Sample Nursing Care Plan: The Client with Cushing Syndrome Due to Long-term Use of Corticosteroids

Mrs. Fitzpatrick is a twenty-eight-year-old woman who was diagnosed with Crohn's Disease ten years ago. Since that time, she has been taking 10 mg of prednisone twice a day. Due to the long-term use of this corticosteroid medication, she has developed many of the signs and symptoms of Cushing's Syndrome, i.e., weight gain, elevated blood pressure, moon face, muscle weakness, elevated blood pressure and edema. Her lab tests show a serum sodium level of 150 mEq/L and a serum potassium level of 3.0 mEq/L. She has requested assistance from the nurse on dealing with the effects of fluid retention and muscle weakness which have resulted from her long-term use of corticosteroids.

Nursing Diagnosis 1: Fluid volume excess related to sodium and water retention as evidenced by elevated blood pressure, weight gain, edema, and hypernatremia.

Goals	Nursing Interventions	Rationale	Evaluation
Mrs. Fitzpatrick will exhibit a decrease in signs and symptoms of fluid excess within one week.	Assess dietary intake that may contribute to fluid retention, i.e., amount of fluid and salt intake.	Liquids consumed and foods eaten affect fluid retention.	Mrs. Fitzpatrick has demonstrated a decrease in the signs and symptoms of fluid retention. Her blood pressure is now in the 135–140/75–80 range. She has lost seven pounds in the past week and the edema in her legs has decreased. She was observed sitting with her legs in a dependent position and when reminded to keep them elevated whenever possible, she responded, "I'll have to work on remembering to do that more consistently."
	Weigh client daily at the same time, wearing similar clothing and using the same scale.	Daily weight provides a basis for monitoring the effectiveness of nursing interventions.	
	Teach client to restrict fluid intake.	Restricting fluids prevents fluid retention.	
	Teach client and family methods to reduce sodium intake, i.e., do not add salt to foods, substitute spices, such as lemon, mint, basil, vinegar, and so on, check labels for sodium content and avoid canned and frozen foods.	Reducing sodium intake reduces fluid retention.	
	Teach client and family methods to promote blood return to the heart, i.e , elevate legs on a stool or ottoman when sitting, avoid crossing legs or ankles, avoid restricting clothing, such as knee-high socks and recommend wearing antiembolic stockings.	Elevating legs above the level of the heart and avoiding restricting garments enhance blood return.	

| | Teach client and family to check skin on a daily basis for any signs of breakdown and report any abnormal findings to physician. | Detecting signs of skin breakdown in the early stages allows for institution of treatment before the condition becomes severe. | |

Nursing Diagnosis 2: Knowledge deficit (foods high in potassium) related to lack of exposure as evidenced by request for information.

Goals	Nursing Interventions	Rationale	Evaluation
Mrs. Fitzpatrick will verbalize an understanding of foods high in potassium and methods to incorporate them in her diet.	Assess client's prior knowledge of foods high in potassium. Assess client's dietary habits and food likes and dislikes. Teach client and family the foods high in potassium, such as oranges, raisins, bananas, apricots, avocados, potatoes, and beans. Encourage client to develop methods to incorporate foods high in potassium in her regular eating routine.	Assessing prior knowledge establishes a basis for identifying needed teaching. Assessing regular eating habits and likes and dislikes provides a foundation for incorporating dietary changes. Knowing which foods are high in potassium will increase their use in meals and snacks. Development of a plan to incorporate dietary changes enhances behavioral changes.	Mrs. Fitzpatrick related an understanding of the methods to add foods high in potassium to her diet and now eats at least two foods high in potassium each day.

CALCIUM

Calcium (Ca^{++}) plays an essential role in bone and teeth integrity, blood clotting, smooth, skeletal and cardiac muscle functioning, and nerve impulse transmission. Vitamin D is required for absorption of calcium in the GI tract. Most calcium in the body is located in bone and teeth tissue. Only about 1 percent is found in serum. In blood, it is found both in an ionized form and bound to albumin. Normal adult ionized serum calcium level is between 4.5 and 5.6 mEq/L. Total serum calcium concentration is a measurement of both the ionized concentration and the calcium bound to albumin. The normal adult level ranges between 9.0 and 10.5 mg/dL. For the elderly, values may be slightly less.

▶ HYPOCALCEMIA

A person with a total serum calcium concentration < 9.0 mg/dL or an ionized serum calcium level < 4.5 mEq/L has hypocalcemia. Possible critical value = < 6 mg/dL and is related to tetany. Along with an inadequate intake of dietary calcium and vitamin D, a variety of pathological conditions can lead to hypocalcemia. These include hypoparathyroidism, renal failure, malabsorption, administration of large amounts of citrated blood, alkalosis, and acute pancreatitis.

▶ *Medical/Surgical Management*

▶ *Medical*

Treatment involves oral supplements of calcium and vitamin D. Vitamin D is needed to promote absorption of calcium in the GI tract. For more acute conditions, intravenous administration of calcium gluconate is required.

▶ *Nursing Process*

Assessment

Subjective Data   Client history often reveals previous pathological fractures, a diagnosis of osteoporosis, tingling or numbness of extremities or around the mouth, muscle cramping, or nausea.

Objective Data   Physical symptoms include carpopedal spasms, vomiting, and diarrhea. In severe cases, laryngeal spasms which can lead to airway obstruction, seizures, bleeding, and cardiac arrhythmias develop. Two classic tests for hypocalcemia are positive Chvostek's sign and Trousseau's sign. To perform the Chvostek's test, gently tap the facial nerve just in front of the earlobe below the zygomatic process. In clients with low calcium levels, this results in immediate spasms of the cheek muscles. Trousseau's sign involves decreasing the blood flow to the nerves of the hand. It may be done by constricting the wrist or by inflating a blood pressure cuff on the upper arm. Carpal spasms indicate a positive Trousseau's sign.

The serum albumin level should be measured for clients with hypocalcemia since a low serum albumin level causes the total serum calcium concentration level to be low also.

▼ ▼

Possible nursing diagnoses for a client with hypocalcemia may include:

Nursing Diagnoses	Goals	Nursing Interventions
▶ *Therapeutic regimen, ineffective management of, related to insufficient knowledge of methods to maintain normal calcium levels.*	The client will describe methods to promote calcium intake.	Encourage clients to take calcium supplements, as ordered by the physician, and to increase their dietary intake of calcium-rich foods. These include milk, cheeses, yogurt, broccoli, spinach, breads, and juices.
	The client will have a serum calcium level within normal limits.	Monitor calcium intake and lab reports for serum calcium level.
▶ *Injury, high risk for, related to possibility of hypocalcemic tetany.*	The client will not be injured because of hypocalcemic tetany.	Monitor client for muscle cramps, twitching of the muscles, and convulsions.

▶ *Evaluation*

Each goal must be evaluated to determine how it was been met by the client.

▲ ▲

▶ HYPERCALCEMIA

A person with a total serum calcium level > 10.5 mg/dL or ionized serum calcium level > 5.6 mEq/L has hypercalcemia. Possible critical value = Total serum calcium level > 14 mg/dL with normal serum albumin level. Generally, three separate determinations are made before a diagnosis of hypercalcemia is made. Often hypercalcemia is a symptom of an underlying disease. A number of conditions, such as metastatic bone tumors, Paget's disease, acromegaly, and hyperparathyroidism, increase bone reabsorption and thereby foster the release of calcium into circulating blood. Increased calcium absorption may be caused by increased levels of vitamin D and parathyroid hormone. Excess dietary intake or use of calcium-containing antacids may also cause hypercalcemia.

▶ Medical/Surgical Management

▶ Medical

Mild cases are treated by encouraging fluid intake and limiting calcium intake. In severe cases, calcitonin is used to promote a calcium shift from serum into bone tissue. IV fluids and furosemide (Lasix) may be ordered to facilitate excretion of circulating calcium. Thiazide diuretics, such as hydrochlorothiazide (Hydro DIURIL), are never used with hypercalcemia because they make the condition worse.

▶ Nursing Process

Assessment

Subjective Data Client history may reveal a lack of appetite, constipation, bone pain, nausea, thirst, and lethargy.

Objective Data Physical symptoms include vomiting, decreased muscle tone, polyuria, lethargy, irritability, confusion, and pathological fractures. Long-term immobility may be a contributing factor. If the condition persists for a period of time, renal stones may develop.

▼ ▼

Possible nursing diagnoses for a client with hypercalcemia may include:

Nursing Diagnoses	Goals	Nursing Interventions
▶ Therapeutic regimen, ineffective management of, related to insufficient knowledge of methods to maintain normal calcium levels.	The client will describe methods to reduce calcium intake.	Encourage clients to drink 3000 to 4000 mL of fluids per day to dilute serum calcium concentration.
	The client will have a normal serum calcium level.	Monitor intake and output and lab reports for serum calcium level.
▶ Physical mobility, impaired, related to pathological fractures.	The client will maintain mobility.	Teach client to avoid any sudden movements and to use assistive devices, such as a cane or a walker.
▶ Injury, high risk for, related to renal stone formation.	The client will not have renal stone formation.	Teach client to avoid foods high in calcium and to have daily physical activity.
		Encourage client to drink plenty of fluids.
		Monitor I&O.

▶ Evaluation

Each goal must be evaluated to determine how it has been met by the client.

▲ ▲

MAGNESIUM

Most magnesium (Mg^{++}) is found in intracellular fluid and in bone, muscle and soft tissue combined with calcium and phosphorus. Blood serum contains only about 1 percent. Magnesium activates enzymes that are catalysts for reactions between phosphate ions and ATP. It is associated with body temperature regulation, neuromuscular contractions, and synthesis of protein. Magnesium is excreted primarily by the kidneys. If a magnesium deficiency develops, the body will conserve magnesium at the expense of excreting potassium.

There is a close relationship between magnesium, calcium, and potassium. All are found in intracellular fluids. Low level of one results in low levels of the others. Normal adult serum magnesium concentration ranges between 1.5 and 2.5 mEq/L.

▶ HYPOMAGNESEMIA

A person with a serum magnesium level < 1.2 mEq/L has hypomagnesemia. Possible critical level = < 0.5 mEq/L. The critical level seldom happens because of the supply available from bone and the kidney's ability to conserve magnesium. It may occur secondarily with other conditions. A decreased magnesium level occurs in clients with alcoholism, hypoparathyroidism, prolonged malnutrition, malabsorption, and hyperaldosteronism. Heavy use of diuretics, aminoglycosides (gentamicin sulfate [Garamycin]), cyclosporin (Sandimmune) and cisplatin (Platinol) may cause hypomagnesemia.

▶ Medical/Surgical Management

▶ Medical

Treatment involves promotion of foods high in magnesium, such as fish, seafood, meats, green vegetables, and whole grains. Oral magnesium salts may cause diarrhea. In severe cases, intravenous administration of magnesium sulfate may be required. Since a low magnesium level often coexists with low calcium and potassium levels, management is often focused on replacement of multiple electrolytes. Clients taking

digitalis must also be monitored for digitalis toxicity that develops with hypomagnesemia.

▶ Nursing Process

Assessment

Subjective Data   Client history may reveal a history of alcohol abuse, ulcerative colitis, a recent episode of diarrhea, paresthesia, muscle cramps, the use of loop diuretics, (furosemide [Lasix]), or aminoglycoside antibiotics, (gentamicin sulfate [Garamycin] or tobramycin sulfate [Nebcin]).

Objective Data   Physical symptoms include facial tics, tremors, ataxia, hypotension, confusion, tetany, and convulsions. Chvostek's sign and Trousseau's sign are both positive.

Laboratory tests often reveal low serum calcium and potassium levels also. ECG may reveal tachycardia and cardiac arrhythmias.

▼ ▼

Possible nursing diagnoses for a client with hypomagnesemia may include:

Nursing Diagnoses	Goals	Nursing Interventions
▶ *Therapeutic regimen, ineffective management of, related to insufficient knowledge of methods to maintain normal magnesium levels.*	The client will describe methods to promote magnesium intake.	Teach client foods high in magnesium, such as fish, seafood, green vegetables, and whole grains.
	The client will have a serum magnesium level within normal limits.	Monitor lab reports for serum magnesium level.
▶ *Injury, high risk for, related to IV magnesium replacement.*	The client will not be injured by IV magnesium replacement.	Observe client closely for signs of neuromuscular irritability and cardiac arrhythmias.
		When IV magnesium sulfate is being administered, carefully monitor the client for a sudden drop in blood pressure, slowed respirations (less than 12 per minute), weak deep-tendon reflexes, and urine output of less than 30 cc/hr.
		Monitor for digitalis toxicity, i.e., vomiting, headache, heartbeat abnormalities, and visual color distortions.

▶ Evaluation

Each goal must be evaluated to determine how it has been met by the client.

▲ ▲

▶ HYPERMAGNESEMIA

A person with a serum magnesium level > 2.5 mEq/L has hypermagnesemia. Possible critical level = > 3.0 mEq/L. Hypermagnesemia rarely occurs if kidney function is normal. Increased magnesium levels are associated with ingestion of magnesium antacids (Maalox, Mylanta) or laxatives (milk of magnesia [MOM], magnesium citrate [Citroma]), hypothyroidism, uncontrolled diabetes mellitus (ketoacidosis), Addison's disease, and renal failure.

▶ Medical/Surgical Management

▶ Medical

Treatment involves decreasing magnesium intake, increasing fluid intake, and promoting urine excretion.

Diuretics are often used. In severe cases, hemodialysis may be necessary to restore a normal magnesium level.

▶ Nursing Process

Assessment

Subjective Data Client history may reveal the overuse of magnesium-containing antacids or laxatives or renal failure. Often client verbalizes feeling tired most of the time, being thirsty, and nauseated.

Objective Data Physical symptoms include decreased blood pressure and respirations, vasodilation, flushing, cardiac arrhythmias, and weak or absent deep-tendon reflexes. Hypermagnesemia may progress to coma and cardiac arrest.

Assess lab tests for high calcium and potassium levels. Peaked T waves may be present on ECG.

▼ ▼

Possible nursing diagnoses for a client with hypermagnesemia may include:

Nursing Diagnoses	Goals	Nursing Interventions
▶ Therapeutic regimen, ineffective management of, related to elevated magnesium level.	The client will have a serum magnesium level within the normal range.	Monitor lab reports for serum magnesium level.
	The client will describe methods to reduce magnesium intake.	Teach clients with hypermagnesemia to avoid magnesium antacids and laxatives.
▶ Injury, high risk for, related to alteration in neuromuscular functioning.	The client will not be injured because of high magnesium level.	Monitor client's vital signs, deep-tendon reflexes and I&O. Report to the physician a decrease in these signs. This may indicate impending development of cardiac arrhythmias.
		Promote urine excretion and administer diuretics as ordered.

Evaluation

Each goal must be evaluated to determine how it has been met by the client.

▲ ▲

CHLORIDE

Chloride (Cl^-) is a major electrolyte in extracellular fluids. It functions in combination with sodium to maintain osmotic pressure and is found most commonly combined with sodium as a salt. Therefore, when the sodium level is low, so is the chloride level. The reverse is also true. The main route of excretion is through the kidneys.

Chloride also assists in maintaining acid-base balance. When the carbon dioxide level increases, bicar-

bonate shifts from the intracellular compartment to the extracellular compartment. Chloride, in an effort to maintain hemostasis, moves into the intracellular compartment. The kidneys selectively excrete chloride or bicarbonate ions depending on the acid-base balance.

Normal adult serum chloride level ranges between 100 and 110 mEq/L. Since hypochloremia and hyperchloremia are so closely associated with sodium imbalances, the causes and symptoms are similar. They are rarely considered, except as part of a larger electrolyte problem.

PHOSPHATE

Phosphate (PO_4^{--}) is an intracellular electrolyte. The majority is found in bone and teeth, with some in muscle and nerve tissue. There is a close relationship between phosphate and calcium. It exists in an inverse relationship. As one increases the other decreases. Phosphate level is regulated by calcium level, parathyroid hormone, and intestinal absorption. Normal adult serum phosphate level ranges between 1.8 and 2.6 mEq/L. Clients with a lower level have hypophosphatemia. Clients with a higher level have hyperphosphatemia. The phosphate level is always evaluated in relationship to the calcium level to have a better idea of what is happening.

Hypophosphatemia occurs in clients who have hyperparathyroidism, hypercalcemia, severe burns, chronic alcoholism, malabsorption, or starvation. It can also develop during the treatment phase of severe protein-calorie malnutrition due to the overuse of simple carbohydrates.

Assessment data includes irritability, apprehension, muscle weakness, numbness, confusion, seizures, and coma. Changes in white blood cells may result in the development of infections. Treatment focuses on replacing the deficit magnesium.

Carefully assess clients at risk for developing hypophosphatemia for possible signs and symptoms. Clients and family members should be taught the importance of handwashing and other methods of preventing infection.

Hyperphosphatemia develops primarily in clients with renal failure. It may occur in cancer clients receiving chemotherapy or individuals with a high magnesium intake.

Symptoms of an elevated serum phosphate level are associated with the consequential low serum calcium levels (See hypocalcemia). Treatment focuses on correcting the causative disorder.

Teach clients to avoid phosphate-containing antacids or laxatives and foods high in phosphorous, such as dairy products, kidneys, sardines, sweetbreads, whole grains, nuts, dried fruits, vegetables, and many soft drinks. Instruct to watch for the signs and symptoms of hypocalcemia.

NURSING CARE OF CLIENTS RECEIVING FLUID AND ELECTROLYTE REPLACEMENTS

Fluids and electrolytes may be replaced orally, via tube feedings, through the administration of intravenous solutions or by total parenteral nutrition.

Oral Fluid and Electrolyte Replacement

Oral replacement is the preferred route for conscious clients who have normally functioning gastrointestinal and urinary systems and who are not experiencing nausea, vomiting, or severe electrolyte losses.

Clients requiring additional fluids are placed on an encourage fluids regimen which promotes the intake of between 1500 and 3000 mL of fluids per day. Those requiring specific electrolyte replacements are taught about dietary sources or given oral supplements. A number of products, such as Gatorade® and Pedialyte®, are specifically designed to replace water and electrolytes.

Tube Feedings

Tube feeding may be the preferred method of replacing fluids, nutrients, and electrolytes for clients who are unable to eat due to oral or upper GI tract surgery or neurological conditions that interfere with swallowing, such as strokes or myasthenia gravis. Most tube-feeding formulas are isotonic and easily tolerated. If additional electrolytes are necessary, they may be added to the enteral feedings.

A client receiving tube feedings should be weighed daily. Tube maintenance includes regular instillation of water, at least 30 to 50 mL every four to eight hours, to assure patency of the tube. The length of the tube exiting the body and placement of the tube should be checked each shift. A client with a tracheostomy often has tube feedings also. This individual is especially prone to fluid loss through breathing. Additional water should be instilled on a regular basis, as ordered by the physician.

Standard Intravenous Solutions

A variety of standard intravenous solutions are currently available. Some physicians prefer to use basic solutions like 5 percent dextrose in water (D5W), normal saline or 5 percent dextrose and half strength normal saline in water (D5½NS) and then have individualized electrolyte replacement added for their clients. Other physicians utilize prepared standardized dextrose, electrolyte, and water solutions. Ringer's lactate is an example of such a solution.

Regardless of the type of solution being administered, the nurse must carefully assess the client for signs of fluid deficit or excess. Even though a client is receiving IV solutions, the daily amount may be inadequate. On the other hand, if the solution is infused too fast, the client may develop fluid overload.

Total Parenteral Nutrition

Parenteral nutrition is used for a client with a dysfunctional or nonfunctional GI system. Total parenteral nutrition (TPN) or hyperalimentation is a method of intravenously administering formulas of glucose, amino acids, electrolytes, minerals, vitamins, and water. Fats are included as a supplement to the formula and given separately through a y-connection. Solutions with less concentrated formulas can be administered via a peripheral vein. This is called peripheral parenteral nutrition (PPN). Higher concentrations are extremely irritating to veins. Since most TPN solutions are highly concentrated formulas, a central venous line is commonly used. PPN may be administered to clients in combination with oral intake or tube feedings, depending upon client needs. Daily weight and regular assessment of the IV site, and assessment for signs of fluid, electrolyte, and acid-base imbalances are essential components of nursing care.

BASIC PHYSIOLOGY OF ACID-BASE BALANCE

Maintenance of the acid-base balance is essential to ensure homeostasis within the body. Hydrogen ion concentration regulates the acidity of body fluids. **pH** is the mathematical measurement of hydrogen ion concentration in solution. An increased concentration of hydrogen ions make fluids more acidic, while a decreased concentration make them more alkaline. The normal range of pH for body fluids is between 7.35 and 7.45. When values fall below 7.35, **acidosis** develops. When values rise above 7.45, **alkalosis** develops (see Table 14-3). Arterial blood gases (ABGs) are used to measure acid-base balance (see Table 14-4). Numerous conditions and diseases can alter acid-base balance. The ramifications are often more devastating than the contributing cause.

Acid-base Regulatory Mechanism

Acid-base balance is regulated by chemical **buffer systems**, the lungs and the kidneys. Tests used and normal values are:

PCO_2 = 40 mmHg
pH = 7.35–7.45
Bicarbonate (HCO_3) = 24 mEq
Carbonic Acid (H_2CO_3) = 3% of PCO_2 or 3% x 40 = 1.2 mEq

Chemical Buffer Systems

Chemical buffers in the blood are the most rapid feedback mechanism for correcting alterations in extracellular fluid pH. The chemical buffers work within a fraction of a second to prevent excessive changes in the hydrogen ion concentration. They function by either removing or releasing hydrogen ions to restore balance. The major chemical buffer system is the bicarbonate (HCO_3^-) - carbonic acid (H_2CO_3) system. Carbonic acid is measured indirectly by PCO_2. It is always 3 percent of PCO_2. Bicarbonate level is measured by serum bicarbonate. Twenty parts of bicarbonate is necessary for each one part of carbonic acid to maintain a normal pH (see Figure 14-4). There are three other buffer systems: phosphate, protein, and hemoglobin, but these are not measured in evaluating acid-base balance. The kidneys regulate the number of bicarbonate ions and the lungs regulate the amount of carbon dioxide (CO_2).

Lungs

Carbonic acid (H_2CO_3) is broken down into carbon dioxide (CO_2) and water (H_2O). The lungs, under the control of the nervous system, regulate the amount of CO_2 circulating in the blood by speeding up or slowing down respirations. When the concentration of hydrogen is high, the rate and depth of respirations increase in an effort to remove the excess quantity of

Table 14-3

pH LEVELS & EFFECTS ON ACID-BASE BALANCE		
pH		**H⁺ Concentration**
7.8	Death	Fatally Low
	Alkalosis	Abnormally Low
7.45–7.35	Acid-Base Balance	Within Normal Range
	Acidosis	Abnormally High
7.0	Death	Fatally High

Table 14-4

ARTERIAL BLOOD GASES		
	Normal Adult Values	**Critical Values**
pH	7.35–7.45	< 7.2 or > 7.6
PCO_2	35–45 mmHg	< 20 or > 70 mmHg
PO_2	80–105 mmHg	< 40 mmHg
HCO_3^-	22–26 mEq/L	< 10 or > 40 mEq/L
O_2 Saturation	95%–100%	< 75%
Base Excess	–2 to +2	< –3 or > +3

Bicarbonate-carbonic acid buffer system

$$H_2O + CO_2 \rightleftharpoons H_2CO_3 \rightleftharpoons H^+ + HCO_3^-$$
(lungs)   (kidneys)

FIGURE 14-4 Bicarbonate-carbonic acid buffer system.

CO_2, thereby restoring normal hydrogen ion concentration. When the hydrogen ion concentration is low, respirations slow down to retain CO_2.

Kidneys

The kidneys are the slowest but the most effective mechanism for adjusting acid-base balance. They either increase retention or excretion of hydrogen (H^+) and bicarbonate ions (HCO_3^-) to restore balance.

▶ ACIDOSIS

Acidosis develops when there is an excess accumulation of acid or a decreased amount of alkali in body fluids. It may be either metabolic or respiratory.

▶ METABOLIC ACIDOSIS

Metabolic acidosis results from retaining too much acid (H^+) or by losing too much bicarbonate (HCO_3^-). Conditions that can lead to metabolic acidosis include diabetics experiencing insulin deficiency, lactic acid accumulation from cardiac arrest, renal failure, salicylate poisoning, diarrhea, dehydration, shock, and starvation. Untreated it results in coma and death.

▶ Medical/Surgical Management

▶ Medical

Treatment depends upon identifying the underlying causes and correcting them. For example, if the condition is due to lack of insulin, as in the case of diabetic metabolic acidosis, insulin is given. If the condition is due to renal failure, dialysis may be required. Administration of sodium bicarbonate, either orally in mild cases or intravenously in more severe cases, promotes restoration of normal acid-base balance. Lost fluids and electrolytes need to be replaced.

▶ Nursing Process

Assessment

Subjective Data   Client history may reveal a lack of appetite, headache, nausea, and abdominal pain.

Objective Data   Respirations increase in depth and rate (Kussmaul's respirations) in an effort to blow off CO_2. Hypotension and an abnormal heart rate develops. The skin becomes cold and clammy. Vomiting may occur. Neuromuscular weakness and irritability develop due to the exchange of hydrogen ions for the potassium ions within the cells. CNS symptoms such as disorientation, confusion, and coma may develop.

Laboratory tests reveal arterial blood gases with a pH below 7.35, bicarbonate level below 22 mEq and a PCO_2 less than 35 mmHg. The serum potassium level often exceeds 5 mEq/L and the chloride level is elevated.

▼ ▼

Possible nursing diagnoses for a client with metabolic acidosis may include:

Nursing Diagnoses	Goals	Nursing Interventions
▶ *Injury, high risk for, related to change in level of consciousness.*	The client will demonstrate behaviors to reduce risk factors and protect self from injury.	Assess level of consciousness frequently. If weakness and/or confusion is present, monitor client closely. Keep side rails up.
▶ *Fluid volume deficit, high risk for, related to excess loss of fluids.*	The client will verbalize an understanding of causative factors to reduce risk of volume deficit.	Provide good oral care frequently for client comfort. Administer IV fluids, as ordered, to replace lost fluids and electrolytes. Rapid administration of sodium bicarbonate puts clients at risk for rebound alkalosis, hypokalemia, and hypocalcemia. Carefully assess the client for early signs of the development of these conditions. Monitor ABGs and electrolyte values to determine the effectiveness of therapy.

(continued)

▶ Evaluation

Each goal must be evaluated to determine how it has been met by the client.

▲ ▲

▶ *RESPIRATORY ACIDOSIS*

Respiratory acidosis is the result of an increase in carbonic acid due to the failure of the lungs to adequately eliminate CO_2. It may be either acute or chronic. Acute respiratory acidosis may be caused by a variety of respiratory disorders, such as pneumonia, acute bronchial asthma, atelectasis, pulmonary edema, or as a consequence of conditions that slow down normal breathing, such as prolonged effects of anesthesia, head injuries, drowning, or drug overdose. Chronic respiratory acidosis is a result of long-term respiratory conditions, such as chronic obstructive pulmonary disease, emphysema, bronchial asthma, and cystic fibrosis.

▶ *Medical/Surgical Management*

▶ *Medical*

Treatment will depend upon the cause and whether the condition is acute or chronic. Bronchodilators and oxygen may help improve the causative respiratory conditions. Antibiotics are given if pneumonia develops. If breathing does not improve, mechanical ventilation may be required.

▶ *Nursing Process*

Assessment

Subjective Data   Client history may reveal recent breathing problems, lethargy, an occipital headache, and restlessness. Symptoms of chronic respiratory acidosis are more subtle, such as a dull headache and weakness.

Objective Data   Physical symptoms of acute respiratory acidosis include difficulty breathing and decreased respirations. Cardiovascular symptoms develop, i.e., tachycardia, dysrhythmias, hypertension, and a flush face. Neuromuscular effects include muscle twitching and weakness. Respiratory acidosis leads to CNS symptoms such as disorientation, confusion, and coma.

In acute respiratory acidosis, arterial blood gases show a pH less than 7.35 and a PCO_2 above 45 mmHg. With chronic respiratory acidosis, pH may be normal or slightly below normal with an increased PCO_2. Bicarbonate (HCO_3^-) remains normal until the kidneys have time to compensate. Serum potassium will be elevated above 5 mEq/L.

▼ ▼

Possible nursing diagnoses for a client with respiratory acidosis may include:

Nursing Diagnoses	Goals	Nursing Interventions
▶ *Breathing pattern, ineffective, related to hypoventilation.*	The client will regain effective breathing pattern.	Elevate the head of the bed. Teach and encourage the client to take deep breaths and prolong the expiratory phase. Encourage clients to cough up mucus.
▶ *Injury, high risk for, related to use of oxygen or sedatives for chronic obstructive disease.*	The client will demonstrate behaviors to reduce risk of potential injury.	Ensure adequate hydration to help liquefy the secretions. Suctioning may be necessary for some clients. Teach client and family safety measures that must be followed when oxygen is in use.

▶ Evaluation

Each goal must be evaluated to determine how it has been met by the client.

▲ ▲

▶ *ALKALOSIS*

Alkalosis occurs when there is excess accumulation of alkali or loss of acid in body fluids. It may be either metabolic or respiratory.

▶ *METABOLIC ALKALOSIS*

Metabolic alkalosis results from an increase in bicarbonate or a decrease in hydrogen ion concentration. The bicarbonate level increases when excessive amounts are taken in, such as in the form of baking soda to relieve gastric upset or via IV solutions. The level also elevates when hydrogen and chloride ions are removed from extracellular fluids. This occurs as a consequence of excessive vomiting or prolonged NG suctioning. Hypokalemia can also lead to metabolic alkalosis. When the serum potassium level is low, potassium shifts from intracellular to intravascular fluid. Hydrogen ions move into cells to maintain the electrical balance. This results in a state of low hydrogen concentration in the intravascular fluid (metabolic alkalosis). Prolonged use of nonpotassium sparing diuretics can cause this type of acid-base imbalance.

▶ *Medical/Surgical Management*

▶ *Medical*

Treatment depends upon the cause. IV fluids with the appropriate electrolyte additives are ordered, usually sodium chloride or potassium chloride. Sedatives and tranquilizers are limited, since they depress respirations.

▶ *Nursing Process*

Assessment

Subjective Data   Client history may reveal nausea, anorexia, tingling and numbness of extremities, headache, and lethargy.

Objective Data   Physical symptoms of hypocalcemia develop, although the serum calcium level is normal. Muscle weakness, hyperactive reflexes, tremors, or tetany are noted. Respirations become slow and shallow to conserve carbon dioxide. CNS symptoms include a change in level of consciousness and confusion.

Arterial blood gases reveal a pH more than 7.45, bicarbonate more than 26 mEq/L and PCO_2 more than 45 mmHg. Serum calcium, potassium, and chloride are decreased.

▼ ▼

Possible nursing diagnoses for a client with metabolic alkalosis may include:

Nursing Diagnoses	*Goals*	*Nursing Interventions*
▶ *Injury, high risk for, related to neuromuscular irritability and possible tetany.*	The client will not have injury related to the neuromuscular changes of metabolic alkalosis.	Protect the client from falls and injury related to possible convulsions. Administer medications and IV fluids as ordered. Use saline solutions rather than water for NG tube irrigations. Administer ordered antiemetics to control vomiting before acid-base imbalances develop.
▶ *Knowledge deficit, related to use of bicarbonate-containing antacids.*	The client will relate an understanding of the consequences of taking bicarbonate-containing antacids.	Teach client not to use baking soda or bicarbonate-containing antacids for relief of gastric upset.

▶ *Evaluation*

Each goal must be evaluated to determine how it has been met by the client.

▲ ▲

▶ RESPIRATORY ALKALOSIS

Respiratory alkalosis is due to a decreased level of carbonic acid. The major cause of respiratory alkalosis is hyperventilation which results in a rapid abnormal loss of carbon dioxide. Anxiety, fever, salicylate poisoning, and overvigorous mechanical ventilation can all lead to hyperventilation.

▶ Medical/Surgical Management

▶ Medical

Treatment is aimed at correcting the cause of the hyperventilation. Sedatives may be necessary.

▶ Nursing Process

Assessment

Subjective Data   Client history may indicate severe anxiety and numbness and tingling of fingers and toes.

Objective Data   Physical symptoms include elevated blood pressure, sweating, dry mouth, and confusion. Convulsions may occur in severe cases.

Arterial blood gases reveal a pH above 7.45, $PaCO_2$ below 35 mmHg, and the serum bicarbonate level is normal. It takes the kidneys a few days to compensate and hyperventilation does not last long enough for this to happen except when a mechanical respirator is improperly adjusted for a long period of time.

▼ ▼

Possible nursing diagnosis for a client with respiratory alkalosis may include:

Nursing Diagnoses	Goals	Nursing Interventions
▶ *Anxiety related to actual or perceived threat to personal situation.*	The client will verbalize having less anxiety.	If anxiety has precipitated the hyperventilation, assist the client in identifying the cause of the anxiety. Often verbalization of concerns diminishes their magnitude.
		Maintain eye contact and instruct the client to take slow, even breaths.
		Have the client breathe into a paper bag held over the nose and mouth. In doing so, the client rebreathes the exhaled CO_2.
		Limit the time clients are encouraged to take rapid deep breaths, such as during labor, and have the client resume a normal breathing pattern.

Evaluation

Each goal must be evaluated to determine how it has been met by the client.

▲ ▲

▶ **CASE STUDY**

Mr. G. R. Calahan is a sixty-seven-year-old retired Army captain who lives with his wife in an apartment over their son's hardware store in a small Midwestern town. Due to behavioral changes throughout the course of the day, his family brought him to the emergency room of the local hospital.

Other than surgeries for an inguinal hernia and hemorrhoids, he has been in good health. Four months ago, during his annual visit to the doctor, his blood pressure was elevated. The diuretic pill prescribed has kept his blood pressure within normal limits. He eats a well-balanced diet, does not smoke, but does like a beer when he is hot. He and his dog go for a two-mile jog each day.

Despite the high humidity and temperature in the nineties, he and his dog went for their usual morning exercise. He had a bowl of oatmeal, a grapefruit, two cups of coffee, and his medication before jogging. When he returned home, he complained of being weak and tired. He apologized for not getting the air conditioner fixed the day before but promised to do it right after his nap. He told his wife he did not feel like eating lunch. He drank a beer to quench his thirst before lying down. Twice he got up to urinate. The second time he almost fell because he was so dizzy. When his son came to visit during the evening meal, he noticed his father was becoming confused and decided to take him to the emergency room.

Serum blood tests revealed elevated

(continued)

The following questions will guide your development of a Nursing Care Plan for the case study.

1. Identify factors that contributed to Mr. Calahan's fluid volume deficit.

2. What changes in vital signs should the nurse expect to find in a client with a fluid volume deficit?

3. Why are elderly clients especially prone to fluid imbalances?

4. Discuss why Mr. Calahan's hematocrit is elevated.

5. Identify two nursing diagnoses and goals for Mr. Calahan.

6. Relate three nursing interventions for a client with a fluid volume deficit.

   An IV of D5NS at 125 cc/hr was started in the ER and he was admitted to a medical unit for future evaluation. When he arrived on the unit, one hour-and-a-half after entering the hospital, the IV site showed no signs of infiltration and 100 cc remain in the bag.

7. Identify a priority nursing diagnosis for Mr. Calahan based upon this information.

8. Identify three nursing interventions the nurse should implement.

9. Relate criteria to use to evaluate the effectiveness of nursing care.

10. Identify client teaching to aid in preventing fluid volume deficit during periods of high atmospheric temperature and humidity.

▶ *CASE STUDY (continued)*

hematocrit, electrolytes, and BUN. Although he had been urinating large quantities earlier in the day, he could only produce 30 cc of very concentrated urine in the ER. Specific gravity was 1.025. Mr. Calahan was diagnosed with dehydration.

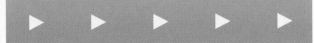 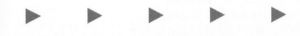

SUMMARY

- Maintenance of fluid, electrolyte, and acid-base balances is essential to ensure homeostasis within the body.
- Body fluids are located either in intracellular or extracellular compartments.
- Osmosis, diffusion, filtration, and active transport are methods that facilitate movement of fluids and electrolytes between extracellular and intracellular compartments.
- ADH, aldosterone, glucocorticoids, parathyroid hormone, and thyrocalcitonin are hormones that regulate fluid and electrolyte balances.
- Age, atmospheric conditions, and exercise affect fluid and electrolyte balances.
- Environmental factors, personal behaviors, psychological influences, therapeutic modalities, and diseases can potentiate fluid deficits or excesses.
- Clients with hyponatremia, hypokalemia, hypocalcemia, hypomagnesemia, hypochloremia, or hypophosphatemia need to be taught methods to increase their intake of these serum electrolytes.
- Oral supplements, tube feeding, or intravenous solutions are utilized to replace lost fluids and electrolytes.
- A wide variety of factors can lead to the development of acidosis or alkalosis.
- The four types of acid-base imbalances are metabolic acidosis, respiratory acidosis, metabolic alkalosis, and respiratory alkalosis.

Review Questions

1. The largest percentage of fluid in the body is located:

    a. in the blood vessels.
    b. in extracellular fluid.
    c. in interstitial spaces.
    d. within the cells.

2. Diffusion is the movement of:

    a. substances across cell membranes with the aid of chemical energy.
    b. a solute from an area of high concentration to an area of low concentration.
    c. water from an area of low solute concentration to one of high solute concentration.
    d. water and substances due to hydrostatic pressure.

3. Which of the following foods is high in potassium?

    a. cooked carrots
    b. dried cereals
    c. bananas
    d. potato chips

4. Clients with hypocalcemia should be encouraged to eat more:

    a. broccoli.
    b. chicken.
    c. dried fruits.
    d. potatoes.

5. A pH of 7.41 indicates:
    a. metabolic acidosis.
    b. impending coma.
    c. respiratory alkalosis.
    d. normal ph.

6. Respiratory acidosis develops as a result of:
    a. chronic obstructive pulmonary disease.
    b. diabetes mellitus.
    c. hyperventilation.
    d. nasogastric suctioning.

7. Diabetics who forget to take their insulin are prone to develop:
    a. metabolic alkalosis.
    b. respiratory alkalosis.
    c. metabolic acidosis.
    d. respiratory acidosis.

Critical Thinking Questions

1. How do you maintain fluid balance?

2. How would you feel having tube feedings?

MEDICAL TERMINOLOGY

Hyper-	an excess of
Hypo-	a deficiency of
hypercalcemia	an excess of serum calcium
hypocalcemia	a deficiency of serum calcium
hyperchloremia	an excess of serum chloride
hypochloremia	a deficiency of serum chloride
-natremia	serum sodium
hyperkalemia	an excess of serum potassium
hypokalemia	a deficiency of serum potassium
hypermagnesemia	an excess of serum magnesium
hypomagnesemia	a deficiency of serum magnesium
hyperphosphatemia	an excess of serum phosphorus
hypophosphatemia	a deficiency of serum phosphorus

News Flash

The concentrated form of potassium chloride, supplied in 20 mEq per 20 mL vials, has been associated with more lethal medication errors than any other drug. Fatalities have occurred when it has been erroneously given IV push or added to an existing IV solution without thoroughly agitating the solution prior to administration. Government agencies, manufacturers, and hospitals have instituted guidelines to prevent potential dangers. Pharmaceutical companies have been mandated to package the concentrated form in black-capped vials. The print on the labels has been enlarged and includes the warning "Must Be Diluted." Based on regulator agency recommendations, many hospitals have removed this concentrated form of potassium from nursing units. Instead, a 100 mL diluted solution is available. Physicians have been advised to avoid using the term "IV push" or "IV bolus" when ordering potassium intravenously. Hospital pharmacies have been given the sole responsibility of adding KCl to all IV solutions. Despite these changes, fatal errors continue to occur (Davis, 1995).

Nurses need to be especially cognizant of the inherent dangers when administering potassium chloride intravenously. Carefully follow the "5 rights" of medication administration. Read all labels. Never give IV push. Administer in a diluted form. Agitate solutions prior to hanging to ensure the concentrate has been mixed throughout. Never give faster than 20 mEq/hour. Failure to follow these guidelines can have deadly consequences to the client.

UNIT
5

Special Topics
of Medical-Surgical Care

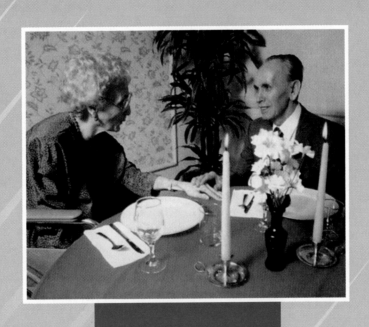

CHAPTER

15

Oncology Nursing

Celinda Kay Leach

LIST OF DISORDERS

- ▶ Lung Cancer
- ▶ Colorectal Cancer
- ▶ Breast Cancer
- ▶ Gynecological Cancers
- ▶ Prostate Cancer
- ▶ Testicular Cancer
- ▶ Skin Cancer
- ▶ Leukemia
- ▶ Lymphoma

LEARNING OBJECTIVES

Upon completion of this chapter the learner should be able to:
- Define key terms.
- Explain how the behavior of cancer cells differs from normal cells.
- Describe the role of the nurse in cancer detection.
- Discuss three medical treatments for cancer.
- Describe four complications that can occur in advanced cancer.
- Discuss ways the licensed practical/vocational nurse can aid the client coping with cancer.

▶ KEY TERMS

alopecia
antineoplastic
ascites
benign
biologic response modifiers
biopsy
bone marrow suppression
cachexia
carcinogen
carcinoma
chemotherapy
curative
differentiation
extravasation
leukemia
lymphoma
malignant
metastasis
neoplasm
oncology
palliative
radiotherapy
reconstructive
sarcoma
tumor markers
vesicants

▶ *MAKING THE CONNECTION*

INTRODUCTION

One in three Americans will develop some type of cancer during their lifetime. It is the second leading cause of death in the United States. Cancer can develop in individuals of all races, gender, ages, socioeconomic status, or culture. It is not a single disease but a group of more than 100 different diseases that can occur in any tissue or organ of the body.

According to the American Cancer Society, in the 1930s less than one in five cancer clients was alive five years after treatment. In the 1940s one in four survived five years. Today, four of ten people diagnosed with cancer will be alive in five years. Survival rates are influenced by the type of cancer, the progression of the disease at diagnosis, and the response to the treatment.

INCIDENCE

Women develop cancer more often than men although a greater number of men actually die from the disease. Incidence and mortality rates are usually higher for African Americans than for Anglo Americans. The incidence of cancer is higher in the elderly population than in any other age group. In men, the most common cancers are skin, prostate, lung, and colorectal; in women, they are cancers of the skin, breast, colorectal, lung, and uterus (see Figure 15-1).

PATHOPHYSIOLOGY

Cancer is a disease characterized by neoplasia, an uncontrolled growth of abnormal cells. Unlike normal cells that reproduce in an orderly manner and grow for a purpose, cancer cells develop rapidly, undiscriminatingly, and serve no useful function as they grow at the expense of healthy tissue. Abnormal growths may be **benign** or **malignant**.

Benign tumor cells form not cancerous and are usually harmless. They grow slowly, are encapsulated, well-defined, and do not spread to neighboring tissues. They are associated with a favorable prognosis unless their location interferes with vital functions.

Malignant tumor cells form irregular-shaped masses with fingerlike projections. They usually multiply quickly and spread to distant body parts by way of the bloodstream or the lymph system. This process is called **metastasis**. Patterns of metastasis will differ depending on the type of cancer. **Neoplasms** can be found in any body tissue but most frequently occur in those cells that repair themselves quickly.

Cancers are usually named according to the site of the primary tumor or the type of tissue involved. There are four main classifications of cancer according to tissue type:

(1) **lymphomas** (cancers originating in infection-fighting organs)
(2) **leukemias** (cancers originating in blood forming organs)

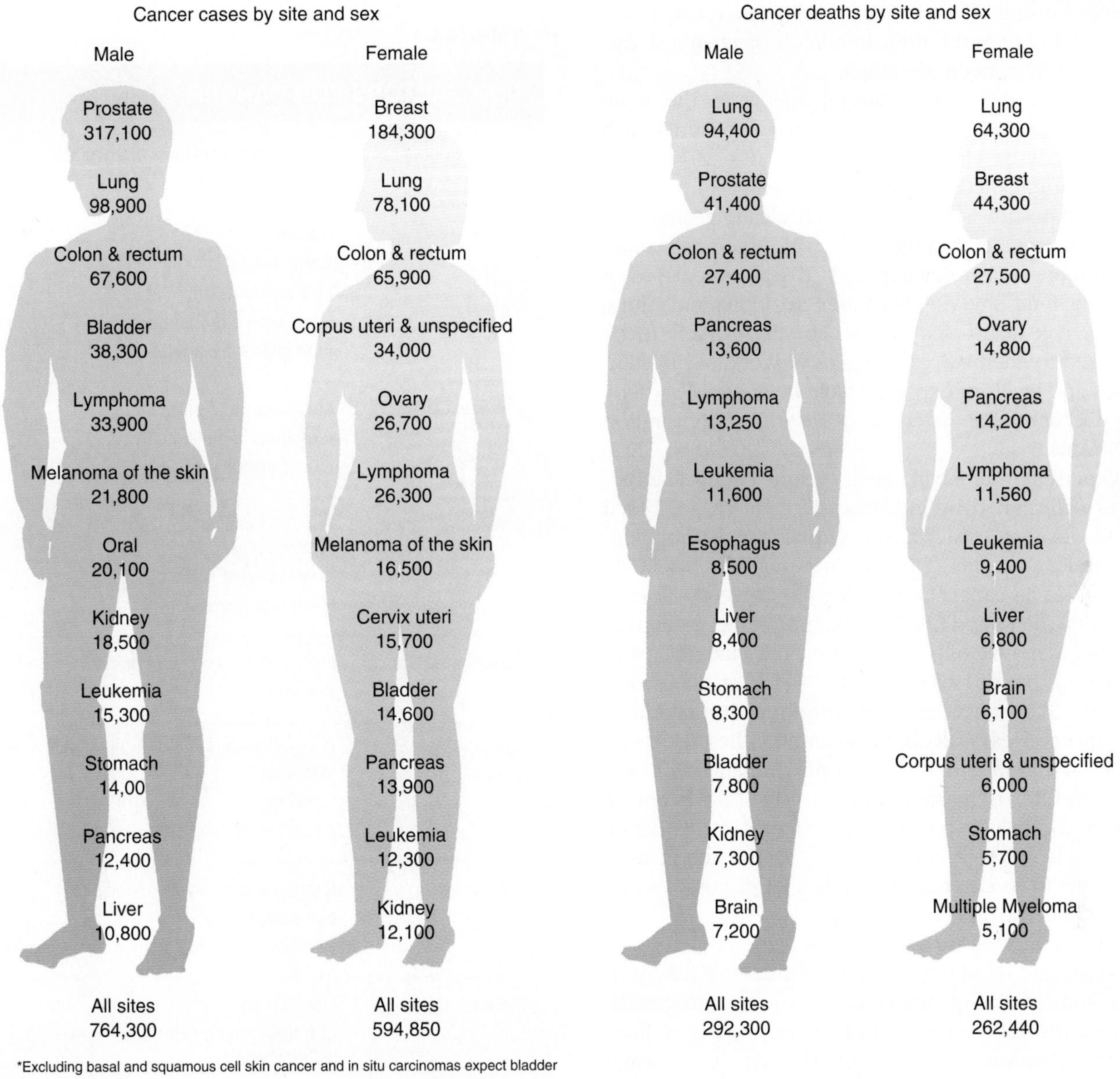

Cancer cases by site and sex

Male	Female
Prostate 317,100	Breast 184,300
Lung 98,900	Lung 78,100
Colon & rectum 67,600	Colon & rectum 65,900
Bladder 38,300	Corpus uteri & unspecified 34,000
Lymphoma 33,900	Ovary 26,700
Melanoma of the skin 21,800	Lymphoma 26,300
Oral 20,100	Melanoma of the skin 16,500
Kidney 18,500	Cervix uteri 15,700
Leukemia 15,300	Bladder 14,600
Stomach 14,00	Pancreas 13,900
Pancreas 12,400	Leukemia 12,300
Liver 10,800	Kidney 12,100
All sites 764,300	All sites 594,850

Cancer deaths by site and sex

Male	Female
Lung 94,400	Lung 64,300
Prostate 41,400	Breast 44,300
Colon & rectum 27,400	Colon & rectum 27,500
Pancreas 13,600	Ovary 14,800
Lymphoma 13,250	Pancreas 14,200
Leukemia 11,600	Lymphoma 11,560
Esophagus 8,500	Leukemia 9,400
Liver 8,400	Liver 6,800
Stomach 8,300	Brain 6,100
Bladder 7,800	Corpus uteri & unspecified 6,000
Kidney 7,300	Stomach 5,700
Brain 7,200	Multiple Myeloma 5,100
All sites 292,300	All sites 262,440

*Excluding basal and squamous cell skin cancer and in situ carcinomas expect bladder

FIGURE 15-1 Leading sites of cancer incidence and death 1996 estimates. (*Reprinted from American Cancer Society Cancer Facts and Figures, 1996*)

(3) **sarcomas** (cancers originating in connective tissue such as bone)
(4) **carcinomas** (cancers originating in epithelial cells)

The exact mechanism that causes cancer is unknown but most authorities believe that cancer develops from a combination of causes rather than a single factor. Environmental, genetic, and viral factors have been implicated as **carcinogens**, or cancer-causing agents. These agents are thought to alter the DNA in the cell nucleus.

RISK FACTORS

A number of risk factors, such as environmental, genetic, and viral, may increase an individual's chances of developing cancer. These factors are discussed below.

Lifestyle Factors

The first demonstration of an environmental carcinogen was noted by Percival Pott in 1760 when he recognized that chimney sweeps had a very high rate of scrotal cancer because they were exposed to cancer-causing oils in soot which was rubbed into their clothing. Since then hundreds of chemical carcinogens have been identified.

Many of the cancer-causing agents in the environment are related to occupational exposures such as asbestos or vinyl chlorides. The risk of workers developing cancers is greatly increased if occupational exposure is combined with cigarette smoking. Tobacco may act synergistically with other substances to promote cancer development. Exposure to asbestos and cigarette smoking increases an individual's lung cancer risk nearly sixty times. For those likely to be exposed to chemical carcinogens at work, safety standards and levels of exposure have been established by the Occupational Safety and Health Administration (OSHA).

Other environmental agents include chemical exposures determined by individual lifestyle choices such as the use of tobacco, sun exposure, alcohol consumption, and diet. Smoking accounts for about 30 percent of all cancer deaths. It is associated with cancer of the head and neck, esophagus, lungs, pancreas, and bladder. Overexposure to the sun's ultraviolet rays over long periods of time is the cause of many skin cancers. Skin cancer accounts for about 10 percent of all cancers. Heavy alcohol consumption has also been implicated in mouth, throat, esophageal and liver cancers. Alcohol is hypothesized to cause 5 percent of cancer deaths. Despite the epidemiological evidence linking alcohol to cancer, the exact carcinogen in alcohol is yet to be determined. Table 15-1 discusses some risk factors for cancer.

Dietary factors are also thought to be related to 40 to 60 percent of all environmental cancers. While findings from studies of cancer and diet are controversial, current research suggests an increase in dietary fiber may help prevent colon cancer (Hansen, 1995). Some studies have suggested that obesity is a significant risk factor for breast, colon, endometrial, and prostate cancers. Studies have also shown that salt-cured, smoked, and nitrite-cured foods are risk factors for cancer of the stomach and esophagus. Food substances that may reduce cancer risk include cruciferous vegetables (cabbage, broccoli, cauliflower, brussels sprouts, kohlrabi) and possibly vitamins A, E, and C and selenium. Some foods have been found to contain carcinogens in the forms of additives or as byproducts of storage. On the basis of current knowledge, the American Cancer Society has offered dietary guidelines to reduce cancer risk (see Table 15-2). The effects of carcinogenic agents are usually dose dependent. The larger the dose or the longer the duration of exposure, the greater the risk of cancer development. It is estimated that 80 percent of all cancers may be associated with environmental exposures and might be prevented if exposure is avoided (see Table 15-3).

Table 15-1

RISK FACTORS FOR CANCER

Breast Cancer	Positive family history (immediate female relatives)
	High-fat diet
	Obesity
	Early menarche
	Late menopause
	Long-term estrogen therapy
	First child after age 30
Cervical Cancer	Multiple sexual partners
	Exposure to genital herpes
	Exposure to human papilloma virus
Colorectal Cancer	Positive family history (immediate relatives)
	Low-fiber diet
	History of rectal polyps
Esophageal Cancer	Heavy alcohol consumption
	Smoking
Lung Cancer	Positive family history (immediate relatives)
	Smoking
	Asbestos exposure
Skin Cancer	Exposure to ultraviolet sunlight
	Fair complexion
	Work with coal, tar, pitch, or creosote
Stomach Cancer	Family history
	Diet heavy in smoked, pickled, or salted foods
Testicular Cancer	Undescended testicles
	Mothers took hormones during pregnancy

Genetic Factors

There are some families who have a high incidence of certain types of cancer. Fortunately, familial tendencies are rare and probably account for less than 5 percent of all cancers. Breast cancer, for example, occurs more frequently in women whose mothers, grandmothers, or sisters have had the disease. Cancers of the breast, colon, stomach, prostate, lung, ovary, and leukemia may show inherited patterns. Therefore, relatives of persons with these cancers need careful monitoring.

Table 15-2

DIETARY GUIDELINES TO REDUCE THE RISK OF CANCER

- Limit fat intake to 20% to 30% of total calories.
- Increase fiber.
- Limit alcohol consumption to no more than one or two drinks per day.
- Eat foods high in vitamin A and vitamin C such as, leafy green and yellow vegetables, and fresh fruits.
- Eat more cruciferous vegetables (a group of vegetables named for their cross-shaped blossoms) such as, broccoli, cabbage, brussels sprouts, turnips, and rutabagas.
- Limit foods containing nitrites (preservative found in some processed meats).
- Reduce intake of red meat.

Table 15-3

REDUCE CANCER RISK WITH A HEALTHY LIFESTYLE

- Do not smoke or use tobacco in any form.
- Avoid overexposure to the sun.
- Eat a healthy diet. (See Table 15-2.)
- Get plenty of exercise.
- Have a physical examination on a routine basis, including a mammogram, Pap smear, testicular, and colon examination.
- Get plenty of sleep (six to eight hours per night).
- Keep weight within normal limits.
- Practice self-examinations faithfully and see your physician if you have any questions.
- Know and follow health and safety rules at the workplace.

Viral factors

Viruses have been linked to a number of cancers but their exact role is unclear. They are thought to incorporate themselves into the genetic structure of the cell. Herpes simplex II virus and some of the human papillomaviruses that are transmitted sexually are known to predispose women to cervical cancer. Reducing the number of sexual partners and better hygiene can reduce the risk of contracting the virus.

DETECTION

When cancer does develop, the earlier it is detected the more likely it is to be controlled. In some cases diagnosis can be made before symptoms become apparent. Cancer is usually found by an individual who notices a warning sign or by a health care provider during a checkup. A cancer checkup is recommended every three years for persons ages twenty to thirty-nine and annually for those age forty and over. Risk assessment is the first step in cancer prevention. The cancer examination should include a medical history of exposures to environmental agents and a comprehensive family history.

If cancer is suspected due to early or late symptoms, diagnostic studies will be ordered. The diagnostic studies to be performed will depend on the suspected primary or metastatic site of the cancer and include laboratory studies or blood tests, radiologic studies, endoscopy, cytology, and biopsy. Nurses must be able to give brief descriptions of such tests as well as assist in client preparation.

Although no one blood test can establish a cancer diagnosis, some malignancies do alter the chemical composition of the blood. Specialized laboratory tests have been developed for **tumor markers**. Tumor markers are specific proteins, antigens, genes, hormones, or enzymes released by cancers. They are not 100 percent accurate as benign processes can also cause an elevation, thus they are more useful in monitoring response to treatment or detecting a relapse.

COMMON DIAGNOSTIC TESTS

The following is a table of the commonly used diagnostic tests for clients who present with symptoms of cancer.

Test	Explanation/Normal Values	Nursing Responsibilities
LABORATORY TESTS & BLOOD STUDIES		
Acid Phosphatase	Acid phosphatase is an enzyme found in highest concentrations in the prostate gland. Elevated levels are seen in clients with prostatic cancer that has metastasized to other body parts. If tumors are treated successfully, levels will decrease. Rising levels may indicate a poor prognosis. Adults 0.11–0.60 U/L	Tell the client that no food or drink restrictions are associated with this test. Apply pressure to venipuncture site. Observe the site for bleeding.
Alkaline Phosphatase	Alkaline phosphatase is an enzyme found in many tissues. The highest concentrations are found in the liver, biliary tract, and bone. Detection is important for determining possible liver and bone cancers. Adults 30–85 ImU/mL	Tell the client that no food or drink restrictions are associated with this test. Apply pressure to venipuncture site. Observe the site for bleeding.
Bence Jones Protein	Bence Jones proteins are immunoglobulins typically found in the urine of clients with multiple myeloma. They may also be associated with tumor metastases to the bone and chronic lymphocytic leukemia. Normal = No Bence Jones proteins present in urine.	Instruct the client to collect an early morning urine specimen of at least 50 mL. Instruct the client not to contaminate specimen with toilet paper or stool.
CA-15-3	CA-15-3 (cancer antigen) is a tumor marker available for monitoring breast cancer. Since benign breast or ovarian disease can also cause elevations it has limited use in diagnosis. Normal <22 U/mL	Tell the client no fasting is required. Apply pressure to venipuncture site. Observe the site for bleeding.
CA-19-9	CA-19-9 (cancer antigen) is a tumor marker used primarily in the diagnosis of pancreatic carcinoma. Normal <37 U/mL	Tell the client no fasting is required. Apply pressure to venipuncture site. Observe the site for bleeding.
CA-125	CA-125 (cancer antigen) is a tumor marker especially helpful in making the diagnosis of ovarian cancer. 0-35 U/mL	Tell the client no fasting is required. Apply pressure to venipuncture site. Observe the site for bleeding.

Test	Explanation/Normal Values	Nursing Responsibilities
CEA	CEA (carcinoembryonic antigen) was thought to be a specific indicator of the presence of colorectal cancer but has been found in clients with a variety of carcinomas. It is especially useful in monitoring treatment response in breast and gastrointestinal cancers and is occasionally the first sign of tumor recurrence. Normal <5 ng/mL	Tell the client no fasting is required. Apply pressure to venipuncture site. Observe the site for bleeding.
PSA	PSA (prostate-specific antigen) is an antigen detected in all males; levels increase with prostatic cancer. It is more sensitive and specific than the acid phosphatase. Normal <4 ng/mL	Tell the client no fasting is required. Apply pressure to venipuncture site. Observe the site for bleed ing.
Stool for occult blood (Guaiac)	Fecal occult blood screening studies may be utilized as an indicator for possible colorectal cancer. Negative for blood	Explain the method of stool collection to the client. Instruct not to mix toilet paper or urine with specimen. Wear gloves when obtaining and handling specimen.
Serum Calcitonin	Serum calcitonin is a hormone secreted by the thyroid gland and in response to elevated serum calcium levels. Elevated levels can also be seen in people with cancer of the lung, breast, pancreas, and thyroid. males <19 pg/mL females <14 pg/mL	Tell the client an overnight fast is required. Water is permitted. Apply pressure to venipuncture site. Observe the site for bleeding.
RADIOLOGIC STUDIES		
X-ray Studies	Allow for the visualization of internal structures, may be site specific (mammogram) or visualize entire organ systems. Frequently used to detect lung and gastrointestinal cancers. Contrast agents such as iodine or barium may be used where visualization is difficult such as the gastrointestinal tract, gallbladder, liver, and urinary tract.	Follow agency protocol for client preparation when x-ray studies are ordered.
Computerized Axial Tomography (CT Scan or CAT Scan)	Provides a three-dimensional cross sectional view of tissues. Computer constructed picture interprets densities of various tissues. Most useful for viewing tumors in the chest, abdominal cavity, and brain.	Explain procedure. NPO if dye to be used. Remove all objects from hair for head scan. Body scan may or may not require special preparations.

(continued)

Test	Explanation/Normal Values	Nursing Responsibilities
Magnetic Resonance Imaging (MRI)	Provides sectional images using magnetic fields. Especially useful for studying tumors where bone hampers visualization by x-ray or CT scans such as tumors of the central nervous system.	Explain procedure. No food or beverage restrictions. Have client empty bladder, test could take 60 or more minutes. Remove all metal objects from person. If client has metal implants, this test cannot be used. Assess if client is claustrophobic.
Scans (Radioisotope Test)	Rely on a radioactive substance or isotope being taken up by the part of the body being examined. Organ sites most frequently studied are the liver, spleen, lungs, heart, urinary tract, thyroid, and brain. The radioactive substance is given orally or intravenously by the nuclear medicine department.	Explain procedure. Client must lie still for 30-60 minutes. Machine makes clicking noise at times. Liver & spleen—no special preparation; lungs—no special preparation; heart—NPO; kidney—hydrate as ordered; thyroid—no special preparation; brain—no special preparation.
Ultrasound	A source of high frequency ultrasound waves is sent into the body and echoes are recorded as they strike tissues of different densities, producing an image or photograph. Useful in distinguishing between cystic and solid masses. Most often used to assess the pelvis, heart, and abdomen.	Explain procedure. Most ultrasound tests need no special preparation. Pelvic sonogram—client should have a full bladder. Abdominal sonogram—client usually NPO and needs bowel preparation. Gall bladder sonogram—NPO for 12 hours and a fat-free diet the evening before test.

INVASIVE DIAGNOSTIC TECHNIQUES

Test	Explanation/Normal Values	Nursing Responsibilities
Endoscopy	Permits visual examination of internal structures of the body with specially designed instruments. The observation may be done through a natural body opening or through a small incision. A **biopsy** (removal of sample tissue) of suspicious areas may then be done for further study.	Explain procedure. NPO except for sigmoidoscopy. Sigmoidoscopy—liquid diet for several days. Laxative and then cleansing enema.
Cytology	The study of cells and fluids obtained from various organs by scrapings, brushings, or needle aspiration. Cytologic smears, such as the Pap smear, are routinely done to study cells from the female genital tract. Cytologic smears showing evidence of a malignancy are followed by a biopsy to provide a more comprehensive diagnosis.	Explain procedure for obtaining cells and fluids for study. Follow agency protocol for client preparation.
Biopsy	Removal of sample tissue for microscopic study. Tissue may be quickly frozen or placed in formalin before it is chemically stained and thinly sliced for analysis. The frozen section takes only a few minutes and is often completed while a client is still in surgery. The permanent section takes 24 to 48 hours to complete but is the most accurate means of establishing a cancer diagnosis. Tissue biopsy is essential to confirm the type of cancer, the amount of lymph node involvement, and whether the cancer was successfully removed.	Explain procedure. Follow physician's orders and/or agency protocol for client preparation.

KEY ABBREVIATIONS

The following abbreviations and acronyms are used in this chapter:

ABMT	autologous bone marrow transplantation
ACS	American Cancer Society
ALL	acute lymphocytic leukemia
BSE	breast self-examination
CLL	chronic lymphocytic leukemia
CCS	cell-cycle specific
CCNS	cell-cycle nonspecific
DIC	disseminated intravascular coagulation
EVAD	explantable venous access device
IFN	interferon
IVAD	implantable vascular access device
NCI	National Cancer Institute
NHL	non-Hodgkin's lymphoma
Pap	Papanicolaou smear
PCA	patient controlled analgesia
PIC	peripheral indwelling catheter
SCC	spinal cord compression
SVCS	superior vena cava syndrome
TSE	testicular self-examination
UV	ultraviolet radiation

STAGING OF TUMORS

Staging determines the extent of the spread of cancer. The TNM classification proposed by the American Joint Commission on Cancer is one of the most frequently used systems. The *T* refers to the anatomic size of the primary tumor, *N* is the extent of lymph node involvement, and *M* denotes the presence or absence of metastasis. Staging is important because it affects decisions about treatment modalities and additionally helps predict overall prognosis.

GRADING OF TUMORS

Normal body cells have individual characteristics so they can perform different body functions. This process is called **differentiation**. Cancer cells that retain many of the identifiable tissue characteristics are termed well differentiated. Cancer cells having little similarity to the tissue of origin are undifferentiated. Tumor grading is based primarily on the degree of differentiation of malignant cells. Grading evaluates tumor cells in comparison to normal cells. Pathologists determine tumor cell grades by using Roman numerals I through IV; the higher the grade, the worse the prognosis. Thus, a grade I tumor is the most differentiated

and a grade IV is the least differentiated. Tumors containing poorly differentiated cells are more aggressive in growth and may display uncharacteristic behaviors. This client has a poorer prognosis. Grading criteria varies for different neoplasms.

TREATMENT MODALITIES

After cancer is diagnosed, staged, and graded, a medical treatment plan will be developed. The most common treatment methods used today are surgery, radiation therapy, or **chemotherapy** (use of drugs). These methods may be used alone or in combination.

Surgery

Surgery is the oldest form of cancer treatment and still remains the common method of treatment today. It can be classified as **curative**, **palliative**, or **reconstructive**.

The goal of curative surgery is to excise all of the tumor, the involved surrounding tissue, and the regional lymph nodes. Surgery is most often curative in early stage cancers such as cervical, breast, or skin cancer. The first commonly used surgical procedure for treating cancer was the radical mastectomy, a procedure developed by a surgeon named Halsted in the early 1900s. In women whose cancer was localized to the breast, this operation was curative. Fortunately a radical approach to operable tumors is no longer routinely used.

Unfortunately since 70 percent of clients show evidence of metastasis at diagnosis, cure is not always possible, and palliative surgery may be necessary. This surgery is effective in relieving symptoms in more advanced stages of cancer. It is usually performed in an attempt to relieve complications such as obstructions, or to surgically interrupt nerve pathways for intractable pain. It may also be used to insert special access devices or to place tubes for enteral nutrition.

Reconstructive surgery may follow curative or radical surgery. The goal is to produce a better return of function or a better cosmetic effect. Reconstructive surgery to areas such as the head and neck, breast, and extremities can minimize deformity. The surgery may be done at one time or it may be done in stages.

Radiation Therapy

Radiation therapy is the second most common method of treating cancer. Although radiation occurs naturally, it was not recognized until 1895, when Wilhelm Roentgen discovered that x-rays (rays of unknown origin) could penetrate solid materials.

Radiation therapy uses high-energy ionizing radiation to kill cancer. Ionizing radiation has the ability to penetrate tissue cells and deposit energy within them. This intense energy causes breakage in chromosomes within the cell, thus preventing the ability to replicate. Cell death may occur hours, days, or even years after treatment, depending on the rate of mitosis.

The goal of radiation therapy is to eradicate malignant cells without causing harm to healthy tissues. Some cells are more sensitive to radiation than others. More vascular, better oxygenated cells and those that divide rapidly are the most sensitive.

It is estimated that radiation therapy is used to treat more than half of all people with cancer at some point during their illness. It may be used alone or as an adjunct to other therapies. As a single treatment modality it is most often used when the disease is localized. Preoperative radiation is frequently used to reduce the tumor mass before surgery. Postoperative radiation therapy is frequently used to decrease the risk of local recurrence following surgery. Some chemotherapeutic drugs increase the sensitivity of cancer cells to radiation and are used together. Radiation therapy can be classified as curative or palliative. It is frequently used to palliate symptoms of metastases such as pain.

The unit dose of measuring radiation is called a rad or radiation absorbed dose. The actual dosage given is determined by factors such as sensitivity of the tumor, tissue tolerance, and the amount of tissue to be irradiated. There are two types of radiation therapy, external and internal radiation.

External Radiation

External radiation or teletherapy is given with special equipment that can deliver high energy radiation. The kind of machines used will depend on the type and extent of the tumor. Linear accelerators are most commonly used.

Treatments are usually given on an outpatient basis, divided over many days or weeks. Customized shielding blocks may be created to protect healthy tissues and immobilization devices may be used to maintain the exact position for each treatment. Dyes or tattoos may be used to designate reference points on the skin. Care must be taken not to remove these markings during bathing. Clients should be instructed that they will be alone during the treatment and must lie absolutely still. A treatment is usually painless and typically lasts one to three minutes depending on the number of areas involved.

Nursing care should be directed toward client teaching, safety, and carrying out interventions that provide relief of side effects. Undesirable side effects that are most likely to occur include varying degrees of skin reactions and gastrointestinal discomforts such as abdominal cramping, diarrhea, loss of appetite, and

fatigue. Treatments have a cumulative effect and may produce symptoms after the therapy is completed.

Internal Radiation

Internal radiation delivers radioactive isotopes directly within the body. Isotopes commonly used for these purposes include: cobalt[60], iridium[192], iodine[125], phosphorus[32], cesium[137], gold[198], and radium[226]. Clients treated with internal sources of radiation can be a source of radioactivity. Isotopes may be introduced into the body via sealed or unsealed sources.

Sealed sources involve encapsulating radioactive elements in special containers. These containers take many forms such as tubes, wires, needles, seeds, or capsules. They are implanted close to the cancer cells hoping to give a highly concentrated dose. The implants may be temporary or permanent depending on the site and the type of isotope used. Bed rest will usually be required to prevent dislodging. Body fluids are not radioactive since sources are sealed. Radioactive implants are commonly used in the treatment of cancers of the tongue, lip, breast, vagina, cervix, endometrium, rectum, bladder, and brain.

Personnel caring for clients with sealed sources must be familiar with the hazards of radiation. Generally, the degree of exposure is dependent on three factors:

1. the distance between the individual and the source
2. the amount of time an individual is exposed
3. the type of shielding provided

Client care should be modified based on these principles as shown in Figure 15-2.

Radioactive isotopes can also be placed in suspensions or solutions as unsealed sources of radiation.

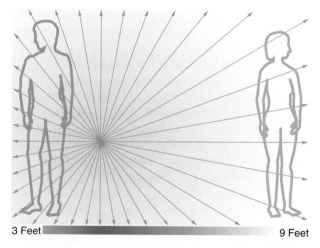

3 Feet   9 Feet

FIGURE 15-2 Radiation dose decreases with distance. (*Courtesy of the U.S. Nuclear Regulatory Commission*)

They may be given orally, parenterally, or instilled into intrapleural or peritoneal spaces. The most common unsealed elements used are iodine[131], phosphorus[32] and gold[198].

Some unsealed radioactive elements are eliminated in body secretions, thus special precautions should be taken. Agency policies and procedures must be followed closely. Unsealed sources are not usually radioactive as long as sealed sources. Clients are discharged when isotope levels are reduced to designated safe margins.

A universal symbol has been developed to indicate the use of radiation. Presence of the symbol notes the need for caution in order to prevent contamination with or undue exposure to radiation (see Figure 15-3).

Chemotherapy

Chemotherapy may be used to cure, prevent, or relieve cancer symptoms. The term *chemotherapy* means using chemical therapy or drugs to kill cancer cells. The idea to use drugs was developed during World War II, after discovering that nerve gas could cause **bone marrow suppression**.

The goal of **antineoplastic** drugs is to destroy all malignant cells. To understand how anticancer drugs work, one must have a basic understanding of the cell cycle.

A cell cycle is a series of steps that all cells undergo while they reproduce. Each step is called a phase. The phases include:

- *Step 1* - G_1 phase—cell manufactures enzymes needed to form DNA
- *Step 2* - S phase—DNA synthesis occurs
- *Step 3* - G_2 phase—Specialized DNA proteins and miotic spindles are made
- *Step 4* - M phase—Mitosis occurs

Almost all anticancer drugs kill cancer cells by affecting DNA synthesis or function, but they will vary how they exert their activity within the cell cycle. Most chemotherapeutic drugs are classified as cell-cycle specific (CCS) or cell-cycle nonspecific (CCNS).

Cell-cycle specific drugs (CCS) attack the cancer cells when they enter a certain phase of reproduction. These agents are most effective against rapidly growing tumors. Many of the drugs are "schedule dependent" because they produce a greater cell kill when given in multiple, repeated doses.

Cell-cycle nonspecific drugs (CCNS) can destroy cancer cells in any phase of the cell cycle, whether resting or reproducing. These drugs are used for large tumors that have fewer actively dividing cells. These drugs are not schedule dependent, but rather dose dependent. Dose dependent indicates that the number of cells destroyed is determined by the amount of drug given.

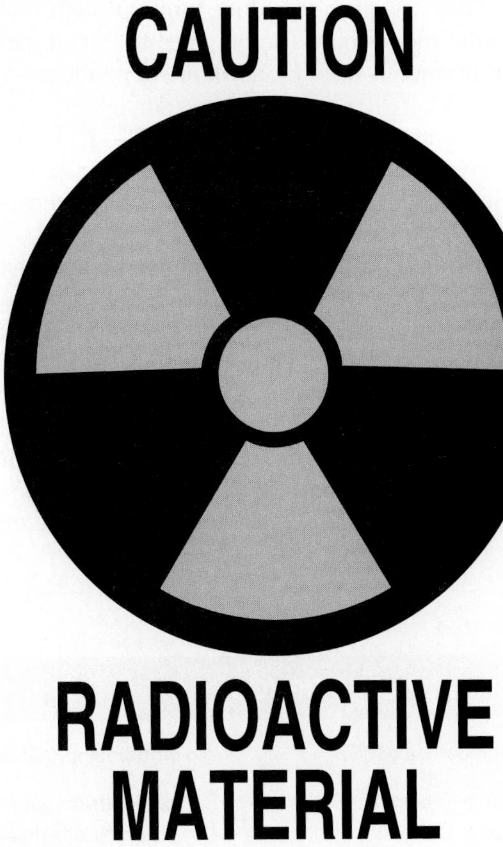

CAUTION

RADIOACTIVE MATERIAL

FIGURE 15-3 Universal symbol for radiation.

Anticancer agents are cytotoxic and destroy both normal and abnormal cells. They are most effective against cells that reproduce rapidly, such as those in bone marrow, gastrointestinal lining, hair follicles, and the ova and sperm. The drugs work best against cancer in its earliest stages, as cells multiply at their most rapid rate at the beginning of the disease.

Common drug classifications for chemotherapeutic agents include:

1. Alkylating agents (CCNS)—act by causing breaks in DNA strands, preventing mitosis.
2. Antimetabolites (CCS)—block essential enzymes necessary for DNA synthesis or become incorporated into the DNA and RNA so that a false message is transmitted.
3. Antibiotics (CCNS)—disrupt DNA transcription and inhibit DNA and RNA synthesis. Antitumor antibiotics are not used for infections since they are highly toxic.
4. Nitrosureas (CCNS)—inhibit DNA and RNA synthesis.
5. Vinca alkaloids (CCS)—bind to proteins during M phase, causing the cell to lose the ability to divide.
6. Hormones (CCNS)—alter the environment of the cell by affecting the cell membrane's permeabil-

ity. They are given to reduce tumor growth. (Antihormones may also be given to inhibit natural hormones used by hormone-dependent tumors).

7. Miscellaneous agents (CCS or CCNS)—act by a variety of mechanisms. (For example, L-asparaginase [Elspar] acts by inhibiting protein synthesis.)

Many of these drugs are given in combination with or after radiation or surgery to achieve maximum effect. They are usually given intermittently over an extended period of time. Drug resistance can occur.

The most common routes of administration are oral and intravenous. A few drugs may be given topically, subcutaneously, or intramuscularly. Recently, other methods have been introduced to increase the local concentration of the drug at the tumor site. These may be injected intrathecally or instilled intracavitarily. Table 15-4 lists some commonly used drugs.

Caring for a client receiving chemotherapy requires special knowledge and skill beyond basic nursing. Before preparing and giving anticancer drugs, the nurse must become familiar with agency protocols. Since many of the drugs are carcinogenic, protective equipment must be worn by the nurse during preparation and administration. All personnel involved in any aspect of handling chemotherapeutic agents should receive instructions regarding the known risk of such drugs, proper use of protective equipment, spill procedures, and medical policies covering personnel who are pregnant. Additionally, personnel handling blood, vomitus, or excreta from clients who have received chemotherapy within the prior forty-eight hours should wear disposable latex gloves and dispos-

Table 15-4

COMMONLY USED DRUGS

Antimetabolites (CCS)	Antibiotics (CCNS)	Antihormonal Agents (CCNS)
cytarabine (Cytosar)	dactinomycin (Cosmegan)	flutamide (Eulexin)
fluorouracil (Adrucil)	doxorubicin hydrochloride (Adriamycin)	tamoxifen (Nolvadex)
methotrexate (Mexate)	daunorubicin (Cerubidine)	goserelin acetate (Zoladex)
6-mercaptopurine (Purinethol)	mitomycin (Mutamycin)	
	mithramycin (Mithracin)	
	bleomycin (Blenoxane)	
Vinca Plant Alkaloids (CCS)	**Hormones (CCNS)**	**Nitrosureas (CCNS)**
vincristine sulfate (Oncovin)	testosterone (Histerone, Testoderm)	carmustine (BiCNU)
vinblastine sulfate (Velban)	megestrol acetate (Megace)	lomustine (CeeNU)
	medroxyprogesterone acetate (Depo-Provera)	
	diethylstilbestrol (DES)	
Alkylating Agents (CCNS)	**Corticosteroids**	**Miscellaneous Agents**
busulfan (Myleran)	dexamethasone (Decadron)	L-asparaginase (Elspar)
chlorambucil (Leukeran)	prednisone (Deltasone)	procarbazine hydrochloride (Matulane)
cisplatin (Platinol)	hydrocortisone sodium succinate (Solu-Cortef)	etoposide (VePesid)
cyclophosphamide (Cytoxan)		
mechlorethamine hydrochloride (Mustargen)		
melphalan (Alkeran)		
thiotepa (Thiotepa)		

Frequently Used Combinations

CMF ± P	cyclophosphamide, methotrexate, 5-fluorouracil, and prednisone
CAMP	cyclophosphamide, doxorubicin (Adriamycin), methotrexate, and procarbazine
CAE	cyclophosphamide, doxorubicin (Adriamycin), and etoposide
CVP	cyclophosphamide, vincristine and prednisone
FAC	5-fluorouracil, Adriamycin and Cytoxan
MOPP	mechlorethamine hydrochloride (Mustargen), vincristine (Oncovin), procarbazine, and prednisone

able gowns. Contaminated linen should be placed in specially marked laundry bags according to agency procedures.

Careful attention must also be given to intravenous administration. Leakage of chemotherapeutic drugs from the vein into the surrounding tissues during infusion is called **extravasation**. This is a potential problem as most of these drugs are irritating to the tissues. It is especially serious if the drugs being administered are **vesicants** (see Table 15-5). These agents are so irritating that they can cause blistering and even necrosis. All sites must be monitored carefully. Pain, swelling, redness, and the presence of vesicles are signs of extravasation. Additional signs include:

- The first symptom is usually a burning feeling at the site or along the vein.
- Blood return is absent or sluggish.
- Redness usually occurs six to twelve hours later.
- The client may experience pain.

Table 15-5

VESICANT DRUGS

• dactinomycin	(Cosmogen)
• daunorubicin HCl	(Cerubidine)
• doxorubicin HCl	(Adriamycin)
• mechlorethamine HCl	(Mustargen)
• mytomycin	(Mutamycin)
• vinblastine sulfate	(Velban)
• vincristine sulfate	(Oncovin)

- The client may experience swelling.
- Diffuse hardening may occur.

If extravasation does occur, the drug must be stopped immediately and protocols for treatment initiated.

Chemotherapy may also be administered by explantable venous access devices (EVAD) or implantable vascular access devices (IVAD) as shown in Figures 15-4A and B.

Explantable devices are special catheters that may be used for short- and long-term use. They may be inserted peripherally or centrally via the subclavian or jugular vein, and terminate in the superior vena cava or right atrium. Long-term central venous catheters are used when a prolonged course of therapy is expected. They are surgically threaded to an exit site in the chest and sutured in place.

Implantable devices consist of a self-sealing silicone rubber septum enclosed in a metal or plastic port that is attached to a silicone catheter. The port is implanted under the skin. The catheter is surgically threaded subcutaneously into the right atrium. The system is accessed by a needle puncture through the skin into the port's septum.

These devices are especially useful when clients have poor veins, require multiple venipunctures, or long-term therapy. They can also be used to administer blood products, total parenteral nutrition, and other medications. Many models are commercially available.

Improved infusion techniques, control of symptoms such as nausea and vomiting, and cost containment restrictions have reduced hospitalizations. Teaching clients and family members to monitor side effects in the home care setting is an essential function for the **oncology** (study of tumors) nurse. Some important points to emphasize are the following:

- Inspect the skin daily for any signs of rash or dermatitis, which may signal hypersensitivity to a drug.
- Report loss of taste or tingling in face, fingers, or toes, which may signal peripheral neuropathy.
- Report signs of dizziness, headache, confusion, slurred speech, convulsions, which may be signs of CNS toxicity.

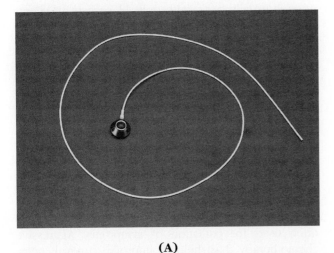

(A)

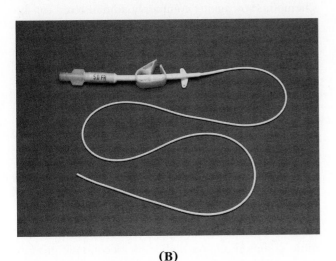

(B)

FIGURE 15-4 Explantable/implantable devices: **(A)** Mini-Vital Port; **(B)** Peripherally inserted venous catheter. (*Courtesy of Cook Incorporated, Bloomington, IN*)

- Report signs of unusual bleeding or bruising, fever, sore throat, or mouth sores, which may signal developing myelosuppression.
- Report signs of jaundice, yellowing of eyes, clay-colored stools or dark urine, which may signal developing hepatic dysfunction.
- Report a continued cough or shortness of breath, which may signal developing pulmonary fibrosis.

Clients should also be advised that readjusting lifestyle may be necessary to cope with the side effects of chemotherapy. They should be instructed to pace themselves according to their energy levels and allow time for rest throughout the day. Between treatments it is also important to note that they may not have the same amount of energy they did before the treatment. While many clients do not have any adverse effects, others may experience a life-threatening toxicity. Nursing care of the client receiving chemotherapy requires not only a thorough understanding of the drugs used to destroy the cancer but also skills in helping clients and families cope with the side effects.

Biologic Response Modifiers

Biologic response modifiers (BRMs) are agents that stimulate the body's natural immune system to control and destroy malignant cells. Most BRMs are still being evaluated in trial studies. Biotherapy is used after surgery, radiation, and chemotherapy have removed the bulk of the tumor. Some agents currently being investigated include interferons, monoclonal antibodies, interleukin-2, tumor necrosis factor, BCG, and colony stimulating factors. Side effects are usually less severe than those seen in chemotherapy. They may include fever, malaise, myalgias, and headaches. Anaphylactic reaction can occur.

Bone Marrow Transplantation (BMT)

Bone marrow transplantation is used for cancers that respond to high doses of chemotherapy or radiation therapy. The treatment involves aspirating and storing a fraction of bone marrow, exposing the client to high dose drug therapy or total body irradiation, and then reinfusing the bone marrow after the treatment is complete.

Bone marrow can be obtained from one of three possible sources. The client can be transplanted with his or her own marrow (autologous), marrow taken from an identical twin (syngeneic), or that taken from a histocompatibly matched donor, preferably a sibling (allogeneic).

According to Otto (1991), the cost of BMT is high. Client expenses may range from $100,000 to $200,000.

The average length of hospital stay is thirty-five to forty days. Complications can be life threatening and include infection, bleeding, GI effects, renal insufficiency, veno-occlusive disease (deposits of fibrin obstruct venules of liver), and graft-versus-host disease (new bone marrow cells recognize environment as foreign and try to destroy the host). Clients undergoing autologous BMT do not experience graft-versus-host disease.

▶ SELECTED CANCER DISORDERS

▶ LUNG CANCER

According to the American Cancer Society, lung cancer is the leading cause of cancer death for men and women. It accounts for 25 percent of all cancer deaths in the United States. Approximately 80 percent of all cases are attributed to cigarette smoking. Prognosis is usually poor, with only 13 percent of clients surviving five years. The four types of primary cancers are squamous cell carcinoma, adenocarcinoma, large cell undifferentiated cancer, and oat cell or small cell carcinoma. The most common sites for metastases are the brain, bone, liver, cervical lymph nodes, adrenal glands, and kidneys. Early detection is uncommon as few symptoms occur at the onset. Chronic cough, dull chest pain, and a change in the odor and volume of sputum are the most common early symptoms. Medical management may consist of surgery, radiation therapy, and chemotherapy, depending on the type and extent of the disease. Surgery is usually indicated for early nonsmall cell carcinomas. Radiation is most often used for palliation of symptoms. Aggressive chemotherapy has helped improve survival rates. Chemotherapy agents commonly administered for the treatment of lung cancer include combinations such as:

- Cyclophosphamide, doxorubicin, methotrexate, and procarbazine
- Etoposide and cisplatin
- Mitomycin, vinblastine, and cisplatin.

▶ COLORECTAL CANCER

Colorectal cancer has the third highest rate of mortality. The American Cancer Society estimates that colorectal cancer caused 56,000 deaths in the United States in 1994. Incidence increases with age. Approximately 94 percent of all cases occur after age fifty. It is more common among higher socioeconomic groups. Etiological factors have not been determined but diets have been suspected. Individuals at greater risk include those with a family history of the disease and those with chronic bowel diseases. Past research indicates that the Guaiac test, a fecal occult blood test, can help reduce colorectal cancer mortality (Mandel, 1993). Symptoms vary according to tumor location. Two-thirds of all colorectal cancers occur in the lower sigmoid colon and the rectum. The most common symptoms are rectal bleeding, followed by bowel changes, abdominal pain or cramping, unexplained weight loss, and anemia. The liver is the most common site of metastases followed by the lung. Prognosis is dependent on the extent of the disease. Surgery is usually the treatment of choice. It is usually done in combination with radiation. Chemotherapy is generally reserved for clients with advanced disease. The drug of choice for treatment is 5-fluorouracil or 5-FU (Adrucil).

▶ BREAST CANCER

Breast cancer is the second major cause of cancer death in women. Statistics indicate one woman in ten will develop breast cancer sometime during her life. The American Cancer Society estimates 182,000 new cases were diagnosed in the United States in 1994. Less than 1 percent of all breast cancers occur in men. According to the 1994 estimates, about 1,000 new cases of breast cancer were diagnosed in men. The five-year survival rate is 93 percent for localized cancer, 72 percent for cancer that has spread regionally and 18 percent for those who have distant metastases. Elderly women have twice the incidence. The key to cure is early detection through physical examination, mammography, and breast self-examination. Most breast malignancies occur in the upper outer quadrant. A painless mass or thickening is the most common presenting symptom. Women at greater risk include those with a strong family history of the disease, early menarche or late menopause, or a first full-term pregnancy after the age of thirty. Other factors are obesity, a high-fat diet, and long-term estrogen therapy. Diagnosis is done by biopsy. Common sites of metastases are bone, liver, lung, and brain. Stages 1 and 2 clients are usually treated by surgery and radiation. Stage 3 clients have a poorer prognosis and are not good candidates for curative surgery. Clients with metastases usually require chemotherapy with or without **radiotherapy**. Common chemotherapy drugs include multiple agents such as cyclophosphamide, methotrexate, and 5FU. Tamoxifen is often administered to women who have estrogen receptor-positive tumors.

▶ GYNECOLOGICAL CANCERS

The incidence of gynecological cancers is increasing. According to Belcher (1992), they account for 15 percent of all cancers in women. Fortunately, most are highly curable if detected early. Most are linked with lifestyle behaviors such as obesity, smoking, sexually transmitted diseases, and early age of first intercourse.

The most preventable gynecological neoplasm is cervical cancer. A major factor in the development of cancer of the cervix is one's sexual habits. Sexually transmitted disease, particularly the human papilloma virus (HPV), is a significant factor. According to Otto (1991), some 15 percent of all women who have genital herpes will develop dysplasia or cancer *in situ*. Other factors associated with cervical cancer include: early age at first intercourse, history of multiple sexual partners, and women whose mothers used diethylstilbestrol (DES) during pregnancy. The most common sign of cervical cancer is abnormal bleeding. The bleeding progresses from a thin, watery, blood-tinged discharge to frank bleeding. Contact bleeding may also occur after intercourse. Advanced disease is indicated by odor, pain in the lower back and groin, difficulty voiding, hematuria, and rectal bleeding. The Pap smear is the key to early detection. Promotion of regular pelvic exams and education regarding risk are essential. Medical management is based on the stage of the disease. (Refer to Chapter 31 for more information on cervical cancer staging.)

Endometrial cancer is the most common gynecological cancer. It occurs primarily in post-menopausal women. Classic symptoms include vaginal bleeding and lumbosacral, hypogastric, or pelvic pain. Women with advanced disease may develop jaundice, **ascites** (excess fluid in peritoneal cavity), respiratory difficulty, and bowel obstructions. Since endometrial cancer occurs mostly in postmenopausal women, estrogen stimulation unopposed by progesterone is thought to be implicated. Prolonged use of estrogen without added progestin during menopause increases the risk of occurrence. There are no tests for premalignant conditions of the uterus. Treatment options include surgery, pre- or postoperative chemotherapy, hormone manipulation, and radiation. Internal radiation implants are typically used for lesions that have extended beyond the pelvic wall. External therapy is often given first to shrink the tumor and increase the effectiveness of the implant. Special applicators are used to insert the radiation source into the pelvis as shown in Figure 15-5.

Ovarian cancer causes more deaths than any other gynecological cancer. It is difficult to detect early, as signs and symptoms do not appear until the disease has advanced. The cause of the disease is unknown. No specific test can be performed for early detection, although CA-125, a possible tumor marker is sometimes utilized in diagnostic evaluation. Symptoms such as nausea, change in bowel habits, urinary frequency, and vague abdominal and pelvic discomfort occur with advanced disease. Unexplained weight gain, especially around the waist, can be a common symptom. Diagnosis usually occurs with an exploratory

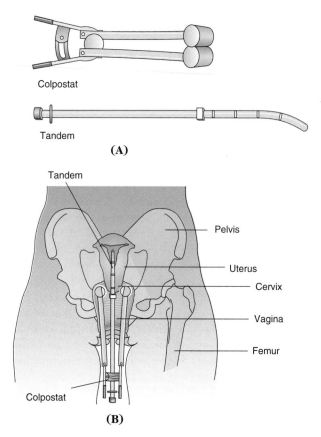

Colpostat

Tandem

(A)

Tandem

Pelvis

Uterus

Cervix

Vagina

Femur

Colpostat

(B)

FIGURE 15-5   Radium implant devices: **(A)** Colpostat and tandem; **(B)** Shows insertion of radium implant device.

laparotomy. Medical management is related to the stage of disease. A total abdominal hysterectomy with a bilateral salpingo-oophorectomy is done for most stages of the disease. Radioactive isotopes may be used after surgery and numerous chemotherapy agents may be tried.

The American Cancer Society indicates the overall five-year survival rate for cervical cancer is 67 percent, endometrial cancer 83 percent, and ovarian cancer 41 percent.

▶ PROSTATE CANCER

Prostate cancer is the second leading cause of cancer deaths in men. According to 1994 estimates by the American Cancer Society, 200,000 new cases were diagnosed. Unfortunately, incidence and mortality are currently increasing. Incidence increases with age as 80 percent of all prostate cancers are diagnosed in men over age sixty-five. Rectal examination and PSA-serum level are the most effective screening tools. Most prostatic cancers are adenocarcinomas, slow growing tumors, that spread via the lymphatics. Early

symptoms include dysuria, a weak urinary stream, and urinary frequency. Treatment depends on the extent of the disease and the age of the client. Radical surgery and radiation therapy may be done. Hormonal agents such as diethylstilbestrol (DES), goserelin acetate (Zoladex) or leuprolide acetate (Lupron) may be used to counteract the production of androgen dependent hormones. Systemic chemotherapy has not proven very effective in the treatment of prostate cancer. However, it may be used for those clients who fail to respond to hormone manipulation. Unfortunately, response is limited. Overall five-year survival rates are 78 percent.

▶ TESTICULAR CANCER

Although testicular cancers account for one percent of all cancer in men, they are the most common cancers in young men between the ages of fifteen and thirty-five. According to Otto (1991), advances in treatment have made a cure rate as high as 90 percent. The etiology is unknown but the incidence is higher in men with undescended testicles and those whose mothers have taken hormones during pregnancy. A small, hard painless lump is usually the first symptom noted. Sensations of heaviness, sudden fluid accumulation in the scrotum, or perineal discomfort can also occur. Monthly testicular self-examination is recommended for early detection. Cisplatin (Platinol) is the chemotherapy drug of choice. It may be used in combination with drugs such as vinblastine sulfate (Velban), bleomycin sulfate (Blenoxane), etoposide VP-16 (VePesid), cyclophosphamide (Cytoxan), doxorubicin hydrochloride (Adriamycin), and dactinomycin (Cosmegen). Surgery and radiation can also be initiated. Fertility issues are a concern.

▶ SKIN CANCER

Skin cancer is the most common form of cancer and the most curable. The most common types are squamous cell carcinoma, basal cell carcinoma, and malignant melanoma. Approximately two-thirds are basal cell carcinomas. Fortunately this type grows slowly and does not metastasize. The American Cancer Society estimates over 700,000 cases of basal or squamous cell cancers occur yearly. The most serious type is malignant melanoma. This cancer represents about 3 percent of all skin cancers but accounts for about 75 percent of skin cancer deaths. An estimated 9,200 deaths will occur in 1994—6,900 from malignant melanoma and 2,300 due to other skin cancers.

The primary risk factor in skin cancer development is exposure to the ultraviolet rays of the sun. Light-haired, fair-skinned, light-eyed individuals are more susceptible. Tanning booths and sun lamps are also sources of ultraviolet rays. The use of sunscreen (SPF 15 or higher) and protective clothing can provide protection. People who work outdoors such as farmers, and those who sunbathe are at highest risk for developing skin cancer.

Other symptoms include changes in the size, color, or surface of moles or birthmarks (see Figure 15-6). Routine self-examination of the skin is recommended for early detection. For more information on skin cancer, refer to Chapter 23, Integumentary Disorders.

▶ LEUKEMIA

The American Cancer Society projected 28,600 new cases of leukemia in the United States in 1994. Although often thought of as primarily a childhood disease, it strikes more adults (26,000) than children (2,600). Leukemia strikes both sexes and all ages. An estimated 19,100 leukemic deaths occurred in 1994.

Leukemia is not a single disease entity, but several diseases involving blood-forming tissues of the body such as the spleen, lymphatic system, and bone marrow. Causes of most cases are unknown. Persons with Down Syndrome and certain other genetic abnormalities have a higher incidence. It has also been linked to excessive exposure to ionizing radiation, chemicals such as benzene, and certain types of viruses.

Fatigue, malaise, weight loss, and anorexia are early

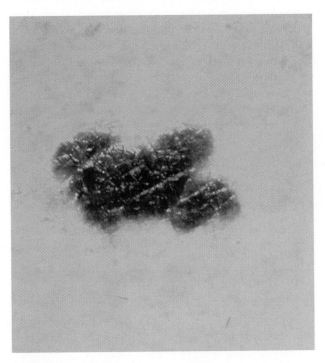

FIGURE 15-6 The signs of melanoma. (*Courtesy of the American Academy of Dermatology.*)

symptoms. Diagnosis is confirmed by blood studies and biopsy of the bone marrow.

Chemotherapy is the most effective method of treating leukemia. Different institutions and different physicians vary the agents used. Typical agents include, L-asparaginase (Elspar), busulfan (Myleran), chlorambucil (Leukeran), cyclophosphamide (Cytoxan), cytarabine (Cytosar-U), daunorubicin (Cerubidine), melphalon (Alkeran), methotrexate (Mexate), prednisone (Deltasone), and vincristine sulfate (Oncovin). Since severe bone marrow suppression is a major problem, transfusions of blood components and antibiotics are used as supporting treatments. Bone marrow transplantation may also be initiated. For more information on leukemia, refer to Chapter 22, Blood and Lymph Disorders.

▶ LYMPHOMAS

Lymphomas are malignancies of lymphoid tissue. They are classified as Hodgkin's disease and non-Hodgkin's lymphoma. The American Cancer Society estimates for 1994 indicate 52,900 new cases of lymphoma, including 7,900 cases of Hodgkin's disease and 45,000 non-Hodgkin's lymphoma. According to Lundquist and Stewart (1994), the classification of lymphomas into these groups is made by the recognition of the Reed-Sternberg cell. Its presence identifies Hodgkin's disease; its absence identifies non-Hodgkin's disease.

Non-Hodgkin's lymphoma is almost four times more common than Hodgkin's disease. It is more prevalent in older adult populations. Clients with immunodeficiency are at increased risk, including those with acquired immunodeficiency syndrome (AIDS) and those undergoing organ transplantation. Signs and symptoms are dependent on the site of involvement. Painless, superficial adenopathy is a common feature. Approximately 80 percent have enlarged cervical lymph nodes but axillary or inguinal nodes may also be enlarged. In contrast to Hodgkin's disease, non-Hodgkin's clients have generalized lymphadenopathy. They may also have symptoms of fever, night sweats, nausea, anorexia, weight loss, back pain, and vague abdominal discomfort. Chemotherapy is the treatment of choice. Early stage disease can also be treated with radiation. The overall survival rate for non-Hodgkin's lymphoma is 52 percent.

According to Erickson (1994), 75 percent of clients diagnosed with Hodgkin's disease will be cured. The cause of Hodgkin's disease is unknown. Diagnosis is made only by biopsy. Clients usually present with painless, superficial adenopathy. The enlarged nodes are usually located in the neck and supraclavicular regions. Fever, night sweats, and weight loss may also be noted. The disease spreads in a predictable pattern, first involving adjacent lymph nodes and viscera, then moving to distant organs such as the liver, spleen, and bone marrow. Early stages are treated with radiation therapy alone. Combination chemotherapy such as (MOPP) mechlorethamine, vincristine sulfate (Oncovin), procarbazine, and prednisone or (ABVD) doxorubicin (Adriamycin), bleomycin, vinblastine, and dacarbazine (DTIC-Dome) are given in cycles.

▶ SYMPTOM MANAGEMENT

Cancer clients undergoing treatment experience a variety of secondary problems. One of the most important responsibilities of the oncology nurse is to develop nursing interventions to manage these problems.

▶ Bone Marrow Dysfunction

Cancer treatments kill both malignant cells and normal cells in bone marrow. Blood counts should be monitored carefully during and after treatment.

A low white cell count increases the risk of infection. A decreased neutrophil count, less than $500/mm^3$, is an indicator that special infection prevention measures should be initiated. Scrupulous handwashing is the most effective method of controlling bacterial infection. Personnel should maintain strict asepsis when changing dressings or doing invasive procedures. Clients should avoid contact with anyone who is ill. Antimicrobial soaps should be used for bathing the clients. The skin and mucous membranes should be inspected daily for signs of infection. Vital signs should be taken every four hours, and the client observed for fever and chilling.

Clients with a platelet count of less than $50,000/mm^3$ should be monitored for bleeding. Their skin should be inspected for bruises or petechiae daily. Shaving should be done with an electric razor. Stool and urine should be monitored for occult blood. The nurse should observe the client for bleeding from the vagina, rectum, nose and mouth, as well as venipuncture sites. If bleeding does occur, pressure should be applied to the site for five minutes. Any bleeding that does not stop in five minutes should be reported. A soft toothbrush may be recommended for oral care. Aspirin should not be given.

▶ Nutritional Problems

Two-thirds of the people with cancer will develop **cachexia**, a marked state of malnutrition. It begins early in tumor development, even before weight loss

occurs. Cachexia appears to be tumor induced. Nutritional problems that contribute to cachexia include anorexia, altered taste sensation, nausea, vomiting, stomatitis, and dysphagia. Anorexia is generally recognized as the major precipitating factor. These problems can be caused by a combination of factors, among which are adverse reactions to drugs, effects of chemotherapy and radiotherapy, tumors obstructing portions of the gastrointestinal tract, emotional distress, or an inability to digest food. Hallmarks of malnutrition are 10 percent or greater weight loss or a serum albumin level less than 3.4 g/dL. Clients unable to take solid food for long periods of time may be given enteral or total parenteral nutrition (TPN).

▶ Anorexia

Anorexia, loss of appetite, is a common complaint. It is generally best for cancer clients to eat small, frequent high-calorie meals. Nurses should attempt to determine the client's likes and dislikes. Highly seasoned foods help increase taste. Clients should be encouraged to eat when feeling best. Weight should be monitored.

▶ Nausea and Vomiting

These usually occur within three to four hours after chemotherapy is administered and may last up to seventy-two hours. According to Camp-Sorrell (1991), antiemetics should be given at least thirty minutes before chemotherapy and continued twenty-four to seventy-two hours afterwards depending on the drug (see Table 15-6). Small frequent feedings of complex carbohydrates may be beneficial. Liquids should be given thirty to sixty minutes before eating. Cool, bland foods are more easily tolerated. Foods with strong odors should be avoided. Frequent mouth care can help remove the taste of chemotherapy so that the client feels like eating.

▶ Altered Taste Sensation

This probably occurs because cancer cells release substances that stimulate bitter taste buds, causing

Table 15-6

COMMONLY USED ANTIEMETICS	
prochlorperazine	(Compazine)
metoclopramide	(Reglan)
trimethobenzamide hydrochloride	(Tigan)
ondansetron hydrochloride	(Zofron)
lorazepam	(Ativan)

some clients to have a bitter or metallic taste in their mouth. Some find they no longer enjoy the taste of red meat and others say they have an aversion to sweets. Tart foods usually enhance flavors. Many foods taste better if they are cold or at room temperature. Plastic utensils, rather than metal ones, may help reduce metallic taste.

▶ Stomatitis

Stomatitis occurs in half of cancer clients receiving treatment. It usually occurs seven to fourteen days after chemotherapy administration and lasts two to three weeks. To minimize stomatitis, assess for early signs and symptoms such as edema, ulceration, erythema, excessive saliva, and infection. If the client is receiving a chemotherapy drug that is known to cause stomatitis (methotrexate, for example) give oral care at least four times a day.

Rough, chewy foods as well as acidic foods should be avoided. Straws are beneficial since food can be taken in the back of the mouth and swallowed. Popsicles and other frozen fruit bars sometimes help numb and lessen pain. Commercial mouthwashes containing alcohol should be avoided. Saline rinses may be helpful. If the client has dentures they should be removed at night. Viscous Xylocaine rinses can be ordered for pain. Lemon and glycerine swabs should not be used since lemon may be irritating to mouth lesions. Teach the client to use a soft bristle toothbrush and to avoid flossing if bleeding or discomfort occurs. The client should avoid tobacco products and alcohol because of their drying effects.

▶ Dysphagia

Dysphagia or difficulty swallowing, occurs with radiation and typically in esophageal cancers.

Artificial saliva may be ordered for severe dryness. A softer diet may be prescribed along with nutritional supplements. Dry foods such as toast can scratch the delicate tissues of the throat. Food pureed in a blender may be easier to tolerate. Clients should take plenty of time to chew and swallow.

▶ Pain

Approximately 60 percent to 90 percent of all individuals with progressive malignancy will experience pain. The pain may be acute but it is more likely to be chronic (greater than three months' duration). Usually, pain does not occur until the advanced stages of the disease are reached. The most common causes of pain are metastatic bone disease, venous or lymphatic obstructions, or nerve compression.

Pain can have profound effects on a cancer client. It can cause anxiety, depression, feelings of helplessness as well as physical discomfort. It can affect the client's sleeping habits, eating patterns, work, family, and social relationships. Ultimately, pain can affect the client's quality of life.

In recent months, the federal government has taken steps toward ensuring that cancer pain can be treated. The Agency for Health Care Policy and Research (AHCPR) has developed Cancer Pain Guidelines for clients, family members, and health care professionals. Some points emphasized by the guidelines include the following:

- Cancer pain can be managed effectively through relatively simple means in up to 90 percent of cancer clients in the United States. Skin patches, slow-release tablets, and client-controlled pumps are now available to complement standard drugs.
- The mainstay of pain assessment is the client self-report. Since there is no test for pain, the nurse must respect the client's report of pain and regard it as the single most reliable indicator. Kohr (1995) recommends using a verbal assessment measurement tool using a scale 0 to 5, a precise description to each number and a pain intensity flow sheet, to monitor medication effectiveness. For example 0–no pain; 1 is mild; 2 is moderate or discomforting; 3, severe or distressing; 4, horrible or incapacitating; and 5 is excruciating or unbearable pain.
- Use the simplest dosage schedules and least invasive pain management modalities first. Nonnarcotics are the first step in the analgesic ladder. They should be tried first for mild to moderate pain. Since much of cancer pain is due to inflammation, many of the nonnarcotics used are potent, anti-inflammatory drugs. These drugs are helpful in pain relief because they inhibit prostaglandins. The release of prostaglandins in tissues causes pain, edema, and inflammation. Anti-inflammatory drugs decrease pain and inflammation.
- Morphine is the most commonly used opioid for moderate to severe pain because it is available in a wide variety of dosage forms, it has well-characterized pharmacokinetics and pharmacodynamics, and is relatively low cost. Morphine can be given orally, subcutaneously, intramuscularly, intravenously, rectally, and intraspinally. It can also be given in sustained-release preparations. Since needs vary with cancer pain, there is no limit to the dosing of morphine. A major reason for inadequate pain control is the exaggerated fear of respiratory depression. This rarely occurs in the cancer client.
- Health care providers should prevent pain rather than trying to treat it. Analgesics work better when given regularly around the clock before pain becomes severe. A major nursing responsibility is to teach the client to request pain medication before the pain becomes severe. When ordered around the

clock, the nurse should not hesitate to wake the client. A combination of drugs often achieve better pain control.

Noninvasive pain relief techniques may also be useful in pain management. They include cutaneous stimulation (heat, cold, massage), transcutaneous electrical nerve stimulation (TENS), relaxation techniques, imagery, and hypnosis. Most of these techniques are inexpensive and easy to perform. They have few side effects and can usually be done in any environment. They also give the client control over the treatment of pain. Although not everyone will be successful with these measures, it is worthwhile to attempt them before using invasive techniques.

If pain control cannot be achieved with noninvasive techniques or medications, neurosurgical procedures such as nerve blocks may be done.

▶ Fatigue

Fatigue may occur as a direct result of the cancer or it may occur because of anemia, chronic pain, stress, depression, insufficient rest, and nutritional intake. The etiology of fatigue is not well understood. It is often related to side effects of medications and treatments such as radiation therapy. Fatigue may contribute to problems of the client complying with the treatment regimen.

Frequent rest periods should be provided for the client. The nurse should assess for the presence and pattern of fatigue. Planning will allow the client to be active during times when energy levels are higher, which may restore a greater sense of control. The nurse should evaluate factors that increase or decrease fatigue, such as nutritional intake. Blood counts should be monitored for anemia.

▶ Alopecia

Alopecia, thinning or loss of hair, may be induced by chemotherapy or radiation treatments. The extent of hair loss depends on the dose and duration of the therapy. Scalp hair is commonly affected but pubic, axillary and facial hair, even eyebrows and eyelashes, may also be affected. The treatments cause hair loss by interfering with the growth processes in the hair follicle. This results in weakening the hair shaft thereby causing the hair to break off at the surface of the scalp. Hair loss usually begins two to three weeks after the initial treatment. Drug induced alopecia is not permanent. Hair usually begins to grow within eight weeks after completing treatment. The color and consistency of the hair may change. While health professionals view alopecia as a minor problem, for many clients it

may pose a major threat to body image. Clients should be encouraged to buy a wig or hairpiece before treatment actually begins so the replacements will match normal hair. Scarfs or bandanas may also be worn to help clients cope with the change in body image.

▶ Odors

Unpleasant odors emanating from the cancer client may be a source of embarrassment. These odors are usually associated with drainage or exudates and incontinence. Fortunately, meticulous nursing care can eliminate most offending odors. Soiled linens, drainage pads, and dressings should be changed immediately. They should be washed or discarded. The client's skin should be washed gently with soap and warm water. Protective creams may be used if the areas are not receiving radiation. Room deodorizers can be helpful but should be used cautiously as many clients experience nausea with such odors. Placing a drop of oil of wintergreen or oil of cloves on a cotton ball near the ventilation system can sometimes add a light freshness to the environment.

▶ Dyspnea

Half of all clients with terminal cancer experience dyspnea. There are many possible causes such as development of fluid in the chest, infection such as pneumonia, fibrosis due to radiation, or anemia. Lungs should be auscultated every four hours. Oxygen may be ordered. Fluid may be drained by an invasive procedure called a thoracentesis. High-Fowler positioning helps maximize ventilation. The nurse should plan care to keep activity to a minimum to balance oxygen requirements with oxygen supply. The oxygen status can be monitored with a pulse oximeter. The nurse should report a sustained reading less than 90 percent. The nurse should avoid pulling the privacy curtain or shutting the client's door unless absolutely necessary since it may reduce air flow and create more anxiety.

▶ Bowel Dysfunctions

Cancer clients frequently exhibit changes in bowel patterns. Constipation, diarrhea, and bowel obstructions are common elimination disorders.

Factors frequently causing diarrhea include radiation therapy, chemotherapy, antibiotics, tube feedings, hyperosmolar dietary supplements, stress, and fecal impactions. Clients can develop fluid and electrolyte imbalances from constant diarrhea. If the client is receiving a chemotherapy drug that is known to cause diarrhea (such as fluorouracil [Adrucil] or doxorubicin hydrochloride [Adriamycin]), encourage a low residue diet. The nurse should instruct the client to avoid foods that stimulate the gastrointestinal tract such as warm liquids and coffee.

The perineum should be kept clean and dry after each loose stool. Anal irritations should be treated cautiously with agents such as heat lamps, ointments, and cornstarch. These may be contraindicated in clients receiving radiation therapy. Signs of fluid and electrolyte imbalance such as thirst, dry mucous membranes, and decreased skin turgor should be noted. The potassium level should be monitored. The nurse should measure and record the amount, frequency, and characteristics of all client bowel movements. Antidiarrheal medications such as Lomotil or Imodium should be given for every loose stool. Sitz baths will help soothe sore or broken-down tissues.

Constipation results from decreased motility of the colon. It is frequently caused by chemotherapy, narcotic analgesic, or lack of activity. Nurses should monitor and record the frequency of the client's bowel movements. Constipation can be an early sign of vincristine toxicity. Fluid consumption may be encouraged and stool softeners given daily. Clients at risk for constipation should be started on a high fiber diet with increased intake of bran and prune juice.

Bowel obstructions occur more commonly in advanced abdominal malignancies. It should always be suspected if the client has received radiation or has adhesions from prior surgeries. Symptoms include nausea, vomiting, and abdominal pain. Surgery may be required to relieve the obstruction.

► Pathologic Fractures

Pathologic fractures are a major problem in cancers that metastasize to bone. These cancers weaken the bone to the point that normal activities can cause painful breaks. Limbs should be supported and handled gently. Special devices such as splints may be used for extra protection. Extreme care should be taken when moving clients. Weight bearing restrictions may be ordered.

► Ascites

Abdominal cancers may cause ascites or fluid to accumulate in the abdomen. Clients may experience abdominal swelling and difficulty breathing. Symptoms may be treated temporarily with an invasive procedure called a paracentesis. A small plastic tube is advanced through the abdominal wall and the excess fluid is withdrawn. Sometimes chemotherapeutic drugs are instilled to try to prevent the fluid from returning. The nurse should visually assess the abdomen. A pro-

truding abdomen may be indicative of ascites as well as intestinal distention and enlarged organs. Abdominal girth should be measured daily at the umbilicus with a tape measure to monitor changes. The abdomen is then auscultated in all four quadrants. Gurgling bowel sounds heard every five to fifteen seconds indicate normal peristalsis. Decreased or absent bowel sounds may indicate peritonitis or paralytic ileus. The presence of fluid accumulation can be confirmed by percussing for shifting dullness. When a large amount of fluid is present the nurse may see fluid waves. Gentle palpation is used to detect pain and tenderness as well as abdominal masses. The nurse should carefully document any abnormal findings.

The nurse should weigh the client daily to monitor weight gain. Fluid consumption may be restricted. Good skin care, especially to the abdomen is essential. Fowler positioning helps maximize ventilation. Clients should be observed closely for electrolyte imbalance if large amounts of fluids are withdrawn by a paracentesis.

► ONCOLOGICAL EMERGENCIES

Medical emergencies occur in approximately 20 percent of advanced cancer clients. Early recognition and treatment can prevent irreversible complications and improve the quality of life. Four complications with which nurses should become familiar are hypercalcemia, spinal cord compression, superior vena cava syndrome, and cardiac tamponade.

► Hypercalcemia

Hypercalcemia occurs commonly and can be a potentially fatal complication if not detected early. It is found most often in clients with malignant tumors that metastasize to bone such as breast cancer. The condition occurs when the tumor destroys bone and the serum calcium level rises greater than 10.5 mg/dL[5]. The kidneys are unable to eliminate the excess calcium.

Early symptoms of hypercalcemia such as nausea, vomiting, constipation, and weakness may be overlooked. Later symptoms such as dehydration, renal failure, coma, and cardiac arrest may develop swiftly.

It is treated aggressively with intravenous normal saline and furosemide (Lasix). This increases the calcium excretion. Clients may also be given drugs to decrease bone reabsorption. The serum calcium levels should be monitored while on Lasix. Clients should be taught early symptoms so they can recognize a recurrence. These clients are also at risk for pathological fractures.

▶ *Spinal Cord Compression*

Spinal cord compression can result in permanent paralysis if not treated promptly. Cancer of the lung, breast, and prostate carry the greater risk of metastasizing to the spinal cord.

The chief symptom of metastasis to the spinal cord is back pain. The discomfort is aggravated by lying down, coughing, or moving. The pain may be relieved by sitting upright.

Treatment is aimed at reducing the tumor size so pressure on the spinal cord can be reduced. Radiation, surgery, and steroids may be given. Pain medications should be given frequently and clients should be supported carefully when transferring.

▶ *Superior Vena Cava Syndrome*

Superior vena cava syndrome is a collection of symptoms caused by an obstruction of the superior vena cava. It occurs more frequently with lung cancer and lymphomas. Typically clients experience dyspnea and swelling of the face and neck. They may also have edema in their upper extremities, chest pain, and a cough. Central nervous system symptoms such as headache, visual disturbances, and alteration in consciousness rarely occur. The goal of treatment is to reduce the tumor size. Radiation is usually ordered along with diuretics. The nurse should administer oxygen as ordered, and provide a calm, restful environment. The client should be encouraged to limit activities and lie in Fowler's position. Respirations should be carefully monitored. Lower extremities should not be elevated as this will increase venous return to an area already engorged.

▶ *Cardiac Tamponade*

Cardiac tamponade is caused by the formation of pericardial fluid, which reduces cardiac output by compressing the heart. Tumor metastasis to the pericardium is associated with cancers of the lung, breast, Hodgkin's disease, lymphoma, melanoma, gastrointestinal tumors, and sarcoma. Frequent symptoms of cardiac tamponade include a rapid, weak pulse, distended neck veins during inspiration, ankle or sacral edema, pleural effusion, ascites, enlarged spleen, lethargy, and altered consciousness. Treatment is aimed at aspirating the fluid constricting the heart (pericardiocentesis). The nurse will need to reassure the client, explain the procedure to remove the fluid and give medication for pain.

▶ PSYCHOSOCIAL PROBLEMS

Perhaps of all cancer problems, none is more challenging than the psychosocial problems clients encounter. The mere diagnosis of cancer invokes fear and misunderstanding. A myriad of emotions may be encountered initially. These may range from deep depression to denial and total refusal of treatment. Anxiety, sadness, and withdrawal are common. Some may feel that the disease is an intended punishment for some misguided deed. Every client will respond to the diagnosis differently, depending on acquired coping mechanisms and support systems.

Research has identified effective and ineffective coping mechanisms. Clients who face their cancer seeking information or sharing feelings tend to cope effectively. Conversely, those who submit to treatment and procedures without questions or who use small talk to avoid threatening issues tend to cope ineffectively.

Cancer not only affects the client but the family is also overwhelmed. The family members' response to the disease will have a significant impact on the client's coping. The client and family must face issues such as loss of control, changes in body image, and financial burdens. Cancer is an expensive illness. Hospitalization, outpatient treatments, and medications are very costly.

The nurse has several roles during this time. The client needs time and space to adjust to the diagnosis. Nurses should be there to offer support and reassurance. They should answer questions but not bombard the client with information. They may interpret information given by the physician, and help the client formulate questions to ask the physician. The nurse should also encourage the client to express feelings concerning fears regarding illness.

The initial treatment is very frightening for most cancer clients. Many have heard the myth that "the treatment is worse than the cure." Nurses can allay anxiety by giving information about the treatment's purpose, adverse reactions, and signs and symptoms to report to the physician. Explaining procedures and answering questions in simple language can help the client and family regain some control. Treatment modalities cause many discomforts, but if the client knows what to expect, the distress can generally be handled. Symptom management is critical to prevent lifestyle disruptions. The client may require special care at home and may feel he is a burden. Family caregivers may be angry that their needs go unmet. Clients may need medical equipment and help with transportation.

The terminal phase forces a complex set of problems. The client and family must face separation and impending death. Some families will demand that extraordinary measures be taken to keep the client alive. Some will search for meaning in life and experience a genuine closeness. Nurses should give the client and family privacy and time to share feelings. Perhaps the only psychosocial support the client needs is to have someone sitting by the bedside. Touch, especially at times when words are hard to find, can be the most comforting intervention one can offer.

As the client's condition deteriorates, physical needs become more pronounced. The nurse should focus on keeping the client comfortable and free from pain. Hospice care is designed to provide spiritual, emotional, and physical support during the final days of illness. The goal of hospice is to keep the client as comfortable as possible. Pain relief and symptom management are stressed. The focus is shifted from cure to care. Care may be given in an institution, but most hospice care is given in the home. Hospice care is medically managed and nurse coordinated. Members of the hospice team typically include a chaplain, physician, nurse, social worker, physical therapist, home health aide, and various volunteers. The team functions to assure that the client's plan of care is carried out and that family members receive adequate

support. The family is instructed in the area of care to be given. Bereavement counseling is offered to help the family deal with loss.

▶ Nursing Process

Assessment

The nurse must carefully gather information from multiple sources to assess the cancer client. The assessment begins with the client interview and assessment to determine subjective/objective data. Vital sign assessment is done along with a head to toe assessment of general systems. During the client interview the nurse will determine the client's perception of illness regarding treatment and prognosis. General health practices are assessed and health concerns are identified. The nurse will review past hospital records along with the current chart. Laboratory reports, biopsy results, treatment modalities, and comments from other health care professionals are perused. The nurse will also interview significant others to determine support systems.

▼ ▼

Possible nursing diagnoses for a client with cancer may include:

Nursing Diagnoses	Goals	Nursing Interventions
▶ Anxiety and fear related to cancer diagnosis.	The client will express anxieties and fears to family and/or health care givers.	Review the client's previous experience with cancer to determine any misconceptions based on past beliefs. Encourage the client to share feelings regarding the diagnosis to help detect coping strategies. Explain hospital routines and focus on the recommended treatment, its purpose, and potential side effects. Accurate descriptions that convey what the client can expect help ease fears associated with the unknown. A calm, reassuring environment can also enhance coping abilities.
▶ Grieving, anticipatory, related to potential loss of body function.	The client will express grief to family and/or health care givers.	Open, honest discussions can help the client cope with the situation. Be aware that mood swings, hostility, and other negative behaviors often occur. Discuss the loss of body function with the client. Ask what the loss of body function means to the client. Encourage the client to seek help and support from close family members.

(continued)

Nursing Diagnoses	Goals	Nursing Interventions
▶ *Nutrition, altered, less than body requirements related to side effects secondary to chemotherapy.*	The client will maintain body weight.	Encourage the client to eat a high-calorie, nutrient rich diet. Supplements may be useful. Some clients may benefit from frequent small meals and snacks. Foods high in protein such as cheese, fish, and poultry are also recommended. Provide oral hygiene before and after meals. Administer antiemetics approximately thirty minutes before meals. Mints, hard candy, and saltine crackers may help if the client complains of metallic taste. Nondietary interventions may include varying the surroundings, using small plates, eating at a table with friends, and minimizing food odors. Monitor intake and output along with daily weight to assess nutritional status.
▶ *Skin integrity, impaired, high risk for, related to chemotherapy and radiation*	The client will maintain skin integrity.	Assess skin frequently for side effects of cancer therapy. (A reddening or tanning effect may develop with radiation. Skin reactions such as rashes, pruritus and alopecia develop with chemotherapy.) Bathe the client's skin with lukewarm water and wash gently with soap. Skin often becomes sensitive during radiation treatments
▶ *Infection, high risk for, related to neutropenia secondary to side effects of chemotherapy.*	The client will remain free from infection.	Monitor vital signs at least every shift. White blood count should be monitored and protective isolation should be instituted if counts fall below 500/mm³. Educate the client, staff, and visitors in all aspects of infection prophylaxis. Thorough handwashing is the most important means of preventing and controlling the transmission of organisms. Since raw fruits, fresh flowers, and vegetables can transmit microbes, they should be eliminated. The client should not be exposed to anyone with an infection, recent vaccination, or recent exposure to a communicable disease. Visitors should be limited.
▶ *Injury, high risk for, related to bleeding tendencies secondary to side effects of chemotherapy.*	The client will prevent injury from bleeding.	Assess the client for signs of bleeding every shift (petechiae, ecchymoses, hematomas, bleeding gums, epistaxis, tarry stools, hematuria, frank bleeding or prolonged bleeding from puncture sites) because transfusions may be indicated. Monitor platelet count. Institute special precautions if the count falls below 50,000/mm³. Apply pressure to all puncture sites for three to five minutes. This prevents prolonged bleeding, which can cause damage to underlying tissues, such as nerves. Instruct the client to use a soft toothbrush or sponge for oral hygiene to prevent damage to oral mucosa which is susceptible to bleeding. Instruct the client to use an electric razor when shaving.

Nursing Diagnoses	Goals	Nursing Interventions
▶ *Fatigue related to analgesics, anemia, stress, and increased metabolism.*	The client will express less fatigue.	Plan frequent rest periods for the client to restore energy and schedule activities when the client has the most energy.
		Monitor nutritional intake as adequate nutrients are necessary to meet energy needs.
		Recognize that weakness places the client at increased risk for injury. Since fatigue may make activities of daily living difficult to complete, assistance may need to be provided.

▶ Evaluation

Each goal must be evaluated to determine how it has been met by the client.

▲ ▲

Sample Nursing Care Plan: The Client with Lung Cancer

Mr. John Smith is a fifty-four-year-old carpenter. He is admitted with pain over his left scapula radiating to the left arm. He describes having dyspnea and admits that he does have a productive cough. He denies any recent weight loss but does acknowledge experiencing extreme fatigue for the last two months. Mr. Smith has been a chronic smoker for twenty years. A chest x-ray reveals an area of density in the left lung. A needle biopsy confirms small cell lung cancer. A CT scan confirms extrathoracic involvement. His physician referred Mr. Smith to an oncologist for palliative chemotherappy. Mr. Smith is to receive his first treatment of cisplatin (Platinol) and etoposide (VePesid). Mr. Smith states that he is not sure about this treatment since it will not cure him and he does not know how he will keep breathing. He has never before been hospitalized.

Nursing Diagnosis 1: Anxiety related to unfamiliar surroundings and uncertainty regarding change in health status as evidenced by Mr. Smith's statement that he is not sure about this treatment and the fact that he has never before been hospitalized.

Goals	Nursing Interventions	Rationale	Evaluation
Mr. Smith will share his feelings regarding his diagnosis and treatment regimen.	Determine what the physician has told Mr. Smith and what conclusions he has reached. Encourage Mr. Smith to share feelings concerning cancer.	Accurate description of the treatment regimen can help decrease fear of the unknown. Verbalization can identify the source of misconception that often increases anxiety.	If the care plan is successful, Mr. Smith will: Share his feelings about his diagnosis and treatment regimen.
Mr. Smith will express less anxiety about being in the hospital.	Maintain frequent contact with Mr. Smith. Explain the hospital routine and what Mr. Smith should anticipate happening to him.	Provides reassurance that Mr. Smith is not alone. An unfamiliar environment increases anxiety.	Have less anxiety about the change in his health status and being in the hospital.

(continued)

Nursing Diagnosis 2 Gas exchange impaired, related to decreased lung capacity and increased secretions as evidenced by dyspnea, productive cough, and dense area in left lung.

Goals	Nursing Interventions	Rationale	Evaluation
Mr. Smith will report less dyspnea.	Monitor pulmonary status by ascultating breath sounds; checking rate, depth and pattern of respirations; evaluating skin color for cyanosis and monitoring pulse oximetry.	Provides information regarding changes of pulmonary status indicating improvement or onset of complications.	Maintain adequate ventilation with oxygen saturation > 90%.
	Position Mr. Smith in Fowler's position.	Promotes expansion of lungs and respiratory muscles.	
	Administer oxygen at prescribed level.	Supplemental oxygen corrects hypoxemia and provides oxygen for metabolic needs.	
	Administer narcotics with caution.	Narcotics can depress the respiratory center.	
	Monitor amount, color, and consistency of sputum.	Changes in sputum suggest infection or change in pulmonary status.	
	Plan care and treatments within Mr. Smith's tolerance.	Oxygen demands increase with activity.	

Nursing Diagnosis 3 Pain related to tumor growth and tissue destruction as evidenced by pain over his left scapula radiating to his left arm.

Goals	Nursing Interventions	Rationale	Evaluation
Mr. Smith will report less pain following pain relief measures.	Provide routine comfort measures such as repositioning and backrub.	Noninvasive pain relief techniques may be helpful in pain management.	Report less pain < 4 on a scale of 0 to 10.
	Teach Mr. Smith to request pain medication as pain begins.	Medication should be administered as soon as pain begins to keep the pain under control.	
	Have Mr. Smith rate pain on an scale of 0 to 10 (0 = no pain and 10 = worst pain).	The scale provides a method of evaluating the subjective experience of pain.	
	Teach Mr. Smith relaxation techniques.	Relaxation may decrease the perception of pain.	

| | Document Mr. Smith's response to the pain control regimen and adjust as needed. | Ongoing assessment of pain relief technique's effect is essential for optimal comfort. | |

Nursing Diagnosis 4 Fatigue related to chronic pain and dyspnea as evidenced by his description of dyspnea and extreme fatigue for two months.

Goals	Nursing Interventions	Rationale	Evaluation
Mr. Smith will report feeling less fatigued.	Plan care to allow for rest periods.	Frequent rest periods help conserve energy.	Exhibit less fatigue by having frequent rest periods daily.
	Assess for related factors such as nutritional imbalances, lack of sleep, and causes of stress.	Identification of contributing factors may reduce fatigue.	
	Have Mr. Smith rate fatigue on a scale of 0 to 10 (0 = not tired, 10 = total exhaustion) throughout a twenty-four hour period.	Identify peak energy and exhaustion times for planning activities to minimize energy output.	
	Teach energy conservation strategies such as plan ahead, set priorities, schedule rest periods, rest before a difficult task.	Conserving energy will decrease physical and psychologic stress.	

Nursing Diagnosis 5 Knowledge deficit related to chemotherapy treatment as evidenced by Mr. Smith's statement of not being sure about this treatment since it will not cure him.

Goals	Nursing Interventions	Rationale	Evaluation
Mr. Smith will increase his knowledge regarding his chemotherapy treatment.	Reinforce the oncologist's explanation of the treatment regimen.	Provides reassurance to Mr. Smith.	Cope adaptively with the chemotherapy regimen.
	Provide written information regarding chemotherapy and symptom management.	Written information provides reinforcement of teaching.	
	Discuss potential hair loss and regrowth with Mr. Smith.	Knowing what to expect decreases anxiety.	
	Explore potential impact of hair loss on Mr. Smith's self-image.	Knowing the impact allows Mr. Smith to plan interventions.	

(continued)

	Suggest the use of wigs and/or hats.	Suggestions can be a starting point for planning.	
	Reassure Mr. Smith that hair loss is a potential side effect of etoposide (VePesid) and is usually temporary.	Knowing the cause may make it easier to accept.	
	Discuss nausea and vomiting as potential side effects of cisplatin (Platinol) and etoposide (VePesid) and assure Mr. Smith that medication will be given to relieve the nausea and vomiting.	Knowing what may happen and that medications will be given relieves anxiety.	
	Discuss the potential for bone marrow depression with Mr. Smith.	Provides Mr. Smith with reasons for what may happen to him.	
	Monitor lab report of Mr. Smith's daily blood count.	Provides information of physiological response to treatment.	
	Advise Mr. Smith to avoid contact with crowds or persons who have any type of infections.	If Mr. Smith's blood count is depressed, he would be more susceptible to any infection.	
	Emphasize frequent handwashing.	Frequent handwashing is one of the best methods to prevent infections.	
	Encourage Mr. Smith to use an electric razor.	There is less chance of cutting himself with an electric razor.	
	Instruct Mr. Smith to report bruising or any bleeding especially from a body cavity as these are potential side effects of cisplatin (Platinol) and etoposide (VePesid).	Mr. Smith will know what to report to his physician.	

Nursing Diagnosis 6 Grieving, anticipatory, related to loss of body function as evidenced by Mr. Smith's statement that he does not know how he will keep breathing.

Goals	Nursing Interventions	Rationale	Evaluation
Mr. Smith will verbalize his loss and develop coping skills as he acknowledges his illness is terminal.	Provide opportunities for Mr. Smith to ventilate his feelings.	Such information helps the nurse detect Mr. Smith's coping strategies that helps him move through the stages of grief.	Resolve the reality of his diagnosis and prognosis.
	Answer all of Mr. Smith's questions honestly.	Open, honest discussions can help Mr. Smith cope with the situation.	
	Encourage Mr. Smith's participation in his care.	Gives Mr. Smith greater sense of control over his life.	
	Encourage family support and visiting by friends.	Assures Mr. Smith that he is not alone and provides time to discuss concerns openly.	
	Utilize appropriate referrals to professionals such as clergy as needed.	Facilitates the grief process and spiritual care.	

▶ **CASE STUDY**

Mr. John Dalton is a seventy-year-old male with a history of cancer of the prostate, which was treated with palliative hormones and radiation. His admitting diagnosis is adenocarcinoma of the prostate with widespread bone metastasis. Mr. Dalton is married and has one grown daughter who often helps with his care. His chief complaint is severe back pain. The physician has ordered intrathecal morphine sulfate and aspirin 10 gr. for pain relief.

The following questions will guide your development of a Nursing Care Plan for the case study.

1. List symptoms typically seen in clients diagnosed with prostate cancer.

2. Identify the population most at risk for developing prostate cancer.

3. List three possible risk factors for prostate cancer.

4. List two types of hormones used in the management of prostate cancer.

5. Discuss why the physician's orders include aspirin along with morphine sulfate. How do non-narcotic analgesics differ from narcotics?

6. Discuss why benzodiazepines should not be used for pain relief.

7. List the subjective and objective data the nurse would want to obtain.

8. When you walk into Mr. Dalton's room he greets you with a smile and continues talking and joking with his daughter. While assessing him, you note that his vital signs are normal. You ask him to rate his pain on a scale of 0 to 10. He pauses to think about it, then rates the pain at 8. In the chart you must record your nursing assessment by circling the appropriate number on the scale. Which number do you think you should circle?

9. Write three individualized nursing diagnoses and goals for Mr. Dalton.

10. Discuss which oncologic emergency Mr. Dalton is most likely to develop.

SUMMARY

- Cancer is the second most common cause of death in the United States.
- Most cancers are curable if treated early.
- Benign neoplasms are localized, encapsulated, and do not spread.
- Malignant neoplasms spread to neighboring tissues via blood and lymph.
- Biopsies are the most accurate diagnostic test for cancer.
- The most common medical treatments for cancer are surgery, radiation, and chemotherapy. They may be used alone or in combination.
- Surgery is the treatment of choice for early cancers.
- Chemotherapy is the treatment of choice for metastatic cancers. It is also the treatment most responsible for increasing the cancer cures in recent years.
- Lung cancer is the leading cause of cancer death in men and women. Eighty percent of all cases are related to smoking.
- Oncology nurses believe that quality of life, not quantity of life, is the ultimate goal for clients living with cancer.

Review Questions

1. The nurse carefully monitors the client's IV chemotherapy. Which is an early indicator that extravasation may be occurring?

   a. the fluid stops infusing
   b. edema is noted at the site
   c. blood returns when the bottle is lowered
   d. burning occurs at the site

2. A breast cancer client states that the doctor says he is going to prescribe hormone therapy. Which of the following hormones would probably be ordered?

   a. thyroxin
   b. parathormone
   c. progesterone
   d. testosterone

3. A cancer client develops a low white cell count. She is placed on neutropenic precautions. Which of the following menu selections would be the best choice?

   a. meat loaf, mashed potatoes, green beans, and fruit gelatin
   b. meat loaf, mashed potatoes, marinated carrots, and a garden salad
   c. meat loaf, mashed potatoes, chef salad, and tapioca
   d. meat loaf, mashed potatoes, green beans, fruit salad, and a cookie

4. As stomatitis develops, which would be the best nursing intervention to encourage?

   a. drink plenty of orange juice
   b. use lemon and glycerine swabs frequently
   c. brush teeth after eating and at bedtime
   d. rinse with commercial mouthwash as needed

5. Which nursing action should be encouraged when clients receive radiation?

   a. wash and dry the skin carefully and apply lotion
   b. tell the client not to bathe while she is receiving radiation
   c. tell the client not to apply deodorants or lotions while she is receiving radiation
   d. wash the skin with soap and apply baby powder

6. Due to excessive vomiting, the oral route of administration is not possible. Which of the following routes should the nurse consider first?

   a. intradermal
   b. rectal
   c. intramuscular
   d. intravenous

News Flash

A study from Sweden shows that tanning lamps and sunbeds increase the risk of developing malignant melanoma, the deadliest form of skin cancer. In a study of more than 1,000 people, those who used sunbeds or sunlamps one to three times a year had twice the risk of developing melanoma as those who never used the machines. Those who use them four to ten times a year had nearly four times the risk. And individuals under 30 years of age had over eight times the risk of melanoma as non-users. Despite studies showing the risk for skin cancer, 1 to 2 million Americans a day continue to use the machines in peak season." ("Tanning Machine Users Reported to Suffer More Melanomas." *Dermatology Nursing,* August, 1994, *6*(4), 280–281.)

MEDICAL TERMINOLOGY

carcin/o-	cancer
-oma	tumor of
carcinoma	a cancerous tumor
sarc/o-	flesh; connective tissue
sarcoma	cancer from or of the connective tissue
lys/o-	breakdown
lysis	a breakdown of cells
meta-	after, beyond
-stasis	controlling or stopping; standing or placing
metastasis	when a neoplasm moves beyond its original place in the body
neo-	new
-plasm	growth, development
neoplasm	a new growth of some kind
onc/o-	tumor
oncologist	a specialist who specializes in the study of tumors or oncology

Critical Thinking Questions

1. How would you respond if you were told you had cancer?

2. What are you doing to prevent cancer in your body?

CHAPTER
16
Caring for the Older Adult

Joan Fritsch Needham

LEARNING OBJECTIVES

Upon completion of this chapter the learner should be able to:
- Define key terms.
- Describe stereotypes associated with older adults.
- List the realities of aging.
- Compare the current biological theories of aging.
- Discuss the current psychosocial theories of aging.
- Describe key factors in health maintenance of the aging adult.
- Identify concerns associated with the aging process.
- Summarize the expected physiological changes of aging.
- Identify common disorders related to aging.
- Discuss nursing interventions for each disorder.

▶ *MAKING THE CONNECTION*

Refer to the topics in the following chapters to increase your understanding of caring for the older adult.

- **Chapter 5, Communications:** Geronotological Considerations, p. 76.
- **Chapter 9, Substance Abuse:** Gerontological Considerations, p. 157.
- **Chapter 13, Perioperative Nursing:** Age, p. 230; Gerontological Consideration, p. 239.
- **Chapter 14, Fluid, Electrolyte, and Acid-Base Balance:** Fluid Volume Deficit, p. 271.
- **Chapter 19, Respiratory Disorders:** Tuberculosis, p. 404; Chronic Obstructive Pulmonary Disease, p. 423.
- **Chapter 20, Cardiac Disorders:** Congestive Heart Failure, p. 481.
- **Chapter 21, Vascular Disorders:** Hypertension, p. 508.
- **Chapter 23, Integumentary Disorders:** Skin Cancer, p. 569; Shingles, Fig 23-6, p. 574

- **Chapter 26, Musculoskeletal Disorders:** Osteoporosis, p. 664; Osteoarthritis, p. 665.
- **Chapter 27, Nervous System Disorders:** Mental Status Examination (Figure 27-4), p. 689; Stages of Alzheimer's Disease (Table 27-6), p. 727.
- **Chapter 28, Sensory Disorders:** Cataracts, p. 760; Glaucoma, p. 762; Macular Degeneration, p. 769.
- **Chapter 30, Diabetes Mellitus:** Non-Insulin Dependent Diabetes Mellitus, p. 831.
- **Chapter 31, Female Reproductive Disorders:** Breast Cancer, p. 868.
- **Chapter 32, Male Reproductive Disorders:** Benign Prostatic Hypertrophy, p. 918.
- **Chapter 34, Digestive Disorders:** Constipation, p. 995.
- **Chapter 35, Urinary Disorders:** Incontinence, p. 1021; Infectious Disorders, p. 1022.

KEY ABBREVIATIONS

The following abbreviations and acronyms are used in this chapter:

AARP	American Association of Retired Persons
AD	Alzheimer's disease
BPH	benign prostatic hypertrophy
BUN	blood urea nitrogen
COPD	chronic obstructive pulmonary disease
ERT	estrogen replacement therapy
HIV	human immunodeficiency virus
IADL	instrumental activities of daily living
NIDDM	non–insulin-dependent diabetes mellitus
NIH	National Institutes of Health
ORIF	open reduction, internal fixation
PVD	peripheral vascular disease
RDA	recommended dietary allowance
RTI	respiratory tract infection
THA	total hip arthroplasty
TIA	transient ischemic attack
UTI	urinary tract infection

INTRODUCTION

Gerontology is the study of the effects of normal aging and age-related diseases on human beings. It is a general term used by all health care and social services disciplines. The specialty practice of caring for older adults was formerly referred to as **geriatric nursing**. Today the preferred term is **gerontologic nursing** to more accurately reflect an emphasis on healthy aging rather than illness. **Senescence** (aging) is a complex phenomenon that begins at conception, continues throughout the lifespan, and culminates with death. The phrase *older adult* is very subjective and usually refers to persons over the age of sixty-five.

The purpose of this chapter is to provide basic information about the process of aging, the physiological and functional changes that occur during aging, and nursing interventions designed to maintain health and prevent illness. Gerontologic nursing is practiced in hospitals, long-term care facilities, the client's home, clinics, and adult day centers. The aging population is steadily increasing and the demand for knowledgeable caregivers is growing.

DEMOGRAPHICS

There were 3.1 million people over the age of sixty-five in 1900. By 1994, there were 33.2 million people in this age group. It is predicted that by the year 2030, the number will reach 70.2 million (Figure 16-1). The most rapid increase is expected to occur in the years 2010 to 2030 when the "baby-boomers" reach age sixty-five.

CULTURAL STEREOTYPES

There are many stereotypes associated with aging and being old. Stereotypes are usually generated in an attempt to categorize people or to set standards that can be applied to large groups of people. As with most stereotypes they are often based on an individual's experience with persons in that group. Stereotypes may be true of some individuals but not of a collective group. Believing stereotypes influences the interactions between the older adult and caregivers. The caregiver may treat the older adult as a child in an old body, calling the person "honey" or "sweetie." This approach is demeaning and strips the individual of dignity. The elderly are a diverse group and deserve respect. They are "survivors" and can teach younger people much about living. Learning from the clients makes caring for older adults a rewarding and satisfying experience. The aging process is very individualized and independent of chronological age. The way in which a person ages is influenced by genetic makeup, the individual's lifestyle, the availability and quality of health care, and socioeconomic status. We do know that aging is universal, progressive, irreversible,

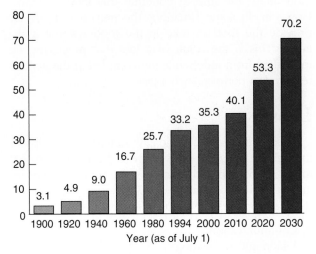

Number of persons 65 +: 1900 to 2030

FIGURE 16-1 Number of persons 65+ 1900–2030. (*From "A Profile of Older Americans," © 1995. The Administration on Aging and the AARP*)

and eventually results in death. There are certain expected physiological changes that occur with aging. However, there is considerable variation in the time of onset, the rate, and the degree of these changes.

MYTHS AND REALITIES

Myths are fictitious ideas. Myths about the elderly are abundant and do not reflect the reality of the aging population. Here are some common myths associated with aging. The following information is from *A Profile of Older Americans* based on data from the United States Bureau of the Census (American Association of Retired Persons [AARP], 1995).

- Myth: Senility is an expected result of aging.
  Reality: Senility is an outdated term once used to refer to any form of dementia that occurred in older people. Dementia is a result of disease and can affect adults of all ages and is not a natural consequence of aging.
- Myth: Incontinence is an expected result of aging.
  Reality: Incontinence is never normal. There are nursing interventions that can prevent or alleviate incontinence in many cases.
- Myth: The elderly are lonely and deserted.
  Reality: Sixty-seven percent of older noninstitutionalized persons live in a family setting. Sixty-six percent of older persons with living children live within thirty minutes of a child. Sixty-two percent have at least weekly visits and seventy-six percent talk on the phone at least weekly with children.
- Myth: Most people spend the last years of their lives in nursing homes.
  Reality: Five percent of the sixty-five and over population live in nursing homes. The percentage increases with age: one percent for persons sixty-five to seventy-four years, six percent of persons seventy-five to eighty-four years, and twenty-four percent of persons eighty-five and over.
- Myth: Older adults are no longer interested in sexuality or sexual activity.
  Reality: Sexuality is a life-long need. The elderly can be and are sexually active, regardless of age (Figure 16-2). Sexual functioning may be affected by changes in the reproductive systems, both sexes are capable of orgasmic experiences. Despite interest and desire, physiological or psychosocial problems may present barriers to sexual activity. In such situations, sexuality without coitus can provide love and intimacy.
- Myth: The elderly are financially impoverished.
  Reality: The median net worth of older households

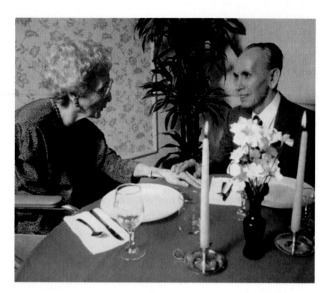

FIGURE 16-2 Sexuality is a life-long need and does not diminish with aging. (*Courtesy of Country Park Health Care Center, Long Beach, CA*)

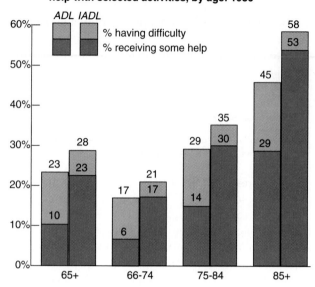

FIGURE 16-3 Percent of older Americans having difficulty and receiving help with selected activities, by age: 1986. (*From "A Profile of Older Americans," c. 1995. The Administration on Aging and the AARP*)

is $73,500. The poverty rate for older persons is 12.9%. Families headed by persons 65+ had a median income of $25,315 in 1992 (AARP, 1993).

- Myth: Sickness and aging are synonymous.
  Reality: In 1993, 28 percent of people over sixty-five assessed their health as poor compared to 8% of individuals under sixty-five. In 1993 there was an average of thirty-four days when usual activities were restricted because of illness or injury. Twenty-three percent of persons living in the community had health related difficulties with one or more ADL (activities of daily living). Twenty-eight percent had difficulty with one or more IADL (instrumental activities of daily living), Figure 16-3. ADL include bathing, dressing, eating, mobility, and using the toilet. IADL include shopping, preparing meals, managing money, using the telephone, and doing housework.

THEORIES OF AGING

At this time, no single theory of aging has been universally accepted by practitioners in gerontology. Aging is a complex issue that must take into account the psychosocial, cultural, and experiential aspects of living. Several biological theories of aging have been presented to explain the physiological and functional changes that are observed in older adults. Psychosocial theories of aging explain the behaviors and social interactions of older adults (Needham, 1993). These theories are summarized in Table 16-1.

SPECIAL CONSIDERATIONS

Maslow (1970) states that life satisfaction is based on needs fulfillment. Basic human needs are universal and are applicable to all age groups. The methods used to meet these needs change throughout life. For example, food is provided and fed to an infant by a significant other. During childhood the food must still be provided by others, but the child is able to self-feed. Adults are expected to provide for their nutritional needs in all respects. During old age, most individuals are able to continue this independence. However, in some situations the person can neither provide the food or take in the food without assistance. This is the result of a loss that precludes the individual from independently completing the actions required to perform such a task.

Losses

Older adults have generally suffered many losses through the years. Some losses are slight and require only minor adaptation. Other losses may have a significant impact on the life of the person. Physiological changes or disease processes may result in losses causing impaired:

- Communication
- Vision and/or hearing
- Mobility
- Cognition
- Psychosocial skills

Table 16-1

THEORIES OF AGING

Biological Theories

Title	Major Premise
Somatic Mutation Theory	Radiation or miscoding of enzymes causes changes in the DNA. Changes associated with aging are the result of decreased function and efficiency of the cells and organs.
Programmed Aging	The lifespan is programmed within the body cells. This genetic clock determines the speed with which the person ages and eventually dies.
Cross-Linkage or Collagen Theory	Collagen is the principal component of connective tissue and is also found in the skin, bones, muscles, lungs, and heart. Chemical reactions between collagen and cross-linking molecules cause loss of flexibility causing diminished functional mobility.
Immunity Theory	The thymus becomes smaller as people age. The ability to produce T cell differentiation decreases. This impairs immunologic functions and results in increased incidence of infections, neoplasms, and autoimmune disorders.
Stress Theory	The occurrence of stress throughout the lifetime causes structural and chemical changes in the body. These changes eventually cause irreversible tissue damage.

Psychological Theories

Title	Major Premise
Activity Theory	Roles and responsibilities change throughout a lifetime. Life satisfaction is dependent on maintaining an involvement with life by developing new interests, hobbies, roles, and relationships.
Disengagement Theory	There is decreased interaction between the older person and others in his/her social system. The disengagement is inevitable, mutual, and acceptable to both the individual and society.
Continuity Theory	Successful methods used throughout life for adjusting and adapting to life events are repeated. Characteristic traits, habits, values, associations, and goals remain stable throughout the lifetime regardless of life changes.

If the impairment is severe, the individual will lose some degree of independence. There is a cascading effect as one loss contributes to another. For example, a person with IDDM loses a driver's license due to impaired vision related to diabetic retinopathy. This restricts the individual's socialization, which, in turn, can increase feelings of loneliness and diminished self-esteem. The spouse may provide caregiving assistance, which allows the individual to remain in the home. If the spouse dies, the individual may have to move to an assisted living facility, thus losing the home as well as the spouse.

Health care professionals need to remember that persons who have lived a long time are survivors. They are often much stronger, more ingenious, and enterprising than they are given credit for. The strengths of each individual must be identified and utilized when planning care (Table 16-2).

HEALTH PROMOTION AND MAINTENANCE

Like all age groups, the elderly can do much to adopt a healthy lifestyle that will add quality to the remaining years.

Personal Hygiene

Being well-groomed enhances the self-esteem of older adults. There are adaptive devices and techniques that can be utilized for those who may need assistance with the activities of daily living. For example, a hand-held shower and a bath chair placed in the tub can simplify the bathing process. Handrails decrease the risk of falling in the tub. Because of the drying of the skin, it may be preferable to bathe or shower only two to three times a week, taking sponge baths in between. A gentle soap should be used sparingly for the bath followed with an application of moisturizing lotion. Instruct the individual to periodically inspect the skin during the bath for indications of skin breakdown, lumps, or changes in moles.

The hair also loses oil secretions. Shampooing once or twice a week is usually adequate. A simplified hair style may be helpful to someone who has difficulty raising the arms. The use of mild shampoos and conditioners enhances the texture of the hair.

Fingernails may become more brittle but require no special care. Keeping the nails short prevents accidental self-injury to fragile skin. Impaired circulation in the lower extremities is common in older adults. Special attention needs to be given to the care of the feet and lower extremities. Toenails frequently become thick and tough. Soaking the feet facilitates nail care. A podiatrist may be needed to cut and trim toenails on a regular basis. Persons with diabetes need explicit instructions on nail care. Follow these guidelines for foot care to avoid injury and impairment:

Table 16-2

EXAMPLES OF IDENTIFIED STRENGTHS OF OLDER ADULTS TO USE WHEN PLANNING CARE

- Cognitively healthy.
- Free of deficits or impairments or has successfully adapted to; is adequately compensating for the deficit or impairment.
- History of healthy lifestyle in regard to diet, sleep, stress management, exercise, and freedom from chemical abuse.
- Adequate functional ability to carry out ADL.
- Free of incapacitating physical discomfort and pain.
- Lives in physically safe environment.
- Feels secure in present environment.
- Knowledgeable and realistic about capabilities.
- Avoids dangerous situations, does not take unnecessary risks.
- Compliant with health care regime.
- Capable of managing own environment.
- Has an intact support system.
- Has satisfying relationships with others.
- Has opportunities for sexual expression.
- Has access to transportation.
- Has adequate functional mobility.
- Has successfully adapted to life changes and crises.
- Has relinquished roles as phases of life require and has replaced them with satisfying new roles.
- Has a pattern of successful mourning for losses.
- Participates in groups: church, community, hobbies.
- Family members respect each other and are willing to give and receive help when necessary.
- Utilizes successful problem-solving skills.
- Seeks information to improve situation.
- Gives evidence of initiative and self-confidence in abilities and judgment.
- Participates in self-care by making decisions and accepting responsibility for decisions.
- Has developed a well-defined value system.
- Accepts what cannot be changed.
- Uses assertive skills successfully.
- Has strong spiritual beliefs and finds comfort and strength in spiritual and religious practices.
- Embraces aging and takes advantage of the positive aspects and adapts to the negative aspects.
- Participates in healthy reminiscing and has few regrets for past life.
- Finds meaning and enjoyment in hobbies and activities.
- Experiences joy in nature, art, and music and has a well-developed sense of humor.

Assessment should include the identification of strengths as well as problems. Strengths are utilized to achieve or maintain optimal physical, mental, and emotional function.

- Discourage the client from using circular garters.
- Discourage smoking because it interferes with circulation.
- Avoid using the knee gatch on the bed.
- Avoid the use of heating pads or hot water bottles. The client may not feel temperatures that are too hot.
- Maintain body warmth. Make sure the client has warm clothes including well-fitting socks. Provide blankets for the bed.
- Prevent injury to the feet:
  - Instruct the client to wear shoes when out of bed.
  - Check to see that the shoes are in good repair and that they fit well.
  - Avoid pressure to the legs and feet from any source.
- Inspect the feet carefully during the bath or if the client complains of any discomfort in the feet. Promptly attend to any signs of inflammation, injury or circulatory problems:
  - Broken skin
  - Color change; redness, white, or cyanotic
  - Heat or coldness
  - Cracking between toes
  - Corns or calluses

The need for adequate oral care does not diminish with aging. Dental problems can result in poor eating habits and inadequate nutrition. Brushing and flossing two to three times daily, seeing the dentist every six months and eating a balanced diet are important for prevention and early detection of dental disease. Inadequate brushing and flossing leads to gingivitis which if untreated, progresses to periodontal disease. Periodontal disease is the major cause of tooth loss in older adults. Bacterial plaque builds up and adheres to teeth. The microorganisms *Treponema microdentium* and *Campylobacter sputorum* are two common causes. Gingivitis (gums bleed and become edematous) results from the penetration of periodontal tissues by bacterial antigens. The disease spreads slowly with destruction of connective tissue and then alveolar bone and periodontal ligaments. Inspect dentures regularly. They may not fit properly due to changes in the mouth. Improperly fitting or damaged dentures can cause ulcers in the mouth. Persons with dentures need to brush the dentures and the gums regularly with a soft brush and a mild cleanser.

Male clients may feel much better with a clean-shaven face. Using an electric razor is safer and simplifies the process. Women may also need attention for facial hair. It is common for older women to note hair on the chin or above the upper lip. Routine shaving of these areas may be necessary.

Dressing may be difficult for clients who have restricted joint motion, paralysis, or limited endurance due to health problems. Many choices are available to make dressing easier such as elastic waists and velcro closures. The client who consistently wears soiled clothing may need assistance with laundry procedures. Investigation may be needed if a client who previously took pride in his/her appearance becomes disinterested and sloppy in appearance. This may be an indication of Alzheimer's disease or other disorders.

Bowel elimination problems can be avoided by:

- Including adequate fiber in the diet
- Adequate fluid intake
- Regular daily exercise
- Developing regular elimination habits

For the client in the hospital or long-term care facility it is helpful to:

- Maintain previous effective habits such as reading on the toilet or drinking warm liquids upon arising
- Assist the client to toilet about thirty minutes after eating to take advantage of the gastrocolic reflex.

Evacuation aids such as laxatives, lubricant, stool softeners, and enemas all have side effects and should be avoided if at all possible.

Increased frequency of urination may be noted in both men and women as they age as a result of the physical changes that occur. It is not uncommon for older adults to self-limit fluid intake due to a fear of being incontinent. This habit is unhealthy and needs to be discouraged. Cases of incontinence need to be assessed to determine the cause and type. The appropriate interventions and treatment can then be implemented.

Exercise

What has previously been accepted as the normal deterioration of old age is now considered the results of disuse through sitting and bed rest. Research indicates that high-intensity, progressive resistance training can improve muscle strength and size in elderly, frail people. Walking and all other maneuvers required for activities of daily living are also forms of beneficial exercise (Tetlow, 1995). Exercise programs should be individually planned and take into consideration the older person's:

- General health status
- Presence of physiological disorders
- Preference for solitary or group activity
- Physical environment
- Financial status

Nutrition

For many older adults cultural heritage, religious rites, ethnic practices, and family traditions are linked with food. The physiological, psychological, sociological, and economic changes of aging can compromise the nutritional status of older adults. The elderly need to follow a balanced diet with lowered intake of sugar, caffeine, fat, and sodium. There are no published guidelines that specifically establish the nutritional requirements of older adults. The Food Guide Pyramid developed by the United States Department of Agriculture (1992) suggests that 1,600 calories may be adequate for some older adults. An active person may require 2,000 to 2,200 calories per day. A sample diet for a day at 1,600 calories would include:

- Bread group — 6 servings
- Vegetable group — 3 servings
- Fruit group — 2 servings
- Milk group — 2-3 servings
- Meat group (ounces) — 5
- Total fat (grams) — 53
- Total added sugars (teaspoons) — 6

The ideal weight and food intake for a specific individual can be determined by a dietician taking into consideration height, ideal weight, and activity level.

The National Institutes of Health (NIH) recommend 1000 mg of calcium a day for both men and women over the age of twenty-five. Postmenopausal women aged fifty to sixty-five years who are not receiving estrogen replacement therapy, need 1500 mg of calcium daily (Yen, 1995). The need to take vitamin supplements depends on the individual's nutritional status and ability to maintain an adequate diet. Supplements should provide the twelve vitamins for which recommended dietary allowances (RDAs) have been set. Individual vitamins should be prescribed by a physician for specific purposes (Yen, 1994).

When poor appetite and weight loss are problems, calorie intake may be increased by:

- Adding nonfat dry milk powder to almost anything liquid; sauces, mashed potatoes, gravy, deserts, cooked cereal, and yogurt
- Offering finger foods
- Emphasizing taste and eye appeal to compensate for diminished smell and taste
- Using whole milk to make foods often made with water like soup and cereal
- Offering the most food at the time of day the client is most hungry; for most people, this is breakfast time
- Offering liquid supplements to provide additional calories and nutrients (Yen, 1994)

Nurses must be knowledgeable about community services available for meeting nutritional needs for the elderly. These include home-delivered meals, group meals at senior food sites, and the food stamp program.

Psychosocial Considerations

Older adults like all individuals have psychosocial needs. Maintaining mental activity and emotional involvement are as necessary as physical activity for overall well-being. It is beneficial to develop hobbies or activities that are interesting and stimulating. These may be of a solitary or group nature. Volunteer work or paid part-time employment can provide feelings of productivity and self-worth. Socialization with other people of all age groups can prevent feelings of loneliness and despair.

Health Care

Older adults need to be aware of factors that affect disease prevention and risk reduction. Knowledge of self-care and participating in screening tests are important components for health maintenance. Nurses can teach their clients habits for healthy living and inform them of signs and symptoms that require medical investigation.

PHYSIOLOGIC CHANGES ASSOCIATED WITH AGING

Overview

The aging process brings with it several physiological changes. Aging and disease are not synonymous and it should be remembered that the disorders described here are not considered normal. However, older adults are at risk for certain disorders due to (1) physiological changes and (2) living longer which increases the chance of acquiring a chronic illness. Many researchers feel that the system changes described here could be diminished or eradicated with lifestyle changes.

Integumentary System

See Chapter 23 for anatomy and physiology of the integumentary system. The following are changes resulting from the aging process:

- Subcutaneous tissue and elastin fibers diminish causing the skin to become thinner and less elastic.
- Eccrine, apocrine, and sebaceous glands decrease in size, number, and function resulting in diminished secretions and moisturization, causing pruritus.

- Body temperature regulation is impaired due to decreased perspiration.
- Capillary blood flow decreases resulting in slower wound healing.
- Blood flow decreases especially to lower extremities.
- Vascular fragility causes senile purpura.
- Cutaneous sensitivity to pressure and temperature are diminished.
- Melanin production is reduced causing gray-white hair.
- Scalp, pubic, and axillary hair thin. Females have increased facial hair on the upper lip and chin.
- Nail growth slows. Nails become more brittle and longitudinal nail ridges form.

Common Disorders Related to Aging/Integumentary System

- Pressure ulcers
- Herpesvirus varicella zoster (shingles)
- Scabies (Scabies is included here because it may be undiagnosed due to dryness and itching of the skin frequently seen in older adults. When diagnosed in residents of long-term care facilities, immediate and thorough action is required to prevent the widespread incidence of the disease.)
- Skin cancer (Skin cancer is included here because the risk of skin cancer increases with age.)

Nursing Interventions/ Pressure Ulcer Prevention

1. Perform a pressure ulcer risk assessment upon admission to the health care system, Figure 16-4.
2. Implement a pressure ulcer prevention protocol for clients at risk for pressure ulcer formation, Table 16-3.

Nursing Interventions/ Herpesvirus Varicella Zoster

1. Treat the pain.
2. Prevent infection.
3. Implement appropriate isolation procedures if client is in a hospital or other health care facility.
4. Monitor for signs of complications.

Nursing Interventions/Scabies

1. Identify the source of the scabies. Place in contact transmission precautions until twenty-four hours after effective treatment.
2. Consider application of scabicide to all clients in facility.

Date of Assessment: _____ Nurse: _____

Pressure Ulcer present on admission: No _____ Yes _____ Stage _____

A score of 11 or more places a client at risk for pressure ulcer formation. Preventive protocol should be established.

Activity		Total	Level of Consciousness		Total
Ambulant without assistance	0		Alert	0	
Ambulant with assistance	2		Slow verbal response	1	
Chairfast	4		Responds to verbal or painful stimuli	2	
Bedfast	6	_____	Absence of response to stimuli	3	_____
Mobility—Range of Motion			**Nutritional Status**		
Full range of motion	0		Good (Eats 75% or more of required intake)	0	
Moves with minimal assistance	2		Fair (Eats less than 75% of required intake)	1	
Moves with moderate assistance	4		Poor (Minimal intake, consistent weight loss)	2	
Immobile	6	_____	Unable/refuses to eat/drink, emaciated	3	_____
Skin Condition			**Incontinence—Bladder**		
Hydrated and intact	0		None	0	
Rashes or abrasions	2		Occasional (less than 2/24 hours)	1	
Decreased turgor, dry	4		Usually (more than 2/24 hours)	2	
Edema, erythema, pressure ulcers	6	_____	Total (no control)	3	_____
Predisposing Disease Process			**Incontinence—Bowel**		
No involvement	0		None	0	
Chronic, stable	1		Occasional (formed stool)	1	
Acute or chronic, unstable	2		Usually (with semi-formed stool)	2	
Terminal	3	_____	Total (no control, loose stool)	3	_____

FIGURE 16-4 Pressure ulcer potential assessment.

3. Apply scabicide according to manufacturer's directions. (Wear gown and gloves.)
4. Apply antipruritic emollient or topical steroid after treatment if prescribed to control itching.
5. Disinfect all clothing and bed linens after treatment is completed. Repeat if retreatment is required.
6. Do client teaching (personal hygiene measures, reporting of signs and symptoms) to prevent further outbreaks.

Nursing Interventions/Skin Cancer

1. Teach cancer prevention methods and skin self-examination to detect lesions early.
2. Provide information regarding treatment in both verbal and written form; surgery, chemotherapy, radiation.
3. Monitor for signs of infection at lesion site.

Neurologic System

See Chapter 27 for anatomy and physiology review of the neurologic system. The following are changes resulting from the aging process:

- Neurons in the brain decrease in numbers resulting in decreased production of neurotransmitters causing reduction in synaptic transmission.
- Cerebral blood flow and oxygen utilization are decreased. These changes result in a need for more time to carry out motor and sensory tasks requiring speed, coordination, balance and fine motor hand movements. In the absence of pathology, intellect and capacity for learning remain unchanged.
- Short-term memory may be somewhat diminished without changes in long-term memory.
- Night sleep decreases due to more frequent and longer wakeful periods.
- Deep tendon reflexes are decreased.

Table 16-3

PROTOCOL FOR CLIENTS AT RISK FOR PRESSURE ULCERS	
Objective	**Interventions**
Relieve Pressure	• Establish positioning schedule. • Place pressure relieving mattresses on bed, cushions on chair. • Teach client wheelchair exercises. • Stand and/or ambulate client in chair frequently. • Use wheelchair for transporting only. • Allow client to sit on bedpan, commode, or toilet for only brief periods. • Check areas of pressure under casts, braces, splints, slings, prostheses.
Relieve Friction and Shearing	• Use turning sheet for positioning in bed and chair. • Keep head of bed lower than 30 degrees unless contraindicated. • Use supportive devices to prevent sliding in chairs. • Use appropriate transfer techniques. • Do not use powder on skin. • Place bed cradle under top covers.
Prevent Moisture/Maceration	• Implement scheduled toileting or bladder retraining program. • Use absorbent incontinent briefs or pads. • Check incontinent clients frequently. Wash and rinse thoroughly. Apply moisture barrier. • Avoid use of plastic/rubber sheets, protectors.
Prevent Spasticity and Contractures	• Avoid quick, rough movements. • Do range of motion exercises at least twice daily. • Assess for synergy patterns when positioning. • Administer oral antispasmodics if ordered.
Maintain Hydration/Nutritional Status	• Assess nutritional status. • Investigate causes of anorexia. • Correct underlying nutritional deficits. • Encourage additional fluids unless contraindicated. • Give high protein supplement if necessary. • Monitor weight weekly.

Continue with routine skin care.
Do skin checks with each position change.

Common Disorders Related to Aging/ Neurologic System

There are many disorders affecting the neurologic system that are not unique to the elderly. However, the risk of acquiring one of these disorders increases with age. One of the most common diagnoses seen among the elderly in long-term care facilities is Alzheimer's disease (AD). AD is one form of **dementia**. Dementia is a clinical syndrome characterized by the loss of intellectual functioning. *The clinical manifestations associated with a dementia are never considered normal aging changes.* Depression is a significant matter in the elderly because of its prevalence and the complexity of differential diagnosis. Transient ischemic attack (TIA) is also more common in the elderly.

Nursing Interventions/ Alzheimer's Disease

1. Before diagnosis, encourage a diagnostic workup including a mental status examination (see Chapter 27).
2. Facilitate orientation in the early stages.
3. Arrange an environment that is therapeutic, consistent, calm, and safe.

4. Implement consistent routines with consistent caregivers.
5. Monitor general health status. Treat any underlying medical problems.
6. Monitor nutritional status.
7. Monitor ability to complete activities of daily living and provide assistance if needed.
8. Build a trusting relationship with the client and the family (significant others).

Nursing Interventions/Depression

1. Assess for signs of physical basis for fatigue: infection, pain, altered nutritional status, shortness of breath upon exertion.
2. Administer treatment for underlying physiological problem if necessary.
3. Provide opportunity to ventilate feelings about past and present life experiences.
4. Establish therapeutic, psychological environment.
5. Establish a therapeutic relationship.
6. Evaluate relationships and assist client to identify persons who can serve as a support system.
7. Involve in activities of daily living, providing assistance and modifying environment if necessary.
8. Plan and encourage intake of nourishing and appetizing diet.
9. Establish small goals for various types of activities including physical exercise.
10. Give opportunities for making simple nonfail decisions.
11. Monitor for sudden changes in behavior and for signs of increased anxiety (pacing, wringing of hands, increased smoking).
12. Assess for verbal or nonverbal signs of suicidal thoughts/intent.

Nursing Interventions/TIA

1. Assess for risk factors for stroke.
2. Explain relationship between risk factors, TIA, and stroke.
3. Provide teaching to assist in reducing risk factors.

Sensory Changes

See Chapter 28 for anatomy and physiology review of the sensory system. The following are changes resulting from the aging process.

Vision

- The lens is less pliable and is less able to increase its curvature in order to focus on near objects causing **presbyopia** (trouble seeing close objects) and decreased accommodation. The lens yellows causing distorted color perception with greens and blues

washing out; warm colors are more distinct. Alterations in the lens causes increased incidence of cataracts.
- Accommodation of pupil size decreases requiring more time to adjust to changes in lighting and decreased ability to tolerate glare.
- Vitreous humor changes in consistency causing blurring of vision.
- Changes in the anterior chamber may cause increased pressure of aqueous humor resulting in glaucoma.
- Lacrimal glands secrete less fluid causing dryness and itching of the eyes.

Common Disorders Related to Aging/Vision

- Presbyopia
- Cataract
- Glaucoma
- Age-related macular degeneration

Nursing Interventions/ Vision Impairment

1. Teach the visually impaired adaptive techniques for activities of daily living.
2. Advise regular examination by an ophthalmologist.
3. Provide preoperative and postoperative care and teaching for clients undergoing cataract surgery.
4. Teach actions, side effects, and administration of eye drops.

Hearing

- The pinna is less flexible and the hair cells in the inner ear stiffen and atrophy. Cerumen increases.
- The number of neurons in the cochlea decreases and the blood supply is less. This causes the tissue in the cochlea to deteriorate and the ossicles degenerate.
- **Presbycusis** is the impairment of hearing in older adults often accompanied by a loss of tone discrimination. High frequency tone loss occurs first.

Common Disorders Related to Aging/Hearing

- Presbycusis

Nursing Interventions/Impaired Hearing

1. Assess for ear pain, drainage, inflammation, abnormalities, surgeries, perforations, or impacted cerumen.

2. Evaluate medication regime and assess for ototoxicity if medication history reveals a risk.
3. Advise testing by an audiologist if above assessments are negative.
4. Monitor care and use of hearing aid.
5. Instruct caregivers and family about communication and socialization with client.

Respiratory System

See Chapter 19 for anatomy and physiology review of the respiratory system. The following are changes resulting from the aging process.

- The muscles of respiration become less flexible causing decreased vital capacity and increased residual capacity of the lungs.
- Decrease in functional capacity results in dyspnea with exertion or stress; usual activity is not affected.
- The cough mechanism is less effective increasing the risk for lung infection.
- Decreased functional capacity results in dyspnea with exertion or stress.
- The alveoli thicken and the number and size of alveoli decrease causing less effective gas exchange. This intensifies deficits in individuals who also have chronic lung disease.

Common Disorders Related to Aging/ Respiratory System

- Respiratory Tract Infection (RTI)
- Chronic Obstructive Pulmonary Disease (COPD)
- Pulmonary Tuberculosis (TB)
  The elderly are vulnerable to TB because of:
  - Ineffective cough reflex and inability to clear the lungs
  - Altered immune system and reduced response to extrinsic antigens in persons over 60 years old and in others with debilitating illnesses
  - Depression of lymphocytes (Moody, 1995)

Nursing Interventions/ Respiratory Tract Infections

1. Advise getting pneumonia vaccine.
2. Advise annual influenza vaccine.
3. Assist client to assume position of comfort.
4. Avoid distention of bladder and bowel which can increase breathing discomfort.
5. Allow adequate time for nursing care.
6. Administer humidified oxygen therapy as prescribed.
7. Administer analgesics and antipyretics as prescribed.

8. Assess for signs of dehydration. Have fluids accessible.
9. Review diagnostic data.
10. Monitor intake and output (I&O). Weigh daily.

Nursing Interventions/COPD

1. Assist client to assume position of comfort.
2. Teach client to use pursed-lip breathing when short of breath.
3. Teach diaphragmatic breathing to use with activity.
4. Teach client to use inhaler correctly.
5. Teach client to cough and clear the airway.
6. Administer chest physical therapy if prescribed.
7. Set up schedule for ambulation and gradually increase distance.
8. Assist with active assistive range of motion exercises.
9. Monitor for signs of infection.
10. Monitor breathing and pulse rate and administer O_2 if necessary during periods of increased activity.
11. Suggest smoking cessation program if necessary.

Nursing Interventions/ Pulmonary Tuberculosis

1. Monitor nutritional intake. Provide supplements if necessary to maintain adequate body weight.
2. Evaluate for risk of HIV infection.
3. Protect from microorganisms transmitted through direct or indirect contact.
4. Provide rest periods throughout the day.
5. Inform client/family regarding need for isolation.
6. Encourage short visits by family.

Reproductive System: Females

See Chapter 31 for anatomy and physiology review of the female reproductive system. The following are changes resulting from the aging process.

- Estrogen production decreases with onset of menopause.
- Ovaries, uterus, and cervix decrease in size.
- The vagina shortens, narrows, and becomes less elastic with thinner lining. Secretions decrease and become more alkaline, resulting in increased incidence of atrophic vaginitis. These changes may result in discomfort during coitus.
- Supporting musculature weakens increasing risk of uterine prolapse.
- Breast tissue decreases and nipple erection is diminished during sexual arousal.
- Libido remains unchanged.

Common Disorders Related to Aging/Female Reproductive System

- Altered sexuality patterns related to physiologic changes and changes in body image
- Risk of breast cancer increases with age

Nursing Interventions/ Female Reproductive System Disorders

1. Establish rapport and encourage client to verbalize feelings and concerns related to self-esteem and sexuality.
2. Complete a sexual history. Implement interventions based on findings.
3. Suggest consulting with physician on estrogen replacement therapy (ERT).
4. Assess mobility, endurance, and strength. Suggest adaptations for sexual activity if necessary.
5. Teach and encourage monthly breast self-examination.
6. Encourage annual clinical examination and mammography.
7. Encourage annual gynecologic examination.

Reproductive System: Male

See Chapter 32 for anatomy and physiology review of the male reproductive system. The following are changes resulting from the aging process.

- Testosterone production decreases resulting in decreased size of testicles.
- Sperm count and viscosity of seminal fluid decreases.
- The penis is less firm during erection. More time is required to achieve erection, delaying achievement of orgasm. There is greater control but less intensity of ejaculation.
- Prostate gland may enlarge.
- Libido remains unchanged.

Common Disorders Related to Aging/ Male Reproductive System

- Altered sexuality related to physiologic changes and changes in body image
- Benign prostatic hypertrophy (BPH)

Nursing Interventions/ Male Reproductive System Disorders

1. Establish rapport and encourage client to verbalize feelings and concerns related to self-esteem and sexuality.
2. Complete a sexual history. Implement interventions based on findings.
3. Assess mobility, endurance, and strength. Suggest adaptations for sexual activity if necessary.
4. Instruct on signs and symptoms of prostate disorders.
5. Encourage annual digital rectal examination of prostate gland. (The use of Prostatic Specific Antigen as a routine screening tool is questionable.)
6. Encourage monthly testicular self-examination.

Musculoskeletal System

See Chapter 26 for anatomy and physiology review of the musculoskeletal system. The following are changes resulting from the aging process.

- Muscle mass and elasticity diminishes resulting in decreased strength and endurance. This decreases reaction time and coordination.
- Bone demineralization occurs, causing skeletal instability and shrinkage of intervertebral disks. The spine is less flexible and spinal curvature is often present.
- Joints undergo degenerative changes resulting in pain, stiffness, and loss of range of motion.

Common Disorders Related to Aging/ Musculoskeletal System

- Osteoporosis
- Degenerative arthritis
- Fractured hip

Nursing Interventions/Osteoporosis

1. Make dietary recommendations for adequate intake of calcium, protein, and vitamin D.
2. Recommend smoking cessation programs if necessary.
3. Advise to avoid alcohol.
4. Advise on use of calcium supplements.
5. Suggest consultation with physician regarding ERT (for females).
6. Instruct on measures to reduce the risk of falling and sustaining fractures.
7. Establish exercise program appropriate to client's capabilities.

Nursing Interventions/Degenerative Arthritis

1. Suggest schedule for alternating periods of rest and activity.
2. Advise weight reduction program if necessary.
3. Establish exercise program with emphasis on gentle stretching and movement of all joints.
4. Advise avoidance of "quackery."
5. Advise on use of pain relieving medications.

Nursing Interventions/Fractured Hip

NOTE: Nursing interventions may vary depending on whether client has open reduction/internal fixation (ORIF) or total hip arthroplasty (THA).

1. Maintain postoperative positioning as appropriate to form of treatment.
2. Prevent complications: skin breakdown, respiratory infection, infection of surgical site, dislocation of prosthesis, or internal fixation device.
3. Instruct on techniques for restoring mobility as prescribed by physical therapist.
4. Instruct on fall prevention. Do home evaluation and make recommendations to provide safe environment.

Cardiovascular System

See Chapters 20 and 21 for anatomy and physiology reviews of the cardiovascular system. The following are changes resulting from the aging process.

- Cardiac output and recovery time decline. The heart requires more time to return to a normal rate after increasing in response to activity.
- The heart rate slows with age.
- Blood flow to all organs decreases. The brain and coronary arteries continue to receive a larger volume than other organs.
- Arterial elasticity decreases causing increased peripheral resistance. This results in a rise in systolic blood pressure and a slight increase in diastolic pressure.
- Veins dilate and superficial vessels are more prominent.

Common Disorders Related to Aging/ Cardiovascular System

- Peripheral vascular disease (PVD)
- Hypertension
- Chronic congestive heart failure

Nursing Interventions/Peripheral Vascular Disease

1. Assess lower extremities for signs of arterial or venous insufficiency.
2. Evaluate factors in lifestyle that may aggravate or advance atherosclerosis such as high-fat diet and little exercise.
3. Teach about disease, treatment, medication actions and side effects, signs of thrombosis.
4. Instruct on care and inspection of lower extremities.
5. Provide instructions on interventions specific to type of PVD/arterial or venous.

Nursing Interventions/Hypertension

1. Evaluate food intake patterns especially for sodium, fats, and cholesterol. Make recommendations based on findings.
2. Recommend smoking cessation program if necessary.
3. Advise to avoid alcohol use.
4. Recommend appropriate exercise program.
5. Discuss relationship of stress to hypertension. Provide resources for learning relaxation techniques.
6. Provide information on medications and importance of compliance with medication regime.
7. Arrange for regular blood pressure checks. Teach client or significant other how to use equipment.

Nursing Interventions/Chronic Congestive Heart Failure

1. Frequently monitor serum digitalis level. Teach signs of digoxin toxicity.
2. Take apical pulse for one minute before administration of digoxin. Notify physician of significant changes.
3. Monitor blood pressure and lung sounds.
4. Monitor electrolyte levels, blood urea nitrogen (BUN), and creatinine levels.
5. Monitor for signs of fluid retention: intake and output, daily weight, shortness of breath, coughing.
6. Teach methods for energy conservation.
7. Encourage to maintain regular physical activity within limits of physical condition.
8. Instruct on use of nitrates depending on type prescribed.

Gastrointestinal System

See Chapter 34 for anatomy and physiology review of the gastrointestinal system. The following are changes resulting from the aging process.

- Tooth enamel thins.
- Periodontal disease increases.
- Taste buds decrease and saliva production is less.
- The gag reflex is less effective increasing the danger of choking.
- Esophageal peristalsis slows and the esophageal sphincter is less efficient. This causes delayed entry of food into the stomach, increasing the risk of aspiration.
- Hiatal hernia is more common.
- Gastric emptying is delayed. Food remains in the stomach longer, decreasing the capacity of the stomach.
- Peristalsis and nerve sensation of the large intestine is decreased contributing to constipation.
- Diverticulosis increases with age.
- Liver size decreases after age 70.
- Liver enzymes decrease, slowing drug metabolism and the detoxification process.
- Gallbladder emptying becomes less efficient. Bile is thicker, cholesterol content is increased. There is increased incidence of gallstones.

Common Disorders Related to Aging/ Gastrointestinal System

- Over/under nutrition
- Constipation
- Dehydration (fluid volume deficit)
- Dental disorders

Nursing Interventions/ Over/Under Nutrition

1. Assess nutritional status, Table 16-4.
2. Provide nutritional instruction based on assessment findings.
3. Advise on community nutrition programs: Meals-on-Wheels, Senior Center Food Sites, Food Pantries, availability of Food Stamp programs.

Nursing Interventions/Constipation

1. Assess food and fluid intake.
2. Make recommendations based on assessment-increased fiber intake, increased fluid intake.
3. Discuss relationship of exercise to bowel activity.
4. Discuss importance of routine for regular bowel elimination.
5. Advise avoiding use of laxatives.

Nursing Interventions/Dehydration

1. Identify reason for dehydration; inadequate fluid intake or excessive fluid output.
2. Identify reason for inadequate fluid intake:
   - Fluids inaccessible due to client's physical limitations—offer fluids on regular basis throughout the day
   - Dislike of water or other available fluids—identify fluid choices
   - Self-restriction of fluid intake related to fear of incontinence—explain relationship of decreased fluid intake to bladder infections—arrange for assistance as needed for toileting
3. Identify reasons for excessive fluid output and treat accordingly.

Table 16-4

DETERMINING ALTERATIONS IN NUTRITION: INFORMATION TO EVALUATE

- Height and weight: Record actual body weight, usual body weight, and ideal body weight. If usual weight has varied significantly from the ideal for several years, the use of height/weight tables may be meaningless. Compare actual body weight with usual body weight to determine present status.
- Review laboratory values: hematocrit, hemoglobin, total iron-binding capacity, total protein, BUN.
- Determine if client is on a weight-loss diet.
- Determine if client was edematous when initially weighed and has lost weight with treatment.
- For client at home-evaluate ability to shop and prepare meals.
- Evaluate mealtime environment for uinpleasant odors, noises, and visual stimuli.
- Evaluate table setting: appealing table cover, centerpiece, colorful dishes.
- Evaluate cognitive status: cognitively impaired clients may be unaware of hunger or be unable to attend to the task of eating.
- Evaluate presence of sensory-perceptual deficits that interfere with eating in clients with central nervous system damage.
- Evaluate ability to pick up utensils and glasses and to get items from table to mouth.
- Evaluate dental/oral status: status of teeth/dentures, gums, presence of oral dryness (xerostomia).
- Determine presence of impaired swallowing.
- Determine if client has distaste for certain food groups.
- Assess knowledge in regard to nutrition and food purchase and preparation.
- Determine if client is taking medications that interfere with taste or food absorption.
- Determine if financial status interferes with food purchasing.
- Determine if history of compulsive eating.

Nursing Interventions/Dental Disorders

1. Teach oral hygiene procedures for flossing and brushing.
2. Inspect mouth regularly for signs of dental disorders.
3. Advise regular dental checkups.

Urinary System

See Chapter 35 for anatomy and physiology review of the urinary system. The following are changes resulting from the aging process.

- Nephrons decrease in number and function resulting in decreased filtration and gradual decrease in excretory and reabsorptive functions of renal tubules.
- Glomerular filtration rate decreases resulting in decreased renal clearance of drugs.
- Blood urea nitrogen (BUN) increases 20 percent by age seventy. The creatinine clearance test is a better index than the BUN of renal function in elderly.
- Sodium conserving ability is diminished.
- Bladder capacity decreases causing increased frequency of urination and nocturia.
- Renal function increases when lying down, sometimes causing a need to void shortly after going to bed.
- Bladder and perineal muscles weaken resulting in inability to empty the bladder. This results in residual urine and predisposes the elderly to cystitis.
- Incidence of stress incontinence increases in females.
- The prostate may enlarge causing frequency or dribbling in males.

Common Disorders Related to Aging/ Urinary System

- Incontinence
- Urinary Tract Infection (UTI)

Nursing Interventions/Incontinence

1. Complete an assessment for bladder management, Figure 16-5.
2. Identify type of incontinence, Table 16-5.
3. Implement appropriate bladder management program, Table 16-6.
4. Implement interventions for total incontinence:
   - prevention of skin impairment
   - use of absorbent incontinent pads or briefs.
5. Identify issues of diminished self-esteem and body image.

Nursing Interventions/ Urinary Tract Infection

NOTE: Elderly persons frequently do not present the usual signs and symptoms of urinary tract infections. Falling or signs of confusion may be the major clinical manifestations.

1. Monitor fluid intake and output. Increase intake unless contraindicated. Offer cranberry juice frequently.
2. Teach to empty bladder completely every three to four hours.

To be completed and reviewed every 90 days or as frequently as needed based on outcome and response.

CLIENT_____ Adm No. _____ Date_____ Diagnoses_____ Birthdate_____

Bladder function: History of infection or other urinary problem._____ Urinalysis:Date_____

Protein___ Glucose__ Ketones__ RBC__ WBC__ Bacteria__ Crystals__ Sp.Gr.__ Culture: Date_____ Result_____

Treatment_____

BUN___ Ser.Creatinine___ Tot.Pro.___ FBS___ To be completed after two week assessment period

Frequency of voiding_____ Average amount_____ Is client aware of need to void?_____ Urgency?_____ Dribbling?_____

Incontinence preceded by laughing, sneezing_____

Medications affecting bladder function/continence_____

Mental status: Short term memory_____ Orientation_____ Able to express self_____

Able to follow directions_____ Reaction to incontinence_____

Hydration baseline: Daily average fluid intake: Days_____ Eve._____ Night_____

Mobility/self care skills: Ambulatory/self_____ Cane_____ Walke_____ Requires assist of 1 or 2_____

Weight bearing_____ Propels self by w/c_____ Transfers self_____ Requires assistance_____

Can manage clothing_____ Cleans self after toileting_____ Washes hands_____

FIGURE 16-5 Assessment for bladder management.

Table 16-5

TYPES OF URINARY INCONTINENCE

Type	Characteristics
Functional	Bladder emptying unpredictable, complete. Incontinence related to impairment of cognitive, physical, or psychological functioning or to environmental barriers.
Urge	Incontinence occurs immediately after the sensation to void is perceived.
Reflex	Related to neurogenic bladder related to central nervous system or spinal cord injury. Bladder fills and uninhibited bladder contractions cause loss of urine.
Stress	Increased abdominal pressure is higher than urethral resistance. Stress associated with coughing or laughing causes incontinence.
Total	Unpredictable, involuntary, continuous loss of urine.

Table 16-6

BLADDER MANAGEMENT TECHNIQUES

Program	Description
Kegel exercises	Used for stress incontinence for cognitively alert persons. Exercises strengthen pelvic floor musculature.
Scheduled toileting	Client is on a fixed schedule of toileting—usually every two hours. Techniques can be used to facilitate voiding and emptying the bladder.
Habit training:	Client is toileted according to individual pattern of voiding. Requires several days to assess pattern.
Bladder retraining	Restores normal pattern of voiding/continence. Requires accurate assessment before establishing schedule with progressive shortening or lengthening of toileting intervals. Client must be cognitively alert.
Prompted voiding	Client is prompted to toilet at regular intervals and is given social reinforcement for appropriate toileting behavior.

3. Teach female clients to:
    - Wipe from front to back after urination
    - Cleanse thoroughly after bowel movement
    - Avoid vaginal sprays, douches, bubble baths, and colored toilet paper
    - Wear underwear made of cotton rather than synthetic fibers
4. Advise to report any signs of bladder infection promptly.
5. Instruct to finish all medication for UTI as prescribed.

Endocrine System

See Chapter 29 for anatomy and physiology review of the endocrine system. The following are changes resulting from the aging process.

- Changes in both the reception and the production of hormones.
- Release of insulin by the beta cells of the pancreas is delayed, causing an increase in blood sugar.
- Changes in the thyroid may lower the basal metabolic rate.

Common Disorders Related to Aging/ Endocrine System

- Non–Insulin-Dependent Diabetes Mellitus (NIDDM)

Nursing Interventions/ Diabetes Mellitus

1. Arrange for consultation with dietitian to assess nutritional status and to provide food management instruction.
2. Teach client procedure for blood glucose testing specific to equipment client will be using.
3. Develop a personal exercise plan based on physical condition, mental status, resources, and interests.
4. Provide information regarding oral hypoglycemic medications.
5. Teach causes, signs, and treatment of hypoglycemia and hyperglycemia.
6. Advise on self-care to avoid impaired skin integrity.

Sample Nursing Care Plan: The Client with Alzheimer's Disease

Mrs. Jane Rodriguez, sixty-four years old, was admitted to the Alzheimer's unit of a long-term care facility. Mrs. Rodriguez was visiting her daughter in another state and wandered away from the daughter's home. She was found sixty miles away, unharmed but completely disoriented. Mrs. Rodriguez had worked as a nursing assistant before she retired. She is a widow and has two children in the same community where the nursing home is located in addition to the daughter in another state. Unless reminded, she does not shower or change clothes. She awakens at least once each night and asks for breakfast.

Nursing Diagnosis 1 Thought processes, altered, related to progressive dementia and characterized by disorientation to time and place, loss of short-term memory, inability to concentrate, and periods of agitation.

Goals	Nursing Interventions	Rationale	Evaluation
Mrs. Rodriguez will remain calm and avoid experiencing agitation and anxiety as a result of the disorientation and memory loss.	Provide Mrs. Rodriguez with clues for orientation: "Good morning, Mrs. Rodriguez, my name is Jean and I will help you today." Avoid putting her on the spot by asking questions she cannot answer such as "Do you know what day this is?"	People in the early stages of Alzheimer's disease may become agitated because their world is always unfamiliar to them. The issue is not whether individuals with a dementia are oriented but whether they can cope with their environment.	Mrs. Rodriguez remained calm showing no signs of agitation or anxiety.
	Place a large sign on her door with her name printed in large letters to help her find her room.	Because of short-term memory loss, it is impossible to remember where her room is or where the bathroom is. If she still recognizes her name, this helps her find her way.	
	Have family bring in snapshots and photos to stimulate reminiscence.	Reminiscing can be a satisfying activity. It is especially helpful if the photos are from an earlier, happier time such as when her children were young. Long-term memory may still be intact allowing her to recall these happier times.	
	Avoid changing her room. Put items back in the same place all of the time.	Consistency in the environment (as well as routine and staff), reduce frustration.	
	Consult with activities staff in planning self-expressive, non-fail activities that require little concentration; painting with nontoxic paints, modeling with nontoxic clay.	Appropriate activities prevent boredom which can lead to irritation. It is important to plan nonstressful, noncompetitive, failure-free activities in order to avoid frustration.	

Nursing Diagnosis 2 Injury, high risk for, related to wandering behavior, impaired judgment, loss of impulse control, and the inability to recognize sensory cues indicating danger.

Goals	Nursing Interventions	Rationale	Evaluation
Mrs. Rodriguez will remain free of injury while retaining as much independence and freedom as possible.	Lock up tools, medicines, and chemicals. Keep only nonpoisonous plants on the unit. Arrange furniture so walkways are open. Pad sharp corners of tables and chests. Cover electrical outlets and hot radiators. Place electrical cords and telephone wires out of reach. Provide assurance during fire drills.	Persons with Alzheimer's disease do not recognize unsafe acts or conditions due to loss of impulse control and loss of judgment. They do not comprehend cause and effect. Unusual activity of any sort increases agitation especially when the noise level is increased.	Mrs. Rodriguez has had no injury.

Nursing Diagnosis 3 Self-care deficits (total) related to memory loss and sensory-perceptual deficits as evidenced by needing a reminder to shower and change clothes.

Goals	Nursing Interventions	Rationale	Evaluation
Mrs. Rodriguez will complete the activities of daily living with minimal assistance, increasing assistance as the disease progresses.	Use verbal cues and hand-over-hand assistance with activities of daily living. Instruct staff to avoid doing tasks that Mrs. Rodriguez can do by herself. Watch for signs of frustration and irritation and intervene when appropriate. Ask family to bring in clothing that is easy to manipulate. Set clothing out in the order it is put on. Consider tub baths rather than showers. Provide privacy, check the temperature of the bathroom and do not leave her alone.	Using these simple techniques can minimize the need for assistance thereby increasing feelings of self-esteem. Dressing is one of the more difficult tasks to accomplish. Appropriate clothing can simplify the activity. Showers are frequently threatening to persons with Alzheimer's disease. Tub baths are also more relaxing.	Mrs. Rodriguez participates in activities of daily living.

(continued)

Nursing Diagnosis 4 Sleep pattern disturbance related to disorientation.

Goals	Nursing Interventions	Rationale	Evaluation
Mrs. Rodriguez will experience fewer periods of wakefulness during the night. If she awakens she will remain calm and free of agitation.	Avoid stimulating activities prior to bedtime. Establish a consistent bedtime routine. Take Mrs. Rodriguez to the bathroom, allowing sufficient time for complete bladder emptying.	Overstimulation prior to bedtime may increase anxiety, preventing sleep.	Mrs. Rodriguez sleeps through the night several times a week.
	Help her with a sponge bath and oral care; give a back rub with warm lotion and slow, smooth strokes.	These activities are relaxing.	
	Provide a light snack with a warm, noncaffeinated beverage and plain, easily digested cracker, cookie, or toast. Be patient and do not rush.	Hunger or overeating can interfere with sleep.	
	Question family concerning previous bedtime routines and sleeping habits.	Individuals may have used specific sleep routines throughout their lifetimes such as: sleeping with a night light, having a window open, playing a radio, or wearing socks to bed.	
	Repeat bedtime routine when Mrs. Rodriguez awakens during night.	Mrs. Rodriguez will think it is time to go to bed.	
	Try a short nap early in the afternoon.	Sundowning may be a result of overfatigue.	
	Avoid the use of sleeping medications.	Sleeping medications are seldom effective and may increase confusion, disorientation, and restlessness.	

▶ CASE STUDY

Mr. Jack Baroni, a seventy-two-year old male, was admitted to the skilled care facility for rehabilitation following an open reduction, internal fixation of the right hip. Mr. Baroni had fallen while going up the stairs of his home suffering an intertrochanteric, comminuted fracture of the right femur. He has no recollection of what caused him to fall. He is married and until his surgery was working part time as a school-crossing guard. While in the hospital Mr. Baroni exhibited mental status changes including disorientation and confusion. His wife reports that he never had this problem previous to the surgery. He is continent of bowel and bladder. Mr. Baroni was in relatively good health until the fall. He and his wife agree that he should return home after rehabilitation is complete.

The following questions will guide your development of a Nursing Care Plan for the case study.

1. Identify specific admission assessments that would be required for Mr. Baroni because of his age and condition.

2. Identify complications for which Mr. Baroni is at risk.

3. List interventions to prevent each complication.

4. Describe possible reasons causing Mr. Baroni to fall.

5. Describe methods for assessing Mr. Baroni's mental status.

6. Describe possible reasons for his altered mental status.

7. Write three individualized nursing diagnoses and goals for Mr. Baroni.

8. List nursing actions related to altered mental status.

9. List four successful outcomes for Mr. Baroni.

10. Develop a teaching plan for Mr. Baroni.

11. List the community resources Mr. Baroni may need after discharge.

SUMMARY

- The elderly population is growing at a rapid speed.
- While there are many stereotypes and myths associated with aging, this age group is very diverse in their characteristics.
- There are many biological and psychosocial theories of aging, none of which have been universally accepted.
- Most people experience a number of losses as they age.
- Health maintenance is as important for older adults as it is for younger persons. A healthy lifestyle can add quality to life.
- There are many changes associated with aging. The disorders commonly seen in the elderly are often the result of pathology and so are not considered

normal. However, the risk of acquiring these disorders increases with age.
- Nurses knowledgeable about aging can plan interventions that will prevent complications for which the elderly are at risk.

Review Questions

1. Which of the following is a true statement?

    a. Everyone eventually becomes senile if they live long enough.

    b. People lose interest in sex as they age.

    c. Most elderly are financially impoverished.

    d. Incontinence is not an expected or normal aging change.

2. The programmed aging theory states that:
   a. stress causes structural and chemical changes in the body that cause aging.
   b. a genetic clock determines the speed with which people age.
   c. changes in collagen are the cause of aging.
   d. the decreasing ability to produce T cell differentiation causes aging.

3. The elderly can avoid respiratory tract infections by:
   a. receiving influenza vaccine each year.
   b. staying inside throughout the winter months.
   c. avoiding exercise.
   d. limiting fluid intake.

4. Research indicates that:
   a. weight bearing exercise is not recommended for the elderly.
   b. high intensity resistance training can improve muscle strength in the elderly.
   c. muscle deterioration in the elderly is to be expected.
   d. walking is the only healthy exercise for the elderly.

5. Aging changes in the skin include:
   a. increase in glandular secretions.
   b. increased capillary blood flow.
   c. increased melanin production.
   d. increased vascular fragility.

News Flash

The Agency for Health Care Policy and Research and the National Institute of Aging conducted a study to compare the effectiveness of telephone and in-person interviews. Two assessment tools were used; the Sickness Impact Profile and the Geriatric Depression Scale. Researchers concluded that telephone administration of health status measures was more convenient and less expensive but may be less useful if the older person had significant hearing, physical, or cognitive impairment. (*From Research Activities, Geriatric Nursing 17(3):103*).

Critical Thinking Questions

1. What do you expect to be like at age 65 and 80?

2. How are the elderly different from young and middle aged adults?

3. How are the elderly the same as young and middle aged adults?

CHAPTER
17

Rehabilitation, Home Health, and Long-Term Care

Joan Fritsch Needham

KEY TERMS

accreditation
adult day care
assisted living
certification
licensure
long-term care facility
Medicaid
Medicare
Medigap insurance
rehabilitation
respite care
subacute care
synergy

LEARNING OBJECTIVES

Upon completion of this chapter the learner should be able to:

- Define key terms.
- List three reasons why there has been a significant change in the growth of nonacute care services.
- Discuss the legal/ethical implications of:
  1. Limiting aggressive health care services (such as rehabilitation or intensive care) for the elderly as a cost saving measure for the preservation of Medicare funds.
  2. Determining nurses' responsibility for accepting decisions made by individuals with questionable mental competency.
- Describe the differences between Medicaid and Medicare.
- Distinguish between licensure, certification, and accreditation.
- Describe the role of the LP/VN as a member of the interdisciplinary health care team in various health care settings.
- Discuss the types of clients that would benefit from participation in a rehabilitation program.
- Identify the responsibilities of the LP/VN in rehabilitation nursing, nursing in long-term care, and in-home care.
- List the various types of long-term care services.

▶ *MAKING THE CONNECTION*

KEY ABBREVIATIONS

The following abbreviations and acronyms are used in this chapter:

ADL	activities of daily living
AHCPR	Agency for Health Care Policy and Research
CARF	Commission on Accreditation of Rehabilitation Facilities
CCRC	continuing care retirement communities
DRG	diagnosis-related group
ECF	extended care facility
HCFA	Health Care Finance Administration
IADL	instrumental activities of daily living
ICF	intermediate care facility
IHCT	interdisciplinary health care team
JCAHO	Joint Commission on Accreditation of Healthcare Organizations
MDS	minimum data set
OBRA	Omnibus Budget Reconciliation Act
SNF	skilled nursing facility

INTRODUCTION

There has been a strong emergence in the last decade of non-acute health care services. The growth of these services is a reflection of several changes occurring in the United States:

- The Tax Equity and Fiscal Responsibility Act of 1983 initiated the Medicare Prospective Payment system and the diagnostic related group (DRG) system. This has resulted in the discharge of clients from acute-care hospitals much earlier. Clients, particularly elderly individuals, often require continuing care.
- Lives are being saved that would have been lost a few years ago. Ongoing health care services are often necessary for these individuals.
- The number of Americans over the age of 65 has tripled in this century. The risk of acquiring a chronic disease increases as individuals age, requiring health care throughout life.
- The cost of acute care has reached critical proportions. Case management is an attempt to contain costs by assisting people in defining their service needs, locating and arranging services, and coordinating the services of multiple providers. The cost of health care can be managed by controlling client access to services (General Accounting Office, 1994).

These changes have resulted in a vast increase in rehabilitation services and long-term care. Long-term care refers to both home and community-based services. There is an intermingling of services under each of these three categories of care. Rehabilitative services for example, may be provided in an acute-care setting, in a rehabilitation hospital, in a long-term care facility, or in the client's home. Home care may provide the same services that would be available in a subacute care nursing facility. Clients of all ages are cared for in these different settings. While many of the clients requiring these services are elderly, there are an increasing number of services specializing in pediatric care.

LEGAL AND ETHICAL RESPONSIBILITIES

The legal basis for the provision of care in long-term care facilities is found in the Omnibus Budget

Reconciliation Act (OBRA) of 1987. This act was legislated after a lengthy study of the care delivery in long-term facilities throughout the country. The major components of the act concern the issues of nursing assistant training, the regulation of the use of physical and chemical restraints, the Minimum Data Set (MDS 2) as an assessment tool, and the legal foundation for residents' rights. Many of the regulations found in OBRA also apply to home health nursing agencies.

The rights of the health care consumer are regulated for both long-term care and home health care. Before receiving services from either, the consumer must be given a copy of these rights and indicate an understanding of their content (Tables 17-1 and 17-2). In addition to OBRA there are many other regulatory acts that affect the delivery of care in the settings described in this chapter. These include the Self-Determination

Act of 1990 (Chapters 18), which is a federal regulation and legislation related to the reporting of client abuse (state regulations).

There is a fine line between what is a legal issue and what is an ethical issue. It is beyond the scope of this chapter to provide answers to the questions arising from such problems. However, these situations are examples of common issues.

1. An eighty-year-old client in the third stage of Alzheimer's disease falls and fractures his hip. Should this client be transferred to a rehabilitation hospital for intensive rehabilitation? If not, what are the alternatives?
2. The staff of a long-term care facility suspects that a client was abused by her son before admission to the facility. The son wishes to take the mother

Table 17-1

RESIDENT'S RIGHTS

This is an abbreviated version of the Resident's Rights as set forth in the Omnibus Budget Reconciliation Act. This document must be given to all residents and/or their families prior to admission to any long-term care facility.

1. **The resident has the right to free choice, including the right to:**
   - choose an attending physician
   - full advance information about changes in care or treatment
   - participate in the assessment and care planning process
   - self-administration of medications
   - consent to participate in experimental research

2. **The resident has the right to freedom from abuse and restraints, including freedom from:**
   - physical, sexual, mental abuse
   - corporal punishment and involuntary seclusion
   - physical and chemical restraints

3. **The resident has the right to privacy including privacy for:**
   - treatment and nursing care
   - receiving/sending mail
   - telephone calls
   - visitors

4. **The resident has the right to confidentiality of personal and clinical records.**

5. **The resident has the right to accommodation of needs including:**
   - choices about life
   - receiving assistance in maintaining independence

6. **The resident has the right to voice grievances.**

7. **The resident has the right to organize and participate in family and resident groups.**

8. **The resident has the right to participate in social, religious, and community activities including the right to:**
   - vote
   - keep religious items in the room
   - attend religious services

9. **The resident has the right to examine survey results and correction plans.**

10. **The resident has the right to manage personal funds.**

11. **The resident has the right to information about eligibility for Medicare/Medicaid funds.**

12. **The resident has the right to file complaints about abuse, neglect, or misappropriation of property.**

13. **The resident has the right to information about advocacy groups.**

14. **The resident has the right to immediate and unlimited access to family or relatives.**

15. **The resident has the right to share a room with the spouse if they are both residents in the same facility.**

16. **The resident has the right to perform or not perform work for the facility if it is medically appropriate for the resident to work.**

17. **The resident has the right to remain in the facility except in certain circumstances.**

18. **The resident has the right to personal possessions.**

19. **The resident has the right to notification of change in condition.**

(As determined by Omnibus Budget Reconciliation Act of 1987 [OBRA])

Table 17-2

CLIENT'S RIGHTS IN HOME CARE

The family receiving home health care services or their families possess basic rights and responsibilities. These include:

The right to:

1. be treated with dignity, consideration, and respect.
2. have their property treated with respect.
3. receive a timely response from the agency to requests for service.
4. be fully informed on admission of the care and treatment that will be provided, how much it will cost, and how payment will be handled.
5. know in advance if you will be responsible for any payment.
6. be informed in advance of any changes in your care.
7. receive care from professionally trained personnel, to know their names and responsibilities.
8. participate in planning care.
9. refuse treatment and to be told the consequences of your action.
10. expect confidentiality of all information.
11. be informed of anticipated termination of service.
12. be referred elsewhere if you are denied services solely based on your inability to pay.
13. know how to make a complaint or recommend a change in agency policies and services.

The responsibility to:

1. remain under a doctor's care while receiving services.
2. provide the agency with a complete health history.
3. provide the agency all requested insurance and financial information.
4. sign the required consents and releases for insurance billing.
5. participate in your care by asking questions, expressing concerns, stating if you do not understand.
6. provide a safe home environment in which care is given.
7. cooperate with your doctor, the staff, and other caregivers.
8. accept responsibility for any refusal of treatment.
9. abide by agency policies which restrict duties our staff may perform.
10. advise agency administration of any dissatisfaction or problems with your care.

home and the mother is in agreement with this plan. The discharge planner learns that the local social services agency had investigated the client's living situation for abuse prior to the mother's admission. The case worker also suspects abuse but could find nothing objective upon which to build a case. Do the nursing staff and social workers of the facility have a legal or ethical obligation to attempt intervention? If so, what actions should be taken?

3. J.B. is a young adult (twenty-three years old) receiving rehabilitation after suffering a traumatic brain injury due to a motorcycle accident. He wishes to make decisions concerning his care and treatment. His mental competency is questionable. However, this has not been legally established and his parents make decisions often in opposition to J.B.'s preferences. What are the legal and ethical responsibilities of the nurse in accepting the decisions of parents versus client?

4. Mr. A. and Mrs. C. are both residents of a long-term care facility. Mr. A. is married and Mrs. C. is a widow. The two have developed an intimate relationship that appears to be mutually satisfying to them both. Both residents are mentally competent and consenting adults. Mrs. A. is troubled by this and expects the staff to intervene. Does the staff have the right to intervene? If so, does this conflict with the resident's rights?

Making Decisions

The solutions to such problems should be a result of shared medical decision making. This process requires knowledge of the client, of the client's condition, and potential for recovery. Most importantly, the question is; what does the client consider to be quality of life? Age of the client should not be the sole criterion used in arriving at a decision. The legal basis for decisions must also be considered. For example, an elderly person who has suffered with a chronic illness for several years is taken to the hospital in acute respiratory distress and goes into cardiac arrest. The client is placed on full life-support. This action may not be in agreement with the family or the staff but it may have a legal basis in the absence of any document from the client (advance directive) stating the client's wishes in situations regarding life-saving measures. (See Chapters 2, Legal Aspects of Nursing, and 18, The Dying Process/Hospice Care in this text.)

SOURCES OF REIMBURSEMENT

Medicare and **Medicaid** have long been traditional sources of reimbursement for non-acute care. All health care providers must be certified by both

Medicare and Medicaid in order to receive payment for services rendered. While virtually all hospitals are certified by both Medicare and Medicaid, many long-term care providers including home health care and skilled care facilities are not. Clients, families, and hospital discharge planners need to be aware of this when planning continuing care.

Medicaid

Medicaid (Title XIX) pays for health services for the aged poor, the disabled, and low-income families with dependent children (Abrams, Beers, & Berkow, 1995). The program is financed by federal and state funds and is administered at the state level. Thus, services provided vary from state to state. Medicaid is currently the primary health financing program for low-income families and disabled individuals. It is a means-tested program, providing funds only when all other financial resources have been exhausted (Buckwalter, 1995). Services covered include inpatient and outpatient hospital care, diagnostic services, physician services, skilled nursing care, and home health services. Medicaid finances health care for 32 million persons at a total annual cost of $125 billion of which $31 billion is spent on the elderly. Of this amount, 73 percent provides long-term care services for 1.4 million elderly persons. Medicaid is the principal source of financial assistance for long-term care. Medicaid pays for skilled home health care in all states and twenty-nine states also cover the optional benefit of personal care in the home. In 1993, 300,000 persons received home health and personal care services at a cost of $2.8 billion to Medicaid (Buckwalter, 1995).

Medicare

In 1965, Medicare (Title XVIII) was signed into law as an amendment to the Social Security Act. Medicare is administered by the federal government through the Health Care Finance Administration (HCFA). Part A covers inpatient hospital care, home health care, and hospice care. Payment may be made for care in a skilled nursing facility. However, there are many restrictions and criteria for coverage frequently changes. Medicare Part B covers partial costs for physician services, outpatient hospital and rehabilitation care, and certain services and supplies not covered by Part A. Medicare is the major source of payment for acute care services for persons over sixty-five years old and for permanently disabled individuals who receive Social Security disability benefits. Thirty-six million people are enrolled in Medicare, 90 percent of whom are over 65 years of age. In 1995, Medicare spent $176 billion accounting for 18 percent of all health care expenditures.

Medicare pays for limited skilled care and rehabilitation services in certified long-term care facilities if the client and the services provided meet specific criteria. Certified home health care agencies may be reimbursed for intermittent visits if the client requires skilled health care by a registered nurse.

Private Insurance

Sixty-six percent of beneficiaries of Medicare purchase Medigap insurance to pay for costs not covered by Medicare. These policies are purchased from private insurance companies. **Medigap insurance** has been restricted by Congress to a basic plan with nine possible expansions (Abrams, et al., 1995). Only 0.2 percent of all long-term care costs are covered by insurance (Fisher, 1995). About 50 percent of costs are paid by the clients and their families, about 3 percent by Medicare and the remainder by Medicaid (Abrams, et al., 1995). Long-term care insurance is a relatively new concept and the benefits vary greatly depending on the insurance company.

LICENSURE, CERTIFICATION, AND ACCREDITATION

There are a number of processes that have been designed to assure the health care consumer that the facility, agency, or service meets minimal standards of care. **Licensure** is mandatory and is regulated by each state. **Certification** is voluntary but is required for any provider who seeks reimbursement from government funds. Since government funding is regulated by the federal government, certification standards are generated by the federal government. **Accreditation** is an additional confirmation of quality and generally indicates that the provider has gone above the minimum standards in the delivery of care and service.

Licensure

All health care facilities must be licensed. Each state has a designated agency (often the Department of Public Health) that is responsible for licensing health care facilities. A team of surveyors visits each facility annually to determine if the facility is in compliance with the rules and regulations of the state. Noncompliance in any area results in severe sanctions and financial penalties to the institution. The facility is given a limited amount of time to correct any deficiencies. In cases where residents' lives or well-being are threatened, the facility may lose its license to operate.

Certification

Certification is required for any facility that chooses to be reimbursed by government funds, Medicare and Medicaid. There are standards that must be met in order for certification to be granted. HCFA contracts with the state agencies to perform this function. In some states the long-term care survey for licensure and certification is done concurrently. Because there are two regulatory agencies (state and federal), the states have adopted the federal regulations and in some cases have exceeded federal regulations. Certification may not be granted if the facility is in noncompliance with regulations. This means the facility will not receive any reimbursement from Medicare or Medicaid funds.

Accreditation

Seeking accreditation is voluntary (not required by law). These organizations issue standards whereas state/federal licensure and certification agencies issue rules and regulations. The Joint Commission on the Accreditation of Healthcare Organizations (JCAHO) has long been accrediting hospitals and skilled nursing facilities. The Commission on Accreditation of Rehabilitation Facilities (CARF) has been accrediting comprehensive inpatient rehabilitation programs since 1966. Facilities like a subacute care unit specializing in rehabilitation may seek accreditation from both commissions (Bailis, 1995).

REHABILITATION

Rehabilitation is a process designed to assist individuals to reach their optimal level of physical, mental, and psychosocial functioning. This goal is accomplished by preventing complications, modifying the effects of the disability, and increasing independence. By so doing, the individual's self-esteem is maximized, thus increasing quality of life (Habel, 1993). Rehabilitation is concerned with increasing the client's ability to complete the basic activities of daily living (ADL) and the instrumental activities of daily living (IADL). ADL include grooming and hygiene, eating, dressing, toileting, and mobility. The IADL include higher level tasks such as household and money management, using the telephone and driving a car. For persons who have limited potential for regaining total independence, the goal is to teach the client to manage his or her own care.

The American Rehabilitation Association estimates that 300,000 Americans return to work each year as a result of receiving rehabilitation services. This employment generates $700 million in federal and state income taxes and saves Medicaid and other insurers $1

to $2 billion. For every dollar spent on rehabilitation, thirty dollars are saved (Huey, 1995).

The Interdisciplinary Health Care Team

The interdisciplinary health care team (IHCT) is an essential component to any rehabilitation process. The client and family are the focus of the team and are encouraged to participate in the planning of care. The degree to which the family participates is determined by the client. The professional members of the team are selected based on the needs of the client. Physical and occupational therapists, a speech/language pathologist, recreational therapists, rehabilitation nurses, the physician, social workers, dietitians, and mental health professionals are usually required to provide services (Figure 17-1).

Each discipline completes an assessment and pools this information at the care planning conference so that a consensus among members (including the client and family) can be reached. The team process avoids both duplication of services and fragmented care. A holistic approach is utilized so that the client's physical, mental, and psychosocial needs will be identified (Wenckus, 1995).

Role of the LP/VN as a Member of the Interdisciplinary Team

Rehabilitation nursing is a specialty practice and requires specialized knowledge, skills, and attitudes. A sound knowledge base in the anatomy and physiology of the neurological, musculoskeletal, gastrointestinal, and urological systems is a prerequisite. The nurse must have excellent clinical skills in the areas of therapeutic positioning, range of joint motion exercises, transfers, ambulation, and activities of daily living. The nurse is responsible for planning measures to prevent complications such as impaired skin integrity and contractures and to implement interventions for dysphagia, incontinence, and other identified problems.

The nurse is a member of the interdisciplinary team and as such may function as caregiver, counselor, coordinator of care, and client advocate (Habel, 1993). The nurse needs an understanding of the roles and responsibilities of each discipline and how the nurse interrelates with each discipline. There is a steady demand for rehabilitation nurses in all settings.

Rehabilitation Settings

Rehabilitation can be conducted in a variety of settings. Rehabilitation begins during the acute stage of

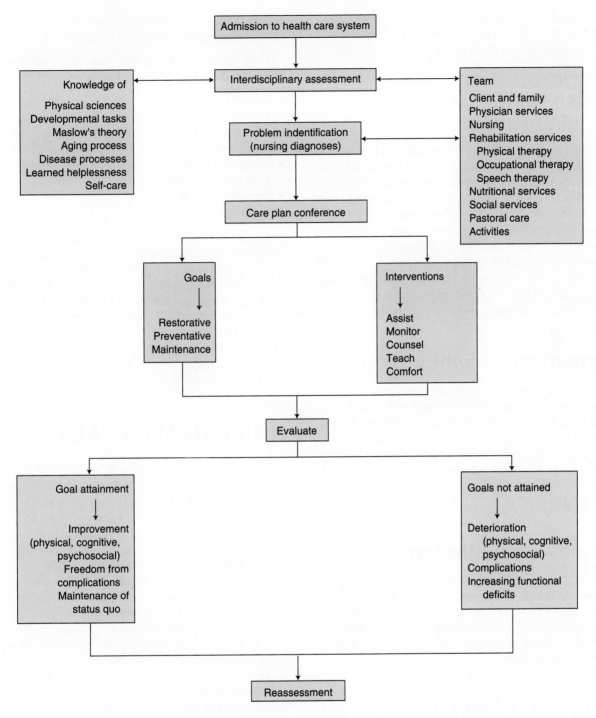

FIGURE 17-1 The interdisciplinary health care team process.

illness when the client's medical condition stabilizes. Continuing rehabilitative services are often needed after discharge from acute care, necessitating transfer to another facility. Decisions about entry into a rehabilitation program should reflect a consensus between the client, family or significant others, physician, and the rehabilitation program. The Agency for Health Care Policy and Research (Gresham, et al., 1995) describes the types of rehabilitation programs.

Hospital Inpatient Program

Hospitals may have a separate rehabilitation unit or services may be available in a free standing hospital specializing in the delivery of rehabilitation services. In either case, the hospitals are staffed by a full range of rehabilitation professionals. Registered nurses and a physician skilled in rehabilitation (physiatrist) are available twenty-four hours a day. Hospital programs are generally more intense and comprehensive than programs in other settings requiring greater physical and mental effort from the client.

Rehabilitation in Skilled Nursing Facilities

Skilled nursing facilities often offer rehabilitation services. The facility may be hospital based or community based. The programs are similar to those offered in hospital settings with a full range of services and health care professionals. Physician coverage varies but professional nursing care is rendered twenty-four hours a day. The program is usually less intense than a hospital program; this may be a benefit to elderly clients with limited energy resources. Families should research the services available because they differ greatly from one facility to the next.

Outpatient Rehabilitation

Outpatient services are offered by hospital-based rehabilitation programs. The intensity may range from occasional visits to three or four visits per week. Day hospital programs are another form of outpatient services but require the client to spend several hours a day for three to five days a week at the hospital. Availability of transportation is a prerequisite for all outpatient programs.

Home Rehabilitation

Some home health agencies provide a full scope of services including nursing, all therapies, and social services. Service is usually provided on an intermittent basis for medically stable clients. The accessibility of services varies greatly depending on the availability of therapists in the area.

Functional Assessment and Evaluation for Rehabilitation

Clients who need rehabilitation are screened before admission to a program. Assessments are completed by health care professionals whose services may be required by the client (Figure 17-2). The purpose of screening is to select the best setting for services. Criteria for admission to a program usually require that the client be:

- Medically stable
- Able to learn

- Able to sit supported for at least one hour a day and to actively participate in the program

Interdisciplinary programs may stipulate that the client has disabilities in two or more areas of function:

- Mobility
- Performance of activities of daily living (ADL)
- Bowel and bladder control
- Cognition
- Emotional function
- Pain management
- Swallowing
- Communication

There are a number of standardized assessment instruments that are designed to evaluate motor function, cognition, speech and language, mobility, and the client's performance of activities of daily living. There are additional tools that identify the client's risk for pressure ulcer formation, and potential for bowel and bladder management for incontinence. Refer to the AHCPR publication Post-Stroke Rehabilitation, Clinical Guideline Number 16 for a complete description of assessment instruments (Gresham, et al., 1995).

HOME HEALTH CARE

Home care encompasses a number of services delivered to persons in their homes and is the fastest growing segment of health care delivery. The total number of home health care agencies increased by 26 percent between 1989 and 1994 (Millea, 1995). Clients are receiving intravenous therapy, ventilator care, parenteral nutrition, and chemotherapy at home. Many agencies have nurse specialists on staff for complicated cases involving wound care, intravenous therapy, diabetes, cardiac, and respiratory care.

Medicare certified agencies provide intermittent care to persons meeting the criteria for care. A registered nurse may call on the client a specified number of times each week to assess the client's condition, supervise the work of other nonlicensed staff, and to deliver skilled nursing care. Nursing assistants are assigned to give personal care, check vital signs, do positioning, transfers, and passive range of motion exercises. In addition to nursing staff, the agency may provide therapists and social workers to serve their clients, also on an intermittent basis. These services are time-limited by Medicare and are not reimbursable if the client is not deemed to require skilled care.

The home health agency may provide or arrange with other vendors for services needed by the client. This may include Meals-on-Wheels, homemaker services for light housekeeping tasks, companion services, transportation for outclient care, intravenous

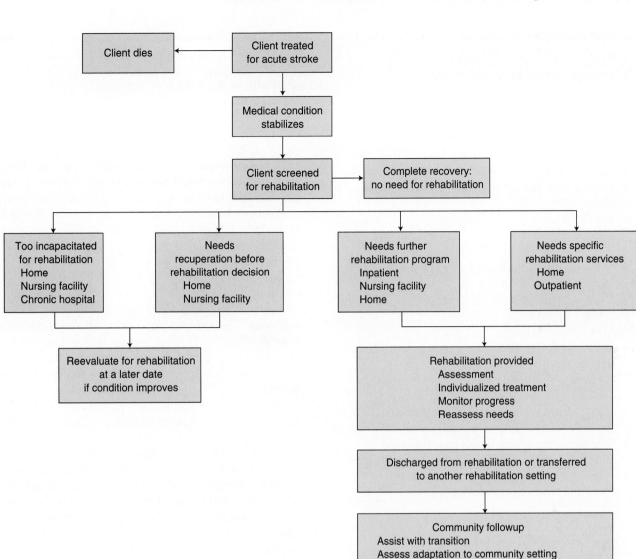

FIGURE 17-2   Assessing potential—stroke rehabilitation.

therapy, pain management, and parenteral nutrition. The home health nurse needs to be aware of the availability of respite care. Family members may need a break from the rigors of caregiving and may need encouragement from the nurse to do so.

Role of the LP/VN as a Member of the Team

Although the role of the LP/VN in home care is expanding, current (1994) statistics indicate that LP/VNs make up the smallest number of home health care professionals. There were 254,643 registered nurses, 34,757 licensed practical nurses, 171,346 home health care assistants, and 48,460 physical therapists (Millea, 1995). The responsibilities of the LP/VN vary between agencies. All nurses working in home care must have excellent assessment skills and a keen ability to identify problems and potential problems. Working with the family may be a greater challenge than meeting the needs of the client. Teaching the client and family is a major responsibility for the home health nurse. The educated client can assume more control. The client with a chronic health problem will have ongoing needs after the home health care is discontinued. Clients and their family caregivers need to know the following:

The disease process

- Complications that may occur
- How to prevent the complications
- Signs and symptoms of the complications
- How to reduce risk factors such as dietary adaptations and exercise programs

Medications

- Actions of medications
- Special administration guidelines such as before or after meals
- Side effects

Special skills

- Drawing up and administration of insulin or other injectables
- Using a blood glucose monitor
- Changing dressings
- Monitoring vital signs
- Use of special client care equipment, adaptive devices, and assistive devices

Documentation

- How to keep records for nurse or physician visit, for example; blood glucose, blood pressure and weight
- Communication with health care providers
- How and when to contact the home health nurse
- How and when to contact the physician
- How and when to contact emergency services

LONG-TERM CARE

Long-term care refers to a spectrum of services provided to individuals who have an ongoing need for health care. Long-term care has traditionally meant a community-based nursing home licensed for skilled or intermediate care. While there is a great demand for this type of care, there is also a market for other levels of health care. It is estimated that by the year 2000, more than 8 million Americans 65 years and older will need some form of long-term care (Diaz,1995). Currently 5 percent of Americans age 65 and over are residents of long-term care facilities. If this figure is broken down by age, statistics reveal that while less than 5 percent of those age 65 are residents, the figure rises to 20 percent for those 85 years and over (AARP, 1995).

Nonacute Care Health Services

The increasing population of elderly persons has resulted in tremendous changes in health care delivery. Housing options are often a component of the package of services available. The least restrictive level of care that is appropriate for the client's needs will generally be the most cost effective.

Long-Term Care Facilities

A **long-term care facility** may be licensed for either intermediate care or skilled nursing care. Long-term care facilities provide services to individuals who are not acutely ill, have continuing health care needs, and cannot function independently at home. Intermediate care facilities (ICF) are not certified for reimbursement from Medicare but may be certified for Medicaid funding. Skilled nursing facilities (SNF) are eligible for certification by both Medicare and Medicaid but not all facilities choose to become certified. These facilities were formerly called nursing homes, rest homes, or convalescent centers. The term *extended care facility* (ECF) refers to any facility that renders care for a long period of time. It has no concrete definition and could refer to either an intermediate or skilled nursing facility. Facilities in every state that receive any government funds from any source are required by law to be in compliance with the OBRA regulations.

Facilities of today bear little resemblance to those of the 1970s and 1980s. A restorative philosophy of care provides direction for the interdisciplinary team. Emphasis is placed on assisting the client (usually called resident) to attain and maintain the highest level of physical, mental, and psychosocial function. A holistic approach is utilized and families are important members of the care team.

A large number of facilities have special units devoted to the care of residents with specific problems. These units may care for persons with Alzheimer's disease, diabetes, respiratory disorders, wounds, and so on.

Subacute Care

Subacute care is a relatively new concept designed to provide services for clients who are out of the acute stage of their illnesses but who still require skilled nursing, monitoring, and ongoing treatments. The clients are not critically ill but do have complex medical needs. Subacute care is intended to fill the gap between the acute care hospital and the traditional long-term care facility (Glosner, 1995).

Subacute care facilities are usually housed in a section of a free-standing long-term care facility. The nurses may have a critical care background or are given additional training to equip them with the skills needed to provide care. Services may include intensive rehabilitation therapies, wound and pain management, care for clients with acquired immunodeficiency syndrome, oncology, postsurgical, intravenous therapy, nutritional support, peritoneal dialysis, ventilator care, and cardiac monitoring. Many subacute care units specialize in one or two of these areas. Clients stay from twenty to thirty days. Efficient discharge planning and client teaching are essential components to the plan of care.

Continuing Care Retirement Communities

Continuing Care Retirement Communities (CCRC) are designed to provide continuing levels of care as the individual's health care needs change. These levels include:

- Independent living in apartments located on the campus—housekeeping services and meals are provided
- **Assisted living**—for persons who need help with the activities of daily living
- Health care—either short-term for persons recovering from a temporary disorder or permanent for long-term illnesses such as Alzheimer's disease. The health care facility of the CCRC may be licensed as either skilled or intermediate

CCRCs usually charge a fee upon entry to the system and a monthly fee thereafter. The client must give proof of adequate financial resources in order to be accepted into the system. In exchange, individuals have the security of knowing that they will receive care for the remainder of their lives. Most CCRCs stipulate that persons must enter the system when they are able to live independently in the apartments. The health care facility of the CCRC may be certified for Medicaid if clients exhaust their financial resources. The health care facility may be certified for Medicare for clients who are qualified to receive such services. Neither Medicare nor Medicaid will pay for the independent living or assisted living sections of a CCRC.

Assisted Living

Assisted living combines housing and services to older persons who require assistance with activities of daily living. Nursing care is not provided. These are persons who cannot live alone but who do not need twenty-four-hour care. It is a less restrictive environment than a long-term care facility and maintains the individual's independence and freedom of choice. This level of care may be offered in a free-standing facility or as a section of a long-term care facility or CCRC as previously described. A monthly fee is charged and covers rent, utilities, housekeeping services, meals, and assistance with ADL (Lasky, 1995). Private funds pay for 90 percent of assisted living expenses. The remaining 10 percent is often rendered by charitable groups that provide funding for the facility.

Adult Day Care

Adult day care centers may be located in a separate unit of a long-term care facility, in a private home, or be free-standing. They provide a variety of services in a protective setting for adults who are unable to stay alone, but who do not need twenty-four-hour care. The centers are generally open from 7:00 A.M. to 6:00 P.M. five days a week, and serve two or three meals a day. A daily or hourly fee is charged with an additional charge for meals. Services may be limited to socialization or may be comprehensive offering modest rehabilitation services and nursing care. Adult day care is often utilized by working persons who have a spouse or parent living with them who cannot be left alone. Fifty percent of clients in day care have some degree of cognitive impairment (Meng, 1995).

Respite Care

Respite care may be offered by adult day care centers, long-term care facilities, or in private homes. It is intended to provide a break to caregivers and may be utilized a few hours a week, for an occasional weekend or for longer vacations. Planned activities, meals, and supervision are included in respite care services.

Foster Care

Some states are investigating the use of foster homes for individuals who cannot live independently but who do not require the services of a health care facility. A person with Alzheimer's disease who is mobile but who is unable to stay alone because of cognitive impairment would be a candidate for foster care. The legal structure is similar to the foster home concept for children.

The Role of the LP/VN in Long-Term Care

There are probably more career opportunities available for the LP/VN in long-term care facilities than in the other types of health care described in this chapter. In a small facility the LP/VN might act as supervisor during the night or evening shifts. In larger facilities the LP/VN might be in charge of one unit with a registered nurse as a house supervisor. The nurse needs sharp assessment skills and a sound ability to make nursing judgments based on assessment findings. The LP/VN may also be expected to supervise and coordinate the work of nursing assistants. The nurse may wish to seek additional course work to acquire supervisory skills.

Sample Nursing Care Plan: The Client With Stroke

Mr. Jason, sixty-five years old, was admitted to a skilled nursing facility following hospitalization for a right cerebral hemisphere stroke. He is unable to purposefully change position without assistance. His gag reflex is weakened, swallowing is delayed, and there is coughing after swallowing. Mr. Jason has smoked for fifty years and is still doing so. Rehabilitation was initiated in the hospital. A feeding tube was put in place with the goal to assist Mr. Jason to regain his swallowing ability so the tube can be removed. Mr. Jason frequently expresses his discouragement with his dependency on the staff. He is married and lives in the community with his wife. Mr. Jason had been retired for one year before the stroke. Mrs. Jason works full time. There are two adult children both of whom live in other states. Mrs. Jason hopes that her husband will regain adequate mobility skills so that she can eventually take him home.

Nursing Diagnosis 1 Physical mobility, impaired related to left hemiplegia and sensory/perceptual deficits as evidenced by inability to purposefully change position of body without assistance.

Goals	Nursing Interventions	Rationale	Evaluation
Mr. Jason will maintain current level of range of motion in all joints.	Change position at least every two hours; place affected extremities out of **synergy**.	Prevent contracture formation and pressure ulcers. Hemiplegic limbs are flaccid immediately after stroke and then become spastic. Synergy patterns, abnormal patterns of movement that result from an overactive stretch reflex due to CNS damage, may develop in response to spasticity, causing contractures. Positioning out of synergy avoids contracture formation.	Range of joint motion is preserved. Complications related to immobility are prevented. Progress in mobilization is achieved; movement in bed, transfers with one to two assists, transfer independently, ambulation.
Mr. Jason will remain free of contractures.	Do passive range of motion exercises twice a day on affected extremities. Assist with active range-of-motion exercises on unaffected extremities. Teach to do self-range-of-motion exercises when condition permits.	Range-of-motion exercises maintain joint mobility and prevent contracture formation. Active and self range of motion exercises will also increase strength and endurance.	
Mr. Jason will begin program of progressive mobilization.	Use bridging techniques to teach Mr. Jason to move in bed: – Client begins in supine position with the knees bent and feet flat in bed. – Instruct client to raise the hips by pressing his heels down.	Using bridging techniques increases the client's bed mobility. The recovery of a client with a stroke is dependent on the cooperative efforts of several interdisciplinary team members.	

	– The nurse stabilizes the affected limb by exerting pressure downward through the thigh just above the knee while assisting the client to lift the pelvis clear of the bed (Galarneau, 1993).		
	Consult with physical therapist about program for progressive mobilization.	The physical therapist is an expert in mobility.	

Nursing Diagnosis 2 Swallowing, impaired related to neuromuscular dysfunction as evidenced by weakened gag reflex, delayed swallowing, and coughing after swallowing.

Goals	Nursing Interventions	Rationale	Evaluation
Mr. Jason will swallow without aspirating.	Consult with speech/language pathologist in regard to video-recorded fluoroscopy for swallowing evaluation.	A video-recorded fluoroscopy is used to make a definitive diagnosis of impaired swallowing. The results of the evaluation provide a basis for interventions suggested by the speech/language pathologist.	There are no signs of aspiration.
	Serve semisolid foods of medium consistency. Use a commercial thickener for liquids. Avoid milk, citrus juices, and water.	These foods require less manipulation in the mouth and allow the client to concentrate on swallowing rather than chewing. Liquids are more manageable when thickened. Water provides minimal sensory stimulation, making it difficult for the client to manage water. Milk and citrus juices stimulate production of saliva.	
	Allow rest period before eating. Position client at 60°–90° angle before, during, and for one hour after eating.	Fatigue increases risk of aspiration.	
	Maintain head in midline with neck slightly flexed.	This position facilitates the passage of food through the pharynx.	

(continued)

	Face the client, avoid haste.	Facing the client allows feeder to evaluate the eating process. If the feeder appears hurried, the client may try to eat faster.	
	Minimize distractions, keep conversation minimal.	The client's attention must focus only on eating.	
	Allow Mr. Jason to see and smell food. Give verbal descriptions. Use regular metal teaspoon, give one-half teaspoon at a time.	Sensory cues promote awareness of eating.	
	Place food on unaffected side of mouth. Teach to hold food in mouth, think about swallowing and then swallow twice.	Buccal pocketing of food in the cheek on the affected side is common after a stroke.	

Nursing Diagnosis 3 Self-esteem, situational, low, related to changes in functional abilities as evidenced by verbal expression of discouragement.

Goals	Nursing Interventions	Rationale	Evaluation
Mr. Jason will verbalize acceptance of self, situation, and lifestyle changes.	Assess for signs of severe or prolonged grieving.	The client needs to grieve the loss of his former self. Prolonged grieving may indicate need for counseling.	Client is progressing through all rehabilitation therapies and presents no signs of prolonged grieving.
	Assess client's interactions with significant others.	Other people may be reinforcing the concepts of helplessness and invalidism.	
	Listen in nonjudgmental fashion to comments about situation.	Each person responds differently to crisis. Being nonjudgmental builds trust and encourages verbalization of thoughts.	

Nursing Diagnosis 4 Injury, high risk for, related to the possibility of having another stroke as evidenced by continuation of smoking.

Goals	Nursing Interventions	Rationale	Evaluation
Mr. Jason will reduce risk factors for repeated stroke.	Monitor blood pressure.	Blood pressure often increases before a stroke.	Must wait to see if Mr. Jason has another stroke.
	Monitor for signs of transient ischemic attack or impending stroke; altered consciousness, hemiplegia, visual problems, impaired speech.	Transient ischemic attacks often occur before a stroke.	
	Consult with dietitian for dietary adaptations; reduced sodium, reduced fat, and cholesterol.	These dietary changes may help prevent a stroke.	
	Encourage Mr. Jason to begin a smoking cessation program.	Smoking increases the risk of a stroke.	
	Teach client and family risk factors of stroke and measures for reducing or eliminating risk factors.	The client and family must know the risk factors of a stroke so they can implement measures to reduce or eliminate them.	
	Teach client and family to identify signs and symptoms of transient ischemic attacks or impending stroke (previously discussed) and to seek immediate medical attention.	The client and family must know the signs and symptoms of transient ischemic attacks or impending stroke so they can seek immediate medical care.	

► *CASE STUDY*

Mrs. Emma James, seventy-two years old, was admitted to Community Hospital for a left below knee amputation. Mrs. James has been an insulin dependent diabetic for thirty-five years. The amputation follows a long and unsuccessful period of treatment for venous stasis ulcers. Mrs. James was transferred from the hospital to a rehabilitation hospital on her fourth postoperative day. After two weeks at the rehabilitation hospital, she was transferred to a skilled care facility near her home for additional rehabilitation and regulation of the diabetes. She is now ready to be discharged to her home. Mrs. James has a prosthesis and is able to ambulate with a walker. She can perform her ADL with minimal assistance. She was on a sliding scale and blood glucose monitoring four times a day while in the long-term care facility. Her physician has now placed her on insulin twice a day with daily blood glucose checks. Her vision is somewhat impaired due to the diabetes. Mrs. James lives alone in a one-story home in a safe residential area. The discharge planner at the skilled care facility has arranged continuing care for Mrs. James through a local home health agency.

The following questions will guide your development of a Nursing Care Plan for the case study.

1. Identify the assessment factors that are most important in planning Mrs. James' care.

2. List the nursing diagnoses that would be applicable to Mrs. James' assessment.

3. Describe the complications for which Mrs. James is at risk.

4. Describe nursing interventions for preventing the complications.

5. What specific actions would you take to prevent a recurrence of venous stasis ulcers?

6. What additional community services does Mrs. James need?

7. What nursing services would you plan to meet her needs; frequency of nurse visits, services from a nursing assistant, other home health services. Which services would each person provide?

8. Describe the outcomes you would expect for Mrs. James.

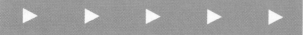

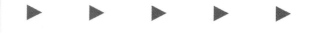

SUMMARY

- There has been a significant increase in the growth of non-acute care settings.
- Medicaid (state and federal funds) and Medicare (federal funds) are major sources of health care payment, especially for the elderly and permanently disabled. The availability of these resources in the future is in jeopardy. Alternative funding sources are being explored by state and federal governments.
- Rehabilitation can be provided in a variety of settings.
- There is a need for the services and skills of the LP/VN in all of these health care services. Experience and additional education may be required for employment in special care settings.

Review Questions

1. One reason for the growth in non-acute care health services is:
   a. the diminishing supply of physicians.
   b. an increase in the number of hospitals in the country.
   c. the cost of acute care.
   d. the increase in Medicare reimbursement.

2. Medicare is a reimbursement system for health care providers that:
   a. is based upon the client's personal financial resources.
   b. is available to persons 65 years of age and over or who have been disabled for two or more years.
   c. pays the full cost of all medical care.
   d. is managed by each state.

3. Subacute care is most often provided:
   a. in a step-down unit of the hospital.
   b. in a special care unit of a skilled care facility.
   c. for clients who are terminally ill.
   d. for clients who require life support.

4. Which of the following clients would be most likely to benefit from rehabilitation services?
   a. Mr. J, sixty-four years old who has had a stroke, is responsive and stable.
   b. Mrs. B, eighty-nine years old, has Alzheimer's disease in the fourth stage.
   c. Miss Z, twenty-six years old, recovering from pneumonia.
   d. Mr. K, fifty-six years old, terminal cancer of the lung.

5. Which of the following is a legal requirement for health care facilities that is controlled by each state?
   a. Accreditation
   b. Certification
   c. Licensure
   d. Provision of free care

6. As a member of the interdisciplinary health care team, the LP/VN must be able to:
   a. participate in the planning of client care.
   b. plan the appropriate diet for clients.
   c. teach the new amputee how to walk with a prosthesis.
   d. provide alternative methods of communication for the client with recent stroke.

7. In the home health care setting it is essential that the LP/VN possess skills in:
   a. advanced intravenous therapy.
   b. respiratory therapy treatments.
   c. physical assessment.
   d. planning and providing speech therapy.

8. In a long-term care facility the LP/VN may serve as the:
   a. charge nurse of a unit.
   b. director of nursing.
   c. clinical nurse specialist.
   d. social worker.

Critical Thinking Questions

1. Imagine what it would be like learning to speak after having a stroke.

2. What are the pros and cons related to working for a home health agency or a long-term care facility?

News Flash

A recent trial has found that service dogs can be trained to assist people with physical disabilities in completing the activities of daily living. The service dogs also provide emotional comfort. After 12 months into the study the people who had dogs needed two-thirds less assistance by home health aides and they needed less help from family members. Service dogs can open and close doors, operate switches, help a person up from a chair or bed, pull a wheelchair, retrieve and carry objects, and drag a person away in an emergency. This study has significant implications for providers of rehabilitation and home health care services (*Source: Journal of American Medical Association, 275(13), 1001–1006, April 3, 1996*).

CHAPTER
18

The Dying Process/ Hospice Care

Joan Fritsch Needham

▶ KEY TERMS

acceptance
advance directives
anticipatory grieving
autopsy
bargaining
bereavement
breakthrough pain
cerebral death
Cheyne-Stokes respirations
coroner
death rattle
denial
depression
durable power of attorney for health care
ethics committee
euthanasia
grief
Health Care Surrogate Law
hospice
life review
Living Will
loss
mortuary
palliative care
Patient Self-Determination Act
post-mortem care
reactive depression
resuscitation
rigor mortis
shroud
terminal illness
thanatology

LEARNING OBJECTIVES

Upon completion of this chapter the learner should be able to:
- Define key terms.
- Cite the dying person's bill of rights.
- Describe the grieving process.
- Identify the key aspects of the Patient Self-Determination Act.
- List the purposes of an ethics committee.
- Describe the hospice philosophy of care.
- Describe factors that influence the family's response to the client's terminal illness.
- Summarize nursing interventions for the care of the dying client.
- Discuss the issue of artificial nutrition for the terminally ill client.
- Describe the procedure for postmortem care.

▶ *MAKING THE CONNECTION*

Refer to the topics in the following chapters to increase your understanding of the dying process and hospice care.

- **Chapter 2, Legal Aspects of Nursing:** Advance Directives, p. 30
- **Chapter 4, Biomedical Ethics:** Organ Donation, p. 59; Euthanasia, p. 63
- **Chapter 5, Communication:** Listening/Observing, p. 71; Therapeutic Communication, p. 71; Communicating with the Terminally Ill Clients and Their Families, p. 78
- **Chapter 6, Cultural Aspects of Health and Illness:** Relationship Between Culture and

Religion, p. 90; Influence of Culture on Beliefs and Practices About Health and Illness, p. 90
- **Chapter 12, Pain Management:** Therapeutic Approaches to Pain, p. 214
- **Chapter 15, Oncology Nursing:** Symptom Management, p. 314; Psychosocial Problems, p. 318
- **Chapter 16, Caring for the Older Adult:** Losses, p. 332
- **Chapter 19, Respiratory Disorders:** Assessment, p. 393

KEY ABBREVIATIONS

The following abbreviations and acronyms are used in this chapter:

DNR	do not resuscitate
HMO	health maintenance organization
MS	morphine sulfate
OBRA	Omnibus Budget Reconciliation Act

INTRODUCTION

Historically, death has been considered as natural as birth, the last stage of life. The last three decades have brought about significant changes in the cultural perception of death. Death represents the earthly end of a life lived. However, in some cases dying and death are no longer simple matters but are issues surrounded by ethical concerns and in some cases legal intervention by the court system. Before the 1970s, nursing textbooks said very little about the dying process. Instructions on physical care for the dying and for the dead were the extent of the information presented. In 1969 Dr. Elizabeth Kubler-Ross made a medical breakthrough when she published *On Death and Dying.* The book was the culmination of many years of research and working with terminally ill clients. **Terminal illness** is defined as one in which cure is not possible and death is expected. **Thanatology** (the science of death) became a legitimate subject in the curriculum of student nurses. This developing interest and concern in the care of the dying soon led to a **hospice** movement. Hospice is a philosophy that focuses on

pain and symptom control and emotional support and counseling for the client, family, and caregivers (Rhymes, 1993).

Just as each person lives a unique life, so does each person die a unique death. Death may be sudden and unexpected caused by heart attack or accident. Death may be prolonged and come after a distressing long-term illness. Death may come quietly for the older person who dies during sleep. And some deaths are planned by those who choose to die on their own terms by suicide.

Health care workers must understand the legal and ethical issues surrounding dying and death. They must also come to terms with their own mortality and feelings about death if they are to provide comfort to dying clients and their families. Health care workers can learn about life from the dying client.

LEGAL CONSIDERATIONS

The **Patient Self-Determination Act** was incorporated into the Omnibus Budget Reconciliation Act (OBRA) of 1990. The act was intended to provide a legal means for individuals to determine the circumstances in which life-sustaining treatment would or would not be provided to them. The individual's choices are validated with advance directives. An **advance directive** means any written instruction, including a **Living Will** or **Durable Power of Attorney for Health Care** that is recognized under state law (Taylor, 1995). The act applies to hospitals, long-term care facilities, home health agencies, hospice programs, and certain health maintenance organizations (HMOs). Anyone entering the health care system through any of these organizations must be given information and the opportunity to complete advance directives if they have not already done so (see Chapter 2, Legal Aspects of Nursing). Persons need to know that in many states, just signing these documents may not be adequate for carrying out their wishes. They may also need to indicate their wishes in regard to artificial feeding, intubation, chemotherapy, surgery, blood transfusions, and transfer to the hospital (for residents in skilled care facilities).

Although the Living Will and Durable Power of Attorney for Health Care are legal documents, they do not preclude the need for **resuscitation** orders (implementation of cardiopulmonary resuscitation and life support measures). The medical record must have a physician's order stating *do not resuscitate* (DNR) if this is in agreement with the client's wishes and with the advance directives. In the absence of such an order, resuscitation will be initiated. The Council on Ethical and Judicial Affairs of the American Medical Association issued this statement on March 15, 1986:

> Life-prolonging medical treatment and artificially or technologically supplied respiration, nutrition, and hydration may be withheld from a client in an irreversible coma even if death is not imminent (Taylor, 1995).

Many states also have a **Health Care Surrogate Law** which is implemented in the absence of advance directives. This law varies from state to state. Basically, it provides a legal means for specific individuals to make decisions for the client when the client can no longer do so. The law has developed a hierarchy of individuals who would act in the interests of the client. The spouse is the first person in the hierarchy, followed by children if there is no spouse.

Donation of organs is another decision that may need to be made by the family if the client has not previously made such arrangements (refer to Chapter 4 for information on organ donation).

Euthanasia is a controversial subject that has received much attention. Euthanasia is defined as the act of taking life in order to relieve suffering. Actively taking measures to end life, usually with the administration of a drug, is considered active euthanasia. Passive euthanasia is sometimes defined as the withholding of treatment. The definition of euthanasia has become somewhat blurred because of the technological ability to maintain life for indefinite periods of time.

Ethics Committees

Hospitals and many long-term care facilities have established **ethics committees**. Their purpose is to protect client interests, provide staff education in ethical analysis, and develop policies for the management

of ethical dilemmas (Mitty, Mathy, Rappaport, & Ramsey, 1996). In some states, long-term care facilities are required to have an arrangement for dispute mediation with regard to issuance of do not resuscitate orders. The Dispute Mediation Committee is an advisory rather than policy-making body and often advises on issues related to the client's advisory capacity (Mitty et al., 1996). This means that when the client is unable to make decisions, the family will be given information upon which to base a decision for the client.

Ethics committees are interdisciplinary and may have attorneys and clergy as members as well as health care providers. Ethical decision making is a complex issue. Ethics committee members must be knowledgeable in areas of legal issues, advocacy, autonomy, economic factors, and obligation (Beckel, 1996).

THE DYING PERSON'S RIGHTS

The person who is dying has a right to expect that health care providers will provide care that will allow death to occur in peace and with dignity. The client has a right to:

- considerate and respectful care.
- be cared for by persons who can communicate openly and honestly.
- freedom from pain and discomfort.
- expect that physical, mental, and emotional needs will be met insofar as is possible.
- participate in the planning of care with the interdisciplinary health care team.
- access to spiritual counseling and direction—they also have the right to refuse spiritual counseling and direction.
- refuse life-extending procedures.
- expect that all communications and records be treated as confidential, except where authorized or required by law.
- expect complete information concerning diagnosis and treatment.
- express grievances related to care and treatment to the appropriate individuals.

GRIEF

Grief is a natural and normal process that is experienced with **loss**. Grief is a mourning process (**bereavement**) for what was and what will be as a result of the loss. The loss of health, the loss of independence, the loss of a loved one are all situations that kindle a grieving response. The terminally ill client may have experienced a number of losses throughout the illness, each one a reminder that the ultimate loss of life itself will eventually follow.

Dr. Elisabeth Kubler-Ross authored *On Death and Dying* in 1969 after two-and-a-half years of interviewing dying clients. Dr. Kubler-Ross learned that clients who know they are dying go through a series of coping mechanisms in their struggle to reach acceptance of an inevitable outcome. Clients do not always experience the stages in an organized manner, moving in an orderly fashion from one stage to the next. Most individuals fluctuate between stages even after reaching acceptance. Some clients may never reach a period of acceptance. The stages described by Dr. Kubler-Ross are denial and isolation, anger, bargaining, depression, and acceptance (Table 18-1).

Denial and Isolation

Upon becoming aware of a terminal illness, the first response is generally, "Oh, no, it can't be me." **Denial** serves as a shock absorber when reality is too harsh to comprehend. Denial is a healthy and normal approach to a painful and distressing situation. Some clients deal with denial by "doctor shopping" (this comment does not mean that second opinions are not sometimes necessary) or by insisting that there must have been a mix-up or mistake in the diagnostic tests. Others may use denial by simply avoiding the issue. They go about their daily routines as though nothing in their lives has changed. Most people, given the time will eventually move through denial. However, they may continue to use denial from time to time. They cannot face death

all the time, so it must be set aside so that life can be lived.

A client may be selective in using denial. For example, the client may use denial with certain family members or friends because he/she is trying to protect that person from the truth.

Anger

Eventually, denial gives way as the client realizes the truth; "yes, it is me." The next question may be "why me?" as the client attempts to deal with feelings of anger, rage, envy, and resentment. This stage is very difficult for family and caregivers. The anger may be displaced on anyone, everyone, the environment, and the health care system. Whatever is done is not the right thing. Families may be greeted with silence or with outbursts of anger. Their response may be anger, guilt, or despair. Loved ones need to know that the client's anger is a normal response and is not directed at them but at the situation. The client needs to deal with the anger in order to move past this stage. Professional counseling may be needed if the anger persists and the family and client are not coping with the situation.

Bargaining

The client who was angry at God for letting this terrible thing happen, may now attempt to enter into an arrangement with God to postpone the inevitable con-

Table 18-1

STAGES OF THE DYING PROCESS		
Stage	**Response**	**Description**
Denial/isolation	"Oh, no, it can't be me."	Reality is too harsh to comprehend. Denial is normal response.
Anger	"Why me?" Displays rage, fury, resentment.	Anger may be displaced on anyone, everyone, the environment.
Bargaining	"God, if you just let me live long enough to see my first grandchild I will not ask for anything more."	Attempting to postpone death. Client usually sets self-imposed limitations.
Depression	"Yes, it is me and I will lose everything and everyone that is near and dear to me."	Reality has set in. Reactive depression is response to present circumstances. Anticipatory grieving is a preparation for approaching losses.
Acceptance	"I will take each day as it comes. I am ready for whatever lies ahead."	Client may sleep more, limit visitors to a few special people, communicates with moments of silence with loved ones. Continues to need hope for comfort and dignity.

clusion by **bargaining**. This reaction is similar to that of a child who is not getting what he wants. He may become angry, shouting and stomping his feet. After being sent to his room, the anger wears off and he may then resort to negotiating; "If I clean my room, can I ?" The bargaining of the terminally ill client is an attempt to postpone and usually has self-imposed limitations. For example, the client will ask to live just long enough to see her first grandchild in exchange for a promise to perform some service for the church. Most clients bargain in silence or in confidence with their chaplain. Caregivers who have cared for terminally ill clients will agree that it is not uncommon for a client to live long enough for some special event (a wedding or birth), only to die shortly afterwards.

Depression

Depression is the response to the overwhelming number of losses the client is experiencing. Body image may be devastated by the loss or deformity of a body part. The client is unable to meet his role commitments as spouse, parent, employee, friend. Concerns increase as the client realizes that the cost of the illness may be placing great financial burdens on the family. Unfortunately clients sometimes feel abandoned as persons who were once friends begin to visit less and less, sometimes severing ties with the client even before death.

Persons suffering depression from losses are suffering a **reactive depression**, an expected response to the present circumstances. The client may verbalize his feelings and benefit from active interventions on the part of various health care disciplines. These clients need support, reassurance, and encouragement.

Another type of depression is associated with **anticipatory grieving**. It does not result from past losses but is a consequence of approaching losses. Depression is a mechanism that must be used to facilitate acceptance. The client will eventually lose everything and everybody that he loves. The client must be allowed to express his sorrow. There is little need for verbalization on the part of the caregiver. Silent acceptance, holding a hand, and listening are effective interventions. The persons around the client should be cautioned to avoid attempts to try to cheer the client, or to use phrases, like "don't worry." The client needs to deal with it in his own way in order to reach acceptance.

Acceptance

Clients, given enough time (not a sudden, unexpected death) and assistance, will eventually reach the stage of **acceptance**. Acceptance of the inevitable outcome is not a case of resignation or giving up. Neither is it a happy time. The client is almost void of feelings. He has worked through denial, resolved the feelings of anger, bargained with God, and experienced depression through anticipatory grieving. The client may sleep more, not to avoid reality but because sleep is needed to fill a physical and emotional need. The client may limit visitors to a few people with whom he feels safe and comfortable. The most significant form of communication at this time is moments of silence. The client needs hope; not hope for cure or recovery, but hope for comfort and dignity. The client needs to know that he will not be abandoned and that he will be kept comfortable. The family needs as much support and understanding as the client. If the client has reached acceptance and the family has worked through their grief, this can be a time of peace and serenity. The relationships between family members may become closer than ever. The family knows they have done everything they could do to make the client's last weeks as physically and emotionally comfortable as possible.

Age-Related Reactions to Grief

Persons of all ages generally experience the same feelings and emotions as they progress through a terminal illness. Elderly clients may welcome death if they have been ill for a long time, especially if they have outlived everyone who was near and dear to them. Persons of any age who have endured a long illness may view death as a release from their suffering. While they may not have chosen to die at this time in their lives, they no longer wish to continue life as it is. Older adults faced with death have had time to complete the accomplishments and developmental tasks that most people take for granted. Even older adults (and people of any age), may find it difficult to reach acceptance if they have unfinished business that has not been settled. When the end of life is near, many people achieve satisfaction from **life review**. Life review is a form of reminiscence in which the client is attempting to achieve integrity. It may cover the entire life span although not always in a chronological course. Life review is most successful when done on a one-to-one basis with a therapeutic listener (Haight & Burggraf, 1992). The listener must be prepared to manage the emotional reactions that may occur if the client has painful moments from the past that need to be resolved.

The age of the client may have a direct influence on the family's reaction to grief. The illness and loss of a spouse brings many lifestyle changes. The surviving spouse may become a single parent and become burdened with many additional responsibilities. The impending loss of companionship and love leaves a yearning for what will never be again.

Losing a child is one of the most devastating life events a family can experience. The family grieves for the young child who will never become an adult. Each birthday is marked by wondering what the child would look like and what the child would be doing if death had not intervened. Older persons who lose an adult child also mourn. The older adult who is ready to let go of life may wonder why the child who was in the prime of life was taken. The child's spouse may have excluded the parents from participation in decision making or caring for their child during illness and death. The parents may wonder if they will be able to continue a relationship with their grandchildren.

Unresolved Grief

It is unfortunate that sometimes a dying person is unable to come to terms with the illness and never reaches acceptance. There are situations when anger prevails throughout the course of the illness. Family members are bewildered and distressed as they try to do anything that will please the client. The anger presents a barrier to meaningful communication diminishing the possibility for a peaceful death. Some clients may not overcome depression, slowly withdrawing more and more from everyone around them.

Families too may carry the weight of unresolved grief. They may be suffering from guilt; "Did I do enough?" "Why didn't I insist that he go to the doctor sooner?" They may be angry at the dead person for "leaving them" too soon. For the survivors unresolved grief may eventually present itself through physical manifestations or stress related illnesses. The nurse can be beneficial in these situations.

- Listen to the family's concerns and expressed feelings.
- Be nonjudgmental.
- Assure the family that their feelings are normal and that it is helpful to express these feelings.
- Continue to be a "safe" person to whom the family can vent their emotions.

CARE SETTINGS FOR THE DYING CLIENT

People die in their homes, in hospitals, and in long-term care facilities. A hospice may or may not be involved in the care of the client. The hospice movement began in the United States in the mid-seventies with the opening of Hospice Incorporated in New Haven, Connecticut. Medicare provides coverage for many services and has extended hospice settings to include skilled care nursing facilities. Medicare mandates participating providers to provide:

- Grief and bereavement services to clients and caregivers
- Nursing and physician services as needed
- Drugs and biologicals on a 24-hour basis
- All other covered services on a 24-hour basis as needed to ease client pain and to manage the terminal illness

Hospice has higher staff-to-client ratios and believes in **palliative care**, treating symptoms and providing comfort rather than extending life. The relief of suffering is a primary objective. Suffering encompasses more than physical pain and agony. Fear, loss of hope, and lack of meaning in life are all forms of suffering. Clients receiving hospice services are expected to be in the terminal stages of illness with less than six months to live. While cancer is a common diagnosis for hospice clients, services are also provided to persons with end stage renal disease, heart failure, stroke, AIDS, chronic pulmonary disease, Alzheimer's disease, and Parkinson's disease.

THE DYING CLIENT'S FAMILY/FRIENDS

Relationships between the dying client and significant others have usually evolved through a period of time, weathering various types of crises. Each family group has its unwritten rules, its leaders and followers, and its methods for coping with crises. The family's equilibrium is threatened by the impending death. If family members have limited coping skills and inadequate support systems, they need assistance and guidance from the caregivers. The rules and coping mechanisms used by the family may not always coincide with the values and beliefs of the staff.

Loved ones may also go through a period of denial because the truth is too painful to accept. They may request that the client not be given information regarding the diagnosis and may interfere with the dissemination of information that the client needs in order to make informed decisions for care. The family needs to be informed that caregivers are there to support the client and that lying is not appropriate if the client asks specific questions (Taylor & Ferszt, 1994).

Buried conflicts between family members may emerge during times of crisis. Each person's former relationship with the client as well as the affiliation between each family member will influence the response of the individuals to the situation. Unresolved guilt, anger, and resentment may rise to the surface. One child may have shouldered the responsibility of caring for the ill parent. The parent may focus anger on this child if nursing home placement becomes necessary. The child who visits once a year may disagree with the decision but offer little assistance and no practical alternatives to the sibling.

It may be difficult for the client and family members to let go of the anger and resentment. A child who was abused may fear that forgiving the parent will mean approval of the act. A family member may want to see justice done and feels the client should also feel the hurt (Ufema, 1995). Anger may be directed at the client for leaving the family by dying; the family blames the client for "not taking care of him/herself."

Each family member will grieve the approaching death in his/her own way. The nurse needs to be supportive and nonjudgmental. The family needs to know that the staff cares about them as well as the client. Regardless of their feelings, their lives will never be the same.

The relationship with the family does not always end with the client's death. Staff members may attend visitations, funerals, or memorial services. If a hospice was involved, the family may participate in a bereavement support program. If the client had been a resident in a long-term care facility, family members may return to visit other residents with whom they became acquainted.

NURSING ASSESSMENTS AND INTERVENTIONS

Terminally ill clients are given palliative care (supportive care). The major goal for care is the physical, emotional, and mental comfort of the client. Many dying clients do not fear death but are anxious about a painful death or dying alone. A primary concern of palliative care is to help the client feel safe and secure. The nurse can do much to increase the client's feelings of safety by being there when needed. Holding the client's hand and listening are therapeutic measures. Ufema (1994) suggests asking the client three questions: "What do you want?" From whom do you want it?" and "When do you want it?" The client needs to know that he has the nurse's support as an advocate for his care and well-being.

Pain

The assessment and relief of pain are major concerns (see Chapter 12, Pain Management). Pain is a subjective, personal experience and the client is the best judge of the severity of the pain. The client needs to know that caregivers accept and believe complaints of pain and that they will intervene to prevent and alleviate the pain. Medication needs to be given around the clock and not "as needed." A nonnarcotic analgesic may be effective in early stages for mild intermittent pain. As the pain increases, the client will need to be started on morphine, titrated at increments until adequate pain relief is achieved without severe side effects. Ask the client to rate the pain from 0 to 10 with 0 being no pain and 10 being severe pain. Titrating the analgesic dose and interval means finding the lowest dose and longest interval of a drug that relieves pain. The dosage that should be used is the one that controls the pain to the satisfaction of the client with minimal side effects. For some clients this may be 10 mg PO morphine sulfate (MS) every four hours. For other clients it may be 480 mg MS IV per hour. The question for the nurse is what dose can be safely given? There is no maximum number of milligrams that apply to every individual. The nurse must monitor the client's responses for pain rating and respiratory rate. For example, 10 mg MS given IM may give pain relief, but if the respiratory rate drops from 12 to 6 per minute, lower the next dose. If the same dose given to another client provides minimal relief and the client is alert with no change in respirations, increase the next dose (McCaffery & Beebe, 1989).

Monitor the client for **breakthrough pain**. This is sudden, acute, temporary pain that is usually precipitated by a treatment or procedure or unusual activity of the client. A supplemental dose of medication is required. If the precipitating factor is known (dressing changes for example), a dose should be given 30 to 60 minutes before the procedure.

Adjuvant therapy may be effective. Nonsteroidal anti-inflammatory agents are beneficial for bone metastases; tricyclic antidepressants and anti-seizure medications for neurogenic pain and steroids for headaches related to cerebral edema (Rhymes, 1993). Nonpharmacologic techniques can be used with medication. Relaxation techniques, guided imagery, massages, and repositioning may enhance the action of the medications.

Fluids and Nutrition

The refusal of food and fluids is almost universal in dying clients. It is believed that the client is not feeling thirst and hunger. The issue of permitting dehydration in terminally ill clients is often met with great resistance. However, the literature supports the concept that forced nutrition has questionable value and may even exacerbate the client's condition (Taylor, 1995). Artificial nutrition often increases the client's agitation, increases the use of limb restraints and increases the risk of aspiration pneumonia (Rhymes, 1994). Hospice nurses have indicated that withholding artificial nutrition is not painful. In every situation the client's own wishes must always take precedence. If the comatose client has not previously made his wishes known, family members must be given accurate and truthful information. For the person in irreversible coma, withholding of artificial nutrition does not cause death; rather, it allows life to take its natural course (Taylor, 1995). Several professional groups have issued statements regarding artificial nutrition and hydration. The American Medical Association, the American Dietetic Association, and the American Nurses Association agree that it is legally, ethically, and professionally acceptable to discontinue nutritional support of the terminally ill (Taylor, 1995).

Physical Care

Physical care of a dying client serves three purposes: it prevents painful and costly complications; it may increase the client's feeling of physical comfort and well-being; it provides caregivers the opportunity to give "hands-on" care, giving the client a sense of security and love. Families should be encouraged and invited to participate in the client's care if they desire to do so.

Care of the Mouth, Eyes, and Nose

Oral discomfort is the only documented side effect of dehydration in the terminally ill client (Taylor, 1995). The administration of oxygen and mouth breathing increase the need for meticulous oral care. Caregivers can use saliva substitutes and moisturizers to alleviate discomfort. If the client is able, the regular use of toothpaste and toothbrush may be adequate. Lemon-glycerine swabs or mouth washes are effective for dependent clients. The tongue needs the same attention as the rest of the mouth with gentle brushing. Offer ice chips and sips of favorite beverages frequently. Apply petroleum jelly to the lips. Oral care must be given every two to three hours to maintain the client's comfort. The eyes may become irritated due to dryness. Artificial tears can alleviate this discomfort. Use a cotton ball and gently wipe from inner to outer canthus (one wipe per cotton ball) to remove any discharge. The nares may become dry and crusted. Oxygen given by cannula can also irritate the nares. Apply a thin layer of water soluble jelly. Avoid applying the elastic strap of the oxygen cannula too tightly.

Mobility

As the client's condition deteriorates, mobility decreases. The client becomes less able to move about in bed or to get out of bed and requires more assistance. Physical dependence increases the risk of complications related to immobility. Attentive nursing care will prevent the onset of these complications which increase client discomfort and the cost of care.

Reposition the client at least every two hours. Keep in mind that the client may have other disorders that contribute to discomfort such as arthritis or lung disease. Maintain body alignment and use pillows and other supportive equipment as needed. Use positioning techniques to facilitate ease of breathing. Perform passive range of motion exercises at least twice a day to prevent stiffness and aching of the joints. The client may prefer to be assisted into a reclining type of chair at intervals throughout the day. Use transfer techniques that are safe for both the client and caregivers. Using a wheelchair can increase the client's environmental space, giving the client more control.

Skin Care

The prevention of pressure ulcers is a priority. Pressure ulcers are painful, can cause secondary complications such as sepsis, and are costly to treat. Regular repositioning and passive range of motion exercises are two preventive measures. In addition, keep the skin clean and moisturized. Bed baths are adequate if the client cannot get into the tub or sit in a shower chair. Inspect the skin once or twice daily, paying attention to pressure points and areas where skin surfaces rub together. Gentle massages with soothing lotion are comforting.

Bowel and Bladder Care

Constipation may occur due to pain medications and lack of physical activity. Fluids and foods with high fiber content can be effective preventive measures for clients with adequate oral intake. Constipation can also be alleviated by maintaining a scheduled time for bowel elimination and administering suppositories if necessary. A commode has arms and can be padded and may therefore be more comfortable than using the toilet. The client may become incontinent of bladder and bowel. Check the client frequently, clean the skin with peri-washes and apply moisture barrier with each incontinent episode. Incontinent panties may increase the client's comfort, especially when out of bed. Indwelling catheters are never a first choice for care. However, for some clients the need for frequent cleaning, the discomfort of using a bedpan, or getting out of bed on the toilet or commode may cause agonizing pain. In these circumstances the benefits of a catheter greatly outweigh the risks.

Grooming

For many clients, maintaining a well-groomed appearance is important. When the client can no longer make requests or give directions for care, caregivers should presume that the client would prefer to look neat and clean. Shave male clients daily and remember that older females frequently have chin hairs that need removal. Clean and trim fingernails and toenails regularly. If a female client has always taken pride in manicured, polished nails, try to continue this procedure. Combing and brushing hair not only improves appearance, it is also a comforting and relaxing activity for many people.

Dressing and undressing may become a cumbersome, frustrating, and fatiguing activity. The client who spends time up and about may choose attractive pajamas, housecoats, dusters, or exercise suits. Advise individuals who may be purchasing clothing for the client to select items that are loose-fitting, have few fasteners, and are washable.

Other Comfort Measures

The client may require other nursing interventions to ease the dying process. Oxygen is frequently ordered for labored breathing. Suctioning may be needed for removal of secretions the client is unable to swallow.

Physical Environment

A soothing physical environment can do much to increase the client's comfort. Soft lighting enhances vision without the discomfort of harsh, glaring light. Comply with the client's wishes if a night light is requested. If possible offer the client the opportunity to have the bed or a chair near a window to increase the range of the environment. As the client's circulation becomes more sluggish, body temperature will fall. Lightweight comforters will increase warmth without adding uncomfortable weight. Avoid environmental odors with adequate ventilation, daily cleaning of the room, removal of leftover food, and frequent linen changes. Noise can be distracting and anxiety provoking. Comply with the client's wishes in regard to the use of radio and television. Remove the telephone from the room if the client finds the ringing disturbing.

Equipment

For the client at home, the nurse can make suggestions that will increase the client's comfort and ease the workload of the caregivers. This equipment can be rented and may qualify for payment by Medicare or private insurance.

- An electric hospital bed with overhead trapeze to give the client more control of the environment
- A commode to extend the client's independence in elimination
- A lifting device to facilitate getting the dependent client out of bed
- Remote control if the client enjoys television
- Portable telephone

- Shower chair in the bathtub with hand-held shower
- Comfort devices such as special mattresses for the bed and cushions on the chair
- Overbed table for eating or hand activities
- Comfortable chairs close to the bed to facilitate visits of family and friends

CLINICAL SIGNS OF IMPENDING DEATH

No one can predict how long a client will be in the terminal stages of illness. A client may exhibit signs of impending death and then rally to live for several more days. It is not uncommon for clients to endure until a member of the family arrives for a last good-bye. The client who has had a long and troublesome illness may be ready to go but needs "permission" to die; a loved one to say "it's okay, you can go now." A client may not wish to die when others are present and will wait to take the last breath until everyone has left the room.

Even when death is expected, it is never easy for the family. The family should be thoroughly informed in simple terms about what will happen.

- Physical changes that will occur
- Pronouncement of death
- Post-mortem care
- Removal of body by funeral director

If the client will die at home (an expected death), the family needs to:

- Have a list of telephone numbers readily available
- Have the name of the funeral director and telephone number
- Know who to call; physician or hospice nurse or funeral director
- Know who not to call (ambulance and emergency services)
- Record time of death
- Record last medications given
- Record condition of client during the last few hours
- Record the last time the client was seen by the nurse

Impending death is signaled by a slowing of body functions and loss of control of bowel and bladder. Breathing may become labored with **Cheyne-Stokes respirations** noted. These are described as periods of apnea alternating with periods of dyspnea. Fluid in the lungs may result in a breathing sound called the **death rattle**. The extremities become colder, pale, and mottled (cyanotic discoloration). The skin becomes moist and cool. Blood pressure and temperature drop and the pulse becomes rapid and weak. Pupils do not respond to light. Verbal response may be weak or absent.

The care of the client does not cease during this final stage of life. Continue the nursing actions previously described. Tell the client in brief simple terms what is happening as care is rendered. Allow the family to continue their participation if that is their wish. Caution family members that the dying client can hear even in the absence of verbal response.

There may be other indications that death is near. The client may report seeing angels (Ufema, 1995) or hearing beautiful music. These experiences should be accepted as a natural step in the process of dying. When the final breath is taken, the heart stops beating. Within a few minutes, **cerebral death** occurs and brain activity ceases.

Rigor mortis occurs within a few hours of death. It is a temporary stiffening of the body that results from the chemical changes that occur in the muscle tissue. After twenty-four hours, rigor mortis disappears.

POST-MORTEM CARE

Post-mortem care is the care given immediately after death. Before the client dies, caregivers should know if:

- The death is considered a coroner's case. (The **coroner** is an elected county official who is responsible for determining the cause of death.)
- An **autopsy** (examination of the body by a pathologist) is to be performed. Generally, any invasive devices are left in place if an autopsy is to be performed such as feeding tubes, catheters, and intravenous devices. The funeral director must know if an autopsy is to be performed.
- The client has made arrangements for organ donation.
- The client has made arrangements for donation of the body to science.
- The client has made pre-burial arrangements with a specific funeral director.

Regulations regarding these issues vary from state to state. Each health care facility should have policies and guidelines for each of these situations. The procedure for post-mortem care may vary among institutions. To give basic post-mortem care:

- Treat the body with respect and dignity.
- Bathe the body and put on a clean gown—place an incontinent pad under the client's hips.
- Remove dressings and tubes (these may need to be left in place if an autopsy is scheduled).
- Place the client in body alignment with the extremities straight.
- Place dentures in the mouth if the client normally wore them.
- Comb the client's hair.

Some health care facilities have morgue kits that contain identification tags, plastic bags for personal belongings, a chin strap, and a **shroud**. A shroud is a covering for the body. Follow the procedure of the facility. After the body is prepared, give the family uninterrupted time to spend with the client. Accept the grief displayed by the family. The person who was the most stoic throughout the client's dying may be the most emotionally upset when death occurs. The family member who seemed the least equipped to deal with death may become the strong one. In some cases the family may simply feel relief that the struggle for their loved one is at last over. There may be family members who have no more tears to shed. They have done their crying and grieving throughout the illness and now feel at peace.

In the hospital or skilled care facility, the body may be taken to a morgue until it can be transported to a **mortuary** (funeral home). In some institutions, the body will remain in the room until the funeral director arrives.

Sample Nursing Care Plan: The Client with a Terminal Illness/ Cancer of the Lung

Mrs. O'Riley is a widow, seventy-eight years old. She was diagnosed with cancer of the lung six months ago. After a right lower lobectomy, she was discharged to a local skilled care facility with plans to go home after completing her treatment. Mrs. O'Riley was transported to a cancer center for radiation therapy. After completing the treatments she resisted the idea of going home and discharge plans were discontinued. Mrs. O'Riley's condition is deteriorating. She now requires pain medication, is frequently short of breath with dyspnea and needs moderate assistance with activities of daily living because of fatigue. She frequently grimaces and says "Oh, it hurts." Her nutritional intake is marginal because of difficulty swallowing. Mrs. O'Riley is in bed most of the day, getting up only to use the commode. She has two adult children and three grandchildren who live nearby and visit often. They are willing to help their mother get her affairs in order but she resists their efforts. The family very much wants to make their mother's remaining time comfortable and as serene as possible. However, Mrs. O'Riley sometimes defies their attempts to do so.

Nursing Diagnosis 1 Pain, chronic, related to disease progression as evidenced by verbal statements and body language, now requiring pain medication.

Goals	Nursing Interventions	Rationale	Evaluation
Mrs. O'Riley will verbalize relief from pain.	Give analgesics as ordered.	Regular doses of medication are more effective than waiting until the pain begins.	Mrs. O'Riley's body language and verbal statements indicate freedom from pain.
	Ask client to rate pain on a scale of 0 to 10 with 0 being no pain and 10 being severe pain, to assess the need for beginning morphine. Give morphine as ordered, titrated at increments until adequate pain relief is achieved.	Morphine is the drug of choice for severe cancer pain. The client should begin morphine as soon as it is necessary.	
	Monitor for signs of sudden, acute, temporary pain (breakthrough pain). If the precipitating factor is known, give medication 30 to 60 minutes before the event. For unpredictable breakthrough pain, give the medication as soon as possible.	Breakthrough pain is often precipitated by activity or stress and requires supplemental medication.	

(continued)

| | Assure Mrs. O'Riley that the nurses will help her manage the pain and keep it under control. Give back massages and reposition as necessary for comfort. Assist with progressive relaxation techniques if client agrees. | Clients need reassurance that everything possible will be done to manage the pain. | |
| | Monitor bowel elimination. | Pain medication may cause constipation. | |

Nursing Diagnosis 2 Breathing pattern, ineffective, related to diminished lung function as evidenced by dyspnea and shortness of breath.

Goals	Nursing Interventions	Rationale	Evaluation
Mrs. O'Riley will be free from moderate or severe dyspnea.	Teach breathing exercises and effective coughing techniques.	Breathing exercises and coughing techniques enhance gas exchange in the alveoli.	Mrs. O'Riley breathes with ease. Dyspnea does not interfere with activities.
	Allow adequate time for physical activities. Postpone activity if dyspnea present. Provide as much assistance as needed.	Physical exertion increases dyspnea.	
	Administer low flow oxygen if blood gases indicate the need.	Oxygen will ease the effort to breathe but will not be effective unless blood gases indicate the need.	
	Encourage to drink eight to ten glasses of fluid each day.	Adequate fluid intake liquifies respiratory secretions and promotes hydration.	
	Humidify the air with a cold-water vaporizer.	Moisturized air enhances breathing.	
	Assess for signs of respiratory tract infection.	The client is high risk for respiratory infection.	

(continued)

Nursing Diagnosis 3 Nutrition, altered, less than body requirements, related to loss of appetite and impaired swallowing as evidenced by diminished oral intake.

Goals	Nursing Interventions	Rationale	Evaluation
Mrs. O'Riley will maintain present body weight.	Encourage to drink milk and eat milk products. Advise avoiding foods with temperature extremes, spicy or acidic foods, foods that are hard, crunchy, or coarse. Include high-fiber foods that are easy to swallow such as cooked prunes, prune juice, and whole-grain cereals with milk.	Milk and milk products coat the mucous membrane making eating more comfortable.	Mrs. O'Riley maintains adequate food and fluid intake and expresses interest in eating.
	Talk with the family to see if there are special foods they can bring in.	Foods can have many meanings and emotions attached to them aside from nutritional value.	
	Administer pain medication thirty to sixty minutes before meals.	Pain destroys appetite.	
	Assess oral mucosa daily—assist with mouth care at least twice daily. Use a soft-bristle toothbrush and nonirritating toothpaste. Instruct to rinse with a solution of 500 mL water, 1/2 teaspoon salt, and 1/2 teaspoon sodium bicarbonate every four hours. Use Toothettes™ if the brush causes bleeding. Avoid commercial mouthwashes containing alcohol. Lubricate lips with petroleum jelly.	Inadequate nutrition can cause stomatitis, resulting in painful ulcerations. Poor condition of the mouth will depress appetite.	
Mrs. O'Riley will participate in meal planning.	Discuss food choices. If possible, ask before the meal what foods sound good at that time.	Client is more likely to eat foods that sound good to her at the time.	
Mrs. O'Riley will establish a regular pattern of defecation.	Assist to commode every morning thirty minutes after breakfast. Provide physical comfort and privacy.	Regular use of commode helps establish a regular pattern of defecation.	Mrs. O'Riley has regular bowel elimination without intervention.

Nursing Diagnosis 4 Fatigue related to multiple factors due to cancer as evidenced by verbalization of overwhelming lack of energy.

Goals	Nursing Interventions	Rationale	Evaluation
Mrs. O'Riley will verbalize alleviation of fatigue.	Monitor comments and behaviors indicative of fatigue by observing physical appearance, breathing patterns, level of activity, food and fluid intake, and mental status.	Care can be postponed when manifestations of fatigue are observed.	Mrs. O'Riley is able to participate in activities that are meaningful to her.
	Assess and correct environmental factors such as noise and excessive heat.	Environmental factors can prevent or interrupt rest and sleep.	
	Establish a structured schedule of alternating rest periods and activity. Help with active assistive range of motion exercises at least twice daily. Assist to ambulate once or twice a day within the limits of tolerance. Suggest sitting up in a comfortable chair for several short periods during the day.	Exercise within the client's tolerance will help reduce tension and facilitate rest and sleep. Alternating rest and activity avoids overfatigue.	
	Rearrange schedule when special activities are planned, giving priorities to such activities as family visits.	The client has the right to decide how she wishes to use her energy resources.	
	Schedule night procedures such as repositioning and skin care to be done when medication is administered.	Careful planning will avoid the need to awaken the client unnecessarily.	

(continued)

Nursing Diagnosis 5 Skin integrity, impaired, high risk for as evidenced by inadequate nutritional status and physical inactivity.

Goals	Nursing Interventions	Rationale	Evaluation
Mrs. O'Riley will be free from skin impairment.	Implement pressure ulcer prevention protocol.	Pressure ulcers can be prevented even though the client is at high risk to develop them.	Mrs. O'Riley has no skin impairment.

Nursing Diagnosis 6 Coping, individual, ineffective, related to terminal illness as evidenced by inability to communicate effectively with family members and to accept their help.

Goals	Nursing Interventions	Rationale	Evaluation
Mrs. O'Riley will express her feelings openly.	Consult client on all aspects of care, giving adequate information. Provide opportunities to express feelings. Acknowledge feelings, let client know that crying and grieving are beneficial. Listen for clues indicating unfinished business that needs attention. Encourage the process of life review.	The client needs to be given as much control as she wishes to have. Letting the client express her feelings will validate those feelings—she needs to know her feelings are normal and expected. There may be something in the client's past that needs to be resolved before she can successfully cope with the business of dying. Life review is a process of reflection and pondering of one's past and accepting one's life as having had value and meaning.	Mrs. O'Riley is at ease with herself.
Mrs. O'Riley will maintain a satisfying relationship with her family.	Encourage family visits. Provide privacy.	Families need privacy to feel freedom to express their emotions.	

▶ CASE STUDY

Mrs. Jason is seventy-six years old with a history of heart failure. She has been hospitalized twice within the last year and was critically ill both times. Both times she was discharged to her home. A home health nurse and a nursing assistant make intermittent visits to monitor her condition and to help with her activities of daily living. Her husband manages the household chores. Mrs. Jason's condition is deteriorating as the shortness of breath becomes more severe. Her energy level is easily depleted and it is getting more difficult for her to get out of bed. The family is concerned because Mrs. Jason does not have any advance directives. Any attempt to bring up the subject is met with avoidance and a change of subject.

The following questions will guide your development of a Nursing Care Plan for the case study.

1. List the clinical manifestations you would expect Mrs. Jason to experience.

2. Identify four nursing diagnoses to utilize in planning her care.

3. Describe several nursing interventions for implementing palliative care.

4. Describe appropriate interactions with the family to ease their concerns.

5. Explain why you think Mrs. Jason and her family could benefit from hospice services.

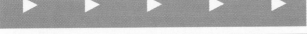

SUMMARY

- Each person dies a unique death.
- Each person has a right to die in peace and dignity.
- Grief is a normal and natural process.
- Most clients who know they are dying go through a series of coping mechanisms in their struggle to reach acceptance of impending death.
- The Patient Self-Determination Act provides a legal means for individuals to determine the circumstances in which life-sustaining treatment will, or will not be given.
- Most health care facilities have Ethics Committees.
- The hospice philosophy can be used with a dying client in any care setting.
- The family and friends of the dying client are also suffering and grieving.
- Palliative care is rendered to the dying client.
- There are specific signs of death but it is not possible to determine exactly when death will occur.

Review Questions

1. Anticipatory grieving is a process of:
   a. suffering from past losses.
   b. acknowledging impending death.
   c. denial of impending death.
   d. acceptance of what is inevitable.

2. The purpose of the Patient Self-Determination Act is to:
   a. serve as an order for "do not resuscitate."
   b. provide a means for disposing of one's worldly goods.
   c. provide an opportunity for making one's wishes known in the event the client is unable to voice his/her wishes.
   d. appoint a legal guardian for the client.

3. The basic premise of supportive care is to:
   a. implement life-extending measures.
   b. provide emotional, physical, and mental comfort.
   c. avoid addiction to narcotics.
   d. speak to the client about organ donation.

4. The hospice philosophy of care believes in:
   a. pain and symptom control.
   b. free care for all dying clients.
   c. providing artificial nourishment when the client no longer wishes to eat.
   d. transferring the client to the hospital when death is imminent.

5. Signs of impending death include:
   a. slower pulse rate.
   b. increased blood pressure.
   c. Cheyne-Stokes respirations.
   d. flushed skin.

Critical Thinking Questions

1. Discuss pros and cons of advance directives.

2. Will you make use of advance directives?

3. How do you feel about caring for a dying client?

News Flash

The American Geriatrics Society recently announced that tools are needed to measure the quality of care provided to people when death is imminent. When quality indicators are developed, the information can be used for selection of health care providers. The society has called for measurements in nine specific areas: physical and emotional suffering, family burden, patient and family satisfaction, advance planning, aggressive care near death, bereavement, survival time, provider continuity and skill, and support of function and autonomy. (*From McKnight's Long-Term NEWS [1996]. 17(6),26*)

UNIT
6

Oxygenation and Perfusion

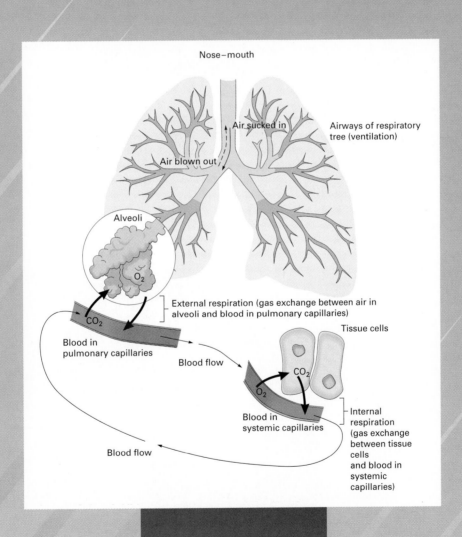

Nose–mouth

Air sucked in

Airways of respiratory tree (ventilation)

Air blown out

Alveoli

O_2

External respiration (gas exchange between air in alveoli and blood in pulmonary capillaries)

CO_2

Blood in pulmonary capillaries

Blood flow

Tissue cells

CO_2

O_2

Blood in systemic capillaries

Internal respiration (gas exchange between tissue cells and blood in systemic capillaries)

Blood flow

CHAPTER
19
Respiratory Disorders

Janet Leah Joost

▶ KEY TERMS

adventitious breath sounds
audible wheezes
bronchial breath sounds
bronchovesicular breath sounds
carina
caseation
cavitation
chemoreceptors
crackles
diffusion
empyema
external respiration
hypoxia
internal respiration
liquefaction necrosis
lung stretch receptors
perfusion
pleural effusion
pleural friction rub
primary tubercle
respiration
sibilant wheezes
sonorous wheezes
status asthmaticus
surfactant
ventilation
vesicular breath sounds

LEARNING OBJECTIVES

Upon completion of this chapter the learner should be able to:
* Define key terms.
* Describe components of a complete respiratory assessment.
* Describe the assessment of the client with a thoracotomy tube.
* Identify normal parameters for common respiratory diagnostic studies.
* Discuss the etiology, medical/surgical management, and nursing care for respiratory disorders.
* Prepare a nursing care plan for a client with a respiratory disorder.

▶ *MAKING THE CONNECTION*

Refer to the topics in the following chapters to increase your understanding of respiratory disorders:

* **Chapter 10, Nursing Assessment:** Percussion, p. 174; Auscultation, p. 175; Thoracic Assessment, p. 179
* **Chapter 15, Oncology Nursing:** Lung Cancer, p. 310; Dyspnea, p. 316; Ascites, p. 317

* **Chapter 20, Cardiac Disorders:** Myocardial Infarction, p. 478; Decreased Function and Failure of Cardiac System, Congestive Heart Failure, p. 481; Cor Pulmonale, p. 486
* **Chapter 21, Vascular Disorders:** Venous Thrombosis/Thrombophlebitis, p. 495
* **Chapter 22, Blood and Lymph Disorders:** Anatomy and Physiology Review, p. 518; Blood, p. 518

INTRODUCTION

Respiratory disorders account for millions of the dollars spent in the United States health care arena. From loss of time on the job due to the common cold to providing care for those with chronic respiratory disorders, the cost of respiratory disease is staggering. This chapter presents the various respiratory disorders with the focus on the nursing process.

ANATOMY AND PHYSIOLOGY REVIEW

Respiration

Respiration provides the body with a means of gas exchange. This process is necessary to supply cells with oxygen to carry on metabolism and to remove the carbon dioxide produced as a waste by-product. There are two types of respiration: **external respiration** and **internal respiration**. External respiration is the exchange of gases between the atmosphere and the lungs. Internal respiration is the exchange of gases at the cellular level (see Figure 19-1). The primary purpose of the pulmonary system is external respiration. This function is dependent upon the adequacy of ventilation, perfusion, and diffusion. **Ventilation** is the movement of gases into and out of the lung. **Perfu-**

sion refers to the flow of blood through the vessels of a specific organ or body part. **Diffusion** is the movement of gases across the alveolar capillary membrane from areas of high concentration to areas of lower concentration. Factors that affect ventilation, perfusion, and diffusion will affect external respiration. These factors are described in Table 19-1.

Table 19-1

FACTORS AFFECTING VENTILATION, PERFUSION, AND DIFFUSION		
Ventilation	a)	Position—dependent areas receive majority
	b)	Lung volume—low volume results in shunting to lung apices
	c)	Disease—bronchial constriction decreases, airway collapse decreases
Perfusion	a)	Position—dependent areas receive majority
	b)	Hypoxia—results in vasoconstriction and decreased perfusion
	c)	Blockage—results in decreased or absent perfusion to distal areas
Diffusion	a)	Alveolar capillary membrane—alterations may occur in thickness and permeability of membrane

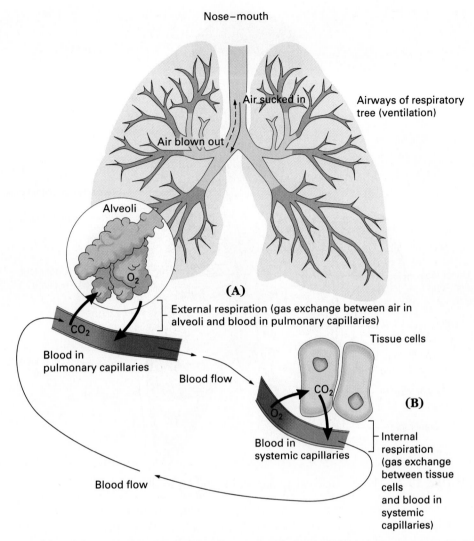

FIGURE 19-1 **(A)** External respiration illustrating the properties of ventilation, perfusion, and diffusion. **(B)** Internal respiration.

The Thoracic Cavity

The chest cage is a closed compartment bounded on the top by the neck muscles and at the bottom by the diaphragm, as shown in Figure 19-2. The walls of the chest cage are formed by the ribs and intercostal muscles laterally, the thoracic vertebrae posteriorly, and the sternum anteriorly. The inside of the chest cage is called the thoracic cavity. Contained within the thoracic cavity are the lungs. The lungs are cone-shaped, porous organs separated from the other chest organs by the mediastinum. The lungs lie free, except for their attachment to the heart and trachea, and are encased in the pleura, a thin, transparent double layered serous membrane lining the thoracic cavity. The layers of the pleura are the parietal pleura, which lies adjacent to the chest wall and the visceral pleura, which adheres to the surface of the lungs. The area between the two pleura is known as the pleural space.

The pleural space contains approximately 5 to 20 cc of serous fluid (pleural fluid) that allows the layers of the pleura to slide on each other, yet hold together. The pressure within the pleural space is less than that of outside air. This difference in pressure creates a suction that prevents the lungs from collapsing on exhalation. However, if the pleura is penetrated the difference in pressure pulls outside air into the pleural space and the underlying lung tissue collapses.

The right lung is larger than the left and is divided into three sections, or lobes, the upper, middle, and lower. The left lung is divided into two lobes, upper and lower (see Figure 19-2). Each lobe of the lung is further divided into smaller sections called segments. The right lung has ten segments; the left lung has nine segments. The upper portion of the lung is referred to as the apex (plural, apices). The lower portion is called the base. The lungs possess a dual blood supply. Bronchial circulation begins with the bronchial artery

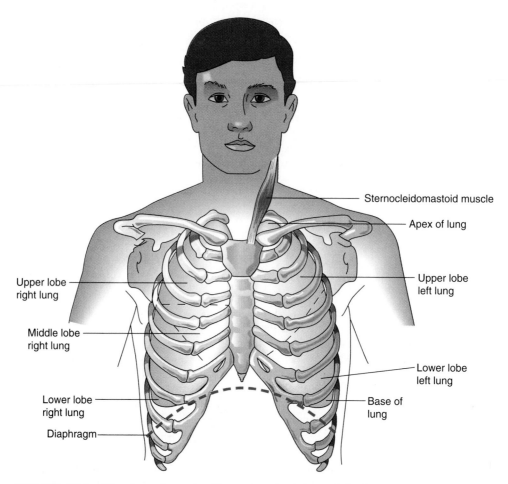

FIGURE 19-2   The thoracic cavity illustrating the lobes of the lungs.

that provides the passageways of the lungs with blood to meet nutritional needs. Bronchial circulation terminates when the venous blood enters the pulmonary veins. This dilutes the oxygen content in the pulmonary vein a small amount. Pulmonary circulation is the route by which blood is delivered to the alveoli for gas exchange.

The Conducting Airways

The conducting airways are tubelike structures that provide a passageway for air as it travels to the lungs. These are the nasal passages, mouth, pharynx, larynx, trachea, bronchi, and bronchioles (refer to Figure 19-3). The conducting airways are lined with epithelial tissue containing serous glands, mucous-secreting Goblet cells, and hairlike projections called cilia. The mucus of the Goblet cells with the cilia form a mucociliary blanket that serves to protect the respiratory system from invasion by foreign particles. The constant upward motion of the cilia propels the mucociliary blanket toward the pharynx where any foreign matter may be expectorated.

The nasal passages are the preferred route for air to enter the respiratory tract. In addition to its function of filtering inspired air, the nasal passages are richly supplied with blood vessels that warm and moisten the air. An alternate route for air to enter is the mouth. When the nasal passages are obstructed or the body has an increased need for air, the mouth may be utilized. Breathing through the mouth, however, reduces the ability to filter, warm, and moisten inspired air, because the mouth lacks cilia and the abundant blood supply. Connecting the nasal passages and mouth to the lower parts of the respiratory tract is the pharynx. The pharynx is divided into three parts: the nasopharynx, the oropharynx, and the laryngopharynx. The pharynx, located behind the oral cavity, serves as a passageway for both inspired air into the larynx and ingested food passing into the digestive system. At the distal portion of the pharynx is the larynx, also known as the voice box.

The larynx is composed of four cartilage structures: the uppermost thyroid cartilage (Adam's apple), the cricoid cartilage which lies at the lower edge, the epiglottis (a leaf-shaped structure that covers the larynx when swallowing), and the glottis (the triangular space between the vocal cords when they are relaxed). The larynx is an enlarged part located at the upper end of the trachea and at the lower end of the pharynx. It is the passageway for air entering and leaving the trachea and contains the vocal cords. The trachea, commonly known as the windpipe, is a tube composed of connective tissue mucosa and smooth muscle supported by C-shaped rings of cartilage extending from the top of the trachea into bronchi. The trachea is 2.0 to 2.5 centimeters in diameter (about one inch) and 10 to 12 centimeters in length (4 to 6 inches). The trachea terminates by branching into two tubes: the right and left primary bronchi. They are somewhat smaller in diameter than the trachea and each passes into its respective lung. The point at which the trachea divides is called the **carina**, which is a cartilaginous ridge between the two bronchi. An abundant nerve supply to the carina provides further protection against entry of foreign matter into the lungs. Stimulation of the carina results in bronchospasm and cough. The primary bronchi accompanied by the pulmonary vessels and nerves enter the lung through a groove called the hilum and then branch into smaller bronchi.

The right bronchus is wider and more vertically positioned than the left. This difference in positioning allows foreign matter to enter the right bronchus more easily than the left. Within the lungs, the bronchi branch off into increasingly smaller diameter tubes until they become the terminal bronchioles. These branch further forming alveolar ducts that end in numerous saclike, thin walled structures called the alveoli. Collectively the alveoli and the alveolar ducts within resemble a cluster of grapes. The branching makes this portion of the respiratory tract resemble an inverted tree giving rise to the term bronchial tree (see Figure 19-3).

Initially, the bronchi are a continuation of the structure of the trachea, smooth muscle supported by cartilage rings. As they branch, the bronchi lose their cartilage rings which give way to a spiral layer of smooth muscle alone. Within the inner surface of the bronchioles lie the mast cells that play an important role in allergen response by releasing histamine. The terminal bronchioles form the alveolar ducts.

Respiratory Tissues

The respiratory tissues perform the function of gas exchange. These structures are the alveolar ducts and the alveoli. While each is supplied with a means for gas exchange, the alveoli are the primary site at which gas exchange occurs. The alveolar ducts are smooth muscular tubes containing abundant alveolar macrophages to remove foreign particles (i.e., bacteria). The alveoli into which the alveolar ducts terminate consist of interconnected spaces with thin walls, or septa,

occupied by a network of capillaries, the alveolar capillary membrane.

The alveoli contain two specialized types of cells. Type I alveolar cells are flat squamous epithelial cells across which gas exchange occurs. Type II alveolar cells produce a substance called **surfactant**. Surfactant coats the inner surfaces of the alveoli that reduces the surface tension of pulmonary fluids, allows gas exchange, and prevents the collapse of the alveoli. Each lung contains about 300 million alveoli. It is estimated that the alveoli of the lungs, if flattened out, would cover a surface area the size of a tennis court.

Neuromuscular Control of Respiration

Unlike the heart muscles, the respiratory muscles must receive continuous neural stimuli to function. Regulation of respiration is integrated by neurons located in the pons and medulla of the brain. The control of respiration is influenced by involuntary (automatic) and voluntary components. Involuntary components include **chemoreceptors, lung stretch receptors**, and impulses from other sources. Chemoreceptors monitor the levels of carbon dioxide and oxygen and the acidity/alkalinity (pH) of the blood. Normally, chemoreceptors initiate respiration in response to rising levels of carbon dioxide in the blood. With certain chronic pulmonary disorders, such as emphysema, chemoreceptors become more responsive to low levels of oxygen. This becomes significant when administering oxygen to persons whose drive to breathe is dependent on low levels of oxygen in the blood. Lung stretch receptors monitor the patterns of breathing and prevent overexpansion of the tissues. Many other sources send impulses to the respiratory center which act in an involuntary manner. For example, if a person becomes frightened or angry, the respiratory rate increases in response to stimuli from the autonomic nervous system. Voluntary components of respiratory control integrate breathing with acts such as talking and speaking.

The diaphragm acts as the primary muscle of respiration. During inspiration, the diaphragm contracts and flattens out in response to stimuli from the respiratory center, increasing the length of the thoracic cavity. At the same time, the intercostal muscles contract, elevating the ribs, and increasing the diameter of the thoracic cavity. The total thoracic space increases, reducing the pressure within the thoracic cavity. The pressure within the thoracic cavity then becomes negative in relation to that of atmospheric pressure and air moves into the thoracic cavity. Upon expiration, the respiratory center signals the diaphragm and intercostal muscles to relax. The thoracic cavity returns to its original size. Aided by the elastic recoil of the lungs, the decrease in size of the thoracic cavity increases pressure and air moves out of the lungs.

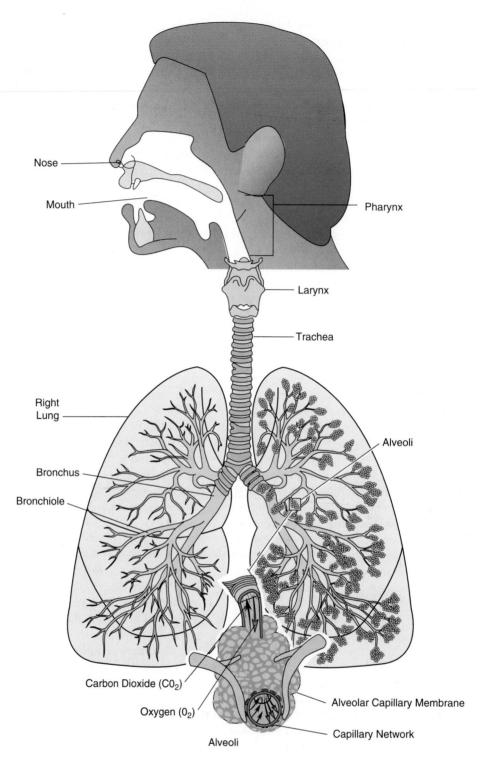

Nose

Mouth

Pharynx

Larynx

Trachea

Right Lung

Alveoli

Bronchus

Bronchiole

Carbon Dioxide (CO$_2$)

Oxygen (O$_2$)

Alveoli

Alveolar Capillary Membrane

Capillary Network

FIGURE 19-3 Structures of the respiratory tract with an inset of an alveolus.

Gas Exchange

Gas exchange occurs at the alveolar capillary membrane. Venous blood from the right ventricle is pumped into the pulmonary arteries and travels to the alveolar capillary network. Here, blood in the alveolar capillaries is exposed to the inhaled air. Due to the higher concentration of oxygen within the alveoli, oxygen diffuses into the blood within the alveolar capillary network. The majority of oxygen binds to the iron atoms of the hemoglobin molecule in the red blood cells. Approximately one to three percent of oxygen dissolves into the blood plasma. The exchange of carbon dioxide also occurs within the alveoli. Most of the carbon dioxide formed as a by-product of cellular metabolism, diffuses into the red blood cells. There carbon dioxide (CO_2) is hydrated and changed into carbonic acid (H_2CO_3) due to the presence of carbonic anhydrase. The carbonic acid dissociates into hydrogen ions (H^+) and bicarbonate ions (HCO_3^-). The hydrogen ions combine with hemoglobin and the bicarbonate ions enter the blood plasma. Hemoglobin that has been reduced (the oxygen has been removed) combines with about 15 percent to 25 percent of the carbon dioxide. Within the alveolar capillary network, the carbon dioxide detaches from hemoglobin and diffuses into the alveolar space. Carbon dioxide is removed from the alveolar space when exhalation occurs. The blood within the pulmonary capillary network is now oxygenated and travels to the heart via the pulmonary veins. From this point, oxygenated blood is sent to the body via the aorta and the arterial network.

ASSESSMENT

Refer to Chapter 10 for information regarding physical assessment.

Respiratory Terminology

To understand the assessment of the respiratory system the student needs to be familiar with related terminology (see Table 19-2).

History

Nursing assessment begins with a complete history. The client should be questioned regarding allergies, occupation, lifestyle, and health habits such as smoking. The client who smokes needs to be evaluated for the amount of tobacco smoked daily and length of time he/she has smoked. Symptoms such as dyspnea, decreased exercise tolerance, and cough need to be explored in depth. Following a complete history, the nurse completes a physical assessment of the client.

Inspection

Physical assessment of the respiratory system starts with inspection. The nurse notes the client's color, level of consciousness, and emotional state. Respirations are observed as to their rate, depth, quality, rhythm, and respiratory effort required to breathe. Symmetry of chest wall movement is noted. The nurse observes for use of accessory muscles to aid breathing.

Table 19-2

RESPIRATORY TERMS

Term	Definition
eupnea	normal breathing
apnea	cessation of breathing, may be temporary in nature
dyspnea	labored or difficult breathing, may be normal if associated with exercise
bradypnea	abnormally slow breathing
tachypnea	abnormally rapid breathing
orthopnea	discomfort or difficulty with breathing in any but an upright sitting or standing position
anoxia	deficiency of oxygen
hypoxia	synonym for anoxia, lack of adequate oxygen in inspired air such as occurs at high altitude
hypoxemia	insufficient amount of oxygen in the blood; may be due to respiratory, cardiovascular, or anemia related disorders
cyanosis	bluish, grayish, or purplish discoloration of the skin due to abnormal amounts of reduced (oxygen-poor) hemoglobin in the blood; is not always a reliable indicator of hypoxia
acrocyanosis	cyanosis of the fingertips and toes; often due to vasomotor disturbances associated with vasoconstriction
circumoral cyanosis	bluish discoloration encircling the mouth
oxygen saturation	refers to the amount of oxygen combined with hemoglobin
Kussmaul's respirations	abnormal respiratory pattern characterized by irregular periods of increased rate and depth of respiration; most often seen with diabetic ketoacidosis
Biot's respirations	abnormal respiratory pattern characterized by irregular periods of apnea alternating with short periods of respiration of equal depth; most commonly seen with increased intracranial pressure
Cheyne-Stokes respirations	abnormal respiratory pattern characterized by initially slow shallow respirations increasing in rapidity and depth followed by a gradual decrease until respiration stops for 10 to 60 seconds, the pattern then repeats itself in the same manner

The position the client assumes provides information as to respiratory status.

Percussion and Palpation

The next steps in the respiratory assessment are palpation and percussion. These are normally done by the registered nurse or physician. Through the use of palpation and percussion, areas of varying densities in the lung can be detected. The density of lung tissues changes with disease states such as pneumonia, pneumothorax, and pleural effusion.

Auscultation

Auscultation provides a great deal of information about respiratory status. See Chapter 10 for the areas that need to be auscultated. The listener needs to assess breath sounds at each location for the length of a complete inspiration and expiration. Breath sounds are assessed for duration, pitch, and intensity.

Normal Breath Sounds

Bronchial breath sounds are heard over the sternum under normal circumstances. These loud, high-pitched sounds last longer during expiration than during inspiration. When heard in areas other than the sternum, bronchial breath sounds indicate fluid, exudate, or compression of lung tissue. **Bronchovesicular breath sounds** are heard over the anterior one-third of the chest near the sternum and also around the scapula posteriorly. Bronchovesicular breath sounds have a medium pitch and intensity. Inspiration and expiration are of equal duration. Bronchovesicular breath sounds may be heard in the periphery of the lung when consolidation and fluid are present.

Vesicular breath sounds are heard over the majority of the lungs. These breath sounds are soft and low in pitch. Vesicular breath sounds are best heard during inspiration and may be inaudible during expiration.

Adventitious Breath Sounds

Abnormal breath sounds are called **adventitious breath sounds**. Adventitious breath sounds include: **sibilant wheezes**, **sonorous wheezes**, **crackles**, and **pleural friction rubs**. Sibilant wheezes are high-pitched, whistlelike sounds that may be heard on inspiration or expiration. Sibilant wheezes are present when the airways become obstructed or narrowed as in bronchospasm. Sonorous wheezes are loud coarse sounds that are lower in pitch than sibilant wheezes. Sonorous wheezes are more frequently heard on expiration and may reflect obstruction due to secretions blocking the airway. Crackles are popping noises created as air moves through fluid. Crackles may be heard on inspiration and expiration. Crackles are indicative of fluid accumulation in the lungs associated with conditions such as congestive heart failure. Pleural friction rubs are grating noises best heard on inspiration often associated with inflammation of the pleura. Absence of breath sounds indicates critical disorders like pneumothorax and acute respiratory failure. With atelectasis the breath sounds may be diminished or absent.

COMMON DIAGNOSTIC TESTS

The following is a table of the commonly used diagnostic tests for clients with respiratory disorders.

Test	Explanation/Normal Values	Nursing Responsibilities
Hemoglobin	Measures the grams of hemoglobin present in a deciliter (100 cc) of whole blood	Explain the test to the client and that a blood sample is required. Samples may be drawn from a finger of a child or the heel of an infant.
Arterial Blood Gases (ABGs)	Direct measurement of the pH, pO_2, pCO_2 and calculated measurement of HCO_3 and SaO_2 from samples of arterial blood. pH = expresses the acidity or alkalinity of the blood. PaO_2 = partial pressure of oxygen in the blood. $PaCO_2$ = partial pressure of carbon dioxide in the blood. HCO_3 = bicarbonate ion concentration in the blood. SaO_2 = arterial oxygen saturation. The oxygen content of the blood expressed as a percent of the oxygen carrying capacity of the blood.	Explain that an arterial sample of blood is required. Arterial punctures cause more discomfort than venous. The client is instructed not to move. Assess the adequacy of collateral circulation. Samples must be placed on ice after drawing to prevent dissociation of oxygen from hemoglobin. Apply firm pressure to the site for a minimum of 5 minutes or until all bleeding stops.

Test	Explanation/Normal Values	Nursing Responsibilities
	Compare results to normal values: pH 7.35–7.45 PaO_2 80–100 mmHg $PaCO_2$ 35–45 mmHg HCO_3 22–26 mmHg SaO_2 > 95% (at sea level)	
Pulse Oximetry	Noninvasive means of measuring oxygen saturation utilizing a light beam. SaO_2 > 95% (at sea level)	Explain the procedure to the client. Assess peripheral circulation as this may alter results. Place the sensor on the earlobe, fingertip, or pinna of the ear. Keep sensor intact until a consistent reading is obtained. Observe and record readings. Report measurements below 95% to the physician.
Pulmonary Function Tests (PFTs)	A group of studies used to evaluate ventilatory function. Measurements are obtained directly via spirometer or calculated from the results of spirometer measurements. Measurements included are: Tidal volume = amount of air inhaled and exhaled during a normal respiration. Inspiratory reserve volume = amount of air inspired at the end of a normal inspiration. Expiratory reserve volume = amount of air expired following a normal expiration. Residual volume = amount of air left in lungs after maximal expiration. Vital capacity = total volume of air that can be expired after maximal inspiration. Total lung capacity = total volume of air in the lungs when maximally inflated. Inspiratory capacity = maximum amount of air that can be inspired after normal expiration. Forced vital capacity = capacity of air exhaled forcefully and rapidly following maximal inspiration. Minute volume = amount of air breathed per minute.	Explain the procedure to the client. PFTs should not be done within one to two hours following a meal. Bronchodilators may be used during the study. After the test monitor respiratory status. Avoid activity and allow for rest following the test as it may be fatiguing.
Chest x-ray	Provides a two-dimensional image of the lungs without using contrast media. Used to detect the presence of fluid within the interstitial lung tissue or the alveoli, tumors or foreign bodies, and the presence and size of pneumothorax. The size of the heart can also be determined by chest x-ray.	Explain the test to the client. If appropriate inquire if the client may be pregnant to avoid exposure of the fetus to x-ray. The client will be required to stand for various views. If the client is unable to stand views may be obtained in a sitting position or a portable x-ray may be obtained. The client is instructed to inspire deeply and hold their breath.
Ventilation-perfusion Scan	Assesses ventilation and perfusion of the lungs. Most often used to detect the presence of pulmonary emboli.	Explain the procedure to the client. Assess for allergy to iodine and shellfish. Radioactive contrast media will be introduced via an intravenous access and inhalation of radioactive gas. The client will be required to hold their breath for short periods as images are obtained. A written consent may be required according to facility policy.

(continued)

Test	Explanation/Normal Values	Nursing Responsibilities
Pulmonary Angiography	Assesses the arterial circulation of the lungs. Most often used to detect pulmonary emboli.	Explain the procedure to the client. Assess for allergy to iodine or shellfish. Inform the client that an arterial puncture is required usually of the femoral artery. Injection of the dye may cause a flushing or warm sensation due to vasodilation. After the study, assess the arterial puncture site frequently for evidence of bleeding. Assess vital signs and respiratory status. The client may be required to lie flat for up to 6 hours if the femoral artery is used for access. A written consent is required per facility policy.
Bronchoscopy	Direct visual examination of the bronchi utilizing a fiber optic scope. Used to remove foreign bodies, for aggressive pulmonary cleansing, and to obtain sputum and tissue specimens.	Explain the procedure to the client. The client must be NPO for at least 6 hours prior to the test. If ordered, preprocedure sedation is administered. An intravenous access will be obtained and sedation given during the procedure via this route. Following the procedure, assess vital signs and respiratory status frequently. Assess the client for unusual amounts of bleeding. Sputum may be blood tinged initially following the procedure. The client should be maintained in a side lying position until the gag reflex returns. No food or fluids should be ingested until the client is fully awake and has a gag reflex. A written consent is required per facility policy.
Sputum Analysis	Sputum samples are examined for the presence of bacteria, fungi, molds, yeasts, and malignant cells. Appropriate antibiotic therapy is determined via culture and sensitivity studies.	Explain the procedure to the client. Specimens are best obtained early in the morning to prevent contamination due to ingested food or fluids. Instruct the client to breathe deeply and cough. A specimen originating from the lower respiratory tract is required. If necessary, pulmonary suctioning may be used to induce such a specimen. Sputum should be expectorated into the appropriate container. Specimens should be delivered to the laboratory as soon as possible.
Computerized Axial Tomography (CAT scan)	Provides two-dimensional views of the lungs. Superior to chest x-ray for soft tissue visualization.	Explain the procedure to the client. The client will be required to hold still for up to 30 minutes at a time. The client is placed within a scanning chamber which rotates around them. Written consent may be required according to facility policy.
Thoracentesis	Provides fluid for diagnostic purposes, obtain biopsy, instill medications, removes fluid for client comfort and safety.	Explain the procedure to the client. Have client sign consent for procedure. The client should be placed in an upright sitting position, leaning forward. Have client rest arms on an overbed table to facilitate this position. Explain to the client that the area will be anesthetized prior to the procedure. Instruct the client to hold as still as possible during the insertion of the thoracentesis needle. Assist the physician during the procedure. Deliver specimen to the laboratory as soon as possible. Observe the thoracentesis site for bleeding following the procedure. Assess breath sounds before and after the procedure. Report absent breath sounds immediately.

Test	Explanation/Normal Values	Nursing Responsibilities
Magnetic Resonance Imaging (MRI)	Provides detailed views of the lung utilizing magnetic resonance of the atoms of the body. Provides greater tissue discrimination than chest x-ray or CT scans.	Explain the procedure to the client. Assess the client for the presence of metal objects within the body (i.e., shrapnel, cochlear implants, pacemakers). The client will be required to lie still for up to 20 minutes at a time. The client will be placed within a scanning tunnel. Sedation may be required if the client has claustrophobic tendencies. Inform the client the magnet will make a loud thumping noise as images are obtained. Provide earplugs as necessary. As the test may require up to 2 hours to perform have the client void prior to entering the scanning tunnel. Written consent may be required per facility policy.

KEY ABBREVIATIONS

The following abbreviations and acronyms are used in this chapter:

ADL	activities of daily living
AFB	acid-fast bacillus
APTT	activated partial thromboplastin time
ARDS	adult respiratory distress syndrome
ASO	antistreptolysin O
BCG	bacillus Calmette-Guerin
CHF	congestive heart failure
COLD	chronic obstructive lung disease
COPD	chronic obstructive pulmonary disease
CVA	cerebrovascular accident
INR	international normalized ratio
NSAIDs	nonsteroidal anti-inflammatory drugs
PPD	protein purified derivative
PT	prothrombin time
TB	tuberculosis
TPN	total parenteral nutrition

► INFECTIOUS/ INFLAMMATORY DISORDERS

► INFECTIOUS/ INFLAMMATORY DISORDERS OF THE UPPER RESPIRATORY TRACT

Infectious and inflammatory disorders of the upper respiratory tract are common and usually self-limiting. Table 19-3 summarizes the various types of disorders associated with infection and inflammation of the upper respiratory tract. Among the causal factors of infectious and inflammatory disorders are various viruses and bacteria such as rhino viruses, influenza viruses, streptococci, and pneumococci. Group A *beta-hemolytic streptococci* infections of the upper respiratory system are associated with serious sequelae such as rheumatic fever. Long-term consequences of rheumatic fever may include rheumatic carditis, valvular damage, and nephritis. Allergic reactions frequently play a role in the development of sinusitis and pharyngitis. Laryngitis is correlated with irritation due to factors such as pollution, smoking, and excessive use of the voice. Breathing cold air decreases local immune responses of the respiratory tract. This fact coupled with closer contact with others during winter months leads to an increased incidence of acute upper respiratory tract inflammatory disorders.

The signs and symptoms that occur with acute upper respiratory tract infection or inflammation are a

Table 19-3

UPPER RESPIRATORY TRACT INFECTIONS OR INFLAMMATORY DISORDERS	
Disorder	**Etiology**
rhinitis (coryza, common cold)	virus
allergic rhinitis	exposure to allergens
sinusitis	bacterial (streptococci, pneumococci) or virus
pharyngitis	bacterial or viral
tonsillitis	bacterial (streptococci most common)
laryngitis	irritation due to excessive use of voice, exposure to irritants (i.e., cigarette smoke) and extension of rhinitis

result of the inflammatory process. Early signs and symptoms include general malaise, low-grade fever, localized redness, and edema of affected tissues. With viral disorders, symptoms such as joint pains are common. Furthermore, the client may complain of nasal or sinus congestion and often a headache. Drying of the mucous membranes and edema cause local discomfort such as sore throat. Cough and nasal or sinus discharge may occur. Secretions that are thick and purulent indicate bacterial infection.

▶ Medical/Surgical Management

▶ Medical

The majority of clients with acute upper respiratory tract infectious or inflammatory disorders are treated in a clinic or office setting. Unless the disorder becomes chronic or bacterial infection occurs, treatment is symptomatic. When infection is suspected, specimens for culture and sensitivity are obtained and appropriate antibiotic therapy is initiated. Disorders that develop into chronic conditions (i.e., tonsillitis) may require surgical intervention to remove or drain affected tissues.

▶ Pharmacological

Nonprescription antipyretic, analgesic, anti-inflammatory medications may be used to reduce discomfort, fever, and inflammation. Examples of such medications are acetaminophen (Tylenol), ibuprofen (Advil), and acetylsalicylic acid (Aspirin). Antitussives to suppress cough and allow for rest may be used such as dextromethorphan hydrobromide combinations (Comtrex, Dimetane-DM, Rondec-DM) or hydrocodone bitartrate (Hycodan) preparations. To aid in removal of secretions, expectorants, such as guaifenesin (Robitussin, Humibid L.A.) are used. Bacterial infections are treated with various antibiotics according to culture and sensitivity studies. Some of the more common antibiotics used are erythromycin base (E-mycin, PCE Disperstab), ampicillin (Omnipen), amoxicillin (Amoxil),

cefaclor (Ceclor), and cephalexin monohydrate (Keflex). Comfort measures such as saline gargles may be useful.

▶ Diet

Fluids are encouraged to liquefy secretions and hydrate dry mucous membranes. Nausea may occur if secretions are swallowed versus expectorated. The client should be encouraged to cough up all secretions and dispose of them properly. With severe coughing, emesis may occur. The client should be encouraged to rest prior to meals and may require an antitussive to reduce coughing.

▶ Activity

Normally, activity is not affected. The client who is infectious should be encouraged to avoid contact with others. Strenuous activity should be avoided to reduce oxygen requirements and decrease coughing.

▶ Nursing Process

Assessment

Subjective Data This includes information about present signs and symptoms, onset of symptoms, exposure to allergens or infected individuals, and frequency of the disorder. Common symptoms include sore throat, dyspnea, and headache.

Objective Data This includes fever, visual inspection of the oropharynx for presence of inflammation, redness, edema, and drying of the mucous membranes. Secretions are evaluated for their color, viscosity, amount, and odor. The client may have hoarseness and a cough. Culture and sensitivity studies may reveal a causative organism and serve to guide antibiotic therapy. If infection with group A *beta-hemolytic streptococci* is suspected, an ASO (anti-streptolysin O) titer may be done to reveal the presence of antibodies formed in reaction to this bacteria. Nonspecific diagnostic studies include elevated white blood cell counts and erythrocyte sedimentation rates.

▼ ▼

Possible nursing diagnoses for a client with an upper respiratory infectious or inflammatory disorder may include:

Nursing Diagnoses	Goals	Nursing Interventions
▶ Knowledge deficit related to signs and symptoms of respiratory bacterial infection, potential allergens, and antibiotic therapy.	The client will be able to state the signs and symptoms of bacterial infection.	Educate the client regarding signs and symptoms indicating a respiratory bacterial infection, such as purulent or green-colored secretions, and fever.
	The client will be able to identify individual potential allergens.	Assist the physician in allergy testing. Teach the client to avoid those things that precipitate an allergic response.
	The client will complete entire course of antibiotic therapy.	Instruct client to complete the entire course of antibiotics.
▶ Airway clearance, ineffective, related to nasal secretions.	The client will verbalize a decrease or absence of nasal congestion.	Teach client to blow nose and not snuffle secretions back up into nose.

▶ Evaluation

Each goal must be evaluated to determine how it has been met by the client.

▲ ▲

▶ PNEUMONIA

Pneumonia is inflammation of the bronchioles and alveoli. It can result from bacteria, virus, mycoplasm, fungus, or parasite invasion. Pneumonia can also be caused by aspiration, oversedation, or inadequate ventilation. Pneumonia remains a common cause for hospitalization and often a cause of death particularly among the elderly. Under normal circumstances, the alveolar macrophages are able to remove foreign matter. When confronted with overwhelming numbers of virulent microorganisms, this protective mechanism fails. The invading organism irritates the wall of the alveoli. In response to this irritation, the alveolar wall secretes exudate (an accumulation of fluid in the pulmonary passageways). Eventually the alveoli fill with the exudate creating consolidation. The presence of the exudate within the alveoli also interferes with gas exchange. Risk factors for the development of pneumonia include immobility, depressed cough reflex (i.e., due to anesthesia or CVA), alterations in respiratory function (i.e., COPD), advanced age, and numerous other chronic debilitating conditions (i.e., CHF, diabetes mellitus). Common bacterial causes of pneumonia are *Streptococcus pneumoniae, Pneumococcus, Staphylococcus aureus, Klebsiella pneumoniae,* and *Pseudomonas aeruginosa.* Chemical pneumonia is due to entry of irritating substances into the pulmonary passageways. A common source of chemical pneumonia is the aspiration of gastric contents. Inhalation of irritating substances can result in a chemical pneumonia. A common, serious viral source of pneumonia is the *Cytomegalovirus.* The *Cytomegalovirus* affects those clients with compromised immune status such as those taking immunosuppressant medications or those with acquired immunodeficiency syndrome (AIDS). *Pneumocystis carinii* pneumonia also occurs in the immunosupressed client. The invading organism with *Pneumocystis carinii* pneumonia is thought to be a protozoan. The infecting microorganisms that cause pneumonia are spread by airborne droplets or direct contact with infected individuals or carriers. Pneumonia is now classified according to the causative factor rather than the area of the lung affected as was done in the past. The right middle and lower lobes are affected by pneumonia more frequently than the right upper and left lobes of the lungs due to the anatomy of the right bronchus and the effects of gravity.

A high fever of sudden onset is often the presenting complaint of the client. The elderly client, however, may be seriously ill and have only a low-grade fever. Productive cough of abnormally thick and discolored sputum occurs frequently. Associated respiratory symptoms include dyspnea, coarse crackles, and diminished breath sounds. The majority of clients complain of pleuritic chest pain. This type of pain is stabbing in nature and increases with inspiration. Pain occurs due to irritation of the pleura lying adjacent to the affected alveoli. In the case of bacterial pneumonia, the white blood cell count increases and may go as high as 40,000/mm³. Pneumonia caused by viruses or mycoplasms may result in normal or lowered white blood cell count. Chest x-ray will reveal consolidation in the affected areas. Bacterial pneumonia is more likely to produce isolated areas of consolidation on chest x-ray, while viral and chemical pneumonia appear as more diffuse areas of consolidation. Arterial blood gases (ABGs) may reveal a decrease in PaO_2 or oxygen saturation due to interference with gas exchange. Pulmonary function tests are usually within normal limits unless the client has an underlying pulmonary disorder such as emphysema.

▶ Medical/Surgical Management

▶ Medical

Clearing the airways of exudate and maintaining adequate oxygenation are the goals of treatment for pneumonia. Postural drainage and percussion may be ordered to aid the client in mobilizing secretions (see Figure 19-4). Aerosol or nebulization treatments may also be utilized. Medications are often added to aerosol or nebulization treatments as discussed with pharmacological management of pneumonia. The client is encouraged to cough and deep breathe, particularly following respiratory treatments. Incentive

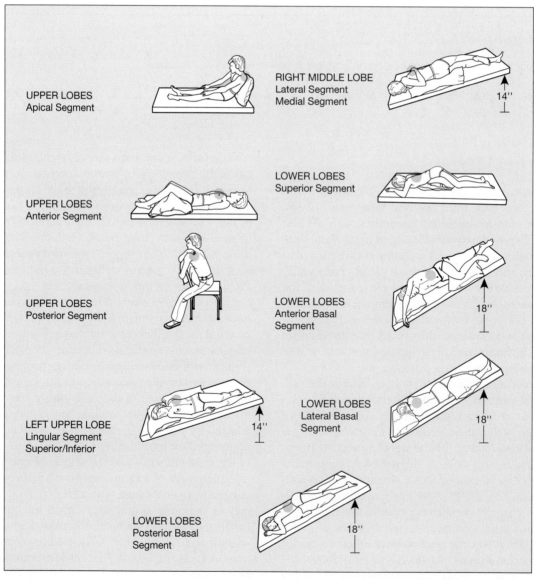

UPPER LOBES
Apical Segment

UPPER LOBES
Anterior Segment

UPPER LOBES
Posterior Segment

LEFT UPPER LOBE
Lingular Segment
Superior/Inferior

LOWER LOBES
Posterior Basal
Segment

RIGHT MIDDLE LOBE
Lateral Segment
Medial Segment

LOWER LOBES
Superior Segment

LOWER LOBES
Anterior Basal
Segment

LOWER LOBES
Lateral Basal
Segment

FIGURE 19-4 Positions which facilitate the drainage of the lobes of the lungs may be used with percussion.

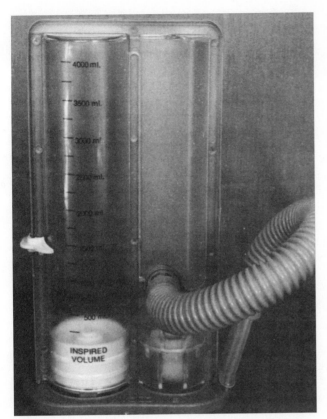

FIGURE 19-5 An incentive spirometer. This one is a Sherwood Medical Voldyne incentive spirometer.

spirometry may be ordered to aid the client when coughing and deep breathing are inadequate (see Figure 19-5). If the client is unable to mobilize secretions, suctioning of the respiratory tract is indicated. When secretions are overwhelming, the physician may perform a bronchoscopy in order to remove them. Intravenous fluids may be utilized to maintain adequate hydration, especially in the presence of fever. Adequate hydration promotes liquefaction of respiratory secretions and thus aids in their removal. Pulse oximetry or ABGs are done to assess the level of oxygenation. Supplemental oxygen is used when oxygenation is inadequate. Refer to Figure 19-6 and Table 19-4.

▶ Pharmacological

The treatment of choice for bacterial pneumonia is specific pharmacological therapy. A sputum specimen for culture and sensitivity should be obtained prior to initiating antibiotic therapy. Once a specimen is obtained, the physician may start therapy with a broad spectrum antibiotic. A specific antibiotic will be started if laboratory data indicate resistant microorganisms. Antiviral agents, such as acyclovir sodium (Zovirax), are utilized for serious viral pneumonia. Prophylactic antibiotic therapy is often utilized for viral pneumonia

to prevent a secondary bacterial infection. Bronchodilators, such as albuterol (Ventolin), and mucolytic agents, such as acetylcysteine (Mucomyst) are administered via aerosol or nebulization by the respiratory therapist or nurse to promote opening and clearing of the airways. Expectorants, such as guaifenisin (Robitussin), may be given orally. Cough suppressants and pain relievers, especially those containing narcotics such as codeine sulfate, are administered with discretion as they may further inhibit the ability to clear the airways.

Client teaching should include pertinent medication information, individual risk factors, measures to prevent spread of infection (i.e., cover cough, dispose of tissues) and methods to avoid future infection (i.e., avoid crowds, obtain vaccine if at risk).

▶ Diet

The client with pneumonia is encouraged to force fluids as this aids in the liquefaction of respiratory secretions. Small frequent meals that are nutritionally balanced are preferred. Respiratory treatments that promote coughing should be avoided immediately before meals to avoid nausea and vomiting associated with vigorous coughing.

▶ Activity

Bed rest or limited activity for the client with pneumonia to avoid client fatigue is recommended.

▶ Prevention

Pneumococcal vaccine (Pneumovax 23), a vaccine to prevent infection by *Streptococcus pneumoniale* should be given to clients at risk to develop pneumonia. It is recommended for all elderly persons.

Table 19-4

SUPPLEMENTAL OXYGEN DEVICES AND OXYGEN CONCENTRATIONS PROVIDED		
Device	Flow Rate	Oxygen Concentration
nasal cannula	1–6 L/min.	20–40%
simple mask	8–10 L/min.	40–60%
reservoir masks	6–10 L/min.	60–100%
venturi mask (used to control oxygen concentrations for the COPD patient)	4–8 L/min.	24–40%

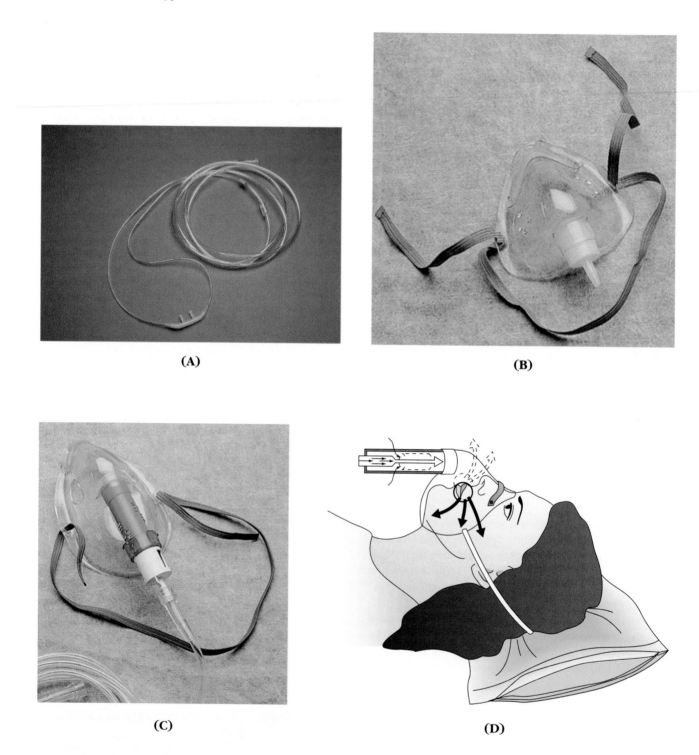

(A)

(B)

(C)

(D)

FIGURE 19-6 Supplemental oxygen devices. **(A)** A nasal cannula; **(B)** A simple mask; **(C)** A reservoir mask; **(D)** An illustration of a Venturi mask.

▶ Nursing Process

Assessment

Subjective Data Data gathered in the history includes: the onset, duration, and severity of cough; the color, amount, and odor of sputum, if present; the onset and duration of elevated temperature; and the presence or absence of night sweats.

Objective Data Assess the client's level of consciousness. Evidence of respiratory embarrassment such as dyspnea, orthopnea, tachypnea, and cyanosis may be present. Upon auscultation the lung fields have moist crackles or diminished breath sounds. In the event of obstruction of the airways sibilant wheezes occur. Vital signs including temperature are taken prior to and following drug therapy. This provides information as to the severity of the illness and the efficacy of treatment. The color, amount, viscosity, and odor of sputum is noted.

▼ ▼

Possible nursing diagnoses for a client with pneumonia may include:

Nursing Diagnoses	Goals	Nursing Interventions
▶ Airway clearance, ineffective, related to inability to remove airway secretions.	The client will have clear breath sounds to auscultation.	Encourage the client to breathe deeply and cough a minimum of every two hours.
		Teach use of the incentive spirometer to encourage lung expansion.
		Administer aerosol and nebulizer treatments as ordered.
		Provide percussion and postural drainage in conjunction with respiratory treatments as ordered.
		Provide bronchial suctioning for debilitated or comatose clients to remove sputum and mucous plugs.
		Assess breath sounds and respiratory rate prior to and following respiratory procedures to evaluate their effectiveness.
		Encourage fluids to liquefy thickened secretions.
		Assist clients who are able to sit up or ambulate three to four times daily.
		Turn the client on bed rest every two hours.
		Administer medications as ordered.
		Provide oral care several times a day.
▶ Gas exchange, impaired, related to inflammatory changes in alveolar capillary membrane.	The client will have an oxygen saturation of 95 percent or greater.	Monitor pulse oximetry and or arterial blood gases.
		Administer supplemental oxygen as ordered.
▶ Activity intolerance related to hypoxia secondary to pneumonia.	The client will be able to complete ADLs and activity as ordered without complaints of fatigue.	Encourage the client to complete ADLs according to their ability and the physician's order.
		Alternate periods of activity and care with periods of rest to avoid client fatigue.

▶ Evaluation

Each goal must be evaluated to determine how it has been met by the client.

▲ ▲

▶ *TUBERCULOSIS*

Pulmonary tuberculosis (TB) is an infection of the lung tissue with *Mycobacterium tuberculosis*. Infection with the tubercle bacillus can occur in other parts of the body, but with less frequency. Other parts of the body that may be affected include bones, joints, gastrointestinal and genitourinary tracts, nervous system, skin, and lymph nodes. In the case of pulmonary tuberculosis, the tubercle bacilli are inhaled into the lungs. Whether or not infection occurs is dependent upon: the host's susceptibility, the virulence of the tubercle bacilli, and the number of bacilli inhaled. Tuberculosis is not as highly contagious as once thought. Prolonged exposure to the bacilli is needed to produce an infection. In addition, persons with uncompromised immune systems are able to combat the bacilli and do not develop the disease itself. Those at risk for tuberculosis include persons suffering from malnutrition, those living in crowded conditions, persons with compromised immune status, and health care workers providing care to high risk individuals.

Once inhaled in sufficient numbers the tubercle bacilli cause an inflammatory response within the alveoli of the lung. A small nodule, called a **primary tubercle**, containing tubercle bacilli forms within the lung tissue. The body attempts to isolate these primary tubercles and forms a fibrous outer coating. The fibrous surface interferes with the blood supply and nutrition to the primary tubercle. In time the interior of the tubercle becomes soft and mushy, a process known as **caseation**. At this point the tubercles may become calcified or **liquefaction necrosis** may occur. In the case of liquefication necrosis, the tubercle liquefies and the fluid may be coughed up. A cavity is formed at the previous tubercle site. This condition is known as **cavitation** or cavitary disease.

Following the advent of antitubercular medications in the 1950s the incidence of TB decreased dramatically. In recent years, however, TB has been occurring with increased frequency. In addition, forms of TB are now occurring that are resistant to conventional drug therapy. Some of the factors that may be responsible for the increase in TB cases are: increased numbers of persons with compromised immune systems (many AIDS clients suffer from TB), increased mobility of the world's population (immigrants from areas of high incidence moving to areas of low incidence), IV drug abuse, increased numbers of those with poor access to health care, and increased numbers living in impoverished conditions.

Symptoms of tuberculosis develop gradually following infection. The nurse should suspect tuberculosis if the following symptoms are present: low-grade fevers that occur in the afternoon, persistent cough, hemoptysis, hoarseness, dyspnea on exertion, night sweats, fatigue, and weight loss. Due to the body's attempt to fight the infection, lymph nodes may be enlarged.

The Mantoux skin test is the preferred method of screening for tuberculosis. For the Mantoux test 0.1cc of purified protein derivative (PPD) of killed tubercle bacilli is injected intradermally on the inner forearm. The test is evaluated by measuring the area of induration (palpable swelling) that occurs forty-eight and seventy-two hours following injection of the killed tubercle bacilli. The area of induration, which indicates a positive reaction, is dependent upon the risk factors for TB of the individual being tested. Those at highest risk, such as persons infected with the HIV virus or those with recent close contact with a person infectious with TB, are considered to have a positive reaction if the area of induration is 5 mm or more (see Figure 19-7). Individuals with no risk factors for TB are considered to have a positive reaction if the area of induration is 15 mm or greater. A positive skin test, however, only indicates that the client has been exposed to and developed antibodies against the tubercle bacillus.

A negative reaction does not rule out the possibility of TB. Individuals at high risk, such as those infected with HIV and have a compromised immune status, may not have a positive reaction because they are unable to develop antibodies. Immediately following exposure to TB, a skin test may react falsely negative since it can take up to ten weeks for an infected individual to develop antibodies to react to the killed tubercle bacilli. An additional skin test may be done in a week. If the second TB test is positive, the client's history is reviewed for the presence of symptoms suggesting TB and further evaluation is indicated.

Chest x-ray and sputum specimens are utilized to confirm a diagnosis of TB. Sputum is tested for the presence of acid-fast bacilli, or AFB. The sputum specimen is collected when the client arises in the morning. This prevents contaminating the specimen with

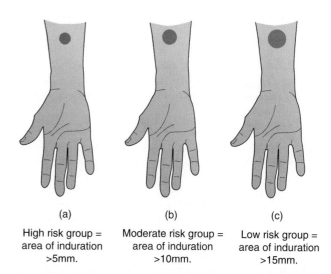

(a) High risk group = area of induration >5mm.

(b) Moderate risk group = area of induration >10mm.

(c) Low risk group = area of induration >15mm.

FIGURE 19-7 Scale showing positive tuberculin skin tests according to risk group.

ingested food and liquids. In most instances, three specimens collected on consecutive days and testing positive for AFB indicate a positive diagnosis of TB. Confirmation of a TB diagnosis is made if the TB bacilli grow in a culture. Individuals who are unable to produce sputum, including children and the elderly, may have stomach contents aspirated for the purpose of AFB testing. Chest x-ray may reveal the presence of primary tubercles in the lung. Areas of calcified lesions and cavitation are also revealed on x-ray.

▶ Medical/Surgical Management

▶ Medical

The majority of clients are treated briefly in the hospital with long-term treatment continuing at home. While hospitalized, the client should be placed in an isolation room with negative air pressure (one in which the flow of air is into the room and air outflow is exhausted directly to the outside and not recirculated to other rooms.). The doors and windows of the client's room must be kept closed to maintain control of air flow. Caregivers should wear particulate respirator masks as standard isolation masks do not prevent *Mycobacterium tuberculosis* from passing through to the wearer.

The Centers for Disease Control and Prevention recommend periodic TB skin testing for health care personnel. Health care workers with low risk for developing TB, those who have contact with less than six TB clients in a year, should be tested yearly. Health care workers who have had contact with five or more TB clients within the last year should be tested every six months. Any health care worker who is exposed to clients in a variety of settings (i.e., ambulance personnel) or who deal with a transitory client population should be tested every three months.

▶ Surgical

In the past, surgical intervention involving the removal of affected lung tissues was common. With the advent of effective chemotherapy (treatment with drugs), surgical intervention is now rarely utilized.

▶ Pharmacological

Active tuberculosis is treated with a combination of medications. Three medications, rifampin (Rifadin), isoniazid (Laniazid), and pyrazinamide (Pyrazinamide), are given for a period of two months. This is followed by a regimen of rifampin and isoniazid for four additional months. The combination of three drugs is given initially to rapidly decrease the number of active bacilli and prevent the development of drug resistance. Long-

term therapy is required as TB bacilli have long periods of metabolic inactivity. Those clients with bone and joint infections, meningitis, or resistant forms of TB will need to be treated with isoniazid and pyrazinamide for longer periods. HIV-positive clients require a seven-month regimen of isoniazid and pyrazinamide. Prophylactic treatment of the HIV-positive client with isoniazid is indicated from then on. Ethambutol hydrochloride (Myambutol) and streptomycin sulfate are included in the treatment of TB if the infecting organism is resistant to one of the three medications normally used to treat TB. Infection with a multidrug resistant form of TB requires the use of medications such as, kanmycin (Kantrex), capreomycin sulfate (Capastat Sulfate), and cycloserine (Seromycin). The client is considered noninfectious following three negative AFB sputum specimens. At this point the client may return to work and other normal activities. Prophylactic treatment of high risk individuals is recommended to reduce their chances of developing the disease following their exposure.

▶ Diet

The client with TB often suffers from nutritional deficits in addition to the tuberculosis. Correction of these deficits is necessary to assist the client in overcoming the disease process. Dietary management is based upon the type of deficiency present. A well-balanced diet is encouraged for all clients with TB. Fluids are encouraged to aid in the liquefaction of respiratory secretions.

▶ Activity

Activity is restricted based upon the client's tolerance. The client who is severely compromised from a respiratory standpoint may be placed on bed rest. If the client's condition allows, activity is encouraged as it promotes lung expansion and aids in the removal of static secretions. The client in isolation whose condition permits it, may ambulate in the hallways as long as a particulate respirator mask is worn by the client while outside of the room.

▶ Prevention

Prevention of tuberculosis is by far preferred. In areas where the disease remains endemic, a vaccine containing attenuated tubercle bacilli, BCG (bacillus Calmette-Guerin), is recommended. One disadvantage of the vaccine is that individuals receiving it test positive to the tuberculin skin test. Also, lifelong immunity to the disease has not been proven with the use of the vaccine to date. Other measures that decrease the likelihood of developing TB include: adequate nutrition, housing, health care access, and treatment of individuals with or at risk for TB.

▶ Nursing Process

Assessment

Subjective Data   Certain groups of individuals are at higher risk to develop TB, such as those who: are infected with HIV, have close contact with persons known or suspected to have TB, are immigrants from areas in which TB remains prevalent (for example, Africa and Asia), are residents of institutions (such as long-term care facilities or prisons), are intravenous drug users or alcoholics, have certain medical conditions, such as diabetes mellitus or chronic renal failure, and have been infected with the TB bacilli within the last two years. The history includes questions about the presence of signs and symptoms of TB, such as night sweats, dyspnea on exertion at rest in late disease, anorexia, loss of muscle strength, and fatigue. Pleuritic pain occurs when the pleura is involved.

Objective Data   This includes weight loss, persistent, low-grade fever, and persistent cough. The cough may be nonproductive early in the disease. Later the cough is productive of thick, purulent sputum. Eventually, hemoptysis occurs. Auscultation of the breath sounds reveals coarse crackles. In the presence of cavitary disease, the breath sounds are diminished or absent in the affected areas. Sputum is observed as to amount, color, odor, and consistency.

▼ ▼

Possible nursing diagnoses for a client with tuberculosis may include:

Nursing Diagnoses	Goals	Nursing Interventions
▶ Breathing pattern, ineffective, related to pulmonary infectious process.	The client will have color and respiratory rate within normal limits and no complaints of dyspnea.	Assess the client's color, respiratory rate, and respiratory effort.
		Auscultate the breath sounds.
		Administer and evaluate the results of the TB skin test.
		Obtain sputum specimens for AFB. Note the amount, color, and viscosity of the sputum.
		Plan care activities to allow the client uninterrupted periods of rest.
		Assist the client in assuming the position that aids respiratory effort most.
		Administer medications as ordered.
		Encourage fluids if not otherwise contraindicated.
▶ Infection, high risk, for transmission related to viable bacilli in respiratory secretions.	The client will verbalize ways to prevent the transmission of the tubercle bacillus.	Instruct client to cover the mouth or nose when coughing or sneezing.
		Double bag secretions and dispose of them as infectious waste.
		Use disposable items when giving care.
		Thoroughly clean and disinfect nondisposable articles.
		Teach the client and family how to contain and dispose of secretions and contaminated articles in the home setting.
		Test everyone who has been in close contact with the client without protective measures for TB.
		Instruct family members and/or significant others to eliminate or reduce the number and length of intimate contacts, such as kissing, with the client.
		Teach the client and family to clean articles, such as eating utensils, used by the client thoroughly prior to use by others in the household.

Nursing Diagnoses	Goals	Nursing Interventions
		Be aware of risk when caring for the client with TB and take adequate precautions.
		Follow Standard Precautions and Airborne Precautions.
		Wear a particulate respiratory mask when giving care to the client.
		Activities that increase the likelihood of exposure to the tubercle bacilli, such as sputum induction, require the use of face and/ or eye shields as well as the wearing of the particulate mask.
		Plan care activities to limit prolonged exposure to the client even when wearing appropriate barriers.
▶ Knowledge deficit related to disease process and its treatment.	The client will verbalize an understanding of the disease process and its treatment.	Teach client and family about the basic pathophysiology of TB, how the infection is contracted, who is at risk to develop an infection, the signs and symptoms of TB infection and complications that may arise.
		Present medication information regarding the actions, side effects, and untoward effects of the drugs being administered.
		Teach the client signs and symptoms of adverse drug reactions to report to the physician.
		Emphasize the necessity of long-term therapy to cure TB.
		Inform the client and family that symptoms decrease and are often gone long before the organism is eliminated from the body.
▶ Compliance, altered, related to long-term treatment.	The client will continue medication regimen for the prescribed length of time.	Include the client and family in making decisions about the care when appropriate.
		Allow the client some choices to make him an active participant and increase personal responsibility and accountability. Visits from public health or home care nurses may be necessary to monitor the client for compliance.
		Explore the reasons for noncompliance with the client and family.
		Based upon information obtained, identify strategies to increase compliance.
		Refer the client unable to afford the cost of medications to agencies, such as the local health department, for assistance.
		Monitor client suffering from adverse medication effects.
		If the client continues to be noncompliant, directly observed therapy may be required. Directly observed therapy involves sending the nurse or another health care worker to the client to administer the medications and observe that they are taken.

▶ Evaluation

Each goal must be evaluated to determine how it has been met by the client.

▲ ▲

Sample Nursing Care Plan: The Client with Tuberculosis

Mr. Stuart is an eighty-seven-year-old male admitted to the hospital with a chief complaint of productive cough and fatigue. Four months ago, Mr. Stuart was placed in a long-term care facility due to his inability to care for himself at home following his wife's death one year ago. Since admission to the long-term care facility, Mr. Stuart has lost 15 pounds. The nurses at the facility report that Mr. Stuart has experienced progressive fatigue, dyspnea on exertion, cough, night sweats, and anorexia. Initially, his cough was nonproductive, but it is now productive of moderate amounts of thick, purulent sputum that is occasionally streaked with blood. Vital signs are: temperature 99.8°F, pulse 108, respirations 26, and blood pressure 138/86. A TB skin test done at the long-term care facility one week ago was evaluated as negative. Sputum specimens for AFB reveal the presence of active tubercle bacilli. Chest x-ray is positive for TB. White blood cell count is 13,000 mm^3. Auscultation of breath sounds reveal crackles in the right lower half of the lung. Mr. Stuart says, "I don't understand why I don't breathe good and what all this fuss is about."

Nursing Diagnosis 1 Breathing pattern, ineffective, related to pulmonary infectious process as evidenced by dyspnea on exertion and productive cough.

Goals	Nursing Interventions	Rationale	Evaluation
Mr. Stuart will have respiratory rate, oxygen saturation, and color within normal limits and no complaints of dyspnea.	Assess initially and periodically Mr. Stuart's respiratory status including color, respiratory rate, respiratory effort, oxygen saturation, breath sounds, level of consciousness, cough, and sputum.	The initial assessment provides a data base from which the plan of care may be formulated and by which the effectiveness of treatment may be evaluated. Subsequent assessments provide a means of detecting changes in Mr. Stuart's condition. This allows for the evaluation of the effectiveness of interventions and modification of the plan of care.	Mr. Stuart verbalizes a decrease in dyspnea and cough. Mr. Stuart's color, respiratory rate, and oxygen saturation are within normal limits.
	Assist Mr. Stuart in assuming the position which most aids respiratory effort.	An upright, high or semi-Fowler's position displaces the abdominal organs downward allowing for greater ease of respiration and expansion of the lungs.	
	Alternate care activities with periods of rest.	Alternating care with periods of rest allows Mr. Stuart to compensate for the increased oxygen demand required by activity.	
	Encourage activity within Mr. Stuart's tolerance and per physician's orders.	Activity promotes expansion of the lungs.	
	Encourage fluids.	Fluids promote the liquefaction of respiratory secretions thus aiding in their removal	

Administer medications for fever as ordered.	Fever increases cellular metabolism which requires water. Thus fever that persists can lead to dehydration which will hinder the removal of respiratory secretions.		
Administer oxygen as ordered to maintain an SaO_2 of 95 percent or greater.	Oxygen saturations of 95 percent or greater are necessary for optimal cellular function.		
Administer antitubercular drugs as ordered.	Antitubercular drugs decrease the number of viable tubercle bacilli and thus decrease respiratory secretions.		

Nursing Diagnosis 2 Infection, high risk for, spread related to viable bacilli in secretions as evidenced by AFB in sputum.

Goals	Nursing Interventions	Rationale	Evaluation
Mr. Stuart will verbalize those situations that allow for the transmission of the tubercle bacilli and the means to prevent their transmission.	Place Mr. Stuart in a negative air pressure, private room. Door must remain closed at all times. Place Airborne Precaution signs on the door indicating Mr. Stuart has an infectious process and asking visitors to see nursing personnel prior to visiting. Instruct visitors to wear an N95 respirator when in Mr. Stuart's room, to limit the length of the visit, to avoid intimate contact with Mr. Stuart, such as kissing, and to wash their hands when leaving the room.	A negative air pressure private isolation room is required to prevent the transmission of the tubercle bacilli in air that has been circulated into and out of Mr. Stuart's room. Informing the public of the infectious disease process is necessary to prevent inadvertent contact and exposure. The nature of the infection is not revealed publicly to maintain client confidentiality. Visitors are informed of precautions to take to prevent exposure to the tubercle bacilli.	Persons exposed to Mr. Stuart have been tested for TB. Those with TB are being treated. No further unprotected exposures to Mr. Stuart will occur.
	Instruct Mr. Stuart to cover his mouth and nose when coughing and sneezing.	Covering the nose and mouth will aid in the containment of the tubercle bacilli sprayed out with coughing and/or sneezing.	
	Instruct Mr. Stuart to cough up secretion in tissues and to place these tissues in a plastic bag. Dispose of contained secretions as infectious waste.	Containment and proper disposal of infectious secretions aids in preventing the spread of the tubercle bacilli.	

(continued)

	Inform the long-term care facility and family/significant others of the positive results of the AFB studies. Instruct those persons who have been exposed to Mr. Stuart to have a TB skin test. Refer them to appropriate resources. Staff and clients exposed at the long-term care facility will probably be tested by the facility itself. Family and significant others may be tested by their own health care providers or the local health department.	Known exposure to the active tubercle bacilli necessitates testing to identify individuals who may have become infected.	
	Observe Standard Precautions and Airborne Precautions.	Compliance with Standard Precautions and Airborne Precautions decrease the likelihood of transmission of the tubercle bacilli (and other infectious diseases) to staff and other clients.	
	Wear a fitted N95 respirator when in Mr. Stuart's room.	A fitted, N95 respirator is necessary to prevent the inhalation of tubercle bacilli that are able to pass through a simple surgical mask.	
	Plan care activities to limit the length of time in close contact with Mr. Stuart.	Prolonged exposure to the tubercle bacilli, even when taking precautions, increases the likelihood of infection.	

Nursing Diagnosis 3 Knowledge deficit, related to disease process and its treatment as evidenced by client statement: "I don't understand why I don't breathe good and what all this fuss is about."

Goals	Nursing Interventions	Rationale	Evaluation
Mr. Stuart will verbalize an understanding of the disease process and the required medication regimen.	Assess Mr. Stuart's present level of knowledge regarding TB and its treatment.	Provides a data base regarding Mr. Stuart's present level of knowledge regarding TB and its treatment. Client education can then be individualized to build and expand upon that knowledge base. Misinformation can be also be corrected.	Mr. Stuart verbalizes his individual treatment regimen and the purpose of the regimen. Mr. Stuart demonstrates medication administration accurately. Mr. Stuart reports adverse effects of medication

Provide information in small amounts using a variety of approaches (i.e., verbal, written, videos).	Providing information in small amounts increases the likelihood of learning by not over-whelming Mr. Stuart with information. Providing information in a variety of media increases the likelihood of learning by supply-ing stimuli to the various senses (sight, sound, and touch).	to health care personnel to allow for early intervention.
Encourage and allow time for Mr. Stuart to ask questions.	Provides a means for Mr. Stuart to clarify information as well as a means for the nurse to evaluate learning and correct misconceptions.	
Have Mr. Stuart demon-strate medication administration regimen by setting up a day's dose of medications as ordered.	Demonstration of psychomotor skills reinforces learning and provides the nurse with a means to evaluate the effectiveness of teaching.	
Have Mr. Stuart verbalize signs and symptoms of adverse medication effects which should be reported to the staff of the long-term care facility and/or the physician.	Verbalization provides a means of evaluating the effectiveness of teaching. Mr. Stuart needs to be informed of those signs and symptoms that require further evaluation and follow-up by health care personnel.	
Have Mr. Stuart verbalize the length of treatment required for TB and the rationale for the length of treatment.	Provides a means to evaluate the effec-tiveness of teaching. This allows for the reinforcement of material taught, the correction of misinfor-mation, and the revision of the teaching plan.	

▶ *PLEURISY/PLEURAL EFFUSION*

Pleurisy is a painful condition that arises from inflammation of the pleura. This pleuritic pain is sharp and stabbing in nature. Pain increases with inspiration as the irritated pleura rub over one and the other. Inflammation of the pleura occurs with many disorders, such as viral infections, cancer of the lung, trauma, tuberculosis, congestive heart failure, and pulmonary embolism. The inflamed pleura secretes increased amounts of pleural fluid into the pleural space creating a **pleural effusion**. As fluid accumulates within the pleural space, it compresses the lung tissue (see Figure 19-8). Collapse, or atelectasis, results if left untreated. Those areas of collapsed lung tissue are unable to take part in gas exchange decreasing oxygenation. **Empyema** is a condition in which the pleural exudate becomes infected.

The primary manifestation of pleurisy is pain upon inspiration as described above. Signs and symptoms of pleural effusion are dependent upon the amount of lung tissue compressed and the source of the effusion. With large pleural effusions, the mediastinum shifts toward the unaffected side. MRI or CT imaging studies are useful in detecting pleural effusions, particularly small ones. A chest x-ray will show pleural effusions of 250 cc or more. Culture and sensitivity studies will identify the presence and type of infection if empyema is suspected. The client with empyema will also have an elevated temperature and white blood cell count.

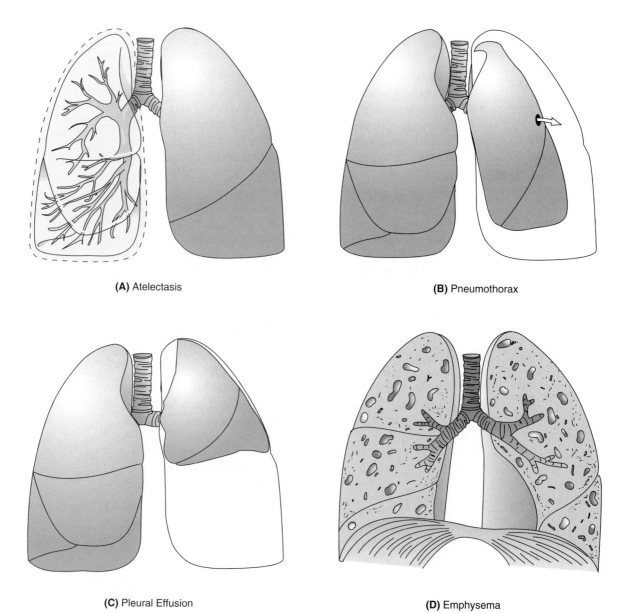

(A) Atelectasis

(B) Pneumothorax

(C) Pleural Effusion

(D) Emphysema

FIGURE 19-8 **(A)** Atelectasis of the right lung; **(B)** Pneumothorax of the left lung; **(C)** Pleural effusion of the left lung; **(D)** Emphysema.

▶ Medical/Surgical Management

▶ Medical

Treatment of pleurisy is aimed at eliminating the underlying cause, maintaining adequate oxygenation to the tissues, and preventing complications such as atelectasis and pneumonia. Adequacy of oxygenation is evaluated by means of arterial blood gases and/or pulse oximetry. Supplemental oxygen is given to maintain an oxygen saturation of 95 percent or greater. Respiratory treatments to aid lung expansion such as incentive spirometry are used.

▶ Surgical

Larger pleural effusions require a thoracentesis be performed by the physician to remove accumulated fluid (see Figure 19-9). After anesthetizing the overlying tissues, a large bore needle is placed into the pleural space. Fluid is removed and may be sent to the laboratory for diagnostic purposes (i.e., culture, cytology). If fluid accumulation continues to present a problem, as with empyema, a thoracotomy tube is placed by the physician into the pleural space to drain fluid continuously. Following administration of local anesthetics, the physician places a large bore catheter into the pleural space. This catheter is attached to an underwater seal drainage device (refer to Figure 19-10). Numerous commercial devices are available for this purpose. The underwater seal drainage device prevents the negative pressure within the pleural space from pulling air into the pleural space and allows for the drainage of accumulated fluid or air. In addition, most devices also include a chamber to which suction may be applied to assist in the removal of fluid or air from the pleural space. Following insertion of a chest tube, a chest x-ray is done to evaluate its placement and effectiveness.

▶ Pharmacological

If a pleural effusion is small and does not interfere greatly with respiratory function, diuretics are used to promote removal of fluid from the pleural space. Furosemide (Lasix) and bumetanide (Bumex) may be given for this purpose. If empyema is present specific therapy is used once the causative agent is identified. Relief of pain is a high priority. Analgesia that also decreases inflammation is preferred. Ketorolac tromethamine (Toradol) and other NSAIDs are often used. Severe pain will require narcotics such as morphine sulfate or meperidine (Demerol). If inflammation is extensive, corticosteroids such as hydrocortisone sodium succinate (Solu-Cortef) are utilized.

▶ Activity

The client's activity is limited to prevent fatigue. The client on bed rest is placed in a high Fowler's position to assist respirations.

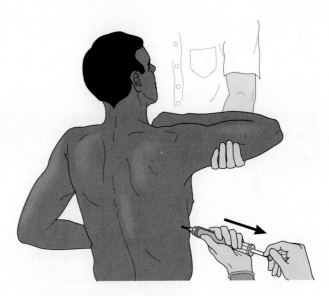

FIGURE 19-9 Thoracentesis.

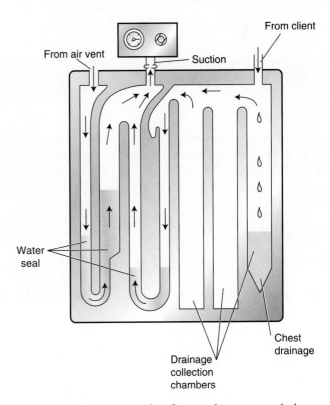

FIGURE 19-10 Example of an underwater seal chest drainage device.

▶ *Nursing Process*

Assessment

Subjective Data A nursing history is obtained from the client regarding onset, duration, and severity of symptoms. The client usually describes chest pain that increases with each inspiration and difficulty breathing.

Objective Data Assess the client's level of consciousness. Evaluate the client's color, respiratory rate, and effort. Abnormalities in vital signs are noted. The breath sounds over the areas of involvement are diminished or absent. A pleural friction rub may be audible. Dyspnea, cyanosis, and hypoxia occur proportional to the severity of the condition. If a chest tube is in place the amount and color of drainage are assessed.

▼ ▼

Possible nursing diagnoses for a client with a pleural effusion may include:

Nursing Diagnoses	*Goals*	*Nursing Interventions*
▶ *Pain, acute, related to inflammation of the pleura.*	The client will verbalize a decrease in the level of pain using a scale of 1 to 10.	Administer pain medications as ordered. Assist the client in attaining the position that allows for greatest comfort. Elevate the head of the bed. Provide diversional activities.
▶ *Gas exchange, impaired, related to ineffective breathing pattern.*	The client will maintain an oxygen saturation of 95 percent or greater, a respiratory rate of 14–22, and have clear breath sounds.	Provide supplemental oxygen as ordered. Encourage the client to breathe deeply or use the incentive spirometer as ordered. Administer diuretics and anti-inflammatory medications as ordered. Assist the physician with the thoracentesis or placement of a thoracotomy tube. Collect specimen for culture and sensitivity and other studies at this time.
▶ *Self-care deficit related to mobility restriction.*	The client will increase self-care activities as mobility increases.	Assist the client with hygiene and self-care needs. Encourage participation in self-care activities within the limits of the physician's orders.
▶ *Activity intolerance related to hypoxia secondary to pleural effusion.*	The client will increase activity without complaints of fatigue.	Activities should be staggered with periods of rest. Plan activity around therapies to avoid fatigue.

▶ *Evaluation*

Each goal must be evaluated to determine how it has been met by the client.

▲ ▲

▶ ACUTE RESPIRATORY TRACT DISORDERS

▶ ATELECTASIS

Atelectasis refers to the collapse of a lung or a portion of a lung. The most common cause of atelectasis is airway obstruction. A bronchiole becomes blocked with secretions and the alveoli distal to it collapse (refer to Figure 19-8A). Airway obstruction of this nature is common after surgery and with immobility problems. Anesthesia, pain, narcotics, and immobility work in combination to cause hypoventilation and the retention of secretions. Atelectasis also occurs with compression of lung tissue as is the case with pleural effusion or pneumothorax. An insufficient level of surfactant results in increased recoil properties of the lungs leading to atelectasis. Hypoventilation can cause atelectasis and atelectasis increases hypoventilation.

Signs of respiratory distress are proportional to the amount of lung tissue involved. When large areas of the lung are involved, orthopnea or cyanosis may develop. Breath sounds are diminished or absent over collapsed areas. Late in the disease process chest wall movement decreases on the affected side. Oxygenation decreases as demonstrated by arterial blood gases or pulse oximetry. Pulse and respiratory rate increase as the heart and lungs work harder to meet the body's oxygen needs. Trapped secretions are a rich growth medium for microorganisms. An elevated temperature indicates secondary infection (pneumonia). Chest x-ray studies reveal the areas of collapse. Bronchoscopy is used for direct visualization of the area of obstruction and to obtain specimen for diagnostic purposes (see Figure 19-11).

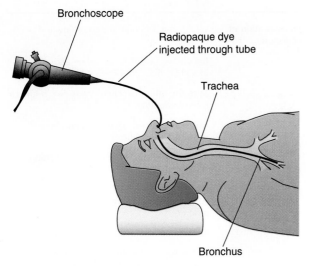

Bronchoscope

Radiopaque dye injected through tube

Trachea

Bronchus

FIGURE 19-11   Bronchoscopy.

▶ Medical/Surgical Management

▶ Medical

The physician will order various measures to promote expansion of the lungs. Incentive spirometry and deep breathing and coughing exercises are ordered. Postural drainage with percussion aids in the removal of any static secretions. If the client is unable to cough up static secretions, suctioning of the respiratory tract is done. Bronchoscopy may be done by the physician to remove secretions and obtain specimens. Arterial blood gases or pulse oximetry are utilized to evaluate the need for supplemental oxygen. Oxygen is administered to maintain an oxygen saturation of 95 percent or greater.

▶ Surgical

Clients with pneumothorax or pleural effusion as the underlying cause of atelectasis require removal of trapped air or fluid via thoracentesis or placement of a thoracotomy tube (refer to pleural effusion and pneumothorax). Atelectasis resulting from the growth of a tumor requires surgical removal of the tumor.

▶ Pharmacological

Adequate pain control aids the client, particularly the surgical client, in being able to breathe deeply and cough. Client-controlled analgesia or a routine schedule of pain medications may be used to provide effective pain management. Aminophylline (Aminophyllin) and other bronchodilators may be used to open the airways. Mucolytic agents such as guaifenisin (Humibid) are used to liquefy respiratory tract secretions. Bronchodilators, such as albuterol sulfate (Ventolin) and mucolytics such as acetylcysteine (Mucomyst) may also be administered via updraft or nebulizer treatments. The client with an infection requires treatment with an appropriate antibiotic such as ciprofloxacin hydrochloride (Cipro).

▶ Diet

Unless otherwise contraindicated, fluids are encouraged to promote liquefaction of static respiratory secretions.

▶ Activity

Activity promotes lung expansion. Immobile clients are turned a minimum of every two hours and assisted to do range of motion exercises. Surgical clients may do leg exercises as well as deep breathing and coughing. Ambulation is recommended if the client's condition allows. If the client is unable to walk sitting up in a chair is encouraged. Rest periods are planned between activities to prevent fatigue.

▶ *Nursing Process*

Assessment

Subjective Data   Clients who smoke or those who are immunocompromised or with known chronic respiratory or cardiovascular diseases present an increased risk for the development of atelectasis. Question the client about the onset, duration, and severity of symptoms such as pain, cough, and dyspnea. The client may complain of or show signs of air hunger, shortness of breath, fatigue, and anxiety.

Objective Data   Assess the client for changes in the level of consciousness, an early sign of decreased oxygenation. Periodically evaluate the client for dyspnea, tachypnea, cyanosis, and restlessness. Assess vital signs frequently with particular attention to respiratory rate and effort. Auscultation reveals diminished or absent breath sounds over the areas of atelectasis. Crackles or sonorous wheezes may be heard if pneumonia develops. Note objective indicators of pain such as facial grimacing, in addition to subjective questioning. The effectiveness of the client's cough is assessed. A productive cough is evaluated for amount, color, consistency, and odor of secretions.

▼ ▼

Possible nursing diagnoses for a client with atelectasis may include:

Nursing Diagnoses	*Goals*	*Nursing Interventions*
▶ *Knowledge deficit, related to the complications of surgery and/or immobility.*	The client will verbalize the purpose of deep breathing, coughing, and activity following surgery and demonstrate deep breathing and coughing.	Teach all preoperative and immobile clients to cough and breathe deeply at least every two hours. Have the client demonstrate coughing and deep breathing to assure that learning has occurred. Teach the surgical client to splint the surgical incision to minimize discomfort that might occur with coughing and deep breathing. Instruct clients at risk for the developing atelectasis in the use of incentive spirometry. Emphasize the importance of early ambulation and activity to promote lung expansion.
▶ *Gas exchange, impaired, related to decreased alveolar-capillary surface.*	The client will have an oxygen saturation of 95 percent or greater, a respiratory rate of 14 to 22 and clear breath sounds.	Establish a schedule for coughing and deep breathing. Encourage clients to ambulate and/or sit up in a chair three to four times daily. Turn the immobile client every two hours or more frequently. Assess the client's vital signs and breath sounds periodically. Encourage fluids if the client's condition allows. The nurse or respiratory therapist administers respiratory treatments as ordered. Administer medications as ordered. Assess secretions (sputum) for color, amount, consistency, and odor.

Nursing Diagnoses	Goals	Nursing Interventions
▶ *Activity intolerance, related to hypoxia secondary to atelectasis.*	The client will complete activity without complaints of shortness of breath, dyspnea, or fatigue.	Encourage some activity to promote lung expansion.
		Alternate periods of activity with rest to avoid overtiring the client.
		Provide assistance with ADLs as the client's condition requires.
		Place the client in a high or semi-Fowler's position to aid lung expansion.
		Position client on the unaffected side.

▶ Evaluation

Each goal must be evaluated to determine how it has been met by the client.

▲ ▲

▶ PULMONARY EMBOLISM

Pulmonary emboli develop when a bloodborne substance lodges in a branch of a pulmonary artery and obstructs flow. A common source of pulmonary embolism is deep vein thrombophlebitis. Other sources of emboli are air from IV infusions, fat from long bone fractures, and amniotic fluid. Pulmonary emboli rarely develop before adulthood. As age increases, the risk for pulmonary emboli is greater due to the development of arteriosclerosis and other vascular changes associated with aging. Other factors increasing the risk for pulmonary emboli are heredity, smoking, peripheral vascular disease, diabetes mellitus, and use of oral contraceptives. The size and location of the emboli determines the severity and outcome of the condition. Emboli interfere with gas exchange to the pulmonary circulation distal to the emboli. As a result hypoxemia occurs. The client complains of breathlessness and dyspnea. Pulse oximetry or arterial blood gases will demonstrate the degree to which oxygenation has been affected. Obstruction of a main branch of a pulmonary artery can result in lung infarction and necrosis.

All clients at risk for pulmonary emboli should be observed for signs and symptoms of deep vein thrombosis, such as localized calf tenderness or swelling. Measures to prevent thrombus formation should be utilized for these individuals. Any signs of thrombophlebitis are reported to the physician immediately.

Signs and symptoms of pulmonary emboli are abrupt in onset. The client is anxious and restless. Sudden, sharp chest pains of a pleuritic nature develop. Dyspnea and cough with hemoptysis occur. Venous return is diminished resulting in jugular venous distention. The client becomes diaphoretic. A low-grade fever develops in response to inflammation. A high temperature is indicative of lung infarction. Diagnosis of pulmonary emboli is accomplished by a ventilation/perfusion lung scan. Arterial blood gases show hypoxia and respiratory alkalosis. In severe cases, pulmonary angiography is done to find the exact location of the clot.

▶ Medical/Surgical Management

▶ Medical

As indicated above, preventive measures are instituted for the client at risk to develop deep vein thrombosis. Following surgery antiembolism stockings and early ambulation are indicated. Supplemental oxygen is given to increase oxygenation when hypoxia occurs. The underlying cause of the pulmonary emboli is treated when identified.

▶ Surgical

In severe cases, the physician may elect to remove the clot via an embolectomy. This procedure is usually done at the time of angiography. Clients who experience successive episodes of pulmonary emboli may require a venacaval plication. This surgical procedure involves placing a sieve-like device in the inferior vena cava to catch emboli before they enter the pulmonary circulation.

▶ Pharmacological

The client at risk to develop deep vein thrombosis and/or pulmonary emboli may be treated with enoxaparin sodium (Lovenox). Lovenox is often used in the postoperative client to prevent clot formation. Once pulmonary emboli have occurred anticoagulation is ordered to prevent the formation of further clots. Initially heparin (Hep-Lock) is used to establish anticoagulation. Heparin is administered parenterally either by the intravenous or subcutaneous route. Once adequate anticoagulation is established, heparin therapy is followed by warfarin sodium (Coumadin) therapy. Coumadin is given orally and may be used long term on an outpatient basis. If the clot is large or lies in a branch of a main pulmonary artery, fibrinolytic therapy may be utilized. Fibrinolytics lyse or dissolve the clot versus inhibiting the formation of new clots. Examples of fibrinolytic agents are alteplase (Activase) and streptokinase (Streptase). These agents may be administered intra-arterially at the site of the clot or intravenously to achieve a systemic effect. Narcotic analgesics such as morphine are ordered to control pain.

▶ Activity

Activity is encouraged to prevent the formation of clots. Once a clot has formed, however, the client's activity will be restricted to prevent the clot from moving and becoming an embolus. Activities such as sitting, crossing the knees, or prolonged bending at the hips are to be avoided as these promote venous stasis.

▶ Diet

Fluids are encouraged to prevent hemoconcentration leading to clot formation. Unless contraindicated, fluids should be encouraged for the client at risk to develop pulmonary emboli.

▶ Nursing Process

Assessment

Subjective Data   The client's history is obtained to identify potential risk factors for the development of pulmonary emboli. Ask the client about the onset, duration, and severity of symptoms. Shortness of breath, dyspnea, and severe pleuritic chest pain are abrupt in onset. Evaluate pain as to onset, location, duration, severity, and character.

Objective Data   Monitor pulse oximetry measurements that reflect oxygenation. The client's respirations are rapid and shallow. Pallor progressing to cyanosis develops as oxygenation decreases. The client becomes diaphoretic. A change in the level of consciousness or increased anxiety may be the first indications of a pulmonary embolus. The pulse increases in response to anxiety and as an attempt to supply oxygen to the body's cells. Blood pressure may increase or decrease in response to hypoxia, anxiety, and pain. Temperature may be elevated in response to inflammation and tissue necrosis. Upon auscultation breath sounds may or may not be decreased. The jugular veins are distended.

▼ ▼

Possible nursing diagnoses for a client with pulmonary emboli may include:

Nursing Diagnoses	Goals	Nursing Interventions
▶ Gas exchange, impaired, related to alteration in pulmonary circulation.	The client will maintain an oxygen saturation of 95 percent or greater, have a respiratory rate of 14 to 22 and have color within normal limits.	Assess the client for indications of decreasing oxygenation.
		Auscultate breath sounds every four hours or more often.
		Assess peripheral pulses and capillary refill.
		Encourage deep breathing and coughing.
		Provide supplemental oxygen to maintain oxygen saturation > 95% or as ordered.
		Administer subcutaneous heparin as ordered.
		Once anticoagulation is established, administer Coumadin as ordered.
		Encourage fluids, unless contraindicated, to prevent hemoconcentration.

Nursing Diagnoses	Goals	Nursing Interventions
▶ Pain, acute, related to decreased perfusion of lung tissue.	The client will state pain is decreased using a scale of 1 to 10.	Administer pain medication as ordered. Assist the client in assuming a position of comfort. If possible, place the client in a high Fowler's position to aid respiratory effort.
▶ Injury, high risk for, related to anticoagulation/fibrinolytic therapy.	The client will be free of abnormal bleeding and maintain hemoglobin and hematocrit within normal limits.	Assess for evidence of bleeding. Monitor lab reports for APTT, INR, and PT and hemoglobin and hematocrit levels. Evaluate blood pressure and pulse for signs of bleeding, i.e., rapid pulse and low blood pressure. Check stool and for occult blood. Assess gums for bleeding. Use soft toothbrush for brushing the teeth to avoid trauma. Monitor menstrual flow in the female client. Teach client signs and symptoms of bleeding, avoidance of activities that might induce trauma, foods and medications to avoid while taking anticoagulants, especially Coumadin, and the purpose and times for blood tests.

▶ Evaluation

Each goal must be evaluated to determine how it has been met by the client.

▲ ▲

▶ PULMONARY EDEMA

Acute pulmonary edema is a life-threatening condition characterized by a rapid shift of fluid from plasma into the pulmonary interstitial tissue and the alveoli. As a result gas exchange is markedly impaired. Pulmonary edema can occur as a result of severe left ventricular failure (i.e., following myocardial infarction), rapid administration of intravenous fluids, inhalation of noxious gases, or with opiate and barbiturate overdoses.

The hallmark of acute pulmonary edema is a cough producing a copious amount of frothy blood-tinged sputum, often appearing pinkish. The client rapidly becomes dyspneic, orthopneic, and cyanotic. Anxiety ranging from restlessness to panic occurs. Heart and respiratory rate increase. Progressive crackles are heard in the lung fields when auscultating the lungs. Initially, fine crackles are present in the posterior bases of the lung. As pulmonary edema progresses, the crackles become increasingly coarser, louder, and more diffuse. Wheezes are present with significant obstruction of the airways by fluid. Left untreated the client deteriorates rapidly as oxygenation decreases.

▶ Medical/Surgical Management

▶ Medical

The goals of medical management are to remove fluid from the alveoli and pulmonary interstitial space, prevent further influx of fluid, and improve oxygenation. Arterial blood gases and pulse oximetry are used to assess oxygenation. Supplemental oxygen is administered when hypoxia is present per physician's order.

▶ Pharmacological

A diuretic such as furosemide (Lasix) is given to increase urinary output. When the pumping force of the left ventricle is impaired, a digitalis preparation, i.e., digoxin (Lanoxin) is given to improve the contractile force of the myocardium. To prevent further influx of fluid into the lungs, venous pooling is enhanced. This also decreases the workload on the heart by limiting venous return. Morphine is used to promote vasodilatation and thus venous pooling and to relieve anxiety. Bronchodilators, such as aminophylline (Aminophyllin) are administered to dilate airways obstructed with fluid.

▶ Activity

The client is placed on bed rest to reduce the workload of the heart and lungs. High Fowler's position aids respiratory effort and enhances venous pooling. Activities are increased slowly according to the physician's order and the client's ability to tolerate activity.

▶ Diet

The physician may order a diet restricted in sodium to prevent fluid retention. Intake and output as well as daily weight are done to monitor fluid balance.

▶ *Nursing Process*

Assessment

Subjective Data The nurse needs to be aware of those conditions that predispose the client to pulmonary edema. The client may describe feeling anxious, breathless, and fatigued.

Objective Data Auscultate the breath sounds for the presence of crackles. Increasingly coarse and diffuse crackles are reported to the physician. Assess the client's level of consciousness, respiratory rate, effort, and color. Dyspnea, tachypnea, cyanosis and/or pallor may be present. Oxygenation is assessed via pulse oximetry or arterial blood gases. A productive cough may be present. Symptoms of congestive heart failure such as rapid weight gain and peripheral edema may precede pulmonary edema. The pulse may be rapid and weak. Blood pressure may increase in response to anxiety and decreased oxygenation.

▼ ▼

Possible nursing diagnoses for a client with pulmonary edema may include:

Nursing Diagnoses	Goals	Nursing Interventions
▶ *Gas exchange, impaired, related to fluid in the lung tissue.*	The client will maintain an oxygen saturation of 95 percent or greater, have respiratory rate and color within normal limits, normal blood gases and clear breath sounds.	Place the client in high Fowler's or orthopneic position. Assess oxygenation continually via arterial blood gases or pulse oximetry and provide supplemental oxygen to maintain an oxygen saturation of 95 percent or greater or per physician's order. Assess respiratory rate, breath sounds, heart rate, and blood pressure frequently administer respiratory treatments as ordered. Assist the client with activities to reduce the typical workload on the heart and lungs by alternating activity with periods of rest to avoid client fatigue. Administer medications as ordered and evaluate the effectiveness of each. Monitor lab reports for electrolyte values.
▶ *Fluid volume excess, related to altered tissue permeability.*	The client's weight will return to normal.	Weigh client daily. Monitor intake and output. Assess the client frequently for peripheral edema. Provide the client with a low salt diet. Administer diuretics per order and evaluate their effectiveness. Monitor lab reports for electrolyte values. Monitor the rate intravenous fluids are given. Teach client and family signs and symptoms of fluid excess, information about the medications taken, and dietary modifications.

▶ *Evaluation*

Each goal must be evaluated to determine how it has been met by the client.

▲ ▲

▶ *ADULT RESPIRATORY DISTRESS SYNDROME (ARDS)*

Adult respiratory distress syndrome (ARDS) is a life-threatening condition characterized by severe dyspnea, hypoxemia, and diffuse pulmonary edema. The condition usually follows a major assault on multiple body systems or severe lung trauma. Underlying causes include trauma, sepsis, coronary artery bypass surgery, major thoracic or vascular surgery, renal failure, severe pulmonary infections, inhalation lung injuries, and acute drug poisoning. ARDS is also called noncardiogenic pulmonary edema, shock lung, progressive pulmonary congestion or traumatic wet lung. The term *adult respiratory distress syndrome* more accurately describes the pathophysiology underlying this condition.

During the initial assault on the body, the pulmonary capillary membrane is damaged. The damaged membrane allows fluid to leak from the vascular system into the pulmonary interstitial tissue and the alveoli themselves. Gas exchange is severely impaired due to the damage to the pulmonary capillary membrane and the presence of fluid in the alveoli. The surfactant is rendered inactive resulting in the collapse of the alveoli, and gas exchange is further reduced. Hypoxemia develops, and is resistant to conventional oxygen therapy.

The client with ARDS is critically ill as reflected in the signs and symptoms. Severe dyspnea, tachypnea, and cyanosis are present. Arterial blood gases will show a PaO_2 less than 70 mmHg, $PaCO_2$ more than 35 mmHg, bicarbonate ion less than 22 mEq/L and a pH elevated at first, then steadily decreases. The ABGs and pulse oximetry reveal severe hypoxemia and progressive respiratory and metabolic acidosis. On auscultation, the lung fields are filled with diffuse coarse crackles and sonorous wheezes. The client will have a productive cough of blood-tinged sputum. Chest x-ray will show widely scattered infiltrates often referred to as a "white out."

▶ *Medical/Surgical Management*

▶ *Medical*

The client with ARDS is cared for in the intensive care unit. The underlying cause of ARDS is found and treated, until that time supportive care is given. Mechanical ventilatory support is necessary with multiple systems often being supported as well. A mechanical ventilator allows the percentage of oxygen, pulmonary pressure, and lung volume to be controlled (see Figure 19-12). Oxygenation is monitored with arterial blood gases and pulse oximetry. Respiratory secretions are removed by frequent bronchial suctioning.

▶ *Pharmacological*

Pharmacological therapy includes corticosteriods such as hydrocortisone sodium succinate (Solu-Cortef) or methylprednisolone sodium succinate (Solu-Medrol) in high doses. Furosemide (Lasix) and other diuretics are given to increase urinary output. Aminophylline (Aminophyllin) is administered to open the bronchi. While the client is on the mechanical ventilator, pancuronium bromide (Pavulon), is given to

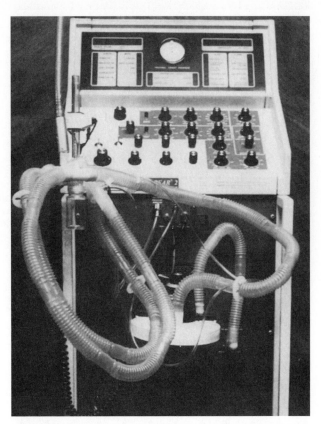

FIGURE 19-12 A mechanical ventilator. This is a BEAR 2 volume ventilator.

suppress the client's own respiratory effort. Blood pressure can fall dangerously low and vasopressors such as dopamine hydrochloride (Intropin) may be required to maintain the blood pressure within acceptable ranges.

▶ Activity

The client with ARDS will be on bed rest. Special beds that provide movement and pressure adjustment are used to prevent the complications associated with immobility.

▶ Diet

Total parenteral nutrition (TPN) may be given to the client, especially during the acute phase of the illness. When possible the gastrointestinal tract is used for nutrition through enteral feedings.

▶ Nursing Process

Assessment

Subjective Data The client history is gathered from family members or significant others as the client is usually too ill to communicate.

Objective Data Assess the client's level of consciousness and response to stimuli. Observe the client for restlessness and anxiety. Assess vital signs frequently, every fifteen minutes or more often if the client is critically ill. Heart rate is increased and arrhythmias may be present. Blood pressure is usually low. The rate, rhythm, and respiratory effort are assessed for signs of dyspnea, nasal flaring, cyanosis, tachypnea, and other indications of respiratory distress. Arterial blood gas and pulse oximetry values are assessed to evaluate oxygenation and acid/base balance. Diffuse coarse crackles and wheezes are heard throughout the lung fields.

▼ ▼

Possible nursing diagnoses for a client with ARDS may include:

Nursing Diagnoses	Goals	Nursing Interventions
▶ Gas exchange, impaired, related to pulmonary capillary membrane damage.	The client will have an oxygen saturation of 95 percent or greater, arterial blood gases within normal limits, and respiratory rate and effort within normal limits.	Provide adequate oxygenation and ventilation as ordered. Monitor arterial blood gases and pulse oximetry to evaluate oxygenation and acid/base balance. Assess the client's respiratory rate and effort and auscultate the lungs frequently. Suction the respiratory tract as necessary to remove excess secretions. Provide oral care frequently.
▶ Anxiety, related to the condition and mechanical ventilation.	The client will verbalize a decrease in anxiety if able or have less objective signs of anxiety such as restlessness, facial grimacing.	Describe care and purposes to the client. Allow rest periods between activity to decrease overwhelming the client with stimuli. Plan care to allow for uninterrupted rest. Allow family and significant others to visit and participate in care as appropriate. Assess the client for signs of sensory overload/deprivation.

▶ Evaluation

Each goal must be evaluated to determine how it has been met by the client.

▲ ▲

ACUTE RESPIRATORY FAILURE

Acute respiratory failure is not a disease entity in and of itself. The term is used to refer to conditions in which there is a failure of the respiratory system as a whole. This condition occurs as a result of the client's literally becoming too tired to continue the "work" of breathing. Mechanical ventilatory support is required during the acute phase. Clients with preexisting pulmonary conditions coupled with acute respiratory tract infections are at risk to develop acute respiratory failure.

CHRONIC RESPIRATORY TRACT DISORDERS

CHRONIC OBSTRUCTIVE PULMONARY DISEASE (COPD)

Chronic obstructive pulmonary disease (COPD), also called chronic obstructive lung disease (COLD), describes a broad category of respiratory conditions with a variety of etiologic factors. COPD is characterized by chronic airflow limitation. Changes within the lungs lead to a narrowing of the bronchial airways, excessive mucous secretions within the airways, and an increase in the size of the airways distal to the terminal bronchioles (the alveoli) thus causing air to be trapped. The conditions most often associated with COPD include: asthma, emphysema, chronic bronchitis, and bronchiectasis.

ASTHMA

Asthma is a condition characterized by intermittent airway obstruction arising from response to a variety of stimuli. The epithelial lining of the airways responds by becoming inflamed and edematous. Bronchospasm occurs in the smooth muscles of the bronchi and bronchioles. Secretions increase in viscosity. Elastic recoil is decreased. All of these changes result in a reduction of the diameter of the airways and cause difficulty of inspiration. Over time, the changes may become chronic and chronic obstructive pulmonary disease (COPD) results. Some clients who develop the disease in childhood have spontaneous recovery. Asthma may be classified as intrinsic or extrinsic. Extrinsic asthma is caused by substances outside the body that precipitate the asthma response. Intrinsic asthma is diagnosed when no extrinsic factor can be determined. The asthma response in intrinsic asthma is the result of internal factors. Allergies, environmental factors such as air pollution, heredity, exercise, and psychological factors have been indicated in predisposing an individual to asthma. An asthma attack that does not respond to treatment and persists is known as **status asthmaticus**.

The hallmark of an asthma attack is sudden onset of wheezing, increasing dyspnea, and chest tightness. Mild asthma is usually controlled by medication. Severe asthma attacks usually occur at night. Wheezing with severe attacks may be audible to the unaided ear. Expiratory wheezes are common as air attempts to escape through the narrowed airways. Both inspiratory and expiratory wheezes may be heard. The respiratory rate rises initially but as the client tires the rate may decrease. Nasal flaring and costal and sternal retractions may be present, particularly in the young client. The client will use accessory muscles to assist respiratory effort. Cough occurs as the respiratory secretions become thick and plug the airways. Cyanosis and a decrease in oxygen saturation occurs. The heart rate is elevated and blood pressure may increase. The client is anxious and may complain of a sense of impending doom. This is thought to be due to release of catecholamines. Values of arterial blood gases indicate hypoxia and respiratory acidosis. Chest x-ray shows hyperinflation of the lungs. Pulmonary function tests will reveal an abnormal flow rate and lung volume. Apnea and sudden death can occur in minutes with a severe asthmatic attack.

Medical/Surgical Management

Medical

In addition to medications, treatment for asthma may include manipulating known triggers. The client with allergies avoids specific antigens such as animal hair, pollens, and dietary factors, which might bring on an attack. Controlling psychological stressors aids some asthmatics. Routine physical exercise is beneficial in treating exercise induced asthma. The asthmatic should be told to avoid other respiratory irritants, such as cigarette smoke and air pollution. Asthmatic children often experience a reduction in the number and severity of asthmatic attacks as they age. Those who develop asthma later in life, however, develop more symptoms as they age.

Pharmacological

The primary treatment for an acute asthmatic attack is pharmacological. A combination of medications is used to open the narrowed airways. Medications used to dilate the bronchi include bronchodilators, such as aminophylline (Aminophyllin) and terbutaline sulfate

(Brethine, Bricanyl); beta agonists, such as epinephrine (Primatene Mist) and albuterol sulfate (Ventolin), and anticholinergics such as atropine sulfate and ipratropium bromide (Atrovent). Corticosteroids, such as prednisone (Delatsone), are utilized to decrease inflammation. Mucolytic agents, such as acetylcysteine (Mucomyst), aid in liquefying secretions. Supplemental oxygen is given when indicated.

▶ Diet

Adequate fluid intake should be maintained.

▶ Activity

Incorporate several rest periods into the day. Relaxation techniques can be used to manage anxiety.

▶ Nursing Process

Assessment

Subjective Data A detailed history is taken regarding exposure to triggering stimuli and past asthmatic attacks. The onset, duration, and severity of symptoms such as dyspnea is obtained.

Objective Data Evaluate the effectiveness of ventilation. Wheezes are evaluated as to their duration, location, and the phase of respiration in which they occur (i.e., inspiration). Wheezing heard without the aid of a stethoscope is called **audible wheezes**. Respiratory rate, depth, and rhythm, position assumed, respiratory effort, and client color are evaluated. Monitor pulse oximetry or lab reports of arterial blood gases to determine oxygenation and acid/base balance. If sputum is produced it is assessed as to its color, amount, viscosity, and odor.

▼ ▼

Possible nursing diagnoses for a client with asthma may include:

Nursing Diagnoses	Goals	Nursing Interventions
▶ Breathing pattern, ineffective, related to narrowed airways.	The client will have respiratory rate and color within normal limits, clear breath sounds to auscultation, and arterial blood gases or pulse oximetry within normal limits.	Assist the client in assuming a position that facilitates ventilation. Administer medication as ordered. Assist the client with use of inhalers and aerosol treatments. Assess oxygenation via arterial blood gases or pulse oximetry as ordered. Administer supplemental oxygen as ordered. Assess the client's respiratory rate, effort, and color frequently. Auscultate the lung fields for presence of wheezes. If sputum is produced note its color, amount, viscosity, and odor. Assess vital signs frequently. Unless otherwise contraindicated encourage fluid intake to promote liquefaction of respiratory secretions.
▶ Knowledge deficit related to asthma, its treatment, and individual triggers for attacks.	The client will verbalize the pathophysiology of asthma an understanding of its treatment, including the medications taken, their purposes, and side effects. The client will also identify individual triggers and a means to avoid these triggers.	Teach client about the disease process. Teach client and family the purpose, effect, adverse effects, and side effects of all medications taken, especially the use of inhalers and respiratory aerosol equipment. Assist client to establish a medication schedule to encourage taking the medications regularly and on time.

Nursing Diagnoses	Goals	Nursing Interventions
		Instruct the client to use the inhaler prior to meals.
		If the client is taking steroids, teach to rinse mouth after using the inhaler to avoid fungal infection.
		Encourage exercise for all asthmatic clients as it increases respiratory reserve and improves overall physical condition.
		Assist client to identify triggering stimuli and ways to avoid them.
		Teach client and family signs and symptoms of asthma attacks and respiratory tract infections.
		Teach client to avoid crowded areas and close contact with persons with infections.
▶ *Anxiety, moderate, related to perceived threat of dying.*	The client will verbalize a decrease in anxiety.	Provide the client with explanations for all care.
		Provide care in a calm, unhurried manner.
		Plan care to allow the client uninterrupted periods of rest.
		Allow the client to make decisions regarding cares if possible.
		Provide the client with opportunities to discuss his or her anxiety with staff, family, or significant others.

▶ Evaluation

Each goal must be evaluated to determine how it has been met by the client.

▲ ▲

▶ CHRONIC BRONCHITIS

Bronchitis is an inflammation of the bronchial tree accompanied by hypersecretion of mucous. The condition becomes chronic if an individual has an infection with a productive cough at least three months a year for two consecutive years. Constant irritation of the bronchi results in hypertrophy of the mucus secreting glands. The bronchioles fill with exudate and subsequent infections are common. Eventually the alveoli adjacent to the bronchioles become damaged and fibrosed. Environmental factors, especially cigarette smoking, play an important part in the development of chronic bronchitis. Certain individuals may have a hereditary predisposition to developing chronic bronchitis. Exposure to cold, damp air with repeated respiratory infections has been indicated as a cause of chronic bronchitis.

The client usually has a history of recurrent respiratory infections, dyspnea, cyanosis, and chronic or recurrent cough with copious amounts of sputum. Often, that sputum is purulent or green in color. Over the course of time the chest wall configuration becomes slightly distended. There are coarse crackles present throughout the lung fields. The breath sounds may be diminished or absent over the periphery of the lung fields. Elevation of pulmonary artery pressure results in an increased workload for the right ventricle and signs and symptoms of right-sided congestive heart failure occur, such as peripheral edema and fatigue. Arterial blood gases reveal an increased $PaCO_2$ and decreased PaO_2. The red blood cell count is elevated (polycythemia) with an increase in the hemoglobin and hematocrit also. The increase in the amount of red blood cells and hemoglobin is an attempt by the body to compensate for the lower oxygen levels. Chest x-ray shows hyperexpansion of the lungs. When congestive heart failure occurs, the chest x-ray also shows an enlarged heart.

▶ *Medical/Surgical Management*

▶ *Medical*

The goals of medical treatment are to decrease symptoms of irritation of the airways, decrease airway obstruction due to secretions and inflammation, prevent infection, maintain oxygenation, and increase the client's exercise tolerance. Respiratory therapy includes the use of updraft (nebulizer) and aerosol treatments with percussion and postural drainage. Humidification of inspired air helps to liquefy secretions. Supplemental oxygen is administered based upon arterial blood gas or pulse oximetry measurements. The neurological response to breathe becomes altered in some chronic bronchitis clients so that the stimulus to breathe is initiated when the blood level of oxygen falls versus when the level of carbon dioxide rises. Consequently, when the level of oxygen in the blood is relatively high in relation to the level of carbon dioxide, the client and the stimulus to breathe are depressed. When this occurs, carbon dioxide rises to a dangerous level and further depresses the CNS. When supplemental oxygen is necessary, it should be maintained at the lowest possible flow rate to maintain oxygenation and prevent depression of the client's respiratory drive. The client with chronic bronchitis and congestive heart failure is evaluated for signs of fluid overload. Daily weight and intake and output are monitored.

▶ *Pharmacological*

Bronchodilators, such as theophylline (Theo-Dur), oxtriphylline (Choledyl), terbutaline sulfate (Brethine), and ipratropium bromide (Atrovent) are given to open the airways. Inhalation or aerosol treatments with bronchodilators such as albuterol (Ventolin) or metaproterenol sulfate (Alupent) are often used in conjunction with oral medications to control symptoms. Prednisone (Meticorten), a corticosteroid, is given as short term therapy with acute exacerbations. If steroids are required on a long-term basis they may be given by inhalation to avoid some adverse systemic effects. Examples of inhalation forms of steroids are beclomethasone dipropionate (Beclovent) and triamcinolone acetonide (Azmacort). In addition to agents that open the airways, medications that liquefy respiratory secretions are administered. Acetylcysteine (Mucomyst) may be given by inhalation. Mucolytic medications such as guaifenesin (Humibid LA) may be given orally. If infection occurs, broad spectrum antibiotics are given such as cephalexin monohydrate (Keflex), cefaclor (Ceclor), erythromycin base (E-Mycin), and penicillin V potassium (Pen-Vee K).

Immunization against influenza viruses and *streptococcus pneumoniae* are recommended.

The client with chronic bronchitis, who also suffers from congestive heart failure, will receive medications to aid the function of the weakened heart. Digoxin (Lanoxin) is given to strengthen the force of the contraction of the heart muscle. Diuretics, such as furosemide (Lasix), are given to increase the urinary output. Supplemental potassium chloride (K-Dur, Kay-Ciel elixir) is administered if the client's level of potassium decreases due to the effect of the diuretic.

▶ *Diet*

The client is encouraged to eat a well-balanced diet. If the client has congestive heart failure as well as chronic bronchitis, sodium intake is restricted. Unless contraindicated fluids are encouraged.

▶ *Activity*

Activity is restricted to decrease the workload of the heart and lungs. With acute exacerbations, the client is placed on bed rest. The level of activity is then slowly increased based upon the client's ability to tolerate activity.

▶ *Rehabilitation*

Programs consisting of breathing exercises and graded exercise regimes are utilized to assist the client in achieving the maximum level of activity tolerance. The client is taught breath retaining exercises such as: coughing techniques, pursed lip breathing, and diaphragmatic or abdominal breathing. Graded exercise regimens are similar to those used for cardiac rehabilitation. The client is monitored from a respiratory standpoint while exercising. The goal is to increase the client's capacity for all activities of daily living.

▶ *Nursing Process*

Assessment

Subjective Data Obtain a thorough past medical history. Inquire about the onset, duration, and severity of symptoms. The client may describe fatigue and difficulty breathing.

Objective Data Assess for changes in the level of consciousness or mental status. Note the client's color, respiratory rate, and effort. Observe the position the client assumes to aid respiratory effort. Note the use of accessory muscles. Review arterial blood gases or pulse oximetry. Auscultate the lung fields for crackles and diminished breath sounds. Note the color, amount, viscosity, and odor of sputum. Specimens are obtained for culture and sensitivity if indicated. Assess vital signs frequently. The pulse may be elevated and irregular. Blood pressure may be elevated or decreased.

An elevated temperature indicates the possibility of infection. Assess the client for peripheral edema, neck vein distention, and rapid weight gain.

▼ ▼

Possible nursing diagnoses for a client with chronic bronchitis may include:

Nursing Diagnoses	Goals	Nursing Interventions
▶ Airway clearance, ineffective, related to thicker and increased amounts of respiratory secretions.	The client will have color, respiratory rate, and arterial blood gases within normal limits.	Assess level of consciousness, mental status, vital signs, respiratory effort, and color frequently.
		Auscultate the breath sounds frequently.
		Assess sputum for its amount, viscosity, color, and odor.
		Assist the client in assuming the position that aids respiratory effort most, usually an upright position.
		Administer oxygen and respiratory treatments as ordered and assess their effectiveness.
		Evaluate the results of diagnostic and laboratory tests and notify the physician of abnormalities.
		Obtain sputum specimens as ordered.
		Alternate care with periods of uninterrupted rest.
		Administer medications as ordered.
		Provide the client with a well-balanced diet.
		Unless otherwise contraindicated, encourage fluids.
		Assess the client for signs and symptoms of congestive heart failure, i.e., fine crackles heard on auscultation, peripheral edema, weight gain, and fatigue.
		Report any signs and symptoms of congestive heart failure to the physician.
▶ Activity intolerance related to hypoxia.	The client will complete activity without complaints of shortness of breath, dyspnea, or fatigue.	Plan care to allow the client periods of rest to avoid fatigue.
		Avoid activity immediately before and after meals.
		Assist the client in assuming the position in which breathing is easiest.
		Assist the client with activities of daily living if needed.
▶ Knowledge deficit, related to chronic bronchitis, its treatment and prevention.	The client will verbalize signs and symptoms to report to the physician, safety precautions to take with medication and equipment, medication and respiratory treatment regimen, and types of (breathing) techniques to assist breathing.	Teach client to avoid respiratory infections, maintain adequate nutrition, increase fluid intake, and maintain adequate rest.
		Instruct the client regarding the purpose, expected effects, and side effects of medications. ▶

(continued)

Nursing Diagnoses	*Goals*	*Nursing Interventions*
		Teach the client to administer respiratory treatments and medications prior to eating, to aid in breathing.
		If the client is taking steroids, instruct to rinse his mouth following administration of inhalers.
		Teach the client to self-administer oxygen.
		Provide information regarding the use of equipment and safety measures for equipment.
		Refer the client to an established respiratory rehabilitation program if available.
		If such a program is not available, instruct the client in breathing techniques.
		Encourage regular exercise within the client's limits.
		Encourage the client to obtain immunization against influenza viruses and *Streptococcus pneumoniae*.

▶ Evaluation

Each goal must be evaluated to determine how it has been met by the client.

▲ ▲

▶ EMPHYSEMA

Emphysema is a complex and destructive lung disease. The airways become fibrotic and lose their elasticity resulting in a narrower lumen. Airflow is impeded as it leaves the lungs (i.e., expiration). The alveoli distal to these airways are then overdistended with trapped air (refer back to Figure 19-8). Rupture of the alveoli wall may occur. The alveolar capillary membrane is destroyed with a loss of available area for gas exchange to occur. Emphysema is the leading cause of respiratory death in the United States. Cigarette smoking is the most common cause of emphysema. Other factors, such as air pollution and exposure to occupational respiratory irritants have been identified as contributing to the development of emphysema. Deficiency in alpha-1-antitrypsin is a familial disorder that leads to the development of emphysema. Alpha-1-antitrypsin is an enzyme that inhibits the activity of the enzyme elactase, which breaks down lung tissue.

Emphysema develops slowly over a period of years. The client or a family member notes increasing dyspnea with activity. Dyspnea at rest eventually occurs. The dyspnea corresponds to the degree of hypoxia, which is usually mild at rest, but becomes more severe with activity. In advanced stages of the disease, hypoxia is evident even at rest. Sputum produced is scant and mucoid in nature, unless an infection is present. When infection is present, a cough with production of purulent sputum occurs. The client's complexion appears ruddy, or reddish in color. The chest becomes barrel-shaped as the chest cage enlarges to accommodate distended lung tissues. The respiratory rate is elevated. The expiratory phase of respiration becomes increasingly difficult. Accessory muscles are used to aid respiratory effort. Bronchial breath sounds are heard in the periphery of the lungs due to destruction of the alveoli. As the disease progresses, the breath sounds become diminished and eventually absent over the periphery of the lungs. Arterial blood gases reveal varying degrees of hypoxia depending on the severity of the disease. Hypercapnia, or retention of carbon dioxide, is not as likely as with chronic bronchitis. The extra effort required to breathe increases the metabolic needs resulting in weight loss. Chest x-ray reveals hyperinflated lung tissue and a flattened diaphragm, which has been displaced by distended lung tissues. Pulmonary function studies reveal a decrease in expiratory volume. Polycythemia and elevation of the hemoglobin and hematocrit occur in response to prolonged hypoxia.

▶ Medical/Surgical Management

▶ Medical

The goals of treatment are to prevent further damage to the lung tissues, maintain adequate oxygenation, prevent infection, and improve the client's activity tolerance. The client who smokes should stop, or, at least, decrease the number of cigarettes smoked daily. Supplemental oxygen is given to maintain oxygenation. The client with advanced emphysema and more severe, chronic hypoxia may be maintained at PaO_2 of 55 to 59 mmHg and/or oxygen saturation of 90 percent or greater. As in chronic bronchitis, the client with emphysema is given supplemental oxygen at the lowest possible flow rate to avoid respiratory and CNS depression.

▶ Pharmacological

The client with emphysema receives many of the same medications used to treat chronic bronchitis. To open airways that have become fibrotic, theophylline and similar preparations are used. Steroids may be required with exacerbations. The emphysemic client usually does not need mucolytic agents, unless infection occurs. Antibiotics are used to treat and prevent respiratory tract infections. The client should receive immunizations against influenza and *Streptococcus pneumoniae*. The client who smokes may use nicotine polacrilex gum (Nicorette [gum]) or nicotine transdermal system (Nicoderm) to aid in smoking cessation.

▶ Diet

The client with emphysema requires a diet high in carbohydrates to supply the energy necessary for breathing. If a negative nitrogen balance exists due to the client's using muscle tissue to provide energy, a diet high in protein is ordered. Dietary supplements, such as Ensure, may be needed to supply the necessary calories and nutrients. Unless contraindicated, fluids are encouraged.

▶ Activity

The client is placed on bed rest. The level of activity is increased based upon the client's oxygenation. Oxygen saturation is evaluated periodically as the activity level is increased to determine the effect of activity on oxygenation.

▶ Rehabilitation

The client with emphysema will benefit from a respiratory rehabilitation program. The client is taught breathing exercises similar to those taught to the client with chronic bronchitis. A graded exercise program is also used for the client with emphysema. Group programs that aid in smoking cessation are useful for the client who smokes.

▶ Nursing Process

Assessment

Subjective Data Included in the history is information regarding when dyspnea occurs, those factors that exacerbate dyspnea, and those factors that relieve dyspnea.

Objective Data If cough is present, the client is assessed for other indications of infection such as elevated white blood cell count and fever. The cough is evaluated as to onset, duration, and severity. Any sputum produced is assessed for color, amount, viscosity, and odor. Assess vital signs frequently. An elevated pulse may indicate hypoxia and/or infection. Auscultate the lungs for the presence of adventitious, diminished, or absent breath sounds. Observe the position the client assumes to aid respiratory effort. Note the client's color, respiratory rate, effort, and use of accessory muscles to aid breathing. Evaluate the client's nutritional status by weighing the client and measuring nutrient and calorie intake. Review the results of laboratory and diagnostic tests.

▼ ▼

Possible nursing diagnoses for a client with emphysema may include:

Nursing Diagnoses	Goals	Nursing Interventions
▶ *Gas exchange, ineffective, related to destruction of the alveoli.*	The client will have a respiratory rate, color, and blood gases within normal limits.	Assess the client's level of consciousness and mental status.
		Frequently evaluate the client's respiratory rate, effort, and color.
		Evaluate oxygenation via arterial blood gases and/or pulse oximetry.
		Assess the effect of activity on oxygenation, particularly when activity is being increased.
		Provide supplemental oxygen as ordered.
		Auscultate the lungs and report abnormalities to the physician.
		Assess the client's vital signs: heart rate and temperature elevations may indicate infection. An elevated pulse can also indicate hypoxia.
		Review the results of diagnostic and laboratory tests and report abnormalities.
		Assist the client in assuming the position that most aids breathing.
		Administer medications and respiratory treatments as ordered.
▶ *Activity intolerance, related to hypoxia.*	The client will complete activity without complaints of fatigue or dyspnea.	Assist the client with activities of daily living and hygiene needs.
		Plan care and treatments to allow the client uninterrupted periods of rest.
		As activity progresses, assess the effects of activity on oxygenation.
		Allow the client to rest prior to and after meals.
		Assist the client in assuming the position that offers the most comfort and aids respiratory effort.
		Instruct the client in breathing techniques, such as pursed-lip breathing.
▶ *Knowledge deficit, related to emphysema and its treatment.*	The client will verbalize signs and symptoms to report to the physician, safety precautions to take with medication and equipment use, medication and respiratory treatment regime, and (breathing) techniques to aid respiration.	Teach client and family signs and symptoms to report to the physician, including the signs and symptoms of infection.
		Instruct in the use of inhalers and aerosol treatments.
		Provide the client with information about the purposes, effects, side effects, and untoward effects of medications.
		Review measures to avoid infection, such as immunization, with the client and family.
		Encourage the client to participate in a smoking cessation program, if available.
		Present information about available respiratory rehabilitation programs.

Nursing Diagnoses	Goals	Nursing Interventions
▶ Nutrition, altered, less than body requirements, related to increased energy requirements to maintain respiration.	The client will achieve or maintain a weight within normal limits for height.	Assess the client's weight and evaluate in relation to client's height.
		Evaluate the client's diet for nutritional adequacy.
		Review the client's food likes and dislikes.
		Provide a well-balanced diet based upon the client's likes and dislikes.
		Provide nutritional supplements as ordered.
		Avoid activities prior to meals that might reduce appetite, i.e., enemas, and so on.
		Administer medications and respiratory treatments prior to meals to aid in breathing.

▶ Evaluation

Each goal must be evaluated to determine how it has been met by the client.

▲ ▲

▶ BRONCHIECTASIS

Bronchiectasis is a chronic dilation of the bronchi. The main causes of this disorder are infection with pulmonary tuberculosis, chronic upper respiratory tract infections, and complications of other respiratory disorders of childhood, particularly cystic fibrosis. The bronchi become distended and eventually lose their elastic recoil properties. The mucociliary blanket's function is impaired and secretions become thicker. Secretions accumulate in the bronchi offering a media for infection. As with chronic bronchitis and emphysema, airflow is hindered reducing gas exchange.

The client with bronchiectasis complains of a frequent or chronic productive cough. Other complaints include: dyspnea, weight loss, and fatigue. Sputum is thick. When infection is present, the sputum is purulent. Crackles, which clear with coughing, are heard scattered throughout the lungs fields. Upon the client's arising in the morning, the crackles are more prominent. Accessory muscles are used to aid respiration. Over a period of time, right-sided congestive heart failure develops and symptoms such as peripheral edema occur. Arterial blood gases reveal elevated $PaCO_2$, decreased PaO_2, and respiratory acidosis. Sputum analysis will reveal if infection is present, the causative organism, and resistance or sensitivity to specific antibiotics. Polycythemia and elevation of the hemoglobin and hematocrit levels are demonstrated in the complete blood count. Chest x-ray shows slight hyperinflation of lung tissue and, in the presence of congestive heart failure, cardiomegaly. The respiratory flow rate decreases and lung volume increases as demonstrated by pulmonary function studies. Table 19-5 compares chronic bronchitis, emphysema, and bronchiectasis.

▶ Medical/Surgical Management

▶ Medical

Medical treatment is aimed at removing respiratory secretions, eliminating and preventing infection, and maintaining adequate oxygenation. Percussion and postural drainage are used to aid in removing secretions. Aerosol and updraft respiratory treatments may be ordered prior to percussion and drainage. If the client is unable to remove secretions, bronchial suctioning is performed. The physician may opt to do a bronchoscopy for the removal of especially tenacious and copious secretions. Arterial blood gases and/or pulse oximetry are evaluated to assess the need for supplemental oxygen. Daily weight and I&O are done to detect signs of congestive heart failure. Pulmonary function studies are performed to evaluate the severity of lung damage. Genetic studies and genetic counseling are indicated for the family and client with cystic fibrosis.

▶ Pharmacological

Acetylcysteine (Mucomyst) and other mucolytic agents are given to promote liquefaction of respiratory secretions. Antibiotics are ordered to treat and prevent

Table 19-5

SIGNS AND SYMPTOMS OF CHRONIC BRONCHITIS, EMPHYSEMA, AND BRONCHIECTASIS			
	Chronic Bronchitis	**Emphysema**	**Bronchiectasis**
History	recurrent respiratory infections, chronic cough	insidious onset, dyspnea on exertion to dyspnea at rest	cystic fibrosis, recurrent respiratory infections
Cough	chronic or recurrent productive cough	present with infections	frequent or chronic productive cough
Sputum	frequent copious, purulent, green	scanty mucoid unless infection present	thick, tenacious secretions, sometimes purulent
Weight	slight or no weight loss	weight loss common	weight loss or failure to gain is common
Appearance	cyanosis common, "blue bloater"	ruddy complexion, "pink puffer"	clubbing of fingernails
Chest Configuration	slight overdistention	overdistention prominent, "barrel chest"	slight overdistention
Breath Sounds	coarse crackles	bronchial breath sounds in peripheral lung fields, diminished or absent in late disease	crackles
Edema	peripheral edema common, especially ankles	infrequent	peripheral edema in late disease
Right-sided CHF, (Cor Pulmonale)	frequent complication	infrequent	frequent complication late in disease
CO Retention, (Hypercapnea)	common	unlikely	common in late disease
Hypoxemia	maybe severe	usually mild especially at rest	maybe severe in late disease and with infection
Dyspnea	progressive dyspnea	dyspnea on exertion to dyspnea at rest usually presenting symptom	dyspnea with respiratory infection and late disease
Accessory Muscles Used for Respiration	yes	yes	yes
Polycythemia	late in disease	yes	yes in late disease
Respiratory Failure	common	may occur	common

infection. The client is immunized against influenza and *Streptococcus pneumoniae* by the pneumococcal vaccine (Pneumovax 23). Bronchodilators are indicated to open the fibrotic airways. Inflammation is treated with steroids such as prednisone (Meticorten), orally, and/or beclomethasone dipropionate (Beclovent) via inhalation. The client with cystic fibrosis is required to take pancreatic enzymes, pancrelipase (Pancrease capsules, Cotazym capsules) to replace those absent with this disorder. If congestive heart failure occurs, the client is treated with digoxin (Lanoxin), diuretics furosemide (Lasix), and potassium supplements as indicated.

▶ Diet

The diet should be high in carbohydrates and calories to provide energy for breathing. Protein is supple-

mented if needed. Dietary supplements, such as Ensure, may be required. Fluids are encouraged, unless otherwise contraindicated. Sodium is restricted in the diet of the client with congestive heart failure. The diet for the client with cystic fibrosis is restricted in fats.

▶ Activity

During acute exacerbations or with serious infection, activity is limited. The client is placed on bedrest. Progressive increase in activity is made depending upon the client's tolerance.

▶ Rehabilitation

Respiratory rehabilitation and graded exercise programs are useful in the treatment of bronchiectasis.

Regular exercise is encouraged, particularly for the pediatric client with cystic fibrosis.

▶ Nursing Process

Assessment

Subjective Data Information to be ascertained in the history is: history of recent and past respiratory tract infections, history of or exposure to tuberculosis or other respiratory infections, and family or client history of cystic fibrosis. The onset, duration, and severity of symptoms, such as dyspnea and cough, are noted.

Objective Data The client may display a change in the level of consciousness. Dyspnea, tachypnea, and cyanosis may be present. To aid respiratory effort the client may assume the orthopneic position and use accessory muscles. Heart rate may be elevated in response to hypoxia and/or infection. An elevated temperature and purulent sputum indicate infection. Below normal weight and muscle wasting are seen in the client with chronic disease. Secretions within the airways creates crackles on auscultation. Evaluate the results of diagnostic and laboratory data. Note signs and symptoms of congestive heart failure, i.e., peripheral edema, weight gain.

▼ ▼

Possible nursing diagnoses for a client with bronchiectasis may include:

Nursing Diagnoses	Goals	Nursing Interventions
▶ Airway clearance, ineffective, related to increased and viscous respiratory tract secretions.	The client will have clear breath sounds and respiratory rate, color, and arterial blood gases within normal limits.	Observe the client's level of consciousness, color, respiratory effort, use of accessory muscles, and the position the client assumes for ease of respiration. Assist the client in assuming the position that aids respiratory effort most. Assess vital signs. Auscultate the lung fields. Alternate care with periods of rest. Evaluate sputum for amount, color, viscosity, and odor. Administer medications and respiratory treatments as ordered. Obtain arterial blood gases or pulse oximetry per order. Supply supplemental oxygen as indicated. Provide the client with the prescribed diet, including supplements. Unless contraindicated, encourage fluids to aid in liquefying secretions.
▶ Knowledge deficit, related to bronchiectasis, the underlying cause and treatment.	The client will verbalize the basic pathophysiology of bronchiectasis; the underlying cause of her/his bronchiectasis; medication and respiratory treatment schedules; the purpose, actions, side effects and adverse effect of medications, signs and symptoms to report to the physician, use of respiratory equipment, safety precautions to take with medications and equipment, and (breathing) techniques to aid breathing.	Provide information about the pathophysiology of bronchiectasis and the underlying cause, if identified. Discuss the course and purpose of treatment. Present information about respiratory treatments and the use of respiratory equipment. Instruct client how to perform percussion and postural drainage.

Nursing Diagnoses	*Goals*	*Nursing Interventions*
		Encourage prevention and early detection and treatment of respiratory infections.
		Review signs and symptoms of respiratory infection.
		Teach which information to report to the physician.
		Provide information on medications, including the purpose, action, side effects.
▶ *Nutrition, altered, less than body requirements, related to increased energy requirements to maintain respiration.*	The client will achieve or maintain a weight within the ideal for height.	Provide an environment conducive to eating.
		Avoid treatments and therapies that fatigue the client or are painful prior to meals.
		Assess the client's likes and dislikes.
		Provide the prescribed diet based upon the client's likes and dislikes.
		Administer medications and respiratory therapies that aid breathing prior to meals.
		Assess the client's weight and compare to the ideal weight for the client's height.
		Assess the client's nutritional intake and evaluate for adequacy.
		Provide dietary supplements as ordered.

▶ Evaluation

Each goal must be evaluated to determine how it has been met by the client.

▲ ▲

▶ CHEST TRAUMA

▶ PNEUMOTHORAX/ HEMOTHORAX

Normally, there is no space between the visceral and parietal pleura. They are held together by surface tension. Thus, the pleural space is a closed compartment with a pressure that is negative when compared to that within the lungs or to the atmosphere. When the integrity of the pleura is interrupted, air moves from the atmosphere or from the lungs between the pleura creating a space. This condition is known as a pneumothorax (refer back to Figure 19-8). The lung tissue underlying the pneumothorax is compressed and thus unable to expand fully. If the pneumothorax is large enough, the underlying lung tissue collapses as a result of this compression. Pneumothorax may occur following blunt chest trauma, as in a motor vehicle accident, penetrating chest trauma, such as knife or gunshot wounds, or surgery involving the thoracic cavity.

A pneumothorax may be referred to as open,

closed, spontaneous, or tension. A closed pneumothorax occurs when there is no communication between the pleura and the external environment. One example of a closed pneumothorax would be that associated with blunt trauma to the chest. In this instance, a broken rib may pierce the pleura and lung allowing air to enter between the pleura. Conversely, an open pneumothorax exists when there is direct communication between the external environment and the pleural space. Spontaneous pneumothorax is a condition in which pneumothorax occurs without an obvious underlying cause. Tension pneumothorax refers to a life-threatening condition in which air enters the pleural space with inspiration, but is unable to exit with expiration. The air continues to accumulate in the pleural space, compressing the underlying structures. If left untreated a tension pneumothorax will collapse the lung and encroach upon the structures on the opposite side. All of the structures within the mediastinum, the heart, aorta, and vena cava, are affected. Without intervention tension pneumothorax results in cardiopulmonary arrest. Tension pneumothorax is often associated with mechanical ventilation. The pressure exerted by the ventilator on compromised lung tissue interrupts the integrity of the pleura. Air continues to enter the pleural space, but is unable to exit, as mechanical ventilation continues. In the case of pneumothorax associated with trauma or surgery, bleeding of adjacent vessels into the pleural cavity often results. Blood within the pleural space is referred to as a hemothorax. When accompanied by air the condition is called a hemopneumothorax.

The severity of injury and the amount of lung tissue affected determine the signs and symptoms the client exhibits. Clients with a small pneumothorax may be asymptomatic or complain of minor dyspnea. Those with a significant pneumothorax may exhibit signs of severe respiratory distress. Dyspnea, tachypnea, orthopnea, and cyanosis may be present. Oxygenation is impaired. Pleuritic pain is common. Breath sounds are absent in the area of the pneumothorax. In the case of tension pneumothorax, the structures of the mediastinum will shift to the unaffected side as more and more air accumulates in the pleural space. The client with an accompanying hemothorax will evidence signs and symptoms of shock associated with blood loss.

▶ Medical/Surgical Management

▶ Medical

In order for the affected lung to reexpand, the air and/or blood must be removed from the pleural space. When the blood loss associated with a hemothorax is significant, fluid and blood replacement may be necessary.

▶ Surgical

A thoracotomy tube, or chest tube, is inserted by the physician into the pleural space to drain air and fluid and allow the lung to reexpand. To drain fluid and air, the tube is placed in the midaxillary line at approximately the fifth intercostal space. To remove air, the tube is placed in the anterior chest at the midclavicular line, fourth intercostal space. The thoracotomy tube is connected to an underwater seal drainage device. Numerous commercial devices are available for this purpose (refer back to Figure 19-10). The underwater seal is necessary to prevent the negative pressure within the pleural space from pulling more air in through the chest tube itself. A drainage chamber is included to allow for removal of any fluid or blood within the pleural space. In addition, most devices also include a chamber to which suction may be applied to assist in the removal of air and fluid from the pleural space. Following insertion of the chest tube, a chest x-ray will be done to assure its proper placement and to

assess reexpansion of the lungs. The underlying cause of the hemopneumothorax will then need to be treated.

Spontaneous pneumothorax that recurs may require a pleural cortication to prevent further episodes. This surgical procedure involves roughing the adjacent surfaces of the visceral and parietal pleura in the hopes that scar tissue formed increases adhesion between the two surfaces. To render emergency treatment for a tension pneumothorax that is severely compromising the function of the heart and lungs, a large bore needle is placed into the anterior chest at the fourth intercostal space. Following this, a thoracotomy tube will be inserted until the lung(s) are fully reexpanded and to prevent a recurrence.

▶ Pharmacological

To control pleuritic pain narcotic analgesics, such as morphine sulfate or meperidine (Demerol), are prescribed. Analgesia may be given orally or parenterally as indicated by the severity of the pain. Prior to insertion of a thoracotomy tube, intravenous narcotics may be given prophylactically. Tissues adjacent to the area of pneumothorax are injected with local anesthetics prior to inserting a thoracotomy tube.

▶ Activity

The presence of a pneumothorax or a thoracotomy tube does not in itself call for restricting the client's activity. If hypoxia results from compromised breathing, activity restrictions are necessary. The presence of other injuries or conditions may also result in restricting activity. Once the client is adequately oxygenated and stable, activity is encouraged to promote expansion of the lungs.

▶ Diet

A well-balanced diet with sufficient amounts of protein for healing to occur is encouraged. The client with other injuries and conditions may require total parenteral nutrition or enteral feedings.

▶ Nursing Process

Assessment

Subjective Data Gather information about the source of the pneumothorax. Ask the client about previous pneumothoraces, recent chest injury, falls, or severe coughing. The client often describes being very anxious.

Objective Data Assess the client's level of consciousness and mental status. Observe the client's chest wall movement, color, and respiratory effort. Chest wall movement is decreased on the affected side. When a large pneumothorax is present, the trachea shifts toward the unaffected side. Dyspnea and cyanosis may occur. The cough is forceful and nonproductive. Respiratory rate and heart rate are elevated. Blood pressure may be elevated due to the presence of pain and anxiety or the blood pressure may be hypotensive due to blood loss. The breath sounds are diminished or absent over the affected areas. Assess the location, duration, and severity of pain. Once inserted, chest tubes are assessed for their function, patency, and amount and character of drainage.

▼ ▼

Possible nursing diagnoses for a client with pneumothorax may include:

Nursing Diagnoses	Goals	Nursing Interventions
▶ *Breathing pattern, ineffective, related to decreased lung expansion.*	The client will have a respiratory rate and color within normal limits and clear breath sounds in affected area.	Monitor the amount and character of drainage from the chest tube.
		Observe fluctuations in the water seal chamber, called tidaling, which indicates the tube has been placed in the pleural space.
		Investigate the absence of tidaling as it can indicate the lung may be fully reexpanded or that the tube itself may be occluded or kinked.
		Observe for the presence of bubbling in the water seal chamber which indicates an air leak.
		Assess the connections and chest tube to determine the presence of leaks.
		If none are present, notify the physician as to the possibility of an air leak within the client's lungs.
▶ *Pain, acute, related to pleural space irritation.*	The client will verbalize a decrease in pain on a 1 to 10 scale.	Assist the client in assuming the position that aids respiration the most. The majority of clients find this is the orthopneic position.
		Assess vital signs and respiratory status.
		Unless otherwise contraindicated, encourage fluids.
		Monitor intake and output to evaluate fluid balance.
		Include any drainage from the chest tube in the client's output.
		Encourage the client to cough and deep breathe to prevent further respiratory complications.
		Administer pain medications as ordered.
		Be aware that respiratory depression is possible with narcotic medications.
		Provide diversional activities.

▶ *Evaluation*

Each goal must be evaluated to determine how it has been met by the client.

▲ ▲

▶ NEOPLASMS OF THE RESPIRATORY TRACT

▶ BENIGN NEOPLASMS

A benign tumor or cyst in the lung shows sharply defined edges on an X-ray. Peripheral tumors usually have no symptoms. Bronchial tumors may cause obstruction, infection, or atelectasis.

▶ LUNG CANCER

Malignant tumors (carcinomas) of the lung may originate within the lung itself or may result from metastasis from other tumor sites (i.e., breast, colon, or kidney). The incidence of lung tumors is on the rise (Rosdahl, 1995). Men, especially those over 40 years of age, are more likely to suffer from lung cancer. However, the incidence of lung cancer among women is rising more rapidly than that for men (Harkness & Dincher, 1996). Tobacco smoking is one of the most common causal factors for lung cancer (Rosdahl, 1995). Air pollution and exposure to carcinogens, such as asbestos, are also factors that increase a person's risk for developing lung cancer.

The majority of lung cancers may be classified into three cell types. Squamous cell carcinomas, the most common form of lung cancer, and adenocarcinomas arise from the epithelial cells of the lung. Oat cell, undifferentiated small cell, carcinoma has the poorest prognosis and is the least common. Prognosis for lung cancer is dependent upon the size of the tumor when diagnosed and the specific cell type.

Most lung cancers are relatively silent, meaning that symptoms develop late in the course of the disease. Peripheral lesions generally have few symptoms. Initially, the client may complain of a chronic cough or wheezing. Central lesions cause obstruction and erosion of the bronchi. As the tumor grows and occludes the air passages, the client may experience shortness of breath, dyspnea, and blood-tinged sputum. Pain is a relatively late occurring symptom, indicating the tumor has grown to significant size to put pressure on adjacent nerves and other structures. While some tumors may be seen on chest x-ray, many are not detected. CAT and MRI scans are more reliable studies when assessing soft tissue structures. To confirm diagnosis, the physician will order cytology studies on specimens collected via bronchoscopy, needle biopsy, or mediastinoscopy. Lung scans are occasionally useful in diagnosis. Prior to initiating treatment, the client is evaluated for metastatic disease using bone and total body scans.

▶ Medical/Surgical Management

▶ Medical

Treatment of lung cancer depends on the type and stage of the lung cancer. Most clients are diagnosed too late for a surgical cure.

▶ Surgical

Surgical intervention involves the removal of the tumor and adjacent lung tissue. Pneumonectomy is the removal of an entire lung. A lobectomy is the removal of a lobe of a lung. Segmental resection is the removal of a segment of a lung. The client will have a thoracotomy tube on the operative side. Radiation and chemotherapy are often used in conjunction with surgery. The incidence of lung tumor recurrence is high.

▶ Pharmacological

The specific type of chemotherapy used is dependent upon the cell type and the extent of tumor growth. Oat cell carcinoma is treated with chemotherapy alone or in combination with radiation.

▶ Prevention

The number one means of preventing lung cancer is to avoid smoking or to cease smoking. People should also avoid the second-hand smoke of others. Many efforts to decrease the number of individuals smoking are presently being encouraged throughout the United States. Unfortunately, the rate of teen smokers remains relatively high. Also, the rate of tobacco use in some foreign countries has risen dramatically as tobacco producers attempt to make up for lost profits in the United States. Other means to avoid developing lung cancer include avoiding exposure to high concentrations of pollutants, such as carbon monoxide, supporting efforts to decrease air pollution on the whole, and protecting oneself in the workplace/school from exposure to carcinogens, such as asbestos.

▶ Nursing Process

Assessment

Subjective data The client's history is reviewed for history of smoking, exposure to carcinogens, and other causative factors. Gather information regarding the onset, duration, and severity of symptoms. The client may report hoarseness, chronic cough, pain, and shortness of breath. Pain is assessed as to its location, character, duration, and severity.

Objective Data The color, amount, consistency, and odor of sputum are noted. Prior to surgery, the nurse may hear wheezing or decreased breath sounds on the affected side. Following surgery, breath sounds are diminished to absent on the affected side. The amount and color of drainage from the thoracotomy tube are monitored. The wound is assessed for hem-

orrhage and infection. Respiratory rate and effort may be increased. Pulse rate may be increased due to a variety of factors including decreased oxygenation, hemorrhage, and infection. Hypotension occurs with significant blood loss. A high blood pressure may indicate pain, anxiety, or other underlying pathology such as essential hypertension.

▼ ▼

Possible nursing diagnoses for a client with lung cancer may include:

Nursing Diagnoses	Goals	Nursing Interventions
▶ Breathing pattern, ineffective, related to disease process.	The client will have a respiratory rate and color within normal limits.	Monitor the client's level of consciousness, vital signs, color, and respiratory effort frequently.
		Auscultate the breath sounds.
		Stagger activities with periods of rest to prevent overtaxing the client's reserves.
		Assess the wound for evidence of hemorrhage and infection.
		Evaluate the chest tube for tidaling, bubbling, and patency.
		Note character of chest tube drainage.
		Include drainage from the chest tube in the client's output.
		Assist the client in assuming the position that maximizes respiratory effort most.
		Position the client in semi-Fowler's position or lying on the affected side.
		Assess oxygenation and provide supplemental oxygen as indicated.
		Monitor lab reports for blood gas levels.
▶ Pain, related to lung cancer.	The client will state pain is decreased on a scale of 1 to 10.	Administer pain medication as ordered.
		Monitor for respiratory depression.
		Provide for diversional activities.
		Assist the client in assuming a position of comfort.
▶ Grieving, anticipatory, related to prognosis and perceived separation from significant others.	The client will be able to express to significant others and/or staff feelings related to diagnosis and prognosis.	Aid the client in expressing feelings of grief related to the diagnosis.
		Hope should not be eliminated, but false hope should not be encouraged.
		Assist family members and significant others in coping with their feelings.
		Allow the client and family time to express their feelings.

▶ *Evaluation*

Each goal must be evaluated to determine how it has been met by the client.

▲ ▲

▶ CANCER OF THE LARYNX

Cancer of the larynx is more common among men than women (Harkness & Dincher, 1996). Risk factors for cancer of the larynx include smoking, chronic alcohol abuse, chronic laryngitis, and overuse of the voice.

Cancer of the larynx is relatively asymptomatic. The client may experience hoarseness or difficulty speaking above a whisper. If this persists for more than two weeks, medical care should be sought. Difficulty swallowing is sometimes present. Larynx pain radiating to the ear or feeling a lump in the throat are often signs of metastasis.

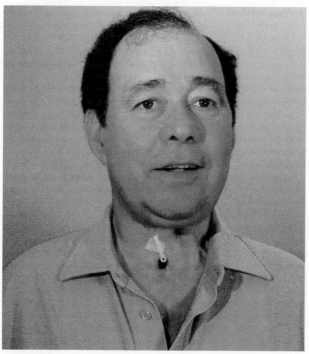

FIGURE 19-13 Laryngeal stoma for a permanent tracheostomy.

▶ Medical/Surgical Management

Treatment is determined by the extent of tumor growth.

▶ Surgical

Surgical removal of the larynx, a laryngectomy, is used to treat cancer of the larynx. If the cancer has spread to surrounding tissues, a simple or radical neck dissection may be required. Radiation may be used as an adjunct to surgery or as primary treatment if the tumor is detected in the early stages. Following surgery, a permanent tracheostomy is necessary to allow air to enter the respiratory tract (see Figure 19-13). A small incision is made into the trachea below the Adam's apple and a plastic tube is inserted.

▶ Nursing Process

Assessment

Subjective Data Assessment of the client with cancer of the larynx includes taking a history as to the onset, duration, and severity of symptoms such as hoarseness or laryngitis and alcohol and tobacco use. The client may describe ear pain, difficulty breathing and swallowing.

Objective Data The client's respiratory status is evaluated for other respiratory problems that may accompany cancer of the larynx, such as COPD. Examine sputum for the presence of blood.

▼ ▼

Possible nursing diagnoses for a client with cancer of the larynx may include:

Nursing Diagnoses	Goals	Nursing Interventions
▶ *Communication, impaired verbal, related to removal of the larynx.*	The client will be able to communicate needs.	Before surgery, establish a means to communicate to be used afterwards. If available, a manual or computer word/picture board works well.
		Keep call light by client's bed.
		Avoid mouthing communications as it is frustrating to the client and is time consuming.
		Ask questions that only require a yes or no answer.
		Refer the client to the local support group (Lost Chord Club) or the American Cancer Society.
		Talk to the client and explain all procedures.
▶ *Airway clearance, ineffective, related to tracheostomy tube.*	The client will have respiratory rate and color within normal and clear breath sounds to auscultation.	Suction frequently following surgery to remove static secretions.
		Provide routine tracheostomy care.
		Provide small, frequent feedings of liquid or pureed food to prevent choking.
		Assist client to turn, cough, and deep breathe two to four times an hour.
		Teach client stoma protection.
		Auscultate lung sounds.
		Assess respirations two to four times an hour if secretions are copious.
		Keep head of the bed elevated.
		Provide extra humidity.
▶ *Knowledge deficit related to tracheostomy care.*	The client will verbalize precautions and safety measures for a tracheostomy; how to use equipment, how to suction the respiratory tract, how to change a tracheostomy tube, and actions to take in an emergency.	Teach the client and family how to suction the respiratory tract, care for the tracheostomy, and use respiratory equipment.
		Instruct the client and family what to do in case of an emergency, such as plugging of the tracheostomy tube with secretions.
		Advise client not to swim and to avoid aspirating water when showering or bathing.
		Suggest that the client avoid extremely cold temperatures. If the tracheostomy site is covered for warming or cosmetics purposes, the covering must be of a porous material without frayed or loose threads.
▶ *Grieving, anticipatory, related to diagnosis and potential outcome.*	The client will express feelings related to diagnosis and related losses to significant others and/or staff.	Provide time for the client to discuss grieving.
		Allow the client time to communicate needs.
		Planning before surgery, a means of communication does much to support and aid the client.
		Provide the client and family with time alone.
		Refer the client and family to available community and support groups.

▶ Evaluation

Each goal must be evaluated to determine how it has been met by the client.

▲ ▲

▶ DISORDERS OF THE NOSE

▶ EPISTAXIS

Epistaxis is hemorrhage of the nares or nostrils. It may be either unilateral, which is most common, or bilateral. Epistaxis may be of a primary origin due to drying of the nasal mucosa, local irritation, or trauma. Or, the hemorrhaging may be secondary to uncontrolled hypertension or coagulopathies (i.e., thrombocytopenia, anticoagulant therapy). The diffuse vascularity and proximity of blood vessels to the surface of the nasal mucosa make the nares a susceptible avenue for hemorrhage. Blood loss can be minimal to severe. With significant blood loss hypovolemic shock occurs.

▶ Medical/Surgical Management

▶ Medical

The client with epistaxis usually arrives at an urgent care facility or emergency room following unsuccessful attempts to stop the bleeding. Signs of airway obstruction or aspiration will require immediate attention. The goals of treatment are to stop bleeding, identify the cause, and prevent recurrence. Nosebleeds are usually responsive to compression of the nares. Firm pressure should be maintained for five minutes. If bleeding persists, the client is instructed to blow the nose and clear the nasal passages. Pressure is then resumed for a full ten minutes. Epistaxis that continues following these measures will require more aggressive treatment. Bleeding sites that cannot be visualized require packing. Sterile nasal packing is inserted following application of a local anesthetic. In severe cases, a nasostat is inserted. This device resembles a Foley catheter and provides direct compression to the site of bleeding via the balloon. As this procedure is painful, local anesthesia is used prior to placing the nasostat. Clients with severe nose bleeds may require

fluid and blood replacement to avoid hypovolemic shock. Persistent or recurrent epistaxis may require surgical ligation of the artery supplying the area.

▶ Pharmacological

Sites of bleeding that can be visualized are cauterized by the physician. Silver nitrate sticks are used for cauterization. Hemostasis may also be accomplished by packing the affected nostril with epinephrine 1:1000 on cotton packing.

▶ Nursing Process

Assessment

Subjective Data The client needs to be questioned about the onset, precipitating events, duration, and frequency of epistaxis. Inquire about associated symptoms such as nausea, vomiting, headache, and lightheadedness. The client with an occult, or hidden bleed, may complain of needing to swallow frequently.

Objective Data Blood flow is evaluated for amount, consistency, color, and rate (or severity). Overt bleeding from the nose may be present. This bleeding can vary in flow from a continuous drip to a pulsating stream of blood. The client who has an occult epistaxis should have the posterior oropharynx visually examined by the nurse or physician to assess blood flow. Vomiting may be present. A lowered blood pressure and rapid heart rate are signs of hypovolemic shock. Conversely, the client with uncontrolled hypertension demonstrates an abnormally high systolic blood pressure. Pediatric clients should be assessed for the presence of foreign bodies and/or local trauma from inserting objects into the nares. Prothrombin time (PT), activated partial thromboplastin time (APTT), international normalization ratio (INR), and other clotting studies will be abnormal with underlying coagulopathies. Decreased red blood cell count, hemoglobin, and hematocrit are evidence of significant bleeding.

▼ ▼

Possible nursing diagnoses for a client with epistaxis may include:

Nursing Diagnoses	Goals	Nursing Interventions
▶ Gas exchange, impaired, related to airway obstruction.	The client will have a respiratory rate, color, and blood gases within normal limits.	Place the client in high-Fowler's position with the head bent slightly forward.
		Instruct the client to breathe through the mouth and allow the blood to escape freely from the nose into a container. This aids in preventing obstruction of the airway and swallowing of blood.
		Monitor the client for signs and symptoms of airway obstruction.
		Assess the client's respiratory rate, effort, and color.
		Auscultate the breath sounds.
		Administer supplemental oxygen as indicated by pulse oximetry or arterial blood gases.
		Monitor pulse oximetry and lab reports of arterial blood gases.
▶ Aspiration, high risk for, related to epistaxis.	The client will develop no complications related to aspiration.	Place the client in the position described above to aid in preventing aspiration of blood.
		Assess the client for signs of aspiration, such as choking, coarse crackles on auscultation, or elevated temperature.
		Suction the respiratory tract via the oral route to remove secretions and blood.
▶ Fluid volume deficit, related to blood loss.	The client will maintain adequate fluid volume.	With a gloved hand, compress the nares as described above.
		If bleeding continues following these attempts, prepare to assist the physician with procedures such as cautery or insertion of nasal packing.
		Administer medications to control the blood pressure as ordered.
		Once hemostasis has been established the clots formed should not be removed or dislodged as this will lead to recurrence of the bleeding.
		Frequently evaluate the blood pressure and pulse of the client who shows signs of volume depletion.
		Assess for orthostatic hypotension as a way to measure volume depletion. A decrease in the systolic blood pressure greater than 10 mmHg when the position is changed from lying to sitting or standing indicates hypovolemia.
		Administer IV fluids as ordered.

▶ Evaluation

Each goal must be evaluated to determine how it has been met by the client.

▲ ▲

▶ **CASE STUDY**

Mrs. White is a seventy-seven-year-old female with a history of smoking two to three packs of cigarettes a day for the last sixty years. Mrs. White has been diagnosed with COPD for the past four years. She has required supplemental oxygen at 2 liters/ min. for the last eighteen months. Three days ago Mrs. White was admitted with a chief complaint of increasing dyspnea on exertion and a productive cough of thick green-yellow sputum. She states that she does not know why she is coughing up this awful stuff.

Physical examination of Mrs. White this morning revealed: vital signs of T = 101.5°F., P = 124, R = 38, BP = 168/74; sonorous and sibilant wheezes upon expiration in the posterior lung fields with superimposed coarse crackles heard in the right posterior lower lung field. She is unable to ambulate to the bathroom or complete other ADLs due to the dyspnea. Chest x-ray showed a large area of consolidation in the right lower lobe. Sputum culture is still pending.

The following questions will guide your development of a Nursing Care Plan for the case study.

1. List the clinical manifestations that indicate Mrs. White is experiencing an infection concomitant with her COPD.

2. Explain why COPD predisposes a client to respiratory infection.

3. Explain why the physician will increase Mrs. White's oxygen flow to 3–4 liters/minute.

4. List the subjective and objective data the nurse should obtain during the nursing assessment.

5. Write three nursing diagnoses and client goals that would be pertinent to Mrs. White's care.

6. Prioritize the above diagnoses with the first being the highest priority.

7. Describe client outcomes that would indicate Mrs. White's treatment and nursing care regimen are successful.

▶ ▶ ▶ ▶ ▶   ▶   ▶   ▶   ▶   ▶

SUMMARY

- The primary function of the respiratory system is external respiration, or the exchange of gases between the atmosphere and the lungs. This occurs at the capillary membrane of the alveoli.

- Pneumonia is an infection of the lungs in which infection secretions accumulate in the air passages and interfere with gas exchange. Clients with chronic pulmonary disorders and those with problems of immobility are at greater risk to develop pneumonia.

- Pulmonary tuberculosis in an infection of the lung tissue caused by the *Mycobacterium tuberculosis*. Treatment of tuberculosis requires the long-term administration of pharmacological agents. Noncompliance with the treatment regimen is a concern when caring for the client and family with tuberculosis.

- A common respiratory tract disorder associated with the administration of anesthetic agents and immobility is atelectasis. Clients at risk are encouraged to cough and breathe deeply to aid in preventing atelectasis.

- Obstruction of a pulmonary artery by a bloodborne substance is known as pulmonary embolism. Deep vein thrombosis is a common source of pulmonary emboli.

- COPD is a collective term used to refer to chronic disorders of the lungs in which the air flow is limited into or out of the lungs. COPD is associated with asthma, chronic bronchitis, emphysema, and bronchiectasis.
- Traumatic disorders of the respiratory tract include pneumothorax and hemothorax. The lung tissue underlying a pneumothorax or hemothorax is compressed and eventually collapses.
- Cigarette smoking is indicated as a major causative factor in the development of respiratory disorders, such as lung cancer, cancer of the larynx, emphysema and chronic bronchitis.

Review Questions

1. The physician orders oxygen to be delivered to the client with COPD at 2 to 3 liters because:

   a. no client ever requires more than 2 to 3 liters of oxygen.
   b. the client requests it.
   c. a higher flow rate may suppress the client's drive to breathe.
   d. 2 to 3 liters is the maximum flow a nasal cannula can deliver effectively.

2. A particulate respirator mask is used by the nurse caring for a client with tuberculosis because:

   a. regular masks allow the tubercle bacilli to pass through.
   b. this mask is more comfortable for long-term use.
   c. this type of masks allows the nurse to be in close contact with the client for prolonged periods of time.
   d. there is no need for this type of mask when caring for clients with TB.

3. Bronchodilators are used to treat bronchiectasis in order to:

   a. dilate airways that are in bronchospasm due to an antigen-antibody reaction.
   b. dilate airways that have lost their elasticity.
   c. bronchodilators are contraindicated for use in bronchiectasis.
   d. dilate airways that are chronically narrowed.

4. Incentive spirometry is used to measure the amount of air that:

   a. is exhaled in one minute.
   b. is inspired in one minute.
   c. is inspired with one inhalation.
   d. is exhaled with one exhalation.

5. Asthma is characterized by:

   a. chronic narrowing of the airways.
   b. intermittent airflow obstruction.
   c. chronic dilation of the airways.
   d. fibrosis of the alveoli.

6. The client with a pneumothorax experiences hypoxia due to:

   a. the entry of air into the thoracic cavity.
   b. compression of the lung tissue underlying the pneumothorax.
   c. there is no impairment in the client's ability to exchange gases.
   d. a lack of surfactant.

Critical Thinking Questions

1. What can an individual do to have a healthier respiratory system?

2. How would COPD affect a person's lifestyle?

3. Explain the occurence of polycychemia and elevated HgB and Hct and hypoxia.

News Flash

Helium is again being utilized to aid oxygen transport through constricted airways. Prior to the advent of effective bronchodilators, helium was often mixed with oxygen to assist its transport to the alveoli. This practice ceased when bronchodilators became widely used. Nitrogen, the gas present with oxygen in the atmosphere, replaced helium. Mechanical ventilators in particular, use a mixture of nitrogen and oxygen to deliver oxygen to the client. Recent trials have shown that when helium is used rather than nitrogen, its lighter molecular weight allows the gaseous mixture to travel more easily through constricted airway passages (i.e., asthma attacks) (Ritchie & Hagel, 1994).

Medical Terminology

alveol/o-	tiny cavity
alveoli	refers to saclike structures of the terminal airways
bronch/o-	(major branch of) windpipe
bronchus	refers to large airways immediately below trachea
bronchiol/o-	little (branch of) bronchus
bronchioles	refers to smaller airways that branch off of bronchi
nas/o-	pertaining to the nose
nasal	adjective, refers to the nose or from the nose
pharyng/o-	referring to the pharynx
pharyngitis	inflammation of the pharynx
pleur/o-	refers to the pleura
pleurisy	inflammation of the pleura
pneum/o-	pertaining to the lungs
pneumonia	inflammation of the lungs
pneumon-	pertaining to the lungs
pneumonitis	inflammation of the lungs
rhin/o-	pertaining to the nose
rhinitis	inflammation of the nose
sinus	pertaining to the sinuses
sinusitis	inflammation of the sinuses
spir/o-	refers to breathing
spirometry	measurement of the amount of air moved into and/or out of the lungs
thorac/o-	pertaining to the thorax
thoracentesis	to remove fluid from the thorax, specifically the pleural cavity
trache/o-	pertaining to the trachea, windpipe
tracheal	adjective, refers to the trachea
ventil/o-	meaning to blow
ventilation	movement of air, specifically the movement of air into and out of the lungs

CHAPTER
20
Cardiac Disorders

Gena Duncan

▶ KEY TERMS

angina pectoris
annulus
arteriosclerosis
ascites
atherosclerosis
automatic implantable cardioverter-
   defibrillator
cardiac catheterization
cardiac cycle
cardiac output
cardiac tamponade
depolarization
dyspnea
echocardiogram
ejection fraction
heart sound
hepatomegaly
hypertrophies
orthopnea
palpitation
paroxysmal nocturnal dyspnea
percutaneous balloon valvuloplasty
pericardial friction rub
pericardiocentesis
repolarization
stent
stroke volume
thallium scan
transesophageal echocardiography (TEE)

LIST OF DISORDERS

▶ Cardiac Dysrhythmias
Inflammatory Disorders
▶ Rheumatic Heart Disease
▶ Infective Endocarditis
▶ Myocarditis
▶ Pericarditis
▶ Valvular Heart Diseases
Occlusive Disorders
▶ Arteriosclerosis
▶ Atherosclerosis
▶ Angina Pectoris
▶ Myocardial Infarction
Decreased Function and Failure of Cardiac System
▶ Congestive Heart Failure
▶ Cor Pulmonale

LEARNING OBJECTIVES

Upon completion of this chapter the learner should be able to:
• Define key terms.
• Describe the anatomy and physiology of the heart.
• Relate laboratory results to heart conditions.
• Describe basic heart dysrhythmias.
• Explain the pathophysiology of heart conditions.
• Describe nursing interventions in caring for clients with heart conditions.

▶ *MAKING THE CONNECTION*

Refer to the topics in the following chapters to increase your understanding of cardiac disorders:

- **Chapter 8, Health Maintenance:** Make a Genogram, p. 129; Prevent Common Health Problems, Heart Disease, p. 130; Stress, p. 131
- **Chapter 10, Nursing Assessment:** Thoracic Assessment, p. 179
- **Chapter 12, Pain Management:** Assessment, p. 211; Principles of Administering Analgesics, p. 215
- **Chapter 14, Fluid, Electrolyte, and Acid-base Balances:** Fluid balance, p. 271; Electrolyte Balance, p. 275

- **Chapter 19, Respiratory Disorders:** Anatomy and Physiology Review, Respiration, p. 388; The Thoracic Cavity, p. 389; Gas Exchange, p. 392; Pulmonary Embolism, p. 417; Chronic Obstructive Pulmonary Disease (COPD), p. 423
- **Chapter 22, Blood and Lymph Disorders:** Anatomy and Physiology Review, Blood, p. 518
- **Chapter 30, Diabetes Mellitus** Chronic Complications of Diabetes, p. 842

INTRODUCTION

Since 1900, heart disease has been the leading cause of death in the United States every year except in 1918 ("Heart and Stroke Facts: 1996 Statistical Supplement," American Heart Association, 1996). Approximately 1.5 million Americans experience a myocardial infarction each year with 500,000 of the occurrences ending in death (Linton, Matteson, & Maebius, 1995). Congestive heart failure is a contributing factor in approximately 250,000 deaths each year ("Heart and Stroke Facts: 1996 Statistical Supplement," American Heart Association, 1996).

Even though these facts are astounding, the death rate for cardiovascular disease has been declining in the last fifteen years. This is due to public education in modifying and decreasing risk factors such as smoking, high-fat diets, and minimal exercise.

This chapter reviews the anatomy and physiology of the heart. Laboratory tests, pathophysiology, medical management, and nursing interventions related to cardiac conditions are discussed with an emphasis on decreasing cardiac risk factors and improving lifestyles.

ANATOMY AND PHYSIOLOGY REVIEW

The heart is about the size of a fist and weighs less than one pound. Even though the heart is relatively small, its proper functioning is necessary for life. The heart is located in the lower anterior area of the mediastinum with the apex near the diaphragm. In an average lifetime, the heart will pump 80 million gallons of blood.

Function

The function of the circulatory system is to provide oxygen, nutrients, and hormones to the cells of the body and remove carbon dioxide and waste products of cellular metabolism from body cells. Body temperature is maintained by the circulatory system distributing heat throughout the body that has been produced by the metabolic activity of muscles and other body organs. Body cell needs are met by the blood pumped to them by the heart.

Structure of the Heart

The heart consists of three layers; endocardium, myocardium, and epicardium. The endocardium is the inner endothelial lining of heart chambers and valves. The myocardium is the thickest part of the heart and consists of cardiac muscle. The epicardium consists of a visceral layer and a parietal layer. The visceral epicardium attaches to the myocardium and is the outer layer of the heart. The parietal epicardium forms the inner layer of a double walled sac called the pericardium that surrounds the heart.

The heart is a hollow muscular organ containing four chambers that fill and empty of blood with each contraction (**depolarization**) and recovery phase (**repolarization**) of the cardiac muscle. The upper chambers are the atria and the lower chambers are the ventricles (Figure 20-1). When the atria contract, blood is forced into the ventricles. Contraction of the right ventricle pumps blood into the pulmonary arteries and on to the lungs (pulmonary circulatory system). Contraction of the left ventricle pumps blood into the aorta and out to the entire body (systemic circulatory system). The myocardium of the left ventricle is thicker than the right ventricle as more force is needed to pump blood throughout the body to meet the body's oxygen demands.

There are four sets of valves in the heart; tricuspid, bicuspid (mitral), pulmonary, and aortic. One end of fibrous cords called chordae tendineae are attached to the cusps of the tricuspid and mitral valves and the other end is attached to papillary muscles on the walls of the ventricles. The chordae tendineae keep the valves from inverting when the ventricles contract, thus preventing blood from flowing back into the atrium. The pulmonary and aortic valves prevent blood from flowing back into the ventricles from the pulmonary artery and aorta during repolarization.

Circulation of Blood

Blood enters the heart through veins and leaves the heart through arteries. With the contraction of the right ventricle, blood is forced through the pulmonary valve into the pulmonary artery. Blood circulates through the pulmonary circulatory system where carbon dioxide is exchanged for oxygen in the lungs. The blood then returns to the left atrium through the pulmonary veins providing oxygenated blood for systemic circulation. When the left ventricle contracts, blood is forced

through the aortic valve into the aorta beginning systemic circulation. Blood is distributed throughout the body by smaller arteries, arterioles, and capillaries. In capillary beds, oxygen, carbon dioxide, nutrients, water, and waste products are exchanged between blood and body tissues. From capillaries, blood flows into venules, veins, and returns to the right atrium of the heart through the inferior and superior vena cava.

Each time the heart beats, the ventricle pumps 60–80 cc of blood. The volume of blood pumped by the ventricle with each contraction is called **stroke volume**. The volume of blood pumped by the left ventricle per minute is known as **cardiac output** and averages 5 liters for an adult at rest. Stroke volume multiplied by the pulse rate yields the cardiac output. If the heart has a strong ventricular contraction, more blood will be pumped by the heart into the systemic circulatory system. Therefore, cardiac output has a direct effect upon the volume of arterial blood being circulated.

Coronary Arteries

Coronary arteries supply nutrients and oxygen to the muscle tissue of the heart. The two coronary arteries are the right coronary artery and the left coronary artery, which branch off the aorta (Figure 20-2). The right coronary artery divides into the posterior

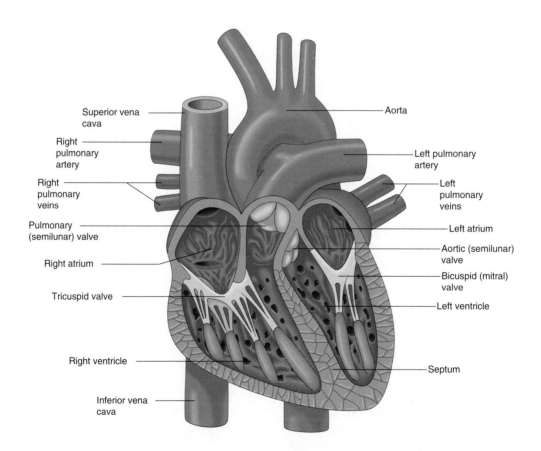

FIGURE 20-1 Internal view of the heart showing pulmonary arteries and veins.

descending artery (interventricular artery) and the marginal artery. The left coronary artery divides into the anterior descending artery and the circumflex artery. The right coronary artery supplies blood to the anterior area of the right and left ventricles, the posterior area of the right ventricle, the AV node, and the posterior section of the interventricular septum. The left anterior descending (LAD) artery supplies blood to the anterior section of the interventricular septum, anterior area of the left ventricle, and the lateral aspect of the left ventricle. The circumflex artery nourishes the left atrium and ventricle.

Conduction System

The specialized cardiac muscle cells are capable of conducting electrical impulses from one part of the heart to another. For the heart to beat regularly in a rhythmic sequence, electrical impulses follow a set pattern called the conduction system of the heart. The conduction system consists of the sinoatrial node (SA node), atrioventricular node (AV node), bundle of His, bundle branches, and Purkinje fibers. The electrical conduction system controls the heartbeat (refer to Figure 20-4 later in this chapter for an illustration of this process).

Since the SA node initiates electrical impulses that cause the heart to beat, it is called the pacemaker of the heart. The SA node is located in the superior aspect of the right atrium. Electrical impulses from the SA node pass through the muscle fibers of the right and left atria causing the atria to contract almost simultaneously. Atrial impulses are transmitted to the AV node located in the lower part of the right atrium. There is a short delay in the impulse at the AV node that allows the atria to complete their contraction and empty the blood into the ventricles. The electrical impulse is transmitted from the AV node into a group of specialized conduction fibers. The group of fibers is called the atrioventricular (AV) bundle or the bundle of His. Once the impulse leaves the AV node, it travels down the fibers of the bundle of His into the interventricular septum. The fibers separate into right and left bundle branches dividing into smaller and smaller branches, called Purkinje fibers. These terminate in the ventricular muscle causing the ventricles to contract. When an impulse has completely gone through the conduction system of the heart and the ventricles have contracted, a **cardiac cycle** has been completed.

There are two normal **heart sounds** called S_1 and S_2. They yield a sound like "lubb-dubb." S_1, or the "lubb," is the sound of the mitral and tricuspid valves closing simultaneously. It is heard on the left fifth intercostal space. S_2, or the "dubb," is the simultaneous closing of the pulmonary and aortic valves. S_2 is heard on the

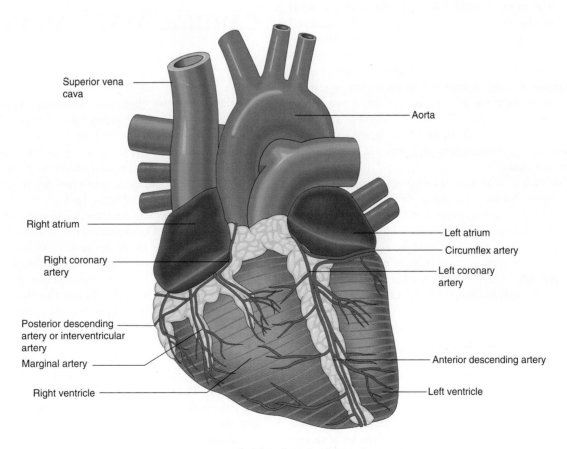

FIGURE 20-2   Coronary arteries supply blood to the heart tissue.

right second intercostal space. There is a slight pause after the "lubb-dubb" is heard (again, refer to Figure 20-4). It is not uncommon for some children to have an S_3 sound, which is produced by blood rapidly entering a partially filled ventricle. If this sound persists after the age of thirty, it is considered abnormal. Clients with congestive heart failure may have a third sound known as S_3. This low-pitched sound occurs after the S_2 sound, or the "dubb," making the heart sound like the word "Kentucky (lubb-dubb-by)." The S_3 sound has also been described as a gallop.

HEALTH HISTORY

The nurse has three goals when obtaining a health history from a client. The goals are to identify present and potential health problems, identify possible familial and lifestyle risk factors, and involve the client in planning long-term health care.

The nurse should interview the client in a caring, calm, relaxed environment. A relationship of trust needs to be established between the nurse and the client. A trusting relationship can be developed if the nurse listens attentively to the client's concerns.

It is important for the nurse to determine the onset of the symptoms, the predisposing factors that cause the symptoms, and the client's treatment of the symptoms. The nurse should ask if the client has noticed any other bodily changes that occur or have occurred at the same time as the main symptoms. Special attention should be given to the client's activity level or limitations in activity. When asking about dietary habits, the nurse should determine if there has been an increase or decrease in appetite. Asking about sleeping habits will help evaluate the client's ability to sleep, the need for the trunk of the body to be supported with pillows when sleeping, or the need to sleep in a chair.

Risk factors that have been associated with coronary artery disease and other cardiac conditions are familial factors, aging, gender, diabetes mellitus, high-fat diet, cigarette smoking, oral contraceptives, postmenopause, and stress. Advancing age, male gender, and familial history of chest pain or myocardial infarctions are risk factors that cannot be altered. However, risk factors such as diet, smoking, contraceptive methods, and stress can be modified.

Research shows that diets high in saturated fat, sugar, and calories lead to cardiac problems. A person with a cholesterol level above 300 mg/dL is four times more prone to develop coronary artery disease than a person with a level of 200 mg/dL (Phipps et al., 1995). Limiting fat to 30 percent or less of caloric intake, increasing fiber, and balancing caloric intake to maintain optimum weight greatly reduces the chances of devel-

oping a cardiac problem. Cigarette smoking increases the chances of coronary artery disease two-and-one-half times when a person smokes two or more packs of cigarettes a day (Monahan et al., 1994). Oral contraceptives elevate serum lipid levels, increase systolic blood pressure, and affect clotting factors predisposing the person to clot formation. If a woman smokes and takes oral contraceptives, she has five times the chance of developing coronary artery disease above one who does not smoke (Monahan et al., 1994).

Research shows that stress also plays a role in coronary artery disease. Stress factors associated with a lower socioeconomic level and a job with little autonomy may predispose one to cardiac conditions. There is some controversy as to whether the characteristics of the type A personality are stressors leading to cardiac disease. Learning ways to reduce stress produces a healthier heart.

The nurse has a two-fold objective in directing the client toward a healthier lifestyle. The first objective is to educate the client about risk factors present in his life. The second objective is to determine what risk factors the client would like to modify. Once this has been determined, the nurse can assist the client in establishing goals and determining actions to achieve the goals.

CARDIAC ASSESSMENT

Subjective Data

The typical concerns expressed by a client with heart problems are chest pain, dyspnea, edema, fainting, palpitations, diaphoresis, and fatigue. When a client states they have chest pain, it is important to determine the onset of the pain, situation occurring at the onset of pain, location and radiation of pain, severity of chest pain, duration, past episodes of chest pain, and methods used to alleviate pain.

There are several types of **dyspnea** the client may be experiencing. Exertional dyspnea occurs when a person participates in moderate activity and becomes short of breath. This occurs in the early stages of heart failure and indicates that the heart is not able to meet the demands of the body during moderate activity. **Orthopnea** is when a client has difficulty breathing and must sit upright or stand to relieve the dyspnea. This occurs in a more advanced stage of heart failure. **Paroxysmal nocturnal dyspnea** is when a person suddenly awakens, is sweating, and having difficulty breathing. This usually occurs two to five hours after the person has fallen asleep. The nurse needs to ascertain the level at which the person is having difficulty breathing.

A client may have fainting spells for various physical and psychological reasons. In cardiac clients, fainting occurs because of decreased cardiac output that causes a decreased blood flow to the brain.

A client may describe a "fluttering" or "pounding" sensation in the chest. This is known as **palpitations**. If these sensations occur during exercise it is a sign that the heart is having to work harder to meet the demands of the body. Palpitations may also be caused by anxiety, ingestion of a large meal, lack of adequate rest, or a large intake of caffeine.

A cardiac client usually will experience fatigue because the heart is not able to keep up with the daily demands of the body. Often the fatigue will increase throughout the day. Frequent rest periods will help alleviate some of the fatigue.

Objective Data

To perform a head-to-toe assessment on a cardiac client, carefully assess the skin, neck veins, respirations, heart sounds, abdomen, and extremities. The skin should be observed for cyanosis in the earlobes, lips, fingers, and feet. Assessment of skin turgor could give an indication of fluid volume. If the skin is dry and has poor turgor, the client may be dehydrated from diuretics. If a client has distended neck veins when the head of the bed is at a 45° angle or higher, he may be experiencing right-sided heart failure. The nurse should assess the quality of respirations for rate and ease of breathing. Observe for dyspnea and coughing. Heart sounds are assessed for the normal S_1 and S_2 sounds. If the typical lubb-dubb is heard, the valves are closing properly. A pericardial friction rub may be heard if the client has pericarditis. This is an extra sound heard as the heart rubs against the pericardial sac. The sound will be a short, high-pitched squeak. While listening to the heart, palpate the radial

pulse to account for every heartbeat. If a heartbeat is heard through the stethoscope but not felt in the radial pulse, the heart has decreased cardiac output to the extremities. If the abdomen is distended, the client may have **ascites**, which is excess fluid in the abdomen. After the heart and lung sounds have been assessed, check the peripheral pulses. Pulses on both sides of the body should be checked at the same time to determine adequate bilateral perfusion. It is important to check pedal pulses in both feet to determine blood flow to each foot. Pulse amplitude can be rated on a scale of 0 to 4.

> 0 = absent
> 1+ = diminished but palpable
> 2+ = normal
> 3+ = full, increased
> 4+ = bounding

Literature gives various scale ratings for pulse amplitude so documentation should be according to the scale used in the local facility.

If the hands and feet are cold or have mottling, this could indicate decreased cardiac output. Capillary refill should be assessed in the fingers and toes. To check for capillary refill, squeeze the fingernails or toenails so they blanch. Color should return to the fingernails and toenails within 3 seconds if perfusion is adequate.

If the feet, ankles, or legs have edema present this should also be noted. According to Beare & Myers (1994), edema can be assessed by a rating scale of 1 to 4 (Figure 20-3).

A client can gain 10 pounds before edema can be detected. It is important that fluid volume be assessed daily on cardiac clients with edema problems. This can be done by having the client weigh daily. The weight is to be taken on the same scale, the same time of day, and wearing the same amount of clothing.

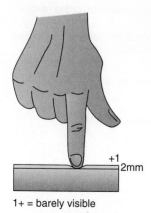

1+ = barely visible

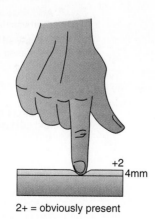

2+ = obviously present

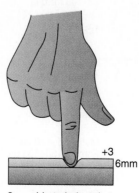

3+ = able to indent, but rebounds when finger removed

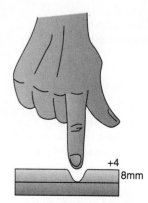

4+ = indentation remains when finger removed

FIGURE 20-3 Edema rating scale.

COMMON DIAGNOSTIC TESTS

The following is a table of the commonly used diagnostic tests for clients with cardiac disorders.

Test	Explanation/Normal values	Nursing Responsibilities
LABORATORY TESTS		
Arterial blood gases	Indicates respiratory and metabolic functioning. pH = 7.35–7.45 PCO_2 = 35–45 mmHg HCO_3^- = 21–28 mEq/L PO_2 = 80–100 mmHg O_2 saturation = 95%–100%	This test is done by a physician, lab technicians, respiratory therapists, or specialty nurses. The blood sample is drawn in a syringe containing heparin. After the specimen has been obtained, rotate the syringe to mix the blood and heparin. The blood sample is placed on ice and taken immediately to the lab. Apply pressure to the arterial site for 3 to 5 minutes or 15 minutes if client is on an anticoagulant. Assess site for bleeding.

Complete blood count (CBC)
 	
White blood cells (WBC)
Red blood cells (RBC)
 	
Hemoglobin (Hg)
  males
  females
Hematocrit (Hct)
  males
  females
	Indicates oxygen carrying capacity of blood and presence of infection.
	5,000–10,000 mm³
	4.2–5.4/mm³
	
	13.5–17.5 g/dl
	12–16 g/dl
	
	40–54%
	37–47%
		Client is not fasting or NPO.
		
		Elevated in MI and bacterial infections.
		Elevation indicates compensation for hypoxemia.
		Elevated in CHF.
		If less than 5 g/dl may lead to heart failure.

Culture and sensitivity (C&S)	Determines presence of microorganism and determines antibiotic that will kill or inhibit growth of microorganism. Normal value is negative for microorganism growth.	Blood sample is done before administration of antibiotics. Assists in diagnosis of bacterial endocarditis.
Electrolytes Sodium (Na) Potassium (K) Chloride (Cl) Carbon dioxide (CO_2) Magnesium (Mg)	Test determines blood electrolyte levels. 136–145 mEq/L 3.5–5 mEq/L 98–106 mEq/L 22–30 mEq/L 1.5–2.5 mEq/L	Client is not fasting or NPO. Na and K are necessary for cardiac electrical conduction. Acid-base imbalances can cause cardiac dysrhythmias. Decreased levels can cause dysrhythmias; decreased in CHF.
Cardiac enzymes Serum aspartate aminotransferase AST (formerly serum glutamic oxaloacetic transaminase, SGOT) Creatine kinase CPK (CK) CK isoenzymes CK-MM (muscle) CK-BB (brain) CK-MB (heart)	Test indicates possible tissue damage if elevated. Males 7–21 u/L Females 6–18 u/L Males 55–170 u/L Females 30–135 u/L Present in skeletal muscle brain/lungs heart muscle 100% 0% (0% >5% in MI)	Client is not fasting or NPO. Pattern of elevated levels of AST, CPK, and LDH is indicative of MI. Elevation of an isoenzyme indicates damage to tissue in a specific organ; CK-MB is specific for myocardial cells.

Test	Explanation/Normal values	Nursing Responsibilities
Lactic dehydrogenase LDH	70-180 mg/dL or 95-200 u/L	When LDH_1 value is greater than LDH_2 value it is indicative of an acute MI. LDH_5 is elevated with CHF.
LDH isoenzymes LDH_1 LDH_2 LDH_3 LDH_4 LDH_5	* 17.5–28.3% * 30.4–36.4% * 18.8–26% * 9.2–16.5% * 5.3–13.4% * % of total LDH	
Serum lipids (lipid profile) cholesterol	Blood lipid produced in the liver that forms bile salts to assist in the digestion of fat <200 mg/dL	Elevated in hyper-cholesterolemia; if elevated increase risk of CAD, hypertension, and MI.
High density lipoprotein (HDL)	30–70 mg/dL	
Low density lipoprotein (LDL)	60–160 mg/dL	
Very low density lipoprotein (VLDL)	25%–50%	
triglycerides	40–150 mg/dL	Elevated level in CAD; level increases when LDL level increases.
Erythrocyte sedimentation rate (ESR, Sed rate test)	Nonspecific test indicating presence of inflammation. Male = up to 15 mm/hr Female = up to 20 mm/hr (Westergen method)	Elevated levels indicate MI and bacterial endocarditis. Decreased levels indicate CHF and angina.
Glucose	Determines blood glucose level. 70–100 mg/100 mL	Client may have water. Do not administer insulin until after blood test is completed. Increased in diabetes mellitus, acute stress, and MI.

OTHER DIAGNOSTIC TESTS

Test	Explanation/Normal values	Nursing Responsibilities
Cardiac biopsy	This procedure is done during a cardiac catheterization. A tissue sample is taken from the apex or septum to determine toxicity from drugs, inflammation, or rejection from a heart transplant.	Same preparation as for a cardiac catheterization. After the procedure observe the client for symptoms of a perforation, such as chest pain, decreased blood pressure, or dyspnea.
Cardiac catheterization (cardiac angiogram, coronary arteriogram)	A catheter is passed into the right and/or left side of the heart to determine oxygen level, cardiac output, and pressure within the heart chambers.	Assess the client for allergies to iodine or shellfish. The client is to fast for 6 hours prior to the test, but medications can be taken with sips of water. Inform the client of the possibility of feeling warm or flushed during the test. After the procedure, assess the peripheral pulses every 15 minutes for 2 to 4 hours or according to physician's orders. Note the color, temperature and pulse quality in the extremity below the catheter insertion site. Instruct the client to keep the involved extremity straight for 6-8 hours.
Chest x-ray	Detects size, as to enlargement or hypertrophy, and displacement of the heart within the chest. Lung congestion may indicate heart failure.	Instruct the client to remove all metal objects from the chest and neck area and wear a hospital gown that does not have snap closures.

(continued)

Test	Explanation/Normal values	Nursing Responsibilities
Cardiac positron emission tomography scan (cardiac PET scan)	Radioactive tracers are injected intravenously prior to the test. Nuclear imaging is used to confirm tissue that has a good blood supply and tissue that has become impaired due to a lack of blood.	Instruct the client not to have caffeine for 18 hours and not to smoke 4 hours prior to the test. The client is NPO except for medications with water from 10 P.M. the evening before the test. A signed consent is needed. Encourage the client to drink fluids after the procedure so the radioactive material will be excreted quicker.
Echocardiogram	An ultrasound of the heart to determine hypertrophies, cardiomyopathies, or congenital defects. Very helpful in diagnosing valve abnormalities and pericardial effusion.	Explain the procedure to the client and assure the client that there is no discomfort during the procedure. Some pressure may be felt on the chest wall from the transducer.
Electrocardiogram (EKG or ECG)	Electrodes are placed on the skin to record wave patterns of the electrical conduction of the heart. Determines myocardial damage, rhythmic disturbances, and hyperkalemia.	Explain the procedure to the client. Inform the client that the test is painless.
Holter monitor	A client wears a portable EKG that monitors and records the electrical conduction of the heart for a period of 24 hours. The heart rhythm is compared to client activities.	Instruct the client to engage in normal daily activities and keep a journal of symptoms experienced in performing these activities.
Magnetic resonance imaging (MRI)	The test provides three-dimensional imaging of soft tissue structures and is important in evaluating coronary artery disease and pericardial disease. The client is placed in an electromagnetic cylinder.	Evaluate the client for claustrophobic tendencies since they will be surrounded by a cylinder. No metal objects are to be worn. Inform the client that various sounds will be heard during the procedure and ear plugs may be worn. Generally the sounds are not intolerable. The test may take one hour to complete.
Pericardiocentesis	Fluid is removed from the pericardial sac for analysis or to relieve pressure.	Inform the client that the procedure will be done under a local anesthetic. Pressure may be felt when the needle is inserted. The client will be in a semi-Fowler's position during the procedure and attached to an EKG monitor. Postoperatively take vital signs every 15 minutes and monitor the EKG rhythm.
Pulse oximetry	A noninvasive procedure in which a transdermal clip is placed on a finger or earlobe to detect the arterial oxygen saturation.	Explain the procedure to the client and record the oxygen saturation.
Radionuclide angiography (Multiplegated radioisotope scan, multi-gated acquisition scanning, MUGA)	A radioisotope is injected to evaluate the function of the left ventricle. The ejection fraction (a comparison of the volume of blood pumped by the left ventricle to total volume of blood left in the ventricle) is measured.	A signed permit is usually needed.
Stress test	An EKG is done as the client exercises to evaluate the effects of exercise on the heart. Often the client is asked to walk on a treadmill in which the incline is elevated at various times throughout the test. The test is used frequently with clients who have CAD.	Explain the procedure to the client. Encourage the client to wear good walking shoes during the test.

Test	Explanation/Normal values	Nursing Responsibilities
Technetium pyrophosphate scanning	The test is important in diagnosing acute myocardial infarctions with the best accuracy obtained at 48 hours after the client experiences symptoms suggestive of an infarct. A tracer or radioisotope, which is injected intravenously, accumulates in the damaged or infarcted tissue and are called hot spots.	Inform the client to avoid smoking, caffeine, or alcohol 3 hours before the test. The test will take 45 to 60 minutes.
Thallium scan (myocardial perfusion scan)	A radioactive tracer (thallium 201) is injected and accumulates in myocardial tissue that is well perfused. The tracer has a decreased accumulation in myocardial tissue that is not well perfused and these areas are called "cold spots." The client may be asked to do exercise such as ride a bike, during the test to evaluate the perfusion of myocardial tissue during exercise.	Inform the client to be NPO 3 hours prior to the test.

KEY ABBREVIATIONS

The following abbreviations and acronyms are used in this chapter:

AICD	automatic implantable cardioverter-defibrillator
AST	aspartate aminotransferase
AV	atrioventricular
CAD	coronary artery disease
CAHD	coronary artery heart disease
CHF	congestive heart failure
CK or CPK	creatine kinase or creatine phosphokinase
EKG	electrocardiogram
HDL	high-density lipoprotein
IABP	intra-aortic balloon pump
LAD	left anterior descending
LDH	lactic dehydrogenase
LDL	low-density lipoprotein
MI	myocardial infarction
NSR	normal sinus rhythm
PAC	premature atrial contractions
PSVT	paroxysmal supraventricular tachycardia
PTCA	percutaneous transluminal coronary angioplasty
PVC	premature ventricular contraction
SA	sinoatrial
TEE	transesophageal echocardiography
VAD	ventricular assist device
VF	ventricular fibrillation
VT	ventricular tachycardia

▶ CARDIAC DYSRHYTHMIAS

▶ Normal Sinus Rhythm

The electrical conduction of the heart begins with the sinoatrial (SA) node (Figure 20-4). The SA node is located in the superior section of the right atrium. From the SA node, the electrical impulse spreads in wave fashion stimulating both atria. The electrical impulse spreads through the atria similar to the ripples from a pebble dropped in water.

The electrical impulse spreading across both atria yields a P wave on the EKG. Thus the P wave represents the electrical activity causing the contraction of both atria.

After the atria contract, the electrical impulse then reaches the atrioventricular (AV) node. When the electrical impulse reaches the AV node it pauses for approximately one-tenth second, which allows blood to enter both ventricles. The electrical impulse then starts down the AV bundle, also called the bundle of His, which divides into right and left bundle branches in the interventricular septum. The electrical impulse continues from the right and the left bundle branches to the Purkinje fibers. The Purkinje fibers transmit the electrical impulse to the myocardial cells causing contractions of the ventricles. On an EKG the QRS complex represents the electrical impulse as it travels through the AV node, bundle of His, bundle branches, Purkinje fibers, and myocardial cells terminating with the ventricles contracting. The Q wave is not always present on the EKG strip.

There is a pause after the QRS complex. The pause is called the ST segment. The ST segment represents the period between the contraction and the beginning of the recovery or repolarization of the ventricular muscles. The T wave represents the repolarization of the ventricles (Figure 20-4).

After the repolarization of the ventricles, the entire cycle begins all over again at the SA node. In this way the P wave, QRS complex, and T waves are repeated with each heartbeat. Figure 20-5 shows an EKG strip of normal sinus rhythm.

▶ Dysrhythmias

A dysrhythmia is an irregularity in the rate, rhythm, or conduction of the electrical system of the heart. The dysrhythmia can occur in the atria, ventricles, or any part of the conduction system. Specialized cells in the

heart muscle have the ability to generate an electrical impulse. Under certain conditions these cells start sending impulses to other cells in the heart causing irregular beats called ectopic beats. The most common causes of dysrhythmias are coronary artery disease (CAD) and myocardial infarction (MI). Other causes of dysrhythmias are electrolyte imbalances and drug toxicity.

Symptoms of a client experiencing a dysrhythmia can vary from asymptomatic to cardiac arrest. The client may experience fainting, seizures, fatigue, decreased energy levels, exertional dyspnea, chest pain, and palpitations.

▶ Bradycardia

Sinus bradycardia is a heart rate of 60 beats/minute or less (Figure 20-6). Causes of sinus bradycardia are myocardial ischemia, electrolyte imbalances, vagal

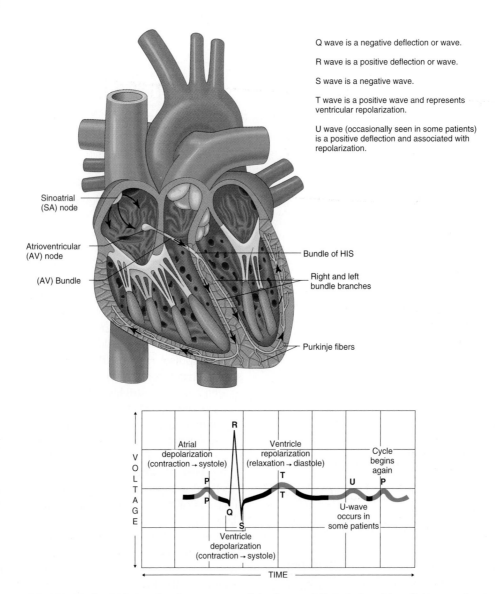

FIGURE 20-4 **(A)** Conduction system of the heart. **(B)** Relationship of the conduction system to an EKG strip. **(C)** Relationship of S_1 and S_2 heart sounds to an EKG strip.

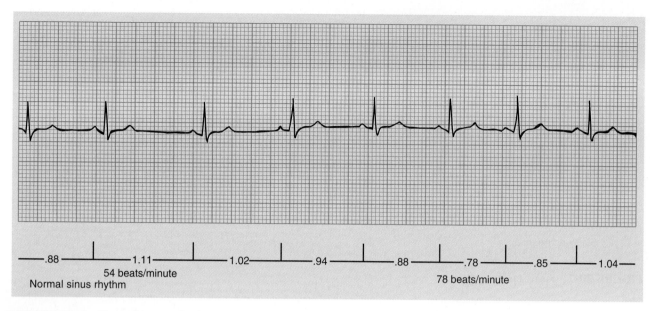

—.88—|—1.11—|—1.02—|—.94—|—.88—|—.78—|—.85—|—1.04—

54 beats/minute   78 beats/minute

Normal sinus rhythm

FIGURE 20-5   Normal sinus rhythm.

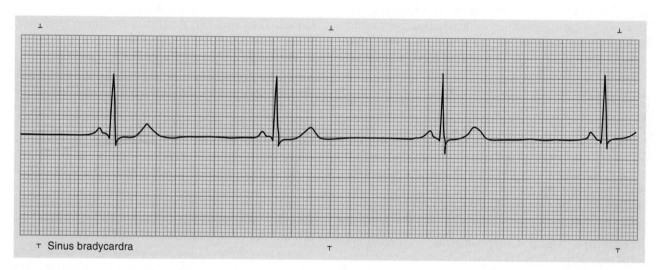

⊤ Sinus bradycardra

FIGURE 20-6   Sinus bradycardia.

stimulation, heart blocks, drug toxicity, intracranial tumors, sleep, and vomiting. An advantage of bradycardia is increased preload (the volume of blood the heart has to pump with each contraction), which provides increased stroke volume and increased blood supply to the heart through the coronary arteries. The treatment for bradycardia is the administration of atropine. Some clients with bradycardia may require a permanent pacemaker.

► Tachycardia

Tachycardia is a sinus rhythm with a ventricular rate ranging from 100 to 150 beats/minute (see Figure 20-7). Causes of tachycardia are exercise, emotional stress, fever, medications, pain, anemia, thyrotoxicosis, peri-

carditis, heart failure, excessive caffeine, and tobacco. When the ventricles are beating at this rate, there is limited time for the ventricles to fill with blood. This causes a decreased amount of blood to be pumped to the coronary arteries and throughout the body. The client may experience anginal pain. The treatment for sinus tachycardia is dependent on the cause. If the cause is stress or anxiety, the client is treated for anxiety. Sometimes the heart rate will slow spontaneously. At other times, medications such as beta blockers, calcium channel blockers, and digitalis are needed. Tachycardia may also be treated with Valsalva maneuver and carotid sinus massage. When performing the Valsalva maneuver the client is instructed to take a deep breath and bear down as if having a bowel movement. Carotid sinus pressure or massage is done

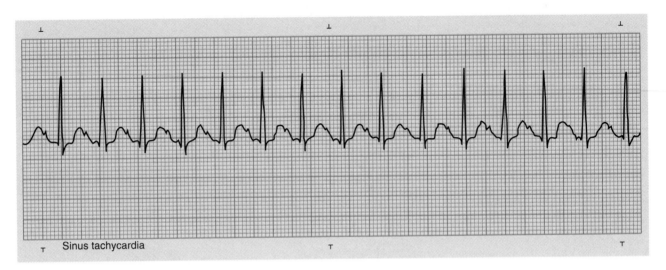

Sinus tachycardia

FIGURE 20-7 Sinus tachycardia.

by a physician or a nurse with special skills to perform the procedure. Carotid sinus pressure or massage is done by applying pressure or massaging the carotid sinuses in the neck below the jaw bone. When this area is massaged, there is a reflex vagal stimulation causing vasodilation that slows the heart rate.

▶ Atrial Dysrhythmias

Atrial dysrhythmias occur from disturbances in the electrical conduction in the atria resulting in premature beats or abnormal atrial rhythms. Common causes for atrial dysrhythmias are myocardial infarction, congestive heart failure, electrolyte imbalances, emotional stress, and drugs.

Premature Atrial Contractions A premature atrial contraction (PAC) is an ectopic impulse not originating in the sinoatrial node, but rather in the atrial tissue. This causes an atrial depolarization to occur earlier in the cycle than expected. Thus the term *premature atrial contraction*. This dysrhythmia is also known as premature atrial complexes (PACs) or atrial premature beats (APBs).

PACs often do not cause the client to experience physical symptoms depending on how often they occur. Generally they are benign and occur several times a day in healthy individuals. If their occurrence causes an increase or decrease in the pulse rate, they should be evaluated. PACs can be a symptom of myocardial ischemia, developing congestive heart failure, digitalis toxicity, hypokalemia, or an inflammatory condition. Stress, caffeine, and smoking can also cause PACs. PACs can be the first indication that more serious atrial dysrhythmias could occur if not treated properly.

If PACs are occurring because of serious underlying problems they should be medically managed with antidysrhythmic drugs such as quinidine and procain-

amide hydrochloride (Procan SR). If stress is the cause of PACs, the nurse can assist with stress reduction techniques. The client may desire counseling to assist with stress reduction. The client is encouraged to decrease or eliminate caffeine intake and stop smoking.

Atrial Tachycardia Atrial tachycardia is an ectopic impulse that causes the ventricles to contract at the rate of 140 to 250 beats per minute. This is sometimes referred to as a supraventricular dysrhythmia meaning the impulse causing the dysrhythmia is occurring above the ventricles. This dysrhythmia can occur as a continuous rhythm or as short, sudden eruptions that start and end spontaneously.

Atrial tachycardia occurs with hypokalemia, digitalis toxicity, and ischemia. Potassium supplements are given if the cause of the dysrhythmia is hypokalemia. If increased levels of serum digitalis is the cause, digitalis is withheld until the level returns to normal. The client may not experience digitalis toxicity as easily if the serum potassium level is maintained at a high normal level. Phenytoin sodium (Dilantin sodium) may be given as an antiarrhythmic to control the digitalis toxicity. An artificial pacemaker may be surgically inserted to regulate the atrial tachycardia dysrhythmia.

Paroxysmal Supraventricular Tachycardia Paroxysmal supraventricular tachycardia (PSVT) was previously called paroxysmal atrial tachycardia (PAT). PSVT is a rapid atrial beat accompanied by an abnormal conduction in the AV node. The dysrhythmia occurs suddenly (paroxysmally) and is usually initiated by a premature beat. PSVT can stop as abruptly as it begins.

PSVT is a common dysrhythmia in children and young adults and may not be indicative of heart disease. It can be caused by myocarditis, caffeine, alcohol ingestion, smoking, and stress. PSVT may also be present in clients with coronary artery disease, mitral valve prolapse, and acute pericarditis.

The client needs to be taught vagal stimulation procedures such as the Valsalva maneuver and carotid sinus pressure or massage, which usually stops the dysrhythmia. If these measures do not work, digoxin (Lanoxin) and propranolol hydrochloride (Inderal) are the drugs of choice. Occasionally cardioversion may be needed to stop PSVT.

Atrial Flutter   Atrial flutter, a rapid contraction of the atria, yields a heart rate of 250 to 350 beats per minute. The EKG displays a sawtooth wave pattern (see Figure 20-8). The AV node attempts to block some of the atrial impulses but usually the ventricles are also contracting at a rate of 300 beats per minute. This causes a decreased blood supply to the body because the atria and ventricles are unable to fill with blood when they are contracting at such a fast rate. This dysrhythmia requires immediate intervention.

Underlying causes of atrial flutter are coronary artery disease, pulmonary embolism, mitral valve dis-ease, acute myocardial infarction, and cardiomyopathy. The client may experience palpitations or go into cardiac shock depending on the underlying cause. If atrial flutter occurs during an MI or with congestive heart failure, it is a sign of poor prognosis.

Medications of choice for atrial flutter are digoxin (Lanoxin) which slows the rate and antiarrhythmic agents such as quinidine or procainamide hydrochloride (Procan SR). Calcium channel blockers such as verapamil (Calan) and nifedipine (Procardia) may be given to block the impulses at the AV node. If the atrial flutter is not controlled with medications, cardioversion can be done. Refer to cardioversion later in this chapter.

Atrial Fibrillation   Atrial fibrillation is an erratic electrical activity of the atria, resulting in a rate of 350 beats/minute to 600 beats/minute (Figure 20-9). Atrial depolarization is so uncoordinated during the dysrhythmia that the atria quiver rather than contract. The

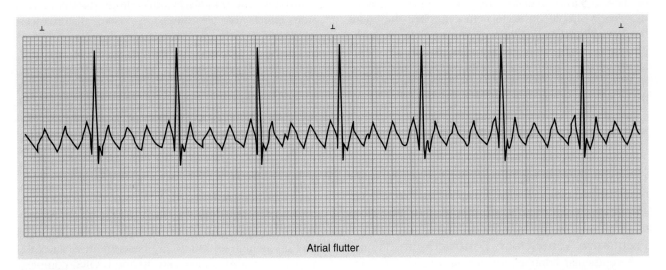

Atrial flutter

FIGURE 20-8   Atrial flutter.

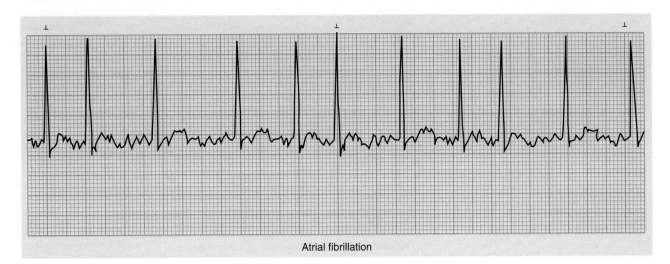

Atrial fibrillation

FIGURE 20-9   Atrial fibrillation.

AV node is bombarded with impulses and randomly transmits the impulses to the ventricles causing varied irregular contractions of the ventricles. The underlying cause of the dysrhythmia is of an organic nature such as mitral conditions, CAHD, acute MI, hypertensive heart disease, and hyperthyroidism. Since the atria are not contracting properly, blood is allowed to pool in the atria. This predisposes the person to thrombi forming on the walls of the atria. The clots can dislodge and travel to the brain, lungs, and other parts of the body. Most clients take an aspirin daily to prevent clot formation.

Once the underlying condition is treated, atrial fibrillation may stop. However, it is usually treated with quinidine or procainamide hydrochloride (Procan SR) and digoxin (Lanoxin). A calcium channel blocker, verapamil (Calan) and nifedipine (Procardia), or beta blocker, atenolol (Tenormin) or timolol maleate (Blocadren), can be used for a short time to slow the heart rate. If the dysrhythmia cannot be controlled with medication, cardioversion may be necessary. Cardioversion should be done with caution if the client has been digitalized. Digitalization causes the heart to be sensitive to cardioversion and the heart may fibrillate from the cardioversion. Anticoagulants should be used before the client undergoes cardioversion so a thrombus is not released into the system.

▶ *Ventricular Dysrhythmias*

Ventricular dysrhythmias originate in the ventricles. They are more life threatening than other dysrhythmias because the ventricles supply blood to the lungs and the body. These dysrhythmias need to be treated promptly.

Premature Ventricular Contractions Premature ventricular contractions are also known as ventricular premature beats (VPBs). PVCs arise from ectopic beats in the ventricles and are the most common ectopic beats. PVCs can easily be identified on the EKG because of the wide, bizarre QRS complexes (see Figure 20-10). There are no P waves preceding the QRS complex.

PVCs may occur in the healthy individual; in fact, the number of PVCs increase as one ages. However, the more pertinent PVCs occur because of underlying heart conditions.

Coronary artery disease is the most common cause of PVCs. Clients with an acute MI should be monitored closely for PVCs as more serious dysrhythmias may occur. Other causes of PVCs are myocardial ischemia, CHF, electrolyte imbalances, digitalis toxicity, anxiety, exercise, hypoxia, caffeine, and excessive alcohol consumption.

The most common pharmacological treatment for PVCs is lidocaine hydrochloride (Xylocaine HCl). Initially lidocaine is given as an IV bolus and then titrated according to the client's response. Once the PVCs are controlled oral antidysrhythmic drugs may be given. Side effects of lidocaine are visual disturbances, headache, seizures, and respiratory depression.

Other medications used to treat PVCs are procainamide hydrochloride (Procan SR), quinidine, disopyramide phosphate (Norpace), bretylium tosylate (Bretylol), and magnesium sulfate. Antidysrhythmic doses may need to be reduced with the elderly who may have hepatic or renal impairment. Administering oxygen may increase the oxygen perfusion to the myocardial tissue and decrease the frequency of premature beats.

Ventricular Tachycardia Ventricular tachycardia (VT) is the occurrence of three or more consecutive PVCs. The ventricular rate is 100 beats/minute and may go as high as 140 to 240 beats/minute. The EKG reveals a wide, abnormally shaped QRS complex. Underlying conditions in which VT occurs are car-

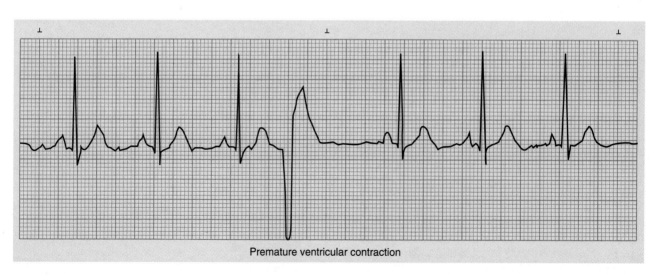

Premature ventricular contraction

FIGURE 20-10 Premature ventricular contraction.

diomyopathy, hypoxemia, digitalis toxicity, and electrolyte imbalance.

The two types of VT are sustained and nonsustained. Sustained VT last for more than thirty seconds and nonsustained last less than thirty seconds.

During VT, the client will have a low blood pressure, weak or absent peripheral pulses, body weakness, and may become unconscious. The ventricle is beating so rapidly that it is unable to fill with blood or eject blood properly. This causes blood to back up in the pulmonary circulation leading to pulmonary congestion.

It is important that VT be treated promptly because a ventricular tachycardia rhythm may lead into ventricular fibrillation, a life-threatening dysrhythmia. The client is given oxygen and an intravenous line is inserted if one is not already in place. The drug of choice is procainamide hydrochloride (Procan SR) given intravenously because it slows the electrical conduction in the ventricle. Lidocaine hydrochloride (Xylocaine HCl) is given if PVCs occur with myocardial ischemia or infarct. If the VT is not controlled with medications, the client may be cardioverted or defibrillated.

Cardioversion is the delivery of a synchronized electrical shock to change a dysrhythmia to a rhythm that will circulate more blood to the body tissues and improve oxygenation of the tissues. The electrical shock is set to be delivered on the R wave as a shock during ventricular depolarization may cause ventricular fibrillation. Cardioversion is done as an elective or emergency treatment. Electrodes are placed to the right of the sternum below the clavicle and at the apex of the heart. The electrodes are lubricated with a special gel or placed on normal saline pads. An electrical current is delivered through the electrodes. The client is NPO for eight hours prior to an elective cardioversion. Diuretics and digitalis preparations are withheld twenty-four to seventy-two hours before the cardioversion since the myocardium cells are less responsive to convert to a normal rhythm or may develop a serious dysrhythmia after the cardioversion. Anticoagulants and oral antiarrhythmics are still given before cardioversion. Anticoagulants are given so a thrombus is not released into the system. The client is given a sedative such as diazepam (Valium) or midazolam hydrochloride (Versed) intravenously before the procedure. The client's vital signs and EKG strip are monitored closely for the first hour after the cardioversion and then as ordered by the physician.

Defibrillation is the delivery of an unsynchronized electrical shock during an emergency situation such as a cardiac arrest to convert the life-threatening dysrhythmia or arrhythmia to a more stable sinus rhythm. The electrical current depolarizes the myocardium and allows the heart's pacemaker to reestablish a normal sinus rhythm. Defibrillation is done by a physician or a nurse who has had special education to handle emergency situations. Paddles are lubricated with a special gel or normal saline pads are applied to the skin where the paddles will be placed. The paddles are placed to the right of the sternum below the clavicle and at the apex of the heart. When the electrical shock is delivered to the client, everyone stands clear of the bed to prevent them from also receiving the electrical shock. More than one electrical shock may be delivered in an attempt to convert the rhythm.

If conservative measures do not control the VT and the client has periodic episodes of VT, an **automatic implantable cardioverter-defibrillator** (AICD) is implanted in the client (see Figure 20-11). This device senses the dysrhythmia and automatically sends an electrical shock directly to the heart to defibrillate it.

One type of AICD has leads that are attached to the heart muscle. The pulse generator that initiates the shock is placed in a pocket of subcutaneous tissue in the abdominal wall. The pulse generator is powered by lithium batteries. Another type of AICD has an endocardial lead that is guided through a vein into the right side of the heart. The pulse generator may be placed under the skin below the collarbone or in the abdomen.

The AICD detects VT and ventricular fibrillation (VF) through the leads attached to the heart muscle. Once VT or VF are detected, an electrical shock is sent from the pulse generator. The AICD is capable of delivering three more shocks to the heart muscle if the heart does not return to normal sinus rhythm (NSR). Usually clients are converted to NSR with the first shock. Complications following the insertion of a AICD are atelectasis, pneumonia, pneumothorax, thrombus, and a seroma at the generator site.

Ventricular Fibrillation   The most common cause for VF is CAD. VF is a disorganized, chaotic quivering of the ventricles. The ventricles are unable to contract and no blood is ejected into the circulatory system. The EKG reading is a series of jagged, unidentifiable waves (see Figure 20-12). The client will not have a pulse, blood pressure, or respirations. This dysrhythmia is serious. Aggressive measures must be taken to initiate CPR and defibrillate the client immediately.

Ventricular Asystole   Ventricular asystole is represented by a straight line on the EKG (see Figure 20-13). The ventricles are not contracting and the client is in cardiac arrest. The client loses consciousness and has no pulse or respirations. Aggressive treatment should be initiated within one minute to prevent chemical changes within the body that jeopardize recovery. CPR is started and the client is defibrillated. Atropine sulfate and epinephrine are given intravenously.

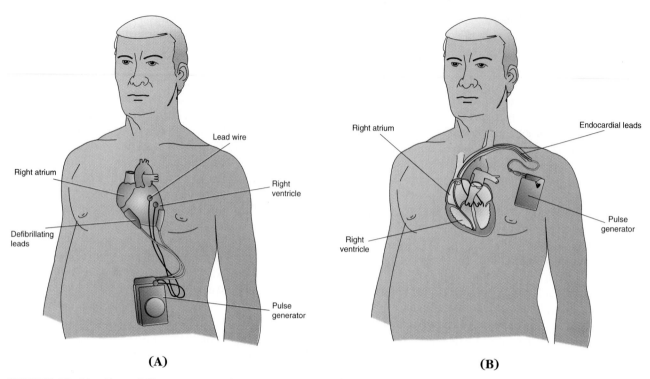

(A)   **(B)**

FIGURE 20-11   Two different types of automatic implantable cardioverter-defibrillators (AICD). **(A)** AICD has pulse generator implanted in the subcutaneous tissue of the abdomen with lead wires and a defibrillating lead going to the heart. **(B)** AICD with pulse generator implanted below the collarbone with endocardial leads positioned in the heart through a vein.

▶ Atrioventricular Blocks

In atrioventricular blocks the electrical conduction is interrupted to some degree between the atria and ventricles at the AV node. The extent of interruption is classified as first degree, second degree, or third degree.

First Degree AV Block   In first degree block the impulse is delayed in traveling through the AV node. The impulse eventually reaches the ventricles, but is delayed. On the EKG the PR interval is longer than 0.02 seconds (see Figure 20-14). There are no physical symptoms or treatment for first degree block.

Second Degree AV Block   In second degree block some of the impulses pass through the AV node to the ventricles and others are blocked. When the impulse is blocked, the EKG reveals an extended PR interval that is not followed by a QRS complex. There are two types of second degree blocks, type I (Wenckebach or Mobitz I) and type II (Mobitz II). Type I AV block is usually caused by a drug toxicity and is treated by withholding the drug. Type I may also occur with an acute inferior wall myocardial infarction. Type II is more serious than type I and indicates a blockage in the conduction in the bundle of His or the bundle branches (see Figure 20-15). Type II block occurs most often in clients with an acute anterior septal wall myocardial infarction and may be followed by third degree AV block. A temporary pacemaker may be

inserted until the conduction pattern is stabilized. If the dysrhythmia persists a permanent pacemaker may be implanted. Symptoms include irregular pulse, vertigo, and weakness.

Third Degree AV Block   Third degree heart block is when no impulses are able to pass from the atria through the AV node to the ventricles. The atria and ventricles beat independently of each other. The P waves and QRS complexes on the EKG have no relationship to each other (Figure 20-16). The causes of third degree block are myocardial ischemia, drug toxicity, and electrolyte imbalances. Atropine sulfate may be given to improve conduction through the AV node. A permanent pacemaker is usually required to control the dysrhythmia.

A pacemaker is a battery-operated device that stimulates the myocardium to contract. It consists of one or two lead wires that are attached to the endocardium or epicardium of the right atrium, right ventricle, or both, and a pulse generator. The purpose is to regulate the heart rate and increase cardiac output. Pacemakers are used for bradycardia, tachycardia, myocardial infarction, and heart block.

There are two types of pacemakers, temporary and permanent. The temporary pacemaker is used until a condition improves or until a permanent pacemaker is inserted. With a temporary pacemaker, the pulse generator remains outside of the body. The permanent

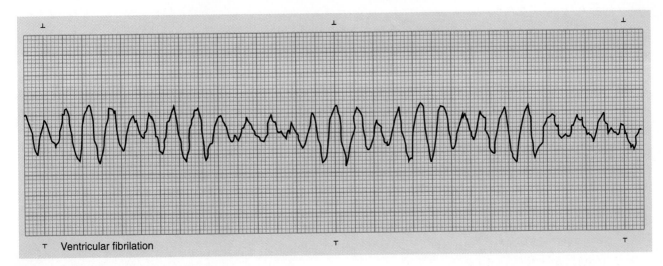

FIGURE 20-12 Ventricular fibrillation.

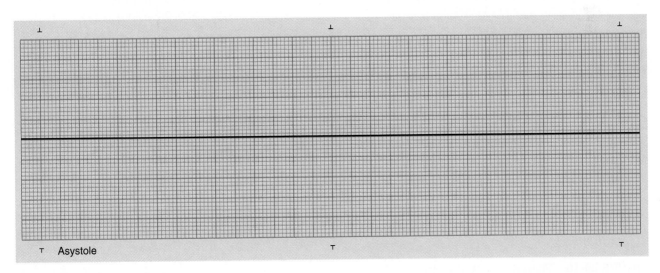

FIGURE 20-13 Asystole.

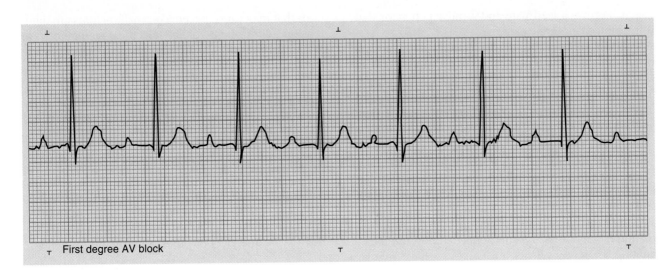

FIGURE 20-14 First degree AV block.

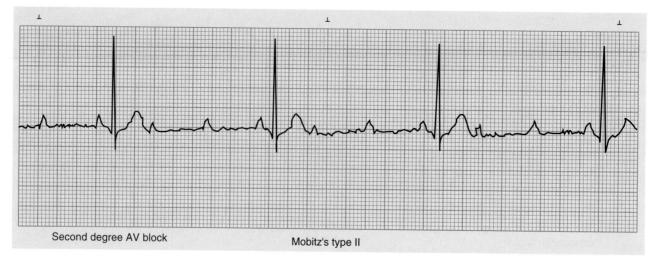

Second degree AV block   Mobitz's type II

FIGURE 20-15   Second degree AV block: Mobitz's type II.

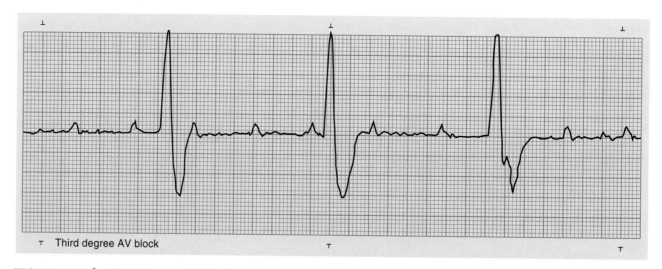

T Third degree AV block   T   T

FIGURE 20-16   Third degree AV block.

pacemaker has a lead wire and a pulse generator that is implanted under the skin.

Pacemakers are also transcutaneous, transvenous, or implantable. The transcutaneous pacemaker has an electrode placed on the skin and delivers the stimuli through the skin. A transvenous pacemaker has a wire that is threaded through a vein into the heart. The implantable pacemaker has wires threaded through a vein to the heart and the pulse generator is implanted subcutaneously, usually under the right clavicle.

An EKG of a client with a pacemaker shows the impulse from the pulse generator by a pacemaker spike, a vertical line before each QRS on the EKG strip.

Before discharge, teach clients to take accurate apical and radial pulses. Inform clients to report dizziness, fainting, or fever. Clients are taught to have regular pacemaker checks or transtelephonic monitoring in which an EKG strip is sent by phone to a designated hospital. The client should wear a medical identification tag indicating the presence of a pacemaker. Situa-

tions that may cause pacemaker malfunctions are high-tension wires, high-voltage electrical generators, or MRIs. The client should also avoid contact sports. Pacemakers may activate airport security alarms.

▶ Medical/Surgical Management

▶ Pharmacological

Dysrhythmias originating in the atria are treated with a digitalis preparation while dysrhythmias originating in the ventricles are treated with lidocaine hydrochloride (Xylocaine HCl) or other antiarrhythmic agents.

▶ Diet

The client is usually placed on a low-fat, low-cholesterol diet. Caffeine consumption is restricted.

▶ *Nursing Process*

Assessment

Subjective Data Inquire if the client has experienced palpitations, lightheadness, nausea, dyspnea, anxiety, fatigue, or chest discomfort.

Objective Data If a client is experiencing dysrhythmias, check the heart rate, blood pressure, and respirations. While listening to the apical pulse and respirations, listen for abnormal heart sounds and monitor the breath sounds for crackles. The presence of crackles indicates the lungs are filling with fluid. Observe the skin for pallor and cyanosis. Urine output may decrease.

▼ ▼

Possible nursing diagnoses for a client with dysrhythmias may include:

Nursing Diagnoses	Goals	Nursing Interventions
▶ *Cardiac output, decreased, related to inadequate electrical conduction.*	The client will have adequate cardiac output.	Apply electrodes for telemetry monitoring. Balance activity with rest periods. Monitor the vital signs during activity and at rest. Listen to the apical pulse, especially noting rate and rhythm. Elevate the extremities so they are not in a dependent position. Perform cardiac resuscitation as needed.
▶ *Anxiety, related to fear of potential diagnosis, treatment regimen, and death.*	The client will relate fears of potential cardiac problems.	Care for the client in a calm, confident, and efficient manner. Remain with the client and explain procedures and treatments. Encourage client input regarding the care. Encourage the client to verbalize concerns about the dysrhythmia and potential future complications. Teach the client relaxation activities.
▶ *Knowledge deficit, related to electrical conduction of the heart and treatment methods.*	The client will describe electrical disorder and treatment methods.	Explain medication administration times, action, side effects, and symptoms that need reporting. Provide written instructions to the client and family. Explain symptoms of dysrhythmias such as fatigue, edema, palpitations, lightheadness, nausea, dyspnea, and anxiety. If a pacemaker is needed, explain the purpose, insertion procedures, and home care. Include the family in all the teaching sessions.

▶ *Evaluation*

Each goal must be evaluated to determine how it has been met by the client.

▲ ▲

INFLAMMATORY DISORDERS

▶ RHEUMATIC HEART DISEASE

Rheumatic heart disease is a complication from ineffective treatment of rheumatic fever. Rheumatic fever is a systemic inflammatory disease that occurs two to three weeks after an untreated pharyngitis caused by the group A *beta-hemolytic streptococcus*. Symptoms of rheumatic fever are a mild fever, polyarthritis, carditis, chorea, and a rash. The endocardium, myocardium, and epicardium can become inflamed with the most damage occurring in the mitral valve. The mitral valve becomes insufficient or stenosed because of adhesions on the chordae tendineae and valve leaflets. Mitral prolapse may result.

Once a person has had rheumatic fever they are more prone to having it again. It is treated with intravenous antibiotics, anti-inflammatory agents, corticosteroids, and strict bed rest. The main goal is to treat the inflammation, prevent cardiac complications, and prevent the recurrence of the disease. These clients are placed on prophylactic antibiotic therapy prior to dental procedures or invasive surgery.

▶ INFECTIVE ENDOCARDITIS

Infective endocarditis is an inflammation or infection of the inside lining of the heart, particularly the heart valves. The etiology of inflammatory endocarditis is a collagen-vascular disease or rheumatic fever. Infective endocarditis is caused by bacteria, fungi, or rickettsia. As the microorganisms invade the valves, they form fibrinous substances called vegetations. Vegetations cause scar tissue on the valves so they become hard and brittle and do not close properly. When the valve is incapable of holding the blood in the appropriate chamber, blood seeps into the next chamber. The valve is said to be insufficient. Sometimes the vegetations cause the valve flaps to grow together resulting in a narrowing of the opening. This is called a valvular stenosis. The mitral valve is more frequently affected than the other valves. When the mitral valve is affected it is termed mitral insufficiency or mitral stenosis.

Historically, rheumatic fever was the common cause of endocarditis. More recently, endocarditis is a risk factor for IV drug users, immunosuppressed clients, and clients with valvular heart disease.

The client with endocarditis will have a fever, heart murmur, splenomegaly, and petechiae on the conjunctiva, palate, buccal mucosa, and distal extremities. There are two forms of endocarditis: acute and subacute. Symptoms of acute endocarditis are elevated temperature, tachycardia, pallor, diaphoresis, and symptoms of a systemic infection, such as temperature of 103°F and shaking chills. Clients with subacute endocarditis have low-grade fever, malaise, weight loss, and anemia. Clients with both types of endocarditis may have murmurs and symptoms of congestive heart failure, such as dyspnea, peripheral edema, and pulmonary congestion.

Endocarditis is diagnosed by the client's history and symptoms. A **transesophageal echocardiography (TEE)** can confirm the diagnosis of endocarditis by allowing ultrasonic imaging of the cardiac structures through the esophagus. The erythrocyte sedimentation rate (ESR) and WBC are elevated. A blood culture and sensitivity is done to determine the causative organism and to determine the most effective antibiotic.

▶ Medical/Surgical Management

▶ Surgical

Surgical repair or replacement of a valve is done in severe cases.

▶ Pharmacological

Clients are treated with antibiotics intravenously. The antibiotics are usually continued for two to six weeks. The most commonly used antibiotics are penicillin V potassium (V-Cillin K), vancomycin hydrochloride (Vancocin) and gentamicin sulfate (Garamycin).

▶ Diet

The client is given a well-balanced nutritious diet to help his or her body fight the infection.

▶ Activity

The client is placed on bed rest to decrease the workload of the heart. A calm, quiet environment should be provided.

▶ Preventive Treatment

Clients who have previously had endocarditis or have a mitral valve prolapse are more prone to develop endocarditis. They should take antibiotics prophylactically before having dental work, genitourinary, or gastrointestinal invasive procedures. Clients prone to develop endocarditis should take amoxicillin trihydrate (Amoxil) one hour before the procedure and again after the procedure.

► Nursing Interventions

Administer oxygen as needed. Take the blood pressure and pulse before and after activity to monitor toleration. Assess apical pulse for rate and rhythm and listen to breath sounds for adventitious sounds. Balance activity with rest periods. If a client is on vancomycin hydrochloride (Vancocin) or gentamicin sulfate (Garamycin), monitor the BUN and creatinine levels as both of these drugs are nephrotoxic.

► MYOCARDITIS

Myocarditis is an inflammation of the myocardium of the heart. Lymphocytes and leukocytes invade the muscle fibers of the heart causing the chambers to enlarge and the muscle to weaken. This can lead to congestive heart failure. Myocarditis is caused by bacteria, viruses, fungi, or parasites. It can also be an autoimmune reaction such as in the conditions of rheumatic fever or lupus erythematosus. Usually the cause is a virus. Recently myocarditis has been more prevalent in clients with AIDS.

Acute myocarditis presents itself with flulike symptoms of fever, pharyngitis, myalgias, and gastrointestinal complications. The client will also have chest pain and should be monitored for signs of congestive heart failure. A **pericardial friction rub** is often heard if the pericardium becomes involved. The friction rub is a "squeaky" sound heard through the stethoscope when the two inflamed pericardial surfaces rub together with the contraction of the heart.

Myocarditis diagnostic symptoms are nonspecific. They include elevated ESR and elevated LDH, CK, and SGOT levels. The diagnosis of myocarditis can be confirmed with an endomyocardial biopsy.

► Medical/Surgical Management

► Pharmacological

Digitalis preparations are given to prevent congestive heart failure. Broad spectrum antibiotics are also given to fight the infection. Anti-inflammatory agents may be given to decrease the inflammation. Oxygen is administered as needed.

► Activity

The client is placed on bed rest. This decreases the workload of the heart.

► Nursing Interventions

Monitor for symptoms of congestive heart failure or pericarditis. The client is placed in a semi-Fowler's position. A quiet environment and frequent rest periods are important for the client. A pulse oximeter is applied to monitor oxygen saturation.

► PERICARDITIS

Normally there are 30–50 milliliters of fluid in the pericardial sac. The fluid lubricates the heart and allows it to move freely within the pericardium. Sometimes pericardial effusion will occur in which several milliliters of excess fluid will slowly develop within the pericardial space. If the fluid slowly accumulates, the sac will expand to accommodate the excess fluid. However, **cardiac tamponade** will result if the fluid rapidly increases and hinders the functioning of the ventricle. The S_1 and S_2 sounds are often muffled and hard to hear with fluid accumulation.

When the pericardium becomes inflamed, the condition is called pericarditis. Causative organisms are a virus, bacteria, fungus, or parasite. Inflammation can also occur from rheumatic or collagen-vascular conditions like systemic lupus erythematosus. The most common cause of pericarditis is idiopathic, meaning no known cause. Symptoms of pericarditis are precordial pain (pain on the anterior surface of the chest over the heart) and a pericardial friction rub. The pain may radiate to the neck, back, or abdomen and become worse when the client coughs or lies on his left side. If the client sits erect and leans forward, the pain is relieved.

With inflammation, scar tissue develops in the pericardial sac. Heart movement is limited by the scar tissue and cardiac failure results.

► Medical/Surgical Management

► Medical

A **pericardiocentesis** is done to aspirate the excess fluid from the pericardial sac. A needle is inserted through the chest wall into the pericardial space.

▶ Surgical

If fibrotic scar tissue in the pericardium hinders heart performance, a pericardiectomy or pericardial window may be done. Pericardiectomy is removal of the pericardium. When a pericardial window is done, a section of the parietal pericardium is cut and tacked back onto itself allowing fluid to escape from the pericardial sac.

▶ Pharmacological

Clients are given antipyretics, analgesics, and anti-inflammatory agents. The infection is combated with antibiotics. Clients may also be given a digitalis preparation and diuretics to improve the pumping action of the heart and decrease fluid retention.

▶ Nursing Interventions

Assess apical pulse and blood pressure. Monitor the EKG for dysrhythmias. Assess for signs of cardiac tamponade such as decreased pulse and blood pressure, muffled heart sounds, increased respirations, restlessness, and oliguria. Administer oxygen as needed. Assist the client to a position of comfort. Administer analgesics, antibiotics, and anti-inflammatory agents as ordered. Encourage the client to verbalize concerns and fears. Provide nursing care with confidence and a caring attitude.

▶ VALVULAR HEART DISEASES

Valvular heart disease occurs when the valves do not open and close properly. A thickening of the valve tissue, causing the valve opening to be narrow, is called valvular stenosis. Valvular insufficiency is the inability of the valve to close completely. When the valve does not close completely, blood leaks back into the chamber from which it was just pumped. This is called regurgitation (see Figure 20-17)

▶ Stenosis and Insufficiency

The definition, symptoms, diagnostic findings, medical management, and nursing interventions for various valve conditions are covered in Table 20-1.

▶ Medical/Surgical Management

▶ Medical

Clients with valvular heart disease are to take antibiotics prophylactically before any dental procedures and genitourinary or gastrointestinal invasive procedures.

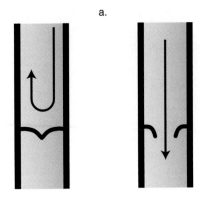
a.

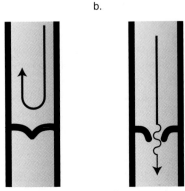
b.

Scar tissue thickens valve preventing it from opening the whole way

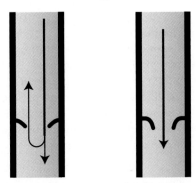
c.

Scar tissue causes the valve to harden and pull apart, preventing it from closing completely and allowing blood to leak backwards

FIGURE 20-17 **(A)** Normal valve. **(B)** Stenosed valve. **(C)** A leaking valve.

▶ Surgical

When the activities of a client with valvular heart disease become curtailed because of decreased cardiac output and the symptoms can no longer be controlled by medical means, surgery may be done. The type of

Table 20-1

MITRAL AND AORTIC VALVULAR STENOSIS AND INSUFFICIENCY

Valvular Condition	Definition	Symptoms	Diagnostic Findings	Med-Surg Management	Nursing Intervention
Mitral stenosis	The diseased valve becomes narrowed and the leaflets thickened preventing blood from freely flowing from the left atrium into the left ventricle.	Gradual onset of symptoms; exertional dyspnea, fatigue, orthopnea, paroxysmal nocturnal dyspnea, murmur. **Later symptoms:** peripheral edema, atrial fibrillation, jugular venous distention, hepatomegaly, abdominal distention, hypotension, thrombus from blood pooling in the left atrium.	**Chest x-ray:** hypertrophy and enlargement of left atrium and right ventricle. **EKG:** atrial fibrillation. **Echocardiogram:** fusion of valve leaflets, enlarged left atrium, decreased blood flow through valve.	**Medical management:** diuretics, digitalis, anticoagulants antidysrhythmics, prophylactic antibiotics for invasive procedures, low-sodium diet, semi-Fowler's position, activity restrictions as needed. **Surgical management:** commissurotomy, percutaneous balloon mitral valvuloplasty, mitral valve replacement.	Encourage rest periods, administer oxygen, elevate head of bed, reposition frequently to decrease pressure points, elevate legs, low-sodium diet, monitor for signs of right and left-sided heart failure, teach stress reduction techniques, daily weight.
Mitral insufficiency	The valve leaflets become hard and do not close completely. Blood backs up in both the left atria and ventricle causing both chambers to hypertrophy.	Gradual onset of symptoms: exertional dyspnea, palpitations, fatigue, atrial fibrillation, loud murmur and gallop.	**Chest x-ray:** hypertrophy and enlargement of left atrium and left ventricle. **EKG:** atrial fibrillation.	**Medical management:** same as mitral stenosis. **Surgical management:** valvuloplasty, mitral value replacement.	Same as mitral stenosis, teach exercise modification.
Aortic stenosis	The valve cusps become hard and calcify due to rheumatic fever, syphilis, a congenital anomaly, or the aging process	Syncope, exertional dyspnea, arrhythmias, angina, murmur, and gallop, sudden death may occur. **Later symptoms as the disease progresses:** paroxysmal atrial tachycardia orthopnea.	**Chest x-ray:** enlargement of left ventricle, calcification of aortic valve. **EKG:** hypertrophy of left ventricle inverted T wave echocardiogram fusion of valve leaflets, regurgitation	**Medical management:** same as mitral stenosis. **Surgical management:** percutaneous balloon aortic valvuloplasty, aortic valve replacement.	Same as mitral stenosis.
Aortic insufficiency	The valve cusps become so hardened they do not close completely. The blood no longer flows through the vessel but backs up into the left ventricle.	Palpitations, chest pain, exertional dyspnea, nocturnal angina, dizziness, fatigue, decreased activity, intolerance, paroxysmal nocturnal dyspnea, visible pulsation of the neck veins, murmur, lung congestion.	**Chest x-ray:** hypertrophy and enlargement of left ventricle.	**Medical management:** same as mitral stenosis. **Surgical management:** aortic valve replacement.	Same as mitral stenosis, teach exercise modification.

surgery performed will depend on the client's overall condition and on the involved valve.

For the mitral valve, surgery alleviates the symptoms, but it does not cure the condition. Surgeries frequently have to be repeated. A commissurotomy is done for mitral stenosis. In this surgery the valve leaflets are surgically separated. For mitral regurgitation or insufficiency, a valvuloplasty is becoming the treatment of choice. A percutaneous mitral valvuloplasty is a repair of perforated cusps or torn chordae tendineae. The risk of a thrombus is less with valvuloplasty than with grafts or prosthetic valves. An annuloplasty, a repair of the **annulus** or valvular ring, can also be done. The annulus is tightened with a purse-string suture or an annular ring. The mitral valve is replaced when other repair measures are not feasible.

Aortic valves are not repaired and are only replaced if the symptoms cannot be controlled by medical means. The preferred treatment for a client with an aortic stenosis is percutaneous aortic valvuloplasty. This treatment is often used in elderly or high risk surgical clients. A **percutaneous balloon valvuloplasty** can be done in the cardiac catheterization laboratory and no anesthesia is required. A catheter is advanced to the affected valve and a balloon is inflated in the stenosed valve. The narrowed valvular space is expanded by the balloon leaving a wider opening. Later, larger balloons may be used to expand the opening as needed.

There are two types of replacement valves: mechanical and biological. The mechanical valves are the caged-ball valve or the tilting-disk valve (see Figure 20-18). There is a higher risk of a thromboembolism with a caged-ball valve. Clients remain on anticoagulant therapy with both types of valves. The biological valves come from calves, pigs, or humans. The disadvantage of the biological valves is tissue degeneration and calcification of the valve.

▶ Mitral Valve Prolapse

Mitral valve prolapse is an extension of mitral insufficiency in which the valve leaflets, chordae tendineae, and papillary muscle become damaged. The valve leaflets flip back into the left atrium when the left ventricle contracts. This condition affects more women then men. Often the client remains asymptomatic. The symptoms that a client may experience depends on how seriously the mitral valve is affected. Sometimes they may experience palpitations and fatigue due to a decreased cardiac output. They also may experience angina, dizziness, and syncope. Some clients have panic attacks. Often a click or murmur can be heard.

▶ Nursing Process

▶ Assessment

Subjective Data Review past medical history for conditions such as rheumatic fever or streptococcal infections. Inquire if the client has experienced any dyspnea, palpitations, fatigue, cough, lightheadedness, or numbness and tingling in the extremities.

Objective Data Take the vitals signs and listen to the apical pulse for rate, rhythm, murmurs, and S_3 sounds. Listen to the breath sound for adventitious sounds. Check for edema, jugular distention, and cyanosis. Check equality of peripheral pulses and do a Homan's sign as dysrhythmias may produce clots.

▼ ▼

Possible nursing diagnoses for a client with cardiac valvular disorders may include:

Nursing Diagnoses	Goals	Nursing Interventions
▶ Cardiac output, decreased, related to structural changes in valves.	The client will have increased cardiac output.	Administer oxygen as needed. Balance activities with rest periods. The pulse should return to the baseline pulse within ten minutes of activity. If it does not, it is an indication of excessive activity. Discourage smoking and refer clients to support groups to assist them to stop smoking. Encourage the use of Nicoderm or Nicorette gum while attempting to stop smoking if ordered by the physician.

(continued)

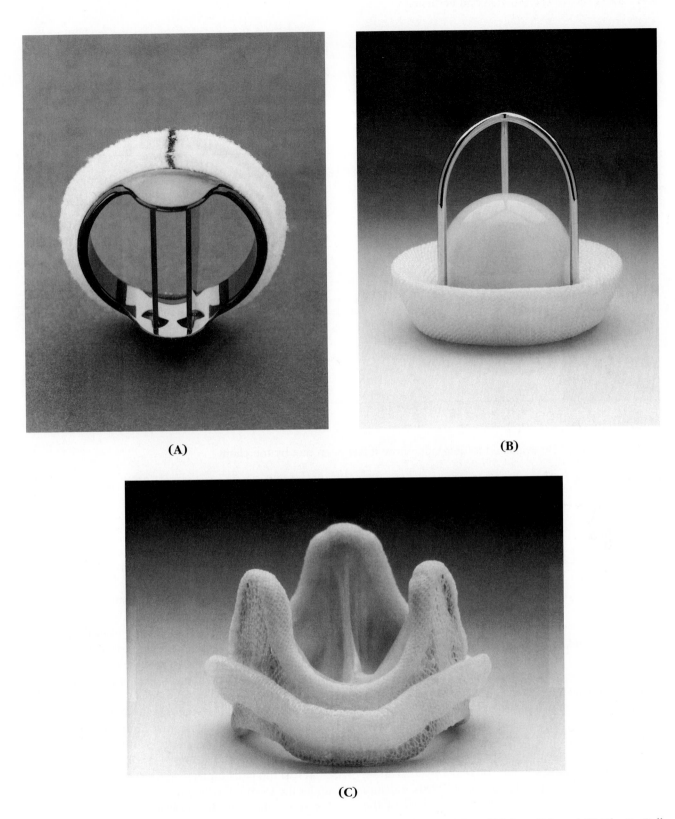

FIGURE 20-18 Types of artificial valves. **(A)** St. Jude® Mechanical Heart Valve; **(B)** Starr-Edwards™ Silastic Ball Valve, Model 1260 Aortic; **(C)** Carpentier-Edwards® Bioprosthesis, Model 2625 Aortic. (*A. Courtesy of St. Jude Medical, Inc. All Rights Reserved; B and C Courtesy of Baxter Healthcare Corporation, Edwards CVS Division*)

Nursing Diagnoses	Goals	Nursing Interventions
▶ *Fluid volume excess, related to decreased cardiac output.*	The client will have no edema.	Administer diuretics as needed.
		Support the extremities and do not let them be in a dependent position.
		Encourage the client to maintain a low-sodium diet.
▶ *Anxiety, related to fear of diagnosis and potential life changes.*	The client will list ways to cope with stressors.	Calmly explain the procedures before doing them.
		Encourage the client's input to decisions regarding care.
		Assist the client and the client's family in identifying ways to cope with stressors.
		Teach relaxation techniques.
▶ *Knowledge deficit, related disease process and treatment.*	The client will relate the disease process and needed self-care management.	Explain the valvular disease process, medication actions, dosage times, and medication side effects to report.
		Refer the client and family members to the dietitian for low-sodium diet instructions.
		Encourage the client to begin an appropriate exercise program.

▶ *Evaluation*

Each goal must be evaluated to determine how it has been met by the client.

▲ ▲

▶ *OCCLUSIVE DISORDERS*

▶ *ARTERIOSCLEROSIS*

Arteriosclerosis is a vascular narrowing and hardening of arteries. A buildup of lipids, collagen, and smooth muscle cells narrows the inner lining of the vessel (Sommers, 1994). Blood flow through the vessel is decreased causing decreased perfusion to body cells beyond the narrowed or hardened area.

There are three types of arteriosclerosis: atherosclerosis, calcific sclerosis, and arteriolar sclerosis (Sommers, 1994). **Atherosclerosis** is a fatty deposit on the inner lining, the tunica intima, of vessel walls. The fat deposit is called plaque. In calcific sclerosis, calcium deposits are on the middle layer of the wall of the arteries, the tunica media. Hypertension causes a thickening of the arterioles and is called arteriolar sclerosis. With these conditions, vessels lose their elasticity resulting in various conditions, such as arteriosclerotic heart disease, angina, myocardial infarction, stroke, and peripheral vascular disease.

▶ *ANGINA PECTORIS*

When coronary arteries lose elasticity or become narrow due to plaque collection, the heart muscle receives less blood and oxygen. Physical exertion, emotional stress, smoking, exposure to extreme cold, heavy meals, or an arterial spasm may cause a temporary inadequate blood and oxygen supply to the heart. Myocardial ischemia and angina pectoris result. Myocardial ischemia is a temporary inadequate blood and oxygen supply to the myocardial tissues. When this temporary condition occurs, the person experiences chest pain or **angina pectoris** (angina).

At first the person may experience a squeezing pain under the sternum, which radiates to the left shoulder. For some, the pain may radiate to the right shoulder, jaw, or ear. The discomfort may vary from a mild discomfort to an immobilizing pain. Anginal attacks usually increase in frequency and severity over time. The severity of the condition depends on the amount of collateral circulation that has developed.

Collateral circulation develops as larger vessels

gradually narrow or harden. Blood that normally passes through the larger vessels is shunted into surrounding smaller vessels. These vessels enlarge in an attempt to supply blood to the affected area. Collateral circulation increases the blood supply to tissues that suffer from an inadequate blood supply.

Hicks (1994) states that 70 percent of people experiencing ischemic attacks do not experience angina. These people may be having a silent myocardial infarct or ischemia. Symptoms indicative of silent ischemia are chest pressure or heaviness, restlessness, shortness of breath with increased respiratory rate, a sensation of epigastric fullness with noisy belching, numbness or tingling in both arms or shoulders, physical or mental fatigue, and dizziness. The person may also experience a change in sleep patterns and mental alertness. The person may state that he "feels funny."

According to Hicks (1994), researchers are not sure why some clients do not experience pain with silent ischemia and MI. Some possibilities that have been proposed are some people have decreased or altered pain perception. These people may culturally be able to endure more pain, or have higher levels of endorphins that diminish pain sensations, or previously had an MI or cardiac surgery, or be denying any sensation of myocardial pain.

Two other types of angina are unstable angina and Prinzmetal's angina. Unstable angina occurs at rest or with minimal exertion and is not relieved with nitroglycerin. This client is more susceptible to myocardial infarction and sudden death. Prinzmetal's angina is caused by a coronary artery spasm and occurs at rest.

The diagnosis of angina is made after reviewing the client's history, lifestyle, laboratory tests, and stress tests. Cholesterol, low-density lipoprotein (LDL), and high-density lipoprotein (HDL) levels are evaluated. Angina pectoris can be diagnosed by a stress test, thallium scans, or a coronary arteriogram. During a stress test, the heart is placed under stress through increasing physical activity on a treadmill or exercise bicycle. The increased oxygen demand of the body puts an extra load on the heart causing electrocardiogram changes and sometimes pain. Thallium and multi-gated acquisition scanning (MUGA) scans evaluate the blood supply to the myocardial tissue and determine how well the left ventricle is functioning. A coronary arteriogram shows a narrowing or occlusion of the vessels of the heart.

Angina frequently occurs in men over fifty. There is a high incidence of angina pectoris in clients with hypertension and diabetes mellitus.

Medical/Surgical Management

▶ Medical

Treatment for angina includes measures to increase the blood supply to the affected area. This can be accomplished by rest and vasodilation medications.

Silent ischemia is treated in the same way symptomatic ischemia is treated. The client needs to be educated about cardiac risk factors, the importance of following the prescribed medical regime, and maintaining regular physical check-ups.

▶ Surgical

A percutaneous transluminal coronary angioplasty (PTCA) may be done if only one coronary artery is involved and if the atherosclerotic material is small and has not hardened. When a PTCA is done, atherosclerotic matter is pressed against the walls of the coronary vessels to improve circulation to myocardial tissue supplied by that coronary artery (see Figure 20-19). A guide wire is inserted to the stenosed area and a special balloon-tipped catheter is placed in the narrowed sclerotic area. When the balloon is inflated, the atherosclerotic material is pressed against the wall of the vessel. The vessel, now open, allows more blood to flow to the myocardial tissue. During this procedure, a piece of the atherosclerotic material may break off and occlude the vessel. If this occurs, the client would have to undergo immediate coronary bypass surgery. Other complications of the procedure are occlusion of the vessel because of a vascular spasm or vessel rupture.

An intracoronary **stent** may be implanted into a stenosed vessel to prevent the vessel from collapsing and to keep the atherosclerotic plaque pressed against the vessel wall. A stent is a tiny metal tube with holes in it (see Figure 20-20). The procedure is sometimes done when a vessel collapses after a PTCA or in place of a PTCA. The stent is tightly wrapped around a balloon catheter. When the balloon catheter has been threaded through a vessel to the stenosed area, the balloon is inflated and the stent expands and presses the plaque against the vessel wall. The stent remains in the vessel and the catheter is withdrawn.

Sometimes a transcatheter ablation is done to break up the atherosclerotic areas with a laser. The sclerotic material is broken into pieces smaller than blood cells and excreted through the kidneys.

With a coronary atherectomy, an atherectomy catheter is inserted into the affected coronary vessel to the atheroma (fatty deposit in the vessel wall). The cut-

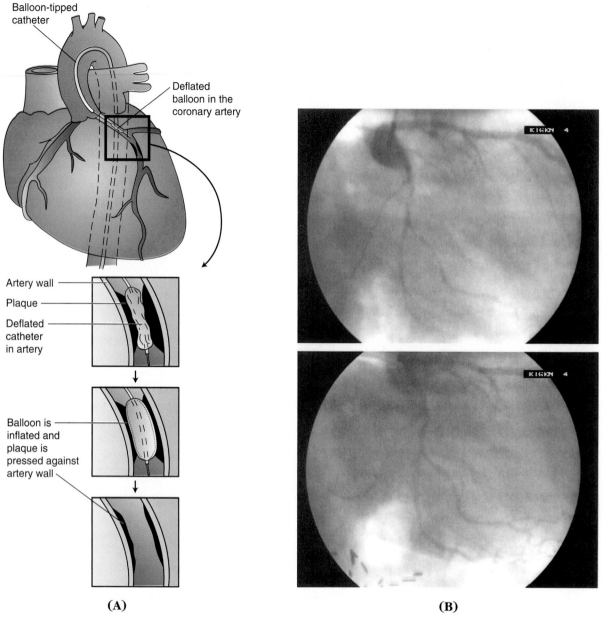

(A)   **(B)**

FIGURE 20-19 **(A)** Demonstration of the function of a balloon-tipped catheter during a percutaneous transluminal coronary angioplasty procedure. **(B)** X-ray of an angioplasty showing a blocked artery and revascularization of the vessel after the angioplasty. (*Courtesy Ken Hicks, Fort Wayne, IN*)

ter on the catheter shaves the plaque from the wall of the vessel (see Figure 20-21). Depending on the type of catheter, the shavings may be saved in the end of the catheter, suctioned out or shaved so small they pass through the capillary circulation without damage to the body.

If a coronary artery bypass is done, the internal mammary artery, the saphenous vein, or an accordion type of synthetic graft material is used. The vein or synthetic material is grafted to the aorta and passed beyond the obstruction in the coronary vessel (see Fig-

ure 20-22). The graft provides an increased blood supply to the affected myocardium. The client then experiences reduced angina and has an increased tolerance for activities.

▶ *Pharmacological*

Vasodilators, such as nitroglycerin tablets, cause the blood vessels to dilate thus providing an increased blood supply to body tissues. The client may not need as much analgesic medication if beta-blockers are

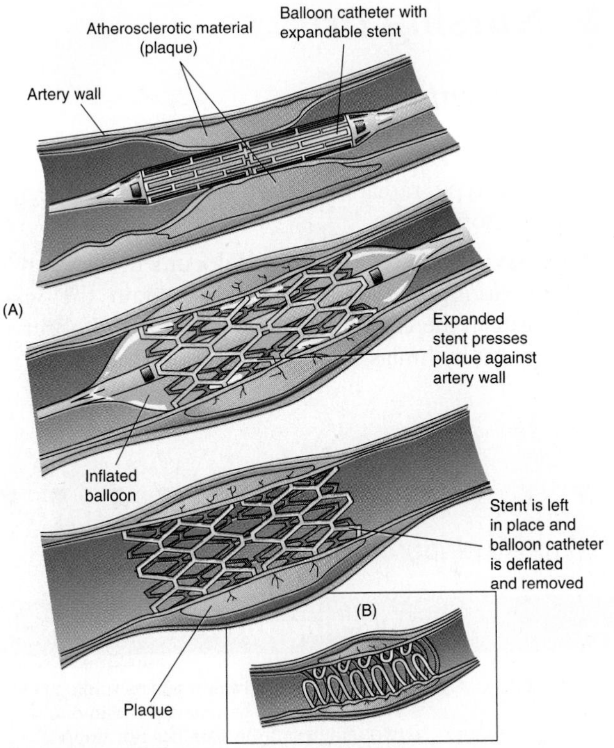

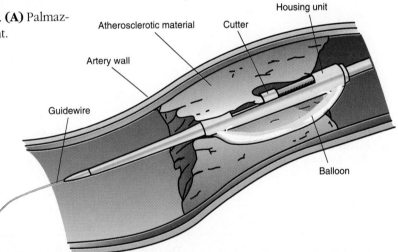

FIGURE 20-20 Placement of stent in artery. (A) Palmaz-Schatz stent. (B) Gianturco-Roubin ex-Stent.

given. Beta-adrenergic blockers and calcium channel blockers slow the heart rate and decrease the oxygen demand of the heart. Calcium channel blockers also dilate vessels and decrease spasms of the coronary vessels. All these measures provide an increased blood supply to the myocardium.

▶ Diet

The client is placed on a low-fat, low-cholesterol, salt-restricted diet. Sodium restriction may vary from no salt to 4 grams daily depending on the ability of the client's kidneys to excrete excess sodium.

▶ Activity

Rest decreases the oxygen demands of the body so the heart does not have to work as hard to meet the body needs, therefore, the blood supply requirements of the heart are decreased.

FIGURE 20-21 The Simpson Coronary AtheroCath cuts the atherosclerotic material (plaque) away from the artery wall.

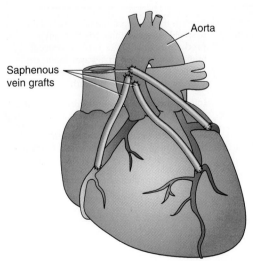

FIGURE 20-22 Coronary artery bypass with a saphenous vein.

▶ *Preventive Treatment*

To prevent coronary artery disease resulting in angina, it is recommended that a person limit fat intake to 30 grams or less per day and exercise three to five times a week for at least twenty minutes. Simple activities such as parking a car a farther distance from an entrance to increase walking distance, or taking the stairs instead of the elevator improves circulation and helps decrease cholesterol levels. Activities such as gardening or housework are also good.

▶ *Nursing Process*

Assessment

Subjective Data   Ask the client to describe the pain as to type, radiation, onset, duration, and precipitating factors.

Objective Data   Observe and document the client's actions during the anginal attack. Obtain the vital signs. Attach the client to an EKG monitor and observe for any dysrhythmias.

▼ ▼

Possible nursing diagnoses for a client with angina may include:

Nursing Diagnoses	Goals	Nursing Interventions
▶ *Pain related to decreased oxygen supply to the myocardium.*	The client will experience decreased episodes of angina.	Administer nitroglycerin tablets sublingually. The pain should be relieved within one to two minutes. If the pain has not stopped after three doses five minutes apart, notify the emergency personnel.
		Once the acute situation is over, administer nitroglycerin as ordered. It is supplied in ointment, transdermal patch, and extended-release capsules.
		Administer other medication such as beta blockers or calcium channel blockers as ordered.
▶ *Anxiety related to perceived threat of death or change in lifestyle.*	The client will relate concerns and practice stress reduction techniques.	Assist the client in learning to decrease personal expectations and live within personal activity limitations.
		Emphasize the importance of getting adequate rest and stopping before becoming too exhausted.
▶ *Knowledge deficit related to disease process, medications and treatment regimen.*	The client will explain the disease process, medication actions, dosage times and side effects, and self-care practices.	Explain the cause of angina. Teach the client to avoid stressful situations that may produce angina. Other ways to prevent angina are to sleep in a warm room, eat smaller proportions at mealtimes, and not exercise outside in cold weather.
		Inform the client to carry nitroglycerin at all times in a tightly closed container.
		Nitroglycerin may cause orthostatic hypotension, so inform the client to change positions slowly after taking the medication.
		Encourage the client to start and maintain a regular exercise program as recommended by the physician.

▶ *Evaluation*

Each goal must be evaluated to determine how it has been met by the client.

▲ ▲

Sample Nursing Care Plan: The Client Scheduled for a Cardiac Catheterization

Todd Taylor, a forty-year-old white male, is the vice-president of a small company. He has been working long hours and been under pressure to close an account with a local firm. He smokes a pack of cigarettes a day and often eats fast foods on the run. Recently, he has been experiencing chest pressure, numbness and tingling in both arms and has become dizzy twice when climbing stairs. After receiving a call from his boss firmly urging him to get the account settled this week, he suddenly experienced a severe squeezing pain in his chest that lasted a minute or so. The pain was severe enough to make him stop working. When he met his wife for lunch and related the story to her, she urged him to see their doctor. He finally agreed after much persuasion. When his doctor was notified of the symptoms Todd was having, she scheduled him for a cardiac catheterization. Todd and his wife, Sherry, are both anxious about the test. Todd asked the nurse how long it would take to do the procedure and how long it would be before they would get the results. Sherry asked the nurse to explain how this procedure is done.

Nursing Diagnosis 1 Anxiety related to fear of cardiac catheterization results as evidenced by anxious behavior and asking questions about the procedure.

Goals	Nursing Interventions	Rationale	Evaluation
Todd will relate concerns about the procedure to his wife and the nurse caring for him.	Encourage Todd and Sherry to share their concerns about the procedure.	Only expressed concerns can be alleviated.	Todd shared his concerns about the cardiac catheterization with his wife and nursing personnel.
	Allay fears by giving appropriate explanations.	Explaining how the procedure is done will prepare Todd and Sherry for the procedure and make them have more of a sense of control.	
	Offer to call the chaplain, their pastor, or priest.	Increases Todd and Sherry's support system.	

Nursing Diagnosis 2 Knowledge deficit related to cardiac catheterization procedure as evidenced by asking the nursing personnel questions about the procedure.

Goals	Nursing Interventions	Rationale	Evaluation
Todd will explain the purpose of the exam, how the procedure is done and his responsibilities concerning the procedure.	Explain the purpose of the cardiac catheterization in terms Todd and his wife can understand.	Increases their understanding of the procedure and decreases their anxiety.	Todd related the purpose of the exam, how it was done, and his responsibilities before the exam.
	Explain how a cardiac catheterization is done and provide a video if available.	Provides verbal and visual explanation of the cardiac catheterization procedure and offers opportunity to clarify questions Todd and Sherry may have.	

▶ *MYOCARDIAL INFARCTION*

A myocardial infarction (MI) is the leading cause for sudden death in men and women (Sommers, 1994). According to Goldman (1994), 40 to 50 percent of MI clients die in the first twenty days. In the United States 650,000 persons die each year from myocardial infarctions. The most common cause for myocardial infarction is atherosclerosis.

A myocardial infarction is caused by an obstruction in a coronary artery resulting in necrosis (death) to the tissues supplied by the artery. The obstruction is usually due to atherosclerotic plaque, a thrombus, or an embolism. The area most commonly affected is the left ventricle.

Obstruction of a large coronary artery damages the myocardial tissue and affects the pumping efficiency of the heart. A client's prognosis is better if a small coronary artery or arteriole is obstructed and there is good collateral circulation to the heart. If a large vessel is obstructed and the client does not have sufficient collateral circulation, the client may die immediately.

The typical symptoms of an MI are feelings of chest heaviness or tightness that progresses to a severe gripping pain in the lower sternal area. The pain is not relieved by rest or nitroglycerin. The client becomes short of breath (dyspneic), diaphoretic, and anxious. Frequently the client becomes nauseated and vomits. The pulse will be irregular, rapid, and weak and the blood pressure will be low. The skin will be pale and then turn cyanotic.

According to Hicks (1994), half of the people who have an MI do not experience the typical symptoms of an MI and may not notice or experience any symptoms. An EKG confirms that a person has experienced a silent MI. There will be an abnormal Q wave that is more than 1 mm wide and is one-third to one-fourth the height of the R wave. The abnormal Q wave may last for months or years and then disappear. If a person experiences mild symptoms of a silent MI, the MI could go undetected for years or forever.

Even though a person may not experience the typical MI symptoms, the condition can still be serious or fatal. Complications such as heart failure and stroke may also occur.

When the right coronary artery and the branches supplying the posterior area of the heart are affected, it is referred to as a posterior myocardial infarction. The right coronary artery is involved in 30 to 40 percent of the cases. An anterior myocardial infarction or anteroseptal myocardial infarction involves the left coronary artery and branches affecting the anterior and upper section of the left ventricle. The left anterior descending (LAD) artery is involved in 40 to 50 percent of the cases (Goldman, 1994). Branches of the LAD artery affect the septum. A transmural infarction extends through the entire thickness of the myocardium.

A myocardial infarction can be diagnosed by client symptoms, electrocardiogram tracings, cardiac enzyme values, and a radioactive isotope scan. When an MI is evolving, the EKG would have an elevated ST segment which eventually changes into an inverted T wave. Cardiac enzymes are creatine kinase (CK) or creatine phosphokinase (CPK), lactic dehydrogenase (LDH), and aspartate aminotransferase (AST), previously known as serum glutamic oxaloacetic transaminase (SGOT). The pattern of the rising and falling values of CK, LDH, and AST are significant in diagnosing a myocardial infarction. The CK level rises within three to six hours of the infarct, peaks within twelve to eighteen hours, and returns to normal in three days. The higher the CK level rises the greater the damage to the heart and the longer the level peaks the more serious the prognosis. AST value increases in six hours, peaks in twelve to fourteen hours and returns to normal in three to four days. LDH level peaks in seventy-two hours and slowly returns to normal in eleven to fourteen days. The CK and LDH enzymes can be broken down into isoenzyme (a fragment of an enzyme) fractions of the total values of CK and LDH. A CK-MB fraction, which measures an isoenzyme specific to the cardiac muscle, rises in three to six hours of the onset of a myocardial infarct, peaks in eighteen to twenty-four hours and returns to normal in seventy-two hours. CK studies are done as soon as the client is admitted and every eight hours until four samples have been obtained. A CK-MB fraction above 5 percent indicates myocardial damage. LDH isoenzymes, LDH_1 and LDH_2, are also specific to heart muscle. LDH studies are done on admission and every eight to twelve hours for twenty-four hours. According to Olbrych (1993), the LDH_1 value rises higher than the LDH_2 value within twelve to forty-eight hours in 80 percent of clients after an MI. This is called the "LDH flip." An LDH_1 of more than 40 percent is indicative of myocardial damage.

During the first three days after the infarction, the client may have a low-grade fever and an increased white cell count. The infarcted heart tissue is soft and necrotic. It is incapable of responding to electrical stimuli. Life-threatening dysrhythmias are most likely to occur at this time. Four to seven days after the infarction, the infarcted tissue is at the softest and weakest. An aneurysm, or ballooning effect, can occur on the wall of the ventricle with the potential of rupturing at this time. There is a possibility of the ventricle rupturing from the time of the infarct to two weeks after the infarct. Collateral circulation begins forming around the edges of the infarct but it will be two to three weeks before the collateral circulation will function effectively. Two to three months will pass before the heart muscle will regain maximum strength.

▶ Medical/Surgical Management

▶ Medical

Medical/surgical management focuses on reducing the workload of the heart, relieving pain, improving tissue perfusion, preventing complications, and further tissue damage. Immediately after an MI, a client is admitted into a coronary care unit. The client's heart is constantly monitored for dysrhythmias. The client's vital signs are monitored by an arterial line for hemo-dynamic monitoring or a noninvasive blood pressure monitoring system (Sommers, 1994).

Three dysrhythmias that may occur following an MI are ventricular fibrillation, bradycardias, and tachycardias. Ventricular fibrillation is treated by defibrillation. Atropine and, if needed, a temporary pacer may be inserted for bradycardias. Two tachycardias that may occur are atrial fibrillation and ventricular tachycardia. Atrial fibrillation is treated with digoxin (Lanoxin) or amiodarone hydrochloride (Cordarone). Ventricular tachycardia is treated with lidocaine or cardioversion. If dysrhythmias continue, magnesium may be given.

Medical complications that can occur following an MI are acute left ventricular failure, cardiogenic shock, pericarditis, embolism and/or thrombosis, and cardiac rupture. The health care team must closely monitor the client for signs of these complications.

▶ Pharmacological

Oxygen will be given by a Venturi mask or nasal cannula. Morphine sulfate is given intravenously to control the pain. Nitrates are also given intravenously or sublingually to relieve pain and dilate coronary arteries. Sedatives may be given to help calm and relax the client. Stool softeners are given to prevent straining with stools.

Thrombolytic therapy is sometimes used within three to six hours of the myocardial infarction to dissolve a clot blocking an artery. Medications such as streptokinase (Streptase), anistreplase (Eminase), and tissue plasminogen activator (Activase) are used. A possible complication from thrombolytic therapy is bleeding. Bleeding problems are rare but the nurse should be alert for symptoms of hemorrhaging in the gastrointestinal tract (hematemesis and tarry stools), retroperitoneum (low back pain and numbness in lower extremities), or cerebrum (headache, vomiting, and confusion).

▶ Diet

Fluids are usually offered during the acute stage as desired. When solid food is resumed, the client is placed on a low-calorie, low-cholesterol, salt-restricted diet. The client may tolerate small frequent feedings better than three large meals. Caffeine and extreme hot and cold foods are avoided.

▶ Activity

It is vital the client receive little stimuli to provide physical, mental, and emotional rest. The less stimuli the client receives, the less demands will be placed upon the heart. Procedures need to be explained in simple terms so the client will understand the care being provided by the health care team.

The client is usually limited to bed rest during the first twenty-four hours and progressed to sitting in a chair by the second day. If pain returns or other complications occur, the client should be confined to bed rest. Early ambulation is encouraged to prevent thrombosis. During and after each activity, the client's tolerance is assessed by monitoring the heart rate for an increase of 20 beats/minute, checking for a decrease in systolic blood pressure, and observing for dyspnea and dysrhythmias. Verbal and nonverbal statements of fatigue and chest pain are assessed.

Before the client is dismissed, low-intensity exercise tests may be done to determine types of activities in which the client may engage at home. When the client is able to climb two flights of stairs, sexual activity may be resumed.

▶ Preventive Treatment

Two important measures that can be taken to prevent myocardial infarctions are exercise and diet. A regular aerobic exercise schedule of twenty to forty minutes three times a week is effective in increasing DLs, lowering cholesterol and LDL levels, and increasing collateral circulation. A diet of no more than 30 grams of fat a day helps prevent atherosclerosis.

▶ Nursing Process

Assessment

Subjective Data Inquire as to medications the client has taken including over-the-counter medications, anticoagulants, and thrombolytic medications. Assess the client's pain as to onset, duration, intensity, location, radiation, and precipitating factors. Ask client to describe the symptoms. Keep in mind that not all persons having angina or an MI will experience or state having pain. Some may describe feelings of chest heaviness, indigestion, or "something not right." Explore these statements with the client and have them explain their sensations in more detail.

Objective Data   The nurse's assessment will include vital signs, skin changes, breath sounds, and EKG rhythm strips. Monitor the vital signs for an irregular, decreased, or increased pulse or a decreased or elevated blood pressure. Watch for pallor, cyanosis, diaphoresis, or vomiting. Assess the client for cool clammy skin, numbness, tingling, or confusion which indicates decreased oxygenation of the tissues. Listen to the breath sounds for lung congestion. Monitor the EKG for dysrhythmias. Notice if the client is grimacing, clenching his hands, or clutching his chest. Watch closely for these symptoms as activities are increased. Inquire as to the client's ability to perform activities of daily living.

▼ ▼

Possible nursing diagnoses for a client with myocardial infarction may include:

Nursing Diagnoses	Goals	Nursing Interventions
▶ Cardiac output, decreased, related to damaged heart tissue.	The client will have increased cardiac output.	Encourage bed rest until the condition is stabilized. Administer oxygen per mask or nasal cannula at 2 to 4 liters per minute. Start an IV so medications such as morphine and antidysrhythmics can be administered. If beta-blockers are administered, the nurse should closely monitor for a drop in heart rate and blood pressure. Constantly monitor the client for dysrhythmias. Place a rhythm strip on the chart at least once a shift. Administer medications as prescribed by the physician.
▶ Pain, acute, chest, related to decreased oxygenation of myocardial tissue.	The client will verbalize decrease in frequency and intensity of chest pain.	Observe for verbal and nonverbal signs of pain such as grimacing, diaphoresis, or increased heart rate. Ask the client to rate the pain on a scale of 0 to 10, 0 being no pain and 10 extreme pain. Administer analgesics as ordered.
▶ Activity intolerance related to decreased circulation to body tissues.	The client will increase activities with decreased symptoms of angina, dyspnea, cyanosis, and dysrhythmia.	Place objects within reach of the client. Balance activity with rest periods. Assist the client and partner to discuss their fears and feelings candidly about resuming sexual activity.
▶ Anxiety, moderate, related to concern about disease process and future socioeconomic status.	The client will verbalize situations that are causing stress.	Encourage the family and client to verbalize their feelings. Provide a quiet, calm environment to relax the client and family. Provide the client with periods of uninterrupted rest. Administer sedatives to help the client relax. Since the myocardial client may be in denial, be aware of denial symptoms such as attempting to conduct business over the phone while hospitalized or statements that the pain is really nothing.

Nursing Diagnoses	Goals	Nursing Interventions
▶ Constipation, high risk for, related to opiate analgesics and bed rest.	The client will have soft bowel movements.	Administer stool softeners to prevent straining or bearing down with defecation.
		Provide privacy when the client is defecating. Use of a bedside commode may require less energy than using a bedpan.
		Encourage adequate fluid intake to prevent hard stools and offer fruit juices.
		Encourage the client to choose foods high in fiber.
▶ Knowledge deficit related to disease process, medications, diet, and plan for recovery.	The client will verbalize understanding of disease process, diet, activity, and medications.	Begin teaching at the moment of admission. Instruct the client to inform the nurse of any chest pain or shortness of breath.
		During hospitalization, teach the client about the anatomy and physiology of the heart, what physiologically happened to the heart to cause the myocardial infarction, importance of exercise, diet instructions, actions and side effects of medications, importance of not smoking, and stress reduction.

▶ Evaluation

Each goal must be evaluated to determine how it has been met by the client.

▲ ▲

▶ DECREASED FUNCTION AND FAILURE OF CARDIAC SYSTEM

▶ CONGESTIVE HEART FAILURE

Congestive heart failure (CHF) is often the final stage of many other heart conditions. A weakened muscle wall from a myocardial infarction or a heart that has been stressed over a period of time to meet metabolic needs of the body can cause congestive heart failure. Congestive heart failure develops when the heart is no longer capable of meeting the oxygen needs of the body. The heart is literally failing. The muscle of the left ventricle **hypertrophies** (increases in muscle mass) and often the ventricular chamber enlarges in an attempt to meet the oxygen needs of the body.

Both the right and left ventricles act as pumps. Each of these pumps can fail separately resulting in two types of heart failure: right-sided heart failure and left-sided heart failure. Heart failure usually begins on the left side. Some of the causes of right-sided failure are untreated left ventricular failure, right ventricular myocardial infarction, chronic obstructive coronary disease, cor pulmonale, and pulmonary valve stenosis. Left-sided failure is caused by left ventricular myocardial infarction, aortic valve stenosis, prolapsed valve complications, and hypertension. Notice that right- and left-sided failure are caused by a defect of the ventricle or an increased resistance ahead of the ventricle in the blood flow, causing an increased workload for the involved ventricle.

When left-sided heart failure occurs, the left ventricle is not able to completely empty of blood or effectively pump blood out through the aorta to the body systems. Usually the right ventricle continues to pump adequate quantities of blood. This causes blood to back up in the left ventricle, left atrium, and pulmonary veins. The lungs become congested with fluid as fluid leaks through the capillaries and fills air spaces in the lungs. The client becomes cyanotic, dyspneic, restless, and coughs up blood-tinged sputum. The breath sounds have moist crackles. Often the client has tachycardia with low blood pressure because the heart is not able to pump sufficient blood to meet the body's demands. The client may have decreased urinary output because enough blood is not being pumped through the kidneys. As the blood oxygen level decreases, the client becomes confused.

As the right side of the heart fails, blood becomes

congested in the inferior vena cava causing edema first in the extremities and then in the trunk of the body. As the condition progresses, the client experiences edema of the ankles, lower legs, thighs, and finally in the abdomen. The excess abdominal fluid causes the client to be anorectic. **Hepatomegaly** (enlargement of the liver) and splenomegaly (enlargement of the spleen) develop. The jugular veins in the neck become distended when the client is sitting or standing and pitting edema occurs in the lower extremities. Refer back to Figure 20-3. Oliguria occurs as decreased amounts of blood are pumped through the kidneys.

In the early stages of congestive heart failure, the client experiences fatigue, dyspnea with slight exertion, pedal edema, and a slight cough with a small amount of expectoration. The client may also have paroxysmal nocturnal dyspnea.

▶ *Medical/Surgical Management*

▶ *Medical*

Left-sided failure is diagnosed by a chest x-ray. The chest x-ray is done to directly visualize the left ventricle and check for evidence of lung congestion. The client's past medical history and present symptoms are evaluated. An EKG is done and arterial blood gases are evaluated. The client's oxygen saturation level is also monitored by pulse oximetry. Depending on the seriousness of the client's condition, a pulmonary artery catheter may be inserted to determine left ventricular function.

Right-sided failure is diagnosed with the same diagnostic exams as left-sided failure such as chest x-ray, EKG, arterial blood gases, and O_2 saturation monitoring. However, the symptoms of edema, hepatomegaly, and neck vein distention are significant diagnostic evidence.

▶ *Surgical*

Goals for treating congestive heart failure are to improve circulation to the coronary arteries and decrease the workload of the left ventricle. Two mechanical methods of doing this are the insertion of an intra-aortic balloon pump and the use of a ventricular assist device (VAD). An intra-aortic balloon is threaded through the femoral artery to the descending aorta (see Figure 20-23). The pump is synchronized with the contractions of the left ventricle so the balloon inflates during diastole and deflates during systole. Inflation of the balloon increases the blood flow to the coronary arteries, thus increasing oxygenation of the myocardium. Deflation of the balloon allows the

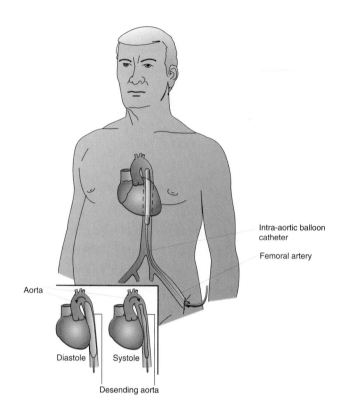

Intra-aortic balloon catheter

Femoral artery

Aorta

Diastole   Systole

Desending aorta

FIGURE 20-23 Intra-aortic ballon pump increases circulation to the coronary arteries and decreases the workload of the left ventricle.

left ventricle to pump blood to the body tissues with less peripheral resistance.

The left ventricular assist device has a cannula that takes blood from the left atrium to the aorta bypassing the ineffective left ventricle (see Figure 20-24). This gives the left ventricle time to rest and heal. The same process can be done for the right ventricle or both ventricles.

A surgical procedure for left ventricular failure is still in the experimental stages. It involves wrapping the latissimus dorsi muscle around the heart and stimulating it with electrical impulses (see Figure 20-25). The latissimus dorsi muscle assists the damaged ventricle in contracting and improves cardiac output. According to Bove (1995), three out of ten clients die within a year of this surgery and one in ten die on the operating table. Candidates for this surgery must have 40 percent of the left ventricle destroyed. Client's with pacemakers or AICDs are not able to have this surgery because the muscle wrap may damage the leads of the pacemaker or AICD or interfere with the placement of the leads to stimulate the latissimus dorsi muscle.

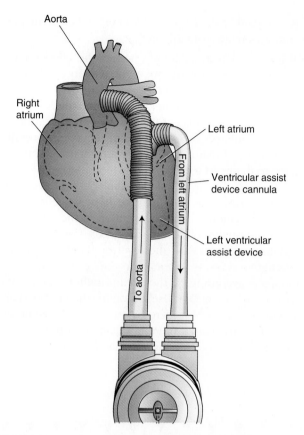

FIGURE 20-24 The cannula of a ventricular assist device takes blood from the left atrium to the aorta, bypassing the ineffective left ventricle.

► Pharmacological

The client with CHF will receive diuretics to decrease fluid retention and a digitalis preparation to increase the strength and contractility of the heart muscle. Vasodilators are given so the blood will stay in the peripheral vessels and not return to the heart, thereby decreasing the possibility of an overload on the heart. Morphine sulfate is given in the acute phase to control pain and decrease anxiety.

► Diet

A daily weight and strict intake and output is necessary to assess fluid volume. Sometimes fluid intake is limited. The client is generally on a low-sodium diet.

► Activity

Activity orders will depend on the client's activity tolerance. The client's activity may vary from strict bed rest to ambulation depending on the severity of the condition. Visitation privileges may be monitored to provide rest periods. According to Swearingen (1994), activity intolerance may be noted if the client's heart rate is above 120, respirations are above 20 and the blood pressure increases 20 mmHg from the resting blood pressure level.

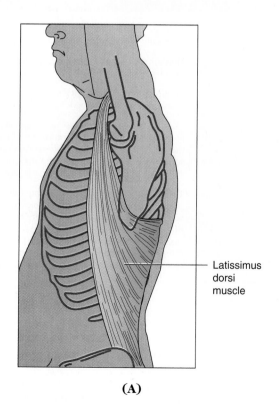

(A)

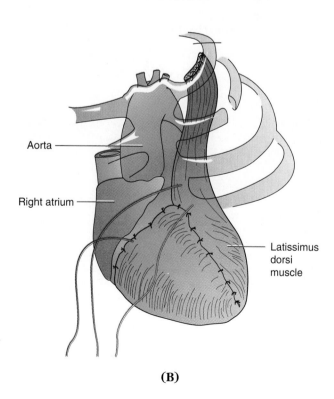

(B)

FIGURE 20-25 Cardiomyoplasty: the latissimus dorsi muscle is wrapped around the heart.

► *Preventive Treatment*

According to Sommers (1994), 50 to 75 percent of clients with CHF have coronary artery disease. The most common cause of CHF is left ventricular failure after a myocardial infarction. To prevent CHF following coronary artery disease, a diet low in fat, high in fiber, and balanced in caloric intake to maintain optimum weight is recommended. Stress reduction and a regular exercise program will also decrease the risk of developing CHF. Clients developing CHF from congenital heart defects may not be able to prevent the prognosis of CHF, but following the prescribed medical regimen may prevent the early development of CHF.

► *Nursing Process*

Assessment

Subjective Data   Inquire if the client has recently experienced more dyspnea, orthopnea, fatigue, anxi-ety, or pain. Ask if there has been difficulty in performing activities of daily living.

Objective Data   Carefully assess the client's level of consciousness to determine circulation of blood to the brain. Check skin color for cyanosis or pallor. Assess skin turgor to help determine the level of hydration. Jugular distention will give an indication of the functioning level of the right ventricle. Carefully listen to the breath sounds for adventitious sounds. Listen to the heart tones for normal or abnormal S_1 and S_2 sounds. If the client has CHF, an S_3 sound may also be heard. Bowel sounds may be hypoactive depending on the amount of fluid retention in the abdomen. Check the quality of peripheral pulses, skin color, and capillary refill to assess the level of circulation to the extremities. Assess edema in the extremities and abdomen according to the edema rating scale (refer back to Figure 20-3). Closely monitor the client's daily weight for possible increase from fluid retention. Notify the physician if there is a gain of more than two pounds in one day. Monitor I&O and especially watch for oliguria.

▼ ▼

Possible nursing diagnoses for a client with congestive heart failure may include:

Nursing Diagnoses	*Goals*	*Nursing Interventions*
► *Cardiac output, decreased, related to mechanical failure of heart muscle.*	The client's vital signs will remain stable.	Take an apical pulse on all cardiac clients, especially checking the rate and rhythm. Monitor the client's heart rate and rhythm by telemetry. Administer diuretics, digitalis, and vasodilators as prescribed. Closely monitor the electrolytes, especially the potassium level, as diuretics can deplete the potassium level. Administer potassium supplements as ordered to keep the potassium serum level within the normal level. Take the apical pulse before giving a digitalis preparation. If the heart rate is below 60, withhold the medication and notify the physician. In some institutions the heart rate can drop to 50 before the physician is notified if the client is taking a calcium channel blocker or beta-blocker along with digitalis.
► *Gas exchange, impaired, related to decreased cardiac output and pulmonary edema.*	The client will breathe without the assistance of oxygen and be oriented.	Provide oxygen by mask or nasal cannula at 2 to 6 liters/minute to assist in the oxygen needs of the body. Elevate the head of the bed to a semi-Fowler's or Fowler's position to relieve pressure on the diaphragm. Apply a pulse oximeter and monitor the oxygenation status. If the pulse oximeter is ≤90%, notify the physician.

Nursing Diagnoses	Goals	Nursing Interventions
▶ *Fluid volume excess related to decreased cardiac output and decreased renal output.*	The client will have no edema of the extremities.	Encourage elevation of the client's legs, not letting them hang in a dependent position. Monitor daily fluids by obtaining an accurate intake and output. Take a daily weight at the same time each day, on the same scales, and with the client wearing the same type of clothing. If the client is on a fluid-restricted diet, offer hard candies to quench the thirst.
▶ *Activity intolerance related to edema, dyspnea, and fatigue.*	The client will balance activity with rest periods.	Schedule nursing care so the client is given frequent rest periods with minimal interruptions at night. Teach the client to take frequent rest periods and to stop activities before becoming tired. Monitor the client's vital signs for an increase or decrease in heart rate or blood pressure, especially after periods of activity. Have an occupational therapist assist the client in energy saving methods. Instruct the client to call the physician if he becomes more dyspneic, fatigued, has less activity tolerance, or gains or loses weight when at home.
▶ *Skin integrity, impaired, high risk for, related to edema, inactivity and poor tissue perfusion.*	The client's skin will be pink, warm, and dry with prompt capillary refill.	Check bony prominences frequently for skin breakdown and massage reddened areas. Turn the client every two hours and use air mattresses to prevent pressure points. Teach the client not to wear knee-high hose or restrictive clothes that may hinder venous return. Support hose or plexipulse machines may be used to increase venous return.
▶ *Anxiety, moderate, related to change in health status, lifestyle changes, or fear of death.*	The client will relate concerns and fears to others.	Explain procedures to the client and family members. Assist the family in identifying stress factors. Refer the client to a local support group such as American Heart Association or Mended Hearts, Inc.
▶ *Knowledge deficit related to disease process, medications, diet, and plan for recovery.*	The client will state knowledge of disease process, medications, diet, and plans for recovery.	Make arrangements for a dietitian to explain the sodium- and/or fat-restricted diet to the client and significant family members. Explain that small frequent feedings, rather than three large meals a day, help prevent feeling distended and dyspneic. Suggest adding seasonings and spices to foods to make them more palatable when salt is restricted. Teach the client to read the labels on the seasonings for sodium content. If taking digitalis, teach the client how to take a pulse accurately before taking the daily dose. Teach the route, dosage, administration times, and side effects of each of the medications when the client is given the prescriptions.

▶ *Evaluation*

Each goal must be evaluated to determine how it has been met by the client.

▲ ▲

COR PULMONALE

With this condition, the heart is affected because of a lung condition that interferes with the exchange of carbon dioxide and oxygen in the alveoli. The carbon dioxide level increases in the blood. For some unknown reason, the pulmonary arteries vasoconstrict causing pulmonary hypertension. The right ventricle is forced to pump against increased pulmonary pressure. The right ventricle enlarges and finally weakens in the attempt to pump blood into the lungs. The symptoms the client experiences and medical and nursing care are the same as for right-sided heart failure.

CARDIAC TRANSPLANT

Cardiac transplantations are done for cardiomyopathy, end-stage coronary artery disease, and valvular disease. Recipients are evaluated for emotional stability, minimal disease involvement, and a good support system. The heart donor and the recipient's tissues are matched.

The transplant is performed by removing the recipient's heart except for posterior sections of the atria. The posterior sections of the atria are removed from the donor's heart and then the heart is sutured to the recipient's posterior atria.

The recipient must remain on an immunosuppressant medication for the remainder of life so the donor heart will not be rejected. Some immunosuppressant medications are azathioprine (Imuran), cyclosporine (Sandimmune), antithymocytic globulin, ATG (Atgam), antilymphocytic globulin (ALG), rapamycin, and FK 506 (Prograf).

▶ CASE STUDY

Mr. Lance Jeffers, a fifty-five-year-old truck driver, was admitted to the emergency room with a feeling of heavy squeezing pressure in his sternal area. The pain is radiating to his left shoulder. He is diaphoretic, short of breath, and nauseated. He states the sternal pain came on suddenly while watching a football game. He had been mowing his yard and decided to rest. The emergency physician gives Mr. Jeffers a nitroglycerin tablet and connects him to an EKG monitor. Cardiac enzymes with isoenzyme fractions and a chest x-ray are requested STAT. Morphine sulfate 2 mg is given intravenously. The EKG shows no Q waves, a depressed ST wave, and T wave changes. Oxygen is given by mask at 4 liters/minute. Mr. Jeffers' apical pulse is 102 and his blood pressure is 130/88. A cardiac catheterization with fluoroscopy is ordered to determine the patency of the coronary blood vessels and functioning of the heart muscle. Three hours after admission, crackles are heard in the lungs, the $CK_2(MB)$ is elevated, and the LDH_1 is higher than the LDH_2.

The following questions will guide your development of a Nursing Care Plan for the case study.

1. List symptoms/clinical manifestations, other than Mr. Jeffers', a client may experience when having a myocardial infarction.

2. List two reasons morphine sulfate was given to Mr. Jeffers.

3. List two other diagnostic tests that may have been ordered for Mr. Jeffers.

4. List subjective and objective data a nurse would want to obtain about Mr. Jeffers.

5. Write three individualized nursing diagnoses and goals for Mr. Jeffers.

6. Mr. Jeffers is moved from the critical care unit. List pertinent nursing actions a nurse would do in caring for Mr. Jeffers related to:

    oxygenation
    cardiac output
    comfort/rest
    activity
    medications
    teaching

7. List resources specific to locale that could assist Mr. Jeffers in his cardiac rehabilitation.

8. List teachings that Mr. Jeffers will need before his discharge.

9. List at least three successful client outcomes for Mr. Jeffers.

SUMMARY

- The function of the heart is to pump blood through the vascular system. Blood is the medium by which oxygen and nutrients are provided to the body cells and carbon dioxide and waste products are removed from the body cells
- The volume of blood pumped into the circulatory system depends on the cardiac output.
- The coronary arteries supply blood to the heart. If the blood flow through these vessels becomes diminished or occluded, ischemia to the heart tissue occurs resulting in angina or a myocardial infarction.
- Typical symptoms experienced by a person with cardiac problems include chest pain, dyspnea, edema, fainting, palpitations, diaphoresis and fatigue.
- A lipid profile and cardiac enzymes, including the CK and LDH isoenzymes, provide diagnostic information as to the risk of heart disease and the occurrence of a myocardial infarction.
- Cardiac catheterization provides information on the patency of the heart vessels, pressure in the chambers, oxygen saturation in the chambers and vessels, and cardiac output.
- Heart tissue perfusion is determined by radioactive tracer scans, the technetium pyrophosphate scanning, and the thallium scan.
- A dysrhythmia is an irregularity in the rate, rhythm, or conduction of the electrical system of the heart.
- Inflammatory or infectious conditions of the heart include endocarditis, myocarditis, and pericarditis. Endocarditis may cause valvular heart disease with the possibility of the valve needing to be surgically repaired (valvuloplasty) or replaced with a mechanical (caged-ball valve or tilting-disk valve) or biological valve from a calf, pig, or human.
- Arteriosclerosis and atherosclerosis cause a narrowing and occluding of vessels and are the primary causes of angina and myocardial infarction.
- Surgical treatment for angina includes a PTCA, intracoronary stent, transcatheter ablation, or coronary artery bypass.
- Nursing interventions for a client who has experienced a myocardial infarction are close monitoring of the vital signs, monitoring EKG rhythms, administering morphine, nitroglycerine, beta-blockers and calcium blockers as ordered, explaining medical and nursing procedures, and progressively increasing activity as ordered.
- Congestive heart failure is often the final stage of many other heart conditions in which the heart is no longer able to fulfill the demands of the body and is literally failing.
- Nursing interventions for CHF are monitoring vital signs with each client activity, administering digitalis, diuretics, and vasodilators as ordered, administering and observing the effects of oxygen, weighing the

client daily, obtaining accurate I&O, and teaching healthy lifestyle changes.

Review Questions

1. The volume of blood pumped by the left ventricle per minute is:
   a. stroke volume.
   b. cardiac output.
   c. ejection fraction.
   d. cardiac cycle.

2. A coronary artery disease risk factor that can be modified or altered is:
   a. age.
   b. gender.
   c. stress.
   d. familial history.

3. The nurse may assist in relieving the chest pain of a client with pericarditis by having the client:
   a. lie flat and turn on the right side.
   b. lie flat and turn on the left side.
   c. sit in a semi-Fowler's position.
   d. sit erect and lean forward.

4. To assess a client with right-sided heart failure, the nurse would:
   a. listen for a pericardial friction rub.
   b. listen for a muffled S_1 and S_2 heart sound.
   c. check for distended neck veins with the bed at a 45° angle.
   d. assess for radiation of the squeezing sensation under the sternum.

5. A diagnostic test for a myocardial infarction is:
   a. cardiac enzymes.
   b. arterial blood gases.
   c. cardiac biopsy.
   d. pulse oximetry.

6. It would be important to teach a client with angina to:
   a. take antibiotics before having dental work.
   b. carry nitroglycerin tablets at all times.
   c. perform Valsalva maneuver daily.
   d. massage the carotid sinuses in the neck.

7. A client with the diagnosis of a myocardial infarction has just been admitted to the ER. To relieve chest pain the physician orders:
   a. amoxicillin (Amoxil).
   b. ibuprofen (Motrin).
   c. digoxin (Lanoxin).
   d. morphine sulfate.

8. A cardiac dysrhythmia that has an erratic electrical activity of the atria resulting in a rate of 350 beats/minute to 600 beats/minute is:

    a. atrial fibrillation.
    b. bradycardia.
    c. ventricular asystole.
    d. third degree AV block.

9. A nursing intervention to improve cardiac output is:

    a. encouraging the client to verbalize fears.
    b. teaching the side effects of new medications.
    c. a referral to a dietitian for low-sodium diet instructions.
    d. administer oxygen per physician orders.

10. The most appropriate nursing diagnosis for a client with coronary artery disease is:

    a. decreased cardiac output.
    b. social isolation.
    c. fatigue.
    d. altered nutrition.

Critical Thinking Questions

1. What lifestyle changes could a person take to decrease the risk factors for a myocardial infarction?

2. List and explore the ethical issues of a heart transplant.

3. Imagine being given the diagnosis of a myocardial infarction. What would be the next three things written on a "to do" list?

Medical Terminology

arterio-	pertaining to an artery
arteriectomy	surgical removal of part of an artery
athero-	pertaining to fat
atherosclerosis	fatty deposits in the arteries
cardio-	pertaining to the heart
cardiomegaly	enlargement of the heart
-emia	pertaining to blood
leukemia	a malignancy characterized by a progressive increase of abnormal leukocytes
myo-	muscle
myoplasty	surgical repair of a muscle

News Flash

A study by Brodsky at the University of California found giving magnesium along with Lanoxin to clients with new-onset atrial fibrillation caused the ventricular rate to slow. All ten clients in their study responded with a decreased ventricular rate compared to four of eight clients in the group receiving placebos (*Nursing 94, December, Research roundup*).

At the University of Washington Medical Center, Coyne conducted a study on postop coronary angiogram clients. When the head of the bed was gradually elevated to 60 degrees over a four-hour period, the client required less pain medication and had less upper and lower back pain than in clients having the head of the bed raised the customary 15 degrees or less for four hours. There also was no statistically significant difference in complications between the two groups (*Nursing 94, December, Coronary angiography: Heads up.*).

The Second International Study of Infarct Survival Collaborative Group found that MI clients who received 300 mg of aspirin within twenty-four hours of the onset of their symptoms had a significantly decreased mortality rate than those who do not receive aspirin within twenty-four hours. After the initial dose, clients daily received lower doses of aspirin. (Goldman, 1994)

CHAPTER 21
Vascular Disorders

Gena Duncan

▶ KEY TERMS

AB index
Allen's test
aneurysm
baseline level
Brodie-Trendelenburg's test
    (Trendelenburg's test or retrograde
    filling test)
embolus
hemolysis
Homans' sign
necrosis
peripheral resistance
phlebitis
phlebothrombosis
plethysmography
reflux
sclerotherapy
stasis dermatitis
thrombectomy
thrombophlebitis
thrombosis
thrombus
varicosities
vasoconstrict
vasodilate
vein ligation
vein stripping
Virchow's triad

LIST OF DISORDERS

▶ Venous Thrombosis/Thrombophlebitis
▶ Varicose Veins
▶ Buerger's Disease (Thromboangiitis Obliterans)
▶ Raynaud's Phenomenon/Disease
▶ Aneurysm
▶ Hypertension

LEARNING OBJECTIVES

Upon completion of this chapter the learner should be able to:
• Define key terms.
• Describe the anatomy and physiology of the peripheral vessels.
• Relate laboratory results to peripheral vascular conditions.
• Explain the pathophysiology of peripheral vascular conditions.
• Describe nursing interventions in caring for clients with peripheral vascular conditions.

▶ *MAKING THE CONNECTION*

Refer to the topics in the following chapters to increase your understanding of vascular disorders.

- **Chapter 10, Nursing Assessment:** Vital Signs, p. 176; Skin Assessment, p. 178; Musculoskeletal and Extremity Assessment, p. 183
- **Chapter 14, Fluid, Electrolyte, and Acid-base Balances:** Fluid Balance, p. 271

- **Chapter 20, Cardiac Disorders:** Anatomy and Physiology Review, Function, p. 447, Circulation of Blood, p. 448; Arteriosclerosis, p. 472
- **Chapter 22, Blood and Lymph Disorders:** Anatomy and Physiology Review, Blood, p. 518

INTRODUCTION

The peripheral vascular system consists of a network of vessels that delivers blood from the left side of the heart, through the body, to the right side of the heart. The purpose of the vessels is to supply body tissues with oxygen and nutrients and to remove carbon dioxide and other waste products from body tissues. Risk factors that affect the integrity of the vessels are high-fat diet, obesity, smoking, inactive lifestyle, and diabetes mellitus.

ANATOMY AND PHYSIOLOGY REVIEW

The peripheral vascular system consists of arteries, arterioles, capillaries, venules, and veins. The arteries carry oxygenated blood away from the left side of the heart to the body tissues and the veins carry deoxygenated blood back to the right side of the heart. The capillaries connect the arterioles to the venules. In the capillaries oxygen, nutrients, minerals, and hormones move from the blood to the body cells and carbon dioxide and waste products move from the body cells into the blood. The venules and veins contain 60 to 70 percent of the body's total blood volume.

Arterioles and Arteries

The arteries are thick-walled tubes consisting of three layers or tunics as illustrated in Figure 21-1. The inner layer is called the tunica intima and consists of a single layer of smooth endothelial cells. The middle layer is the tunica media and is composed of smooth muscle cells. The smooth muscle layer of the artery receives nerve stimulation from the sympathetic nervous system. The suppleness of the smooth muscle allows the vessel to **vasoconstrict** (decrease in diameter) and **vasodilate** (increase in diameter). The outer layer, the tunica adventitia or tunica externa, consists of a con-

nective tissue sheath with some of its collagen fibers fusing with those of the surrounding tissue to hold the vessels in place. The elastic connective tissue allows the artery to expand and recoil with each contraction of the ventricle as an increased volume of blood is pumped through the vessel. The arteries have thick walls so they can withstand the increased pressure from the left ventricle pumping blood through the body.

The arteries divide and branch into smaller vessels called arterioles which are smaller arteries. The same three layers are present in the walls, but as the arterioles approach the capillaries their walls become thinner. The outer layer is reduced to a very thin layer of connective tissue.

Capillaries

Capillaries are very tiny thin vessels that connect the smallest arterioles with the smallest venules. They have only one layer of endothelial cells whose cell membranes are the semipermeable membrane that allows oxygen, nutrients, carbon dioxide, and waste products to be exchanged between the tissues of the body and the blood.

Venules and Veins

Venules are small vessels that emerge from the capillaries and gradually increase in size. As the venules increase in size, they eventually form veins.

Veins have three layers or tunics like the arteries but the middle layer of a vein is thinner having less smooth muscle and elastic tissue. This allows the walls of the veins to dilate more easily. Endothelial flaps, called valves, are on the inside lining of veins. The valves open and close with each contraction of the surrounding muscles. The purpose of the valves is to assist the blood in returning to the heart. Blood is held by the valves at a certain level until the skeletal muscle contractions cause the blood to move higher in the vein. Refer to Figure 21-2 for clarification of the action of vein valves.

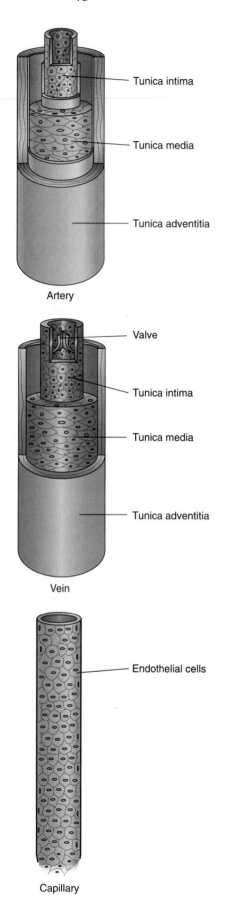

Artery

— Tunica intima

— Tunica media

— Tunica adventitia

Vein

— Valve

— Tunica intima

— Tunica media

— Tunica adventitia

Capillary

— Endothelial cells

FIGURE 21-1 Tunic layers of each vessel.

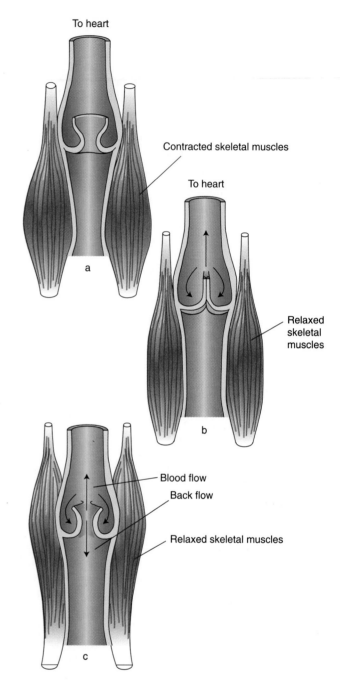

To heart

Contracted skeletal muscles

To heart

Relaxed skeletal muscles

Blood flow

Back flow

Relaxed skeletal muscles

FIGURE 21-2 The contraction of skeletal muscles applies pressure to veins and assists with the circulation of blood. **(A)** Valves in the veins hold the blood at a certain level in the vein. **(B)** Valves prevent the backflow of blood. **(C)** Incompetent valves allow a backflow of blood.

ASSESSMENT

Assessment of the peripheral vascular system also includes an assessment of the cardiac system, since the two systems often have a direct affect on each other. Assessment of the cardiac system is explained in Chapter 20.

Subjective

The nurse obtains a thorough history of the client's past illnesses and asks about the present symptoms being experienced. The nurse should do a thorough pain assessment on a client with peripheral vascular diseases, asking what causes the pain and what relieves the pain. The pain is noted and documented as to type (aching, cramping, sharp, throbbing), occurrence (with exercise and at rest), and location (hands, abdomen, lower back, thigh, calf or foot).

Objective

Assessment of the peripheral vascular system includes assessment of five Ps; pain, pulse, pallor, paresthesia, and paralysis (Linton et al., 1995).

Assessment of rate, rhythm, and quality of peripheral pulses gives an indication as to the perfusion of the extremities. (Refer to Chapter 20 for assessment of the peripheral pulses.) It is important to compare the two extremities to determine that the pulses are the same in both extremities.

Decreased circulation to an area can result in coolness in the ischemic area, pallor, paresthesia, and paralysis. Paresthesia (decreased sensation in an area) and paralysis result from a lack of oxygenated blood and nourishment to the nerves. Symptoms of paresthesia are numbness and tingling.

The nurse observes the color of a client's extremity. If an artery in the leg is occluded, the foot and/or leg becomes reddish in color when the leg is in a dependent position and pale when elevated. As the ischemia progresses, the leg and/or foot becomes mottled. The skin is smooth and shiny. If the veins are occluded, the foot and/or leg becomes cyanotic when in a dependent position and has a normal coloration when elevated. Often the anterior area of the lower leg and ankle have a brown pigmentation with venous involvement.

Clients with decreased circulation to the extremities have hardened and brittle nails. The leg will be cool if there is an arterial circulatory problem but warm if there is a venous circulatory problem. Observe for skin ulcerations around the ankles and toes.

Observe the client's ankles for **stasis dermatitis**, an inflammation of the skin due to decreased circulation. Waste products that normally are carried away in the circulatory system, remain in the tissues causing pruritus and irritation of the skin. At first, the ankle area is reddened and edematous, then vesicles form and start oozing. The skin becomes crusted, thickened, and brown in color.

Allen's test is a simple exam to evaluate the arterial circulation of the hands. As the client places a hand in the lap and makes a tight fist, the nurse places pressure on the ulnar artery to occlude it. The client is asked to open the fist and pressure is released from the ulnar artery. If the artery is not occluded, the color will promptly return to the palm of the hand. If the artery is occluded, the palm will remain pale. The procedure is repeated to check the radial artery.

A positive Homan's sign is present in 10 to 20 percent of deep vein thrombosis (DVT) cases (Hickey, 1994). To test for the **Homans' sign**, the nurse dorsiflexes the client's foot. If there is pain in the calf of the leg or behind the knee, the Homan's sign is positive and may indicate the presence of a venous clot.

The **Brodie-Trendelenburg's test**, also called **Trendelenburg's test or retrograde filling test**, is used to test the ability of the venous valves to hold blood at a certain level in the vein and not allow the blood to retrograde or **reflux** (flow backward to the previous location). The nurse performs the Brodie-Trendelenburg test by having the client lie supine and elevate one leg 90 degrees for thirty seconds. A tourniquet is placed snugly above the knee, but not so tightly that an arterial pulse cannot be felt. The client then stands and after twenty to thirty seconds, the tourniquet is released. The veins should fill from distal to proximal. If the veins promptly fill from proximal to distal, the venous valves are not able to hold the blood at the proper level in the vein.

COMMON DIAGNOSTIC TESTS

The following is a table of the commonly used diagnostic tests for clients with vascular disorders.

Test	Explanation/Normal values	Nursing Responsibilities
Prothrombin Time (PT)	Normal values = 11–12.5 seconds Normal values when on anti-coagulant therapy = 1 1/2–2 times the normal value	Make sure the blood specimen has been drawn before the daily dose of Coumadin. Instruct the client that alcohol intake may increase the PT count and a diet high in fat may decrease the level. Salicylates, sulfonamides, and Aldomet may increase the PT count. Digitalis and oral contraceptives will decrease the levels. Instruct the client not to take any medication without notifying the doctor as the medication may affect the PT results.
Partial Thromboplastin Time (PTT) also called Activated Partial Thromboplastin Time (APTT)	APTT normal values = 30–40 seconds PTT normal value = 60–70 seconds When on anticoagulant therapy, the client's normal value is 1.5–2.5 times the control value.	If the client is receiving intermittent heparin doses, the APTT is drawn 30–60 minutes before the next Heparin dose. If heparin is given continuously, the blood specimen can be drawn at any time. If the APTT is greater than 100 seconds, the client is at risk for bleeding and the physician is notified. The antidote for heparin is 1 mg of protamine sulfate for every 100 units of the heparin dose. Antihistamines, vitamin C, and salicylates prolong the PTT time.
International Normalized Ratio (INR)	Normal value = 2–3 (2.5–3.5 for a client with a mechanical prosthetic heart valve) The INR is more accurate than the PT to monitor warfarin (Coumadin) therapy.	The daily warfarin (Coumadin) dose is given after blood has been drawn for the INR.
Platelet Count	Adult normal value = 150,000–400,000/mm^3 Serious levels = <50,000 and >1 million/mm^3 The test measures the number of platelets per cubic milliliter of blood.	Instruct the client that strenuous exercise and oral contraceptives increase the platelet level. Instruct the client that aspirin, acetaminophen, and sulfonamides decrease the platelet levels.
Doppler Ultrasound	Normal findings = audible "swishing" sound of the doppler when placed over vessel. There should be less than 20 mm Hg pressure in the lower extremity when compared to pressure in the upper extremity. The test determines patency of veins and arteries in conditions such as arterial occulusive disease, arteriosclerotic disease, or Raynaud's disease. An AB index is obtained by dividing the blood pressure reading in the ankle by the blood pressure reading in the arm (brachial artery). This is known as the ankle-to-brachial arterial blood pressure. A normal AB index is 0.85 or greater.	Explain to the client that the procedure is painless. Clothing is removed from the extremity being evaluated. The client is not to smoke 30 minutes prior to the exam because nicotine causes vasoconstriction of the vessels. Conductive or acoustic gel is removed from the skin after the test is completed.

(continued)

Test	Explanation/Normal values	Nursing Responsibilities
Arterial Plethysmography (pulse volume recorder)	Normal values = normal arterial pulse waves The test determines arteriosclerotic disease in the upper extremities and occlusive disease in the lower extremities. The test is done by applying 3 BP cuffs to an extremity. The BP cuffs are connected to a pulse volume recorder which records the amplitude of each pulse wave. If there is a decrease in the amplitude of the pulse wave, an occlusion is in the artery proximal to the BP cuff. A decrease of 20 mm Hg of pressure indicates arterial occlusion. The test is not as reliable as arteriography but also does not have the risks of an arteriogram. (see Cardiac chapter for reference to arteriography).	Explain to the client that the test is painless. The client is to lie still during the test. The client is not to smoke for 30 minutes prior to the test. Clothing is removed from the extremity where the test will be completed.
Venous Plethysmography (cuff pressure test)	Normal values = return of volume pressure to preocclusion value within 1 second after deflation of occlusion cuff The test assists in determining patency of veins. A delay in the return of preocclusion volume indicates venous obstruction. Two blood pressure cuffs are placed on the extremity, one proximally (occlusion cuff) and one distally (recording cuff). The cuffs are attached to pulse volume recorders. The occlusion cuff is inflated to 50 mm Hg pressure to occlude the venous flow of blood. The recording cuff is inflated to 10 mm Hg pressure. The pulse volumes are recorded and then the occlusion cuff is rapidly deflated. The pulse volume of the extremity should return to the preocclusion volume within 1 second if there is no occlusion in the venous system. A delay in the return of volume pressure is indicative of a thrombus. The test is often done in conjunction with a doppler ultrasound. The test is not as reliable as a venogram (See the cardiac chapter for reference to venogram).	Same instructions as for arterial plethysmography

KEY ABBREVIATIONS

The following abbreviations and acronyms are used in this chapter:

AAA	aortic abdominal aneurysm
APTT	activated partial thromboplastin time
DVT	deep vein thrombosis
HTN	hypertension
INR	International Normalized Ratio
ISI	International Sensitivity Index
PT	prothrombin time
PTT	partial thromboplastin time
t-PA	tissue plasminogen activator

▶ VENOUS THROMBOSIS/ THROMBOPHLEBITIS

The terms *phlebitis, thrombosis, phlebothrombosis* and *thrombophlebitis,* are often used interchangeably even though each word has a separate meaning and etiology. **Phlebitis** is an inflammation in the wall of a vein without clot formation. The formation of a clot in a vessel is a **thrombosis** and a formed clot that remains at the site where it formed is a **thrombus**. If the thrombus moves, it would become an **embolus**, a mass such as a blood clot or an air bubble, that circulates in the bloodstream. **Phlebothrombosis** is the formation of a clot because of blood pooling in the vessel, trauma to the vessel's endothelial lining, or a coagulation problem. With phlebothrombosis, there is little or no inflammation in the vessel. **Thrombophlebitis** is the formation of a clot due to an inflammation in the wall of the vessel.

In 1846, Virchow listed three factors leading to the formation of a clot. These are known as **Virchow's triad**. The three factors are pooling of blood, vessel trauma, and a coagulation problem. Risk factors for thrombi formation are prolonged bed rest, leg trauma, oral contraceptives, obesity, varicose veins, hip fractures, and total hip and knee replacement.

There are two types of thrombi, a superficial thrombus and a deep vein thrombus. A superficial vein thrombus is a clot in a superficial vein such as the saphenous vein in the leg. A DVT can form in the deep veins of the arms, pelvic area or legs, but the legs are the most common site. Leg veins in which clots form are the femoral, popliteal, iliac, and deep veins of the calf.

Phlebitis can either form spontaneously or as a result of trauma. IV catheters or cannulas, IV medications such as potassium or antibiotics, or direct trauma to a vein can cause phlebitis. A clot may then form as red blood cells pass over the damaged area, rupture, and start the clotting process.

A phlebitis may manifest as a reddened streak over a vein. If a clot is in a superficial vein, the site becomes reddened, warm, tender, and swollen. The nurse may be able to palpate a hardening in a section of the vein. There may be no symptoms with a deep vein thrombus, or there may be warmth and tenderness at the site, unilateral edema of the affected extremity, positive Homans' sign, dilation of superficial veins, and cyanosis of the foot. The client may say the leg feels "tight" or "heavy." If the clot is in the calf of the leg, the calf may feel tender. If the swelling restricts the arterial blood flow, the leg may be cool and pale. If there are obvious clinical signs of a thrombosis, Homans' sign should not be assessed as the clot may be dislodged and become an embolus. A complication of a DVT is a pulmonary embolus that results in approximately 50,000 to 60,000 deaths each year in the United States (Beare & Myers, 1994). Symptoms of a pulmonary embolus are sudden and severe chest pain, dyspnea, and tachypnea. Emboli may travel and block other vessels in the heart, brain, or peripheral vessels. These conditions are covered in respective chapters.

▶ *Medical/Surgical Management*

▶ *Medical*

A superficial phlebitis or thrombus should be assessed and may need no further treatment. Warm soaks may be applied to the affected area. Aceta-minophen or a nonsteroidal anti-inflammatory drug is given for pain. Elevating the extremity decreases swelling and improves venous return. Some doctors recommend the application of an elastic support hose. If a DVT has been diagnosed, the client is placed on bed rest. Once the client improves and becomes ambulatory, below the knee compression stockings are recommended. Figure 21-3 shows a picture of compression stockings.

▶ *Surgical*

If a clot has formed in a large vein and all conservative methods have failed, the clot may be removed surgically. This procedure is called a **thrombectomy** and is performed only if the tissue in the area becomes ischemic or gangrenous or if the client has a history of thromboemboli.

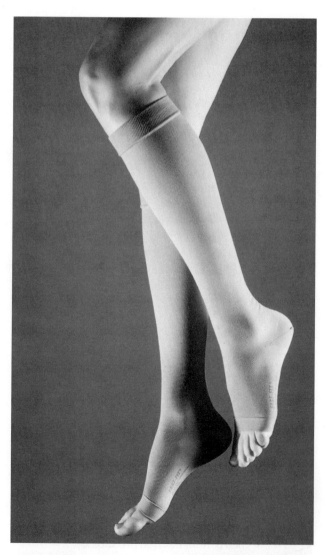

FIGURE 21-3 Elastic support hose improves a client's venous return. (*Courtesy of Beiersdorf-Jobst, Inc., Charlotte, NC*)

Another surgical procedure is a vena cava interruption surgery (venacaval plication) in which a Greenfield vena cava filter or umbrella filter is placed in the inferior vena cava to prevent thromboemboli from traveling from the lower extremities to the lungs, heart, or brain. Refer to Figure 21-4 for a view of these filters and their placement in the vena cava. The procedure is done on clients with a history of pulmonary emboli.

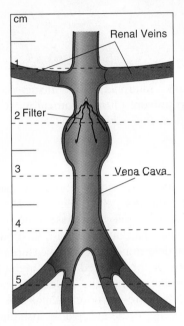

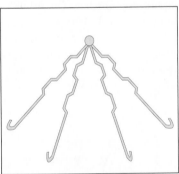

Greenfield filter

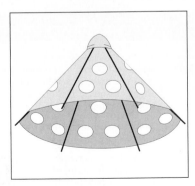

Umbrella filter

FIGURE 21-4 Filters placed in the vena cava prevent an embolus from traveling to the lungs, heart, or brain.

▶ *Pharmacological*

If a client is at risk for a thrombus or phlebitis, anticoagulant therapy can be initiated. A prophylactic heparin dose is given. Enoxaparin injection (Lovenox), a low-molecular-weight heparin, is used prophylactically after hip replacement surgery. Lovenox is started within 24 hours after surgery and is given subcutaneously twice daily for seven to ten days. Lovenox should be used cautiously with clients on oral anticoagulants.

If a clot forms, the client is immediately started on heparin as an IV bolus and then followed with a continuous IV drip of heparin. Before heparin is started, a partial thromboplastin time (PTT) or activated partial thromboplastin time (APTT) and a platelet count are drawn by the laboratory to establish a baseline level. The heparin dose is regulated by the PTT or the APTT. For effective heparin therapy, the client's PTT or APTT level should be two and one-half times the baseline. A **baseline level** is a value at a particular time that will serve as a reference point for future value levels.

Clients are generally given heparin subcutaneously or intravenously in an acute setting. Since warfarin sodium (Coumadin) is taken orally, a client may be discharged on Coumadin. Because of rapid hospital discharges, clients are often started on Coumadin the next day after heparin has been initiated. Once the Coumadin dose is regulated, heparin is stopped.

After the initial Coumadin dose, the daily Coumadin dose is regulated by the prothrombin time (PT) or the International Normalized Ratio (INR). A PT level of 1.3 to 1.6 times the hospital laboratory control value indicates effective Coumadin therapy. By converting the PT to the INR, a more standardized PT report is provided. The laboratory converts the PT to an INR by dividing the client's PT by the laboratory's control PT and raising it to the power of the International Sensitivity Index (ISI). The ISI is determined by the manufacturer of each lot of thromboplastin that is used to perform the test. For a client on Coumadin, an INR of 2 to 3 indicates a therapeutic level. The client generally remains on Coumadin for three to six months.

Thrombolytic drugs, urokinase (Abbokinase), streptokinase (Streptase) and tissue plasminogen activator, t-PA (Alteplase), are used locally and systemically if there is a massive DVT. Streptokinase should only be used on the same client once every six months. If the client has had a recent streptococcal infection, urokinase is given rather than streptokinase because antibodies are present in the blood that will make the streptokinase ineffective (Beare & Myers, 1994). The main complication in a client receiving thrombolytic drugs is bleeding. Heparin and Coumadin are given after the thrombolytic drugs to prevent thrombi formation.

▶ *Diet*

Adequate hydration is important for clients at risk for thrombi. This can be accomplished orally or intravenously.

▶ *Activity*

During the acute stage, the client is placed on bed rest to prevent the clot from dislodging and embolizing. The leg is elevated to improve venous return and decrease swelling.

▶ *Preventive Treatment*

Prevention is the best way to treat a DVT. Early ambulation, adequate hydration, alternating pneumatic compression devices, prophylactic anticoagulants, elevation of legs, leg exercises, and deep breathing exercises, all contribute to the prevention of thrombi. Figure 21-5 shows an alternating pneumatic compression device. The client's leg should never be massaged as a clot could be dislodged and become an embolus.

▶ *Nursing Process*

Assessment

Subjective Data Ask the client if there has been any recent injury to the extremity, if the affected area is tender to touch, or if there have been clots previously. Also ask if the client has had any chest pain, dyspnea, tachycardia, or hemoptysis.

Objective Data IV sites are checked at least once a shift to see if a phlebitis or reddened area is developing at the insertion site. If a positive Homan's sign is

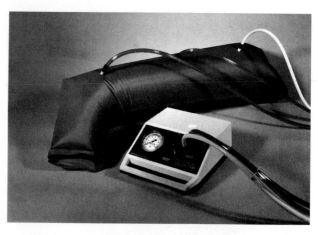

FIGURE 21-5 Alternating pneumatic compression devices help prevent thrombi formation. (*Courtesy of Beiersdorf-Jobst, Inc., Charlotte, NC*)

detected during an assessment, the nurse should notify the physician and not perform another Homan's sign until a clot has been ruled out. Assess the skin for redness, tenderness, hardness, or warmth. Both legs are measured to determine baseline measurements. The circumference of the affected leg is measured every shift to determine an increase or decrease in swelling. Peripheral pulses are obtained as baseline data and charted according to the acceptable institutional scale (refer to Chapter 20, Cardiac Disorders). Peripheral pulses should be checked every four hours and more frequently if the client experiences increased pain in the leg, cyanosis of the foot or extremity, or increased swelling. These are signs of an occlusion.

▼ ▼

Possible nursing diagnoses for a client with a venous thrombosis may include:

Nursing Diagnoses	*Goals*	*Nursing Interventions*
▶ *Tissue perfusion, altered peripheral, related to decreased blood flow and/or clot formation.*	The client will have adequate tissue perfusion.	Elevate the client's entire affected leg when on bed rest to improve venous return. When elevated, the leg should be slightly flexed at the knee with a pillow under the thigh and calf.
		Apply elastic support or intermittent pneumatic compression stockings on the client.
		If the client has received thrombolytic or anticoagulant drugs, assess for signs of bleeding which include hematuria, bruising, bleeding from the gums, and blood in the stool.

Nursing Diagnoses	Goals	Nursing Interventions
▶ *Pain related to inflammatory process.*	The client will state absence of pain.	If the client has a phlebitis, apply warm moist soaks to the affected area.
		Administer acetaminophen or a nonsteroidal anti-inflammatory as ordered for discomfort.
▶ *Anxiety related to possibility of the clot becoming an embolus.*	The client will express anxiety about possible embolus.	Instruct the client on the importance of maintaining bed rest so as not to dislodge the clot. Allow or encourage client to discuss the possibility of embolus formation.
		If the affected area is close to the groin, notify the physician because the clot could become dislodged and move to the lung.
▶ *Knowledge deficit related to disease process and risk factors.*	The client will list measures to prevent thrombus formation.	For clients at risk for thrombus, encourage active range of motion (ROM) exercises while the client is on bed rest or relatively inactive.
		Before discharge, instruct the client to drink 2 to 3 quarts of water per day, not to sit with legs crossed, elevate both legs when sitting, avoid sitting or standing for extended periods, and to wear support hose. When standing the client should shift weight frequently and occasionally stand on tiptoes to stimulate the calf muscle to pump blood.
		Instruct client to notify the physician immediately if he or she experiences leg pain, tenderness or swelling, difficulty breathing, or chest pain.
		Instruct client on anticoagulant therapy to take the medication at the same time each day, maintain appointments to have the PT or INR level checked, watch for signs of bleeding and avoid aspirin or drugs containing aspirin because it increases the clotting time. A physician should be notified if abdominal pain occurs as this could indicate internal bleeding.

▶ Evaluation

Each goal must be evaluated to determine how it has been met by the client.

▲ ▲

▶ VARICOSE VEINS

Varicose veins, also called **varicosities**, are visibly prominent, dilated, and twisted veins. Veins in the lower extremities are more frequently involved, but the veins in the esophagus (esophageal varices) and anus (hemorrhoids) can also be affected. Usually it is the saphenous vein that is affected in the leg. Women are more prone to varicose veins than men (Beare & Myers, 1994). Risk factors for developing varicose veins are a familial tendency, congenital abnormalities, pregnancy, obesity, constrictive clothing, and occupations that require periods of prolonged standing. Pregnancy and obesity cause more pressure in the veins of the legs.

The causes of varicose veins are incompetent valves and veins that have lost their elasticity. The wall of the vessel is weakened from a lack of elastin or collagen and is unable to support the normal pressure of the blood in the vessel. The vein dilates as the blood in it flows backward. As the walls of the vein dilate, the valves become incapable of holding the blood and allow blood to leak backward through the space between the valves. Refer to Figure 21-2C.

There are two classifications of varicose veins, primary and secondary. Primary varicose veins involve the superficial vessels and occur gradually. The vein, exposed to excessive pressure for a period of time, is no longer able to withstand the pressure against its wall by the blood and starts dilating. Secondary varicose veins involve the deep veins and are due to phlebitis or a thrombus.

Clients with superficial vein involvement may be asymptomatic except for dilation of veins. If deeper veins are involved the client may experience ankle and leg swelling, pain, a "heavy" sensation or a "tired" feeling in the affected leg, muscle aches and cramps, especially during the night. Later, possible complications are leg ulcers, stasis dermatitis, embolus, or more thrombi formation.

▶ Medical/Surgical Management

▶ Medical

Varicose veins are treated with conservative measures such as elastic support hose, elevation of the legs when sitting, not crossing legs, and ankle and leg exercises (see Figure 21-6).

▶ Surgical

In more severe cases, varicose veins can be ligated (tied off) or stripped. **Vein stripping** involves intro-

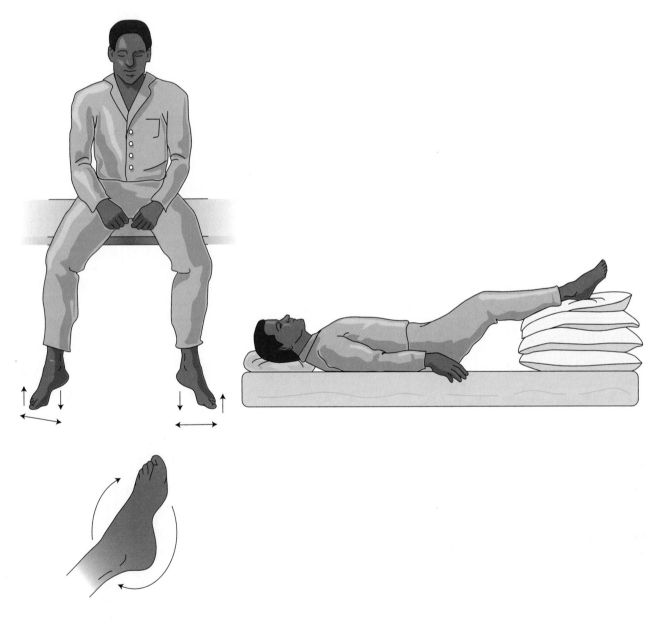

Circular motion

FIGURE 21-6 Exercises to improve circulation to the lower extremities.

ducing a wire into a vein. The wire has collapsible claws on the end. As the wire is withdrawn, the claws expand and strip the walls of the vein. This measure is used when there is a threat of thrombus or leg ulcers. **Vein ligation** is tying off an involved section of a vein with suture.

Another treatment method used with smaller veins or at the same time as vein ligation and stripping is **sclerotherapy**. This treatment involves injecting a chemical into the vein, causing the vein to become sclerosed (hardened) so blood no longer flows through it. A compression bandage or elastic stocking is applied to the extremity for four to five days. The client wears support hose for five more weeks. Complications of the procedure are **necrosis** (tissue death) at the injection site, vasospasm, allergic responses, and **hemolysis** (destruction of red blood cells).

▶ Pharmacological

Analgesics are given for leg discomfort.

▶ Activity

The client is encouraged to exercise regularly. Walking is a very good exercise to improve circulation because the blood circulates faster in response to an increased heartbeat. Muscles in the legs also apply pressure to the veins forcing the blood upward toward the heart. Ankle exercises such as rotating the ankle in circular motions also improves circulation.

▶ Preventive Treatment

Clients with a familial tendency of varicose veins are encouraged to elevate their legs 6 to 10 inches on a small stool when sitting in a chair. Frequent position changes and not standing in one spot for extended times also improve circulation.

▶ Nursing Interventions

Assist the client in elevating the legs above the heart when in bed or elevating the feet 6 to 10 inches on a pillow or stool when sitting in a chair.

The client may be on anticoagulants to prevent clot formation. Administer warfarin sodium (Coumadin) at the same time each day. It is important for the client to maintain regularly scheduled PT level checks.

Client teaching includes instruction in the application of support hose. The hose are to be applied after the legs have been elevated for an extended time, ten to fifteen minutes, so the venous blood drains from the legs. Application before getting out of bed in the morning is ideal. The hose are not folded or rolled down from the top as this would act like a tourniquet causing pooling of blood. The hose are to be smooth on the legs as wrinkles or creases may cause extra pressure leading to stasis or pooling of blood or pressure ulcers. The hose are removed daily so the leg can be washed and dried before reapplication. Instruct the client not to wear constrictive clothing such as knee high socks that restrict blood flow.

After a vein stripping, the client is on bed rest for the first twenty-four hours. Elastic hose are worn continuously for five days to compress the blood into the deeper veins. The client continues to wear compression or support hose for five weeks after the surgery. Administer pain medication thirty minutes before the client ambulates until walking is tolerated without discomfort. Walking and leg exercises are encouraged after the vein stripping.

After sclerotherapy the affected area may be tender and discolored. Most discoloration will disappear in a few weeks, but a darkened pigmentation may last for six to eight months. Repeated sclerotherapy may be needed. Encourage the client to maintain a walking exercise program to improve circulation to the legs.

▶ BUERGER'S DISEASE (THROMBOANGIITIS OBLITERANS)

Buerger's disease is an inflammatory disease of small and medium arteries and veins that leads to vascular obstruction. Inflammation occurs in the adventitia and media layers of the vessels and may affect only a portion of the vessel or the entire vessel. Hands and feet are mainly involved, but the wrists and lower extremities may also be affected. The distal tips of the hands and feet are pale, but as the disease progresses, the hands and feet become reddened when held in a dependent position. At first, pain in the palm of the hand and arch of the foot is the main symptom. Pain becomes more severe with disease progression and, as ischemia affects the nerves, the client may experience numbness, burning, pain when at rest, and decreased sensation in the hands and lower extremities. The dorsalis pedis, posterior tibia, ulnar and radial pulses are weak or absent. Skin color changes, cold sensitivity, ulcers, and gangrene may occur in the later stages.

Buerger's disease occurs in men between the ages of 20 and 40 of Israel, Indian, and Oriental descent. There is a correlation between smoking and Buerger's disease.

▶ Medical/Surgical Management

▶ Medical

The client is encouraged to stop smoking and may be referred to a smoking clinic or seminar. Buerger-

Allen exercises are recommended and explained. Buerger-Allen exercises consist of elevating the legs until they blanch and supporting them at that angle for two to three minutes. The legs are then lowered to a dependent position until they become red and supported at that level for five to ten minutes. The legs are then placed flat on the bed with the client in a supine position for 10 minutes. The exercises are repeated as tolerated by the client.

▶ *Surgical*

A sympathectomy may be done to relieve pain and prevent vasospasm in the affected area. Digits and toes may have to be amputated in the later stages of the disease if gangrene occurs.

▶ *Pharmacological*

Analgesics are given to control pain. Vasodilators are given to increase circulation to the affected area.

▶ *Nursing Interventions*

Nursing diagnoses and interventions are the same as for other obstructive vascular conditions and are described under Raynaud's disease.

▶ RAYNAUD'S DISEASE/PHENOMENON

Raynaud's disease or primary Raynaud's disease is an intermittent spasm of the digital arteries and arterioles resulting in decreased circulation to the fingers and toes. Sometimes the tip of the nose and ears can also be affected. The cause of the condition is unknown but seems to be related to vasospastic disorders, a disturbance with the innervation of the sympathetic nervous system, and angiography complications. During a spasm that lasts approximately fifteen minutes, the fingers become pale, and then cyanotic. As the circulation returns to the fingers, the fingertips become reddened and the person experiences a tingling or throbbing pain in the fingers. Some people only experience pallor and cyanosis. The episode may last one to two hours. Symptoms usually occur when the person is exposed to cold or experiences emotional stress. Gangrene is not common but can occur in the fingertips if the disease has been longstanding. Ulcerations can also occur and are difficult to heal because of decreased circulation in the fingers.

The condition is called Raynaud's phenomenon or secondary Raynaud's phenomenon when it is associated with a connective tissue or collagen vascular disease, medications, or occupational trauma. Raynaud symptoms may occur ten years before the related disease is diagnosed. A two-year history of signs and symptoms with no evidence of underlying disease, especially an autoimmune disease, is necessary for a diagnosis of Raynaud's disease.

Raynaud's is more prevalent in cool, damp climates. It occurs more frequently in women between the ages of 16 and 40 (Linton, et al., 1995). Persons who use vibrating hand tools such as air hammers or grinding wheels or whose hands perform repetitive movements such as typing or playing the piano are also affected. Researchers have also found Raynaud's phenomenon in persons exposed to vinyl chloride which is used in the manufacturing of plastics (Stephenson, 1992).

Diagnostic examinations include a complete blood count, digital blood pressure measurement, digital plethysmography waveforms, and a cold-challenge test. A digital blood pressure of 30 mmHg below the brachial pressure is indicative of a digital artery obstruction. A sedimentation rate, antinuclear antibody, and rheumatoid factor are done to determine the presence of autoimmune diseases. During a cold challenge test, thermistors are placed on the fingers and a baseline temperature is taken. The hands are submerged into ice water for twenty seconds. The temperature is then taken every five minutes until it returns to the baseline level. Hand x-rays determine the presence of subcutaneous calcium deposits and narrowing of bone in the digits. The diagnostic tests distinguish between Raynaud's phenomenon and Raynaud's disease. If a client has unilateral or single digit Raynaud's, an obstruction or emboli is suspected.

▶ *Medical/Surgical Management*

▶ *Medical*

Raynaud's phenomenon is treated conservatively. The client is assessed regularly for symptoms of autoimmune diseases. If the symptoms of Raynaud's are due to a vasospastic disease, relief is best achieved with medications. Biofeedback allows clients to voluntarily control the temperature of their hands (Stephenson, 1992).

▶ *Surgical*

In previous years a sympathectomy was sometimes done to alleviate the client's symptoms. However, clients with connective tissue diseases generally do not receive long-term relief from a sympathectomy and, therefore, a sympathectomy is no longer recommended.

▶ *Pharmacological*

Clients may be given nifedipine (Adalat, Procardia) at night for severe cases of Raynaud's phenomenon. Clients may also take the medication one to two hours before engaging in an outdoor activity during cold weather. They may not need to take the medication during warmer months. Other medications used to improve symptoms in severe Raynaud's phenomenon are diltiazem hydrochloride (Cardizem), verapamil (Calan), nicardipine hydrochloride (Cardene), and captopril (Capoten). Drug therapy improves the symptoms in about two-thirds of the clients (Stephenson, 1992).

Medications that aid in healing finger ulcers are iloprost, a prostaglandin, which is given intravenously and ciprofloxacin (Cipro), an antibiotic. In clinical research at Oregon Health Sciences University, clients with digital ulcers were given pentoxifylline (Trental), which decreases the viscosity of blood and improves the blood flow to peripheral arteries (Whitaker & Kelleher, 1994).

Beta blockers, birth control pills, cold medications, and diet pills cause some clients to have Raynaud's phenomenon. These medications should be substituted or discontinued if they are the source of the symptoms. Chemotherapy drugs such as bleomycin sulfate (Blenoxane) and cisplatin, CDDP (Platinol), also cause secondary Raynaud's.

▶ *Preventive Treatment*

The client is encouraged to avoid exposure to cold, repetitive hand movements, and stressful situations. The client is encouraged to quit smoking and avoid secondary smoke as nicotine is a potent vasoconstrictor. Stress management techniques, for example, biofeedback, may assist in alleviating some distress from the condition.

▶ *Nursing Process*

Assessment

Subjective Data   Obtain a history from the client as to how frequently the vasospastic episodes occur, what symptoms the client experiences, what triggers the episodes, which digits are affected during an episode, and how long the incident lasts. Inquire about daily activities that the client finds difficult such as tying shoes, washing dishes, or handling frozen foods. Obtain a history of occupational activities.

Objective Data   Assess the color, temperature, texture, and appearance of the digits. If the disease is longstanding, the digits may be tapered and the skin shiny in appearance. There may be ulcerated or gangrenous areas on the fingertips.

▼ ▼

Possible nursing diagnoses for a client with Raynaud's disease may include:

Nursing Diagnoses	*Goals*	*Nursing Interventions*
▶ *Tissue perfusion, altered, peripheral, related to vasospasm of peripheral arteries.*	The client will have fewer vasospastic episodes and increased circulation in digits.	Encourage the client to use caution when engaging in activities where he or she may be cut or scratched as healing may be impaired because of decreased circulation.
		If a client has ulcers, wash the areas with soap and water and administer prescribed medications such as ciprofloxacin (Cipro) and intravenous iloprost.
▶ *Pain, acute, related to decreased circulation in digits.*	The client will experience decreased pain as vasospasms are controlled.	Teach client to keep the indoor temperature at a comfortable level to avoid ischemic attacks.
		Encourage client to avoid dramatic changes in environmental temperatures, for example, entering a cold air-conditioned room during hot summer months. Encourage the client to wear woolen or windproof gloves or mittens and layered clothes when exposed to colder temperatures. Mittens may be better than gloves so the fingers can obtain warmth from each other. Chemical warming devices may be used inside gloves and shoes.
		Encourage the client to stop smoking and make a referral to a smoking cessation clinic.
		Teach the client relaxation exercises that may decrease the number of ischemic attacks.

(continued)

Nursing Diagnoses	Goals	Nursing Interventions
▶ *Self-esteem disturbance related to inability of hands to perform activities of daily living.*	The client will learn ways to handle activities of daily living.	Encourage client to use mitts or pot holders when removing items from the freezer or handling cold food to decrease the risk of a Raynaud's episode. Clients can wear mittens or socks to bed. Use of insulated mugs, foam rubber holders, or stemware glasses may reduce ischemic attacks.
		Instruct client to wash vegetables under tepid water instead of cold, to bathe in lukewarm water, and apply lotion regularly to prevent dry and chapped skin.
		Use of gloves when pushing shopping carts or operating some vibrating machines may decrease the cold sensation and soften the vibration.
▶ *Fear related to possible occupational change.*	The client will learn ways to cope with occupational stresses and/or state other occupational opportunities.	Discuss ways to reduce stress.
		Explore other interests, talents, and hobbies in which the client could become employed.
		Teach client that activities, such as playing the piano or typing, can be done in moderation and in warm environments.

▶ Evaluation

Each goal must be evaluated to determine how it has been met by the client.

▲ ▲

▶ ANEURYSM

An **aneurysm** is a localized dilation occurring in a weakened section of an artery's medial layer. The dilatation may extend 1.5 times the normal size of the vessel (Phipps, Cassmeyer, Sands, & Lehman, 1995). Aneurysms are the thirteenth leading cause of death in America (Phipps et al., 1995).

The main cause for aneurysms has previously been attributed to atherosclerosis. Recent research indicates a hereditary lack of elastin in the arterial wall as the most common cause of an aneurysm (Beare & Myers, 1994). The amount of elastin in persons without aneurysms is 12 percent compared to one percent in persons with aneurysms (Beare & Myers, 1994). Another factor indicating a hereditary component is if a person has an abdominal aortic aneurysm (AAA), the risk ratio is 6:1 that a first-degree relative may also develop an aneurysm compared to the general population (Beare & Myers, 1994). Some aneurysms occur because of congenital conditions such as Marfan's syndrome. Others are acquired because of trauma to the vessel wall, infection and/or inflammation, syphilis, or arteritis. Two other possible causes of an aneurysm are an increased turbulence in a section of the vessel and a slower production of smooth muscle cells. A client has a higher tendency to develop an aneurysm if they smoke cigarettes and have hypertension.

Aneurysms can occur in any artery or peripheral vessel, but occur most often in the abdominal aorta. Abdominal aneurysms occur more frequently in men between the ages of sixty and seventy than in women (Beare & Myers, 1994). Other involved vessels are the ascending, transverse, and descending aorta, thoracic aorta, popliteal arteries, and femoral arteries.

Deposits of atherosclerotic plaque on the tunica intima cause a hardening of the vessel and the media layer of the vessel loses elasticity. Atherosclerosis and a lack of elastin in the vessel wall predisposes the vessel to a weakened area which develops into an aneurysm.

There are three types of aneurysms: fusiform, saccular, and dissecting (Figure 21-7). The fusiform is a uniform dilation of the circumference of a vessel. In a saccular aneurysm, one side or section of the vessel balloons out and forms a saclike outpouching on the side of the vessel. A dissecting aneurysm occurs when a tear develops between the intima and the media of a vessel wall and blood enters the torn section. As the blood enters the space between the two layers of the vessel wall, more blood is forced into the area by the high blood pressure in the vessel. The dissecting aneurysm does not circumvent (surround) the vessel but involves only a section of the vessel wall. Approximately 70 percent of the dissecting aneurysms occur in the ascending aorta (Beare & Myers, 1994).

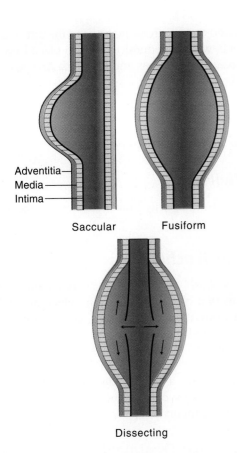

Adventitia—
Media—
Intima—

Saccular   Fusiform

Dissecting

FIGURE 21-7   Three types of aneurysms.

Dissecting aneurysms occur more frequently in the elderly hypertensive client. The complication of dissecting aneurysms is blood that has entered the torn layers may cause the tear to extend and eventually rupture the arterial wall. The rupture is a surgical emergency. Symptoms of a ruptured aneurysm include intense back or abdominal pain, pallor, cool and clammy skin, hypotension, diaphoresis, oliguria, loss of consciousness, and mottling of the abdomen and lower extremities.

Symptoms of an aneurysm depend upon the location of the aneurysm in the body. Aneurysms are often asymptomatic until they start leaking or pressing on other structures. A thoracic aneurysm may press on surrounding structures causing dull upper back pain or deep, scattered chest pain. Pressure on the trachea and bronchus may cause dyspnea, coughing, wheezing, and hoarseness. The client experiences dysphagia from pressure on the esophagus.

The most common location of an AAA is between the renal and iliac arteries. There may be no symptoms from an abdominal aortic aneurysm but as it enlarges and presses on other vessels, organs, and nerves the client may experience abdominal, back, or flank pain. If the AAA presses on the inferior vena cava, the lower

extremities become edematous and cyanotic. The person experiences bloating, abdominal pain, nausea, and vomiting as the AAA presses on the duodenum. If the AAA presses on the lumbar nerves, the person experiences low, dull back pain. The client may feel a pulse in the abdomen when in a supine position. The nurse may palpate a tender, pulsating mass slightly left of the client's umbilicus. Popliteal and femoral aneurysms may cause decreased pedal pulses. Bowel sounds may be diminished because of pressure from the aneurysm and femoral pulses are diminished or absent. An aneurysm is usually diagnosed when a client has an x-ray or ultrasound done for other conditions/symptoms.

▶ Medical/Surgical Management

▶ Medical

An aneurysm usually grows 0.5 cm per year (Phipps et al., 1995). If an aneurysm is less than 4 cm, it is important for the client to maintain frequent follow-up appointments with the physician and have repeated diagnostic testing done every six months to a year. If the aneurysm is between 4 and 6 cm, the size and condition of the aneurysm are carefully monitored with ultrasounds being done every six months. There is some controversy over whether or not a 4 cm aneurysm should be repaired. Some physicians prefer to repair a 4 cm aneurysm rather than take the risk of a rupture and potential mortality (Beare & Myers, 1994). Aneurysms over 5 to 6 cm in size are usually treated surgically because of the risk of rupture and fatality (Sandler, 1995; Phipps et al., 1995). If the client has hypertension, control of the hypertension is the focus of care.

▶ Surgical

Before elective surgery, the status of the client's carotid arteries and peripheral vessels are checked with a Doppler flow analysis (Doppler ultrasound). The client's cardiac status is usually evaluated by a stress test or cardiac catheterization before surgery is scheduled. The surgeon often orders an angiogram, ultrasound, or CT scan of the affected vessel prior to surgery in order to assess the blood supply to the area surrounding the aneurysm. Prior to surgery, it is common to place 4 to 8 units of blood on hold since hemorrhage is a possibility. The surgeon clamps the aorta, removes the section of the vessel involving the aneurysm, and replaces it with a section of the client's saphenous vein or a synthetic graft (see Figure 21-8). Complications that can occur from clamping the aorta are myocardial

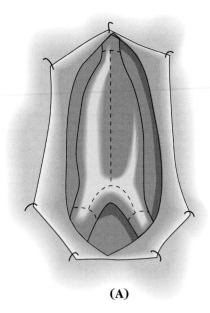

(A)

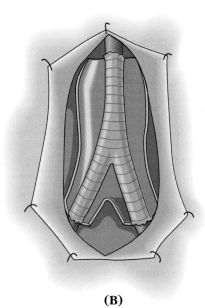

(B)

FIGURE 21-8 **(A)** A dissecting abdominal aneurysm, **(B)** Abdominal aneurysm repaired by a synthetic graft.

infarctions, strokes, and renal damage. Vessels below the repaired aneurysm may become occluded because of decreased blood flow during surgery or from plaque that has broken off from the wall of the vessel. A nasogastric tube may be inserted to decrease pressure on the aneurysm repair site and incision. After surgery, the client may be in an ICU for twenty-four hours with mechanical ventilator assistance in breathing.

▸ Pharmacological

Clients with aortic aneurysms may be given propranolol hydrochloride (Inderal) to decrease the pressure of the blood coming from the heart to the affected vessel. Clients with hypertension will be placed on antihypertensive medications and diuretics. Analgesics are given to control pain.

▸ Diet

There are no dietary restrictions.

▸ Activity

There are no activity limitations with a client who has an aneurysm.

▸ Client Teaching

The client and significant others are taught possible symptoms of a rupturing aneurysm which are sudden pain, the sensation of a tearing or ripping, pallor, diaphoresis, and loss of consciousness. If these symptoms occur, the client will need immediate medical attention.

Aneurysms are a familial disease. Therefore, first-degree relatives are encouraged to have an ultrasound to rule out an aneurysm.

▸ Preventive Treatment

Clients are encouraged not to smoke. Education for the hypertensive client includes the importance of closely monitoring the blood pressure and taking antihypertensive medication as prescribed. Clients are taught the name of the antihypertensive drug and possible side effects.

▸ Nursing Process

Assessment

Subjective Data   Preoperatively, the client may be concerned about an abdominal pulsation when reclining. The client may also have chest, back, abdominal, or flank pain depending on the location of the aneurysm. Postoperatively the nurse listens for statements of pain and assesses the level of pain according to a scale of 1 to 10, or the appropriate scale used in the facility.

Objective Data   If the client has an AAA, palpate the abdomen for a pulsating mass and check vital signs. Be alert for symptoms of bleeding or a rupturing aneurysm. Check the peripheral pulses of the client prior to surgery and document the level of the pulse. Pulses can then be compared preoperatively and postoperatively. Postoperatively, assess the extremities for color, warmth, and peripheral pulses.

▼ ▼

Possible nursing diagnoses for a client with an aneurysm may include:

Nursing Diagnoses	Goals	Nursing Interventions
▶ *Breathing pattern, ineffective, related to abdominal incisional pain.*	The client will have adequate ventilation.	Assist the client to turn, cough, and deep breathe. Assess client's lung sounds. Assist the client in using an incentive spirometer while splinting the incision.
▶ *Tissue perfusion, altered peripheral, high risk for, related to vascular occlusion.*	The client will have well-oxygenated tissues as manifested by strong pulses and the skin remaining pink and warm.	Monitor for symptoms of an occluded vessel (pain, paleness, cyanosis, and coldness). Monitor the warmth, color, and fullness of the peripheral pulses in both extremities and compare them to the preoperative pulses. Assess client's feet for mottling and darkened areas on the toes and soles of the feet. The client will have increased pain in the lower extremity if a vessel becomes occluded. Notify the physician immediately if any of these symptoms occur.
▶ *Fluid volume deficit, high risk for, related to loss of fluid from hemorrhage.*	The client will have adequate fluid volume.	Monitor vital signs closely for signs of hemorrhage. Check the operative site frequently to make sure the dressing is dry. Turn the client to make sure blood is not pooling under the client's body. Monitor for other signs of hemorrhaging. Measure the abdomen for increased abdominal girth indicating internal bleeding. If the client has low back pain, there may be hemorrhaging in the retroperitoneal space. Other symptoms of hemorrhage are lightheadedness, dizziness, and tachycardia. Check for adequate functioning and drainage of the NG tube.
▶ *Tissue perfusion, renal, risk for, related to interruption of blood flow during surgery.*	The client will have a urine output above 25 cc/hour.	Monitor hourly output to make sure the client has at least 25 to 30 cc of urine per hour. For the first twenty-four hours after surgery, administer fluids by a pulmonary artery catheter or central venous line. Fluids may be given by peripheral IV after the first twenty-four hours Assess for edema which could indicate fluid overload or a vessel occlusion

▶ Evaluation

Each goal must be evaluated to determine how it has been met by the client.

▲ ▲

▶ *HYPERTENSION*

Hypertension (HTN), also known as high blood pressure, is defined as an elevated arterial blood pressure. For general purposes, a systolic blood pressure above 140 or a diastolic blood pressure above 90 is indicative of hypertension. A more specific definition of hypertension is an increase, on several readings, of 15 mmHg pressure above the client's normal diastolic and/or systolic blood pressure baseline.

Risk factors for HTN include obesity, African American heritage, psychological stress, oral contraceptives, and smoking. The aging process affects hypertensive tendencies. Hypertension occurs at an earlier age in men than in women until both sexes reach the age of sixty. Familial factors also play a part in HTN as a client whose parents had hypertension is at a higher risk. People in stressful occupations, e.g., air traffic controllers, or in a lower economic status have more of a tendency to have HTN (see Figure 21-9).

When the cause of hypertension is unknown, the diagnosis is "essential hypertension," also called primary or idiopathic hypertension. Ninety-five percent of the clients with hypertension have essential hypertension (Cuddy, 1995). In 5 percent of the cases, the cause of hypertension may be due to another condition within the body such as renal disease, arteriosclerosis, atherosclerosis, hypernatremia (increased sodium in the blood), or prolonged stress (Cuddy, 1995). (The etiology of these conditions is discussed in the next five paragraphs.) When HTN is due to another disease or condition, the diagnosis is secondary hypertension. An easy way to remember the difference between the two diagnoses is to recall that secondary hypertension is secondary to another condition in the body.

Renal diseases may interfere with the flow of blood to the kidneys causing them to release an enzyme called renin. When renin is released, it interacts with plasma proteins forming a vasopressor called angiotensin. Vasoconstriction caused by angiotensin increases the blood pressure because more force is required to get the blood through the vessel. Vasoconstriction causes a decrease in the diameter of the vessel. In contrast, vasodilation increases the diameter of the vessel allowing blood to flow more freely through the vessel with less pressure. Vasodilation decreases vascular or **peripheral resistance** (pressure within a vessel that resists the flow of blood such as plaque buildup or vasoconstriction). Figure 21-10 depicts how renal disease causes hypertension.

Arteriosclerosis causes the vessel walls to have less elasticity, decreasing their ability to expand and recoil. Since the vessel is not able to expand, more pressure is needed to force the blood through the vessel. Atherosclerosis narrows the vessel lumen, or opening, because of plaque buildup along the wall of the vessel. The plaque buildup causes resistance to the flow

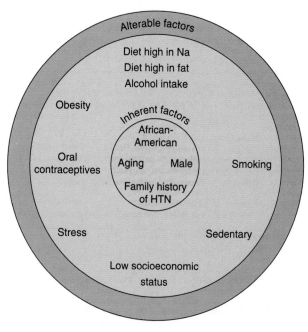

FIGURE 21-9 Risk factors for hypertension. (*Adapted from Beare & Myers,* Factors contributing to hypertension)

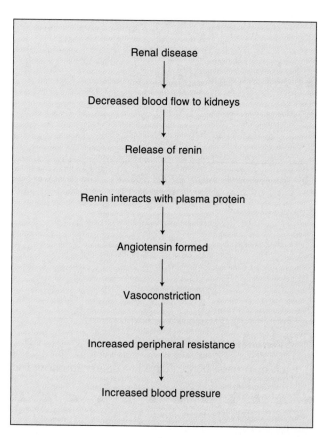

FIGURE 21-10 Pathophysiology of renal disease and hypertension.

of blood through the vessel and more pressure is needed to get the blood through the vessel. Hypernatremia (increased blood sodium) causes vasocongestion. With vasocongestion, the heart must pump with more force, increasing the pressure in the arteries, thus causing HTN.

Stress stimulates the sympathetic nervous system which supplies nerves to the smooth muscles of the arteries, arterioles, veins, and venules. Stimulation of smooth muscles by the sympathetic nervous system causes the vessel to vasoconstrict leading to HTN.

There are four stages of HTN defined as stage 1, stage 2, stage 3, and stage 4. Figure 21-11 shows blood pressure ranges for each stage of hypertension. If the diastolic and systolic pressures are at different stages, then a client eighteen or older is advanced to the next stage. An example is a client with a blood pressure of 162/94. The systolic pressure of 162 is at stage 2 and the diastolic pressure of 94 is a stage 1. The client is in stage 2 hypertension.

Some complications of HTN are cerebral vascular accident (stroke), myocardial infarction, and congestive heart failure. The stroke may be caused from a cerebral thrombosis, embolus, or hemorrhage. A myocardial infarction is caused from the extra workload placed on the heart to force the blood through the system. Congestive heart failure is due to left ventricle hypertrophy and eventual failure when it cannot meet the demands of the body.

Hypertensive crisis is a diastolic BP of 130 mmHg or more and constitutes a medical emergency. The client may manifest symptoms of blurred vision, headache, nausea, vomiting, restlessness, confusion, and retinal hemorrhage. This condition is generally uncommon, but prompt diagnosis and treatment are essential to prevent organ damage.

The client is admitted to the intensive care and the

BP is monitored through an arterial catheter. Parenteral medications such as potent vasodilators, adrenergic inhibitors, and diuretics are given to lower the BP. Antihypertensive medications used to control the crisis are diazoxide (Hyperstat), nitroprusside sodium (Nipride), hydralazine hydrochloride (Apresoline), methyldopa (Aldomet), and phentolamine mesylate (Regitine). Without prompt medical treatment, the client may experience renal failure, cardiac failure, or a cerebral vascular accident.

Conditions that may precipitate a hypertensive crisis are hypertensive encephalopathy, intracranial hemorrhage, cerebral vascular accident, myocardial infarction, eclampsia, pheochromocytoma, or a dissecting aneurysm. Hypertensive crisis may also occur in clients who stop taking their antihypertensive medication.

▶ Medical/Surgical Management

▶ Medical

The physician's main goal in caring for a client with HTN is keeping the blood pressure within normal limits. The regimen is referred to as a stepped-care approach. The first step is to encourage the client to try some diet and lifestyle changes. These include losing weight if the client is more than 15 percent over the optimum weight; limiting sodium, saturated fat, cholesterol, and alcohol intake; exercising on a regular basis; stopping the use of nicotine; and maintaining an adequate intake of calcium, magnesium, and potassium. This step is tried for three to six months and, if the BP returns to normal, these steps would be continued. If the BP still remains high, the second step would be implemented which would be adding a diuretic or a beta-blocker to the client's care regimen. The client would again be evaluated for a period of time, usually two months. If the BP still does not return to less than 140/90 within that time frame, the third step of increasing the drug dosage, trying another drug, or adding a second antihypertensive drug from another class of drugs would be implemented. If the BP is maintained at less than 140/90, the regimen would be continued. If the BP is still high, the last step would be implemented by adding a second or third antihypertensive drug. Often the hypertensive client may not be experiencing any symptoms and does not see the importance of caring effectively for this condition.

Pharmacological

Diuretics are usually the first pharmacological step in treating HTN. Diuretics increase the renal excretion

Four stages of hypertension

Stage	Systolic (mm Hg)	Diastolic (mm Hg)
Normal	< 130	< 85
Stage 1	140 –159	90 – 99
Stage 2	160 – 179	100 – 109
Stage 3	180 – 209	110 – 119
Stage 4	≥ 210	≥ 120

FIGURE 21-11 The four stages of hypertension. (*Adapted from The Fifth Report of the Joint Committee on Detection, Evaluation and Treatment of High Blood Pressure. October, 1992*)

of sodium and water from the body decreasing the total fluid volume. When less fluid is in the body, less pressure or force is needed to pump the blood through the body.

Beta-adrenergic blocking agents such as propranolol hydrochloride (Inderal), timolol maleate (Blocadren), and atenolol (Tenormin) are also given to block the epinephrine and norepinephrine receptor sites. Epinephrine and norepinephrine cause vasoconstriction. Since beta-adrenergic agents block these receptor sites, the vessels will not constrict and the blood will have less resistance flowing through the vessel. Diuretics and antihypertensive medications may cause impotence.

Other medications used to lower blood pressure are alpha$_1$-receptor blockers, angiotensin-converting enzyme (ACE) inhibitors, calcium channel blockers, centrally acting alpha$_2$-agonists, peripherally acting adrenergic antagonists, and direct vasodilators. Refer to Table 21-1 for a list of antihypertensive medications.

▶ Diet

The hypertensive client is encouraged to have a low-fat, low-cholesterol, and low-sodium diet. Restricting sodium intake to 2.3 grams of sodium or 6 grams of sodium chloride a day assists in decreasing blood pressure. Slight lifestyle changes such as avoiding canned foods, carbonated drinks, and most cereals helps decrease sodium intake. The client should have an adequate intake of potassium, magnesium, and calcium. These minerals can be obtained by eating fresh oranges, bananas, broccoli, and collards. Fresh foods are better sources for minerals than frozen foods. Yogurt is a good calcium supplement. The National Committee on Detection, Evaluation, and Treatment of High Blood Pressure recommends that clients with hypertension not consume more than 2 ounces of alcohol at a time and no more than twice a week.

▶ Activity

A regular aerobic exercise regimen assists in lowering blood pressure. The client is to gradually increase the exercise period to 30 to 45 minutes three to five times per week with a pulse rate at 75 percent of the target heart rate (Target heart rate = 220 − age × 0.75). Walking, swimming, and jogging are excellent aerobic exercises.

▶ Preventive Treatment

Measures to prevent hypertension are exercising regularly, decreasing sodium in the diet, maintaining an optimum weight, and decreasing stress in life experiences.

Table 21-1

ANTIHYPERTENSIVE MEDICATIONS

Alpha-adrenergic Blockers
clonidine hydrochloride (Catapres)
doxazosin mesylate (Cardura)
methyldopa (Aldomet)
phentolamine mesylate (Regitine)
prazosin hydrochloride (Minipress)
terazosin hydrochloride (Vasocard, Hytrin)

Angiotensin-converting Enzyme (ACE) Inhibitors
captopril (Capoten)
enalapril maleate (Vasotec)

Calcium Channel Blockers
diltiazem hydrochloride (Cardizem)
nifedipine (Procardia)
verapamil (Calan, Isoptin)

Ganglionic Blocker
trimethaphan camsylate (Arfonad)

Loop Diuretics
bumetanide (Bumex)
furosemide (Lasix)

Potassium-sparing Diuretics
amiloride hydrochloride (Midamor)
spironolactone (Aldactone)
spironolactone with HCTZ (Aldactazide)
triamterene (Dyrenium)

Thiazide Diuretics
chlorothiazide (Diuril)
hydrochlorothiazide (Esdrix, HydroDIURIL)
methyclothiazide (Enduron)
metolazone (Zaroxolyn)

Thiazide-like Diuretic
chlorthalidone (Hygroton)
indapamide (Lozol)

Peripherally Acting Adrenergic Antagonists
reserpine (Serpasil)

Direct Vasodilators
diazoxide (Hyperstat)
hydrolazine hydrochloride (Apresoline)
nitroprusside sodium (Nipride)

▶ Nursing Process

Assessment

Subjective Data Assess the hypertensive client by asking about general lifestyle habits such as smoking, alcohol consumption, exercise routine, dietary intake, and family history of hypertension. Ask if the client has been experiencing dizziness, blurred vision, and headache in the occipital region upon rising in the morning.

Objective Data The basic assessment for HTN is taking the blood pressure. It is important to obtain an accurate BP. Some measures to ensure this are making sure the correct size of BP cuff is used. The bladder of the blood pressure cuff should surround two-thirds of the client's arm. Before taking the blood pressure, the client should rest quietly for five minutes. The blood pressure should be taken in both arms. The client is seated with the arm at heart level and supported. If the client has an elevated BP, wait fifteen minutes and then repeat taking the blood pressure. Observe for a flushed face and epistaxis.

▼ ▼

Possible nursing diagnoses for a client with hypertension may include:

Nursing Diagnoses	Goals	Nursing Interventions
▶ Health maintenance, altered, related to lack of knowledge about lifestyle habits contributing to hypertension.	The client will relate needed changes in lifestyle habits to decrease blood pressure.	Make referrals to the appropriate personnel to teach the client lifestyle changes. These may include a dietitian, stop smoking clinic, fitness center, or stress management seminars. Explain the pathophysiology, risk factors, lifestyle changes, medication actions and side effects, and complications of hypertension. These instructions are important because often the hypertensive client may not be experiencing any symptoms so the importance of caring effectively for this condition is understood.
▶ Noncompliance related to lack of physical symptoms and expense of medication.	The client will keep appointments for regular check-ups and take medications as prescribed.	Regularly inquire about the client's satisfaction of life in regard to the prescribed regimen of diet, exercise, and prescribed medication(s). If the client cannot afford needed medications, refer the client to financial assistant programs. Encourage the client to become an active participant and problem-solver in his treatment as this will give him a sense of control over his condition and care. Encourage the client to record BP readings, weekly weights, exercise activities, and dietary intake as a way of giving him a sense of control and encouraging compliance.
▶ Nutrition, altered, more than body requirements, related to excess caloric intake and excess sodium intake.	The client will maintain weight at no more than 15 percent over optimum weight and have no more than 2.3 grams of sodium per day.	Give basic dietary instructions as stated under medical management or make a referral to a dietitian. Weigh the client at scheduled appointments.
▶ Sexual dysfunction, potential, related to side effects of antihypertensive medications.	The client will state satisfaction with sexual function while taking antihypertensive medications.	Since diuretics and antihypertensive medications may cause impotence, discuss sexual function in an open and candid manner, so the client and spouse will be more open to discuss difficulties in this area.

▶ Evaluation

Each goal must be evaluated to determine how it has been met by the client.

▲ ▲

Sample Nursing Care Plan: The Client with Hypertension

Thomas Liggins, a twenty-eight-year-old African American, is in his last year of law school and is clerking for a prestigious law firm. He and his fiancé are planning to be married as soon as he graduates. During the last week he has had four dizzy spells and has had a headache at the base of his skull upon awakening for the last two days. His father has a history of hypertension, so Thomas is aware that his symptoms may be indicative of high blood pressure. Thomas stops by the clinic on his way home from work and asks the nurse practitioner to check his blood pressure. The nursing assessment has the following data:

Subjective data:

States he has had 4 dizzy spells and has awakened with a headache in the occipital lobe the last 2 mornings. Thomas has been having 1 glass of wine at lunch and 2-3 beers in the evening to relax from the tension of school and work. Most of his meals have been at fast food establishments and have a high fat content. Thomas does not smoke. He used to jog 4 mornings a week but quit when he starting clerking. He has been getting up twice in the night to urinate for the last 3 weeks. He is not taking any medication. Thomas states he is concerned about having hypertension because he does not want to take medication.

Objective data:

T 98.6 P 78 R 16 BP 142/92 Wt 190 (optimum weight 160)

No edema noted in hands, feet, or legs.

The nurse practitioner schedules the following tests for the next morning: cholesterol with lipoproteins, glucose, EKG, repeat BP check.

Nursing Diagnosis 1 Health maintenance, altered, related to lifestyle habits contributing to hypertension as evidenced by high fat diet, lack of exercise, stressful job, and alcohol intake.

Goals	Nursing Interventions	Rationale	Evaluation
Thomas Liggins will change lifestyle habits by engaging in aerobic exercises at least three times a week for thirty to forty-five minutes, stating three ways to reduce stress and limiting alcohol consumption to two ounces twice a week.	Refer Thomas to a dietitian to learn ways to cut fat and sodium in his diet. Discuss ways Thomas can exercise and still meet responsibilities of work, school, and personal and social life. Explain that alcohol consumption should be limited to two ounces of alcohol twice a week.	Knowledge of a low-sodium, low-fat diet will encourage compliance. Thomas will be more willing to exercise if he sees ways that he can still meet responsibilities of life. Knowledge of alcohol content in alcoholic beverages will encourage compliance.	Thomas starts exercising with his fiancé three times a week. Thomas uses breathing techniques and a hot shower to reduce daily stress. Thomas limits alcoholic consumption to one beer a day.

Nursing Diagnosis 2 Nutrition, altered, more than body requirements, related to eating habits as evidenced by 30 pounds overweight and high fat diet.

Goals	Nursing Interventions	Rationale	Evaluation
Thomas Liggins will lose 30 pounds and maintain a low-fat, low-sodium diet.	Refer Thomas to a weight support group.

Encourage Thomas to maintain a weekly weight record and daily intake of fat grams. | It will be easier for Thomas to change life habits if others are encouraging him.

Monitoring personal diet and recording weight weekly promotes self-care and personal involvement in health maintenance. | Thomas and his fiancé are maintaining a diet low in sodium and no more than 30 grams of fat per day. Thomas keeps a weekly record of his weight. |

Nursing Diagnosis 3 Anxiety related to stress of job and possible diagnosis of elevated blood pressure as evidenced by alcohol consumption to relax and statement of not wanting to have hypertension.

Goals	Nursing Interventions	Rationale	Evaluation
Thomas Liggins will state preventive measures to reduce blood pressure.	Identify stress factors in life.

Discuss stress reduction techniques with Thomas.

Discuss risk factors of hypertension.

Explain to Thomas and his fiancé that hypertension is a chronic condition, possibly without symptoms, and with some potentially serious complications. | Thomas may not be aware of some stressors in his life. Action to cope with stressors can only be taken if stressors are identified.

Knowledge of ways to reduce stress will promote compliance.

Knowledge of risk factors will promote identification of risk factors in personal life.

Knowledge of disease process promotes compliance. It is important for client and client's support system to understand disease process so lifestyle changes can be made more easily. | Thomas states four ways to reduce blood pressure. |

▶ CASE STUDY

Lucille Soudin, a sixty-three-year-old female, slipped on a throw rug in her home and fell. She immediately had severe pain in her right hip. Her husband called the emergency service, and she was transferred to the local hospital. Lucille was admitted to the hospital and scheduled for a total hip replacement.

In the evening of the first postoperative day, Lucille stated the calf of her right leg was "hurting." The nurse placed her hand on the area where Lucille indicated there was pain and found the posterior area of the right calf to be warm, reddened, and tender to touch.

The following questions will guide your development of a Nursing Care Plan for the case study.

1. What other assessments should the nurse make before calling the physician?

2. Should the nurse perform a Homans' sign at this time?

3. What orders may the nurse receive from the physician?

4. What medications may have been ordered prophylactically to prevent a thrombus formation? What baseline laboratory results should be obtained before the anticoagulant medications are started?

5. Write pertinent individualized nursing diagnoses and goals for Lucille.

6. List appropriate nursing interventions needed in providing care to Lucille (refer also to Chapter 26, Musculoskeletal Disorders, for total hip replacement postop care.)

7. What information should the nurse include in Lucille's discharge teaching regarding:

    symptoms of another thrombus

    anticoagulant therapy

    elevation and positioning of the extremity

8. List resources specific to locale that could assist in Lucille's rehabilitation process.

9. List successful client outcomes for Lucille.

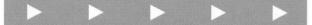 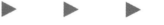

SUMMARY

- The peripheral vascular system consists of arteries, arterioles, capillaries, venules, and veins.
- To assess the peripheral vascular system the nurse assesses pain, pulse, pallor, paresthesia, and paralysis.
- Nursing assessments to determine the patency of the peripheral vascular system are Allen's test, Homans' sign, and Brodie-Trendelenburg's test.
- Three factors leading to the formation of a clot, pooling of blood, vessel trauma and a coagulation problem, are called Virchow's triad.
- A client with a DVT may be asymptomatic or may have warmth and tenderness at the site, edema of the extremity, a positive Homans' sign, cyanosis of the foot, and a sensation of heaviness or tightness in the extremity.
- Treatment for a thrombus includes bed rest, warm soaks, elevation of the extremity, and application of elastic stockings or intermittent pneumatic compression. It is important for the nurse to measure the leg circumference every shift and check peripheral pulses.
- The cause of varicose veins is incompetent valves and veins that have lost their elasticity.
- Primary Raynaud's disease is an intermittent spasm of the digital arteries and arterioles resulting in decreased circulation to the digits.
- Secondary Raynaud's phenomenon is associated with a connective tissue or collagen vascular disease.
- An aneurysm is a localized dilation of a weakened section of the medial layer of an artery.
- According to research, the most common cause of an aneurysm is a hereditary lack of elastin in the arterial wall.
- Symptoms of an aneurysm depend upon the location of the aneurysm in the body and are often asymptomatic until they start leaking or pressing on other structures.
- Hypertension is an elevated arterial blood pressure of 140/90.
- The treatment for hypertension involves a stepped-care approach.

Review Questions

1. The valves are a part of which tunica layer?
   a. tunica intima
   b. tunica media
   c. tunica adventitia
   d. tunica externa

2. A test that a nurse performs to evaluate the arterial circulation of the hands is the:
   a. Homans' sign.
   b. Brodie-Trendelenburg's test.
   c. Allen's test.
   d. venous plethysmography.

3. Instructions to a client on anticoagulant therapy includes:
   a. taking Coumadin twice a day.
   b. watching for symptoms of bleeding.
   c. taking over-the-counter medications as needed.
   d. no dietary or activity limitations.

4. When assessing a client with a possible DVT, the nurse:
   a. routinely does a Homans' sign.
   b. massages the calf of the leg.
   c. gently touches the affected area and checks for warmth.
   d. calls the physician immediately.

5. A varicose vein is more likely to occur in the:
   a. femoral vein.
   b. iliac vein.
   c. popliteal vein.
   d. saphenous vein.

6. A nurse is assigned to care for a client who has just had a hysterectomy. To prevent the formation of a thrombus, the nurse:
   a. encourages the client to lie in bed with the knee gatch activated.
   b. encourages the client to ambulate with assistance according to the physician's orders.
   c. does a Homans' sign as part of the routine postop assessment.
   d. checks peripheral pulses every four hours.

7. A client, admitted with the diagnosis of AAA, states he can feel a pulsation when he lies flat in bed. To assess the pulsation, the nurse would palpate:
   a. the epigastric area.
   b. the right lower quadrant.
   c. one inch above the symphysis pubis.
   d. left of umbilicus.

8. The symptoms a client would most likely experience who has an aneurysm pressing on the inferior vena cava would be:
   a. low dull back pain and a pulsating mass in the abdomen.
   b. dyspnea, wheezing, and hoarseness.
   c. bloating, nausea, and vomiting.
   d. edema in the extremities and possible cyanosis.

News Flash:
White-coat phenomenon

Some people suffer from a phenomenon called white-coat hypertension, which is an elevation in BP readings when a professional in a white coat takes their BP. At first this was believed to be psychosomatic or possibly that it may indicate a client at risk for hypertension. However, recent research has shown that people with white-coat hypertension are at more risk for cardiovascular problems than those whose BP is within the normal ranges during the same circumstances.

The research groups consisted of fifty-eight clients with white-coat hypertension, 113 with hypertension and 88 with normal BP levels. The research showed the white-coat hypertensive clients had more characteristics in common with the hypertensive clients than with subjects with normal BP levels. Some of the common characteristics were more fluctuations in BP levels throughout the day, left ventricular hypertrophy, increased levels of renin and similar levels of aldosterone, insulin, norepinephrine, and LDLs (low-density lipoproteins).

According to these studies, clients with white-coat hypertension are encouraged to take the same preventive measures as clients at risk for cardiovascular conditions. These preventive measures are to maintain weight within 15 percent of optimum weight, monitor serum cholesterol levels, stop smoking, and exercise regularly (*Sources: As cited in* Nursing '95, *1995*).

Hypertension in Middle-aged Men

A research study for three decades followed 3,700 men in the Honolulu Heart Program. The results showed that for every increase of 10 mmHg pressure in the systolic blood pressure there was a 9 percent increase of cognitive impairment in later life. The men had difficulty calculating, communicating, remembering and doing other types of mental functioning. The etiology is attributed to the effect of hypertension on the brain's blood vessels (Rowland, 1995).

9. The first step of the stepped-care approach in treating hypertension is:
    a. changes in lifestyle.
    b. diuretics.
    c. beta-blockers.
    d. adding a second or third antihypertensive.

10. A thirty-two-year-old client has a pulse rate of 72. When she exercises, her target heart rate is:
    a. 122.
    b. 135.
    c. 141.
    d. 157.

Critical Thinking Questions

1. Prepare a teaching strategy to teach the hypertensive client ways to modify the present lifestyle.

2. If a client had hypertension, how would needed lifestyle changes be assessed?

Medical Terminology

angio-	vessel
angiography	a radiographic study of blood vessels after the injection of a radiopaque material
phlebo-	vein
phlebitis	inflammation of a vein
thrombo-	blood clot
thrombosis	abnormal condition in which a thrombus develops within a blood vessel
vaso-	vessel
vasoconstrictive	causing constriction of the blood vessels

CHAPTER 22

Blood and Lymph Disorders

Gena Duncan

► KEY TERMS

bands
blastic phase
combination chemotherapy
erythrocytapheresis
fibrinolysis
hemarthrosis
hematocrit
hematopoiesis
hemolysis
hyperuricemia
induction doses
leukocytosis
leukopenia
maintenance therapy
median survival time
microthrombi
phlebotomy
purpura
reticulocytes
secondary malignancy
sickled
thrombocytopenia

LIST OF DISORDERS

Red Blood Cell Disorders: Anemia and Polycythemia
► Iron Deficiency Anemia
► Hypoplastic (Aplastic) Anemia
► Pernicious Anemia
► Hemolytic Anemias
  • Acquired Hemolytic Anemia
  • Sickle Cell Anemia
► Polycythemia vera

White Blood Cell Disorders
► Leukemia
► Acute Leukemia
► Chronic Leukemia

Coagulation Disorders
► Disseminated Intravascular Coagulation (DIC)
► Hemophilia

Lymph Disorders
► Hodgkin's Disease
► Non-Hodgkin's Lymphoma (NHL)

LEARNING OBJECTIVES

Upon completion of this chapter the learner should be able to:
• Define key terms.
• Relate anatomy and physiology of the blood and lymph systems to disease processes.
• Relate diagnostic test results to the blood and lymph disorders
• Describe nursing interventions in caring for clients with blood and lymph disorders.
• Assist in developing a nursing care plan for clients with blood and lymph disorders.

▶ *MAKING THE CONNECTION*

Refer to the topics in the following chapters to increase your understanding of blood and lymph disorders.

INTRODUCTION

The hematologic system of the body is comprised of blood and blood-forming organs. Blood consists of formed elements (red blood cells, white blood cells, and platelets) and plasma. As blood is pumped through the body, it carries essential substances to the tissues and removes waste products from the tissues. Disorders of the hematologic system usually result from abnormal production or functioning of the cells. Some of these disorders are the result of genetics, environment, or pathogenic organisms.

The lymph system consists of lymph vessels, nodes, and organs. Lymph vessels collect and return lymph fluid to the blood vessels through the right and left lymphatic ducts at the right and left subclavian veins. The functions of the lymph system are to assist with immunity, control edema, and absorb digested fats. The disorders of the lymph system discussed in this chapter are due to malignancies.

Medical management and nursing diagnoses, goals, and interventions are given for each blood and lymph disorder. It is important for the nurse to have a complete understanding of the blood and lymph disorders when providing nursing care to clients.

ANATOMY AND PHYSIOLOGY REVIEW

Blood

The heart pumps 5–6 liters of blood per minute through the circulatory system of an adult. Blood is an aqueous mixture consisting of plasma and cells.

Plasma

Blood plasma is a straw-colored liquid consisting of water, proteins, electrolytes, lipids, carbohydrates, and various other organic and inorganic substances. The formed elements in plasma are red blood cells (RBCs), white blood cells (WBCs), and platelets. The proteins in the plasma are albumin, fibrinogen globulins, RBCs, WBCs, platelets, proteins, and immunoglobulins (gamma globulins) are transported by the plasma throughout the circulatory system.

Red Blood Cells

Red blood cells, also called erythrocytes, are the most numerous blood cells in the body. There are 4.5 to 6.1 million/mm^3 in an adult. RBCs are biconcave disks that do not have a nucleus. They are about the size of the smallest capillary but are flexible and capable of changing shape so they can squeeze through the capillaries.

RBCs in conjunction with the respiratory and circulatory systems accomplish the oxygenation of body tissues. In the capillary bed of the alveoli, blood receives oxygen (O_2) and carbon dioxide (CO_2) is eliminated. The O_2 enriched RBCs (oxyhemoglobin) carry O_2 to systemic capillaries where O_2 is exchanged for CO_2. The carbon dioxide laden blood then returns the CO_2 to the alveoli in the lungs where it is again exchanged for oxygen. The CO_2 is exhaled from the body with each breath. Hemoglobin is a protein in the RBC that carries O_2 and is responsible for the exchange of O_2 and CO_2.

The average life span for a RBC is 120 days. Blood cells originate from a single stem cell that proliferates and differentiates into lymphoid stem cells or blood

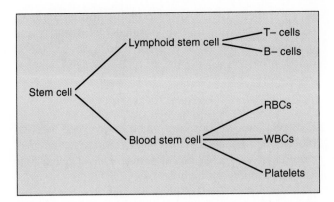

FIGURE 22-1 Origin of blood cells, T-cells, and B-cells.

stem cells (see Figure 22-1). The lymphoid stem cells further divide and differentiate into T-cells and B-cells. The blood stem cells divide and differentiate into RBCs, WBCs, and platelets. The process of blood cell production is called **hematopoiesis**. RBCs are produced daily by the bone marrow according to the demand of the body. When the partial pressure of O_2 drops, a renal hormone, erythropoietin, stimulates the bone marrow to produce more immature RBCs (**reticulocytes**) which are released into the bloodstream. These reticulocytes develop into mature red blood cells. The number of circulating reticulocytes can be used as a diagnostic tool for RBC disorders.

As RBCs age, their outer membrane deteriorates and they are destroyed by large macrophages in the liver and filtered out of the body by the spleen. The iron from heme in the old RBCs is used in the production of new RBCs.

Hematocrit is the percentage of blood cells in a volume of blood. A normal hematocrit is 42 percent to 45 percent of blood volume which means that 42 to 45 percent of a certain amount of blood consists of cells.

White Blood Cells

White blood cells, also called leukocytes, fight infection and assist with immunity in the body. The lifespan of a WBC varies from hours to years depending on the type of WBC. Neutrophils, basophils, and eosinophils live from a few hours to days while the lymphocytes and monocytes live from days to years. The normal WBC count is 5,000 to 10,000/mm³ of blood (Pagana & Pagana, 1995). Another important test for evaluating WBCs is the differential count that measures the number or percentage of each type of WBC in a specific blood specimen. An increased number of WBCs (**leukocytosis**) may signify the presence of an infection, inflammation, tissue necrosis, or leukemia. A decreased number of WBCs (**leukopenia**) may indicate bone marrow failure, a massive infection, dietary deficiencies, a drug toxicity, or an autoimmune disease.

WBCs are classified as granulocytes or polymorphonuclear leukocytes (PMNs) and agranulocytes. The granulocytes have granules (grainy substances) in their cytoplasm, and the agranulocytes do not have granules. Granulocytes are divided into three types: the neutrophils, eosinophils, and basophils. Agranulocytes are classified into two groups, monocytes and lymphocytes (see WBCs under diagnostic laboratory tests). Neutrophils are the most numerous WBCs, making up approximately 60 percent of the total number of WBCs (Linton, et al., 1995). The main function of neutrophils is to digest and kill microorganisms. If a client has an acute infection, the bone marrow is stimulated to produce more neutrophils resulting in an increased circulation of immature neutrophils called **bands**. When an increased production of neutrophils occurs, the process is called a "shift to the left" in WBC production and indicates the presence of an acute infection. An increased number of basophils and especially eosinophils indicate an allergic response in the body.

Monocytes become macrophages, cells that destroy dead and injured cells and bacteria. There are two types of lymphocytes, T-cells and B-cells, which are involved in the body's immune response.

Platelets

Platelets (thrombocytes) are not typical cells but nonnucleated, granular ovoid, or spindle-shaped cell fragments. The normal lifespan of a platelet is approximately ten days (Phipps, et al., 1995). Platelets are active in the clotting mechanism of the body. When platelets flow over a rough or damaged area in a vessel, they adhere to the area and release thromboplastin and clotting factors that start the blood clotting process. They also secrete prostaglandins and serotonin that cause the vessel to constrict which decreases the blood flow through the area. Blood proteins, prothrombin, and fibrinogen, form thrombin and fibrin respectively. The fibrin strands seal the opening or area and a clot is formed (see Figure 22-2).

Blood Types

On the surface of RBC membranes are genetically determined antigens called aggultinogens. The A and B antigens constitute the ABO blood group. If the A antigen is on the RBC membrane, the client has type A blood. If the B antigen is on the RBC membrane, the client has type B blood. If both an A and B antigen are present, the client has type AB blood, and if no antigen is present, type O blood.

Anti-A and anti-B antibodies are present in the serum of every person with type A and type B blood. Type A blood has anti-B antibodies in the serum and type B blood has anti-A antibodies. If a person with

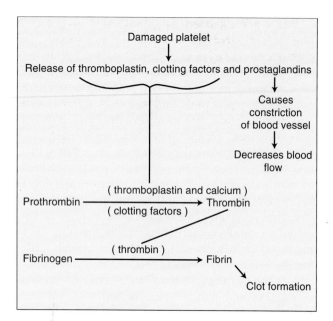

Damaged platelet

Release of thromboplastin, clotting factors and prostaglandins

Causes
constriction
of blood vessel

Decreases blood
flow

(thromboplastin and calcium)
Prothrombin ————————————————→ Thrombin
(clotting factors)

(thrombin)
Fibrinogen ————————————————→ Fibrin

Clot formation

FIGURE 22-2   Clot formation.

type A blood receives type B blood, the anti-B antibodies will attack the infused RBCs and hemolyze (destroy) them. The hemoglobin released when these cells are hemolyzed can lead to kidney damage.

A person with AB blood does not have anti-A or anti-B antibodies. People with AB blood are theoretically universal recipients because they can receive blood from all blood types. Type O blood does not have any antigens that the antibodies can attack. Persons with type O blood can theoretically give blood to persons having any type of blood. Persons with type O blood are called universal donors. The terms universal recipient and universal donor are in theory only because during blood transfusions, blood incompatibilities can occur because of the other types of antigens.

There are fourteen different blood groups and over 100 different antigens. The different blood groups vary in number with different ethnic groups.

Rh Factor

Another factor to consider during blood transfusions is the Rh factor. Persons who have Rh antigens (the D antigen) are Rh positive. Those who do not have Rh antigens on their RBC membranes are Rh negative. Approximately 85 percent of the people have Rh positive blood and 15 percent of the people have Rh negative blood (Lewis, Collier, & Heitkemper, 1996).

If a person with Rh negative blood is exposed to Rh positive blood during a blood transfusion or during childbirth, anti-Rh antibodies form in the blood serum. When a person with Rh negative blood is exposed a second time to Rh positive blood, the anti-Rh antibodies will react with the Rh positive blood and cause hemolysis of the infused blood and a severe blood reaction.

Blood Transfusions

Blood transfusions are given to replace needed blood components because of hemorrhage, anemia, clotting disorders, or blood deficiencies. Transfusable blood products are whole blood, packed red cells, platelets, fresh frozen plasma, and cryoprecipitate. Whole blood is given to increase blood volume and the number of blood components. Packed red cells are given for anemia. Platelets assist in controlling bleeding. Fresh frozen plasma is administered for clotting disorders. Cryoprecipitate corrects fibrinogen deficiencies.

Before blood products are given, the lab does a type- and cross-match to check compatibility between the donor blood type and Rh factor and the client's blood type and Rh factor. The lab also checks all blood products for HIV and hepatitis B and C virus. When obtaining blood from the lab, handle the blood gently so as not to damage the cells. Blood should be administered within thirty minutes of obtaining it from the laboratory refrigerator.

The nurse takes baseline vital signs; temperature, pulse, and blood pressure, before administering the blood product. Once the transfusion is started, take the temperature and pulse after 15 minutes, 30 minutes, and hourly. Take the blood pressure hourly during the transfusion. Blood is generally administered through a peripheral vein using an 18 or 19 gauge cannula. A large cannula is used so the blood cells do not break when passing through the cannula.

Before the transfusion, two nurses check the compatibility of the blood product and the client. The first 50 cc are given within five to ten minutes. Observe closely for a hemolytic blood reaction during this time.

There are three types of blood reactions: hemolytic, febrile, and allergic. Symptoms of a hemolytic reaction include chest pain, dyspnea, flushing, oliguria, hypotension, and shock. It is usually a severe reaction occuring within 15 minutes. The transfusion should be stopped immediately and the physician notified. A client with a febrile reaction would have a temperature above 101.4°F, (often with severe shaking) sweating, and tachycardia. This is usually a mild reaction occuring within 30–90 minutes but may occur up to several hours after the transfusion. An allergic reaction includes symptoms of pruritus, urticaria, and possibly anaphylactic shock. This reaction may be mild or severe and usually occurs within 30 minutes, but may occur up to several hours after the transfusion.

If a client experiences any symptoms of a reaction,

stop the infusion and report the symptoms to the physician. Then follow the protocol of the institution.

Blood should be given within four hours of the start of administration. No medications should be given at the blood administration site during infusion. The only solution given during a blood transfusion is 0.9 percent sodium chloride.

Lymphatic System

The lymphatic system is a separate vessel system. The two main functions of the lymph system are to transport excess fluid from the interstitial spaces to the circulatory system and protect the body against infectious organisms.

Lymph Fluid and Vessels

Lymph fluid is a pale yellow fluid. Fluid and substances move from the plasma through the capillary walls and become interstitial fluid. As fluid accumulates in the interstitial space, pressure within the interstitial space increases. The interstitial fluid then diffuses through the lymphatic vessel wall into the lymph vessel. The flow of fluid is illustrated in Figure 22-3.

Semilunar valves in the lymphatic vessels assist the lymph system in returning the interstitial fluid, which is now called lymph, to the venous system. When the valves do not work properly or the vessels become obstructed, edema occurs. The pumping action or contractions of the skeletal muscles and the rhythmic action of the respiratory muscles assist in the movement of the lymph toward the subclavian veins. The right lymphatic duct drains lymph from the right side of the head, neck, thorax, and arm into the right subclavian vein. The lymph from the rest of the body drains into the left subclavian vein through the thoracic duct.

Lymph Nodes

Lymph nodes are scattered throughout the body along the lymph vessels. Refer to Figure 22-4 for a diagram of the lymph system. They contain dense patches of lymphocytes and macrophages. Lymphocytes act against such foreign particles as viruses and bacteria. Macrophages ingest and destroy foreign substances, damaged cells, and cellular debris. Lymph nodes can be superficial or deep. Those located superficially such as in the neck, axilla, and groin can be palpated especially if they become infected and swollen. The tonsils in the pharynx and Peyer patches in the mucosal lining of the ileum are located deeper within the body and cannot be palpated.

As lymph is collected from body tissues, cancer cells may enter the lymphatic system. When this occurs, the cancer cells may escape into the circulation or to other body tissues, such as the lungs. Wherever the cancer cells collect, more cancer cells may be produced. In this way cancer can spread to other body parts. Lymph nodes are biopsied to check for the spread of cancer. (Refer to Chapter 15, Oncology Nursing for a more in-depth discussion.)

Lymph Organs

The spleen and thymus are lymph organs. The spleen removes old RBCs, platelets, and microorganisms from the blood. Approximately 350 milliliters of blood are stored in the spleen and approximately 200 milliliters can be pumped out within a minute into the body as needed (Thibodeau & Patton, 1993). During an infection, the spleen enlarges to produce and release monocytes and lymphocytes. Lymphocytes in the lymph tissue differentiate into T-lymphocytes (T-cells) and B-lymphocytes (B-cells) (see Chapter 24, Allergies, Immune and Autoimmune Disorders).

In infancy and childhood, the thymus gland is large but decreases in size as one ages. In advanced age, it is replaced with fat and connective tissue. The thymus performs an important role in the special processing and proper functioning of the thymus derived T-lymphocytes (T-cells). The T-cells are actively involved in immunity.

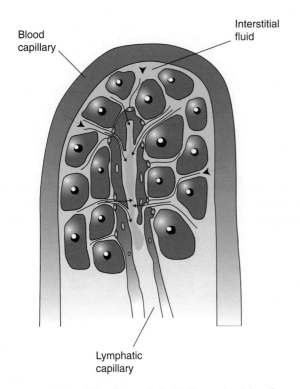

FIGURE 22-3 The flow of fluid from the blood system to the lymphatic system.

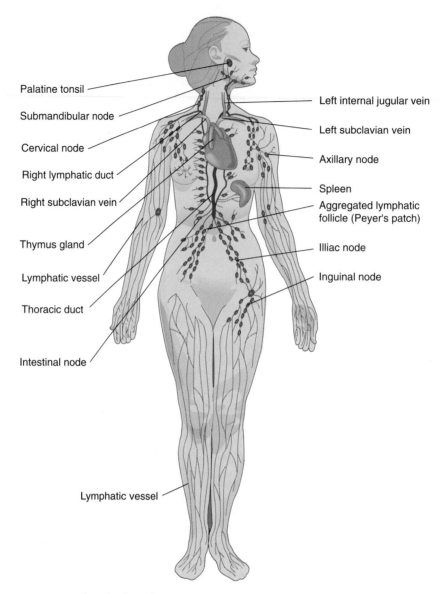

Palatine tonsil

Submandibular node

Cervical node

Right lymphatic duct

Right subclavian vein

Thymus gland

Lymphatic vessel

Thoracic duct

Intestinal node

Lymphatic vessel

Left internal jugular vein

Left subclavian vein

Axillary node

Spleen

Aggregated lymphatic follicle (Peyer's patch)

Illiac node

Inguinal node

FIGURE 22-4 The lymph system.

ASSESSMENT

Subjective Data

Biological data including age, sex, ethnic background, and race is important for many hematological problems. Inquire about the client's occupation and hobbies as there may be exposure to radiation or chemicals. Past military experience is also important, as some military personnel have been exposed to toxic chemicals. Obtain a medication history from the client including prescription and over-the-counter medications. Inquire about recent or recurring infections, night sweats, bleeding problems, previous blood transfusions and if there were any complications.

The neurological functioning is assessed by asking if the client has experienced any cognitive or mental difficulties or numbness and tingling of the extremities. A headache may be indicative of a low erythrocyte count or intracranial bleeding. Ask the client about hearing or vision difficulties.

Ask the client about past surgeries and any complications from surgeries. If the client has had duodenal, gastric, or ileal resection, the absorption of iron and vitamin B_{12} may be affected. Explore alcohol use with the client as alcohol may affect vitamin intake and is caustic to the GI tract. Inquire about the presence of blood in the stool or urine. Ask if the client has experienced anorexia, nausea, vomiting, oral discomfort, or problems with taste perception. A history of dietary intake is helpful when reviewing erythrocyte levels. Inquire if the client has difficulty accomplishing ADLs because of decreased energy.

Objective Data

Start the assessment by obtaining the height, weight, and vital signs. An elevated temperature may indicate an infection. Note recent weight gains or losses.

Laboratory tests are very important when assessing the hematologic and lymph systems. Compare past laboratory tests with present laboratory results.

Palpate the lymph nodes in the neck, axilla, and groin. Normal findings include small (0.5-1.0 cm) nodes that are freely moveable, firm, and nontender. Tender nodes are indicative of inflammation. Hard, fixed nodes may be malignant.

Inspect the skin and extremities for petechiae, bruises, lesions, and brittle nails. Inspect the urine and stool for blood. Note dyspnea, palpitations, an enlarged abdomen, or swollen joints.

COMMON DIAGNOSTIC TESTS

The following is a table of the commonly used diagnostic tests for clients with problems in blood and lymph disorders.

Test	Explanation/Normal Values	Nursing Responsibilities
Partial thromboplastin time (PTT) Activated partial thromboplastin time (APTT)	Measures blood-clotting time in seconds. Norm = APTT 30–40 seconds PTT 60–70 seconds Critical value: APTT > 70 seconds PTT > 100 seconds	A blood specimen is drawn 30 minutes to 1 hour before the next heparin dose if the client is on intermittent heparin therapy, but may be drawn any time if the client is on continuous heparin therapy. Assess any bodily discharge for the presence of blood. The antidote for heparin is protamine sulfate. Antihistamines, vitamin C, and salicylates prolong the PTT time.
Bleeding time	Measures the length of time for a platelet plug to occlude a small puncture wound. Norm = 1–9 minutes (Ivy method) Critical value > 12 minutes	Notify the lab if the client is taking aspirin, anticoagulants, or other medications that may affect the clotting process.
Blood culture and sensitivity	Blood test to determine presence of bacteria. Identifies specific organism and the antibodies to which it is sensitive. Norm = negative	Make sure the specimen is obtained before starting antibiotic therapy. Specimens should be taken to the lab within 30 minutes of obtaining the blood sample.
Coombs' test (direct antiglobulin test)	Detects if immunoglobins are attached to RBCs. Norm = negative	There are several drugs that cause false positives, e.g., ampicillin (Unasyn), captopril (Capoten), indomethacin (Indocin), and insulin.
D dimer test (Fragment D-dimer, Fibrin degradation fragment)	Measures a fibrin split product that is released when a clot breaks. Confirms the diagnosis of DIC. Norm = negative for D dimer fragments	If a client is on thrombolytic therapy, the results of this test would increase.
Erythrocyte Sedimentation Rate (sed rate, ESR)	An exam that measures RBCs that have settled to the bottom of a test tube in a one-hour time frame. Norm = Female 1–20 mm/hr Male 1–15 mm/hr Levels are increased if the client has an inflammation, malignancy, myocardial infarction, and end-stage renal disease.	Explain to the client that a blood sample will be drawn for the test.

(continued)

Test	Explanation/Normal Values	Nursing Responsibilities
Folic Acid (Folate level)	Measures folic acid levels in the blood. Norm = 5–20 ug/mL or 14-34 mmol/L	The test is not fasting. The client is not to drink any alcoholic beverages before the test. The test is drawn before folic acid medications are administered. Phenytoin (Dilantin), primidone (Mysoline), methotrexate, antimalarial agents, and oral contraceptives cause decreased levels.
Hematocrit (Hct)	Measures the percentage of blood cells in a volume of blood. Norm = Male 42–52% Female 37–47% Critical value < 15%	The client does not have to be fasting for the exam. Clients living in high altitudes may have increased levels.
Hemoglobin (Hgb)	Measures the oxygen-carrying capacity of the blood. Norm = Male 14–18 g/dL Female 12–16 g/dL Critical value < 5 g/dL	The client does not have to be fasting for the test.

Hemoglobin electrophoresis	Detects abnormal forms of hemoglobin.
	
	Norm = Hgb S 0%
	        Hgb F < 2%
	        Hgb C 0%
	
	Performed after positive sickle cell test. If the hemoglobin electrophoresis is negative, the client has sickle cell trait. If the hemoglobin electrophoresis is positive, the client has sickle cell anemia.
		If a client has had a blood transfusion within the last 12 weeks, the results of the test may be altered.

Platelet count	Measures the number of platelets per cubic milliliter of blood Norm = 150,000–400,000/mm^3	If the client has a low platelet count, the nurse maintains digital pressure to the puncture site.
Prothrombin time (PT, Protime)	Measures the effectiveness of several blood-clotting factors to clot blood. Norm = 11–12.5 seconds INR = 2.0–3.0 When on anticoagulant therapy the normal values = 1 1/2–2 times the normal values. Critical value = > 20 seconds The critical value if a client is on anticoagulant therapy is > 3 times	Make sure the blood specimen has been drawn before the daily dose of Coumadin. Instruct the client that alcohol intake may increase the PT count and a diet high in fat may decrease the level. Salicylates, sulfonamides, and Aldomet may increase the PT count. Digitalis and oral contraceptives will decrease the levels. Instruct the client not to take any medication without notifying the doctor as the medication may affect the PT results.
Red blood cells (RBCs)	Measures the number of circulating RBCs in a sample of blood. Norm = Male 4.7–6.1 million/mm^3 Female 4.2–5.4 million/mm^3	Client does not have to be fasting for the test. Clients living in high altitudes may have elevated RBC levels.
Schilling test	Determines vitamin B_{12} absorption by the intestine. Differentiates between pernicious anemia and gastrointestinal malabsorption problems. Norm = 8–40% of the radioactive vitamin B_{12} is excreted in the urine within 24 hours	Collect the urine for a 24 to 48 hour period. Laxatives are not given during the test as they decrease the absorption of vitamin B_{12}.

Test	Explanation/Normal Values	Nursing Responsibilities
Sickledex (Sickle cell test)	A screening test to determine the presence of Hgb S. Norm = no Hgbs If the exam results are positive, a hemoglobin electrophoresis test is done.	There are no food or fluid restrictions. Note on the lab slip if the client had a blood transfusion in the past 3 to 4 months.
Total iron binding capacity (TIBC)	Determines the ability of iron to bind to a protein called transferrin. Norm = 250–420 ug/dL or 45–73 umol/L	It is preferred that the client be NPO for 8 hours. A recent blood transfusion and ingestion of a diet high in iron may affect test results. Oral contraceptives increase TIBC levels.

White blood cells (WBCs)
 	
Differential count
 	
Granulocytes
  Basophils
  Eosinophils
  Neutrophils
  Bands
Agranulocytes
  Lymphocytes
  Monocytes
	Measures the number of WBCs in a sample of blood.
	
	Norm = 5,000–10,000/mm^3
	
	Determines the percentage of each type of WBC in a sample of blood.
	
	0.5–1.0%
	1–4%
	55–70%
	3–8%
	
	20–40%
	2–8%
		Aspirin, heparin, and steroids may increase WBC levels.
		
		Physical activity and stress may also increase the number of WBCs.
		
		Antibiotics and diuretics may decrease the number of WBCs.

Bone marrow aspiration	Evaluates how well the bone marrow is producing red blood cells, white blood cells, and platelets. Norm = adequate numbers of RBCs, WBCs, and platelets	Inform the client that they will feel pressure when the physician aspirates the bone marrow. Assess the site for bleeding after the procedure is completed. The client should remain on bedrest for at least 30 minutes after the test.
Gastric analysis, tube and tubeless test	The test determines the amount of hydrochloric (HCl) acid in the stomach. If no HCl acid is present, it indicates the parietal cells are malfunctioning. Parietal cells secrete the intrinsic factor that is essential for vitamin B$_{12}$ absorption. This test is done to diagnose pernicious anemia. Tube test, Norm = basal acid output 2–5 mEq/hr maximal acid output 10–20 mEq/hr Tubeless test, Norm = presence of dye in urine (usually a blue or blue-green coloration)	If the client is having the tubeless test, inform the client of the possibility of a blue or blue-green discoloration of urine. If the client is having the tube test, he is to remain NPO after midnight and is not to smoke prior to the test. A nasogastric tube is inserted prior to the test so gastric contents can be aspirated after the administration of pentagastrin. Antacids, anticholinergics, and cimetidine decrease HCl level. Adrenergic blockers, cholinergics, steroids, and alcohol elevate HCl level.
Lymphangiogram	A contrast dye is injected into the lymph vessels in the hands or feet to examine the lymph vessels and nodes. Used to stage lymphomas and evaluate the effectiveness of chemotherapy and radiation therapy. Norm = Normal-sized lymph nodes with no malignant cells	The dye remains in the lymph nodes for 6 months to a year, so disease progress can be evaluated with an x-ray. A consent form is needed. Inform the client that if a blue-colored dye is used, the skin and urine may have a bluish discoloration. Assess the client's breath sounds after the procedure as lipoid pneumonia is a possible complication if the dye gets into the thoracic duct.

KEY ABBREVIATIONS

The following abbreviations and acronyms are used in this chapter:

ABVD	a combination of chemotherapy drugs (doxorubicin [Adriamycin], bleomycin sulfate [Blenoxane], vinblastine [Velban], dacarbazine [DTIC-Dome])
ALL	acute lymphocytic leukemia
AML	acute myelocytic leukemia
ATG	antithymocyte globulin
CHOP	a combination of chemotherapy drugs (cyclophosphamide [Cytoxan], doxorubicin [Adriamycin], vincristine [Oncovin], prednisone)
CLL	chronic lymphocytic leukemia
CML	chronic myelocytic leukemia
COPP	a combination of chemotherapy drugs (cyclophosphamide [Cytoxan], vincristine [Oncovin], procarbazine [Matulane], prednisone)
CVP	a combination of chemotherapy drugs (cyclophosphamide [Cytoxan], vincristine [Oncovin], prednisone)
DIC	disseminated intravascular coagulation
HD	Hodgkin's disease
HLA	human leukocyte antigen
MOPP	a combination of chemotherapy drugs (mechlorethamine or nitrogen mustard [Mustargen], vincristine [Oncovin], procarbazine hydrochloride [Matulane], prednisone)
NHL	non-Hodgkin's lymphoma
PMNs	polymorphonuclear leukocytes

▶ RED BLOOD CELL DISORDERS: ANEMIA AND POLYCYTHEMIA

Red blood cell disorders discussed in this section are the anemias and polycythemia vera. The nursing process for anemias is presented after the discussion of sickle cell anemia since the nursing diagnoses, goals, and interventions are similar.

Anemia is a common hematopoietic disorder in which the client has a decreased number of RBCs and a low hemoglobin level. The causes for anemia are a decreased production of RBCs, an increased destruction of RBCs, or a loss of blood. The types of anemia discussed in this section are iron deficiency anemia, hypoplastic (aplastic) anemia, pernicious anemia, acquired hemolytic anemia, and sickle cell anemia.

▶ IRON DEFICIENCY ANEMIA

Iron deficiency anemia is the most common type of anemia and occurs when the body does not have enough iron to synthesize functional Hgb. The decrease in iron may be due to a decreased dietary intake, a decreased iron absorption from the gastrointestinal tract, chronic intestinal or uterine blood loss, or an increased bodily need for iron such as during growth periods or pregnancy. More frequent incidents of iron deficiency anemia are in premature or low birth weight infants, adolescent girls, alcoholics, and the elderly. The symptoms are fatigue, loss of appetite, decreased ability to concentrate, and pallor. Clients with chronic anemia may have tachycardia, exertional dyspnea, hypotension, dysphagia, stomatitis, glossitis, and brittle nails. Diagnostic tests of a client with iron deficiency anemia would reveal decreased RBCs, a low Hgb level, a low Hct, a low serum iron, and a high total iron binding capacity (TIBC).

▶ Medical/Surgical Management

▶ Pharmacological

Oral iron preparations are ferrous gluconate (Fergon) and ferrous sulfate (Feosol). These preparations are not given with milk because milk interferes with iron absorption. The administration of iron with meals, with orange juice, or vitamin C rich drinks increases iron absorption. Iron dextran (Imferon), an intramuscular iron preparation, is given by Z-tract technique.

▶ Diet

The treatment for iron deficiency anemia is iron supplements and a diet high in iron. Foods rich in iron are red meats, fish, raisins, apricots, dried fruits, dark green vegetables, dried beans, eggs, and iron-enriched whole grain breads. An increase of vitamin C in the diet assists in the absorption of iron. If the client has a loss of appetite, small frequent snacks may be tolerated better than three large meals.

▶ Activity

Daily activities should be spaced to provide rest periods between times of exercise.

▶ HYPOPLASTIC (APLASTIC) ANEMIA

The bone marrow decreases or stops functioning in a client with aplastic anemia. The client with aplastic anemia has pancytopenia, a drop in the number of red blood cells, white blood cells, and platelets. It develops without a known cause and is thought to be congenital. Secondary aplastic anemia is caused by exposure to chemicals (benzene or airplane glue), radiation, or medications. Some medications that cause aplastic anemia are chloramphenicol (Chloromycetin), mephenytoin (Mesantoin), trimethadione (Tridione), mechlorethamine or nitrogen mustard (Mustargen), methotrexate (Folex PFS), 6-mercaptopurine or 6-MP (Purinethol) and phenylbutazone (Butazolidin). Symptoms include fatigue, weakness, tachycardia, dyspnea, susceptibility to infection, petechiae, gingival bleeding, and epistaxis. Clients with aplastic anemia are extremely ill. Diagnosis is confirmed by a bone marrow aspiration.

▶ *Medical/Surgical Management*

▶ *Medical*

The cause of aplastic anemia is removed if possible. Another treatment is antithymocyte globulin or ATG (Atgam) immunosuppressive therapy which is given to suppress the reaction causing the aplastic anemia and to allow the client's bone marrow to recover. ATG is given daily through a central venous catheter for seven to ten days. If the client has a good response to ATG, his condition will improve in three to six months. The sooner the diagnosis is made and ATG started, the better the prognosis (Brunner, 1995). Transfusions of packed red cells and platelets are also given.

▶ *Surgical*

Bone marrow transplants are done if the client's bone marrow fails to start functioning. Cyclosporine (Sandimmune), an immunosuppressant, is given for a bone marrow transplant to decrease the graft rejection. The best response occurs in a young client who has not previously had a transfusion since transfusions increase bone marrow graft rejection. Bone marrow transplants from a human leukocyte antigen (HLA)-matched sibling donor is the treatment of choice for clients less than forty-five years of age. The treatment of choice for an older adult or a client who does not have a HLA-matched sibling donor is immunosuppression with ATG or cyclosporine. (Bone marrow transplants are discussed in the section on acute myelocytic leukemia.)

▶ *Pharmacological*

Infections are treated with antibiotics. Steroids are also given.

▶ *Preventive Treatment*

If a client is taking medications that cause bone marrow depression, the blood cell count is monitored closely.

▶ PERNICIOUS ANEMIA

The parietal cells of the gastric mucosa secrete a protein, intrinsic factor, that is essential for the proper absorption of vitamin B_{12}. Pernicious anemia is an autoimmune disease in which the parietal cells are destroyed and the gastric mucosa atrophies. Without the secretion of the intrinsic factor, vitamin B_{12} cannot be absorbed in the distal portion of the ileum.

The onset of the disease occurs between fifty and sixty years of age. Pernicious anemia occurs most frequently in those of Northern European and African-American descent. African-American women are especially affected with the disease and often severely. Pernicious anemia can occur in clients who have had a gastrectomy with the section of the stomach removed that secretes the intrinsic factor. A gastric analysis and Schilling test are confirming diagnostic tests.

Pernicious anemia has an insidious onset and it may take several months for the symptoms to be fully manifested. Symptoms include extreme weakness, a sore tongue, numbness and tingling of the extremities, ataxia, dizziness, headache, blurred vision, tinnitus, poor memory, irritability, and loss of bladder and bowel control. The client has decreased sensations to heat and pain because of neurological involvement.

▶ *Medical/Surgical Management*

▶ *Pharmacological*

Topical anesthetics are given to relieve oral discomfort during the acute phase of the disease. Cyanocobalamin or vitamin B_{12} (Rubramin PC) is given IM daily for two weeks and then weekly until the Hct returns to normal levels. Then cyanocobalamin is usually administered monthly for the rest of the client's life. The frequency of administration will depend on the client's symptoms and response to the medication. Oral administration of vitamin B_{12} is not effective because vitamin B_{12} cannot be absorbed without the intrinsic factor. Folic acid or folate (Folvite) is prescribed. The client is encouraged to increase folic acid in the diet by eating green leafy vegetables, meat, fish, legumes, and whole grains. Iron is usually not prescribed because once the condition is corrected with regular administration of cyanocobalamin, erythrocytes are produced and the Hgb returns to normal.

▶ Preventive Treatment

Pernicious anemia is a familial disease. Instruct the client's family about signs of early symptoms and treatment. Clients with pernicious anemia are more susceptible to gastric carcinoma and should be monitored closely for symptoms.

▶ HEMOLYTIC ANEMIAS

The two types of hemolytic anemias are acquired hemolytic anemia and inherited hemolytic anemia (sickle cell anemia). In hemolytic anemias, a **hemolysis** or destruction of RBCs occurs and iron and hemoglobin are released. During a time of hemolysis, RBCs may last only ten days instead of the normal 120 days.

▶ Acquired Hemolytic Anemia

Several causes for acquired hemolytic anemia are an autoimmune reaction, radiation, blood transfusion, chemicals, arsenic, lead, or medications. Sulfisoxazole (Gantrisin), penicillin, and methyldopa (Aldomet) are medications that can cause hemolysis. A substance produced by the bacterium *Clostridium perfringens* can also cause hemolysis. Symptoms may go unnoticed or there may be a severe reaction. Symptoms are mild fatigue and pallor. More severe symptoms include jaundice, palpitations, hypotension, dyspnea, and back and joint pain. Diagnostic tests would reveal a low Hgb and Hct and an elevated LDH. LDH is an enzyme in the heart, liver, kidneys, skeletal muscle, brain, red blood cells, and lungs. As these tissues are damaged, LDH is released into the bloodstream causing an elevated LDH. Hemolysis can also cause a false-positive LDH (Pagana & Pagana, 1995). A positive direct Coombs' test (direct antiglobulin test) assists in determining the antibody causing the anemia.

▶ Medical/Surgical Management

▶ Medical

Treatment is aimed at removing the cause of the hemolytic anemia, if possible. The client may be given blood transfusions or **erythrocytapheresis** (a procedure that removes abnormal RBCs and replaces them with healthy RBCs).

▶ Surgical

The function of the spleen is to destroy RBCs. In severe cases of hemolytic anemia, a splenectomy may be done in an attempt to stop the destruction of RBCs.

▶ Pharmacological

Corticosteroids are administered to decrease the autoimmune response to the foreign antigen. Folic acid may also be given to increase the production of RBCs.

▶ Sickle Cell Anemia (Inherited Hemolytic Anemia)

Sickle cell anemia is also known as either inherited hemolytic anemia or sickle cell disease. It is a genetic disorder in which there is abnormal hemoglobin S rather than hemoglobin A in the RBCs. Sickle cell anemia is caused by a recessive gene that is passed through the generations (see Figure 22-5). The client with one S gene has sickle cell trait (Hb SA), is asymptomatic, but is a carrier of the disease. The client with sickle cell anemia has two S genes (Hb SS) and manifests symptoms.

The condition occurs more frequently in African-Americans with an estimated one of twelve persons being sickle cell carriers (Phipps, et al., 1995). It also occurs in persons from Asia Minor, India, and the Mediterranean and Caribbean areas.

Situations that precipitate sickle cell crisis are dehydration, fatigue, infection, emotional stress, and alcohol consumption. When oxygenation is compromised, the RBCs become **sickled** (crescent-shaped and elongated) and obstruct capillaries and larger vessels (see Figure 22-6). The sickled cells cause circulatory prob-

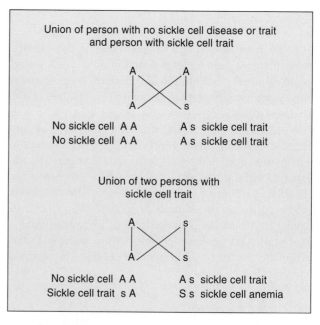

FIGURE 22-5 Inheritance of sickle cell trait and sickle cell disease.

Normal red
blood cell

Sickle-shaped
red blood cell

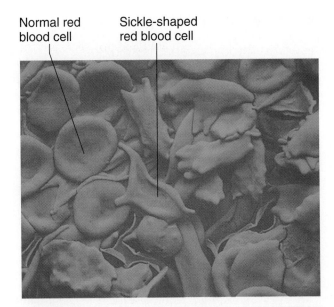

FIGURE 22-6 Blood cells magnified through a scanning electron microscope show normal and sickle-shaped red blood cells. (*Courtesy of Philips Electronic Instruments Company*)

lems by obstructing vessels and rupturing. When the cells obstruct vessels, the area normally supplied by these vessels becomes ischemic and infarcted. The sickled cells are much more fragile than normal cells and rupture more easily. The rupturing of sickled RBCs causes chronic anemia, causing the heart to enlarge in an attempt to circulate more blood for adequate oxygenation of body tissues. Symptoms include fatigue, jaundice, chronic leg ulcers, tachypnea, dyspnea, and arrhythmias. Periodically, the client experiences a sickle cell crisis with symptoms of fever, severe pain, and loss of blood supply to various organs because of obstructed vessels. Areas most frequently affected are the joints, bone, brain, lungs, liver, kidneys, and penis. Joints become painful, swollen, and immobile. The client may experience cerebrovascular accidents, renal failure, pulmonary infarction, shock, and priapism (a continuous, painful erection).

A hemoglobin S blood test (Sickledex) or sickle cell test is done to detect the presence of Hgb S. If Hgb S is present, a hemoglobin electrophoresis is done to distinguish between sickle cell trait or sickle cell disease.

▶ *Medical/Surgical Management*

▶ *Medical*

Medical management of sickle cell disease is still evolving in administration of medications and treat-

ments. Infections are treated promptly with antibiotics. The client is given intravenous fluids (3–5 L/day) to enhance hydration (Brunner, 1995). Skin grafting may be necessary for chronic leg ulcers.

Genetic counseling is recommended for clients with sickle cell trait and sickle cell anemia. There may be more openness to counseling if the counselor is from the same community as the client.

▶ *Pharmacological*

Folic acid or folate (Folvite) is administered daily to assist in the production of RBCs. Cetiedil citrate has an antisickling effect by changing the RBC membrane. Pentoxifylline (Trental) reduces blood viscosity, increases RBC flexibility, and lengthens the time between sickle cell crises. Blood transfusions may be given during a crisis.

Patient-controlled analgesia (PCA) with morphine is effective during a crisis. The client is progressed from narcotics to nonnarcotic analgesics as indicated.

▶ *Preventive Treatment*

Clients with sickle cell disease are encouraged to avoid high altitudes and nonpressurized airplanes. It is important for the client to have adequate fluid intake as dehydration causes a sickle cell crisis. Anesthesia also may cause a sickle cell crisis. All infections should be promptly treated. Sickle cell tests are done on infants to diagnose sickle cell trait or disease.

▶ *Nursing Process*

Assessment

Subjective Data A history of the client's past medical problems is obtained including a history of familial hematopoietic illnesses. Since some anemias may be caused by drugs and environmental conditions, gather information about medications taken and about environmental situations at work and in recreational settings. Ask the client about fatigue, dyspnea with exertion, palpitations, dizziness, pain, petechiae, tingling and numbness in the extremities, blurred vision, and oral discomfort.

Objective Data Obtain the client's weight and vital signs; take the apical pulse and peripheral pulses; listen to the breath sounds; check for sensation and movement in the extremities; check for abdominal tenderness; edema, and the skin for pallor, signs of bruising or jaundice. A thorough assessment of the cardiac system is completed because severe anemia can cause cardiac enlargement and arrhythmias.

▼ ▼

Possible nursing diagnoses for a client with decreased erythrocytes and hemoglobin may include:

Nursing Diagnoses	Goals	Nursing Interventions
▶ *Knowledge deficit related to prescribed treatment regimen.*	The client will relate the prescribed treatment regimen.	Teach the cause of the particular type of anemia and, if possible, ways to avoid the occurrence of that anemia in the future.
		For iron deficiency anemia, teach the importance of taking iron and increasing iron in the diet.
		Instruct clients with pernicious anemia to obtain a vitamin B_{12} injection at regularly scheduled times.
		Teach clients with hemolytic anemias the significance of following the prescribed regimens.
▶ *Activity intolerance related to weakness and fatigue.*	The client will tolerate increased activity.	Assist the client as needed with activities of daily living.
		Teach the client the importance of alternating periods of rest with exercise.
▶ *Tissue perfusion, altered, related to a decreased number of RBCs and decreased oxygenation.*	The client will have adequate tissue perfusion.	Administer oxygen as needed to relieve symptoms of dyspnea.
		Monitor for symptoms of obstructed vessels such as pain, leg ulcerations, abdominal tenderness, dyspnea, confusion, and blurred vision.
		Administer blood products as ordered.
		Monitor the client closely after blood transfusions for possible reactions such as chills, fever, dyspnea, pruritus, wheezing, and pain in the lumbar region.

Evaluation

Each goal must be evaluated to determine how it has been met by the client.

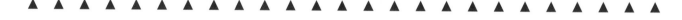

▲ ▲

Sample Nursing Care Plan: The Client with Sickle Cell Anemia

Reggie Thompson, a nineteen-year-old African American, was diagnosed with sickle cell anemia five years ago. Reggie works for a computer company and has been working twelve-hour days to get a system installed. He has felt fatigued lately and decided to relax by playing golf on a warm Saturday morning. After the seventh hole, Reggie experienced dyspnea and tingling and numbness in his legs. After the next hole, he experienced severe pain in his ankles and knees. He was taken to the local medical center where he was admitted. The physician ordered oxygen by nasal cannula, IV fluids, and a PCA pump with morphine sulfate.

Nursing Diagnosis 1 Pain related to occlusion of small vessels by sickled cells as evidenced by severe pain in the knees and ankles.

Goals	Nursing Interventions	Rationale	Evaluation
Reggie Thompson will state pain has been relieved as the analgesic becomes effective.	Assess pain type, location, and intensity.	Other vessels to the brain, heart, lungs, spleen, gallbladder, kidney, and penis may become occluded causing pain.	The morphine in the PCA pump relieved Reggie's pain and oral analgesics were ordered. Reggie recognizes the importance of taking narcotic analgesics only when necessary.
	Monitor analgesic administration by PCA pump.	Analgesic administration is monitored to assess relief from pain.	
	Spport joints and lower extremities with pillows.	Support of joints and lower extremities relieves joint pain.	
	Keep bed linens off of knees and ankles with a bed cradle.	Use of a bed cradle keeps linen from putting pressure on painful areas.	

Nursing Diagnosis 2 Altered tissue perfusion related to a decreased number of RBCs and decreased oxygenation as evidenced by dyspnea and tingling and numbness in his ankles and knees.

Goals	Nursing Interventions	Rationale	Evaluation
Reggie Thompson will experience improved circulation in his extremities as RBCs increase in number.	Elevate the head of the bed and administer oxygen as needed to relieve symptoms of dyspnea.	Lungs can expand more fully if the head of the bed is elevated and oxygen administration increases blood oxygen levels.	Circulation in lower extremities has improved as manifested by prompt capillary refill and strong pedal and popliteal pulses. Extremities are warm to touch.
	Administer IV fluids as ordered.	Adequate hydration decreases the possibility of RBCs sickling.	
	Encourage Reggie to drink eight to ten glasses of water daily.	Dehydration causes RBCs to sickle.	

(continued)

	Monitor for symptoms of obstructed vessels such as pain, leg ulcerations, abdominal tenderness, dyspnea, confusion, and blurred vision.	Since RBCs are sickling, vessels supplying blood to other vital organs can become obstructed.	
	Administer blood products as ordered.	Administration of blood products increases the number of normal RBCs which improves the blood oxygen concentration.	
	Closely monitor for possible blood transfusion reactions such as chills, fever, dyspnea, pruritus, wheezing, and pain in the lumbar region.	Administration of blood products may cause adverse reactions.	

Nursing Diagnosis 3 Activity intolerance related to weakness and fatigue as evidenced by playing only eight holes of golf before occurrence of symptoms.

Goals	Nursing Interventions	Rationale	Evaluation
Reggie Thompson will tolerate activity.	Assist Reggie as needed with activities of daily living.	Assistance with daily activities would conserve energy resources.	Reggie provides periods of rest after each period of activity. He acknowledges that he had been working too hard and not getting enough rest before hospitalization.
	Teach Reggie the importance of alternating periods of rest with activity.	Conservation of energy is important. Impaired circulation to the brain may cause dizziness with ambulation.	

Nursing Diagnosis 4 Knowledge deficit related to prescribed treatment regimen as evidenced by a lack of rest and working long hours.

Goals	Nursing Interventions	Rationale	Evaluation
Reggie Thompson will relate the prescribed treatment regimen before discharge.	Teach Reggie the pathophysiology related to sickle cell disease.	An understanding of the disease process improves compliance with the medical regimen.	Reggie states his RBCs have Hgb S rather than Hgb A and a lack of oxygen causes his RBCs to sickle. Situations that may cause sickling are fatigue, high altitudes, lack of oral fluids,
	Encourage Reggie to take medications as ordered.	Medications will improve circulation and postpone sickle cell crisis situations.	

| | Explain possible effects of alcohol ingestion. | Ingestion of alcohol can cause sudden persistent erections for males with sickle cell anemia. | alcohol ingestion, emotional and physical stress, infection, and anesthesia. He knows the purpose and side effects of each of his medications and the times he is to take them. |
| | Explain the importance of avoiding high altitudes, stressful situations, and the symptoms of infection. | Clients with sickle cell disease should avoid situations that increase oxygen demands. Lack of oxygen can precipitate a sickle cell crisis. | |

▶ POLYCYTHEMIA VERA

Polycythemia vera is a disease in which there is an increased production of red blood cells. Usually the numbers of white blood cells and platelets are also increased. The increased production of cells increases the blood volume and viscosity and decreases the ability of the blood to circulate freely. Polycythemia vera occurs most frequently in the middle-aged and in Jewish men. The etiology of the disease is unknown.

Symptoms are not present early in the disease. As the blood viscosity and volume increase the client experiences headaches, epistaxis, dizziness, tinnitus, blurred vision, fatigue, weakness, pruritus, exertional dyspnea, angina, and increased blood pressure and pulse. The client's complexion becomes ruddy (reddish) and the lips become reddish purple. The client may have petechiae and bruise easily because of a platelet dysfunction. The client is more susceptible to thrombi formation because of the increased viscosity of the blood. The increased destruction of RBCs causes **hyperuricemia** (increased uric acid blood levels).

▶ Medical/Surgical Management

▶ Medical

Polycythemia vera is diagnosed by the red blood cell count, hematocrit, and bone marrow biopsy. Oxygen is administered if the client has difficulty breathing.

The treatment for polycythemia is **phlebotomy**, which is the removal of blood from a vein. Generally 500 to 2000 mL of blood is withdrawn to keep the Hct levels within the normal range. Radioactive phosphorus (^{32}P) and radiation therapy are used to decrease the production of red blood cells in the bone marrow.

Complications that can occur from the disease process are cerebral vascular accident, thrombosis, myocardial infarction, and hemorrhage.

▶ Pharmacological

Antineoplastic drugs such as busulfan (Myleran), chlorambucil (Leukeran), cyclophosphamide (Cytoxan), and mechlorethamine or nitrogen mustard (Mustargen) are also used to decrease bone marrow production. Allopurinol (Zyloprim) is given to decrease the production of uric acid. Pruritus can be relieved with the administration of antihistamines.

▶ Diet

The client is placed on a diet that has increased calories and protein. A diet low in sodium decreases fluid volume. Iron-containing foods should be avoided.

▶ Activity

Activities of daily living may need to be adjusted so the client can have regular periods of rest to relieve fatigue.

▶ Nursing Process

Assessment

Subjective Data Ask about the history of the client's symptoms, especially difficulty breathing, chest pain, dizziness, headache, pruritus, tinnitus, blurred vision, and sensitivity to hot and cold. Assess the nutritional status of the client as there may be an inadequate dietary intake due to GI symptoms of fullness and dyspepsia.

Objective Data Observe the skin for bruises and changes in skin color. Assess the cardiovascular system by checking for distention of neck vessels, listening to the apical pulse, taking radial and pedal pulses, performing a Homans' sign, and checking for edema. Assess the respiratory system by observing for epistaxis and dyspnea and listening to the breath sounds. Assess the central nervous system by checking the pupil response and presence of numbness or tingling.

▼ ▼

Possible nursing diagnoses for a client with polycythemia vera may include:

Nursing Diagnoses	Goals	Nursing Interventions
▶ *Knowledge deficit related to disease process and treatment.*	The client will relate disease process and treatment.	Explain the cause of the disease, possible symptoms, side effects of medications and possible future complications to report. Teach client to report headache, chest pain, dyspnea, or redness, swelling, or tenderness in the arms or legs to the physician or nurse practitioner immediately.
▶ *Tissue perfusion, altered, related to decreased blood circulation.*	The client will have adequate circulation.	Administer oxygen as need for dyspnea. Check vital signs frequently. Perform Homans' sign and signs of thrombi formation (see objective nursing assessment of cardiovascular and central nervous system).
▶ *Injury, high risk for, related to dizziness.*	The client will relate measures to avoid injury.	Encourage the client to change positions slowly to prevent dizziness. Encourage activities of daily living when the client is feeling well. Teach client to avoid activities where bruising or trauma may occur.

▶ Evaluation

Each goal must be evaluated to determine how it has been met by the client.

▲ ▲

▶ WHITE BLOOD CELL DISORDERS

▶ LEUKEMIA

Leukemia is a malignancy of blood-forming tissues in which the bone marrow produces increased numbers of immature white blood cells that are incapable of protecting the body from infections. The increased number of WBCs crowds out the other cells in the bone marrow causing a decreased production of RBCs and platelets. Anemia and bleeding result from the decreased number of RBCs and platelets.

Leukemia has two classifications: acute and chronic. The acute leukemias are subclassified into acute myelocytic leukemia (AML) and acute lymphocytic leukemia (ALL). AML is sometimes known as acute nonlymphocytic leukemia (ANLL). Chronic leukemias are subclassified into chronic myelocytic leukemia (CML) and chronic lymphocytic leukemia (CLL).

Research conducted with the survivors of the Japanese A-bomb indicates a connection between radiation

and AML (Campbell, 1995). Other suspected etiological causes of AML are rheumatoid arthritis clients treated with drugs that suppress the immune system and cancer clients treated with cytotoxic drugs and radiation therapy (Campbell, 1995). This later condition is known as **secondary malignancy**, which means the client had a malignancy, was treated with chemotherapy or radiation therapy, had a period of time with no malignancy, and then developed a second malignant condition. There is a higher risk of ALL occurring in clients with Down's syndrome (Campbell, 1995).

Research has found a link with the Philadelphia chromosome (Ph[1]) and CML (Campbell, 1995). The Philadelphia chromosome is an exchange of genetic information in which a section of chromosome 21 has been dropped and added to chromosome 9. The Philadelphia chromosome is a genetic defect in approximately 90 percent of the clients with CML (RN, 1996). Identification of the Philadelphia chromosome confirms the diagnosis of Philadelphia chromosome positive CML.

Because of the increased production of immature WBCs, clients with acute leukemia generally are fighting persistent infections and have a fever and chills.

The decreased number of RBCs causes symptoms of anemia such as fatigue, pallor, malaise, tachycardia, and tachypnea. The decreased platelet production causes bleeding tendencies and the client will experience petechiae, bruising, epistaxis, melena, gingival bleeding, and increased menstrual bleeding. The client may also experience weight loss, night sweats, and swollen lymph nodes. As the malignant cells invade the central nervous system, the client will experience headaches and visual disturbances. Some clients experience bone pain because the rapid production of WBCs causes cells to become crowded in the bone marrow. Refer to Table 22-1 to see the relationship of leukemia symptoms to laboratory results.

▶ ACUTE LEUKEMIA

Acute leukemias have a rapid onset and must be treated quickly for a good prognosis. ALL usually occurs in children between the ages of two and six and has a more rapid onset than AML. Left untreated, clients with ALL have a **median survival time** (average length of life) of four to six months. Children with ALL have a good prognosis rate with chemotherapy. Approximately 90 percent of the children have complete remissions but only 50 to 70 percent of the adults have complete remissions (Phipps et al., 1995; Monahan et al., 1994).

AML occurs more frequently in adolescence and after fifty-five years of age (Phipps et al., 1995). Untreated, the median survival time for clients with AML is approximately two to three months (Phipps et al., 1995). With chemotherapy, complete remission occurs in approximately 50 to 75 percent of AML clients with a median survival time of two to three years (Phipps et al., 1995).

▶ Medical/Surgical Management

▶ Medical

Diagnosis of acute leukemia is confirmed with a CBC and a bone marrow biopsy. A lumbar puncture determines the presence of malignant cells in the central nervous system. An x-ray, MRI, or CT scan of the chest and skeleton determine the presence of infection and bone marrow tissue involvement.

▶ Surgical

Bone marrow transplants are used with relapsed ALL clients, AML clients under fifty-five, and CML clients. AML clients who have a bone marrow transplant have a 50 to 70 percent cure rate (Campbell, 1995). High doses of chemotherapy and radiation therapy are given to the client to destroy the bone marrow. Leukemic white blood cells and healthy bone marrow cells are both destroyed, placing the client at a high risk for infection and death. Identical human leukocyte antigen (HLA) bone marrow from a sibling, the client, or an antigen matched donor is given intravenously in a manner similar to a blood transfusion. The transfused bone marrow finds its way to the client's bone marrow and starts producing WBCs, RBCs, and platelets. The bone marrow is matched in a process very similar to the process of cross-matching blood. If the client's own bone marrow is used, it is removed from the client, treated with chemotherapy, and then reinfused into the client.

▶ Pharmacological

Initial doses of chemotherapy are called **induction doses**. Small doses of chemotherapy given every three to four weeks to maintain remission are called **maintenance therapy**. Induction doses of chemotherapy for ALL consists of vincristine (Oncovin) and prednisone (Deltasone). Maintenance therapy consists of giving 6-mercaptopurine or 6-MP (Purinethol) and methotrexate or amethopterin (Methotrexate). Usually vincristine (Oncovin) and prednisone (Deltasone) are given periodically with the maintenance therapy.

Leukemic cells can lie dormant in the brain and spinal area because the chemotherapeutic drugs are

Table 22-1

RELATIONSHIP OF LABORATORY TESTS TO LEUKEMIC SYMPTOMS

Lab Result	Overall Symptom	Symptom Manifestation
Immature WBCs	Persistent infections	Fever Chills
Decrease RBCs	Anemia	Fatigue Pallor Malaise Tachycardia Tachypnea
Decrease platelets	Bleeding	Petechiae Bruising Epistaxis Melena Gingival bleeding Increased menstrual bleeding

unable to pass through the blood-brain barrier. Intrathecal (within the spinal canal) administration of methotrexate has decreased recurrences of ALL. Methotrexate is given by a lumbar puncture into the cerebrospinal fluid or through a subcutaneous cerebrospinal reservoir. Sometimes radiation therapy is also used on the brain and spinal area.

AML is treated with chemotherapeutic agents, blood products, and antibiotics. Refer to Table 22-2 for a review of chemotherapeutic agents used in treating leukemia.

▶ *CHRONIC LEUKEMIA*

Chronic leukemia generally occurs in adults with a gradual increase in the white cell count over months or years. Clients treated with oral chemotherapy have a life expectancy of two to ten years with CLL and three to four years with CML (Phipps et al., 1995). The prognosis depends on the severity of the disease at the time of diagnosis.

CLL clients have increased abnormal B lymphocytes with a WBC count between 20,000 and 100,000 (Phipps et al., 1995). CLL can develop at any age but occurs more frequently between the ages of fifty to seventy and has an incident rate three times higher in men than in women (Phipps et al., 1995)

Table 22-2

CHEMOTHERAPEUTIC AGENTS TO TREAT LEUKEMIA	
Leukemia	**Chemotherapeutic Agents**
Acute lymphocytic leukemia (ALL)	vincristine (Oncovin)
	prednisone (Deltasone)
	6-mercaptopurine or 6-MP (Purinethol)
	methotrexate (Methotrexate)
Acute myelocytic leukemia (AML)	daunorubicin HCl (Cerubidine)
	cytarabine or ara-C (Cytosar-U)
	6-thioguanine (Thioguanine)
	doxorubicin HCl (Adriamycin)
Chronic myelocytic leukemia (CLL)	chlorambucil (Leukeran)
	COP (Cytoxan, Oncovin, and prednisone)
Chronic lymphocytic leukemia (CML)	busulfan (Myleran)
	hydroxyurea (Hydrea)
	DAT (daunorubicin, ara-C, thioguanine)

CML occurs most frequently in clients between thirty and fifty years of age with a higher incidence of CML in males (Campbell, 1995). The WBC count ranges from 15,000 to 500,000 (Phipps et al., 1995). Most clients feel good and maintain a relatively normal life until later in the disease process when the chronic recessed phase changes into an intensified stage that resembles an acute phase of leukemia. This acute phase is called a **blastic phase** in which there is an increased production of WBCs. Approximately 50 to 60 percent of the CML cases develop a later blastic phase. When this occurs, the general condition spirals downhill and the client soon dies. The most common cause of death in the leukemic client is viral and fungal pneumonia (Black & Mastassarin-Jacobs, 1993).

▶ *Medical/Surgical Management*

▶ *Medical*

Diagnosis of chronic leukemia is confirmed with a CBC and a bone marrow biopsy.

▶ *Surgical*

In the CML chronic phase, the HLA-identical allogenic bone marrow is given and the client's own treated bone marrow is given in the blastic phase.

▶ *Pharmacological*

Refer to Table 22-2 for a review of chemotherapeutic agents used in treating CLL and CML. Chemotherapy does not extend the quantity of life but seems to give a better quality of life by prolonging the chronic phase. In a recent clinical trial, interferon increased the survival time to sixty-one months as opposed to forty-one months (Campbell, 1995).

▶ *Diet*

The client is on a diet high in protein, carbohydrates, and vitamins. A bland, nonirritating diet prevents oral mucosal irritation.

▶ *Activity*

The decreased RBC level causes the client to have symptoms of anemia that include weakness and increased respirations. It is important for the client to learn methods to conserve energy such as placing frequently used items nearby.

▶ *Preventive treatment*

Clients are encouraged to avoid exposure to benzene and arsenic as there seems to be a connection between these chemicals and leukemia.

▶ Nursing Process

Assessment

Subjective Data Obtain a thorough history of the symptoms the client has experienced. Ask the client or family about chromosomal abnormalities, exposure to chemicals, viral infections, and previous chemotherapy or radiation therapy. Ask the client to describe the location, type, and duration of pain especially in bones or joints. Inquire about symptoms of infection such as the presence of a cough or pain or burning on urination. Obtain a history of bleeding such as epistaxis, gingival bleeding, melena, or hematuria. Fatigue, malaise, and irritability are often described.

Objective Data Assess for signs of infection, bleeding, and chemotherapy complications. Common sites for infection include the mouth, pharynx, lungs, skin, bladder, and perianal area. During chemotherapy the reduced white cell count may stop the formation of pus so infection may manifest as redness, swelling, and pain.

Assessment for bleeding includes monitoring the platelet count as bleeding occurs easily if the platelet count falls below 50,000. Clients can bleed from any orifice so it is important for the nurse to inspect any discharge from the body. Occult blood may be present in the urine and stool.

Chemotherapy complications are nausea, vomiting, and stomatitis. Alopecia occurs one to two weeks after treatments are initiated.

▼ ▼

Possible nursing diagnoses for a client with leukemia may include:

Nursing Diagnoses	Goals	Nursing Interventions
▶ *Knowledge deficit related to disease process and treatment.*	The client will relate treatment methods and possible complications of chemotherapy.	Teach the client to observe for signs of infection and bleeding.
		Review side effects of chemotherapy and radiation with the client, family members, and significant others.
		Explain bone marrow transplant methods.
▶ *Infection, high risk for, related to increased production of immature white blood cells.*	The client will describe ways to prevent infection.	Follow good handwashing techniques.
		Teach proper handwashing to the family and friends who come in contact with the leukemic client.
		Use antimicrobial soaps for the client's daily bath.
		Provide frequent oral care with a soft toothbrush and nonirritating mouthwash to prevent open sores and stomatitis.
		Wash the perianal area after each bowel movement to decrease bacterial contamination and prevent rectal fissures.
		Rectal temperatures and suppositories are avoided.
		Monitor the temperature every four hours for signs of infection.
		Report any temperature over 100°F to the physician.
		Administer antibiotics and antifungals as ordered.
		Closely monitor respiration rates and breath sounds as the client is prone to respiratory infections.

(continued)

Nursing Diagnoses	Goals	Nursing Interventions
▶ *Injury, high risk for, related to decreased production of platelets.*	The client will identify ways to avoid injury and prevent bleeding.	Frequently observe the client for signs of bleeding such as epistaxis, gingival bleeding, petechiae, ecchymoses, hematemesis, enlarged abdomen, hematuria, melena and confusion which can occur from intracranial hemorrhage.
		Administer stool softeners frequently to prevent anal irritation from hard stools.
		Use cotton swabs instead of a toothbrush may be used for oral care.
		Encourage the client to use an electric razor.
		Avoid giving injections as much as possible.
		If a catheter is needed, lubricate it well to avoid trauma to the mucosal lining of the urethra.
▶ *Pain related to enlarged spleen and overcrowded bone marrow spaces.*	The client will implement methods to decrease pain.	Administer analgesics as ordered.
		Since clients have bleeding tendencies, aspirin is not given because of the anticoagulant effect.
▶ *Activity intolerance related to decreased energy sources from disease process.*	The client will list ways to conserve energy.	Encourage the client to plan daily activities so there is a balance of activity and rest.
▶ *Nutrition, altered, less than body requirements related to effects of disease process and chemotherapy on gastrointestinal tract.*	The client will choose nonirritating, high-protein, high-carbohydrate meals and snacks.	Administer antiemetics as ordered to relieve nausea and vomiting.
		Suggest that the client may tolerate small frequent feedings better than three large meals.
		Provide the client with a high-protein, high-carbohydrate diet to prevent infection and provide needed energy.
		Administer vitamin supplements as ordered.
		Teach the client to avoid raw fruits and vegetables as these foods may contain more bacteria than cooked foods.
▶ *Coping, individual and family, ineffective, related to uncertainty about treatment of disease and prognosis.*	The client will identify ways to cope with concerns about disease process.	Inform the client of the possibility of alopecia from therapy treatments.
		Encourage the client to voice concerns and fears related to having leukemia.
		Teach the client, family members, and significant others to monitor and report signs of infection and bleeding.
		Refer to support groups, social workers, and clergy as needed.

▶ *Evaluation*

Each goal must be evaluated to determine how it has been met by the client.

▲ ▲

▶ COAGULATION DISORDERS

▶ DISSEMINATED INTRAVASCULAR COAGULATION (DIC)

Disseminated intravascular coagulation is not a disease in itself but a syndrome that occurs because of a primary disease process or condition. A few of the conditions in which DIC may occur are burns, acute leukemia, metastatic cancer, polycythemia vera, pheochromocytoma, shock, acute infections, septic abortion, abruptio placenta, blood transfusion reactions, and trauma.

DIC is a condition in which there is alternating clotting and hemorrhaging. The primary disease stimulates the clotting mechanism causing many **microthrombi** (very small clots) to form and block the circulation in the arterioles and capillaries. With the formation of the numerous small clots, the body's fibrinolytic process responds in an attempt to stop the clot formation, thus causing hemorrhaging (refer to Figure 22-7). This can be a very serious and potentially fatal condition.

The occlusion of blood vessels from the clots causes infarcts and necrosis of organs and tissues. The kidneys are the most commonly affected organ.

If a client with a predisposing condition develops **purpura** (reddish purple patches on the skin indicative of hemorrhage), bleeding tendencies, or renal impairment, the nurse should assess for DIC. Symptoms of DIC may present as oozing from a venipuncture, mucus membrane, or surgical wound. The oozing may progress rapidly into a hemorrhage within a few hours to a day. The client may have decreased urine output from decreased blood volume or renal infarction.

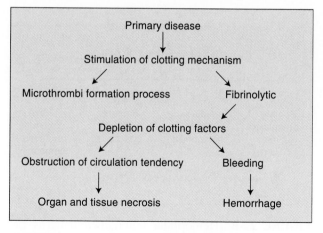

FIGURE 22-7 Pathophysiology of DIC.

▶ Medical/Surgical Management

▶ Medical

DIC is diagnosed by the client's symptoms and laboratory tests. With DIC there is an increased prothrombin time, partial thromboplastin time, thrombin time, and a decreased fibrinogen and platelet count. A laboratory test that confirms the diagnosis is the D dimer which measures a fibrin split product that is released when a clot breaks.

To treat DIC the primary disease or condition must be treated. For example, if the primary disease is an infection, an antibiotic is given. If cancer is the primary disease, chemotherapy is given.

DIC is treated by administering whole blood or blood products to normalize the clotting factor levels. Platelets and packed red cells are given to replace those lost during hemorrhage. Cryoprecipitate or fresh-frozen plasma is given to normalize clotting factor levels.

▶ Pharmacological

Heparin has no effect on the thrombi that are already formed but may be given to prevent the formation of more microthrombi. The administration of heparin is controversial because of the risk of hemorrhage. After thrombi formation has been controlled with heparin, aminocaproic acid (Amicar) can be given to stop the bleeding because it stops the fibrinolysis process. **Fibrinolysis** is the process of breaking fibrin apart.

▶ Nursing Process

Assessment

Subjective Data Ask the client about previous conditions such as infectious processes or cancer. Client statements of joint pain may indicate bleeding into the joint. Also ask the client about recent visual changes.

Objective Data Observe and record amount of bleeding from any wound or body orifice. I&O is monitored closely. Purpura on the chest and abdomen is a common first sign. Abdominal tenderness is often present. Note pulmonary edema, hypotension, tachycardia, restlessness, and absence of peripheral pulses.

▼ ▼

A possible nursing diagnosis for a client with DIC may include:

Nursing Diagnoses	Goals	Nursing Interventions
▶ *Tissue perfusion, altered, related to obstruction of vessels and/or bleeding.*	The client will maintain adequate tissue perfusion.	Monitor vitals signs, peripheral pulses, neurological checks, and urine output.
		Check urine and stool for the presence of blood. Assess for abdominal bleeding by checking for abdominal firmness or rigidity.
		If abdominal bleeding is suspected, measure the abdominal girth every four hours.
		Assess surgical wounds and all body orifices for bleeding.
		Assess color, warmth, sensation, and movement of extremities.
		Elevate extremities to promote venous return and prevent edema formation.
		Avoid giving injections and venipunctures as much as possible.
		Transfer the client with DIC into the intensive care unit for specialized care as ordered.

▶ *Evaluation*

Each goal must be evaluated to determine how it has been met by the client.

▲ ▲

▶ HEMOPHILIA

Hemophilia is an inherited bleeding disorder in which there is a lack of clotting factors. Approximately 20,000 persons in the United States have hemophilia (Beare & Myers, 1994). There are two types of hemophilia: hemophilia A is lacking clotting factor VIII and hemophilia B (Christmas disease) is lacking clotting factor IX. The hemophilia trait is carried on the recessive X chromosome so a mother is asymptomatic but can pass the trait to the son, who then manifests the symptoms of hemophilia (see Figure 22-8). In the male population, hemophilia A occurs at the rate of 1:10,000 and Hemophilia B occurs at the rate of 1:100,000 (Phipps et al., 1995).

There are three classifications of hemophilia: severe (factor level less than one percent of normal), moderate (factor level one percent to five percent normal), and mild (factor level 40 percent of normal). The main symptom of hemophilia is bleeding. The client with severe hemophilia bleeds when there is minor trauma to an area but can also bleed spontaneously. **Hemarthrosis** (bleeding into the joints) occurs most frequently causing pain, swelling, redness, and fever. The client can have spontaneous ecchymoses and bleed from the mouth and gastrointestinal and urinary tracts. The most common cause of death is intracranial hemorrhage. Clients with mild hemophilia will not have

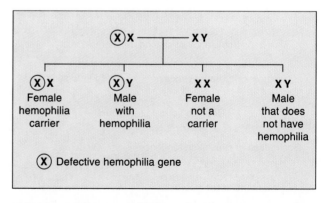

FIGURE 22-8 Hemophilia inheritance patterns between a female hemophiliac carrier and a male without hemophilia.

spontaneous muscle and joint bleeding but will bleed after minor or major surgery. This could prove fatal if the diagnosis is not determined promptly.

▶ Medical/Surgical Management

▶ Medical

Hemophilia is diagnosed by a deficient or absent blood level of factors VIII or IX. The prothrombin time (PT), thrombin time, platelet count, and bleeding time are normal, but the partial thromboplastin time (PTT) is usually prolonged.

The treatment for hemophilia is the administration of clotting factors VIII and IX. Clients with hemophilia A are given fresh frozen plasma and cryoprecipitate which has factor VIII. Clients with hemophilia B are given fresh frozen plasma which contains factor IX. Hemophiliacs, who received blood products before 1984, later often tested seropositive for HIV (Beare & Myers, 1994). This risk has been greatly reduced by heat-treating human-derived Factor VIII. The heat treatment inactivates viruses. Factor IX can also be treated in a similar manner. A genetically engineered product called *recombinant factor VIII* is viral safe and relatively economical in price.

▶ Pharmacological

Desmopressin acetate (DDAVP) and aminocaproic acid (Amicar) can be given to mild hemophiliacs to decrease the fibrinolytic process.

▶ Preventive Treatment

Clients who are carriers or who have the disease are referred to genetic counseling to explore their options regarding having children. Family members or significant others are taught home administration of clotting factors to control bleeding episodes. This way the client does not have to be hospitalized as frequently.

▶ Nursing Process

Assessment

Subjective Data Assess the client for pain. Ask what measures had been used in the past to relieve pain and bleeding.

Objective Data Assess the client for bleeding by checking for petechiae, ecchymoses, hematuria, hematemesis, melena, epistaxis, hemarthrosis, abdominal firmness and rigidity, and frank bleeding. Also note edematous or immobile joints.

▼ ▼

Possible nursing diagnoses for a client with hemophilia may include:

Nursing Diagnoses	Goals	Nursing Interventions
▶ Knowledge deficit related to disease process.	The client will relate symptoms to report and treatment methods if bleeding occurs.	Discuss ways to improve the safety of the client's home environment.
		Encourage the client to use an electric razor and soft-bristled toothbrush.
		Teach family members or significant others administration of clotting factors for prophylactic purposes and if injury occurs.
		Refer for genetic counseling.
▶ Pain related to bleeding into tissues and joints.	The client will remain pain free.	Assess the client for bruising, swelling, and joint discomfort.
		Apply ice and pressure to bleeding sites.
		When a joint is hurting, immobilize it in a flexed position with a supportive device.
		Give analgesics as needed. Aspirin is not given because of the anticoagulant effect.

(continued)

Nursing Diagnoses	Goals	Nursing Interventions
▸ *Injury, high risk for, related to bleeding.*	The client will take precautions to avoid injury.	Transfuse clotting factors as ordered.
		Encourage the client to avoid activities that may cause trauma.
		Emergency medical numbers can be posted in convenient places in case of future need.

Evaluation

Each goal must be evaluated to determine how it has been met by the client.

▲ ▲

▸ LYMPH DISORDERS

A lymphoma is a tumor of the lymph system. Two malignant lymphomas discussed in this chapter are Hodgkin's disease (HD) and non-Hodgkin's lymphoma (NHL). The overview and medical management of each disease will be presented separately. The nursing process for both diseases will be presented together since the nursing diagnoses, goals, and interventions are the same for HD and NHL.

▸ HODGKIN'S DISEASE

Hodgkin's disease is a rare lymphoma that usually arises as a painless swelling in a lymph node. The diagnosis is confirmed when Reed-Sternberg cells are biopsied from the swollen lymph node. The disease occurs twice as frequently in males between the ages of twenty to twenty-four and sixty to sixty-five (Erickson, 1994). Seventy-five percent of clients diagnosed with Hodgkin's disease are cured with appropriate therapy but carry a risk of long-term complications (Erickson, 1994).

The cause of Hodgkin's disease is unknown. Researchers are investigating genetic factors. Some researchers suspect an infectious origin especially in connection with infectious mononucleosis. Other researchers suspect a viral origin associated with the oncovirus and Epstein-Barr virus (Beare & Myers, 1994). Young adults diagnosed with Hodgkin's disease often come from small families, are educated, and in a higher socioeconomic class (Erickson, 1994).

Clients with Hodgkin's disease most commonly have painless enlarged lymph nodes in the neck, in the area above the clavicles, and in the groin. Lymph nodes in the mediastinum may also be enlarged but are not usually diagnosed until the nodes enlarge and press on the mediastinal structures causing dyspnea and a cough. A chest x-ray or a computed tomography (CT) scan confirms the involvement of the mediastinal lymph nodes. Other symptoms are weight loss, anorexia, fatigue, pruritis, fever, chills, night sweats, anemia, **thrombocytopenia** (decreased number of platelets), and lowered resistance to infections.

If a client has painless, enlarged lymph nodes and the symptoms of an elevated temperature, night sweats, pruritus, and weight loss of more than ten percent of the body weight in a six-month period, the prognosis is worse than if only enlarged lymph nodes are present. Hodgkin's disease spreads throughout the body in a predictable pattern. From the site of the original swollen gland, the disease spreads to nearby lymph nodes then to other lymphatic tissue in the body such as the liver, spleen, and bone marrow.

The invasion of other nodes and lymphatic tissue determines the prognosis of the disease. As more tissue is invaded, the disease process moves through different stages and is known as staging (see Figure 22-9). A classification of A or B is added to each stage depending on whether or not the client has symptoms other than swollen lymph nodes. If the client has lymph node enlargement only, he is asymptomatic (A). If he has symptoms other than lymph node enlargement, he is symptomatic (B).

▸ Medical/Surgical Management

▸ Medical

Diagnostic tests to determine the staging of the disease are a history and physical examination, CBC, platelet count, bone marrow aspiration, chest x-ray, abdominal CT scan, and a lymphangiogram.

Localized Hodgkin's disease stages I and IIA are treated with radiation therapy over a four-week period. Eighty-five percent of these clients have a prognosis of being disease free in ten years (Erickson, 1994). Clients with massive mediastinal involvement and those who have relapsed after radiation therapy alone, are treated with radiation therapy and chemotherapy.

During radiation therapy the client may experience symptoms of toxicity which are weight loss, nausea and vomiting, skin reactions, esophagitis, fatigue, and bone marrow suppression. The client's blood count is monitored closely during the therapy treatments to check for infections and bleeding tendencies. If the WBCs drop too low, the client will be more susceptible to infections. Lowered RBCs and platelets cause a bleeding tendency. Long-term complications from radiation therapy include hypothyroidism, radiation pneumonitis, immune system impairment, herpes zoster, and the development of a second cancer.

Generalized Hodgkin's disease, stages IIB, III, and IV, are treated with **combination chemotherapy**, which is administering a series of combined drugs over a set period of time. Serious late complications of chemotherapy are infertility and a secondary malignancy or cancer.

▶ Surgical

Sometimes a laparotomy is done to see if the liver and spleen are involved. The rationale of performing the procedure is being questioned since the overall treatment plan is not altered.

▶ Pharmacological

During radiation therapy antiemetics, such as ondansetron HCl (Zofran), are given for nausea and vomiting. Analgesics can be given for esophagitis discomfort.

Chemotherapy drugs are often given in combinations such as MOPP and ABVD. MOPP combines mechlorethamine or nitrogen mustard (Mustargen), vincristine sulfate (Oncovin), procarbazine HCl (Matulane), and prednisone (Deltasone). ABVD combines doxorubicin HCl (Adriamycin PFS), bleomycin sulfate (Blenoxane), vinblastine sulfate (Velban) and dacarbazine (DTIC-Dome). These drugs are usually administered through an implanted venous port. Allopurinol (Zyloprim) is given to prevent uric acid renal stones caused by the rapid destruction of cells during therapy.

▶ Diet

During therapy the client is on a high-caloric, high-protein diet. An intake of 2500 mL of fluid per day is encouraged to prevent the formation of renal stones.

▶ Activity

Extra rest periods may be necessary to cope with fatigue that occurs with Hodgkin's disease.

▶ NON-HODGKIN'S LYMPHOMA (NHL)

Non-Hodgkin's lymphoma is more common than Hodgkin's disease and is the seventh most common cause of cancer related deaths in the United States. Approximately 35,000 new cases occur each year (Lundquist & Stewart, 1994).

NHL originates from the B lymphocytes and the T lymphocytes. NHL arising from the B lymphocyte occurs in the older adult population while NHL arising from the T lymphocytes manifests in malignant skin diseases such as mycosis fungoides or Sezary syndrome. More men are affected than women. NHL does not have the Reed-Sternberg cell present.

Symptoms of NHL are enlarged tonsils and adenoids and diffuse enlarged painless, rubbery lymph nodes in the cervical, axillary, and inguinal areas. Symptoms of fever, night sweats, and weight loss, are seen in approximately twenty to thirty percent of clients with NHL (Lundquist & Stewart, 1994). About 15 percent of NHL clients have vague gastrointestinal symptoms of nausea, vomiting, and diarrhea.

▶ Medical/Surgical Management

▶ Medical

The diagnosis of NHL is confirmed by a lymph node biopsy. Physicians use a staging system to define the progression of the disease within the body and to determine the appropriate treatment and prognosis of the disease. Two staging systems are the Ann Arbor Staging Classification and the Working Formulation Classification System. The Ann Arbor Staging Classification is used to classify the progression of HD and NHL within the body. (Refer to Figure 22-9 to see the Ann Arbor staging method.) The Working Formulation Classification System divides NHL into three grades: low grade which develops slowly, intermediate grade which develops aggressively, and high grade which

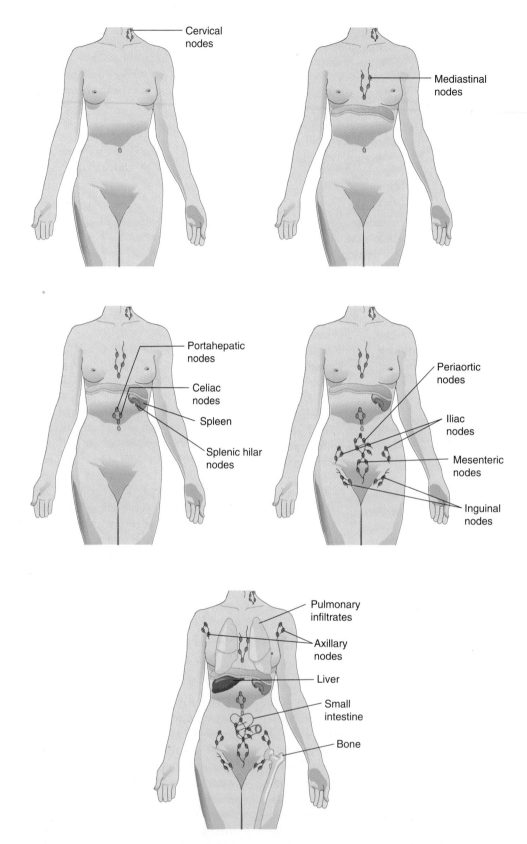

FIGURE 22-9   Staging system for Hodgkin's disease and non-Hodgkin's lymphoma. (*From Lewis, Collier, & Heitkemper (1996), Medical-Surgical Nursing: Assessment and Management of Clinical Problems, 4th ed. St. Louis: Mosby-Year Book, Inc. Reprinted with permission.*)

develops very aggressively. The grading is determined by physical assessment and diagnostic tests.

Low grade NHL treatment is somewhat controversial as some treat it with radiation therapy and others take a more conservative approach and monitor the progress of the disease before treating the symptoms. Intermediate and high grade NHL are treated with a combination of chemotherapy drugs.

▶ Pharmacological

There are three different chemotherapy regimens, CHOP, CVP, and COPP: CHOP combines (cyclophosphamide [Cytoxan], doxorubicin HCl [Adriamycin], vincristine sulfate [Oncovin], and prednisone [Deltasone]); CVP combines (cyclophosphamide [Cytoxan], vincristine sulfate [Oncovin] and prednisone [Deltasone]); COPP combines (cyclophosphamide [Cytoxan], vincristine sulfate [Oncovin], procarbazine HCl [Matulane] and prednisone [Deltasone]).

▶ Nursing Process

Assessment

Subjective Data   Ask if the client is experiencing pruritus, night sweats, weight loss, decreased appetite, fever, fatigue, weakness or chest pain.

Objective Data   The nursing physical assessment consists of weighing the client, taking the vital signs, and assessing for skin infections; dyspnea; cough; voice changes; enlarged lymph nodes in the neck, axilla, and groin; and edema in the extremities. Bone scan shows fractures and tumor infiltration. Review blood tests. Blood tests show hypercalcemia and a positive Coombs' test.

When the client is having radiation or chemotherapy treatments, the assessment includes observing for dysphagia, nausea and vomiting, skin rashes, and alopecia.

Possible nursing diagnoses for a client with Hodgkin's disease and non-Hodgkin's disease may include:

Nursing Diagnoses	Goals	Nursing Interventions
▶ Breathing pattern, ineffective, related to tracheobronchial obstruction from enlarged mediastinal nodes.	The client will complete activities of daily living without dyspnea.	Elevate the head of the bed to assist the client's breathing. Encourage the client to take frequent deep breaths to expand the lungs and prevent infection Assess the client's breathing pattern every shift and as needed for dyspnea.
▶ Infection, high risk for, related to radiation/chemotherapy treatments, decreased WBCs and pruritus.	The client will remain free of infection.	Monitor the lab results for lowered WBC. Teach the client the importance of avoiding situations where there is exposure to infections. Provide cool sponge baths or oral medication to relieve pruritus. Assess the radiated skin areas for redness or breaks in the skin. Because of the possibility of frequent infections, encourage the client to report symptoms of dyspnea, sore throat, and burning or frequency of urination.

(continued)

Nursing Diagnoses	Goals	Nursing Interventions
▶ Anxiety related to disease and therapy treatments.	The client will cope effectively with disease process and therapy treatments.	Listen to the concerns of the client regarding the effect of the disease on lifestyle, family, and finances.
		Encourage the family to express their concerns and discuss effective ways to deal with the diagnosis and treatment.
		Refer the client and family to clergy and social agencies when appropriate.
▶ Nutrition, altered, less than body requirements related to decreased appetite from disease and therapy treatments.	The client will consume an adequate amount of a nutritional diet.	Serve attractive high-caloric, high-protein meals in a pleasant environment.
		Offer six to eight smaller meals throughout the day to decrease a feeling of fullness.
		A soft, bland diet may be more palatable during radiation or chemotherapy treatments.
		Avoid hot, spicy foods as they are caustic to mucous membranes and may lead to infection.
		Encourage an adequate intake of fluids to prevent constipation and renal stones.
		Weigh the client biweekly or more frequently if needed.
▶ Activity intolerance related to fatigue.	The client will balance activity with rest periods.	Teach the client to moderate activities so frequent rest periods can be taken.
		Encourage the client to do range of motion exercises while in bed to maintain muscle strength and tone.

Evaluation

Each goal must be evaluated to determine how it has been met by the client.

▶ CASE STUDY

James Johns, forty-six, owns a hobby shop. He has had a cold for three weeks that has recently settled in his chest. He has been tired lately and takes naps each evening before the evening meal. His wife noticed several bruises on his arms and legs but James could not recall any particular injury. James has gradually lost 10 pounds over the last three months but has not been concerned about it. When James went to the clinic for some antibiotics for his cold, the nurse practitioner completed a physical assessment and ordered a chest x-ray and CBC. The nurse practitioner noticed the WBCs were 250,000/mm³, RBCs 4.2 million/mm³ and the platelets were 100,000/mm³. After several other tests were performed over the next few days, a diagnosis of CML was confirmed.

The following questions will guide your development of a Nursing Care Plan for the case study.

1. List the symptoms occurring in James Johns that are typical of CML.
2. List five other typical symptoms of CML that the case study does not state James had.
3. List other diagnostic tests that could be done to confirm the diagnosis of CML.
4. List subjective and objective data the nurse practitioner would obtain about James Johns.
5. Write three individualized nursing diagnoses and goals for James Johns.
6. List nursing interventions for James Johns.
7. List community resources specific to locale that could assist James and his family during his illness with CML.
8. List discharge teaching the nurse would give to James and his family.
9. List successful client outcomes for James Johns.
10. List chemotherapeutic agents and side effects of the agents that may be prescribed for James.
11. List other medical treatments that may be ordered for James.
12. What measures could the nurse take to meet the emotional needs of James and his family?

SUMMARY

- The main formed components of the blood are red blood cells, white blood cells, and platelets.
- The lymphatic system is composed of lymph vessels that drain lymph into the venous system and lymph nodes that filter microorganisms in the body.
- Sickledex and hemoglobin electrophoresis are diagnostic tests for sickle cell anemia.
- A client with anemia has a decreased number of RBCs and low hemoglobin and hematocrit levels.
- Some of the symptoms of anemia are fatigue, pallor, exertional dyspnea, and tachycardia.

- Clients with polycythemia vera have an increased production of RBCs.
- Symptoms of polycythemia vera are headache, epistaxis, dizziness, tinnitus, blurred vision, fatigue, weakness, pruritus, exertional dyspnea, angina, and increased blood pressure and pulse.
- Polycythemia vera is treated with chemotherapeutic agents.
- DIC is not a disease but a syndrome that occurs because of a client having a primary disease or condition. The primary disease causes the client to alternate between forming many small clots and hemorrhaging.

- Hemophilia is a recessive X chromosome inherited bleeding disorder in which the client is lacking clotting factors. The main symptom is spontaneous bleeding or bleeding due to trauma.
- The two types of malignant lymphomas are Hodgkin's disease and non-Hodgkin's lymphoma. Clients with both types of lymphoma have enlarged lymph nodes.
- Hodgkin's disease is diagnosed by the presence of the Reed-Sternberg cell in the swollen lymph nodes. Non-Hodgkin's lymphoma arises from the B lymphocytes and T lymphocytes and does not have the Reed-Sternberg cell in the lymph system.

Review Questions

1. The diagnostic test for sickle cell anemia is the:
   a. D dimer.
   b. sickledex.
   c. hemoglobin electrophoresis.
   d. Schilling test.

2. For improved iron absorption, a client with iron deficiency anemia takes Feosol with:
   a. milk.
   b. an orange.
   c. water.
   d. processed cheese.

3. A thorough assessment of the cardiac system on a client with sickle cell anemia is important because:
   a. the heart enlarges in an attempt to provide the oxygen needs to the body tissues.
   b. cells sickle more easily in the heart chambers.
   c. more cardiac force is needed to pump RBCs with Hbg S.
   d. they are more prone to bradycardia.

4. Clients with leukemia are prone to infections because:
   a. there are too many WBCs.
   b. the bone marrow is not producing WBCs.
   c. the bone marrow is producing too many cells.
   d. the WBCs are incapable of fighting infections.

5. To treat a leukemic client who has symptoms of a headache and visual disturbances, the physician may order:
   a. prednisone.
   b. penicillin.
   c. methotrexate orally.
   d. methotrexate intrathecally.

6. A nursing action for a client with pernicious anemia is to:
   a. inquire about exposure to radiation and chemicals.
   b. administer cyanocobalamin (vitamin B$_{12}$) as ordered.
   c. teach the importance of increasing iron in the diet.
   d. administer oral vitamin B$_{12}$ as ordered.

7. Nursing care for a client with polycythemia vera includes:
   a. doing a Homans' sign to check for blood clots.
   b. administering folic acid as ordered.
   c. observing for blood in the stool and urine.
   d. observing for petechiae and ecchymotic spots.

8. Symptoms that alert a nurse that a client may have DIC are:
   a. tinnitus and numbness and tingling in the extremities.
   b. jaundice, palpitations, and dyspnea.
   c. purpura, bruising, and decreased urine output.
   d. ruddy complexion, epistaxis, and tinnitus.

9. A client with hemophilia is taught to:
   a. adminster clotting factors as needed.
   b. administer cyanocobalamin (vitamin B$_{12}$) as needed.
   c. maintain a high-caloric, high-protein diet.
   d. report night sweats.

10. Encourage a client with non-Hodgkin's lymphoma to:
    a. use an electric razor.
    b. take folic acid as prescribed.
    c. apply ice and pressure to bleeding sites.
    d. avoid exposure to infections.

Critical Thinking Questions

1. Explain how the symptoms of iron deficiency anemia relate to a decreased red blood cell count and a decreased hemoglobin.

2. Compare the diagnostic tests, symptoms, and treatments stated in the text to an assigned client in the clinical setting.

3. Compare the etiologies and symptoms of iron deficiency anemia, hypoplastic (aplastic) anemia, pernicious anemia, acquired hemolytic anemia, and sickle cell anemia.

Medical Terminology

chromat-	pertaining to a specific color
chromatism	unnatural pigmentation
-cytosis	pertaining to cells
leukocytosis	increase in number of leukocytes
erythro-	red in color
erythroderma	abnormal redness of the skin
hema-	relating to blood
hemargioma	a benign tumor made up of newly formed blood vessels
leuko-	white
leukocytes	white blood cells
macro-	large
macrothrombocytes	large platelets
micro-	small
microthrombi	very small clots
neutro	neutral
neutrophil	most common type of glanulocytic white blood cell
normo-	normal
normochromia	blood possessing normal color and hemoglobin content
-penia	a lack of, insufficent amount
leukopenia	abnormal decrease of white blood corpuscles
-poiesis	production of
hematopoiesis	process responsible for forming both red and white blood
thrombo-	blood clot
thrombosis	formation, development, or existence of a thrombus within the vascular system

News Flash

Interferon alfa-2a (Roferon-A) is a chemotherapeutic agent that increased the survival time to 61 months as opposed to 41 months in a recent clinical trial (Campbell, 1995). Interferon alfa-2a (Roferon-A) has been FDA-approved for CML clients who test positive for the Philadelphia chromosome. The drug is to be used on clients who have had little or no treatment and is administered daily subcutaneously or intramuscularly. Side effects include fever, fatigue, myalgia and chills (*RN, 1995*).

UNIT
7

Body Defenses

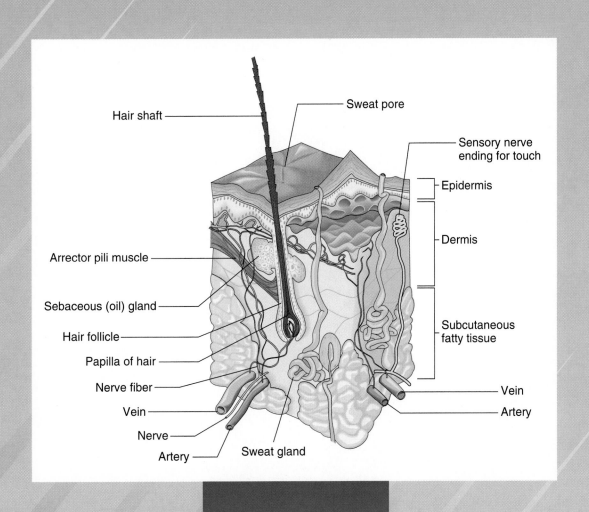

Hair shaft

Sweat pore

Sensory nerve ending for touch

Epidermis

Dermis

Arrector pili muscle

Sebaceous (oil) gland

Hair follicle

Papilla of hair

Nerve fiber

Vein

Nerve

Artery

Sweat gland

Subcutaneous fatty tissue

Vein

Artery

Integumentary Disorders

Margaret Griffin

LIST OF DISORDERS

LEARNING OBJECTIVES

Upon completion of this chapter the learner should be able to:
• Define key terms.
• Describe common disorders of the integumentary system.
• Relate the pathophysiology of each skin disorder.

- Discuss the common diagnostic tests used to differentiate skin disorders.
- State the usual treatment for each disorder.

- Assess the nursing care needs of a client with a disorder of the integument.
- Plan and implement effective nursing care.

▶ *MAKING THE CONNECTION*

Refer to the topics in the following chapters to increase your understanding of integumentary disorders.

- **Chapter 10: Nursing Assessment,** Skin Assessment, p. 178.
- **Chapter 14: Fluid, Electrolyte, and Acid-base Balances,** Fluid Balance, p. 271; Electrolyte Balance, p. 275.

- **Chapter 15: Oncology,** Skin Cancer, p. 312.
- **Chapter 16: Caring for the Older Adult,** Integumentary System, p. 336.
- **Chapter 24: Allergies, Immune, and Autoimmune Disorders,** Systemic Lupus Erythematosus, p. 605.

INTRODUCTION

As an old adage asserts, the health of the skin mirrors the health of the body. Many systemic diseases have skin manifestations. Psychological stress can affect the condition of the skin, and skin rashes can be a complication of drug therapy. As the largest and the most visible system in the body, the integumentary system is vulnerable to injury and is susceptible to a number of primary diseases. It is estimated that skin related problems account for five percent to ten percent of all ambulatory client visits in the United States (Deters, 1992). While the outward appearance of the skin is important for psychological well-being, the healthy, intact status of the skin also is essential for physiologic well-being. Maintaining this status of the integumentary system is, therefore, an important independent nursing function. The focus of this chapter will be to describe common skin disorders, identify the usual treatment modalities for these disorders, and discuss measures that nurses can implement to provide effective nursing care for clients with disorders of the integument.

ANATOMY AND PHYSIOLOGY REVIEW

As the external covering of the body, the skin performs the vital function of protecting internal body structures from harmful microorganisms and substances. The skin is continuous with mucous membranes at external body openings of the respiratory tract, the digestive system, and the urogenital tract. As appendages of the skin, the hair and nails also have protective functions. In addition to its vital protective role, the skin also plays other roles in the normal functioning of the human organism. These roles include participating in the regulation of body temperature, functioning as a sensory organ, helping to maintain fluid and electrolyte balance, producing vitamin D, and excreting certain waste products from the body.

Structure of the Skin

The skin is composed of three layers: the epidermis, the dermis, and the subcutaneous tissue (see Figure 23-1).

Epidermis

The epidermis is a layer of squamous epithelial cells. Most of the cells in the epidermis are keratinocytes that produce a tough, fibrous protein called **keratin**. As new cells are produced in the deep layers of the epidermis, old cells are pushed to the surface of the skin. As these cells move from the deeper epidermal layers to the surface, they undergo a process of keratinization in which they become filled with keratin thus hardening the outer layer of epidermal cells. The keratin creates a barrier that repels bacteria and foreign matter and is impermeable to most substances. The epidermal cells on the palms of the hands and soles of the feet, areas of the body subjected to

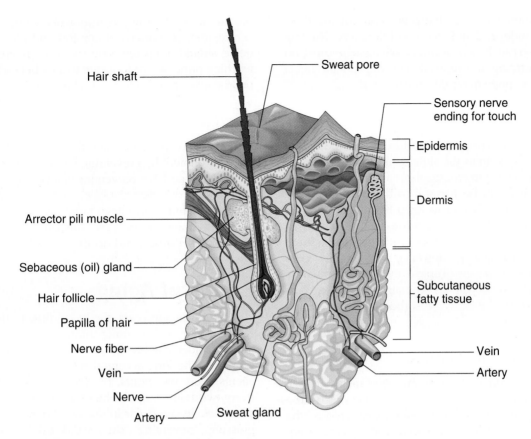

FIGURE 23-1 Cross section of the skin.

increased friction and pressure, contain larger amounts of keratin, resulting in thickened skin and callouses.

The epidermis also contains specialized cells called melanocytes. These cells produce **melanin**, the pigment that gives the skin its color. The more melanin present, the darker the skin color. Moles (**nevi**), pigmented elevations in the skin, are aggregations of melanocytes. In **vitiligo**, melanocytes are destroyed causing milk-white patches of depigmented skin surrounded by normal skin. Exposure to ultraviolet light causes an increase in the production of melanin which provides the skin with some protection against the harmful effects of suntanning.

Dermis

The dermis is dense, irregular connective tissue composed of collagen and elastic fibers, blood and lymph vessels, nerves, sweat and sebaceous glands, and hair roots. The sebaceous glands secrete an oily substance called **sebum** that lubricates the skin, helping to keep it soft and pliable. Sweat glands (eccrine glands) are found in the skin over most of the body surface. Another type of sweat gland, apocrine glands, are concentrated in the axillae, anal region, scrotum,

and labia majora. These glands secrete an organic substance which is odorless at first, but is quickly metabolized by skin bacteria causing the characteristic odor commonly referred to as body odor (Seeley, Stephens, & Tate, 1995). Intradermal injections, such as the TB skin test, are given in the dermis.

Subcutaneous

The subcutaneous tissue is primarily connective and adipose tissue. Here the skin is anchored to muscles and bones. An individual's nutritional status dictates the amount of subcutaneous tissue present. Emaciated persons have very little subcutaneous tissue while obese persons may have several inches of subcutaneous tissue. The amount of subcutaneous tissue is an important factor in body temperature regulation.

Functions of the Skin

Understanding the functions of the skin and contiguous mucous membranes guides the nurse in planning and implementing appropriate nursing care. Because intact, healthy skin and mucous membranes serve as the first line of defense against harmful agents, maintaining skin integrity is one of the most important independent functions of the nurse. Nursing interventions such as providing daily hygiene care and regularly turning and repositioning dependent clients are aimed at preventing skin breakdown.

Protection

The first and most important function of the skin is protection. As long as the skin is intact and healthy, it is a barrier against microorganisms and numerous substances that could be harmful to the individual. Not only is the skin a barrier to keep harmful substances out, it is also a barrier to keep essential substances such as water and electrolytes inside the body. Some fat-soluble substances, however, can readily pass through the epidermis. Topical medications such as nitroglycerin skin patches contain fat-soluble substances that can be slowly absorbed through the skin into the blood.

Temperature Regulation

The body produces heat as a result of metabolism of food. Exercise, fever, or a hot environment can raise body temperature. Through several mechanisms, the skin can either release or conserve body heat to maintain normal body temperature. Radiation is the primary means of heat loss. As body heat increases, arterioles in the dermis dilate, bringing body heat to the skin surface. By the process of radiation, waves of heat from uncovered body surfaces are released to the environment. Layering clothes in winter, for example, helps to prevent excess loss of body heat by radiation. Heat is also lost by conduction. In conduction, heat is transferred from warmer surfaces to cooler ones. Placing a cool washcloth on a client's forehead is an example of using the principle of conduction. The washcloth becomes warmer, the forehead cooler. Evaporation is another way in which excess body heat is lost. As moisture on the skin, either from perspiration or from a tepid sponge bath, evaporates the body is cooled. To conserve body heat, arterioles in the dermis contract to decrease the flow of blood to the skin surface, thus decreasing heat lost by radiation. The phenomenon of "goose flesh" is another method of conserving body heat. Tiny hairs standing on end create a layer of air insulation decreasing loss of body heat to the environment.

Sensory Perception

The skin contains receptors for pain, touch, pressure, and temperature. The sensory receptors help protect the body from environmental dangers as well as providing sensations of comfort and pleasure. The nurse should keep this skin function in mind when teaching principles of foot care to a diabetic client with neuropathy or giving a client a back massage.

Fluid and Electrolyte Balance

The skin helps to maintain the stability of the internal environment by preventing loss of body fluids and electrolytes and by preventing subcutaneous tissues from drying out. Skin damage, such as that occurring with severe burns, results in rapid loss of large quantities of fluid and electrolytes. This can lead to circulatory collapse, shock, and death.

Effects of Aging

With advancing years, the blood flow to the skin is reduced. The skin becomes thinner and is more easily injured. Older skin breaks down easily from prolonged pressure. The long accepted rule of thumb is to turn clients every two hours, but for the ill elderly client, every two hours may not be often enough. Significant skin damage can occur in just one hour of unrelieved pressure. Preventing skin breakdown in the elderly client depends on an accurate assessment of both the client's skin condition and his mobility status.

Loss of subcutaneous tissue causes skin sagging and wrinkling. The activity of sebaceous and sweat glands diminishes, resulting in dry skin and a decreased ability to adapt to changes in environmental temperature. Extremes in temperature pose hazards for older adults. In very hot weather they are susceptible to **hyperthermia**, which can progress to heat stroke. When the core body temperature reaches 106°F, the hypothalamus no longer functions appropriately. Sweating stops, the skin becomes dry and flushed and the person becomes confused and eventually comatose. Each summer elderly persons die from the effects of hyperthermia. Winter puts older adults at risk for **hypothermia**. When the core body temperature drops below 95°F, the client is hypothermic and may be confused and disoriented. As the core body temperature continues to drop, the person becomes comatose. Each winter some older adults will die from severe hypothermia (Seeley et al., 1995).

On the hands and face, melanocytes increase in number causing the age spots commonly seen in older adults. Gray hair occurs from a lack of melanin production. Skin exposed to sunlight ages faster.

Refer to Chapter 16 for more information on the effects of aging on the integumentary system.

ASSESSMENT OF SKIN AND MUCOUS MEMBRANES

Assessing clients with disorders of the integument includes obtaining a health history and performing a physical assessment of the skin, hair, nails, and mucous membranes. The nurse's assessment skills along with an understanding of the anatomy and physiology of the integumentary system ensures a complete, factual data base from which to plan and implement appropriate nursing care. Table 23-1 contains a list of questions to use in obtaining a health history.

Physical Assessment Parameters

There are seven parameters that should be examined when performing a physical assessment of the skin. They are integrity, color, temperature and moisture, texture, turgor and mobility, sensation, and vascularity. Inspection and palpation are the two assessment techniques used when examining the skin. Good lighting is essential for accurate assessment. In Table 23-2 you will find a list of these parameters with the normal and abnormal findings.

Table 23-1

OBTAINING A CLIENT HISTORY OF SKIN PROBLEMS

- When did you first notice this problem?
- Where did the first symptom appear?
- What did the rash/lesion look like when it first appeared?
- Describe what happened in the days/weeks after the first symptom appeared?
- Are the symptoms worse at any particular time? season?
- Have you experienced any itching or burning sensations?
- Are the lesions painful?
- What do you think might have caused this problem?
- Have you ever had a skin problem like this before?
- Has anyone in your family ever had a problem like this?
- What have you been doing to treat this problem?
- What kind of skin care products do you normally use?
- Have you changed any of your usual products/habits/routines?
- Is there anything else you would like to tell me about this problem?

Table 23-2

SKIN ASSESSMENT PARAMETERS

Parameter	Normal	Abnormal
Integrity	Skin intact; no diseased or injured tissue.	Broken skin; open areas such as fissures, ulcers excoriations. Rash or lesions such as papules, nodules, vesicles, pustules, wheals, scales.
Color	Varies with skin type and race. Pink, tanned, olive, brown.	**Pallor**—pale skin, especially in face, conjunctiva, nail beds, and oral mucous membranes. **Cyanosis**—bluish discoloration noticed in lips, earlobes, nail beds. **Jaundice**—a yellowing of the skin; also seen in the sclera. **Erythema**—reddish hue to the skin as in sunburn and inflammation. Palpate for warmth.
Temperature and Moisture	Usually warm and dry, depending on environmental temperature.	Cool, cold, moist, clammy or increased warmth.
Texture	Smooth, soft. Thickness varies in different areas.	Loose, wrinkled, rough, thickened, thin, oily flaking; scaling.
Turgor and Mobility	An assessment of skin hydration. Normally skin moves freely. A pinched fold of skin returns immediately to normal position.	Taut with edema; slack with dehydration. Rigid in some diseases such as scleroderma.
Sensation	Distinguishes hot and cold, sharp and dull, feels changes in temperature and pressure.	Numbness, tingling, insensitive to pressure and sharp objects.
Vascularity	Clear; no discoloration.	**Telangiectasia** (spider veins); **Petechiae** (pin-point hemorrhagic spots); **Ecchymosis** (large, irregular, hemorrhagic areas).

NONPALPABLE

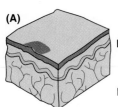

(A)

Macule:
Localized changes in skin color of less than 1 cm in diameter
Example:
Freckle

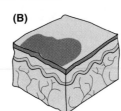

(B)

Patch:
Localized changes in skin color of greater than 1 cm in diameter
Example:
Vitiligo, stage 1 of pressure ulcer

PALPABLE

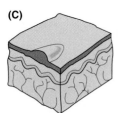

(C)

Papule:
Solid, elevated lesion less than 0.5 cm in diameter
Example:
Warts, elevated nevi

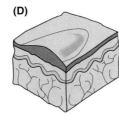

(D)

Plaque:
Solid, elevated lesion greater than 0.5 cm in diameter
Example:
Psoriasis

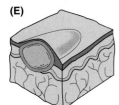

(E)

Nodules:
Solid and elevated; however they extend deeper than papules into the dermis or subcutaneous tissues, 0.5–2 cm
Example:
Lipoma, erythema nodosum, cyst

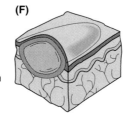

(F)

Tumor:
The same as a nodule only greater than 2 cm

Example:
Carcinoma (such as advanced breast carcinoma); not basal cell or squamous cell of the skin

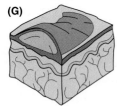

(G)

Wheal:
Localized edema in the epidermis causing irregular elevation that may be red or pale
Example:
Insect bite or a hive

FLUID-FILLED CAVITIES WITHIN THE SKIN

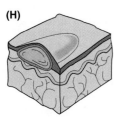

(H)

Vesicle:
Accumulation of fluid between the upper layers of the skin; elevated mass containing serous fluid; less than 0.5 cm
Example:
Herpes simplex, herpes zoster, chickenpox

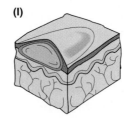

(I)

Bullae:
Same as a vesicle only greater than 0.5 cm
Example:
Contact dermatitis, large second-degree burns, bulbous impetigo, pemphigus

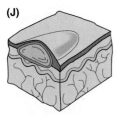

(J)

Pustule:
Vesicles or bullae that become filled with pus, usually described as less than 0.5 cm in diameter
Example:
Acne, impetigo, furuncles, carbuncles, folliculitis

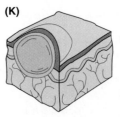

(K)

Cyst:
Encapsulated fluid-filled or a semi-solid mass in the subcutaneous tissue or dermis
Example:
Sebaceous cyst, epidermoid cyst

ABOVE THE SKIN SURFACE

(L)
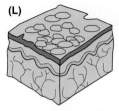
Scales:
   Flaking of the skin's surface
Example:
   Dandruff or psoriasis, xerosis

(M)
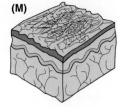
Lichenification:
   Layers of skin become
   thickened and rough as a
   result of rubbing over a
   prolonged period of time
Example:
   Chronic contact dermatitis

(N)
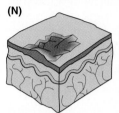
Crust:
   Dried serum, blood, or pus
   on the surface of the skin
Example:
   Impetigo

(O)
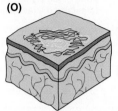
Atrophy:
   Thinning of the skin surface
   and loss of markings
Example:
   Striae, aged skin

BELOW THE SKIN SURFACE

(P)
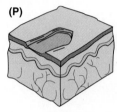
Erosion:
   Loss of epidermis
Example:
   Ruptured chickenpox vesicle

(Q)
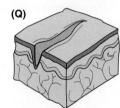
Fissure:
   Linear crack in the epidermis
   that can extend into the dermis
Example:
   Chapped hands or lips,
   athlete's foot

(R)
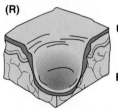
Ulcer:
   A depressed lesion of
   the epidermis and upper
   papillary layer of the dermis
Example:
   Stage 2 pressure ulcer

(S)
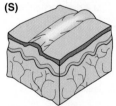
Scar:
   Fibrous tissue that replaces
   dermal tissue after injury
Example:
   Surgical incision

(T)
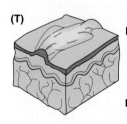
Keloid:
   Enlarging of a scar past
   wound edges due to excess
   collagen formation (more
   prevalent in dark skinned
   persons)
Example:
   Burn scar

(U)
Excoriation:
   Loss of epidermal layers
   exposing the dermis
Example:
   Abrasion

FIGURE 23-2 Types of skin lesions.

Oral mucous membranes normally appear pink and moist. Hair should be smooth, shiny, and resilient. Nails protect the ends of the fingers. They should be smooth and shiny with some flexibility. Thin, dry, brittle nails reflect ill health. Any lesions should be identified according to type and described as to color, size, and location (see Figure 23-2).

Describe the amount, color, odor, and appearance of any drainage that might be present. Document assessment findings clearly, concisely, and completely. Keep in mind that the intent of nursing care is to maintain the integrity of intact skin and to restore damaged skin or mucous membranes to an intact state. Recall that aging changes skin texture, moisture, and mobility requiring increased nursing vigilance to maintain skin integrity. Select daily hygiene products to meet the client's individual skin care needs.

COMMON DIAGNOSTIC TESTS

The following is a table of the commonly used diagnostic tests for clients with integumentary disorders.

Test	Explanation/Normal Values	Nursing Responsibilities
Biopsy	Obtained from a suspicious nodule or plaque by scalpel incision or with a skin punch. Usually to rule out malignancy. Also to establish exact diagnosis.	Let the client know when the test is scheduled. Obtain the necessary equipment. Support the client during the procedure.
Patch Testing	Allergens are applied to normal skin (usually the upper back) under occlusive patches for 48 hours. If the client is allergic to a specific allergen, an erythematous skin reaction occurs.	Clean and dry the skin where the patches are to be applied. Tell the client that the patches must be left in place for the full 48 hours.
Tzanck Smear	Fluid from the base of a vesicle is applied to a glass slide, stained and examined under a microscope. This test is used to diagnose herpes zoster, herpes simplex, varicella, or pemphigus.	Describe to the client how the laboratory technician will obtain the specimen.
Immunofluorescence (IF Testing)	Antigens or antibodies are combined with a fluorochrome dye. IF testing, which may be direct or indirect, detects auto-antibodies and can localize the site of an immune reaction.	Inform the client that the test is scheduled. Answer questions that the client may have about the test.
Wood's Light Examination	Skin and hair are examined by ultraviolet (black light) light in a darkened room. This test diagnoses fungal infections (tinea) of hair and skin.	Reassure the client that the rays are not harmful. Explain the procedure to the client.
Skin Scrapings	The lesion is scraped with an oiled scalpel blade. The cells are then examined under a microscope. This test diagnoses fungal lesions.	Explain the procedure and purpose of the test to the client.
Culture and Sensitivity	Drainage from infected lesions is obtained by sterile swab and incubated in order to identify the causative organism and to determine antibiotic sensitivity.	Obtain the necessary equipment. Explain the procedure. Obtain the specimen. Send to the lab immediately.

KEY ABBREVIATIONS

The following abbreviations and acronyms are used in this chapter:

ADL	activities of daily living
MRSA	methicillin-resistant *Staphylococcus aureus*
ROM	range of motion
SPF	sun protection factor
TPN	total parenteral nutrition

▶ BURNS

Burns are among the most devastating injuries that an individual can suffer. Burns can be painful and disfiguring, requiring long hospitalizations. Many are fatal. Most accidental burns occur in the home and are preventable. Frequently, the burn injury is the result of the individual's own action. Feelings of anger and guilt can complicate recovery. Often the individual suffers self-image disturbances and family relationships can be strained.

▶ Major Causes

By far the greatest number of burn injuries to adults are associated with cigarette smoking and cooking. The elderly are likely to suffer burns by spilling hot liquid on themselves or by catching their clothes on fire as they cook or smoke. Young children are especially prone to burn injuries from spilling scalding liquids on themselves and playing with matches or cigarette lighters. Industrial accidents account for a significant number of burn injuries in young adults.

▶ Severity

Burns are classified according to the depth of the burn and the extent of skin surface involved. First- and second-degree burns are partial-thickness burns. First-degree burns involve only the epidermis. The skin is hot, red, and painful. A sunburn is an example of a first-degree burn. First-degree burns heal in about a week without scarring. Second-degree burns damage the dermis and the epidermis. The skin is red, hot, and painful; blisters form and tissue around the burn is edematous, or swollen with an excessive amount of fluid. Usually, second-degree burns heal in about two weeks without scarring. However, if deep layers of the dermis are involved, healing might take months and scarring can occur. Second-degree burns involving deep layers of the dermis may appear white, tan, or red in color.

When the dermis and epidermis are completely destroyed and deeper tissues are involved, burns are classified as full-thickness burns. Third-degree and fourth-degree burns are full-thickness burns. In third-degree burns all dermal structures are destroyed and cannot be regenerated. Subcutaneous tissue is also damaged. Full-thickness burns can be white, tan, brown, black, charred, or bright red in color. Fourth-degree burns, which extend to the underlying muscles and bones, appear white to black or charred with dark networks of thrombosed capillaries visible inside the wound. Fourth-degree burns occur in explosions and nuclear radiation. Figure 23-3 depicts the various layers of skin involved in burn injuries.

Severely burned individuals generally have both partial-thickness and full-thickness burns. While first and second-degree burns are painful, third- and fourth-degree burns themselves are not painful because of the destruction of sensory nerve endings. The client, however, will still be in severe pain. Body movement causes pain in burned areas; areas of first- and second-degree burns that often surround the full-thickness burns can be quite painful. Skin can regenerate only from the edges of full-thickness burns. Scarring is inevitable. Skin grafting is necessary to promote healing because the section of skin destroyed by the burn cannot regenerate itself.

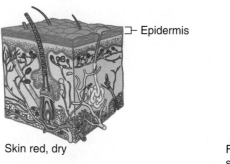
Epidermis
Skin red, dry

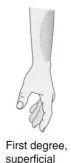
First degree, superficial

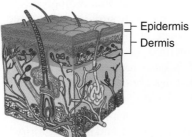
Epidermis
Dermis
Blistered, skin moist, pink or red

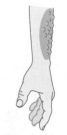
Second degree, partial thickness

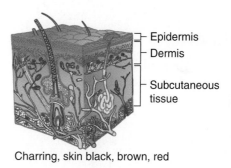
Epidermis
Dermis
Subcutaneous tissue
Charring, skin black, brown, red

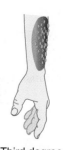
Third degree, full thickness

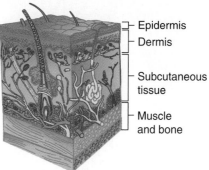
Epidermis
Dermis
Subcutaneous tissue
Muscle and bone
Charring; skin white to black with networks of thrombosed capillaries

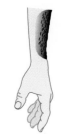
Fourth degree, full thickness

FIGURE 23-3 Skin layers involved in burn injuries.

Prognosis in burn cases depends upon the severity of the burn, the surface area of the body burned and the preinjury health status of the individual. If the client's health status before the burn was good, a burn covering 40 percent of the body will require a minimum of forty days to heal (Fritsch & Yurko, 1995). Elderly burn victims whose physiologic reserves are already reduced as an effect of aging will have an extended recovery period and a greater risk of complications. Documenting the extent of the burn injury can be done by using a burn assessment chart such as the Lund and Browder Chart or the Rule-of-Nines method (Ogden, 1994). The Lund and Browder chart can be used for all ages, from infants through adults. In addition to estimating the body surface area burned, it also includes an estimate of the severity of the burn. The Rule-of-Nines method of estimating the body surface area burned is used for adults. The body is divided into areas that are about 9 percent (or multiples of 9 percent). The head comprises 9 percent (4.5 percent anterior and 4.5 percent posterior). Each arm is 9 percent (4.5 percent anterior and 4.5 percent posterior). The anterior trunk and posterior trunk are each 18 percent. Each leg is 18 percent (9 percent anterior and 9 percent posterior). The genitalia comprise the remaining 1 percent (see Figure 23-4).

▶ *Complications*

Destruction of the skin renders it unable to fulfill its functions. Vast amounts of internal fluids and electrolytes are lost. The ability to maintain body temperature is altered and the individual is susceptible to serious infections. Initially the complications that are the most life threatening are respiratory failure and massive loss of body fluids.

▶ *Smoke Inhalation and Carbon Monoxide Poisoning*

Heat and smoke can cause serious damage to the respiratory tract. Facial burns, singed nasal hairs, and carbon-tinged sputum are signs that the client may have suffered respiratory tract damage (Ogden, 1994). Inhaling heat and smoke in a closed-space fire causes airway inflammation and edema of the respiratory mucosa. The carbon monoxide that is inhaled along with the heat and smoke attaches to hemoglobin, forming the compound, carboxyhemoglobin. A high level of carboxyhemoglobin in the blood means that oxygen is not being delivered to vital body tissues. The client may be stuporous because of cerebral anoxia. Keeping an open airway and administering 100 percent humidified oxygen are essential for treating these two conditions. Intubation is often necessary.

▶ *Shock*

Severely burned clients may suffer both hypovolemic shock (a life-threatening condition caused by massive loss of blood and circulating fluids), and neurogenic shock (a form of shock that occurs when peripheral vascular dilation occurs causing hypoten-

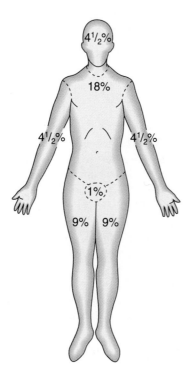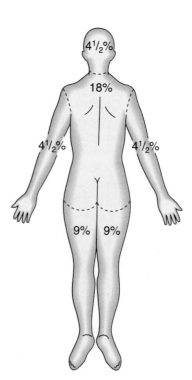

FIGURE 23-4 Rule-of-nines.

sion). Fluids and electrolytes must be replaced as fast as they are being lost. Tremendous amounts of fluids are lost through the burn wounds themselves as well as into surrounding tissues in the form of edema. The fluid loss shock that results can lead to circulatory collapse and renal shutdown. Using the Rule-of-Nines to assess the extent of the burn can be helpful in guiding fluid replacement. Expect at least two large-caliber venous catheters to give large volumes of fluid rapidly.

▶ Infection

Once the client has been stabilized, infection poses a serious risk. *Staphylococcus aureus,* a ubiquitous organism in the environment, is a common cause of infections. Of grave concern is an infection caused by methicillin-resistant *Staphylococcus aureus* (MRSA) because this strain of staphylococcus is resistant to all antibiotics except vancomycin hydrochloride (Vancocin). This antibiotic has serious side effects, especially to the otic nerve and to the liver, and is used only when other antibiotics fail. All persons coming into contact with the client wear gowns, gloves, masks, and caps to help prevent the introduction of organisms such as *Staphylococcus aureus, Pseudomonas aeruginosa* or coliform bacilli into burn wounds. Use sterile technique for wound care and dressing changes. Care of severely burned clients in special burn units reduces the chance of infection because of stringent infection control precautions and a carefully controlled environment.

▶ Medical/Surgical Management

▶ Medical

Immediate Care   Initially medical management of the client involves keeping an open airway, maintaining an adequate level of oxygenation, replacing body fluids and electrolytes, monitoring kidney function, controlling pain, and protecting the burns with sterile dressings to minimize the loss of body temperature and the risk of infection. In cases of severe burns, the client usually requires endotracheal intubation and administration of 100 percent humidified oxygen. A multiport central venous catheter or two large-bore peripheral venous catheters are needed for fluid and electrolyte replacement. A Foley catheter is used and urine output measured hourly to help monitor kidney function. Pain can be controlled with small intravenous doses of narcotics. Emotional and psychological trauma can intensify pain perception. The client will be anxious, not only for his survival, but also about his physical appearance and the effect this injury will have on his family. Prophylactically the client receives tetanus toxoid.

Stabilized Care   Once the client's condition has been stabilized, care focuses on promoting healing, preventing complications, controlling pain, and restoring function. During the recovery phase, preventing infection is an important priority. Burn wounds may require daily cleansing and dressing changes. Because of the nature of the injury, burn wounds contain a large amount of dead tissue along with fluids and proteins, making them highly susceptible to infection even with the best of care. Antibiotics and strict aseptic technique are essential. The dead tissue of full-thickness burns forms a dry, dark leathery **eschar** (a scab of denatured protein) within forty-eight to seventy-two hours. Infection can often begin under the eschar, causing tissue sloughing. Loose eschar must be **debrided** before skin grafting can occur. Debriding, removing dead tissue within the burn wound, can sometimes be done mechanically by hydrotherapy, either by submersion in a whirlpool bath or by placing the client on a spray table and directly spraying the wound with a hose system that controls both the force and the temperature of the solution (Fritsch & Yurko, 1995). Strict aseptic techniques must be followed during these debridement procedures. Burn wounds often require surgical debridement. The base of the wound must be free of infection and necrotic tissue before it can be covered with skin grafts.

▶ Surgical

Grafts   Skin grafts cover the burn wound to promote healing. Four types of skin grafts might be used:

1. Autograft—the client's own skin that is removed from an unburned area and applied to the wound
2. Homograft—skin obtained from a cadaver within six to twenty-four hours after death
3. Heterograft—skin obtained from an animal, such as a pig
4. Synthetic skin substitute—a man-made product that has properties similar to skin (Fritsch & Yurko, 1995). Homografts, heterografts, and synthetic skin substitutes are temporary grafts that facilitate healing. These grafts prevent water, electrolyte, and protein loss. They decrease pain and allow more freedom of movement for the client. When the client's condition is stable and the wound beds have healthy **granulation tissue** permanent closure of the burn wounds is done with autographs. Granulation tissue is a delicate connective tissue consisting of fibroblasts, collagen, and capillaries. It is red in color and provides a base for healing (Seeley et al., 1995). Autografts are taken from areas of healthy skin. They may be either split-thickness grafts or full-thickness grafts. Split-thickness grafts include the

epidermis and part of the dermis. They are not so deep as to prevent regeneration of skin at the donor site. Follow strict aseptic care of both the donor sites and the newly grafted burn wounds to prevent infection.

The application of pressure dressings during the rehabilitative phase reduces the development of hypertrophic scarring, a condition in which the scar becomes elevated and has a "Swiss cheese" appearance (Beare & Myers, 1994). Pressure dressings, which may be elastic wraps, stockinettes, or custom-made pressure garments, must be worn constantly and are to be removed only for daily hygiene care. Full maturation of the burn scar may take one to two years. As the physical wounds heal, so do the emotional and psychological wounds. The client's ability to cope with daily stresses and resume social and work activities coincides with the physical healing process.

▶ Pain Management

Any movement or manipulation of the client is painful. Burn care procedures, such as dressing changes and wound debridement are painful for clients. Many clients become extremely anxious, fearing pain as well as permanent disfiguration and loss of function. Intravenous narcotics, usually morphine, may be ordered ten to fifteen minutes before painful procedures. By decreasing anxiety and fear, daily doses of psychotropic drugs can enhance the effectiveness of pain medications and help the client cope with the prospect of long-term rehabilitation. Use of specialty beds such as alternating air-filled mattresses or fluidized mattresses minimize pressure on skin surfaces, thus promoting comfort. By limiting movement and maintaining normal body alignment, splints also contribute to the client's comfort.

▶ Pharmacological

Treatment of the burn wound with topical agents can decrease infection and promote healing. Common topical agents used are mafenide acetate (Sulfamylon), silver sulfadiazine (Silvadene), povidone-iodine (Betadine), nitrofurazone (Furacin), and antibiotic agents such as neomycin sulfate (Myciguent), bacitracin (Baciguent), and gentamicin sulfate (Garamycin). Mafenide acetate (Sulfamylon) can penetrate thick eschar and is effective against gram-negative and gram-positive organisms, including *Pseudomonas aeruginosa*. Silver sulfadiazine (Silvadene) is effective against many gram-positive and gram-negative organisms as well as *Candida* organisms. It is painless and somewhat soothing, but

may cause a skin rash. Povidone-iodine (Betadine) has broad-spectrum microbial action against a wide variety of bacteria, fungi, yeasts, viruses, and protozoa. Application of povidone-iodine to large open areas could lead to elevated serum iodine levels. Nitrofurazone (Furacin) has broad-spectrum activity and is effective against *Staphylococcus aureus*. It is not absorbed systemically and has a low incidence of sensitivity. Antibiotic ointments are used to decrease infection. Neomycin (Myciguent) and gentamicin sulfate (Garamycin) can be absorbed systemically and have serious side effects of ototoxicity and nephrotoxicity. Bacitracin (Baciguent) has minimal antimicrobial activity, but it is especially useful to prevent drying of the wound. Apply topical agents in a thin layer with a sterile glove. The wound may be left open to the air or covered with a gauze dressing, depending on the properties of the medication and the physician's orders. Application of these medications can be painful because of manipulation of the burned tissue. Administration of pain medication may be necessary before providing wound care. Assess the surrounding skin for any allergic rashes. Silver nitrate therapy, commonly used in the past, is prescribed less often now. Silver nitrate has bacteriostatic effects, lessens pain, and reduces odor, but the dressings must be kept constantly wet. The procedure for dressing changes is involved and painful. Silver nitrate also stains everything it touches (Fritsch & Yurko, 1995).

▶ Diet

Following a moderate to severe burn, the need for calories and protein increases. Actual protein loss occurs with the burn injury itself. Additionally, some protein is metabolized to meet the increased energy requirements brought on by stress. For tissue repair and healing to occur, daily protein needs may increase by two to four times the normal daily protein requirement (Fritsch & Yurko, 1995). Twice the normal caloric requirement may be needed in order to meet the body's energy needs. Supplemental vitamins and minerals are also given.

Initially the client's daily nutritional needs may be met with total parenteral nutrition (TPN) because of a paralytic ileus and gastric dilation. Following a severe burn, decreased enteric circulation leads to slowed or stopped peristalsis. Food and fluids cannot be given orally or by tube feeding until peristalsis is restored. Hearing active bowel sounds is one indication of peristaltic activity in the bowel. Immobility and stress and the negative nitrogen balance brought on by protein catabolism depress appetite. Meeting the client's nutritional needs can be quite a challenge. Six to eight small feedings daily and high protein milk shakes or protein supplements can help meet daily nutritional needs. Involving the family in bringing in favorite foods can also stimulate the client's appetite.

► Activity

Contractures are among the most serious complications of severe burns. They can be prevented with a program of positioning, splinting, exercising and ambulating. Keep the client's body in correct alignment when repositioning her. Use pillows to keep limbs in alignment. Splints can be used on limbs to prevent contractures or to immobilize joints following skin grafting. Range-of-motion exercises maintain joint mobility. Whenever possible, encourage active rather than passive range-of-motion exercises. Active exercise increases circulation, maintains joint flexibility and improves muscle tone. As the client recovers, increase activities of daily living and begin ambulation.

► Aging Considerations

Normal physiologic changes that occur with aging delay recovery and put the older adult at greater risk for complications following a burn injury. As a person ages, the physiologic reserves of organ systems decrease. While the older person may have adequate pulmonary and cardiac functions at rest, the stress of a severe burn can leave his body unable to cope with demands for increased oxygen and increased cardiac output. Renal changes that occur with aging, such as decreased renal blood flow, fewer nephrons, and a decreased glomerular filtration rate, put the older adult at higher risk for kidney failure following a severe burn. With loss of subcutaneous tissue and decreased secretion of sebum, the older person's skin is normally more fragile. Circulation, especially in the lower extremities, may already be compromised. Healing will be delayed. Skin grafting procedures may not be successful because of impaired circulation and impaired tissue nutrition.

► Nursing Process

Assessment

Subjective Data Assess emotional status. Burn clients are likely to be frightened and anxious. Feelings of guilt, anger, and depression are also common following burns. Observe nonverbal behavior as you assess the client. Be especially alert for incongruities in verbal and nonverbal messages. Assess pain level. Ask the client to describe the pain according to location, intensity, and duration. Ask the client to rate the pain on a scale of 0 to 10. Hypoxia or fluid and electrolyte imbalances can cause confusion, disorientation, and decreased level of consciousness. The client may be nauseated.

Objective Data Assess vital signs and level of consciousness. Listen to breath sounds. If the client has a productive cough, note the amount and color of sputum. Black/gray sputum indicates smoke inhalation. Clients suffering from smoke inhalation may also have crackles, wheezing, or diminished breath sounds. Observe burn wounds for signs of infection such as redness, swelling, purulent drainage, and a foul odor. Measure urine output hourly. Monitor intake and output. Obtain a daily weight. Listen to bowel sounds and assess for vomiting. As rehabilitation progresses, continue to assess wounds for signs of healing such as a moist, clean, red wound base and decrease in the size of the wound. Assess the client's mobility status and degree of involvement in his care. Assess daily dietary intake. Monitor laboratory test results:

- Red blood cell counts and hemoglobin levels give information about the body's ability to meet oxygen demands of body tissues and organs.
- Creatinine and blood urea nitrogen as well as the specific gravity of the urine give information about kidney function.
- Total protein and albumin levels yield information about the ability to maintain the volume of circulating fluid as well as information about nutritional status.
- White blood cell counts indicate the presence of infection and the body's ability to fight it.
- Wound culture and sensitivity data indicate the specific organisms causing infection and the specific antibiotics that are effective against these organisms.
- Electrolytes yield information about the homeostasis of body fluids. Alterations in pH and electrolyte levels affect cell function in every body tissue, particularly vital body organs such as the heart and cerebrum.

▼ ▼

Possible nursing diagnoses for a client who presents with a burn injury may include the following. Initially, the greatest dangers to the client will be:

Nursing Diagnoses	Goals	Nursing Interventions
▶ Gas exchange, impaired, related to edema and inflammation of the respiratory tract.	The client will achieve a regular respiratory pattern and oxygen saturation levels >90%.	Monitor the client's vital signs every four hours if stable; otherwise, every one to two hours.
		Listen to breath sounds, especially note respiratory pattern and effort.
		If the client is on continuous oximetry, note the oxygen saturation reading each time vital signs are assessed.
		Assess the client's color and level of consciousness.
		Document assessments and keep the physician informed about the client's condition.
		Elevate the head of the bed 30° to facilitate full chest expansion with each breath.
▶ Fluid volume deficit related to increased capillary permeability with loss of large amounts of fluid through open burn wounds.	The client will maintain electrolytes within normal limits and an hourly urine output >30 mL per hour.	Administer intravenous fluids at the ordered rate.
		Monitor for signs and symptoms of fluid overload such as shortness of breath, crackles auscultated in lung bases, changes in heart rate and/or heart sounds, changes in blood pressure, increased anxiety, or changes in mental status.
		Measure urine output hourly, report hourly outputs below 30 mL to the physician.
		Record intake and output. Involve the client and family in keeping a bedside record of fluid intake.
		Weigh client daily, preferably before breakfast, and in the same type of clothing each day.
		When the client can tolerate oral fluids, set a fluid intake goal for each shift (e.g.,1200 mL during the day; 800 mL during the evening; 500 mL during the night).
		Explain to the client and family the reasons for a high fluid intake.
		Involve family members in helping the client achieve the goal.
		Keep fluids available at the bedside and within dietary restrictions, the client's favorite fluids.
		Monitor for signs and symptoms of electrolyte imbalances such as increased muscle weakness, muscle cramps, cardiac arrhythmias, fatigue, nausea, dizziness.
		Also monitor the client's laboratory results.

During the stabilization and recovery period following a burn, the nursing diagnosis would include:

Nursing Diagnoses	Goals	Nursing Interventions
▶ Infection, high risk for, related to extensive areas of non-intact skin.	The client's burn wounds will exhibit signs of healing without serious or life-threatening infections.	Wear clean gloves when giving client care. Wash hands before and after gloving with an antibacterial skin cleanser. Wear an isolation gown over your uniform when giving client care. Whenever the client's wounds are exposed, wear gown, cap, mask, and sterile gloves. Use sterile technique for wound care and dressing changes. Monitor wound daily for signs of infection: redness, swelling, purulent drainage, pain. Assess for signs of systemic infections. Observe for increased pulse and respirations, decreased blood pressure, and fever. Observe for any changes in mentation such as disorientation and delirium. Note urinary output. Assess for hypoactive bowel sounds. Monitor the client's white blood cell count. Assist client with personal hygiene, and keep noninjured areas of the body clean.

Other nursing diagnoses common to most burn clients include:

▶ Pain related to damaged tissue and nerve endings.	The client will verbalize that pain is controlled at a tolerable level.	Assess for pain every two to four hours by asking client to rate pain level on a scale of 0 to 10. Observe for nonverbal signs of pain. Administer pain medications as ordered, especially prior to wound care or exercise and mobilization activities. Monitor and document response to medications. Implement comfort and diversional measures: a. Reposition client; use pillows or foam supports to keep all body parts in good alignment. b. Teach client to use progressive relaxation exercises or to use guided imagery. c. Encourage the client to use diversionary activities of his choice such as television or music, or place him so that he can see into the hallway.

(continued)

Nursing Diagnoses	*Goals*	*Nursing Interventions*
▶ *Nutrition, altered, less than body requirements, related to increased caloric requirements and difficulty ingesting sufficient quantities of food.*	The client will ingest sufficient calories daily to meet increased metabolic needs.	If the client is currently on TPN or enteral tube feedings, administer the ordered nutrients at the correct rate and closely monitor the client's reaction.
		When oral intake is tolerated, encourage the client to eat 90 percent to 100 percent of daily diet.
		Provide oral hygiene before meals to stimulate salivation and eliminate any bad taste in the client's mouth.
		Give six to eight small feedings daily of the client's favorite foods within dietary restrictions and encourage family members to bring in home-prepared foods and eat with the client.
		When permitted, encourage the client to sit up in a chair for each meal.
		Plan care so that painful procedures are not done immediately before meals. A rest period of twenty to thirty minutes before meals helps the client feel more like eating.
		Determine the time of day when the client feels most like eating and does indeed eat most of his meal and serve the highest calorie/protein nutrients at that time.
		Serve foods attractively and put an occasional small "surprise" on the tray (e.g., a flower, a small, brightly colored seasonal decoration, a funny card) so that the client will look forward to meals.
▶ *Physical mobility, impaired, related to pain and weakness.*	The client will participate in daily activity to maintain joint mobility and prevent contractures.	Perform passive range of motion exercises (ROM) four times a day by supporting the limb above and below the joint and performing exercises slowly and smoothly.
		As the client is able, instruct him to perform active ROM exercises every three to four hours.
		Use small pillows and foam supports to keep the client's body in good alignment.
		Turn and reposition the client every two hours.
		Use splints as ordered by the physician to keep hands, wrists, feet, and ankles in natural alignment and explain the reason for these activities to the client.
		As healing and rehabilitation progress, encourage progressive ambulation and self-care activities.
		Gradually guide and assist the client to resume activities of daily living (ADL).
		Encourage family members to participate in ADLs and provide positive reinforcement as the client becomes involved in his care.

Nursing Diagnoses	Goals	Nursing Interventions
▶ Body image disturbance related to change in physical appearance with loss of body tissues or body parts.	The client will state realistic expectations for recovery and participate in rehabilitation.	Provide time for the client to express feelings (fear, anger, frustration, regret, and depression are commonly expressed by burn clients) and practice active listening.
		Explain the healing process to the client.
		Give the client daily updates on the degree of wound healing and on his progress in rehabilitation.
		Encourage him to look at her wounds, showing her evidence of healing. Stress that wound healing following serious burn injuries proceeds slowly and that complete healing with improved skin appearance may take a year or more.
▶ Family processes, altered, related to the impact of a family member's severe disfiguring injury.	The client and family members will verbalize feelings to professional nurses and each other and will participate in client care.	Involve family members in the client's care and encourage daily visits.
		Encourage family members to express their fears and concerns, especially any feelings of anger, blame, or guilt.
		Guide family members in recognizing and reflecting to the client small step-by-step progress that she makes.
		Maintain an honest, open approach with the client and his family but do not give false reassurance.
		Collaborate with counselor, social worker, and chaplain to help the client and his family cope with his condition.
		Assist the family to appraise the situation and plan for discharge. What is at stake? What is realistic for the future? What can they expect during the rehabilitation phase? What are their choices? Where can they get help?

▶ Evaluation

Each goal must be evaluated to determine how it has been met by the client.

▲ ▲

▶ NEOPLASMS: MALIGNANT

Skin cancer is one of the most common malignant neoplasms in the United States and is the most preventable cancer. Basal cell carcinoma, squamous cell carcinoma, and malignant melanoma are the three most common skin cancers. Exposure to the sun is the leading cause of skin cancer. Skin damage from sun exposure is cumulative. The ability of skin to tan is not fully developed until the teenage years. Most of the long-term skin damage from sun exposure occurs during childhood (Morton, 1993). By age twenty, most adults have already experienced significant skin dam-age; however, it takes ten to twenty years before unprotected sunbathing leads to skin cancer. Regularly using an effective sunscreen product with each sun exposure will protect skin from the damaging and drying effects of the sun. Fair-skinned persons whose skin produces little melanin are at greatest risk of skin damage due to sunlight. Protective measures such as using sunscreen lotions with a sun protection factor (SPF) of at least 15 and avoiding exposure to the midday sun should start in childhood for all persons—not just those persons with minimal melanin production. As a tan develops, switching to a sunscreen lotion with a lower SPF (8 to 12) will provide adequate protection (Morton, 1993).

▶ *BASAL CELL CARCINOMA*

Basal cell carcinoma, the most frequent type of skin cancer, arises from the epidermis. As the disease develops, it extends into the dermis to form an open ulcer. Surgical removal or radiation therapy cures this type of cancer.

▶ *SQUAMOUS CELL CARCINOMA*

Squamous cell carcinoma appears as a nodular lesion in the epidermis. The sun-exposed lower lip is a common site for squamous cell carcinoma. Without treatment it can extend into the dermis and ultimately metastasize to other body tissues, causing death. The lesion may be excised surgically or it may be treated with chemosurgery, which involves application of a dressing with a fixative paste such as zinc chloride. When the dressing is removed, tumor cells trapped in the dressing are removed also. Dressings are reapplied and removed in this fashion until all malignant tissue has been removed (Weaver, 1995).

▶ *MALIGNANT MELANOMA*

In malignant melanoma atypical melanocytes are present in both the dermis and epidermis. Malignant melanoma, the most serious of the three types of skin cancers, usually begins in a preexisting mole (nevus). These moles have an irregular shape. Contrasted to normal moles, they are larger than 6 mm in diameter and do not have a uniform color. Malignant melanoma can metastasize to every organ in the body through the bloodstream and lymphatic system. The incidence of malignant melanoma is increasing in the United States as a result of increased sun exposure. Deters (1992) succinctly summarizes the incidence of malignant melanoma: "Malignant melanoma is the most dangerous of all skin cancers, causing about 2 percent of all cancer deaths. The incidence is doubling every ten years. Melanoma occurs as a result of transformation of precursor lesions . . . The lighter and fairer the skin, the greater the risk. Risk factors include fair skin, red hair, blue eyes, skin that freckles easily, family or personal history of melanoma or dysplastic nevi, and sun exposure. The peak incidence is between twenty and forty-five years of age . . . At present there is no cure." Clearly the best hope of preventing skin cancer lies in education. Limiting sun exposure and using sunscreen products on exposed skin markedly reduces damage from ultraviolet rays and ultimately decreases the risk of skin cancer.

▶ *MYCOSIS FUNGOIDES*

Mycosis fungoides, also known as cutaneous T-cell lymphoma, is a malignant disease involving T-helper cells that have both skin manifestations and multiple organ system manifestations. In the early stages it resembles psoriasis or seborrheic dermatitis. Later, fissures and skin ulcers develop. Pruritus can be severe. Even if the skin condition can be improved with topical steroids and chemotherapeutic agents, the disease is ultimately fatal because of the involvement of vital organ systems (Nicol, 1993). Clients with AIDS can develop mycosis fungoides. Refer to Chapter 25, Immune Disorders, for additional information about mycosis fungoides.

▶ *Medical/Surgical Management*

▶ *Surgical*

Electrosurgery, cryosurgery, and surgical excision are the primary methods of treatment for malignant neoplasms. Electrosurgery uses electric current to destroy and remove malignant tissue. It is best used for small lesions 1 to 2 cm in diameter. Cryosurgery destroys tumor tissue by freezing it. A special type of needle apparatus directs liquid nitrogen through the tumor until a temperature of -40° to -60°C is reached at the base of the tumor (Deters, 1992). In addition, regional perfusion chemotherapy can be used to treat malignant melanomas of the extremities. The circulation of the involved extremity is isolated and a high dose of a cytotoxic drug is perfused directly into the tumor area (Deters, 1992). This method of treating just the area of the malignancy minimizes systemic effects of cytotoxic drugs. Since most skin cancers are treated by excision, client teaching and follow-up care focus on proper wound care to promote healing and prevent infection.

▶ *Nursing Management*

Careful assessment of the client's skin condition can reveal suspicious skin lesions. Clients who have had one skin cancer are likely to have more. Early referral and prompt care can ensure a good prognosis. Clients who have just had skin cancers removed need to be taught good wound care to prevent infection and facilitate healing. All other nursing care should be focused on prevention. Refer to client teaching chart, Table 23-3.

Table 23-3

CLIENT TEACHING CHART FOR SKIN CANCER

Nursing Diagnosis: Health maintenance, altered, related to persistence in maintaining habits of excessive sun exposure.

Goal: Client will adopt practices that reduce excessive sun exposure. Teach/provide the client with the following information:

1. Sunlight is most intense and damaging around midday. Avoid sun exposure between the hours of 11:00 A.M. and 3:00 P.M.
2. Use a sunscreen lotion with a sun protection factor (SPF) of 15 or greater if your skin is fair and burns easily.
3. If your skin is medium in color and tans fairly easily, a sunscreen lotion with an SPF of 10 to 12 can be used safely.
4. Persons with dark brown or black skin have natural pigment protection and do not need sunscreen lotions unless they will be exposed to prolonged midday sun or will be traveling from a northern temperate climate to the tropics. In these instances a lotion with an SPF of 4 to 6 would provide protection.
5. Apply sunscreen lotion 30 minutes before sun exposure. Reapply after every 60 to 80 minutes of sun exposure. Also re-apply lotion after swimming and towel-drying.
6. Continue to use sunscreen lotions even after achieving a light tan. With a light tan, a lotion with a lower SPF can be selected.
7. Apply moisturizing lotions after sun exposure to minimize the drying effects of sunlight.
8. Protect children from sun exposure. Babies under 6 months should not be exposed to direct sunlight. For older children, use protective clothing and sunscreen lotions with a high SPF that have been developed especially for children.

Nursing diagnosis: Health maintenance altered, high risk for, related to knowledge deficit (early signs and symptoms of skin cancer) related to lack of previous exposure to the information.

Goal: Client will list the early signs and symptoms of skin cancer.

Teach/provide the client with the following information:

1. Examine areas of the skin exposed to sunlight regularly. A good time to examine skin is during or after a bath. Look for:
   - A small, waxy-looking nodule with a pearly border.
   - A slightly raised patch that itches, bleeds, crusts, but does not heal.
   - Thick, rough, shallow lesions that may have a raised border and a granular base. These lesions bleed easily and can ulcerate.
   - Changes in the appearance of a mole, such as the ABCDs of malignant melanoma published by the Skin Cancer Foundation (Hill, 1994):
     A - Asymmetry
     B - Border that is irregular and uneven
     C - Color variegation (brown, black, blue, red, white)
     D - Diameter (>5mm)
2. Seek medical attention for any suspicious lesion that changes in size, color, shape, elevation, surface appearance, sensation, or that causes changes in the surrounding skin.

NEOPLASMS: NONMALIGNANT

Benign tumors of the skin include a variety of lesions such as skin tags, **lipomas, keloids,** sebaceous cysts, nevi (moles), and **angiomas**. In general, they do not require medical or nursing intervention except for cosmetic reasons or unless they are subject to continual irritation that might predispose to a break in skin integrity and infection. Lipomas (fatty tumors) or sebaceous cysts (distended sebaceous glands filled with sebum) might cause pressure on surrounding nerves or interfere with normal body function. In these instances they would be surgically removed. A keloid is abnormal growth of scar tissue that is more common among African Americans. Surgical removal is not always successful; healing following surgery can again result in a keloid. Steroids or radiation have been help-

ful in some conditions. Angiomas, commonly known as birthmarks, are vascular tumors involving skin and subcutaneous tissue. They can be raised, bright red nodular lesions (strawberry birthmarks) or dark red/purple patches (port-wine angiomas). Cosmetics can be used to camouflage them. According to Deters (1992), the argon laser is being used on some angiomas with some success.

PSORIASIS

Psoriasis, a chronic inflammatory noninfectious disease of the skin, affects a fairly large segment of the population, especially young adults. The parts of the body most commonly affected are the scalp, hands, arms, knees, lower back, and genitalia (Weaver, 1995) (see Figure 23-5). The exact cause of psoriasis is unknown, although a genetic component may be involved. Emotional stress, infections, trauma, seasonal and hormonal changes trigger exacerbations of psoriasis. It may improve for a while only to recur. This process of subsiding and recurring continues to occur throughout the client's life. Psoriasis is not curable. In psoriasis the process of keratinization has gone awry. Instead of producing cells that provide a natural barrier against harmful substances and microorganisms, abnormal keratinization causes large, red patches covered with thick silvery scales in the outermost layer of the epidermis (Seeley et al., 1995). If these scales are scraped away, bleeding occurs. When fingernails are affected, expect to see pitting and yellow discoloration. Because of the chronic nature of psoriasis, clients can easily fall prey to charlatans who promise miracle cures.

▶ Medical/Surgical Management

▶ Medical

Treatment is directed toward slowing down the rate of cell formation in the epidermis or toward altering the abnormal process of keratinization. Treatment regimens can be effective in reducing the scaling and itching; however, the client must recognize that psoriasis can only be controlled, not cured. Further, the client must be committed to lifetime therapy.

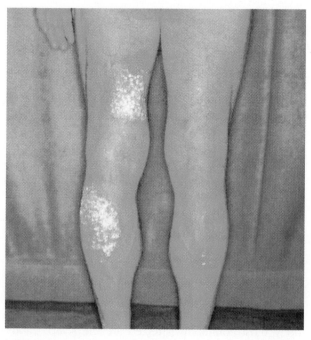

FIGURE 23-5 Psoriasis. (*Photograph courtesy of the Armed Forces Institute of Pathology, negative 74-16637*)

▶ Pharmacological

Keratolytic agents such as salicylic acid preparations and coal tar preparations are applied topically to the lesions. Corticosteroids may also be used to reduce inflammation. Ultraviolet light and methotrexate (Mexate) inhibit DNA synthesis in the epidermal cells, thus slowing down the rate of cell division and the process of abnormal keratinization. Because of its toxicity to the liver, methotrexate is used only in severe cases of psoriasis that do not respond to any other form of treatment. The Goeckerman regimen, which combines the use of coal tar and ultraviolet light, is one of the oldest treatments available, but is effective and is still widely used (Weaver, 1995).

Photochemotherapy is used for severe psoriasis. Photochemotherapy (PUVA) combines the use of methoxsalen (Oxsoralen) with ultraviolet A light waves. The dose of Oxsoralen is based on body weight and must be taken two hours before exposure to ultraviolet A light waves. Oxsoralen is a photosensitizing agent that reacts with ultraviolet A light waves to markedly reduce DNA synthesis, thereby slowing cell division in psoriasis lesions and relieving symptoms. While the treatment is generally effective, the results are not seen immediately. Encourage the client to be patient (Hill, 1994).

Etretinate (Tegison), a compound related to retinoic acid vitamin A, is used in severe psoriasis not amenable to other therapies. It may be used alone or in combination with ultraviolet A light waves. Etretinate has numerous adverse effects, including liver damage and severe birth defects. Monitor the client closely. Women of childbearing age must use effective contraception during treatment and for at least one month after treatment (Karch, 1996).

▶ Nursing Process

Assessment

Subjective Data Psoriasis lesions are generally very visible and likely to make the client feel quite self-conscious as well as very uncomfortable. These clients also tend to suffer self-esteem and body image disturbances, and sometimes depression, because psoriasis requires lifelong treatment. The treatment can be time-consuming, bothersome and from the client's point of view, not completely effective. Encourage the client to verbalize feelings. Assess for itching, burning, or discomfort. Ask the client to describe how he feels. Assess mood.

Objective Data Perform a careful skin assessment, noting the distribution, size, and the appearance of the lesions. Observe for any signs of infection such as redness, swelling, pain, or drainage.

▼ ▼

Possible nursing diagnoses for a client with psoriasis may include:

Nursing Diagnoses	Goals	Nursing Interventions
▶ Therapeutic regimen (individual), ineffective management of, high risk for, related to knowledge deficit of psoriasis and the types of available treatment.	The client will discuss condition and adhere to treatment.	Help the client gain an understanding of psoriasis and comply with the treatment regimen. Support and encourage the client. Explain the purpose of each medication.
▶ Infection, high risk for, related to open lesions.	The client will not get an infection.	Teach the client how to prevent infections.
▶ Body image disturbance related to scaly lesions.	The client will identify positive attributes about self.	Listen actively and encourage the client to express her feelings and frustrations. Reinforce positive behavior. Help the client focus on personal attributes that contribute to effective functioning and a positive self-image.
▶ Self-esteem disturbance or hopelessness related to appearance can occur.	The client will demonstrate behaviors that promote self esteem.	Guide the client in identifying effective coping techniques. Encourage work and social interactions.

▶ Evaluation

Each goal must be evaluated to determine how it has been met by the client.

▲ ▲

▶ INFECTIOUS DISORDERS OF THE SKIN

Given an accessible portal of entry and decreased host resistance, virulent organisms can invade the skin causing inflammation, infection, itching, and pain. Bacteria, viruses, fungi, or parasites can cause infectious disorders of the skin (see Figure 23-6). Treating the client's disease is only one aspect of the treatment plan; preventing the spread of infection is the other. Table 23-4 outlines the disease condition, organism responsible, clinical manifestations of the disease, and the medical management of the disorder.

▶ Nursing Process

Assessment

Subjective Data Ask the client how long he has had the problem, if there is any itching or pain, and what treatment has been used. Assess mood. How is the client reacting to the disease? Clients with infectious disorders of the skin may feel shame or embarrassment because of stigmas attached to some of these conditions.

Objective Data Perform a complete skin assessment. Describe the distribution of the lesions, their size and appearance, and any drainage present. Refer to Figure 23-7.

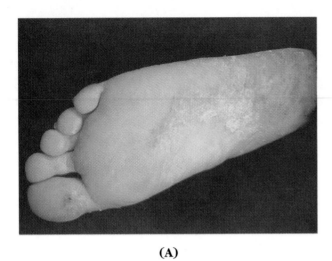
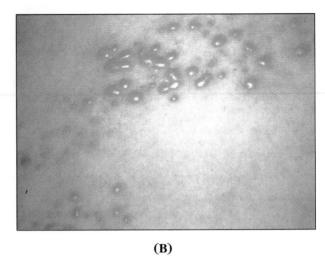

(A)   (B)

FIGURE 23-6 Infectious diseases of the skin. **(A)** Tinea pedis. **(B)** Shingles (herpes zoster). (*Courtesy of the Centers for Disease Control and Prevention, Atlanta, GA*)

Table 23-4

INFECTIOUS DISORDERS OF THE SKIN

Disease	Organism	Clinical Manifestations	Medical Management
Bacterial Infections			
Impetigo contagiosa	*Staphylococcus aureus*	Begins as a small vesicle; becomes a weeping lesion; forms a light brown crust. Usually on the face. More common in children.	Cleanse the affected area at least three times a day. Apply an antibiotic ointment. Occasionally, systemic antibiotics are needed. More common in Spring and Fall. Poor hygiene coupled with warm weather facilitates the spread of the disease.
Carbuncle	*Staphylococcus aureus*	Begins as infected hair follicles in the dermis. Symptoms are redness, swelling, pain. Yellow cores of pus develop. Carbuncles usually occur on the nape of the neck and upper back.	Warm, moist soaks may help "bring the boil to a head." Once the carbuncle ruptures or is incised and drained, pain subsides. Carbuncles tend to recur. The staphylococcus organism may be resistant to topical antibiotics. Systemic antibiotics may be needed. Obese or malnourished person with poor hygiene as well as diabetics are susceptible to carbuncles.
Viral Infections			
Herpes Zoster (shingles) See Figure 23-6B	V-Z (varicella-zoster)	Clusters of small vesicles over the course of a peripheral sensory nerve. Two-thirds of clients have lesions just in the thoracic region. Lesions can occur over the trigeminal nerve, affecting the face, scalp, and eyes. Crusts develop in several days. Symptoms are mild to severe pain, itching, fever, malaise. In older adults, pain can last for months or years.	Acyclovir (Zovirax) is given to clients in severe pain or to immunosuppressed clients. Analgesics help control the pain. Narcotic analgesics are prescribed for severe pain. Antipruritic topical medications decrease the itching. Persons who have not had chickenpox risk contracting the disease if they care for herpes zoster clients with open lesions. Persons susceptible to herpes zoster previously had chickenpox, but only developed partial immunity to it.

Viral Infections (continued)

Herpes Simplex, Type 1 (fever blisters, cold sores)	*Herpes Simplex virus*	Type 1—a cluster of vesicles on an erythematous base occurring most commonly at the corners of the mouth or at the edge of the nostrils. Type 2—lesions in the vagina or cervix of a woman or on the penis of a man. The lesions itch, burn, and frequently break open, forming a crust. Healing occurs in about 10 days.	Topical use of antiviral agents such as acyclovir decreases discomfort. Even with treatment cold sores and fever blisters tend to recur, especially with fever, upper respiratory infections, and stress. Oral administration of acyclovir helps to prevent recurrence of genital herpes.
Warts	Human papillomavirus	Seen as small, painless round papules on hands, face, and neck. On the bottom of the feet, warts grow inward from the pressure and are painful (plantar warts). Warts in the anogenital region itch. Genital warts increase the risk of cervical cancer.	No treatment is indicated for painless warts; they tend to disappear eventually. Plantar warts may be removed by cryosurgery or with locally applied chemicals such as nitric acid. Warts are not highly contagious from person to person, but may be spread on the person's own body by rubbing or scratching. Genital warts are spread by sexual intercourse.

Fungal Infections

Tinea (ringworm) See Figure 23-6A	*microscorim audouini* Tinea capitis (ringworm of the scalp) Tinea corporis (ringworm of the body) Tinea cruris ("jock itch") Tinea pedis (athlete's foot)	Tinea is a superficial infection of the skin, called ringworm because of its circumscribed appearance, typically round, and reddened with slight scaling. Lesions of tinea corporis have a pale center. Itching is common with tinea cruris. Itching and burning occur with tinea pedis.	Tinea is spread easily. "Jock itch" and athlete's foot are more common among men than women. Treat mild infections with a topical antifungal drug such as miconazole nitrate (Micatin) or tolnaftate (Aftate). Severe infections are treated with oral administration of griseofulvin microsize (Grisactin).

Parasitic Infections

Scabies	*Sarcoptes scabiei* (female itch mite)	The itch mite burrows under the skin, lays eggs, and deposits fecal material. Short dark-reddened wavy lines may be seen on hands, wrists, elbows, axillary folds, nipples, waistline, and gluteal folds. Pruritus is severe and can persist for up to three months after treatment. Scratching leads to secondary infection.	Scabies is spread by prolonged contact and is frequently seen in several members of a family. Apply the scabicide, lindane (Kwell), topically to the entire body at bedtime so that the medication remains on the skin 8 to 12 hours. Treat all family members even if they do not have symptoms. Wash all underclothing, bed and bath linens in hot water. Change linens daily.
Pediculosis (lice)	*Pediculus capitis* (head lice) *Pediculus corporis* (body lice) *Phthirus Pubice* (pubiclice)	Eggs, or nits, of pediculosis capitis attach themselves firmly to a hair shaft on the head or in a beard. Nits have a gray, pearly appearance. The pubic louse resembles a tiny crab that attaches itself to pubic hair. Body lice live in the seams of clothing. The bite of the louse causes severe pruritus. Scratching leads to secondary infection.	Lindane is applied topically to the hair as a shampoo or to the body as a cream or lotion. Repeat the treatment again in 8 to 10 days. Wash or dryclean clothing and linens. Disinfect combs and brushes. Vacuum carpets and furniture; then spray with a pediculicide.

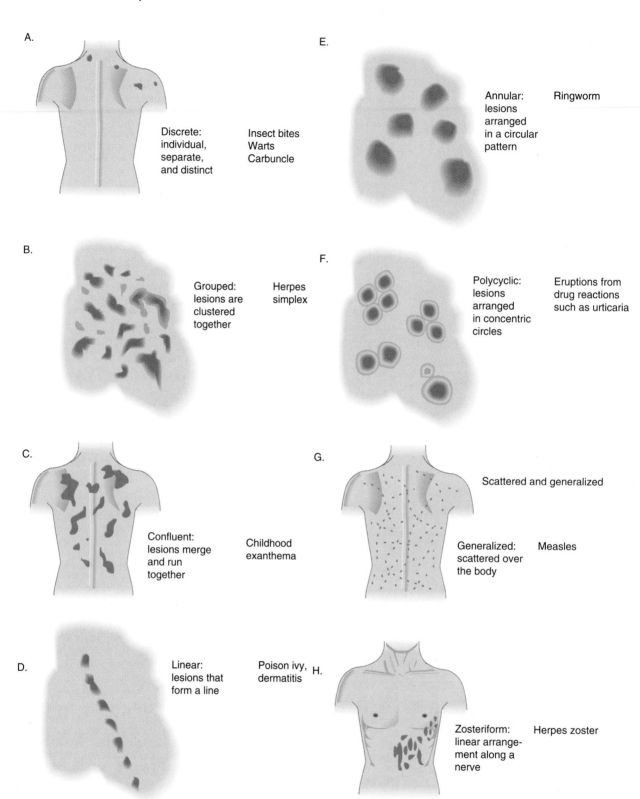

FIGURE 23-7 Types of skin lesions.

▼ ▼

Possible nursing diagnoses for a client with an infectious disorder of the skin may include:

Nursing Diagnoses	Goals	Nursing Interventions
▶ Skin integrity impaired related to invasion of skin structures by pathogenic organisms.	The client will regain skin integrity.	Wear gloves when caring for skin lesions. Cleanse the skin thoroughly, but gently. In the case of bacterial infections or lesions with secondary infections, use an antibacterial soap. Gently remove crusts, scales, and traces of old medication before applying fresh creams or lotions. Administer ordered medications; apply creams and lotions; then monitor their effectiveness. Explain what you are doing and why.
▶ Pain related to itching, burning, and infection.	The client will report less pain.	Instruct the client to keep the environmental temperature cool because warmth increases itching. Cleanse skin lesions with tepid water, not hot. Stress the importance of not scratching the lesions.
▶ Body image disturbance related to unsightly skin lesions, and embarrassment.	The client will verbalize a positive body image.	Encourage the client to ask questions and to talk about feelings. Provide positive reinforcement as the client learns to care for the skin lesions. When possible, suggest ways to camouflage the lesions or minimize their obviousness. When there is no danger of spreading the infection, encourage the client to participate in social and work activities.
▶ Knowledge deficit of effective infection control measures related to lack of familiarity or experience with the infectious skin disease.	The client will describe effective infection control measures.	Since most of these clients are treated in outpatient situations, teach the client the purpose of medications and treatments, the importance of cleanliness, the necessity of carefully and consistently following the treatment protocol, and effective measures to prevent recurrence of the infection in himself as well as measures to prevent the spread of infections to others.

▶ *Evaluation*

Each goal must be evaluated to determine how it has been met by the client.

▲ ▲

Sample Nursing Care Plan: The Client With Scabies

Emma Evans, sixty-eight, has had a skin rash for the past two weeks. The dark red lesions occur mainly on her hands, wrists and elbows, around her nipples, at her waistline, and in her gluteal folds. The itching has become increasingly intense. She has been scratching the lesions, sometimes until they are open and bleeding. Upon examination, some of the lesions are open with small amounts of serosanguineous drainage. Other lesions are scabbed. She lives with her daughter and two teenaged granddaughters. Because the lesions were getting steadily worse, her daughter finally convinced her to seek medical attention. She was horrified when the doctor told her that she had scabies. She had always associated "the itch" with "dirty people who didn't take care of themselves."

Nursing Diagnosis 1 Skin integrity, impaired, related to scratching scabies lesions as evidenced by open lesions draining serosanguineous fluid, scabbed lesions, and client statements of scratching the lesions until they bleed.

Goals	Nursing Interventions	Rationale	Evaluation
Mrs. Evans will follow the prescribed treatment protocol to promote healing of skin lesions and regain skin integrity.	Instruct Mrs. Evans to cleanse lesions carefully using an antibacterial soap and tepid water. Depending upon the condition of the lesions and the severity of the itching, the lesions will need to be cleaned one to three times daily.	Maintaining cleanliness of the skin reduces the number of microorganisms present and decreases the risk of infection. Tepid water does not intensify itching as hot water does.	E. E's lesions are still red, but none are open and draining. Some lesions are still scabbed. No new open lesions have developed. E. E. states that the recommended measures "help," but that the itching is still "pretty bad." Goal of promoting healing of skin lesions is being met. Encourage E. E. to continue outlined protocols. Reassure her that itching will gradually subside as healing progresses.
	Teach Mrs. Evans to apply antipruritic lotions as prescribed by the doctor after cleansing the skin.	Cleansing removes dirt, oils, and microorganisms. Lotion applied to clean skin is more effective. Lotions applied just after bathing help to retain skin moisture. In elderly persons, dry skin causes itching.	
	Instruct Mrs. Evans to keep fingernails short with smooth edges.	Short fingernails with smooth edges are less likely to break the skin if the client does scratch the scabies lesions.	
	Teach Mrs. Evans to press itching lesions, and not to scratch them.	Pressing the skin stimulates nerve endings and can reduce the sensation of itching. Pressing itching skin areas rather than scratching them prevents breaks in the skin which would be portals of entry for microorganisms.	

	Explain that itching can persist up to three months following treatment with the scabicide and that persistent itching does not mean that treatment to kill the itch mite was ineffective.	Skin reaction to the toxins and secretions of the itch mite can persist for up to three months after the itch mites are killed by the scabicide.	
	Keep room temperature between 68° and 72°F and humidity constant at 30 to 35 percent.	Itching is intensified in hot, humid environments. Maintaining room humidity at a constant level decreases drying of the skin and increases comfort.	

Nursing Diagnosis 2 Knowledge deficit (infection control measures) related to lack of familiarity with treatment and prevention protocols as evidenced by client's inability to recognize the skin lesions as infectious and by statements about scabies happening only to people with poor hygiene.

Goals	Nursing Interventions	Rationale	Evaluation
Mrs. Evans will apply the scabicide correctly and state ways to avoid spreading infection to others.	Assess Mrs. Evans' knowledge of scabies, its treatment regimen and infection control measures. Ask specific questions.	Building on knowledge that Mrs. Evans already has provides a frame of reference for the client, which helps her relate new information and integrate it into her behavior.	Mrs. Evans and her family did apply the scabicide as prescribed. The client can describe how scabies are transmitted, but continues to express fear that she will give "this awful thing to somebody." Goal of correctly applying scabicide met. Although Mrs. Evans can state how scabies are transmitted, she still has doubts; hence, the goal of stating ways to avoid spreading the infection to others has only been partially met. Reinforce that even though red skin lesions are still visible, the itch mites were killed by treatment and cannot be transmitted to others even if the client does shake hands, hug, or touch someone else.
	Begin giving information and demonstrating skills the client does not have.	Recognizing that scabies is not a "dirty" disease will help the client feel better about herself.	
	Explain that scabies is transmitted by skin-to-skin contact or by contact with articles freshly contaminated by infected persons and in the United States, infection with scabies affects persons of all social, economic, and age levels.	Teaching that does not "talk down" to the client communicates respect.	
	Stress the importance of following treatment protocol exactly. Review salient points such as: (a) Shower before applying the scabicide; (b) Apply the	Failure to apply the scabicide as directed and/or failure to leave the lotion on the skin for the prescribed length of time will not kill the itch mite.	

(continued)

scabicide to the entire body surface, including skin without scabies lesions; and (c) Apply the scabicide at bedtime so that the medication remains on the skin eight to twelve hours.

Give Mrs. Evans step-by-step written instructions.

Giving the client written step-by-step instructions enhances compliance with the treatment regimen.

Instruct Mrs. Evans to wash hands under warm running water with plenty of soap (preferably an anti-bacterial soap) for at least ten seconds after touching lesions and clean carefully under fingernails while washing hands.

Thorough handwashing is the single most effective means of preventing the spread of infection. Large numbers of bacteria reside under the fingernails.

Advise to not share washcloths, towels, clothing, pillows, or bed linens with other family members.

Disease-causing microorganisms can be spread to well individuals indirectly when their skin comes into contact with contaminated items.

Instruct to wash underclothing, bed and bath linens in detergent and hot water and dry outside in sunlight or in a dryer at the hot setting.

Soap reduces surface tension. When fat or protein substances which shield organisms are broken down, the organisms are exposed to the killing effects of heat. Prolonged exposure to heat or ultraviolet rays from direct sunlight kill microorganisms.

Advise to shower daily, use an antibacterial soap, rinse thoroughly and dry carefully, especially in skin folds and between toes, using a towel and washcloth only once before laundering it.

Regular cleansing reduces the number of microorganisms on the skin. Antibacterial soap further decreases the number of microorgan-isms on the skin. Moisture in skin folds and between toes encourages the growth of microorganisms. Laundering the towel and washcloth after only one use prevents the indirect transfer of the itch mite.

Assess lesions daily for signs of healing. Report any signs and symptoms of infection in secondary lesions such as redness, swelling, pain, drainage (describe characteristics of the drainage) to the physician or clinic.

Early recognition of signs of infection increases the probability of effective treatment with fewer complications.

Teach Mrs. Evans and family members the early signs and symptoms of scabies infection, such as any reddened papules with wavy, threadlike lines visible on the skin around the papules and severe itching, especially at night. Instruct them to assess their skin daily.

Early recognition and treatment of scabies can minimize the severity of the infection.

Nursing Diagnosis 3 Body image disturbance related to unsightly lesions and embarrassment as evidenced by distribution of lesions on exposed skin areas and client statements of being horrified about the diagnosis and associating scabies with "dirty people."

Goals	Nursing Interventions	Rationale	Evaluation
Mrs. Evans will assume self-care of lesions and maintain relationships with family and friends.	Encourage Mrs. Evans to express her feelings about herself and her opinions about scabies.	Allowing the client to express feelings and opinions brings them out into the open where they can be dealt with appropriately.	The client has assumed self-care responsibilities. She does interact with her family, but emphasizes that she "doesn't want to get too close to them until these things are completely gone." She has refused to go to church, social gatherings, or activities outside of the house.
	Provide information to correct any misconceptions she might have.	If the client has any misconceptions, accurate information can dispel them and lead to an improved self-image.	

(continued)

Encourage Mrs. Evans to verbalize the perceptions she has about her family's and friends' feelings about persons with scabies.

Be alert to verbal and nonverbal messages.

Reassure her that she will not infect friends and family members by going places with them, sitting beside them or being in the same room with them for prolonged periods.

Share with Mrs. Evans that wearing long-sleeved cotton blouses or dresses will hide most of the visible lesions.

Explain that by using the scabicide, lindane (Kwell), as directed and by following measures to prevent secondary infection of the scabies lesions, she can expect complete healing of the lesions without any visible scars within a few weeks.

If the client perceives that her friends have derogatory opinions of her, she is likely to socially isolate herself from them.

Nonverbal behavior gives insight into the client's real feelings. Identifying and discussing feelings can lead to behavioral changes.

The client will be unlikely to avoid friends or make disparaging remarks about herself when she realizes that she is not a danger to them.

Covering unsightly skin lesions makes the client less self-conscious and embarrassed. Cotton fabric allows good air circulation. When the skin feels cooler, itching is less intense.

Reassurance that scabies can be cured enhances the client's self-image.

Goal has been partially met in that the client does follow proper procedures when caring for her skin lesions, but has not been met in so far as maintaining relationships is concerned. Encourage the client to talk about her feelings, particularly feelings of embarrassment. Point out to her the evidence that her lesions are healing. Emphasize that symptoms of intense itching, worsening of present skin lesions, and signs of more skin lesions would be present if the itch mites were alive and still spreading. Encourage her to go on at least one outing with her family during the coming week. Reevaluate in one week.

▶ *DERMATITIS*

By definition, dermatitis is an inflammatory condition of the skin. In current usage, eczema has become synonymous with dermatitis, although eczema tends to be used most often to refer to chronic forms of dermatitis. Eczema (or dermatitis) can be caused by allergy, infection, poor circulation, or exposure to chemicals, heat, cold, or sunlight (Seeley et al., 1995).

▶ *Contact Dermatitis*

In contact dermatitis the skin reacts to external irritants such as: (1) allergens like poison ivy or cosmetics; (2) harsh chemical substances like detergents or insecticides; (3) metals such as nickel; (4) mechanical irritation from wool or glass fibers; (5) body substances like urine or feces. Symptoms include pruritus, burning, and erythema. Often a maculopapular rash or a combination of papules and vesicles develop. Scratching the lesions may spread the dermatitis as well as lead to secondary infections of the skin.

▶ Exfoliative Dermatitis

In most cases, the cause of exfoliative dermatitis is unknown. Severe reactions to drugs such as penicillin may sometimes cause exfoliative dermatitis. It may also be associated with other types of dermatitis or lymphoma.

In exfoliative dermatitis inflammation of the skin gradually worsens. Localized symptoms include erythema, severe pruritus, extensive scaling, and loss of skin surface. Exfoliative dermatitis affects the entire body, not just the skin. Systemic symptoms include chills, fever, and malaise. With the loss of large areas of skin surface, the individual has difficulty maintaining body temperature, loses body fluids and electrolytes, and is susceptible to infection. Exfoliative dermatitis can be fatal, primarily because of overwhelming systemic infections and/or massive loss of body fluids and electrolytes. Elderly clients have a greater risk of fatal complications. As body systems age, they are less able to respond quickly and effectively to the stress of illness.

▶ Medical/Surgical Management

▶ Medical

Clients with contact dermatitis can be treated as outpatients. Patch testing may identify a specific allergen that is causing the dermatitis. Taking precautions to avoid the allergenic substance may prevent future cases of contact dermatitis. In some cases of contact dermatitis, application of topical corticosteroids may be all that is needed. When weeping lesions are present, treatment with Burow's solution (1:40 dilution of aluminum acetate) for twenty minutes four times a day relieves symptoms and promotes healing (Weaver, 1995).

When clients are hospitalized with exfoliative dermatitis, medical management is directed toward maintaining fluid balance, preventing infection, decreasing inflammation, and promoting comfort. The client requires intravenous fluids to maintain the volume of circulating fluid, corticosteroids to decrease inflammation, and antibiotics to treat infection. Medicated baths, topical steroids, and mild analgesics may be prescribed to ease the pruritus.

▶ Nursing Management

Similar to other skin disorders, nursing management is directed toward promoting healing, providing com-

fort, preventing infection, and fostering a positive attitude to help the client cope with an altered body image. Nursing diagnoses may include skin integrity, impaired; infection, high risk for; pain; and body image disturbance. These clients will need to know how to care for the lesions, how to prevent infection, how to cope with conditions that alter their physical appearance and psychological well-being, and how to keep their physical discomfort at a tolerable level. Client teaching focuses on identifying and avoiding substances that cause dermatitis. With thinning and drying of the skin secondary to aging, elderly clients are more susceptible to irritants that cause dermatitis. Restoring skin integrity in elderly clients takes longer and requires persistent nursing effort.

▶ PEMPHIGUS VULGARIS

Considered an autoimmune disease, pemphigus occurs worldwide. A rare skin disease, it occurs primarily in persons between the ages of forty and sixty and has a higher incidence among Jewish persons (Weaver, 1995). Characteristics of the disease include large bullae (blisters—1 to 10 cm in diameter) on skin and mucous membranes of the mouth, esophagus, vagina, and rectum (see Figure 23-8).

Oozing and crusting occur after the bullae rupture. These lesions are painful, bleed easily, and heal slowly. The crusts can easily become infected causing a distinctive, foul odor. Untreated, pemphigus is usually fatal. There is no cure.

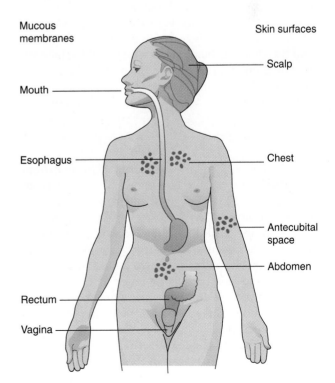

FIGURE 23-8 Sites of pemphigus vulgaris.

▶ *Medical/Surgical Management*

▶ *Pharmacological*

Topical steroids provide some relief, but because of the autoimmune nature of the disease, large systemic doses of corticosteroids are needed to control symptoms. Immunosuppressants such as methotrexate (Mexate) or cyclophosphamide (Cytoxan) given along with corticosteroids are helpful in keeping the corticosteroid dose low enough to avoid serious complications of long-term steroid therapy (Deters, 1992).

▶ Nursing Management

Assess the client's skin, nutritional, and emotional status. With alteration in skin integrity, these clients are at high risk for infection, pain, and body image disturbance. The painful mouth lesions can be a contributory cause of nutritional deficit and fluid volume deficit. Because of pain and altered physical appearance, these clients are at high risk for social isolation. Altered oral mucous membranes is also a common nursing diagnosis. Good mouth care every two to four hours with a non-irritating solution such as normal saline or mild baking soda solution is essential. Air mattresses or high-float (5 to 6 inches) foam mattresses can decrease pressure on skin surfaces, thus promoting comfort. Encourage 2000 to 2500 cc of bland fluids daily. Soft, bland foods help decrease oral discomfort at mealtime. Six smaller feedings a day rather than three large meals can improve overall nutritional intake as well as decrease oral discomfort. Spend time with the client encouraging expression of feelings and providing emotional support. Encourage the involvement of family and friends to decrease the client's fears of rejection because of his physical appearance.

▶ STASIS ULCERS

Poor venous circulation, especially in lower extremities, can lead to a condition known as stasis dermatitis (see Figure 23-9). The skin changes in texture, turgor, and color. The skin develops a brownish discoloration and a brawny induration; i.e., skin in the affected area becomes dry and looks rough; subcutaneous tissue atrophies; and the texture loses its usual resiliency and feels hard to the touch. Body hair is lost in this area of the skin. Pruritus is common. Scratching or small injuries can lead to ulcer formation because of the poor circulation.

Venous stasis ulcers begin as small, tender, inflamed areas above the ankle. Any slight trauma to the area causes an open area that develops into an ulcer. Some edema surrounds the ulcer, which can easily become

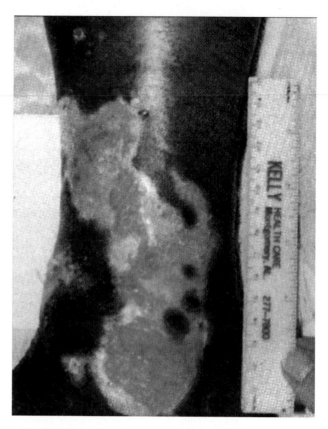

FIGURE 23-9 Venous stasis ulcer. (*Photo courtesy of Carrington Laboratories, Inc., Irving, TX*)

infected, most often with staphylococcus or streptococcus. Healing is very slow. In an effort to decrease venous congestion and improve circulation, varicose veins may be removed. Ulcers that do not heal may require surgery. If diagnostic testing reveals adequate circulation, skin grafting will result in the healing of large venous stasis ulcers. In severe cases that do not respond to treatment, the affected leg has to be amputated.

▶ *Medical/Surgical Management*

▶ *Pharmacological*

For healing to occur, the ulcer must have adequate circulation and be free of infection and necrotic tissue. Usually antibiotics are prescribed. Enzyme preparations such as fibrinolysin and dexsoxyribonucleas (ELASE) or wet-to-dry dressings may be used to debride the ulcer. Normal saline is the solution most often used in wet-to-dry dressings because it is not irritating to healthy tissue. For small ulcers, especially in ambulatory clients, an Unna's boot may be ordered. The "boot" is a special type of gauze impregnated with gelatin, glycerin, and zinc oxide paste that is applied in a spiral fashion around the leg. It hardens around the client's leg providing even, constant support during ambulation. Unna's boot can achieve a 70 percent healing rate (Dennison & Black, 1993).

▶ Diet

A diet high in protein and vitamin C is needed for tissue regeneration. If the client is anemic, include lean meats, whole grains, and green, leafy vegetables.

▶ Nursing Process

Assessment

Subjective Data Assess for pain. Ask the client to describe the pain and rate its severity on a scale of 1 to 10. Is the pain worse with the leg in a dependent posi-tion, or when the client is standing? What helps relieve the pain? Does the skin around the ulcer itch? How long has the client had the ulcer? What, if anything, did the client try to do to treat the ulcer before seeking medical attention?

Objective Data Describe the size and location of the ulcer. Assess the appearance of the ulcer and sur-rounding skin. Observe for necrotic tissue inside the ulcer. It may be yellow and look like thin strands of fibers. The base of the ulcer may have a dark red, "beefy" appearance. Assess the color and appearance of the extremity in both a dependent position and an elevated position. Note any drainage, describing its odor and characteristics. Assess for edema. The lower extremity will look "swollen." Indurated tissue sur-rounds the ulcer. Tissue farther away from the ulcer may "pit" with firm pressure. Assess peripheral pulses.

▼ ▼

Possible nursing diagnoses for a client with a stasis ulcer may include:

▶ *Tissue perfusion, altered, peripheral related to edema and pooling of venous blood.*	Client will follow prescribed measures to improve peripheral circulation.	Encourage client to elevate legs while sitting or when in bed.
		Advise the client to avoid standing for more than a few minutes at a time.
		Advise client to wear elastic stockings when walking and that new stockings should be purchased every few months as continual wear and laundering tend to decrease the elasticity of the stockings. Instruct not to wear garters, tight girdles, or sit with legs crossed.
▶ *Pain, chronic, related to exposed sensory nerve endings and edema.*	Client will report decreased pain after implementing recommended measures.	Encourage client to elevate legs.
		Cleanse ulcer with prescribed solutions.
		Keep ulcer covered with prescribed medications and dressings.
▶ *Infection, high risk for, related to poorly nourished tissue in and around the ulcer and to nonintact skin.*	Client will describe and implement measures to minimize the risk of infection.	Assess the ulcer daily for signs of healing.
		Assess the client's ability to care for the ulcer physically and financially.
		Review diet with the client and instruct as indicated.
		Note the client's hemoglobin level since anemic clients will have difficulty meeting tissue demands for oxygen.
		Encourage foods high in iron such as fortified cereal, lean meats, whole grains, and leafy green vegetables.
		Provide time for the client to talk about his feelings.
		Encourage the client to follow the prescribed regimen faithfully; improvement comes in small increments.

▶ *Evaluation*

Each goal must be evaluated to determine how it has been met by the client.

▲ ▲

▶ *ALOPECIA*

Alopecia, which is baldness or loss of hair, can be caused by illness, malnutrition, effects of certain drugs such as those used in cancer therapy, hormonal imbalances, or diseases that affect the scalp. In men, male-patterned baldness is caused by heredity, excessive levels of male hormones, and aging. If the cause of alopecia is illness or the side effects of drug therapy, alopecia can be reversed. In male-patterned baldness, the loss of hair is permanent. Hundreds of over-the-counter products claim to promote hair growth, but are seldom if ever effective. In some men minoxidil (Rogaine) can promote hair growth, but it must be applied twice daily. Hair growth stops once the drug is stopped. Therapy with minoxidil (Rogaine) can be very expensive. Men who can afford the surgical procedures (often four or more) resort to hair transplant operations. At present, these surgical procedures represent the only "cure" for baldness. As with any surgical procedure, infection is a risk. Teach the client daily wound care using aseptic techniques.

▶ CASE STUDY

Maude Murphy, age sixty-eight, noticed that the skin on the outside of her left lower leg just above the ankle was changing in color and texture. The skin felt rigid and did not move as easily as skin on the upper part of her leg did. Itching was becoming a problem. Inadvertently she would scratch the area, sometimes causing small excoriations. One day she bumped her leg against the rough edge of the outside steps as she was going into the house. The cut was only an inch long and was not very deep. Over the next few weeks she noticed that instead of healing, it was getting bigger and was becoming quite painful. The skin around the wound was red and swollen. The yellow drainage coming from the wound had a bad smell. She had never had this kind of problem before. She did have varicose

The following questions will guide your development of a Nursing Care Plan for the case study.

1. List the clinical manifestations of a venous stasis ulcer.
2. What is the usual medical treatment?
3. List the subjective and objective assessment data that the nurse should obtain from Maude Murphy.
4. Write two to four individualized nursing diagnoses to address these problems.
5. What will be the goals (expected outcomes) of nursing treatment?
6. List appropriate nursing actions for each diagnosis. Include basic nursing care measures. Be specific about client education needs. Address nutrition and pharmacologic implications. Give a rationale for each action.
7. Describe how to evaluate goal achievement for Maude Murphy.

▶ **CASE STUDY (continued)**

veins in that leg, and while she knew that she was uncomfortable if she was standing for long periods, she did not think the problem was serious. When she went to the doctor, he diagnosed a venous stasis ulcer and cultured the drainage. He ordered the following treatment:

1. *Cefaclor (Ceclor) 500 mg p.o. every 8 hours for two weeks. (Culture of the wound identified Staphylococcus aureus).*
2. *Wet-to-dry dressings with normal saline solution. Change every eight hours.*
3. *Bed rest with left leg elevated. May have bathroom privileges and be up for meals.*

The doctor explained that he would be ordering an Unna's boot after the wound was debrided and the infection controlled so that she could be ambulatory, but that even after the Unna's boot was applied, he would want her to have rest periods during the day with her leg elevated. Mrs. Murphy thought she could learn to change the dressings, but she expressed doubt that she could stay in bed most of the time. She was used to being up and active and getting her work done each day.

SUMMARY

- Maintaining intact skin and mucous membranes to protect internal body structures from harmful substances and from invasion by microorganisms is an important independent nursing responsibility.
- Burns are devastating, traumatic injuries that can be prevented.
- In general skin cancers are easily treated, but more importantly, they can be prevented by avoiding excessive sun exposure.
- Treatment of benign skin tumors such as nevi, lipomas, keloids, sebaceous cysts, and angiomas depends on the kind of tumor and its location.
- Psoriasis is a chronic skin condition that can be treated, but not cured.
- Skin infections caused by bacteria, viruses, fungi, or parasites can be effectively treated with medications and supportive nursing care.
- Dermatitis, an inflammation of the skin, can be a contact dermatitis or an exfoliative dermatitis.
- Eczema is a term that is often used for chronic forms of dermatitis.
- Pemphigus is a painful autoimmune disorder that can be treated, but not cured.
- Venous stasis ulcers are more common in older persons, heal slowly, and often recur following a slight injury.
- Alopecia, or baldness, can be caused by illness, drugs, hormonal imbalances, or heredity.

Review Questions

1. The skin has a vital role in the normal functioning of the human organism. That role is:
   a. production of antibodies.
   b. protection from invasion by microorganisms.
   c. support for internal organs.
   d. regulation of cellular oxygenation.

2. The nurse charted that the client's skin was loose, wrinkled, and thin with mild scaling. The nurse was describing:
   a. integrity.
   b. texture.
   c. turgor and mobility.
   d. vascularity.

3. An effective nursing intervention related to the care of open burn wounds that require daily dressing changes would be:
   a. keep the head of the bed elevated 30° with all four side rails up.
   b. set a fluid intake goal of 2500 mL/24 hours (1200 mL during the day; 950 mL during the evening; 350 mL during the night).
   c. wear a cap, gown, mask, and sterile gloves when providing wound care.
   d. weigh daily, preferably before breakfast, and in the same type of clothing each day.

4. The client has lesions on his scalp and on his arms near his elbows. The lesions appear as red patches covered with thick silvery scales. The most likely cause of these lesions is:
   a. herpes zoster (shingles).
   b. pemphigus vulgaris.
   c. psoriasis.
   d. tinea (ringworm).

5. A nursing care plan for a client with an infectious disorder of the skin would include interventions to teach the client:
   a. how to avoid spreading the infection to others.
   b. how to do range of motion exercises to maintain joint flexibility.
   c. ways to conserve energy.
   d. which foods are most likely to cause allergic reactions.

6. Which of the following is a malignant tumor?
   a. angioma
   b. lipoma
   c. melanoma
   d. sebaceous cyst

7. Clients with pemphigus vulgaris often have a nutritional deficit. Which of the following nursing interventions can help improve the client's nutritional intake?
   a. Add spices to foods to improve their taste and aroma.
   b. Drink citrus juices and hot beverages after eating rather than with the meal.
   c. Give mouth care with normal saline or a mild baking soda solution before meals.
   d. Vary the texture of foods from soft and moist to dry and crunchy.

News Flash

Good Skin Hydration: An Infection Control Measure

Microorganisms were the first life forms to inhabit the planet Earth. They still thrive—some at the expense of human beings with whom they share the Earth. Given ideal conditions, microorganisms can multiply at an alarming rate; for example, under ideal laboratory conditions, one pseudomonas bacterium will double every twenty minutes, reproducing to over 1,000,000,000 bacteria in just ten hours (Kovach, 1995). Warm, moist skin folds provide similar ideal conditions for growth of pathogenic organisms. How, then, can we humans best protect ourselves?

Maintaining intact, supple, moist skin is our first line of defense. Dry skin leads to inflammation and excoriation, leaving the person, especially an elderly, or ill, debilitated person, vulnerable to bacterial invasion. When the moisture content of the stratum corneum drops below 10 percent, the epidermis layer of the skin becomes opaque and pale with flaking scales (Kovach, 1995). Without preventive skin care measures such as using nonirritating skin cleansers, patting skin dry, and applying emollients and creams after bathing and at bedtime to maintain moisture above the 10 percent level, small cracks and fissures develop in the skin. Pruritus that accompanies dry skin leads to scratching and subsequent excoriation, giving harmful organisms a portal of entry into the body. Nursing measures that maintain skin hydration thus become infection control measures. (Kovach, 1995)

Medical Terminology

angio-	pertaining to a blood vessel
angioma	a benign tumor with blood vessels
-oma	tumor
lipoma	a benign tumor consisting of mature fat cells
derm-, dermato-	pertaining to skin
dermatitis	inflammation of the skin
nephro-	of or related to the kidneys
nephrotoxic	toxic or destructive to the kidneys
oto-	pertaining to the ear
ototoxic	having a harmful effect on cranial nerve VIII or organs of hearing and balance

Critical Thinking Questions

1. How might a person's self image be affected when the person has a skin disorder on the face or hands?

2. Prepare a teaching plan related to preventing the spread of skin infections.

C H A P T E R

24

Allergies, Immune, and Autoimmune Disorders

Diane R. Behrens

▶ KEY TERMS

allergens
allergic response
anaphylaxis
angioedema
antibodies
antigens
antinuclear antibodies (ANAs)
autoimmune disorder
autologous
cellular immunity
diplopia
exacerbation
histamine
homologous
human leukocyte antigens (HLA)
humoral immunity
hypersensitivity
immune response
immunity
immunotherapy
ptosis
remission
urticaria

LIST OF DISORDERS

▶ Allergies
▶ Anaphylaxis
▶ Blood Transfusions
▶ Organ Transplants
▶ Rheumatoid Arthritis (RA)
▶ Systemic Lupus Erythematosus (SLE)
▶ Myasthenia Gravis (MG)
▶ HIV/AIDS (Acquired Immunodeficiency Syndrome)

LEARNING OBJECTIVES

Upon completion of this chapter the learner should be able to:
- Define key terms.
- Identify three allergic reactions with a systemic response.
- Describe symptoms of anaphylaxis and appropriate first aid.
- Recall common diagnostic tests used to evaluate immunological functioning.
- Discuss the medical/surgical management of clients with immunological disorders.
- Relate signs and symptoms of complications clients with immunological disorders could experience.
- Relate assessment criteria for clients with immunological disorders.
- Identify nursing diagnoses for clients with immunological disorders.
- Describe nursing care for clients with immunological disorders.
- Identify evaluative criteria to determine the effectiveness of nursing care for clients with immunological disorders.

▶ *MAKING THE CONNECTION*

Refer to the topics in the following chapters to increase your understanding of allergies, immune, and autoimmune disorders.

INTRODUCTION

Immunity is the body's ability to protect itself from foreign agents or organisms. This occurs through the complex interaction of the tissues within the immune system. Constant surveillance of cells within the body occurs to differentiate self from nonself. Those identified as nonself are then neutralized or destroyed. Dead or damaged cells are eliminated and homeostasis is maintained. When alterations in the system develop, immunological conditions develop. They may be hypersensitivity responses such as allergies, immunological deficiencies, such as those associated with corticosteroid medications, or **autoimmune disorders**, where the body identifies its own cells as foreign and activates mechanisms to destroy them. Rheumatoid arthritis, systemic lupus erythematosus, and myasthenia gravis are examples of autoimmune disorders.

ANATOMY AND PHYSIOLOGY REVIEW

The human body has a variety of natural physical and chemical mechanisms that enhance immunological functioning. The skin, eyelashes, cilia in the nose and respiratory system, gastric acidity, intestinal mucosa and pH of vaginal mucosa all act to protect against invading organisms. In addition, all body tissues are linked together via lymphatic ducts and blood vessels to the cells and organs of the immune system.

Cells of the Immune System

Leukocytes, white blood cells (WBCs), are vital components of the immune system. Those cells with granules in the cytoplasm are granulocytes, while those lacking them are called agranulocytes (see Figure 24-1). Eosinophils, neutrophils, and basophils are granular leukocytes. Monocytes and lymphocytes are agranular leukocytes. Each has its own unique function. Monocytes travel to the sites of invading organisms and transform into macrophages, capable of ingesting large quantities of microorganisms and damaged cells, a process known as phagocytosis. They also secrete Interleuken-1 which stimulates the activation of specific lymphocytes. Granulocytes, also called polymorphonuclear leukocytes, make up the greatest number of WBCs. Eosinophils come into play during allergic reactions or parasitic invasions. Neutrophils have great phagocytic abilities. Basophils secrete **histamine**, a substance released during allergic reactions, and heparin.

B-lymphocytes, or B-cells, and T-lymphocytes, or T-cells play a vital role in the immune response. B-cells are responsible for **humoral immunity** (see Table 24-1). They stimulate plasma cells to secrete **antibodies** (proteins that react with antigens to neutralize or destroy them) in response to **antigens** (any substance identified by the body as nonself). Antibodies are also called immunoglobulins. IgA, IgD, IgE, IgG, and IgM are common antibodies found in plasma. When an antibody-antigen reaction occurs, the complement system, a complex sequential immunological process, is activated. This system is composed of plasma proteins made in the liver. They alter cell membranes in the antibody-antigen reaction, facilitating the cellular breakdown of the invading antigen, and attract macrophages and granulocytes to the antibody-antigen reaction site. When a B-cell identifies an antigen, it places the characteristics of that antigen in a memory bank. B-cells also produce "memory cells" capable of identifying the antigen, if and when it is introduced to the body again.

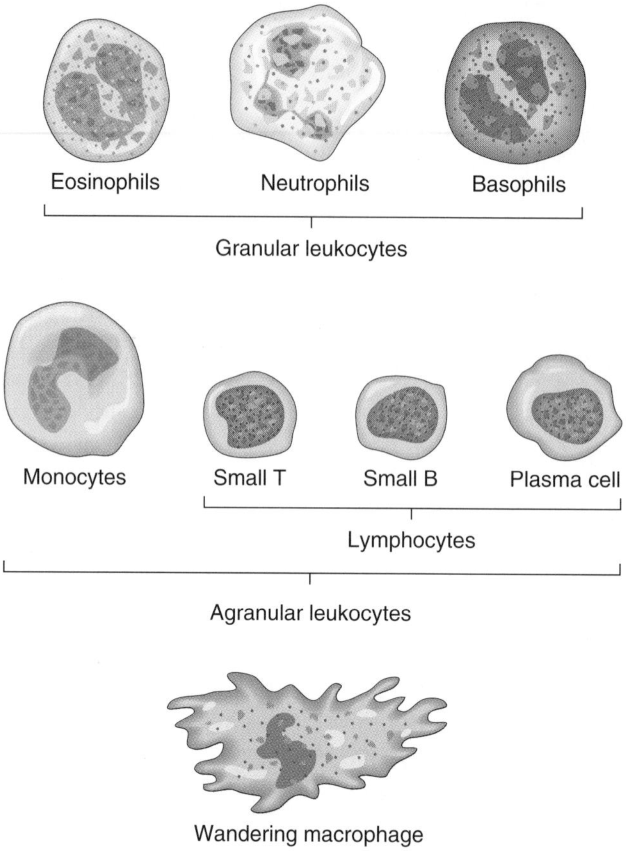

FIGURE 24-1 Cells of the immune system.

T-cells are responsible for **cellular** or cell-mediated **immunity** (see Table 24-1). A number of different T-cells are produced in response to an alien organism. T-helper cells promote B-cell production, while T-suppressor cells decrease or eliminate B-cell production. Killer T-cells attack malignant or viral cells. Cytolytic T-cells destroy antigens. Memory T-cells respond immediately to a repeat invasion of an organism. The combined effort and interaction of these cells promote effective immunological functioning within the body.

Organs of the Immune System

The organs of the immune system are classified as primary or peripheral lymphoid organs. Primary lymphoid organs are bone marrow and the thymus gland. Within bone marrow, stem cells, the parent cells for all blood cells, are produced. The white blood cells mature into either granulocytes, monocytes, or B-lymphocytes. The thymus gland, located in the mediastinal cavity anterior to and above the heart, is responsible for the maturation and differentiation of T-lymphocytes. Peripheral lymphoid organs are lymph nodes, spleen, tonsils, appendix, Peyer's patches of

Table 24-1

HUMORAL AND CELLULAR RESPONSES

Humoral Response (Antibody Response)	Cellular Response (T-cell Response)
• B-lymphocytes become plasma cells, which manufacture antibodies in response to an antigen and release them into the bloodstream.	• Plasma cells are transformed into special T-lymphocyte cells, which detect, attack, and destroy invading antigens.
• Predominant role in response to:	• Predominant role in immune response to:
Bacteria and some viral infections	Viral and some bacteria infections
Allergic reactions	Delayed hypersensitivity (TB testing)
Autoimmune diseases	Transplant rejection
	Graft-versus-host disease
	Fungal and parasitic infections
	Detection and destruction of tumor cells

the small intestines and the liver. Lymph nodes, located throughout the body, connected by an elaborate ductal system, filter lymphatic fluid removing destroyed matter. Enlargement of lymphoid organs indicates an infectious or malignant process is occurring. The spleen serves as a reservoir for macrophages, lymphocytes, and plasma cells. The tonsils, appendix, and Peyer's patches also contain plasma cells and lymphocytes. The Kupffer cells of the liver house monocytes which ingest and destroy foreign organisms in hepatic circulation. See Figure 22-4 on p. 522.

Types of Immunity

There are two types of immunity: natural (innate) and acquired (adaptive) (see Table 24-2). One is born with natural immunity. It is species specific. For example, humans have an innate resistance to distemper while dogs never develop measles or syphilis. Acquired immunity develops after birth and may be active or passive. Acquired active immunity is the result of exposure to the disease itself or its vaccine. As a result, the body develops antibodies and memory cells for the causative microorganism. A repeated exposure results in rapid activation of these components of the immune system and annihilation of the invading agent. Acquired passive immunity utilizes

antibodies produced by another human being or an animal. Injection of these immunoglobulins temporarily prevents developing the disease once exposed. Transmission of antibodies through fetal circulation or injection of immunoglobulin following exposure to hepatitis are examples of acquired passive immunity.

Factors Influencing Immunity

Although the exact physiological mechanisms involved in an immune response are unknown, it has been well documented that a number of factors influence the **immune response** (body's reaction to substances identified as nonself, neutralization of antigen). These include age, sex, nutritional status, stress, and treatment modalities. As one ages, the immune system becomes less effective. Sex hormones affect immunity. Estrogen enhances immunological functioning, while androgen suppresses it. Therefore, women are especially prone to autoimmune diseases, while men are more prone to immunosuppressive disorders. Poor nutritional status and emotional stress lead to increased susceptibility to infections. Radiation therapy and a variety of medications, such as corticosteroids and chemotherapeutic agents suppress the immune system. Nurses need to plan client care incorporating this knowledge.

PHYSICAL ASSESSMENT

Physical assessment of the immune system involves the entire body. The skin and mucous membranes are evaluated for urticaria, inflammation, or bleeding. Superficial head, neck, supraclavicular, axilla, and inguinal lymph nodes are inspected and palpated for redness, tenderness, or swelling. Elevated temperature may indicate infection. Joints need to be evaluated for possible tenderness, swelling, or limited range of motion. Changes in the rate and rhythm of respirations, presence of a cough, or abnormal lung sounds may indicate immunological conditions. Cardiovascular status, including rate, rhythm, arrhythmias, and peripheral vascular circulation must be assessed. Enlarged liver or spleen and gastrointestinal conditions, such as nausea, vomiting, or diarrhea may have an immunological basis. Alterations in vision, hearing, urinary, and neurological function may occur. Assessment of the immune system entails a comprehensive head-to-toe physical examination.

Table 24-2

Natural Immunity	Acquired Immunity	
	Active Acquired Immunity	Passive Acquired Immunity
• Innate immunity • Present at birth • Includes physical and chemical barriers to invading antigens	• Long-term immunity • Antibodies develop as a result of exposure to a disease or vaccine • Antibodies neutralize future invasions of the same antigen	• Temporary immunity • Antibodies obtained from an animal or another human who has been exposed to an antigen • Examples are gamma-globulin or antiserum

COMMON DIAGNOSTIC TESTS

The following is a table of the commonly used diagnostic tests for clients with allergies, immune, and autoimmune disorders.

Test	Explanation/Normal Values	Nursing Responsibilities
Antinuclear Antibodies (ANA)	Antibodies that attack cell nuclei. Positive in 95% of clients with systemic lupus erythematosus. Low levels in clients with mononucleosis, rheumatic, and liver diseases. Adult = negative	No fasting required. Hydralazine and procainamide may increase level. A radioactive scan in the past week may alter results. Inform lab, if applicable.
Complement Assay (Total Complement, C3 and C4)	Decreased levels in autoimmune diseases due to depletion of complement by antibody-antigen complexes. C4 = 15–45 mg/dL C3 = male: 80–180 mg/dL; female: 76–120 mg/dL	No fasting required.
C-reactive Protein Test (CRP)	An abnormal protein appears in the blood of clients with an acute inflammatory process. Used to monitor the progress of clients with autoimmune disorders, such as rheumatoid arthritis. Negative except in pregnancy. More sensitive than ESR.	Some labs may require clients to fast, except for water, 4 to 12 hours prior. NSAIDs, steroids, and salicylates may decrease level. Birth control pill and IUDs may increase levels. Inform lab, if applicable.
Erythrocyte Sedimentation Rate (ESR or Sed Rate Test)	Measures, in mm, red blood cell descent in a normal saline solution after 1 hour. Level increases in inflammatory, infectious, necrotic, or cancerous conditions due to increased protein content in plasma. Used to monitor the course of therapy for clients with autoimmune diseases, such as rheumatoid arthritis. Normal Value Male 1–13 mm/hr Female 1–20 mm/hr	Test should be performed within 3 hours after blood draw. Menstruation or pregnancy may increase level. Ethanbutal, quinine aspirin, cortisone and prednisone may alter results.
Human Leukocyte Antigen DW4 (HLA-DW4)	Present in 50% of clients with rheumatoid arthritis.	No fasting required.
Lupus Erythematosus Test (LE Prep)	Positive in 70–80% of clients with systemic lupus erythematosus. Should be negative. May be positive in clients with rheumatoid arthritis. Used to diagnose and monitor the course of treatment for clients with systemic lupus erythematosus.	No fasting required. May be ordered daily for 3 days. Apresoline, Pronestyl, oral contraceptives, quinidine, penicillin, Aldomet, tetracycline, isoniazid, or reserpine may cause false positive results.
Red Blood Cell Count (RBC Count)	Number of red blood cells per mm of blood. May be low in clients with rheumatoid arthritis. Males: 4.6–5.9 million/mm^3 Females: 4.2–5.4 million/mm^3	No fasting required.
Rheumatoid Factor (RF)	Abnormal protein in serum of about 80% of clients with rheumatoid arthritis. Formed as a result of the reaction of IgM to an abnormal IgG. Also elevated in clients with other autoimmune diseases, such as systemic lupus erythematosus. Normal < 1:20 titer; elderly = slightly increased	No fasting required.

Test	Explanation/Normal Values	Nursing Responsibilities
Total White Blood Cell Count	Number of white blood cells per mm of blood. Elevation is associated with infectious processes. Normal = 4300–10,800/mm³	No fasting required. Exercise, stress, last month of pregnancy, labor, previous splenectomy, and eating may increase levels and alter differential values. Numerous drugs alter results.
Differential Count	Percentage of types of white blood cells in 1 mm of blood.	No fasting required.
Neutrophils	Increase in bacterial infections and trauma.	
-Segs (Mature Neutrophils)	Segs 50–65%	
Bands (Immature Neutrophils)	Bands 0–5%	
Eosinophils	Increased in allergic reactions or parasitic infestation. 1–3%	Decreased levels in clients on corticosteroid therapy.
Basophils	Increased in allergic reactions. Increase during healing periods. 0.4–1.0%	Steroids cause a decrease.
Lymphocytes	Increased in viral infections and others diseases, such as pertussis and TB. Decreased in AIDS. 25–35%.	Steroids cause a decrease.
Monocytes	Increased in chronic diseases, such as malaria, TB, Rocky mountain spotted fever. May be low in clients with rheumatoid arthritis. 4–6%	

KEY ABBREVIATIONS

The following abbreviations and acronyms are used in this chapter:

MG	myasthenia gravis
RA	rheumatoid arthritis
SLE	systemic lupus erythematosus
TENS	transcutaneous electronic nerve stimulator

▶ ALLERGIES

Allergic disorders are the result of an immediate **hypersensitivity** (excessive reaction to a stimulus) reaction of the immune system to **allergens** (a type of antigen commonly found in the environment). Allergens may be inhaled, injected, ingested, or contacted. Upon first exposure to an allergen, IgE antibodies are produced. They adhere to mast cells. When a subsequent exposure occurs, these cells attach to the antigen and activate the release of chemical mediators, such as histamine, bradykinin, and serotonin. These chemicals cause vasodilation, enhanced capillary permeability, and bronchoconstriction (see Figure 24-2). Allergic asthma (see Chapter 19, Respiratory Disorders), atopic allergies, such as allergic rhinitis, drug allergy, food allergy, contact dermatitis, and anaphylaxis are examples of this type of hypersensitivity response.

▶ Allergic Rhinitis

Allergic rhinitis, also known as hay fever or pollinosis, is a common allergy in our society caused by airborne allergens, such as pollen, mold, animal dander, dust, and ragweed. It classically affects the nose, eyes, and respiratory system. Symptoms include nasal congestion, thin, clear, watery discharge, sneezing, itching, swelling, and redness of the eyes. Headaches and ear infections may also develop.

▶ Drug Allergy

Any drug potentially may cause a drug reaction, but common ones include penicillin, cephalosporins,

Allergic response

First exposure

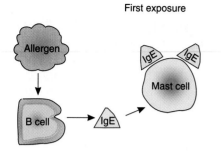

Second or subsequent exposure

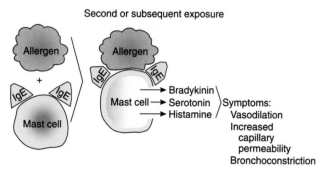

FIGURE 24-2 Allergic response.

insulin, vaccines, and local anesthetics. Reactions vary from mild to severe. Usually symptoms do not occur until the client has taken several doses of the medication, although they can occur at first exposure. The most common reaction is the sudden development of a bright red, itchy rash, often appearing initially on the trunk or arms. Occasionally, a client may develop an anaphylactic reaction.

▶ Food Allergy

Although individuals may be allergic to any edible substance, certain foods, such as milk, fish, chocolate, and nuts, are common allergens that cause diarrhea as a result of immunological reaction in the intestinal mucosa. Headache, nausea, vomiting, rash, itching, and wheezing may also develop.

▶ Contact Dermatitis

Contact dermatitis is caused by soaps, detergents, deodorants, or any allergen that comes in contact with the skin. Redness, rash, itching and/or burning sensa-

tions develop as a result. The extent and severity varies with individuals.

▶ *Medical/Surgical Management*

▶ *Medical*

Medical management of clients experiencing an **allergic response** (reaction to allergen) includes drug therapy to treat symptoms and identification of precipitating agents. Once the allergen/allergens have been identified, **immunotherapy** or desensitization may be used to build up the client's resistance to the allergen. This involves repeated injections of the diluted allergen. Subsequently, decreased levels of histamine are released when exposed to the allergen.

▶ *Pharmacological*

A number of medications are employed to treat the symptoms of an allergic response. Antihistamines counteract the effects of histamine. They may be taken orally, topical or intravenously, depending upon the type of allergic response and urgency for treatment. Nasal decongestants help relieve respiratory symptoms. Topical corticosteroids effectively relieve inflammation associated with contact dermatitis and dermatitis medicamentosa. Oral or injectable forms of corticosteroids may be used either alone or in combination with antihistamines and nasal decongestants.

Skin testing by a physician can determine the causative agents. This is done by either applying special patches or injecting common allergens intradermally under the skin and monitoring the inflammatory response a day or two later.

▶ *Diet*

Individuals allergic to certain foods should be taught to check food labels carefully, be aware of how food is prepared, and not eat any product that could lead to a reaction. This includes restaurant foods and foods prepared in another person's home.

▶ *Activity*

Avoidance of the causative allergen prevents allergic reactions. Activities should be centered around doing this, if at all possible. For instance, individuals who are allergic to pollen may need to stay in air-conditioned environments on those days when the pollen count is extremely high.

▶ Nursing Process

Assessment

Subjective Data A detailed, comprehensive client history should include information about previous allergic reactions, recent foods eaten or medications taken, contact with environmental pollutants, or anything not normally encountered.

Objective Data Physical assessment includes gastrointestinal functioning, respirations, and cardiovascular and neurological status (refer to Chapter 10, Nursing Assessment). It is also important to assess for the presence of **urticaria** and **angioedema**. Urticaria (hives) involves the development of wheals on the outer layers of the skin. Itching, swelling, and redness also occur. Angioedema, also known as angioneurotic edema, is edema of subcutaneous layers and mucous membranes. It is most pronounced in the head and neck areas. Swelling can lead to obstruction of airways and respiratory distress.

▼ ▼

Possible nursing diagnoses for clients with allergies may include:

Nursing Diagnoses	Goals	Nursing Interventions
▶ *Injury, high risk for, related to an allergic reaction.*	The client will identify factors that increase the potential of a reaction.	Assist client in identifying those factors that increase the potential for a reaction.
▶ *Health seeking behaviors related to causative allergen, therapeutic modalities, and/or preventive measures.*	The client will relate methods to avoid exposure to allergens.	Assist client in planning lifestyle changes that will help in avoiding exposure to allergens.
▶ *Knowledge deficit related to lack of information about allergens, treatment, or preventive measures.*	The client will demonstrate an understanding and compliance with therapeutic modalities if a reaction occurs. The client will demonstrate an understanding and compliance with preventive measures to avoid subsequent allergic reactions.	Teach client about allergy treatments and what to do if a reaction occurs.

▶ Evaluation

Each goal must be evaluated to determine how it has been met by the client.

▲ ▲

▶ ANAPHYLAXIS

Anaphylaxis (a systemic reaction to allergens) is the most serious type of allergic reaction. It occurs in individuals who are extremely sensitive to an allergen. Symptoms develop suddenly and can progress to severe levels within minutes. Foods, drugs, hormones, insect bites, blood, and vaccines all are associated with anaphylactic reactions. Shellfish, eggs, nuts, berries, and chocolates are the most common foods involved. Any medication has the potential of causing a reaction, but antibiotics, especially penicillin, insulin, muscle relaxants, and x-ray dyes are the most frequent precipitating agents. Bee, wasp, hornet, and snake bites may also cause anaphylactic reactions.

Symptoms of an anaphylactic reaction vary. They may involve a local or systemic response. In localized reactions, which are seldom fatal, urticaria and angioedema develop at the site. In contrast, systemic anaphylactic reactions may be life threatening. Symptoms involve the skin, GI tract, cardiovascular and respiratory systems. Clients experience peripheral tingling, flushing, fullness in the mouth, throat/nasal congestion, tearing and swelling around the eyes, itching, and cough. In severe cases, laryngeal edema, bronchospasms, severe dyspnea, vasodilation, and cyanosis develop. If untreated, these catastrophic effects lead to respiratory failure, severe hypotension, anaphylactic shock, and death. Therefore, it is crucial symptoms be identified early and treatment initiated immediately. Death can occur in minutes.

▶ Medical/Surgical Management

▶ Medical

Medical management centers around establishing an intravenous line, administering fluids and emergency drugs, and maintaining an airway. Oxygen is provided via nasal cannula or face mask. In severe cases, endotracheal intubation or a tracheotomy may be required.

▶ Pharmacological

Epinephrine is administered subcutaneously as soon as symptoms develop to dilate bronchioles, increase heart contractions and constrict blood vessels. Antihistamines, such as diphenhydramine hydrochloride (Benadryl), blocks the effects of histamine in bronchioles, blood vessels, and the GI tract. Corticosteroids (prednisone [Deltasone], hydorcortisone sodium succinate [Solu-Cortef], methylprednisolone sodium succinate [Solu-Medrol]) are given for their anti-inflammatory effect. Vasopressors, such as norepinephrine bitartrate (Levophed) or dopamine hydrochloride (Intropin) may be needed to increase blood pressures. If bronchoconstriction and spasms are severe, albuterol (Proventil), metaproterenol sulfate (Alupent) and/or Aminophyllin may be administered.

▶ Diet

Clients will be NPO until normal respiratory and circulatory function have been restored.

▶ Activity

Clients will remain on bedrest until vital signs are stable and normal breathing patterns have been restored. Those experiencing severe anaphylactic responses are generally transferred to intensive care units for continued treatment and observation.

▶ Nursing Process

Assessment

Subjective Data Client history may reveal a previous anaphylaxis reaction. The client may describe feelings of uneasiness, anxiety, weakness, itching, dizziness, nausea, peripheral tingling, and a generalized warm sensation throughout the body.

Objective Data Since anaphylaxis is a sudden, unexpected event, nurses must be aware that variations in a client's cardiovascular and respiratory status may be signs of an impending anaphylactic reaction. The first symptoms are sweating, sneezing, tachycardia, hypotension, dysrhythmias, cyanosis, edema of tongue and larynx, wheezing, bronchospasms, vascular collapse, and cardiac arrest. Regularly assessing client's vital signs, cardiovascular, respiratory, and neurological status will detect changes before the severe signs of respiratory distress and impending shock develop.

▼ ▼

Possible nursing diagnoses for clients with anaphylaxis may include:

Nursing Diagnoses	Goals	Nursing Interventions
▶ Tissue perfusion, altered, related to increased capillary permeability and vasodilation.	The client will have adequate tissue perfusion.	Monitor vital signs frequently. Monitor I&O. Place client in Trendelenburg position for hypotension. Administer IV fluids and medications as ordered.
▶ Breathing patterns, ineffective, related to bronchoconstriction, laryngeal edema, and increased secretions.	The client will have effective breathing patterns.	Suction secretions as needed. Administer oxygen and medications as needed.

Nursing Diagnoses	Goals	Nursing Interventions
▶ *Knowledge deficit related to causative allergen, therapeutic modalities, and/or preventive measures.*	The client will relate causative allergen, therapeutic modalities, and preventive measures.	Teach client importance of avoiding allergen.
		Advise client to provide the name of the causative agent and a description of reaction experienced when asked about allergies.
		Encourage client to wear a Medic-Alert bracelet.
		Document on all medical records.
		Teach client and family symptoms of anaphylactic reactions.
		Advise clients allergic to insect stings to carry emergency anaphylactic kits, and teach them how to use.

▶ Evaluation

Each goal must be evaluated to determine how it has been met by the client.

▲ ▲

▶ BLOOD TRANSFUSIONS

Blood components, such as whole blood, packed or frozen RBCs, leukocytes, platelets, and plasma, may be administered to clients when their own bodies are incapable of manufacturing them at a rate required to maintain vascular homeostasis. Any client receiving **homologous** or donor blood products is prone to develop a transfusion reaction. For this reason, some clients are arranging to have their own blood collected, saved, and available for infusion, if needed, during or following elective surgeries. This is known as an **autologous** blood transfusion. Immunological reactions do not develop with this type of blood transfusion. Blood products should be administered slowly for the first half hour since symptoms most frequently occur soon after the infusion is begun.

There are five types of transfusion reactions: febrile nonhemolytic, allergic urticarial, delayed hemolytic, acute hemolytic and anaphylactic. Febrile nonhemolytic reactions are the most common and occur in clients who have had previous blood transfusions. It is the result of an antibody-antigen reaction to WBCs. Symptoms may develop soon after the infusion has started or up to five to six hours after completion. Fever is the classic symptom and may be accompanied by chills, nausea, headache, hypotension, and respiratory problems. Clients who have allergic urticarial reactions develop a skin rash during or within one hour following the transfusion. A delayed hemolytic reaction may occur days to weeks following the transfusion. The client's hemoglobin level falls due to incompatibility of RBC antigens. This type of reaction is often misdiag-

nosed and thought to be related to the condition that created the need for blood replacement rather than a transfusion reaction. An acute hemolytic reaction is potentially a life-threatening situation. Symptoms, resulting from the incompatibility of ABO groups, usually occur during the first fifteen minutes of administration, but can develop anytime during the transfusion. Clients complain of chills, nausea, and back pain. Fever, drop in blood pressure (hypotension), vomiting, hematuria or oliguria may be observed. As the condition progresses, chest pain, dyspnea, anuria, and shock develop. Anaphylactic reactions, although rare, are also life threatening. Symptoms of acute gastrointestinal malfunctioning, cardiovascular and respiratory collapse develop moments after the transfusion has started.

▶ Medical/Surgical Management

▶ Medical

Medical management of clients experiencing a blood transfusion reaction depends on the type of reaction. Treatment of a febrile nonhemolytic reaction includes stopping the blood, infusing normal saline, and treating the symptoms. For clients experiencing an allergic urticarial reaction, slow the transfusion and administer an antihistamine. Usually, this is all that is necessary. Delayed hemolytic reactions often go undetected and untreated. Both an acute hemolytic reaction and anaphylactic reactions are medical emergencies.

The transfusion must be stopped immediately. Normal saline and emergency drugs are given intravenously.

▶ *Pharmacological*

If a febrile nonhemolytic or allergic urticarial reaction occurs, diphenhydramine (Benadryl) and a corticosteroid (hydrocortisone or prednisone) are administered to counteract the immunological response. Antipyretics are ordered to control fever. For life-threatening conditions, emergency medications are employed. (Refer back to Anaphylaxis.)

▶ *Diet*

Clients should not be fed if a reaction is occurring, especially if respiratory symptoms have developed. Aspiration could occur.

▶ *Activity*

Clients should remain in bed until symptoms of the reaction have subsided.

▶ *Nursing Process*

Assessment

Subjective Data   Occasionally, clients will verbalize the feeling of something "not being right" or "something strange is going on in my body" before actual symptoms become apparent. They may have itching, headache, or low back pain.

Objective Data   Clients receiving blood components need to be carefully assessed for any signs of a transfusion reaction, such as fever, chills, or respiratory problems.

▼ ▼

Possible nursing diagnosis for clients with blood transfusions may include:

Nursing Diagnoses	*Goals*	*Nursing Interventions*
▶ *Injury, high risk for, related to infusion of homologous blood components.*	The client will not have injury from infusion of homologous blood products by reporting signs/symptoms of a reaction when first experienced.	Follow protocol for blood products and administration.
		Check the client's identification and the blood product with another nurse.
		If a reaction occurs, stop the transfusion immediately, then call the physician.
		Administer medications as ordered.
		Send the blood tubing and a urine specimen to the lab for analysis.
		Monitor and document the client's condition.
		Teach the client who has a blood transfusion reaction to inform health care providers whenever questioned about allergies.

▶ *Evaluation*

Each goal must be evaluated to determine how it has been met by the client.

▲ ▲

▶ *ORGAN TRANSPLANTS*

Modern technology has made major advancements in the last several decades in the ability to transplant tissues and major body organs. The success of these procedures is directly related to matching antibodies and antigens of the donor and recipient and to the effectiveness of immunosuppressive medications in preventing rejection. Immunosuppressive medications make the client prone to the development of infections and cancers. Clients must have a regular medical check-up, including cancer screening tests.

► Medical/Surgical Management

► Medical

Although blood components are the most common type of tissue transplants, physicians today are capable of transplanting bone marrow, corneal tissue, skin, bone, kidneys, pancreas, hearts, livers, and lungs. Donor tissue and organs come from several sources. Autologous donations are obtained from the recipient themselves, preserved and then readministered at a future date. Bone marrow and blood components often employ autologous donations. Rejection does not occur with this type of transplantation, since it uses the clients' own cells. Homologous donations involve removing tissue or organs from one individual and surgically transferring them to another. They may be from living related donors or living nonrelated donors. Cadaveric donations are harvested from individuals after being pronounced clinically dead. The sooner the transplant occurs, the greater the chance of success. ABO blood groups and **human leukocyte antigen** (HLA), antigens present in human blood, matching is important in preventing rejection when homologous and cadaveric donors are used.

► Pharmacological

A combination of immunosuppressive medications are used to hinder rejection. Steroids (prednisone [Deltasone], methylprednisolone sodium succinate [Solu-Medrol]) decrease the inflammatory response. Cyclosporine (Sandimmune), antithymocyte globulin [equine], ATG (Atgam) and Tacrolimus (Prograf) inhibit T cells. Azathioprine (Imuran) inhibits purine synthesis. Muromonab-CD3 (Orthoclone, OKT 3) prevents acute rejection in kidney transplant clients. Clients taking immunosuppressive medications are especially prone to developing infections. Antibiotics may be prescribed prophylactically.

Steroids cause fluid and sodium retention, low potassium level, elevated blood pressure, moon face, muscle wasting, elevated glucose level, impaired wound healing, mood swings, and masculinization in women. Cyclosporine may be toxic to the kidneys and liver. Imuran may cause hair loss and lower platelet level. OKT 3 also causes fluid retention.

► Diet

Diets are individualized based on client condition. No nutritional alterations are required due to organ transplantation.

► Activity

Activity is dependent upon the type of transplant. Clients who receive a major organ, such as heart, lung, pancreas, or liver are placed in reverse isolation in the hospital setting for at least two weeks. They are carefully observed for signs of rejection. Exposure to others is limited. Once discharged, they are taught to avoid contact with any one who may have an infection and to wear a mask whenever out in public.

► Nursing Process

Assessment

Subjective Data Client history may reveal fear of possible transplant rejection. The client generally describes tenderness at the transplant site.

Objective Data Following transplantation, clients' vital signs, nutritional status, fluid balance, urinary output, mental status, respiratory and cardiovascular functioning need to be carefully monitored. Daily weight should be taken. Wound sites should be checked frequently. Signs of rejection include fever, weight gain, swelling or tenderness at the transplant site.

▼ ▼

Possible nursing diagnoses for clients with organ transplants may include:

Nursing Diagnoses	Goals	Nursing Interventions
► Fear related to possible transplant rejection.	The client will relate less fear regarding rejection.	Allow client to verbalize concerns and develop realistic expectations.
		Set aside time to sit down and talk to the client.

(continued)

Nursing Diagnoses	Goals	Nursing Interventions
▶ *Knowledge deficit related to home care following transplantation.*	The client will discuss signs and symptoms of rejection.	Teach the client and family about signs of rejection and infection.
	The client will demonstrate an understanding of the side effects of immunosuppressive drugs and lifestyle changes to adapt to their effects.	Teach client and family the ramifications of taking immunosuppressive medications. Teach client to watch for side effects and report them to physician.
▶ *Infection, high risk for, related to immunosuppressive medications.*	The client will demonstrate appropriate wound care.	Teach the client and family appropriate wound care.
	The client will be free of infection.	Teach the client to wear a mask whenever out in public. Teach the client the importance of regular check-ups, including cancer screening tests.

▶ Evaluation

Each goal must be evaluated to determine how it has been met by the client

▲ ▲

▶ RHEUMATOID ARTHRITIS

The term *arthritis* refers to inflammation of a joint. There are a number of types of arthritic conditions, depending upon their cause. Rheumatoid arthritis, RA, is an autoimmune disorder. It is believed that abnormal IgG antibodies are produced within synovial joints. Acting as antigens, they react with IgG and IgM antibodies. The specific IgM antibody created is known as the rheumatoid factor (RF). Immune complexes are formed within the joint, causing inflammation, swelling, and increased synovial fluid. As this chronic, systemic condition progresses, surrounding cartilage, tendons, and ligaments become involved. Thickening of synovial tissue eventually leads to calcification of the joint, joint pain, limited mobility, and deformity. Usually, the joints of the hand and wrist are affected initially. As the disease progresses shoulder, elbow, hip, knee, ankle, and cervical spine joints become affected. Other areas of the body where connective tissue is present may also be involved.

Like many other autoimmune diseases, rheumatoid arthritis is more common in women, often initially diagnosed during the later childbearing years. Heredity plays a role in its acquisition. Many clients have the human leukocyte antigen DW4 (HLA-DW4). Hormones also play a role. Women taking oral contraceptives are less likely to develop RA. Clients experience periods of **remission**, a decrease or absence of symptoms, and **exacerbations**, an increase in symptoms. Both physical and emotional stressors lead to increased symptomatology.

▶ Medical/Surgical Management

▶ Medical

Medical management centers around reducing inflammation, relieving pain, maintaining mobility, and promoting general health. Therapeutic regime includes medications, exercise, hot and cold applications, stress management, and/or TENS units.

▶ Surgical

Hip, knee, and finger joints may be surgically replaced. Refer to Chapter 26, Musculoskeletal Disorders, for joint replacement.

▶ Pharmacological

Nonsteroidal anti-inflammatory drugs (NSAIDs), salicylates, corticosteroids, and gold preparations may be used alone or in combination to decrease swelling and reduce pain (see Table 24-3). Because of the large doses required to control inflammation and the long-term use due to the chronicity of this condition, side effects often develop. In severe cases, azathioprine (Imuran), hydroxychloroquine sulfate (Plaquenil Sulfate), D-penicillamine (Depen) or methotrexate sodium (Rheumatrex) may be used. These medications also have serious side effects.

Table 24-3

MEDICATIONS USED TO TREAT RHEUMATOID ARTHRITIS

Drug	Use/Actions	Side Effects	Nursing Interventions
Salicylates Aspirin	Inhibit prostaglandin synthesis resulting in decreased pain. (Analgesia) Antipyretic Anti-inflammatory	GI upset, tinnitus, easy bruising, nausea, prolonged bleeding time.	Instruct client to take with food or take enteric coated aspirin. Report ringing in ears. Do not give to clients on oral anticoagulants. Assess for bleeding bruising.
Nonsteroidal antiinflammatory drugs (NSAIDs) ibuprofen (Motrin, Rufen), naproxen (Naprosyn), phenylbutazone (Butazolidin)	Inhibit prostaglandin synthesis. Reduce joint swelling stiffness. Analgesic and antipyretic properties.	GI irritation, nausea, vomiting, heartburn. GI bleeding and ulceration, dizziness, headache, liver toxicity.	Administer with food. May prolong bleeding time, may require frequent blood count.
Indole analogues indomethacin (Indocin), sulindac (Clinoril)	Analgesic anti-inflammatory effect.	Gastric bleeding, headaches, dizziness, psychiatric disturbances.	Administer with food. Report any bleeding (tarry stools, hematemesis). Avoid giving aspirin.
Corticosteroids prednisone (Deltasone)	Decreases inflammation.	GI irritation, muscle weakness, fluid retention, moon face, muscle wasting, impaired wound healing.	Administer with food. Weigh daily. Monitor BP, sleep pattern, and serum potassium.
Antimalarials hydroxychloroquine sulfate (Plaquenil Sulfate)		Visual disturbances, nightmares, skin lesions, nausea, diarrhea, low blood count.	Monitor CBC and liver function tests.
Gold Salts auranofin (Ridaura)	Anti-inflammatory	Diarrhea, nausea, vomiting, jaundice.	Remind client to keep all physician appointments. Beneficial effects may take 3 months to appear.
Chelating Agent D-penicillamine (Depen)	Palliative when other medications have failed.	Bone marrow depression, fever, rashes, blood dyscrasias, liver toxicity.	Give on empty stomach. Have epinephrine 1:1000 handy for anaphylaxis. Fluids to 3000 mL/day to prevent renal failure.

▶ Diet

Clients need to be taught to eat a nutritious, well-balanced diet. Poorly nourished individuals are prone to infections. For clients with RA, this infection results in exacerbation of symptoms. Foods high in iron are encouraged when RBCs are low.

▶ Activity

Since joint mobility is a major problem, occupational and physical therapists are part of the therapeutic team. Exercises, resting splints, and assistive devices are often employed.

▶ Nursing Process

Assessment

Subjective Data   Client history frequently reveals a gradual development of symptoms, beginning initially with early morning stiffness and pain in finger joints. Eventually, other joints become involved. Fatigue, weight loss, temperature elevations, and anemia develop. Subjective data often includes malaise, loss of appetite, fatigue, and muscle weakness. Information about periods of remissions and exacerbations should be obtained, as well as the clients' understanding and compliance with the treatment regimen.

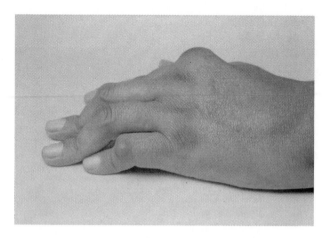

FIGURE 24-3 Arthritic hands. (*Courtesy of the Arthritis Foundation*)

Objective Data Assessment of the hands may reveal the classic deformities associated with RA: boutonniere deformity (fixed flexion of the proximal interphalangeal joint and hyperextension of the distal interphalangeal joint), ulnar drift (deviation of the fingers to the ulnar side of the hand), and swan-neck deformity (fixed flexion of the distal interphalangeal joint and hyperextension of the proximal interphalangeal joint). Figure 24-3 illustrates these changes in the hands.

Assess skin for the presence of ulcers, due to vasculitis, and moveable, subcutaneous skin nodes, known as rheumatoid nodules. Eye tissue may be inflamed. Reduction in tear and saliva production can occur, causing dryness of the eyes, mouth, and mucous membranes. This is known as Sjogren's syndrome. The client may have weight loss and an elevated temperature.

X-rays demonstrate the amount and degree of deformity. There is no specific laboratory test that confirms a diagnosis of RA. Alterations in the following may occur: RBCs decrease, (anemia) as the disease progresses, elevation of WBCs, ESR, antinuclear antibodies (ANAs), C-reactive proteins and platelet count. The rheumatoid factor (RF) is present in about 50 percent of clients in the early stages. This percentage increases as the disease becomes more advanced. HLA-DW4 is present about half of the time

▼ ▼

Possible nursing diagnoses for clients with rheumatoid arthritis may include:

Nursing Diagnoses	Goals	Nursing Interventions
▶ *Pain, chronic, related to swollen, inflamed joints.*	The client will relate appropriate use of anti-inflammatory medications.	Teach client about prescribed analgesics, anti-inflammatory medications.
	The client will relate methods to decrease pain.	Encourage the client to practice relaxation techniques and take warm shower to relieve early morning joint stiffness and pain.
		Use hot and cold packs to decrease muscle spasms.
		Teach client proper body alignment and avoid using pillows under the knees.
		Ask the physician about using TENS unit to control pain (see Chapter 12, Pain Management).
▶ *Mobility, impaired physical, related to pain, edema, and joint immobility.*	The client will demonstrate measures to increase joint mobility.	Teach hospitalized clients to use the overhead trapeze when moving in bed and change position frequently.
	The client will demonstrate use of adaptive devices.	Assist with ROM exercises.
		Maintain planned rest periods.
		Teach client use of assistive devices, such as handrests, tools to pick up objects, or three-legged canes, as needed.
		Check with occupational and physical therapists for available equipment.
		Assist client to use handrails in tub, shower, and toilet; raised toilet seat; and rubber-tipped walker or cane.

▶ *Self-care deficit: bathing/dressing/ grooming related to joint inflammation or deformity.*	The client will bathe, dress, and groom as much as able.	Recommend shoes with Velcro closures. Encourage client to stop and rest when getting tired. Teach self-care using assistive devices, as required. Assist with routine plan for ADLs.
▶ *Fatigue related to chronic inflammatory process.*	The client will state less fatigue.	Explain that fatigue is a common symptom of autoimmune disorders. Allow the client to express feelings about altered lifestyle. Inform client of community services such as Meals on Wheels. Plan rest periods between activities.
	The client will establish priorities for daily activities.	Help identify activities client should perform and what can be delegated. Instruct client to record level of fatigue and activities performed on an hourly basis for twenty-four hours. One method uses 0 to 10 scale (0 = not tired, peppy; 10 = totally exhausted).
	The client will balance daily activities with periods of rest.	Help plan important tasks during high energy periods and distribute difficult ones throughout the week.
▶ *Body image disturbance related to joint deformity and side effects of corticosteroid medications.*	The client will verbalize and demonstrate acceptance of appearance.	Encourage client to express feelings about changes in appearance. Provide an opportunity to discuss feelings with others having the same experience. The Arthritis Foundation can provide help. Accept the individual as a person.
▶ *Infection, high risk for, related to immunosuppressive medications.*	The client will practice appropriate precautions to avoid infection. The client will be free of infection.	Teach client to avoid crowded areas and friends and family with infections.
▶ *Knowledge deficit related to methods to control disease and prevent complications.*	The client will describe disease process, factors contributing to symptoms, and measures to control them. The client will demonstrate health behaviors needed to prevent complications.	Teach client about the disease process, factors that contribute to symptoms, and measures to control them. Encourage exercise of inflamed joints; it may be painful, but it prevents contractures from forming. Inform clients that NSAIDs, salicylates, and corticosteroids should be taken with foods to prevent gastric irritation. Teach stress management techniques to enhance coping skills in dealing with this potentially deforming, chronic, autoimmune disorders.

▶ Evaluation

Each goal must be evaluated to determine how it has been met by the client.

▲ ▲

▶ SYSTEMIC LUPUS ERYTHEMATOSUS

Systemic lupus erythematous (SLE) is a chronic, progressive, incurable autoimmune disease affecting multiple body organs. It is characterized by periods of exacerbation and remission. SLE occurs most commonly in women during their childbearing years and develops three times more frequently in African-Americans and twice as often in Hispanics than in the white population. In clients with SLE, abnormal B-lymphocyte cells produce autoantibodies that destroy body cells. One type, antinuclear antibodies (ANAs), attack the deoxyribonucleic acid (DNA) within cell nuclei. Other types attack red blood cells, white blood cells and platelets, as well as components within cells, such as RNA. Immune complexes are formed, circulate in serum causing inflammation and tissue damage. Production of these autoantibodies is influenced by genetics, medications, infections, stress, and ultraviolet light rays.

No single test is conclusive for a diagnosis. The American Rheumatism Association has established criteria for SLE. If four or more of these criteria are present a diagnosis of SLE is confirmed (see Table 24-4).

Table 24-4

AMERICAN RHEUMATISM ASSOCIATION CRITERIA FOR SYSTEMIC LUPUS ERYTHEMATOSUS

Criterion	Definition
Malar rash	Fixed erythema, flat or raised, over the malar eminences, tending to spare the nasolabial folds
Discoid rash	Erythematous raised patches with adherent keratotic scaling and follicular plugging; atrophic scarring may occur in older lesions
Photosensitivity	Skin rash as a result of unusual reaction to sunlight: noted in patient history or physician observation
Oral ulcers	Oral or nasopharyngeal ulceration, usually painless, observed by a physician
Arthritis	Nonerosive arthritis involving two or more peripheral joints, characterized by tenderness, swelling, or effusion
Serositis	Pleuritis—convincing history of pleuritic pain or rub heard by a physician or evidence of pleural effusion or Pericarditis—documented by ECG or rub or evidence of pericardial effusion
Renal disorder	Persistent proteinuria greater than 0.5 gm/day or greater than 3+ if quantitation not performed or Cellular casts—may be red cell, hemoglobin, granular, tubular, or mixed
Neurologic disorder	Seizures—in the absence of offending drugs or known metabolic derangements, e.g., uremia, ketoacidosis, or electrolyte imbalance or Psychosis—in the absence of offending drugs or known metabolic derangements, e.g., uremia. ketoacidosis, or electrolyte imbalance
Hematologic disorder	Hemolytic anemia—with reticulocytosis or Leukopenia—less than 4,000/mm^3 total on two or more occasions or Lymphopenia—less than 1,500/mm^3 on two or more occasions or Thrombocytopenia—less than 1,000/mm^3 in the absence of offending drugs
Immunologic disorder	Positive LE cell preparation or Anti-DNA: antibody to native DNA in abnormal titer or Anti-Sm: presence of antibody to Sm nuclear antigen or False-positive serologic test for syphilis known to be positive for at least 6 months and confirmed by *Treponema pallidum* immobilization or fluorescent treponemal antibody absorption test
Antinuclear antibody	An abnormal titer of antinuclear antibody of immunofluorescence or an equivalent assay at any point in time and in the absence of drugs known to be associated with "drug-induced lupus" syndrome

Note: Criteria revised in 1982. The criteria are not intended for diagnosis of individual cases. In clinical studies, systemic lupus erythematosus can be indentified if any four or more of the 11 criteria are present, serially or simultaneously, during any interval of observation.

(Courtesy Tan, Eng M., et al. [1982]. The 1982 revised criteria for the classification of systemic lupus erythematosus. Arthritis and Rheumatism. 25(11).1271–1277. This criteria has not changed since 1982.)

▶ Medical/Surgical Management

▶ Medical

Medical treatment is aimed at decreasing tissue inflammation and destruction through the use of antimalarial and corticosteroid medications. During acute exacerbations, plasmapheresis may be used. This treatment modality involves removal of the client's plasma, processing it through a special machine to eliminate various cellular elements, and reinfusing the cleansed plasma. In SLE, autoantibodies are removed.

Since clients with SLE are prone to a variety of complications, they are carefully monitored for renal, cardiac, pulmonary, hematological, and neurological damage. A large percentage of SLE clients eventually develop renal failure, requiring dialysis to maintain life.

▶ Pharmacological

The lowest possible dose of corticosteroid, oral or topical, is used to maintain the client in remission. During periods of exacerbations, higher doses are required. Prolonged use of these medications leads to multiple side effects. Hydroxychloroquine sulfate (Plaquenil sulfate), an antimalarial agent, is used. Although the exact mechanism involved is unknown, it does work effectively in decreasing joint and skin problems. It can lead to the development of retinal toxicity; therefore, clients should have yearly eye exams. Cyclophosphamide (Cytoxan) or azathioprine (Imuran) may be employed to control kidney damage.

▶ Diet

Clients on corticosteroids are prone to developing hypernatremia, hypokalemia, hyperglycemia, and fluid retention. Diets should be low in sodium and glucose and high in potassium. Excessive fluid intake should be discouraged.

▶ Activity

Fatigue is common. Clients should be encouraged to sleep at least 8 hours a night, rest periodically during the day, and reduce exposure to the sun.

▶ Nursing Process

Assessment

Subjective Data   Ask when the disease began, what symptoms have developed, and how they have been treated. Elicit information about medications the client is taking and side effects. Identify activity level and degree of fatigue. Determine client's understanding of the disease process, how lifestyle has changed, and how effectively client is coping. The client may describe having malaise, photosensitivity, pain in joints, irregular menses, irritability, confusion, or hallucinations.

Objective Data   Perform a complete head-to-toe assessment. Most common symptoms include fever, anemia, leukopenia, thrombocytopenia, anorexia, hypertension, respiratory and cardiac infections, renal involvement, enlarged liver and spleen, and skin lesions, especially the classic "butterfly" rash. Table 24-5 illustrates the common clinical manifestations of SLE. Figure 24-4 shows an individual with a "butterfly rash." If exposed to the cold, Raynaud's phenomenon, intermittent attacks of diminished blood supply to fingers, toes, ears, and nose, may develop.

Laboratory tests frequently reveal serum antinuclear antibodies (ANA) and anti-DNA antibodies. Lupus erythematosus cells (LE cells) are present in most clients.

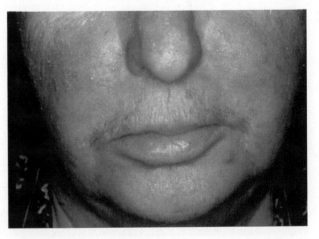

FIGURE 24-4   Butterfly rash. (*Courtesy of the American Academy of Dermatology*)

Table 24-5

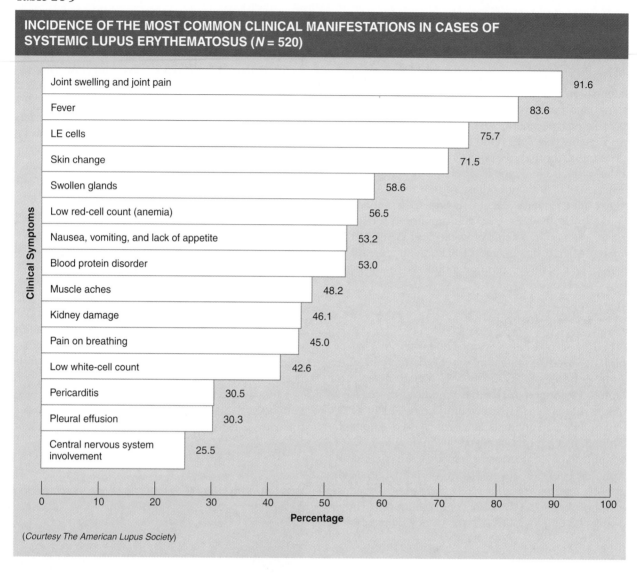

INCIDENCE OF THE MOST COMMON CLINICAL MANIFESTATIONS IN CASES OF SYSTEMIC LUPUS ERYTHEMATOSUS (*N* = 520)

Clinical Symptoms	Percentage
Joint swelling and joint pain	91.6
Fever	83.6
LE cells	75.7
Skin change	71.5
Swollen glands	58.6
Low red-cell count (anemia)	56.5
Nausea, vomiting, and lack of appetite	53.2
Blood protein disorder	53.0
Muscle aches	48.2
Kidney damage	46.1
Pain on breathing	45.0
Low white-cell count	42.6
Pericarditis	30.5
Pleural effusion	30.3
Central nervous system involvement	25.5

(*Courtesy The American Lupus Society*)

▼ ▼

Clients with RA and SLE have common nursing diagnoses of fatigue, impaired mobility, and body image disturbance. Clients with SLE have an additional risk for infection if WBC counts are low. Possible additional nursing diagnoses for a client with SLE may include:

Nursing Diagnoses	*Goals*	*Nursing Interventions*
▶ *Skin integrity, impaired, related to presence of butterfly rash, skin lesions, Raynaud's phenomenon, and/or oral ulcers.*	The client will participate in a plan to promote wound healing.	Teach client to clean and dry area prior to application of topical corticosteroids.
		Warn client that sunlight and ultraviolet rays increase symptoms and tanning sessions are contraindicated.
		Encourage client to wear protective clothing, sunscreen of at least SPF 15 and sunglasses. In cold weather, client should wear a hat and gloves.
		Encourage client in regular oral care to promote healing of mouth sores.

Nursing Diagnoses	Goals	Nursing Interventions
▶ *Knowledge deficit related to adapting lifestyle with treatment and prevention of complications.*	The client will describe disease process, factors contributing to symptoms, and regimen for control.	Teach client effects of disease and methods to control complications.
		Teach stress management techniques.
		Allow client to vent feelings.
		Help plan methods to adapt lifestyle.
		Encourage client to visit the physician on a regular basis to monitor for early symptoms of major organ involvement.
		Advise client to have regular eye exam if taking Plaquenil Sulfate.
		Inform client of community support groups available through the Lupus Foundation of America, Inc. (see Resources).

▶ Evaluation

Each goal must be evaluated to determine how it has been met by the client.

▲ ▲

▶ MYASTHENIA GRAVIS

Myasthenia gravis (MG) is an autoimmune disease characterized by extreme muscle weakness and fatigue due to the body's inability to transmit nerve impulses to voluntary muscles. It is thought that clients with MG develop antibodies that act to decrease the number and effectiveness of acetylcholine receptor sites at neuromuscular junctions. Voluntary muscles are most commonly involved, especially those innervated by cranial nerves. Severity of symptoms vary. In mild conditions known as Group I ocular myasthenia, only the eye muscles are involved. As severity increases, symptoms of Group II generalized myasthenia develop. Facial, neck, skeletal, and respiratory muscles become affected. The thymus gland is enlarged in most clients. It is in this organ where anti-ACH receptor antibodies are produced. MG develops during the middle years, affecting women more frequently in the twenty to thirty age group and men over forty. Periods of remission and exacerbation occur, usually during the first few years.

▶ Medical/Surgical Management

▶ Medical

Medical management involves the use of anticholinesterase medications and plasmapheresis. Plasmapheresis removes anti-ACH receptor antibodies. Since it affords only temporary relief of symptoms, it is used primarily for clients in acute crisis who are not responding to drug therapy or prior to a thymectomy. A client's relief of symptoms is a good indicator of how successful surgery might be.

▶ Surgical

Surgical removal of the thymus gland has been shown to result in marked improvement in most clients.

▶ Pharmacological

Anticholinesterase medications, such as pyridostigmine bromide (Mestinon), neostigmine methylsulfate (Prostigmin), and ambenonium chloride (Mytelase) are prescribed early in the course of the disease and act to increase acetylcholine at the neuromuscular junction. Dosages need to be individually determined. Early side effects of overdosage include nausea, abdominal cramping, vomiting, diarrhea, increased saliva, diaphoresis, and low pulse rate. Variation may occur in muscle group responses for the same client. Steroids are also prescribed to slow down the immunological response.

▶ Diet

Clients need to be encouraged to eat a snack prior to taking anticholinesterase medications to avoid GI irritation. If the client's ability to chew and swallow are affected, the diet may need adjustment.

▶ Activity

Symptoms of MG increase with exercise. Clients should avoid excessive muscular activity and rest periodically throughout the day. ROM exercises, braces, splints, and walkers assist in keeping the client independent.

▶ Complications

Respiratory Distress   Clients need to be carefully monitored for early signs of respiratory distress, such as dyspnea, tachypnea, tachycardia, and diaphoresis.

Myasthenia Crisis   This is an acute emergency characterized increased muscle weakness, difficulty swallowing, chewing or talking, and respiratory distress. It occurs in newly diagnosed clients who are not responding to anticholinesterase medications following infections, surgery, or delivery of a child.

Cholinergic Crisis   This is the result of an overdose of anticholinesterase medications. Physical symptoms of both myasthenic crisis and cholinergic crisis are the same. An edrophonium chloride (Tensilon) test is used to differentiate between the two. Tensilon is administered intravenously. Symptoms of clients experiencing a myasthenic crisis will be relieved within seconds, while those in cholinergic crisis show no response. Atropine is administered to counteract the effects of excessive amounts of anticholinesterase drugs. The treatment goal for both is restoration of normal respiratory functioning and alleviation of symptoms.

▶ Nursing Process

Assessment

Subjective Data   Client describes muscle weakness, fatigue, and possibly difficulty chewing or swallowing.

Objective Data   Assess level of muscle groups affecting the eyes, face, neck, and chest. Look for **diplopia** (double vision), **ptosis** (drooping eyelids) and facial symmetry. Determine if chewing or swallowing is a problem. Assess vocal tones. Carefully listen to breath sounds. Assess level of weakness in arm and legs muscles and muscles used for breathing.

ACH receptor antibody and LE cell tests are often positive. X-rays and CT scans of the thymus gland are used to detect enlargement. Electromyogram (EMG) determines the extent of muscle damage.

▼ ▼

Clients with myasthenia gravis experience problems similar to those with RA and SLE, i.e., fatigue and impaired physical mobility. Although the cause, in this case, is due to weakness of voluntary muscles, client goals and nursing interventions are the same. Additional possible nursing diagnoses for a client with MG may include:

Nursing Diagnoses	Goals	Nursing Interventions
▶ *Breathing patterns, ineffective, related to muscle weakness.*	The client will have normal respiratory rate and rhythm and normal breath sounds bilaterally.	Monitor client's respiratory rate and rhythm and breath sounds frequently.
		Administer oxygen as ordered.
		Elevate head of the bed.
		Notify physician immediately if respiratory problem develops.
▶ *Aspiration, high risk for, related to impaired swallowing.*	The client will not experience aspiration.	Have client eat in a sitting position or with the head of the bed elevated.
		Teach client to chew food well, and swallow only small bites.
		Request a special diet of thickened, soft foods.
		Suction oral secretions as required.
		Teach client to suction secretions as needed.

Nursing Diagnoses	Goals	Nursing Interventions
▶ *Knowledge deficit related to disease process and understanding of methods to control disease and prevent complications.*	The client will describe disease process, factors contributing to symptoms, and regimen for control.	Teach client stress management techniques and methods to avoid infections. Teach clients to take medications at regularly scheduled times to maintain appropriate level.
	The client will practice health behaviors needed to deal with the effects of MG and methods to prevent complications.	Encourage client to wear a MedicAlert bracelet indicating the name and dosage of medications being taken. Refer to the Myasthenia Gravis Foundation for information and support groups (see Resources).
▶ *Urinary elimination, altered, related to decreased muscle control.*	The client will have adequate urine elimination.	Monitor I & O.
		Palpate bladder to determine fullness.
		Establish with the client a regular urine elimination program.
		Catheterize as ordered.
		Provide incontinence aids.
▶ *Communication, impaired, verbal, related to muscle weakness.*	The client will use alternate methods of communication.	Provide paper and pencil or picture board.
		Validate nonverbal communication.

▶ Evaluation

Each goal must be evaluated to determine how it has been met by the client.

▲ ▲

Sample Nursing Care Plan: A Client with Myasthenia Gravis

Mrs. Henry, a twenty-nine-year-old mother of two preschool children, was diagnosed with myasthenia gravis two years ago. Initially, she had double vision and drooping eyelids, but after beginning a course of pyridostigmine bromide (Mestinon) she went into remission. Recently, she has been experiencing facial, neck, and chest muscle weakness and is now admitted to the hospital for evaluation. Occasionally, she has difficulty swallowing and breathing. Her thymus gland is enlarged. She has asked the nurse to teach her some strategies for dealing with this chronic illness.

Nursing Diagnosis 1 Breathing pattern, ineffective, related to difficulty breathing as evidenced by facial, neck, and chest weakness.

Goals	Nursing Interventions	Rationale	Evaluation
Mrs. Henry's respiratory rate and rhythm and breath sounds will remain within normal limits.	Assess Mrs. Henry's breathing patterns q2h. Inform Mrs. Henry to notify the nurse immediately if she begins to develop any breathing difficulties. Notify physician immediately if respiratory problems develop.	Frequent client assessment detects early signs of respiratory distress. Some clients are reluctant to call the nurse and need to be encouraged to do so. When respiratory problems develop, the physician needs to determine the exact cause and if a tracheostomy is needed.	Mrs. Henry's respiratory rate and rhythm have remained within normal limits.

Nursing Diagnosis 2 Aspiration, high risk for, related to impaired swallowing as evidenced by difficulty swallowing.

Goals	Nursing Interventions	Rationale	Evaluation
Mrs. Henry will not experience aspiration.	Position Mrs. Henry to eat in a sitting position. Teach Mrs. Henry the importance of thoroughly chewing food, and swallowing only small bites. Have oral suctioning available at the bedside.	Eating in a sitting position promotes the passage of food into the stomach. Swallowing big bites of food can cause aspiration. If food or secretions become caught in the mouth or throat, suctioning may be required to remove it.	Mrs. Henry has not aspirated. She makes a point of always sitting up when eating.

Nursing Diagnosis 3 Knowledge deficit, related to disease process and understanding of methods to control effects of myasthenia gravis and prevent complications as evidenced by verbalization of need for future teaching.

Goals	Nursing Interventions	Rationale	Evaluation
Mrs. Henry will practice health behaviors needed to deal with the effects of MG and prevent complications.	Assess Mrs. Henry's prior knowledge of MG and methods of controlling the effects of prescribed medications and preventing complications.	Assessing a client prior knowledge provides a basis for planning teaching.	Mrs. Henry and her husband related information about MG, action and side effects of Mestinon, signs and symptoms to watch for, and when to notify the physician. She has obtained a MedicAlert bracelet and has contacted The Lupus Foundation. She plans to attend the next local chapter meeting.
	Include Mrs. Henry and family members in teaching sessions.	Including family members in the teaching session fosters implementation of the teaching in the home setting.	
	Teach Mrs. Henry and family members basic information about MG, the actions of anticholinesterase medication, the need to take it on a regular basis with a snack, side effects of overdose, and the importance of notifying the physician of any signs of respiratory problems or infection.	Information about one's disease, medications, and when to notify the physician is essential knowledge the client and family members need to deal with a chronic illness.	
	Encourage Mrs. Henry to wear a MedicAlert bracelet, which lists her name, diagnoses, and dosage of prescribed medications.	A MedicAlert bracelet provides accurate information to medical personnel in case of an emergency.	
	Provide Mrs. Henry with the address and telephone number of the Myasthenia Gravis Foundation and encourage her to contact them for additional information and support.	Providing a resource for additional information facilitates future attainment of knowledge and possible involvement with a support group.	

HIV/AIDS (ACQUIRED IMMUNODEFICIENCY SYNDROME)

While allergies are hypersensitive immune responses, and autoimmune diseases literally have the body attacking itself, acquired immunodeficiency syndrome (AIDS) is a disease that causes an inadequate immunological response by the body. The human immunodeficiency virus (HIV) may be acquired anytime after conception. Infection results in HIV integration into T4 cells, the progressive decline in the number of T4 cells, and replication of the virus. As this process continues, the client's immune system loses its ability to destroy infectious organisms and malignant cells.

AIDS is rapidly becoming one of the major diseases of the century, affecting all age groups throughout the world. Due to its importance and impact on nursing care, Chapter 25 deals specifically with this devastating immunological disorder.

▶ CASE STUDY

Sharon is a thirty-four-year-old divorced African American woman. Five years ago she was diagnosed with SLE. Recently, she developed a urinary tract infection that has not responded to medication. Yesterday, when she visited her physician, she complained that the pain in her hands and wrists is getting worse. She was admitted to the hospital for evaluation and rehabilitation.

Sharon has three children, ages 16, 12, and 8. Her husband divorced her several years ago. She tells you "He just couldn't take it anymore. He was working full time. When he came home he would have to do all the housework and care for the children." She now lives with her mother. Sharon used to work as an aide in a nursing home, but due to constant fatigue she had to quit.

Upon admission Sharon's vital signs were as follows: temperature 100.6, blood pressure 170/94, pulse 84, respirations 20. Physical exam revealed the presence of a butterfly rash. This is the first symptom she developed. She had hoped it would go away after she started taking prednisone (Meticorten), but it has remained. She

The following questions will guide your development of a Nursing Care Plan for the case study.

1. List signs and symptoms, other than those identified above, that clients with SLE might experience.
2. Since Sharon has a history of long term use of corticosteroids, what side effects might she experience?
3. What diagnostic tests might be ordered to evaluate her arthritic condition?
4. Write three nursing diagnoses and goals for Sharon.
5. Identify nursing interventions to help Sharon deal with the nursing diagnoses identified in number 4.
6. What teaching would be done for Sharon's home care?
7. Identify resources available to help Sharon cope with this chronic condition.

▶ CASE STUDY (continued)

relates that she does not go out in public anymore because everyone stares at her. The assessment revealed that the joints in her hands are stiff; she stated that she has difficulty using her fork.

Initial lab results are:

Urinalysis - Bacteria count greater than 100,000/milliliter
ESR - 24 mm/hr
RBCs - 3.2
WBCs - 15,035
LE Cell Test - Positive
Hemoglobin - 9.2
ANA - Positive

▶   ▶   ▶   ▶   ▶   ▶   ▶   ▶   ▶   ▶

SUMMARY

- The immune system identifies substances as self or nonself and protects the body by neutralizing or destroying foreign organisms.
- The immune system is composed of leukocytes, bone marrow, thymus gland, lymph nodes, spleen, tonsils, appendix, liver, and small intestinal cells.
- Immunity to a disease is either natural or acquired.
- Age, sex, nutritional status, medications, and stress influence the immune response.
- Clients receiving blood transfusions need to be carefully monitored, especially during the first half hour, for signs of a reaction.
- Anaphylactic reactions, which may occur as a result of exposure to foods, medications, blood, or insect bites, can potentially be life threatening.
- Organ transplant clients need to understand the implications of taking immunosuppressive medications.
- Rheumatoid arthritis, systemic lupus erythematosus, and myasthenia gravis are all chronic systemic autoimmune diseases.
- Clients with rheumatoid arthritis need to be taught methods to adapt to the effects of synovial joint inflammation, immobility, and deformity.

- Systemic lupus erythematosus affects multiple body systems.
- Clients with myasthenia gravis experience extreme muscle weakness and fatigue and need to be carefully monitored for signs of respiratory distress, and myasthenic or cholinergic crisis.

Review Questions

1. Ms. Caldwell has just been diagnosed with syphilis and has an order for 1,000,000 units of penicillin I.M. She has no history of allergies to medications. She has never had penicillin. When giving her the injection in the right upper outer quadrant of her buttocks, you note a tattoo. Several minutes after receiving the injection, she tells you she feels anxious and weak. You note she is diaphoretic, scratching her forearm, and is breathing faster than normal. Based upon this assessment data, you would conclude:

   a. she is embarrassed because you saw her tatoo.
   b. she is probably anxious since you know she has a sexually transmitted disease.
   c. her syphilis is getting worse.
   d. these are early signs of an anaphylactic reaction.

2. Which of the following is a potentially life-threatening transfusion reaction?

   a. acute hemolytic reaction
   b. allergic urticarial reaction
   c. delayed hemolytic reaction
   d. febrile nonhemolytic reaction

3. Organ transplant clients living at home and taking immunosuppressive medications, should be encouraged to:

   a. do their grocery shopping on weekends when the stores are busiest.
   b. notify their physician if side effects to their medications develop.
   c. put on a mask as soon as they get up and wear it all day.
   d. stop taking their medications if they develop a respiratory infection.

4. Sensitivity to sunlight, a butterfly rash, and renal failure are symptoms of which of the following conditions?

   a. anaphylaxis
   b. myasthenia gravis
   c. rheumatoid arthritis
   d. systemic lupus erythematosus

5. Rheumatoid arthritis is:

   a. an autoimmune disease characterized by abnormal IgG antibodies.
   b. associated with abnormal B-cell lymphocytes.
   c. curable if the client takes large doses of Plaquenil Sulfate.
   d. the results of a hypersensitivity reaction.

6. Increased muscle weakness, difficulty chewing or swallowing, and shortness of breath in clients with myasthenia gravis are signs of:

   a. cholinergic crisis.
   b. myasthenia crisis.
   c. both cholinergic crisis and myasthenic crisis.
   d. reaction to plasmapheresis.

7. A side effect of corticosteroid medications is:

   a. dehydration.
   b. hypotension.
   c. low glucose levels.
   d. increased susceptibility to infection.

8. Surgical removal of the thymus gland is useful in controlling symptoms of which of the following conditions?

   a. an anaphylactic reaction
   b. myasthenia gravis
   c. rheumatoid arthritis
   d. systemic lupus erythematosus

Medical Terminology

auto-	self
autologous	from the same organism (person)
cyte-	cell
hyper-	excessive
hypersensitivity	an excessive reaction to a stimulus
hypo-	deficient
hypoxia	lack of an adequate amount of oxygen
immuno-	involving the immune system
immunotherapy	treatment to enhance immunological functioning

Critical Thinking Questions

1. What are the lifestyle implications of being diagnosed with a chronic disease such as rheumatoid arthritis or systemic lupus erythematosus?

2. What are the pros and cons about receiving a blood transfusion from a donor?

News Flash: Clients and Nurses are Having Allergic Reactions to Latex Gloves

An operating room nurse switched to vinyl gloves after experiencing severe urticaria to latex. She later required Epinephrine IV to correct the blood pressure drop, rapid pulse, and bronchospasms she developed during the C-section delivery of her child. A pediatric client with a history of periorbital and facial swelling after blowing up balloons started wheezing and became hypotensive during surgery. Both had a systemic allergic reaction to latex.

Although gloves are the most common source of latex exposure in the hospital environment, other items are made of this product. Latex plungers at the end of syringes and stoppers for multidose vials are found on most units. Blood pressure cuffs, stethoscope tubing, manual resuscitation bags, face masks, tourniquets used to start IVs, cloth adhesive tape, urinary catheters, enteral feeding tubes, catheters used for lower GI x-rays, and nasal airways may all contain latex. It is thought that latex particles become airborne and can be inhaled.

Latex, today, must be considered as a possible allergen. Nurses caring for clients suspected of having an allergy to latex should wear vinyl gloves, use equipment made of an alterative substance, if at all possible, and inform other health care providers of the client's allergy. Posting signs on the door and over the bed, furnishing an allergy band, and labeling the chart will ensure this (*Fritsch & Fredrick, 1993*).

CHAPTER
25
HIV Disorders

David K. Miller
Cheryl McGaffic

LIST OF DISORDERS

LEARNING OBJECTIVES

Upon completion of this chapter the learner should be able to:
• Define key terms.
• Explain the modes of transmission related to HIV.
• State risk reduction methods for health care workers.

- Compare and contrast cell-mediated and humoral immunity.
- Discuss diagnostic testing associated with HIV.

- Describe the management of the HIV/AIDS client including medication and diet therapy.
- Assist in formulating a Nursing Care Plan for the HIV/AIDS client.

▶ MAKING THE CONNECTION

Refer to the topics in the following chapters to increase your understanding of HIV disorders:

INTRODUCTION

The Global Programme on AIDS (GPA) estimates that 16 million adults and more than one million children have been infected with the **human immunodeficiency virus (HIV)** since the beginning of the pandemic in 1980 (Global AIDS News, 1994). By the year 2000, it is estimated that there will be 100 million people worldwide infected with HIV. In the United States, there were 513,486 cases of AIDS reported to the Centers for Disease Control and Prevention as of December 31, 1995, and it is estimated that more than one million persons are currently infected with HIV (CDC, 1992, 1995a).

In June 1981, the first description of what would eventually be referred to as **acquired immunodeficiency syndrome (AIDS)** was reported (CDC, 1981). It is important to understand that infection with HIV and AIDS are not the same thing. Studies of the history of HIV infection have documented a wide spectrum of

disease conditions ranging from asymptomatic infection to life-threatening illnesses characterized by severe immunodeficiency, infections, and cancers (CDC, 1992). Most people assume that infection with HIV progresses to AIDS in all cases. It is uncertain whether all persons infected with HIV will progress to AIDS. Thus far, only 35 percent of those infected with HIV have progressed to AIDS (Muma, Borucki, Lyons, & Pollard, 1991). More recently, individuals have been identified who are known to be infected with HIV for more than ten years and have not demonstrated any symptoms of AIDS-related illnesses (Buchbinder, Mann, & Louie, 1993). The different presentations of HIV disease are considered to be a continuum of responses to HIV infection and not separate syndromes.

In the United States, HIV disease is classified according to CD4 T-lymphocyte count and clinical conditions associated with HIV infection. The continuum of HIV infection, as shown in Figure 25-1, includes acute infection, asymptomatic stage, early symptomatic stage,

620 UNIT 7 ▶ Body Defenses

late symptomatic stage, and advanced HIV disease (Flaskerud & Ungvarski, 1995). In general, most persons are able to work and continue their activities of daily living until the late symptomatic stage and advanced HIV disease which is defined as AIDS. In the acute infection stage, severe flu-like symptoms occur in 90 percent of people within one to three weeks after infection. The next stage is the asymptomatic period. Early during the asymptomatic stage, most persons develop positive antibodies to HIV in two to eighteen weeks. Persons can remain asymptomatic for ten years or more; however, other factors such as drug use, sexual activity, and socioeconomic status have hastened progression to later stages of HIV disease (Melnick, et al., 1994; Singer, 1994). The early symptomatic stage develops when the CD4 T-cell count is 500 cells/mm³. The person may experience fever, night sweats, weight loss, and lymphadenopathy. Clinical conditions in this stage include candidiasis (oropharyngeal and vulvovaginal), cervical dysplasia, herpes zoster, pelvic inflammatory disease, listeriosis, and peripheral neuropathy (CDC, 1992). The next stage is the late symp-

tomatic stage. At this stage the infection has reached the CDC criteria for AIDS.

When CD4 T-cell count drops to less than 200 cells/mm³ the client develops **opportunistic infections** and cancers. Opportunistic infections are caused by a wide variety of organisms. Most of these organisms are not pathogenic and rarely cause disease in the person with an intact immune system. The immunocompromised person's immune defense system is so damaged that it is unable to fight off these organisms and cancer cells. At this stage, infections and cancers are generally treatable (Flaskerud & Ungvarski, 1995). The last stage of the HIV continuum is advanced HIV disease. The CD4 T-cell count is less than 50 cells/mm³ persons may have multiple opportunistic infections and cancers that are less likely to respond to treatment.

Current approaches to treatment of HIV infection include the following:

- Medications that inhibit replication of HIV
- Prophylactic medications to prevent development of certain opportunistic infections
- Medications to treat opportunistic infections

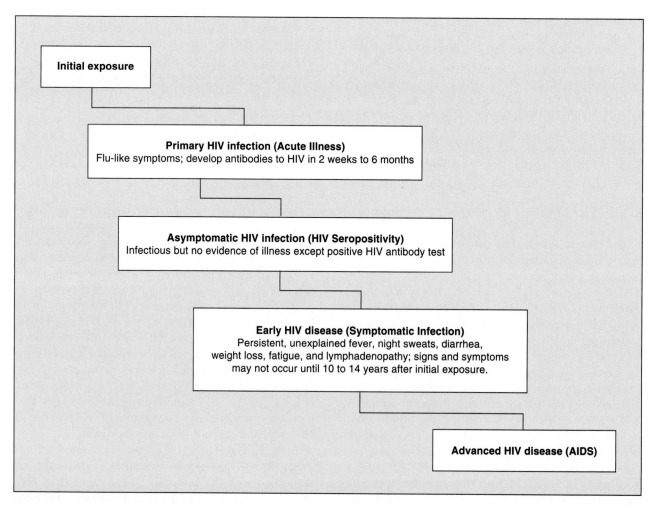

FIGURE 25-1 Continuum of HIV disease.

Until recently, the use of nucleoside analog antiretrovirals (medications that inhibit replication of HIV) such as zidovudine (Retrovir, AZT), didanosine, ddl (Videx) and zalcitabine (Hivid) individually or in combination were the treatment for HIV infection when the CD4 T-cell level was less than 500/mm^3. Although treatment with these nucleoside analogues have been shown to decrease the frequency of opportunistic infections and slow the progression of disease, long-term treatment with these drugs causes strains of HIV to become resistant to them. Three new medications that inhibit replication of HIV, called protease inhibitors have been developed. These protease inhibitors attack HIV at a different stage of the life cycle than the nucleoside analogues. Preliminary results from several large studies suggest that protease inhibitors in combination with nucleoside analogues have slowed progression, decreased amounts of HIV in the blood, and prolonged time until death as compared to traditional treatment with only nucleoside analogues (Collier, et al., 1996).

Prophylactic treatment against opportunistic infections is recommended for persons with a CD4 T lymphocyte count of 200 cells/microliter or less to prevent the most common infections associated with AIDS. Drug therapy to prevent or delay the occurrence of ***Pneumocystis carinii* pneumonia (PCP)**, bacteremia due to ***Mycobacterium avium* complex (MAC)**, and invasive fungal disease are currently recommended (Finkelstein, et al., 1996). Treatment of opportunistic infections, which arise as the immune system progressively weakens, involves a combination of antibiotics, antineoplastic agents, and medications to manage distressing symptoms (diarrhea, loss of appetite, pain) associated with advanced HIV disease.

Demographics of AIDS in the United States

Age

AIDS mainly affects people during the most productive years of their life. In 1993, HIV infection became the most common cause of death among persons ages twenty-five to forty-four (CDC, 1996).

Sex

Trends in HIV-related mortality reflect changes in the demographic patterns of the HIV epidemic. Although more men than women are infected with HIV, the number of AIDS cases in women in the United States has increased by more than 1,000 percent (Cohen & Atwood, 1994). From 1993 to 1994, the death rate for HIV infection for white men did not change, rates for women and black men increased, and the rate for black women ages twenty-five to forty-four surpassed that for white men in that age group (CDC, 1996).

Race

Although whites account for the majority of AIDS cases, African Americans and Hispanic Americans are affected by AIDS in numbers greater than their relative percentages in the population. For example, African Americans constitute 12 percent of the population in the United States, yet they represent 29 percent of reported AIDS cases (Quinn, 1993). Of pediatric AIDS cases, 53 percent are black. Racial differences in death rates for HIV infection probably reflect social, behavioral, and other factors associated with HIV transmission.

Modes of Transmission

HIV is transmitted via exchange of body fluids. These body fluids include blood, blood products, semen, vaginal fluids, and breast milk. Theoretically, HIV is present in sufficient quantities in amniotic fluid, cerebrospinal fluid, pleural fluid, peritoneal fluid, pericardial fluid whereby infection could occur with exchange of these body fluids, particularly in health care settings where contact with these fluids may occur. HIV is not transmitted in saliva, urine, or tears. Certain actions and/or behaviors place people at a higher risk of contracting the virus. Sexual intercourse (anal, oral, vaginal) without using a condom is the most frequently reported risk behavior for infection with HIV. Behaviors associated with increased risk of sexual transmission of HIV by infected persons include unprotected sexual intercourse, multiple sex partners, failure to disclose HIV status, and trading sex for money or drugs (CDC, 1996b). The use of crack cocaine has also been linked to HIV transmission as individuals under the influence of this narcotic are less likely to use preventive measures during sexual intercourse. Injecting-drug use is the second most frequently reported risk behavior for infection with HIV. As of December 31, 1995, 36 percent of AIDS cases were associated with injecting-drug use (CDC, 1996). Until recently, the risk of transmission of HIV from an infected mother to her newborn infant ranged between 14 and 40 percent. A recent government-sponsored study showed that HIV seropositive women who took zidovudine (AZT) during pregnancy and labor, as well as giving zidovudine to the newborn, reduced perinatal transmission to 8.3 percent (Lindberg, 1995).

Prevention

The CDC and the Occupational Safety and Health Administration (OSHA) have developed recommendations to reduce the risk of exposure to blood and body fluids. No risk of transmission exists for the individual who practices sexual abstinence and who does not share needles while injecting drugs. If these are not viable options, the individual can reduce the risk of transmission by using sterilized injection paraphernalia, cleaning injection paraphernalia with full-strength bleach, and by having protected sexual intercourse (using a latex condom). The use of spermicides (nonoxynol-9) with condom use was once recommended. It is now thought that spermicides may increase transmission of HIV through irritation of the rectal or vaginal mucosa (Tierney, 1995).

For the health care worker, the risk of contracting HIV is greatest with percutaneous exposures (needle-stick) to HIV-infected blood. This risk is 0.3 percent or one in two hundred when HIV-infected blood comes in contact with blood or mucous membranes of the health care worker. Personal protective equipment should be worn while caring for all clients to decrease the risk of HIV infection and to decrease the risk of exposure to other bloodborne pathogens such as hepatitis. This equipment includes gloves, gowns, face shields, and masks. This equipment should be worn when there is a reasonable likelihood of contact with any blood or body fluids. These barriers are not necessary for direct care of clients where there is no contact with body fluids (see Table 25-1). All medical sharps, including needles and scalpels, should be discarded immediately into sharps containers (see Figure 25-2). Never reuse or recap needles. These recommendations developed in 1985 were called universal precautions. Universal precautions were intended to protect both the client and the health care worker from exposure to blood and other body fluids. In 1996, after years of research, the CDC updated universal precautions to **standard precautions** (see Figure 25-3). These new guidelines combine previous information from both universal precautions and body substance isolation, and provide new information on protection from drug resistant pathogens and airborne diseases. When using standard precautions, the health care worker is operating under the assumption that all clients, not just those known to have bloodborne diseases such as HIV, are potentially infectious. The Occupational Safety and Health Administration (OSHA) mandates that health care workers follow standard precautions and that their employers provide appropriate resources for them to do so.

ANATOMY AND PHYSIOLOGY REVIEW

Leukocytes or WBCs have a major role in the immune system. They are formed mostly in the bone marrow and partially in the lymph tissue. After formation, they are transported to different parts of the body where they fight infectious organisms. There are six types of WBCs normally found in the blood. They are neutrophils, eosinophils, basophils, monocytes, lymphocytes, and, occasionally plasma cells (Guyton & Hall, 1996). Adults have about 7,000 WBCs/mm³ of blood. Each type is a percentage of the total number of WBCs (see Table 25-2).

The neutrophils and monocytes (which become macrophages) attack and destroy invading bacteria, viruses, and other injurious agents. Eosinophils are responsible for killing parasites and moderating allergic reactions. Basophils play an important role in allergic reactions. There are two types of lymphocytes: B-lymphocytes or B-cells, and T-lymphocytes, or T-cells. These cells are responsible for acquired immunity whereas the other WBCs are responsible for innate immunity.

The acquired immune response in humans can be divided into two broad categories based on the type of cells. In humoral immunity, the body develops circulating antibodies which are important in attacking the invading agent. The B-cells are responsible for this type of immunity. The second type of acquired immunity is called cell-mediated immunity or T-cell immunity. With T-cell mediated immunity, there is a formation of large numbers of activated lymphocytes that are specifically designed to destroy the foreign agent. T-cells include helper cells (CD4), suppressor cells (CD8), and killer (cytotoxic) cells. The CD4 T-helper cells are the major regulators of all immune functions and help in the functions of the immune system in many ways (Guyton & Hall, 1996). The helper cells are very important because they stimulate growth of the suppressor cells, B-cells, and activate macrophages. So either directly or indirectly, the T-helper cells are responsible for the function of other cells in the immune system. Although little is known about the T-suppressor cells, they seem to suppress the function of both the helper and killer cells. The cytotoxic T-cell directly kills microorganisms and at times, even some of the body's own cells. CD4 and CD8 are molecules on the T-helper and T-suppressor cells and are important in understanding how HIV attacks the immune system.

HIV infection affects the immune system and the brain. In the immune system, the main characteristic of HIV infection is progressive depletion of the CD4-T helper cells. The normal ratio of T-helper cells to T-suppressor cells (CD4: CD8 ratio) is 2:1. As immunodeficiency worsens, it is not uncommon for the CD4:CD8 ratio to fall as low as 0:1. The altered T-helper cells causes malfunction of the B-cells and macrophages and leads to collapse of the immune system. HIV also affects the CD4 molecule present on microglial cells in the brain causing memory loss and other brain dysfunctions.

HIV is a retrovirus. Retroviruses use RNA to make DNA copies which then become part of the genetic material of the human cell. It is because this is a rever-

Table 25-1

EXAMPLES OF PERSONAL PROTECTIVE EQUIPMENT USED IN COMMON CLIENT CARE TASKS

Note: There are exceptions to every rule. Use this chart as a guide only. Add personal protective equipment in special situations, such as splashing. Follow your facility policies for use of protective equipment in routine tasks.

Task	Gloves	Gown	Goggles/Face Shield	Surgical Mask
Controlling bleeding (squirting blood)	Yes	Yes	Yes	Yes
Wiping a wheelchair or shower chair with disinfectant solution	Yes	No	No	No
Emptying a catheter bag	Yes	No	Yes, if facility policy	Yes, if facility policy
Serving a meal tray	No	No	No	No
Giving a back rub to a client who has intact skin	No	No	No	No
Giving oral care	Yes	No	No	No
Cleaning a client and changing the bed after an episode of diarrhea	Yes	Yes, if facility policy	No	No
Taking an oral temperature with a glass thermometer (gloves are not necessary with an electronic thermometer)	Yes	No	No	No
Taking a rectal temperature	Yes	No	No	No
Taking a blood pressure	No	No	No	No
Cleaning soiled client care utensils, such as bedpans	Yes	Yes, if splashing is likely	Yes, if splashing is likely	Yes, if splashing is likely
Shaving a client with a disposable razor	Yes, because of the high risk of this procedure for contact with blood	No	No	No
Giving eye care	Yes	No	No	No
Giving special mouth care to an unconscious client	Yes	No, unless coughing is likely	No, unless coughing is likely	No, unless coughing is likely
Washing the client's genital area	Yes	No	No	No
Washing the client's arms and legs when the skin is not broken	No	No	No	No

sal of the usual DNA-to-RNA transcription of genetic information that these viruses are called retroviruses. In the case of HIV, a protein on the virus surface called gp120 attaches to the CD4 molecule. After this, HIV enters the cell and is uncoated. Then through a series of steps, the viral RNA copies itself to make DNA. The DNA then goes to the human cell nucleus, and eventually a new virus emerges from the human cell.

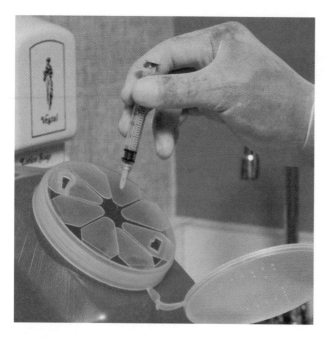

FIGURE 25-2   Sharps container.

Diagnostic Testing

The **enzyme-linked immunosorbent assay (ELISA)** is the basic screening test currently used to detect antibodies to HIV. Viral proteins are immobilized on plastic beads or multiwell trays (Crowe & Mills, 1994). Test serum containing antibodies to HIV will bind to these viral proteins. An enzyme-linked anti-human **antibody** added to the reaction will bind to the complex and can then can be detected. The ELISA is highly sensitive and inexpensive to perform. A sample testing positive is always retested to rule out false positive results and/or technician error. A person who receives a negative test and continues high risk behaviors should consider being retested every three months. Another reason for being retested is the "window period," the time between when a person is infected with HIV and the time it takes for antibodies to HIV to be detected. In most people, this takes from two to eight weeks. Persons who are infected with HIV

STANDARD PRECAUTIONS FOR INFECTION CONTROL

Wash Hands (Plain soap)
Wash after touching blood, body fluids, secretions, excretions, and contaminated items. Wash immediately after gloves are removed and between patient contacts. Avoid transfer of microorganisms to other patients or environments.

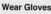

Wear Gloves
Wear when touching blood, body fluids, secretions, excretions, and contaminated items. Put on clean gloves just before touching mucous membranes and nonintact skin. Change gloves between tasks and procedures on the same patient after contact with material that may contain high concentrations of microorganisms. Remove gloves promptly after use, before touching noncontaminated items and environmental surfaces, and before going to another patient, and wash hands immediately to avoid transfer of microorganisms to other patients or environments.

Wear Mask and Eye Protection or Face Shield
Protect mucous membranes of the eyes, nose and mouth during procedures and patient-care activities that are likely to generate splashes or sprays of blood, body fluids, secretions, or excretions.

Wear Gown
Protect skin and prevent soiling of clothing during procedures that are likely to generate splashes or sprays of blood, body fluids, secretions, or excretions. Remove a soiled gown as promptly as possible and wash hands to avoid transfer of microorganisms to other patients or environments.

Patient-Care Equipment
Handle used patient-care equipment soiled with blood, body fluids, secretions, or excretions in a manner that prevents skin and mucous membrane exposures, contamination of clothing, and transfer of microorganisms to other patients and environments. Ensure that reusable equipment is not used for the care of another patient until it has been appropriately cleaned and reprocessed and single use items are properly discarded.

STANDARD PRECAUTIONS FOR INFECTION CONTROL (Continued)

Environmental Control
Follow hospital procedures for routine care, cleaning, and disinfection of environmental surfaces, beds, bed-rails, bedside equipment and other frequently touched surfaces.

Linen
Handle, transport, and process used linen soiled with blood, body fluids, secretions, or excretions in a manner that prevents exposure and contamination of clothing, and avoids transfer of microorganisms to other patients and environments.

Occupational Health and Bloodborne Pathogens
Prevent injuries when using needles, scalpels, and other sharp instruments or devices; when handling sharp instruments after procedures; when cleaning used instruments; and when disposing of used needles.

Never recap used needles using both hands or any other technique that involves directing the point of a needle towards any part of the body; rather, use either a one-handed "scoop" technique or a mechanical device designed for holding the needle sheath.

Do not remove used needles from disposable syringes by hand, and do not bend, break, or otherwise manipulate used needles by hand. Place used disposable syringes and needles, scalpels, blades, and other sharp items in puncture-resistant sharps containers located as close as practical to the area in which the items were used, and place reusable syringes and needles in a puncture-resistant container for transport to the reprocessing area.

Use resuscitation devices as an alternative to mouth-to-mouth resuscitation.

Patient Placement
Use a private room for a patient who contaminates the environment or who does not (or cannot be expected to) assist in maintaining appropriate hygiene or environmental control. Consult Infection Control if a private room is not available.

FIGURE 25-3   Standard precautions. (*Courtesy of BREVIS Corporation, Salt Lake City, UT*)

Table 25-2

PERCENTAGES OF DIFFERENT WBC TYPES	
Neutrophils	55%–70%
Eosinophils	1%–4%
Basophils	0.5%–1.0%
Monocytes	2%–8%
Lymphocytes	20%–40%

and who have not had time for antibodies to be made may test negative but may actually be HIV positive.

A confirmatory test, the **Western blot,** is always employed when the ELISA test is positive. This test is more expensive and takes several days longer to interpret than the ELISA. The Western blot detects antibodies to HIV by passing a current through a gel containing viral proteins to separate antibodies by weight. Results of both the ELISA and Western blot taken together have an accuracy rate of greater than 99 percent.

A third test that is available is the polymerase chain reaction (PCR). The PCR detects HIV-specific DNA. This test is very sensitive and costly. However, the PCR is beneficial in diagnosing HIV serostatus in newborns. Because infants can passively acquire maternal antibodies for eighteen months, the ELISA and Western Blot tests will be positive due to the mother's antibodies present in the infant's blood. The PCR can help distinguish between actual infection in the infant and maternally acquired antibodies.

There are two tasks that the nurse should complete before HIV testing is initiated. The first task is pretest counseling. Very detailed, specific guidelines have been developed for pre- and posttest counseling (American Medical Association, 1988; CDC, 1995a). In general, physicians are responsible for counseling their clients; however, the nurse's role includes clarifying and providing additional information. Essential elements of pre-test counseling should include the following :

- Asking why the client believes the test should be done
- Explaining the meaning of a positive or negative test
- The possibilities of a false-positive test
- Discussing risk reduction and ways to modify behavior
- Confidentiality of test results and state reporting requirements
- Potential benefits of anonymous testing
- Stress often related to test results and possible reactions to learning the results such as depression or anxiety
- Potential negative social consequences of being tested and being seropositive
- Assisting the client in making a decision about testing
- Arranging a return appointment to receive test results.

Assessment of risk-taking behaviors, taking a sexual history, and education about the difference between HIV and AIDS and methods of transmission should also be provided. The interview should begin with open-ended questions and progress with specific, nonjudgmental questions.

The second task is to obtain a signed informed consent (see Figure 25-4). Most states mandate a consent form solely for HIV testing. However, some states now allow verbal consent and a statement of the client's consent signed by the health care provider. The cost of testing ranges from free to $200 depending on the type of facility providing the testing services. Anonymous testing, whereby the client is identified by number only is available in most states. The time it takes to get results varies from a few days to several weeks depending on the testing site.

Posttest counseling should include reviewing the test results, assessing the client's understanding, allowing the client to express feelings, reviewing routes of transmission, assessing the client's psychological condition including the risk for suicide, assessing the client's risk behavior and strategies for reducing risk, and providing information about support groups and national/local resources (American Medical Association, 1988).

COMMON DIAGNOSTIC TESTS

The following is a table of the commonly used diagnostic tests for clients with HIV disorders.

Test	Explanation/Normal Values	Nursing Responsibilities
enzyme-linked immunosorbent assay (ELISA)	Screening test for the presence of antibodies to HIV. Norm = negative	Pre-test counseling. Obtain informed consent. Post-test counseling.
Western blot	Confirmatory test for the presence of antibodies to HIV. Norm = negative	Pre-test counseling. Obtain informed consent. Post-test counseling.

(continued)

PATIENT CONSENT TO RECEIVE
COMMUNICABLE DISEASE BLOOD TEST

I,_____ , am a patient of Dr._____ ("Physician"). My physician/infection control officer has informed me that he/she recommends that I receive a blood test for the virus which is the probable cause of Acquired Immune Deficiency Syndrome ("AIDS").

I understand that the blood tests for the virus which is the probable cause of Acquired Immune Deficiency Syndrome ("AIDS") are not 100% accurate, and that these blood tests sometimes produce false positive or false negative test results. I further understand that the presence of antibodies means that a person probably has been infected with the AIDS virus, but does not necessarily mean that a person will develop AIDS.

I acknowledge the following:
1. That the general nature of my condition has been explained to me.
2. That the above stated test and information regarding the test have been explained to me.
3. I understand that when the blood sample is taken, I may have some slight discomfort at the site of entry of the needle and a small bruise may develop; otherwise there is litttle risk of physical injury.
4. I understand that a positive test does not mean that I have AIDS.
5. I understand that there is a slight chance that I may have the AIDS virus even if my test is negative.
6. I understand that a positive test result could cause psychological stress for me and that a positive test could be used to discriminate against me should it not be kept confidential.
7. That reasonable alternatives to the above stated test have been explained to me.
8. That my consent to the above stated test is voluntary.

I understand that the Physician will notify me of the results of the blood tests and the results will be explained to me. (Place your initials below where applicable)

_____ I authorize the Hospital to furnish my insurance companies and other third party payers with any and all information it has or may hereafter have, either written or oral, pertaining to or in any manner connected with the tests authorized herein, that may aid in payment of any account presented to me or us, jointly or severally, and I further agree that no person, firm or corporation shall be held liable in any manner for furnishing or having furnished such information.

_____ I do not consent to the release of the nature of the test(s) to my insurance company or medical assistance program.

Subject to the foregoing, the Hospital, to the best of its ability, will not disclose the results of this test to others except to the extent required by law or except to the extent such disclosure is required in order to safeguard the well-being of patients and employees at the Hospital or other persons at risk.

On this basis, I authorize the Hospital, Physician and anyone authorized by them to perform the blood test as described, and I understand that my signature below acknowledges:
1. My understanding of the plan described herein;
2. My understanding of the information about AIDS and the blood test that has been given to me;
3. I have been given full opportunity to ask questions to obtain further information;
4. All of my questions have been answered to my satisfaction;
5. My refusal or consent to the testing described is shown by my signature below;
6. That the test results may be disclosed as provided herein.

I consent to the test described herein.

_____   _____
(Patient signature)   (Date)

_____   _____   _____
(Physician/infection control officer signature)   (Date)   (Witness over eighteen years of age)

I refuse the test described herein.

_____   _____
(Patient signature)   (Date)

FIGURE 25-4 Informed consent—Communicable disease blood test.

Test	Explanation/Normal Values	Nursing Responsibilities
polymerase chain reaction (PCR)	Detects HIV-specific DNA (virus). Normal = negative	Explain meaning of test. Follow-up explanation of test results.
CD4 T-cell count	Predictor of HIV progression, baseline taken after positive HIV test. Norm = 500–1000/mm^3 Critical value = <200/mm^3	Explain meaning of test. Follow-up explanation of test results.

KEY ABBREVIATIONS

The following abbreviations and acronyms are used in this chapter:

ABC	antigen-binding capacity
ADC	AIDS dementia complex
AFB	acid-fast bacillus
AIDS	acquired immunodeficiency syndrome
CDC	Centers for Disease Control and Prevention
CMV	cytomegalovirus
CIN	cervical intraepithelial neoplasia
CSF	cerebrospinal fluid
ELISA	enzyme-linked immunosorbent assay
GPA	Global Programme on AIDS
HBV	hepatitis B virus
HCV	hepatitis C virus
HDV	hepatitis D virus
HIV	human immunodeficiency virus
HPV	human papilloma virus
KS	Kaposi's sarcoma
MAC	*Mycobacterium avium* complex
MDR-TB	multidrug-resistant tuberculosis
NHL	non-Hodgkin's lymphoma
OHL	oral hairy leukoplakia
PaCO$_2$	partial pressure of carbon dioxide in the arterial blood
PCP	*Pneumocystis carinii* pneumonia
PPD	purified protein derivative
SaO$_2$	percentage saturation of hemoglobin with oxygen in arterial blood
TB	tuberculosis
TPN	total parenteral nutrition

▶ PULMONARY MANIFESTATIONS

▶ *Pneumocystis carinii* Pneumonia

Pneumocystis carinii pneumonia (PCP) occurs in over 53 percent of clients with AIDS, each episode has a 10 percent mortality rate, and it is the most common opportunistic infection associated with advanced HIV disease (CDC, 1995b). A marked decrease in the number of AIDS clients diagnosed with PCP is due to initiation of prophylactic treatment when the CD4 T-cell count is 200 or less/mm^3. Although *Pneumocystis carinii* is found primarily in the lungs, it has also been reported in the adrenal glands, bone marrow, skin, thyroid, kidneys, and spleen of persons with AIDS.

Clinical signs and symptoms include fever, shortness of breath, nonproductive cough, and crackles. Initial diagnosis is made by chest x-ray, which shows diffuse infiltrates. Fiberoptic bronchoscopy is the procedure of choice to obtain a definitive diagnosis. During the bronchoscopy sputum is obtained to demonstrate the presence of the organism. Saline is inserted into the bronchoscope and specimens are obtained for diagnosis. If the client is unable to tolerate the bronchoscopic procedure, sputum is induced. Sputum induction consists of having the client inhale an aerosolized solution of 3 percent saline. The client is encouraged to cough and expectorate the sputum or the sputum is suctioned by the health care worker.

Current standard treatment for PCP includes either intravenous pentamidine isothionate (Pneumopent, Pentam 300) or sulfamethoxazole-trimethoprim (SMZ-TMP, Bactrim, Septra), given orally or intravenously (Ungvarski, 1991). Oral SMZ-TMP is the treatment of choice; however, approximately one-third of people with AIDS eventually develop hypersensitivity reactions and must switch to pentamidine for primary therapy. Either SMZ-TMP or pentamidine is given for twenty-one days. Prophylaxis against PCP is a therapeutic necessity for all persons infected with HIV when the CD4 T-cell count is 200 or less. Primary prophylaxis refers to therapy for those considered at risk for PCP based on the CD4 count to prevent infection with PCP. Secondary prophylaxis refers to therapy to prevent recurrences in clients who have already had PCP. Current guidelines recommend either oral SMZ-TMP or aerosolized pentamidine for prophylaxis. One double strength (DS) SMZ-TMP three to five times per week is recommended. For those allergic to SMZ-TMP, pentamidine diluted in sterile water administered by a Respigard II nebulizer can be used.

It is very important that proper technique is used when administering aerosolized pentamidine because aerosolized pentamidine may also pose a risk to health care workers administering the medication. Care must be taken to ensure that the nebulizer is properly administered, that large quantities of pentamidine are not released into the air through the mouthpiece and that pentamidine is not administered in poorly venti-lated rooms. Adverse reactions may include a scratchy throat, burning eyes, reduced lung function, and con-junctivitis.

▶ *Histoplasmosis*

Histoplasmosis is an infection caused by the fungus *Histoplasma capsulatum*. The fungus has been iso-lated in bird droppings, dirt from chicken coops, and caves. The spores from the fungus are introduced into the body by inhalation. Histoplasmosis is not specific to the lung. In most clients with HIV disease, histo-plasmosis is **disseminated** (spread out). Histoplasmo-sis should be suspected if the person presents with fever of uncertain origin, cough, and malaise.

The diagnosis is confirmed by culture or biopsy of the bone marrow, blood, lymph nodes, lungs, or skin. Initial treatment of histoplasmosis consists of IV amphotericin B (Amphotericin B) (Muma, Lyons, Borucki, & Pollard, 1994). Oral ketoconazole (Nizoral) can be used for maintenance therapy. The CDC has recently recommended prophylaxis against reoccur-rence of histoplasmosis with itraconazole (Sporanox) (CDC, 1995b).

▶ *Tuberculosis*

Mycobacterium tuberculosis, an acid-fast aerobic bacterium, is the cause of tuberculosis (TB). It is spread through airborne particles and enters the body by inhalation. The particles usually lodge in the apex of the lungs; however, one-half to two-thirds of cases of HIV-associated or AIDS-associated TB involve organs outside the lungs as well (Allen & Ownby, 1991). Tuberculosis is more prevalent in medically under-served populations, foreign-born persons from areas of the world with a high prevalence, homeless persons,

correctional-facility inmates, alcoholics, injecting drug users, the elderly, and people with compromised im-mune systems (CDC, 1994).

Clinical manifestations include fever, night sweats, cough, and weight loss. People with AIDS will com-monly present with a productive cough and pleuritic pain (Allen & Ownby, 1991). Diagnosis is made by a combination of tests: skin testing with purified protein derivative (PPD); examination and culture of sputum, urine, and other fluids; x-rays; and other tests such as IVP.

The Mantoux test is the most common test for expo-sure to TB. The Mantoux skin test consists of injecting 0.1ml of (PPD) intradermally. The Mantoux skin test can detect TB 2 to 12 weeks after exposure. If infection is present, a skin reaction of redness and hardened swelling begins as soon as six hours after injection and reaches maximum size within thirty-six to sixty hours after injection. Induration of 10 mm or greater within forty-eight hours after injection is considered positive for TB. However, a negative reaction does not rule out infection. HIV positive clients with a CD4 count lower than 200/mm^3 may no longer have an immune response to the PPD. The chest x-ray may reveal mid-dle and lower lobe infiltrates. Sputum is obtained by having the client inhale 3 percent sodium chloride, which induces deep coughing. The sample is smeared and stained with an acid-fast stain, then examined under the microscope for acid-fast bacillus (AFB). Other body fluids such as urine, blood, and stool may also be tested for AFB.

The risks of transmission for health care workers are highest during and immediately after procedures that induce coughing (Allen & Ownby, 1991). In the home and health care setting, cough-inducing proce-dures should be performed only in well-ventilated areas. A densely woven, snug-fitting mask (particulate respirator) should be worn by all persons in contact with the person who has TB until the person has received treatment for two to three weeks. Persons with TB should also be taught to cover their mouths while coughing and should wear a particulate respira-tor when they are out of their room for tests.

Outbreaks of multidrug-resistant TB (MDR-TB) have occurred in several states, and the HIV epidemic is contributing to the steady increase of drug-resistant cases. Due to the upsurge of drug-resistant TB, the CDC recommends treating with multiple medications (CDC, 1994). Treatment is provided in two phases. In the initial treatment phase the client receives isoniazid (Laniazid INH), rifampin (Rifadin), pyrazinamide and ethambutol HCl (Myambutol) or streptomycin sulfate for two to six months depending on whether *Myco-bacterium tuberculosis* is identified outside the lungs. In the continuation phase, treatment with two to four of the medications used in the initial phase is indicated for four to six months longer.

▶ Nursing Process

▶ Assessment

Subjective Data Assess client's self-evaluation of own ability to dress, bathe, ambulate, and so on. Assess client's perception of breathlessness.

Objective Data Assess the client's respiratory rate, depth, and breath sounds. Assess for cough (productive or nonproductive), cyanosis, dyspnea, use of accessory muscles, and fever. Monitor arterial blood gases (ABG) results for decreased PaO_2, increased $PaCO_2$ and decreased pH.

▼ ▼

Possible nursing diagnoses for the HIV positive client with pulmonary disorders may include:

Nursing Diagnoses	Goals	Nursing Interventions
▶ Airway clearance, ineffective, related to chronic, unrelieved cough, pain, or viscous secretions.	The client will mobilize secretions effectively.	Administer 2.5 to 3 liters of fluid per day (oral or IV) to decrease thick secretions. Administer medications as ordered to suppress cough and decrease pain. Reposition the client every two hours and PRN.
▶ Gas exchange, impaired, related to inadequate ventilation/oxygenation.	The client will maintain an SaO_2 > 90%.	Administer oxygen as ordered. Encourage the use of incentive spirometer, if not contraindicated.
▶ Breathing pattern, ineffective, related to fatigue.	The client will pace activities to minimize fatigue.	Plan care to allow rest periods.
▶ Anxiety related to perceived breathlessness.	The client will identify factors related to the perception of breathlessness.	Encourage client to talk about feelings of anxiety. Assist client to identify factors related to perceived breathlessness.

▶ Evaluation

Each goal must be evaluated to determine how it has been met by the client.

▲ ▲

▶ GASTROINTESTINAL MANIFESTATIONS

▶ Mycobacterium avium Complex

Mycobacterium avium and *Mycobacterium intracellulare* are two closely related mycobacteria that are grouped together and called *Mycobacterium avium complex* (MAC). For humans, the source of exposure to MAC is contaminated water although it has been isolated from soil, dust, sediments, and aerosols (Muma, Lyons, Borucki, & Pollard, 1994). In persons with AIDS, MAC involvement of the bowel is usually extensive, suggesting that the gastrointestinal tract may be the site of initial infection, with spread to other organs after that. The microorganism can fill the bone marrow and lymph nodes.

The most common symptoms of MAC include chronic fever, malaise, anemia, weight loss, diarrhea, and abdominal pain. Often the client will appear cachectic due to malabsorption. Because the symptoms are nonspecific, MAC is often difficult to distinguish from other AIDS-related infections. MAC is usually disseminated at the time of diagnosis. Diagnosis is made by tissue biopsy and cultures of the lung, bone marrow, lymph nodes, liver, or blood. Treatment for MAC infection may include one or more of the following medications: clarithromycin (Biaxin Filmtabs) to treat disseminated MAC; and a combination of amikacin sulfate (Amikin), azithromycin (Zithromax), ciprofloxacin hydrochloride (Cipro), cycloserine (Seromycin), and ethionamide (Trecator-SC). For persons with AIDS who have a CD4 count of $< 75/mm^3$, rifabutin (Mycobutin) is recommended for prevention of disseminated MAC (CDC, 1995b).

▶ *Cytomegalovirus Colitis*

Cytomegalovirus (CMV) belongs to the herpes virus group. Thus, it shares the same phenomena of latency and reactivation. The virus lies dormant in tissues waiting to be reactivated in the immunocompromised client. It is estimated that 50 to 70 percent of all adults in the United States have antibodies indicating previous infections with CMV. The potential for infection with CMV is increased during two periods: the perinatal period through the preschool years, and later during the sexually active years (Ungvarski, 1992). During birth and early childhood, CMV can be acquired by intrauterine or congenital infection, via vaginal delivery through a contaminated cervix, from breast milk, or from child to child in day care centers. It is hypothesized that in adults, CMV is transmitted via sexual intercourse or kissing as CMV has been isolated from semen, cervical secretions, and saliva. This hypothesis is further supported by the facts that the prevalence of CMV antibody doubles between the ages of fifteen and thirty-five and cases of transfer of CMV from women to men and from men to women have been documented. CMV causes disease by destroying the brain, lung, retina, and liver. CMV infection has been identified in all parts of the gastrointestinal tract from the oral cavity to the perianal area.

Signs and symptoms of CMV include weight loss, fever, diarrhea, and malaise. The diagnosis of CMV is based on microscopic identification of CMV from specific organs such as the brain, lung, liver, or adrenal gland. Ganciclovir sodium (Cytovene) is the drug of choice for treating individuals infected with CMV. Maintenance therapy is required to prevent relapse. Intravenous foscarnet sodium (Foscavir) has been approved by the FDA as an alternative therapy.

▶ *Cryptosporidium* Enteritis

Cryptosporidium is a protozoan that usually infects the epithelial cells that line the digestive tract. Transmission is usually via the fecal-oral route, and can be spread from animal to person as well as person to person. *Cryptosporidium* can also be spread by ingesting contaminated food and water.

Cryptosporidial diarrhea affects 15 percent of HIV-infected clients in the United States (Fegan, 1992). Clinical signs and symptoms include profuse watery diarrhea, from five to twenty stools per day. Abdominal pain, weight loss, abdominal cramping, anorexia, low-grade fever, and malaise may also be present.

Diagnosis is made by identifying the organism in fresh stool specimens. Intestinal biopsy may also be used to identify the organism.

There is no effective treatment for cryptosporidiosis. More than seventy medications have been tried in attempts to alleviate symptoms and find a cure (Fegan, 1992). Antidiarrheals such as diphenoxylate hydrochloride with atropine sulfate (Lomotil), loperamide hydrochloride (Imodium), and opium tincture (Paregoric) should be given on a programmed schedule rather than PRN. Treatment is palliative and focused toward the symptoms. This includes fluid and electrolyte replacement, analgesics, and occasionally the use of total parenteral nutrition. Anticryptosporidial agents are under investigation.

▶ *Hepatitis*

Only three of the five hepatitis viruses are commonly seen with HIV infection (Paar, 1994). These three are hepatitis B virus (HBV), hepatitis C virus (HCV), and hepatitis D virus (HDV). All three viruses have been associated with chronic infection and have similar transmission and risk factors. All three viruses are spread via blood or blood products. Risk factors include exposure to blood or blood products, exposure to contaminated needles and syringes, and multiple sexual contacts.

Signs and symptoms include malaise, weakness, anorexia, nausea, vomiting, and right upper quadrant pain. Abnormalities in bilirubin and hepatic enzymes may also occur. Diagnosis is made by serologic assays identifying antigens and antibodies.

Interferon has been approved for treatment of chronic HBV and HCV. It is currently being investigated for the treatment of HDV. Interferon is taken daily for six months for chronic HBV infection and three times weekly for chronic HCV infection for six months. Response to therapy varies but is decreased with HIV infection. Clients with a CD4 count greater than $400 \ mm^3$ have responded best to this therapy.

▶ *HIV-Wasting Syndrome*

HIV-wasting syndrome is defined as unexplained weight loss of more than 10 percent of body weight associated with either chronic diarrhea or fever (Hoyt & Staats, 1991). Weight loss and malnutrition are related to reduced food intake, malabsorption of nutrients, and altered metabolism of nutrients. Some of the factors related to reduced intake include anorexia, oral or esophageal lesions, nausea, neurologic or psychiatric conditions, fatigue, inadequate finances, and side effects of medications. Nutritional malabsorption is related to injury of the small intestine caused by opportunistic infections or by HIV infection of the cells in the gastrointestinal tract. Opportunistic infections produce fever that depletes the body's energy stores and causes weight loss.

Signs and symptoms of HIV-wasting syndrome are anorexia, diarrhea, nausea, vomiting, changes in taste and smell, and abdominal pain. The criteria for diagnosis include:

- Profound involuntary weight loss, defined as greater than 10 percent of the baseline body weight, plus either
  A. Chronic diarrhea (at least two loose stools per day for more than thirty days, or
  B. Chronic weakness and fever that is present either constantly or intermittently
- The absence of other illnesses such as cancer or cryptosporidiosis that can explain these findings (CDC, 1987).

Symptom control is the major focus for HIV-wasting syndrome. Medications to control nausea and vomiting should be given routinely and not PRN. Treatment of anorexia includes megestrol acetate (Megace) or dronabinol (Marinol). Antimotility drugs such as loperamide hydrochloride (Imodium), luminal acting agents such as kaolin and pectin mixture (Kaopectate), and hormonal agents such as octreotide acetate (Sandostatin) are used to treat diarrhea. Oral nutritional sup-

plements are most frequently used for weight loss. Total parenteral nutrition (TPN) is usually considered a final option except for severe malnutrition because of the risk and expense involved (Hoyt & Staats, 1991).

▶ Nursing Process

Assessment

Subjective Data Ask the client about bowel habits, and what causes and relieves diarrhea. Assess for alcohol consumption since excessive alcohol intake depletes B vitamins and provides no nutrition. Ask the client what activities cause fatigue. Inquire about food likes/dislikes, and food intolerances. Ask the client to describe food intake for the previous three days.

Objective Data Assess the client's skin integrity including temperature, moisture, color, vascularity, texture, lesions, areas of excoriation, and poor wound healing. Assess for fever. Assess the client's weight and daily nutritional intake. Assess laboratory values of nutritional status including serum albumin, total protein, hemoglobin, and hematocrit. Assess stool specimens for ova and parasites.

Possible nursing diagnoses for an HIV positive client with gastrointestinal disorders may include:

Nursing Diagnoses	Goals	Nursing Interventions
▶ Fluid volume deficit related to nausea, vomiting, diarrhea, or inadequate oral intake.	The client will have normal skin turgor and decreased frequency and amount of stools.	Suggest client use hard candy or chewing gum to stimulate saliva production if mouth is dry.
		Encourage client to drink liquids between (not with) meals.
		Monitor intake and output.
		Monitor client for evidence of electrolyte imbalance (hypokalemia, hypochloremia, confusion, muscle weakness).
▶ Nutrition, altered, less than body requirements related to anorexia, dysphagia, inability to prepare or obtain food, ill-fitting dentures, malabsorption, or side effects of medications.	The client will eat 75 percent of prescribed diet and maintain current weight.	Provide the prescribed diet (usually high caloric, high protein) in small frequent meals at room temperature.
		Offer commercially prepared nutritional supplements between meals.
		Administer supplemental vitamins and minerals as prescribed.
		Provide oral hygiene before and after meals.

Nursing Diagnoses	Goals	Nursing Interventions
		Administer antiemetics and antidiarrheals as ordered.
		Weigh client daily.
		Advise client to keep a food diary and a log of exacerbation and remission of signs and symptoms.
		Encourage client to have new dentures made if this is a problem.
▶ *Activity intolerance related to fatigue and/or decreased muscle mass.*	The client will be able to participate in meal preparation.	Allow rest periods while preparing meals.
		Provide the client with community resources for home meal delivery.
		Encourage range of motion exercises and weight bearing mobility.
▶ *Skin integrity, impaired, high risk for, related to diarrhea, malnutrition, decreased mobility.*	The client will maintain skin integrity.	Teach client to avoid large amounts of caffeine and alcohol.
		Monitor stool for presence of blood, fat, undigested food.
		Monitor stool cultures for evidence of new infections.
		Protect the perirectal area by keeping it clean and using compounds such as Aloe Vesta cream.
		Avoid prolonged pressure on bony prominences by a scheduled turning plan.
		If nonambulatory, provide client with a pressure relief mattress.
		Teach client to use nondrying soaps and to pat skin dry.
		Use soft sheets on the bed and avoid wrinkles.
▶ *Body image disturbance, related to severe weight loss.*	The client will express positive feelings about self.	Encourage client to express feelings about self.
		Provide positive feedback.
		Provide client with access to clergy, social worker, HIV counselor, dietitian.
		Encourage client to participate in support groups.

Evaluation

Each goal must be evaluated to determine how it has been met by the client.

▲ ▲

▶ ORAL MANIFESTATIONS

▶ Oral and Esophageal Candidiasis

Oral candidiasis (thrush) is a fungal infection caused by *Candida albicans* (see Figure 25-5). Oropharyngeal fungal infections are common in clients who are immunocompromised. Many clients complain of an unpleasant taste or mouth dryness. Other clinical signs and symptoms include creamy, white "cheesy" intraoral lesions, mucosal tenderness, and painful swallowing. These symptoms may interfere with the client's eating, nutrition, and weight. Diagnosis is established by the presence of the characteristic lesions in the oral

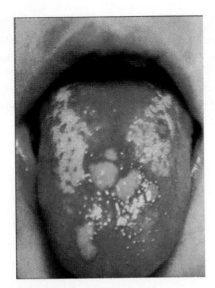

FIGURE 25-5 Thrush.

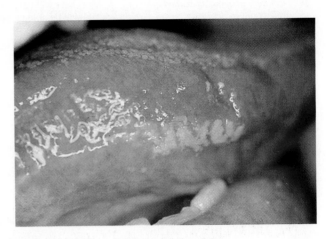

FIGURE 25-6 Oral hairy leukoplakia.

cavity. Microscopic examination of oral or esophageal lesions reveals budding yeast cells.

Treatment includes the use of oral fluconazole (Diflucan). Other medications used to treat candidiasis include ketoconazole (Nizoral), nystatin suspension (Mycostatin), and clotrimazole (Mycelex Troches). Amphotericin B (Amphotericin B) is used to treat disseminated candida infection. The antiulcer drug sucralfate (Carafate) may be used in a slurry form to relieve mouth pain prior to eating.

▶ Oral Hairy Leukoplakia

Oral hairy leukoplakia (OHL) usually appears as a white patch on the lateral borders of the tongue as shown in Figure 25-6. It is caused by the Epstein-Barr virus. The lesions are rarely in other areas of the mouth and are different in appearance from candidiasis. The irregular surface of the lesion appears as projections that resemble hairs and cannot be scraped off. Diagnosis is made by visual inspection of the lesion. OHL is not usually bothersome to the client and may regress spontaneously. No treatment is necessary for most cases of OHL; however, oral acyclovir (Zovirax) may be given to selected clients.

▶ Nursing Process

Assessment

Subjective Data Assess the client's history of symptoms and oral hygiene habits. Ask the client about recent nutritional intake, use of alcohol, tobacco, and current medications.

Objective Data Examine the lips, tongue, buccal mucosal surfaces for lesions, white cheesey patches, bleeding, and assess for difficulty swallowing.

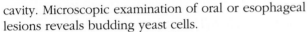

Possible nursing diagnoses for an HIV positive client with oral manifestations may include:

Nursing Diagnoses	Goals	Nursing Interventions
▶ *Oral mucous membrane, altered, related to oral lesions.*	The client will be free from oral lesions.	Administer prescribed medications.
		Frequently assess the oral cavity.
		Instruct client to avoid commercial mouthwashes containing alcohol or glycerine.
		Provide oral hygiene with a small soft toothbrush before and after meals.

(continued)

Nursing Diagnoses	Goals	Nursing Interventions
▶ *Pain with swallowing related to orolesophageal lesions.*	The client will have no difficulty swallowing and will be able to eat without difficulty.	Instruct client to avoid hot, spicy foods, alcohol, citrus juices, and hard foods. Administer medications as ordered.
▶ *Nutrition altered, less than body requirements, related to dysphagia.*	The client will maintain a stable weight.	Provide adequate nutrition. Offer foods that the client can swallow easily. Apply topical agents to control pain before meals. Refer client to dentist and dental hygienist.

▶ *Evaluation*

Each goal must be evaluated to determine how it has been met by the client.

▲ ▲

▶ GYNECOLOGICAL MANIFESTATIONS

▶ *Vaginal Candidiasis*

Vaginal candidiasis is a fungal infection caused by *candida albicans*. It is the most common initial infection occurring in HIV-infected women (American Health Consultants, 1992). Clinical manifestations include a white, clumped-appearing vaginal discharge, vaginal wall inflammation, and vaginal itching. Diagnosis is made by microscopic identification of yeast.

Most cases of vaginal candidiasis are treated with topical antifungal agents such as clotrimazole (Gyne-Lotrimin). For clients who do not respond to treatment with clotrimazole, ketoconazole (Nizoral), or fluconazole (Diflucan) are recommended.

▶ *Cervical Intraepithelial Neoplasia*

Women infected with HIV have a much higher incidence of cervical intraepithelial neoplasia (CIN) than women who are not infected (CDC, 1990). CIN and cancer of the cervix are considered to be on a continuum of abnormal cervical cells, ranging from mild abnormality (Grade I) to severe abnormality and cancer (Grade III). CIN in HIV-infected women progresses more rapidly and is less responsive to standard treatments than in noninfected women. Factors related to increased risk of CIN in HIV positive women include a decreased number of CD4 T-cells and infection with human papilloma virus (HPV) (Vermund, et al., 1991). It is thought that HIV activates HPV, causing cellular abnormalities.

The early stages of CIN have no symptoms. Clinical manifestations of cervical cancer include painless post-coital bleeding, and blood-tinged vaginal discharge. As CIN progresses, back pain, abdominal or pelvic pain, weight loss, anorexia, and leg edema caused by obstruction of lymph nodes may occur. Initial diagnosis is made by Pap smear to determine the presence of abnormal cells. Clients with abnormal Pap smears are referred for cervical biopsy and colposcopy.

Treatment for CIN includes laser therapy, conization, and hysterectomy. Treatment for invasive cervical cancer depends on the stage of the disease and may include chemotherapy, surgery, and radiation.

▶ *Nursing Process*

Assessment

Subjective Data   Ask the client about history of symptoms. Ask the client about bleeding after intercourse, abdominal and pelvic pain, or vaginal discharge.

Objective Data   Assess vaginal discharge for white or blood-tinged secretions. Assess for weight loss and edema.

▼ ▼

Posssible nursing diagnoses for a female HIV positive client with gynecological manifestations may include:

Nursing Diagnoses	*Goals*	*Nursing Interventions*
▶ *Tissue integrity, impaired, related to vaginal mucosal lesions.*	The client will be free of vaginal infections.	Teach the client to have Pap smears every six months.
		Assess the frequency and consistency of vaginal discharge.
		Teach client to keep the vaginal area clean and dry and to wear loose fitting cotton underwear to prevent irritation.
▶ *Body image disturbance related to chronic vaginal infections or surgery, radiation, or removal of cervix.*	The client will verbalize feelings and concerns about body image.	Encourage client to verbalize feelings and concerns about body image.
		Refer client to a support group for women with HIV.

▶ Evaluation

Each goal must be evaluated to determine how it has been met by the client.

▲ ▲

▶ CENTRAL NERVOUS SYSTEM MANIFESTATIONS

▶ AIDS Dementia Complex

The most common central nervous system complication in persons with AIDS is AIDS dementia complex (ADC). ADC is diagnosed in 4 to 15 percent of persons infected with HIV (Britton, 1993). This disorder is chronic and progressive with cognitive, motor, and behavioral dysfunction. ADC is caused by infection of glial cells in the brain with HIV. Signs and symptoms are sometimes vague during the initial stages of ADC. Early signs include poor concentration, forgetfulness, loss of balance, leg weakness, apathy, and social withdrawal. Clients with advanced ADC may exhibit psychotic behaviors and delirium and progress to a catatonic-like state with minimal responsiveness to the environment.

Diagnosis is made by neurological testing of cognitive, motor, and behavioral functioning. Other diagnostic tests include brain imaging to look for cerebral atrophy. Cerebrospinal fluid analysis can show elevated proteins and will exclude other pathogens.

Clients treated with zidovudine (Retrovir) have shown improvement in cognitive and motor skills.

▶ Toxoplasmosis

Toxoplasmosis is caused by the protozoan *Toxoplasma gondii*. Cats and other animals serve as a reservoir for this organism. It is spread to humans by ingestion of oocytes found in contaminated water, soil, or food, especially raw or undercooked meat. After entering the body, *Toxoplasma gondii* reproduces and spreads via the blood or lymph system. A person with an intact immune system may have no symptoms or mild symptoms, and the organism may remain dormant for years. In the immunocompromised person, the infection may be reactivated (secondary) or occur with the ingestion of oocytes from contaminated sources. Clinical signs and symptoms may be vague and nonspecific, or range from a mild headache, fever, and lethargy to poor coordination, seizures, and coma. Diagnosis is made by identification of a lesion through brain imaging (computerized tomography or magnetic resonance imaging), presence of serum antibodies to *Toxoplasma gondii,* and recent onset of a neurologic abnormality.

The treatment of choice is oral pyrimethamine (Daraprim) and sulfadiazine (Microsulfon). Lifelong suppressive therapy of pyrimethamine plus sulfadiazine and leukovorin calcium (Wellcovorin) is required (CDC, 1995b).

Cryptococcal Meningitis

Cryptococcal meningitis is a fungal infection caused by *Cryptococcus neoformans*. Cryptococcus is the most common life-threatening fungal infection associated with AIDS and the third most common central nervous system disease, after HIV encephalopathy and toxoplasmosis (Saag, 1993). This fungus is spread via pigeon droppings and can be found in soil, fruit, and fruit juices. In the noncompromised host, the fungus is inhaled and contained in the lungs. In the immunocompromised host with AIDS, *Cryptococcus neoformans* can be disseminated, remain in the lungs or can infect the brain and meninges. Clinical manifestations include fever, headache, nausea and vomiting, dizziness, photophobia, mental status changes, seizures, and a stiff neck. Diagnosis can be made by visualizing the fungus in cerebrospinal fluid with an India ink stain. Cryptococcal antigen titers in cerebrospinal fluid, urine, or blood can also be used for diagnosis.

Treatment for acute cryptococcal infections includes several medications. Intravenous amphotericin B (Fungizone Intravenous) may given for at least six weeks. Fluconazole (Diflucan) can be given for acute infection. Once treatment for acute infection is complete, lifelong suppressive therapy with oral fluconazole daily is recommended (CDC, 1995b).

Nursing Process

Assessment

Subjective Data Ask the client about forgetfulness, missing appointments, ability to complete activities of daily living, and if there have been any recent falls or accidents. Ask the client's family and significant others about behavior changes such as social withdrawal or unusual behavior.

Objective Data Assess the client for subtle mental status changes such as poor concentration and inability to remember instructions or previous conversations. Assess client for motor impairment such as dropping things, poor coordination or changes in writing ability. Assess the client's ability to remember usual medication schedule. Observe the environment for safety.

▼ ▼

Possible nursing diagnoses for an HIV positive client with central nervous system manifestations include:

Nursing Diagnoses	Goals	Nursing Interventions
▶ *Injury, high risk for, related to impaired coordination.*	The client will have no injuries.	Provide a safe, stable environment. Observe for involuntary movements, muscle weakness, or atrophy of extremities.
▶ *Thought processes, altered, related to impaired judgment secondary to HIV infection in the brain.*	The client will attain highest level of cognitive functioning as is possible.	Assess mental and neurologic status. Evaluate client's emotional, cognitive, and motor skills. Provide cues for reorientation (clock, calendar). Monitor client for adherence to medical regimen.
▶ *Social isolation related to embarrassment about symptoms.*	The client will have contact and interact with significant others.	Inform client and significant others of treatment plan. Encourage client to report persistent headaches, dizziness, seizures, or new symptoms. Provide structured activities and environment to minimize frustration.

Nursing Diagnoses	Goals	Nursing Interventions
		Encourage client to verbalize feelings and concerns.
		Encourage use of a log to document activities.
▶ *Self-care deficit related to inability to perform necessary hygiene, toileting, or feeding without assistance.*	The client will achieve activities of daily living with assistance.	Encourage significant others to assist with activities of daily living.
		Encourage physical closeness between client and significant others.

▶ Evaluation

Each goal must be evaluated to determine how it has been met by the client.

▲ ▲

▶ MALIGNANCIES

▶ Kaposi's Sarcoma

Kaposi's sarcoma (KS) is a cancer of the cells of the lymphatic system. It can occur any place in the body, including internal organs. The first lesions often appear subtly on the face (see Figure 25-7) or in the oral cavity. KS can develop in persons with HIV infection who have a normal CD4 T-cells count. The more immunosuppressed the person is, the more aggressive the spread of KS. Clinical manifestations of KS are red to blue lesions, which are painless, nonblanching, and palpable. These lesions are sometimes mistaken for bruises. Edema in the face, penis, scrotum, and legs can occur as a result of blockages in the lymphatic system. KS can also be found in the GI tract and lungs. Diagnosis is made by tissue biopsy.

Treatment involves a variety of options depending on whether the lesions are local or systemic. Radiation therapy, intralesional therapy with interferon alpha 2a or 2b (Roferon A, Intron A) or vinblastine sulfate (Velban), laser therapy, and cryotherapy are used on single or isolated KS lesions (Kaplan, 1990). For clients with advanced widespread symptomatic disease, single or combination chemotherapeutic regimens include vinblastine sulfate (Velban), vincristine sulfate (Oncovin), etoposide (VePesid), bleomycin sulfate (Blenoxane), doxorubicin HCl (Rubex), and mitoxantrone HCl (Novantrone). Different combinations of these medications are currently being tested in clinical trials.

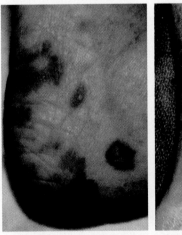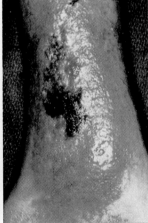

FIGURE 25-7 Kaposi's sarcoma.

Sample Nursing Care Plan: The Client with Kaposi's Sarcoma

Mr. Williams, a twenty-three-year-old singer, is HIV positive. Until recently, Mr. Williams was very active and enjoyed socializing with family and friends. He was diagnosed with Kaposi's sarcoma and has prominent lesions on his forehead and nose. He is unable to make decisions, has called in "sick" to work several times per week, and has not returned telephone calls to family and friends. At his clinic appointment he states how "ugly" his face looks.

Nursing Diagnosis 1 Body image disturbance related to facial lesions as evidenced by the statement "My face looks ugly."

Goals	Nursing Interventions	Rationale	Evaluation
Mr. Williams will express positive feelings about himself.	Provide Mr. Williams opportunities to discuss his feelings.	As Mr. Williams explores his feelings (positive and negative), he may need reassurance that the nurse is willing to listen to all of his concerns.	Mr. Williams was able to discuss his feelings with the nurse and contacted a local AIDS service organization for peer counseling.
	Provide Mr. Williams with information about intralesional treatment.	Providing Mr. Williams with information empowers him to see alternatives to his current situation.	
	Encourage Mr. Williams to contact his local AIDS Service Organization for peer support/counseling.	Interacting with someone who has been through the experience is helpful in adjustment.	
	Assist Mr. Williams in identifying positive aspects of himself.	Identifying positive aspects of himself will enhance Mr. Williams' well-being.	
	Explore possibility of covering lesions with theatrical makeup.	Learning to cover lesions contributes to self-esteem.	

Nursing Diagnosis 2 Coping, individual, ineffective, related to situational crisis of changed physical appearance as evidenced by impaired decision-making ability.

Goals	Nursing Interventions	Rationale	Evaluation
Mr. Williams will verbalize awareness of own coping abilities.	Assist Mr. Williams to identify previous ways of dealing with life problems.	Enables Mr. Williams to identify patterns of successful coping.	Mr. Williams was able to discuss his diagnosis with his pastor.
	Encourage Mr. Williams to evaluate perceptions of his current coping abilities.	Self-awareness leads to new insight and possible solutions.	

| | Assist Mr. Williams in identifying sources of strength. | By identifying sources of strength such as religious beliefs or positive personal attributes, Mr. Williams is able to acknowledge current resources. | |
| | Develop a therapeutic relationship using active listening. | Provides a safe environment for problem-solving. | |

Nursing Diagnosis 3 Social isolation, related to altered physical appearance as evidenced by decreased interpersonal interactions and attendance at work.

Goals	Nursing Interventions	Rationale	Evaluation
Mr. Williams will verbalize willingness to be involved with others.	Develop a written plan of action with Mr. Williams that includes daily contact with others.	Provides Mr. Williams with a reference for action.	Mr. Williams agreed to have face-to-face contact with at least one other person on a daily basis.
	Facilitate Mr. Williams' interactions with others diagnosed with KS.	Provides Mr. Williams with an opportunity to discuss shared problems with others and decreases feelings of aloneness.	
	Involve family members and friends in treatment plan.	Assists Mr. Williams in identifying a network of support and acceptance.	
	Encourage Mr. Williams to explore temporary work arrangements with employer.	Initiating discussions about work-related absences enables Mr. Williams to begin to deal with consequences of social isolation.	

► *Non-Hodgkin's Lymphoma*

Lymphomas are malignant tumors of the immune system. B-cells are the origin of malignancy for the majority of clients with AIDS-related non-Hodgkin's lymphoma (NHL) (Kaplan, 1990). Clinical manifestations are nonspecific and may include fever, night sweats, and weight loss. Confusion, lethargy, and memory loss may be present in persons with CNS involvement.

Diagnosis of NHL is complicated because of the nonspecific symptoms. Examination of tissue is the recommended diagnostic procedure (Kaplan, 1990). There is no standard treatment of NHL. Individualized treatment may include a combination of chemotherapy, antiretroviral agents, prophylaxis against opportunistic infections, and colony-stimulating factors to enhance bone marrow production of blood cells. However, in many clients with advanced HIV disease, treatment of NHL is withheld because it is not tolerated well and may even lead to earlier death.

▶ *Nursing Process*

Assessment

Subjective Data   Ask the client about frequency, onset, and persistence of current symptoms. Ask the client about effect of current symptoms on ability to perform activities of daily living and relationships with others. Ask the client about effect of treatment plan on quality of life.

Objective Data   Assess the skin for lesions. Assess the client for increased frequency, intensity, or reoccurrence of nonspecific symptoms including fever, night sweats, and weight loss.

▼ ▼

Possible nursing diagnoses for an HIV positive client with a malignancy may include:

Nursing Diagnoses	*Goals*	*Nursing Interventions*
▶ *Skin integrity, impaired, high risk for, related to lesions, treatment and/or weight loss.*	The client will maintain skin integrity.	Teach the client to avoid scratching skin lesions and drying soaps and to make sure clothing and linen have been thoroughly rinsed of detergent.
▶ *Body image disturbance related to tumors, treatment, and/or weight loss.*	The client will verbalize feelings about body image and treatment plans.	Identify positive attributes of the client. Convey an open, honest, and caring attitude toward the client. Suggest the use of theatrical makeup to cover lesions.
▶ *Social isolation related to change in appearance.*	The client will maintain usual social interactions, and identify factors that enhance quality of life.	Facilitate the clients interaction with others. Keep client and significant others aware of treatment plan. Encourage significant others to participate in the care of the client. Encourage physical closeness between the client and significant others. Provide the client with access to clergy, social worker, or HIV counselor. Encourage the client to join a support group or obtain peer support. Assist the client in identifying positive coping strategies.

▶ Evaluation

Each goal must be evaluated to determine how it has been met by the client.

▲ ▲

▶ CASE STUDY

Jim Hayes, a thirty-seven-year-old male, suspects that he is HIV positive. He enters the medical unit with chronic symptoms such as fever, night sweats, diarrhea, weight loss, shortness of breath, and a nonproductive cough. On the initial assessment he is alert and oriented, color is pale, temperature 100.6, pulse 92, respirations 36, and blood pressure 140/70. He has generalized lymphadenopathy. Height 5' 11" and his weight is 125 pounds. Jim states that he is not currently taking any medications although he is "familiar" with the drug AZT (Retrovir).

The following questions will guide your development of a Nursing Care Plan for the case study.

1. List symptoms/clinical manifestations, other than Mr. Hayes', that a client may experience when HIV positive.
2. List two reasons AZT (Retrovir) may be initiated for Mr. Hayes.
3. List two diagnostic tests that will confirm the diagnosis of HIV positive.
4. List subjective and objective data the nurse would want to obtain about Mr. Hayes.
5. Write three individual nursing diagnoses and goals for Mr. Hayes.
6. List pertinent nursing actions the nurse would do in caring for Mr. Hayes related to:

   hydration
   fatigue
   nutrition
   oxygenation
   medications

7. List resources that could assist Mr. Hayes with his diagnosis.
8 List teaching Mr. Hayes will need before leaving the medical unit.

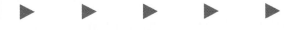

SUMMARY

- HIV is the virus that causes AIDS.
- HIV is transmitted by blood, semen, vaginal fluids, and breast milk.
- All health care workers should follow standard precautions to decrease their risk of exposure.
- HIV affects the T-cells that produce cell-mediated immunity.
- Diagnosis is made by the ELISA and Western blot test. These tests determine the presence of antibodies to HIV, not the virus itself.

- *Pneumocystis carinii* pneumonia is the most common opportunistic infection associated with HIV.
- Drug-resistant TB is on an upsurge. All TB cases should be treated as if they were drug resistant.
- Hepatitis B, C, and D can be co-infections with HIV.
- HIV-wasting depletes muscle mass instead of fat.
- Oral candidiasis can be painful and interfere with the client's nutritional status.
- AIDS dementia complex is a progressive disorder with cognitive, motor, and behavioral dysfunction.
- Kaposi's sarcoma usually begins on the face or in the mouth.

Review Questions

1. Which of the following statements show that the client understands a diagnosis of HIV positive?

    a.   "Being HIV positive means that I have AIDS."
    b.   "Since I am only HIV positive I cannot infect others."
    c.   "Because I am HIV positive I have the virus that causes AIDS."
    d.   "I became infected by donating blood."

2. The drug of choice for treating *Pneumocystis carinii* pneumonia (PCP) is:

    a.   co-trimoxazole (Septra).
    b.   ganciclovir (Cytovene).
    c.   megestrol acetate (Megace).
    d.   fluconazole (Diflucan).

3. The nurse is caring for a client who is experiencing diarrhea and weight loss. Which of the following nursing interventions is appropriate for him?

    a.   encourage fluids with meals
    b.   substitute a milk shake for lunch
    c.   offer small, frequent meals
    d.   suggest he eat more sweets

4. The nurse is caring for a client who asks when AZT (Retrovir) is normally started. Which of the following would be the nurse's correct response?

    a.   when the client becomes symptomatic
    b.   when CD4 level reaches 500/mm³
    c.   after the client's first opportunistic infection
    d.   as soon as the client is diagnosed as HIV positive

5. The nurse is discussing transmission of HIV with a client. Which of the following statements indicates that the client needs more education?

    a.   "I should not share needles with anyone."
    b.   "I can spread the virus through sexual contact."
    c.   "I can no longer donate blood."
    d.   "I should not hug or kiss anyone."

6. The only opportunistic infection that is found when the CD4 cell count is normal is:

    a.   AIDS dementia complex.
    b.   Kaposi's sarcoma.
    c.   *Pneumocystis carinii* pneumonia.
    d.   oral candidiasis.

Critical Thinking Questions

1   How would you tell your family and friends if you were diagnosed HIV positive?

2. How might a person's lifestyle change after receiving a diagnosis of HIV positive?

News Flash

The Food and Drug Administration (FDA) has approved marketing for a test that detects HIV antibodies in saliva. It has not been approved for home use. The test will be sold under the name Ora-Sure. The manufacturer, Epitope, suggests possible uses include community outreach and public health testing programs as well as life insurance screening.

The test involves placing a lollipop-style plastic stick between the lower cheek and gum for two minutes. The device is then placed into a vial and sent to a lab for analysis. The result is sent to the tested person's clinician. A blood test is recommended if a positive result is obtained. The test will sell for $2 to $4, not including the lab work which runs from $3 to $15 (AJN, 1995).

Control, Mobility, and Coordination

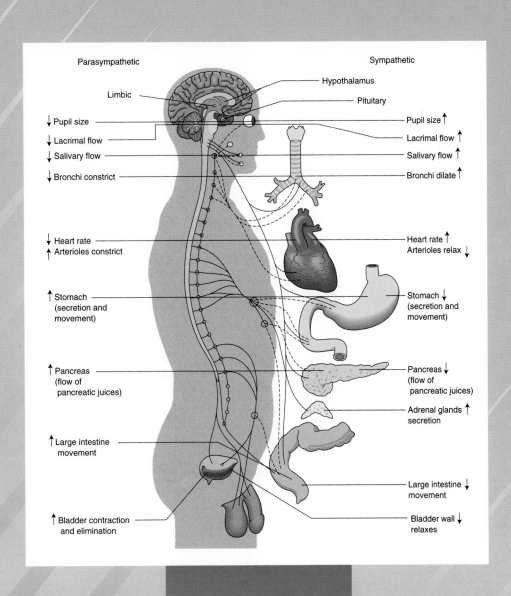

Parasympathetic | Sympathetic

Limbic

Hypothalamus

Pituitary

↓ Pupil size — Pupil size ↑
↓ Lacrimal flow — Lacrimal flow ↑
↓ Salivary flow — Salivary flow ↑
↓ Bronchi constrict — Bronchi dilate ↑

↓ Heart rate — Heart rate ↑
↑ Arterioles constrict — Arterioles relax ↓

↑ Stomach (secretion and movement) — Stomach ↓ (secretion and movement)

↑ Pancreas (flow of pancreatic juices) — Pancreas ↓ (flow of pancreatic juices)

Adrenal glands ↑ secretion

↑ Large intestine movement — Large intestine ↓ movement

↑ Bladder contraction and elimination — Bladder wall ↓ relaxes

CHAPTER

26

Musculoskeletal Disorders

Janet E. Keith

► **KEY TERMS**

amphiarthrosis
arthroplasty
bruxism
closed reduction
contracture
crepitus
diarthrosis
fracture
greenstick fracture
Heberden's nodes
kyphosis
locomotor
lordosis
open reduction
orthopedics
paresthesia
phantom limb pain
scoliosis
subluxation
synarthrosis
tophi
windowing

LIST OF DISORDERS

Musculoskeletal Trauma
► Strains
► Sprains
► Dislocations
► Fractures
► Compartment Syndrome

Inflammatory Disorders
► Rheumatoid Arthritis
► Bursitis
► Polymyositis
► Osteomyelitis

Degenerative Disorders
► Osteoporosis
► Osteoarthritis
► Total Joint Arthroplasty (Hip or Knee
Replacement)

Musculoskeletal Disorders
► Amputations
► Temporomandibular Joint Syndrome (TMJ)
► Carpal Tunnel Syndrome

*Systemic Disorders with Musculoskeletal
Manifestations*
► Gout
► Lyme Disease

LEARNING OBJECTIVES

Upon completion of this chapter the learner should be
able to:
• Define key terms.
• List the diagnostic tests used in the evaluation of
orthopedic disorders and diseases.

- Describe preventive nursing care of the orthopedic client, i.e., positioning, mobility, and so on.
- Identify the various types of casts used in the treatment of orthopedic disorders.
- Describe nursing care of clients with these devices.
- List four types of fractures and their related treatment.

- Discuss the nursing care of the client undergoing a total hip replacement.
- Utilize the nursing process to plan nursing care including physical and emotional needs of the orthopedic client.

▶ *MAKING THE CONNECTION*

Refer to the topics in the following chapters to increase your understanding of musculoskeletal disorders:

- **Chapter 8, Health Maintenance:** Health Promotion, p. 121; Osteoporosis, p. 130; Low Back Pain, p. 130
- **Chapter 10, Nursing Assessment:** Head-to-Toe Assessment, p. 176
- **Chapter 12, Pain Management:** Therapeutic Approaches to Pain, p. 214
- **Chapter 15, Oncology Nursing:** Bone Marrow Dysfunction, p. 314; Pathological Fractures, p. 317

- **Chapter 16, Caring for the Older Adult:** Exercise, p. 335; Common Disorders Related to Aging/Musculoskeletal System, p. 336
- **Chapter 21, Vascular Disorders:** Raynaud's Phenomenon/Disease, p. 502
- **Chapter 24, Allergies, Immune, and Autoimmune Disorders:** Rheumatoid Arthritis, p. 602

INTRODUCTION

Orthopedics is the branch of medical science that deals with the prevention or correction of the disorders and diseases of the musculoskeletal system. It involves the muscles, skeleton, joints, and supporting structures such as ligaments and tendons.

The prime concern of the nurse caring for a client with **locomotor** (moving or ability to move) disorders is the prevention of **contractures** (permanent shortening of a muscle) or deformities. The objective of all caregivers is to maintain good body position, preserve muscle tone, and continue joint motion for the client with acute or long-term therapeutic or rehabilitative needs. Caring for orthopedic clients also requires an understanding of basic principles that apply to all of these clients whether they are in traction, casts, or recovering from surgery.

ANATOMY AND PHYSIOLOGY REVIEW

The musculoskeletal system consists of bones, muscles, tendons, ligaments, cartilage, and joints. When it is functioning properly, the musculoskeletal system allows an individual to stand erect and ambulate. Figure 26-1 identifies the bones of the skeleton.

The skeletal system consists of bones attached to each other by cartilage and strong ligaments. The functions of the skeleton are:

1. To provide the body with structural framework.
2. To act as a protective casing for internal organs such as the brain, heart, and lungs.
3. To allow movement by muscles attached to the skeleton.
4. To store calcium, phosphorus and magnesium and release these minerals when the body requires them.
5. To manufacture blood cells in the red bone marrow.

Bones in the skeletal system are classified as long, short, flat, or irregular. Examples include the humerus, a long bone; finger, short bone; occiput, flat bone, and the vertebrae, irregular bone. Figure 26-2 illustrates these bones.

There are two types of bone. One type of bone is cancellous, which resembles a sponge with spaces and is found in the epiphysis or end of the long bones as well as in all other bones. The other type is cortical bone, which is compact bone and is found in the dia-

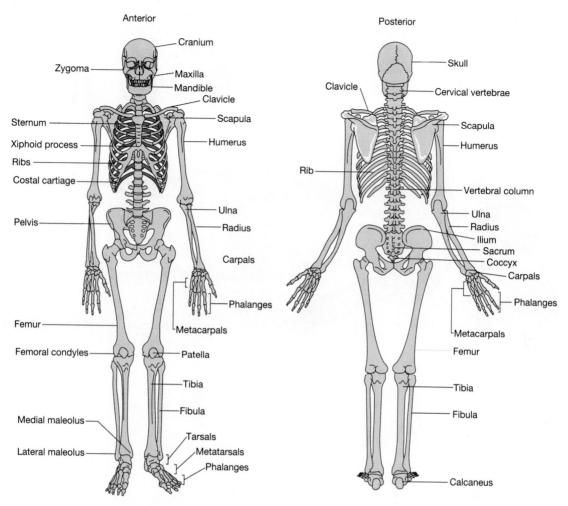

Anterior

- Cranium
- Zygoma
- Maxilla
- Mandible
- Clavicle
- Sternum
- Scapula
- Xiphoid process
- Humerus
- Ribs
- Costal cartiage
- Pelvis
- Ulna
- Radius
- Carpals
- Phalanges
- Metacarpals
- Femur
- Femoral condyles
- Patella
- Tibia
- Fibula
- Medial maleolus
- Lateral maleolus
- Tarsals
- Metatarsals
- Phalanges

Posterior

- Skull
- Clavicle
- Cervical vertebrae
- Scapula
- Humerus
- Rib
- Vertebral column
- Ulna
- Radius
- Ilium
- Sacrum
- Coccyx
- Carpals
- Phalanges
- Metacarpals
- Femur
- Tibia
- Fibula
- Calcaneus

FIGURE 26-1 Anterior and posterior views of the adult human skeleton.

physis or shaft of the long bones. Short bones consist of cancellous bone covered by a layer of compact bone. Flat bones are made of cancellous bone layered between compact bone. Generally, the makeup of irregular bones is similar to that of flat bones.

The muscular system is composed of muscle fibers and tendons innervated by nerves (see Figure 26-3). The muscle fibers vary in size and shape and are arranged according to a muscle's function. The muscles act as motors controlled by nerve impulses from the cerebral cortex. The muscles and the skeleton work together to permit body movement. Muscles are attached to bones by tendons.

The action of muscles is to contract or shorten. Muscles are arranged within the body as opposing pairs to act as antagonists to each other. For example, the biceps flex the forearm and the triceps extend it.

Muscles are surrounded and divided by fibrous envelopes called fascia. In the extremities, the muscles surround and give support to main blood vessels and nerves. Muscles also give support to and keep the body erect as well as give shape to the body.

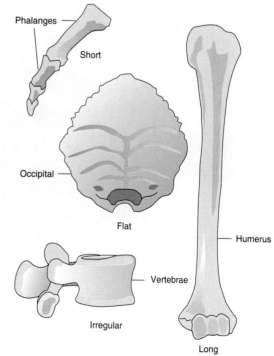

Phalanges

Short

Occipital

Flat

Irregular

Humerus

Vertebrae

Long

FIGURE 26-2 Bone shapes.

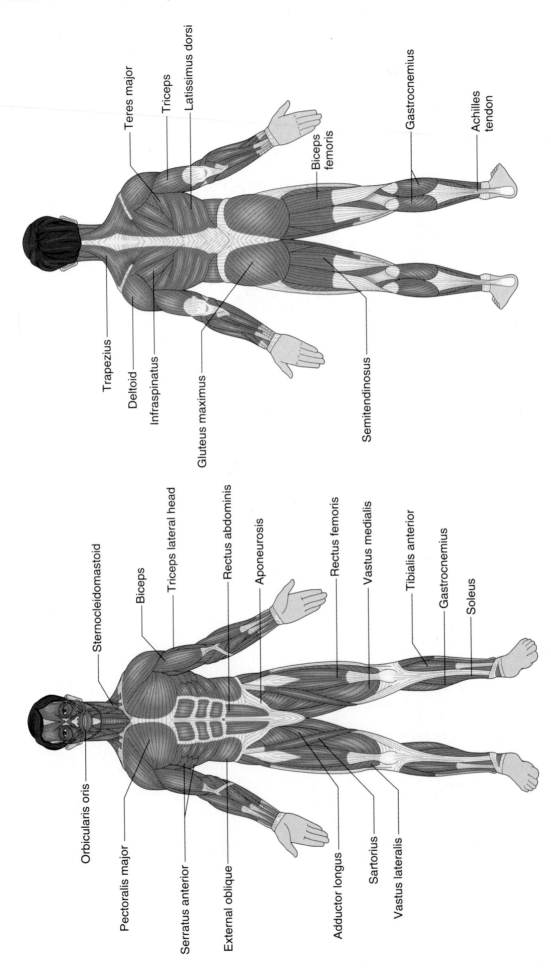

FIGURE 26-3   The muscular system: anterior and posterior views.

Movement of the muscles may be either voluntary or involuntary. Muscles attached to bone can function at the will of the person (voluntary). Involuntary muscles are found within body organs and the actions are not under the person's control. They regulate the physical activity of the organs so the organs can perform their functions. Involuntary muscles are located in the intestinal tract, the pupil of the eye, and in the heart and blood vessels.

A joint is a junction of two or more bones. There are three types of joints: **diarthrosis**, **synarthrosis**, and **amphiarthrosis**. Diarthrosis joints are freely movable joints such as the hinge (ankle), ball and socket (hip and shoulder), pivot (skull and first vertebrae), gliding (wrist), and saddle (thumb). The suture line between the temporal and occipital bones of the skull is an example of an immovable joint (synarthrosis). The ver-

tebrae and pelvic bones separated by fibrous cartilage are called slightly movable (amphiarthrosis). Figure 26-4 illustrates types of joints.

The ends of articulating joints are covered with a smooth articular cartilage. The joint capsule is composed of an outer fibrous layer and an inner synovial layer that secretes synovial fluid. This clear fluid acts as a lubricating fluid for the joints.

Other structures related to the musculoskeletal system include bursa, fascia, tendons, and ligaments. Bursa are sacs filled with fluid that facilitate joint movement by making it possible for muscles and tendons to move or glide over ligaments or bones. Fascia is connective tissue that covers a muscle. Tendons are strong fibrous tissue attaching muscle to bones providing mobility. Ligaments grow out of the periosteum and lash bones together more firmly.

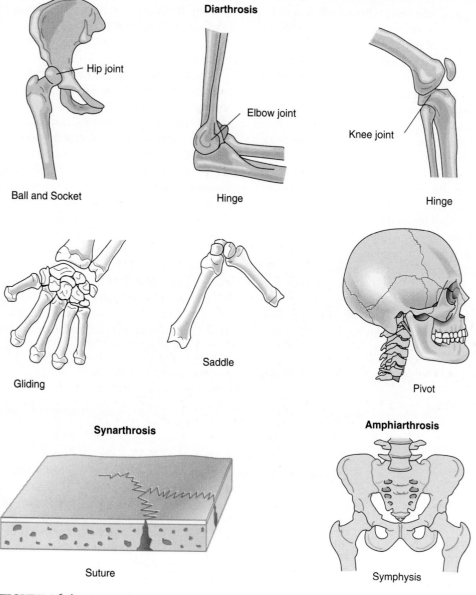

FIGURE 26-4 Joints classified by the degree of movement permitted.

MUSCULOSKELETAL ASSESSMENT

Assessment of the musculoskeletal system ranges from a basic assessment of functional abilities done by the nurse to a complete physical exam by the physician for diagnosis of specific muscle and joint disorders. The extent of the physical exam will depend on the client's complaints, the health history, and any other physical signs or symptoms.

The nurse, in making an assessment, will inspect and palpate to evaluate bone integrity, posture, joint function, muscle strength, and gait. An assessment is also made of the client's ability to perform basic activities of daily living.

The medical history includes information on any past medical or surgical disorders. It also includes any symptoms with relation to onset, duration, or location of discomfort or pain. The nurse should ask if activity makes symptoms better or worse. A family medical history should also be obtained.

Assessment of the bony skeleton includes notation of any deformities, body alignment, abnormal growths due to bone tumors, shortened extremities, amputations, abnormal angulation other than at the joints, and crepitus, a grating sensation or sound.

Assessment of the spine will necessitate exposure of the client's back, buttocks, and legs for adequate visualization. Differences in the height of the shoulders or iliac crests should be noted. Gluteal folds should appear symmetrical. The vertebral column should be straight and perpendicular to the floor with the spine convex through the thoracic portion and concave through the cervical/lumbar portion.

Three common spinal curvatures are: scoliosis, kyphosis, and lordosis. A lateral curving deviation is known as scoliosis. Scoliosis is seen most frequently in schoolage children and adolescents. Kyphosis is seen as an increased roundness of the thoracic spinal curve.

This condition is frequently seen in the older person with osteoporosis. Lordosis is an exaggeration of the lumbar spine curvature as seen in pregnancy as a woman's body adjusts to the center of gravity. These three curvatures are illustrated in Figure 26-5.

Assessment of the articular system includes: range of motion (limited, active, and passive), the stability of joints, deformities and any nodular formation, and pulses in the extremities.

Range of motion (ROM) includes assessment of the client's ability to change position, muscle strength and coordination, and the size of individual muscles. When assessing passive range of motion, the nurse should remember to keep the motion steady and avoid causing any pain.

Joints are examined for excessive fluid. The knee is the most common site for fluid accumulation. Edema and an elevated temperature may be signs of active inflammation in the joint. Normal joint movement is smooth. If there is a snap or crack sound when a joint is passively moved it may be indicative of a ligament slipping over a bony prominence. This sound is called crepitation.

Assess pulse points in the extremities by palpation, assessing for weak or absent pulses. Compare the strength of the pulse in affected extremities with that of nonaffected extremities. Check for skin color, temperature, and the time of capillary refill. Check capillary refill by pressing down on the client's fingernail or toenail for a few seconds, then releasing. Record the amount of time it takes for the client's nail to return to normal color. The color should return immediately (less than two seconds); if a client has an arterial disorder, the color will take longer than two seconds to return to normal.

Deformities may be due to several factors including contractures, dislocations, and subluxation (a partial separation of an articular surface). Nodular formations are produced by musculoskeletal diseases such as gout, rheumatoid arthritis, and osteoarthritis.

COMMON DIAGNOSTIC TESTS

The following is a table of the commonly used diagnostic tests for clients with symptoms of musculoskeletal disorders.

Test	Explanation/Normal Values	Nursing Responsibilities
Radiograph (x-ray)	Most common diagnostic study. Identifies traumatic disorders, i.e., fractures, dislocations, tumors, bone disorders, joint deformities, bone density, and changes in bone relationships. Healing followed/documented. Performed by technician.	Explain procedure. Prepare client as ordered. No specific post procedure care required. Analgesic, especially for arthritic client.

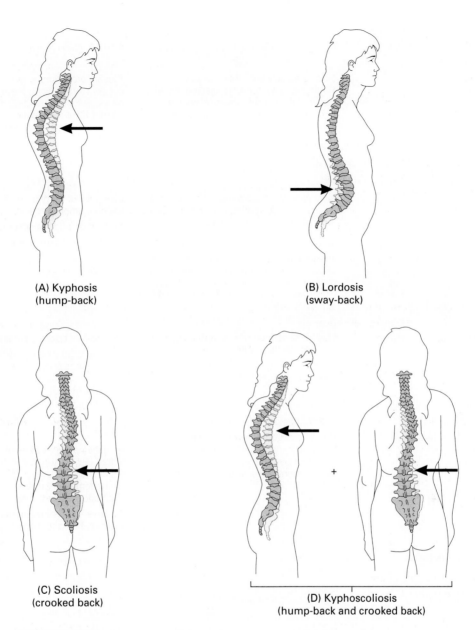

(A) Kyphosis
(hump-back)

(B) Lordosis
(sway-back)

(C) Scoliosis
(crooked back)

(D) Kyphoscoliosis
(hump-back and crooked back)

FIGURE 26-5 Curvatures of the spine.

Test	Explanation/Normal Values	Nursing Responsibilities
Arthroscopy	Endoscopic procedure for direct visualization of a joint. Done in operating room under sterile conditions. Local or general anesthesia.	Do frequent neurovascular checks. Elevate leg. Compression dressing. Administer analgesic for discomfort.
Arthrocentesis	Procedure to obtain fluid from a joint using strict sterile technique. Knee anesthetized, sterile needle inserted into joint space, synovial fluid aspirated. To diagnose infections, crystal induced arthritis, synovitis, inject anti-inflammatory medications. Performed by physician. Takes approximately 10 minutes.	Explain procedure. Consent forms signed. Assess site for edema, pain. Fast if possible. Pressure dressing. Ice.

(continued)

Test	Explanation/Normal Values	Nursing Responsibilities
Arthrogram (graphy)	Radiographic visualization of joint. Radiopaque dye or air is injected into joint cavity to outline soft tissue usually on knee/shoulder joints. Local anesthetic with sterile technique. Performed by physician and takes approximately 30 minutes.	Explain procedure to client. Client signs consent form. Client wears elastic bandage for several days. Check for edema. Give mild analgesic for pain. Monitor for increased pain. No fasting or sedation needed.
Magnetic Resonance Imaging (MRI)	Noninvasive diagnostic scanning technique. Uses magnetic field and radio waves. Detects edema, hemorrhage, blood flow, infarcts, tumors, infections, aneurysms, demyelinating disease, muscular disease, skeletal abnormalities, intervertebral disk problems, and causes of spinal cord compression. Client on platform slid into tube containing magnet. Performed by qualified technologist. Takes approximately one hour.	Explain procedure. Must lie absolutely still. Determine if client is claustrophobic. There will be thumping noises. No fluid or food restrictions. Have consent form signed. Remove all metal objects. Empty bladder. No specific post-procedure needed.
Computed Tomography (CT scan)	May be performed with or without dye injection. Multiple images taken. Clicking noise from machine during procedure. Takes 30 minutes to 1 1/2 hours.	Explain procedure. Consent form signed. Remove wigs, hairpins, clips for head CT. NPO 8 hours prior to scan. Assess for iodine allergy. Observe for signs of anaphylaxis if dye used.
Electromyography (EMG)	Detects primary muscular disorders. Needle electrode inserted into muscle being examined. Measures electrical activity of skeletal muscles at rest and during voluntary muscle contraction.	Explain procedure. Have consent form signed. No caffeine drinks or smoking for 3 hours before test. Assure client that needle will not cause electrocution. Inform client there will be temporary discomfort when needle electrode inserted. Observe site for hematoma or inflammation after test.
Complete blood count (CBC) WBC Hg	Series of tests on peripheral blood 5,000–10,000 Males = 13.5–17.5 gm/dL Females = 12–16 gm/dL	Assess puncture site for bleeding.
Uric Acid serum: urine:	Elevated in gout Males = 2.1–8.5 mg/dL Females = 2.0–6.6 mg/dL 250–750 mg/24 hour	There are no food or drink restrictions. Drugs affecting results: ascorbic acid, diuretics, levadopa, allopurinol, coumadin. Label container with client's name and date/times of collection. Drugs affect: corticosteroids, cytotoxic agents.
Rheumatoid factor (RF)	Used in diagnosis of rheumatoid arthritis Normal value < 1:20 titer; 1:20–1:80 Positive for rheumatoid arthritis and other conditions; > 1:80 positive for rheumatoid arthritis.	No food or fluid restrictions. Collect 24-hour urine specimen.
C-Reactive Protein (CRP)	Usually not present. >1:2 titer positive. Used to monitor acute inflammatory phases of rheumatoid arthritis so early treatment can be initiated.	Client is NPO except for water 8 to 12 hours. Oral contraceptive affect results.
Serum Calcium	9.0–10.5 mg/dL (total)	No food or fluid restrictions. Drugs affecting results: cortisone, antibiotics, antacids, heparin, estrogen, vitamin D.

Test	Explanation/Normal Values	Nursing Responsibilities
Erythrocyte Sedimentation Rate (ESR)	Nonspecific test used to detect inflammatory, neoplastic, infectious and necrotic processes. Males = up to 15 mm/hour Females = up to 20 mm/hour	No food or fluid restrictions. Drugs affecting results: aspirin, cortisone, quinine, methyldopa, oral contraceptives, vitamin A.
Antinuclear Antibodies (ANA)	Reacts with nuclear antigen. Found in blood serum of clients with systemic lupus erythematosus, rheumatoid arthritis, juvenile arthritis, and polymyositis. Negative at 1:20 dilution.	No food or fluid restrictions.

KEY ABBREVIATIONS

The following abbreviations and acronyms are used in this chapter:

ADL	activities of daily living
AKA	above the knee amputation
AROM	active range of motion
BKA	below the knee amputation
CMS	circulation, movement, sensation
CPM	continuous passive motion machine
DJD	degenerative joint disease
NSAIDs	nonsteroidal anti-inflammatory drugs
ORIF	open reduction internal fixation
PROM	passive range of motion
ROM	range of motion
THA	total hip arthroplasty
TKA	total knee arthroplasty
TMJ	temporomandibular joint

▶ MUSCULOSKELETAL TRAUMA

Trauma to the musculoskeletal system may cause a variety of injuries to clients of all ages. Such injuries include strains, sprains, dislocations, fractures, and compartment syndrome.

▶ STRAINS

A strain is an injury to a muscle or tendon due to overuse or overstretching. A strain may be either acute or chronic. An acute strain may be caused when an individual performs unaccustomed exercises vigorously. A chronic strain may develop after repeatedly overusing certain muscles. Individuals suffering acute strains experience sudden severe pain while the onset is gradual in chronic strains with the affected part feeling only stiff and sore.

Chronic strains require no specific treatment, but acute strains will require rest and possibly immobilization. Immediately after the injury cold packs may be applied for twenty- to thirty-minute periods, then removed for one hour for a twenty-four-hour period to reduce any edema. Heat may then be applied for the client's comfort. In the case of a severe strain when the muscle may be completely ruptured, surgical repair may be necessary.

▶ SPRAINS

A sprain is an injury to ligaments surrounding a joint caused by a sudden twist, wrench, or accidental fall. Symptoms include pain, edema, loss of motion, and ecchymosis. X-ray will reveal soft tissue edema but no evidence of joint or bone injury. Immediate treatment includes elevation of the injured part and the application of cold packs. The part may then be immobilized with an elastic compression bandage or a brace. After the edema has decreased significantly, a cast may be applied.

▶ DISLOCATIONS

Dislocations occur when articular surfaces of a joint are no longer in contact. The bones are literally "out of joint." The displaced bone may hinder the blood supply, damage nerves, tear ligaments, or rupture muscle attachments. Traumatic dislocations are considered orthopedic emergencies. Congenital dislocations are present at birth while spontaneous or pathologic dislocations are caused by diseases affecting joints.

Symptoms of a dislocation include localized joint pain, loss of function of the joint, and a change in the length of the extremity and contour of the joint. Diagnosis is based on the symptoms, physical exam, and x-rays. X-rays reveal either a complete or partial separation of the articulating surfaces.

Some dislocations may reduce (go back in place) themselves, while others may require surgical or therapeutic reduction. Reduction accomplished without surgical intervention is called **closed reduction**. Closed reduction requires the manual manipulation of the joint. The physician pulls on the joint with a gradual steady pull rather than a sudden forceful jerking of the joint. This procedure may require either a local or general anesthesia. Reduction requiring surgery is called **open reduction**. Following the reduction the joint may be immobilized by applying a cast or splint. Immobilization may be maintained for three to six weeks. Active range of motion (ROM) exercises are done to adjacent joints not immobilized.

▶ FRACTURES

A **fracture** is a break in the continuity of a bone. Fractures occur when the forces from outside the body become greater than the strength of the bone causing the bone to break. Fractures usually involve soft tissue (edema and bleeding), damaged nerves, and tendons. Most fractures are caused by accidents. These may be the result of direct force, torsion or twisting, or violent contractions of highly developed muscles. Other fractures may be the result of a disease process that weakens the bone. This type of fracture is known as pathologic or spontaneous. Individuals considered high risk for fractures include those who have predisposing bone conditions such as metastatic or primary bone tumors or osteoporosis, poor coordination, diminished vision, dizzy spells, or general weakness.

There are more than ninety different classifications of fractures. Some of the more common types include: greenstick, simple or closed, compound or open, impacted or telescoped, spiral, and comminuted.

A **greenstick fracture** is also considered an incomplete fracture. The continuity of the bone is not completely disrupted but has splintering on one side and bending on the other. This fracture is seen most frequently in children. An uncomplicated fracture in which the skin remains intact is called a closed or simple fracture. The fractured surfaces are not contaminated by outside air. In a compound or open fracture the bone is completely broken. The skin is also broken allowing the bone to protrude and provide a greater chance for infection. An impacted fracture is also called a telescoped fracture. One portion of a bone fragment is forcibly driven into another. A spiral fracture twists around the shaft of the bone. This type of fracture may occur from a twisting force. In a comminuted fracture the bone is splintered into many unaligned fragments. Various types of fractures are shown in Figure 26-6.

Healing time for fractures is affected by the age of the client and the type of injury or any underlying disease process, and may take weeks, months, or even years before the healing is complete. The sequence of healing takes place beginning with the formation of a hematoma, then granulation tissue formation, callus formation, callus ossification, and ultimately remodeling.

Hematoma formation begins with the formation of a clot that serves as a fibrin network. Bleeding comes from ruptured vessels within the bone as well as from tears in the periosteum and adjacent tissues. The hematoma is not absorbed but develops into granulation tissue. Granulation tissue forms a soft tissue callus that surrounds the fracture site and serves as a temporary splint. Callus ossification is the result of deposits of calcium salts in the callus forming rigid bone in excess as a protective measure. The formation of bone binds the bone ends together. Remodeling is completed by osteoclastic activity. Excess bone is gradually reduced and removed by absorption until the original shape

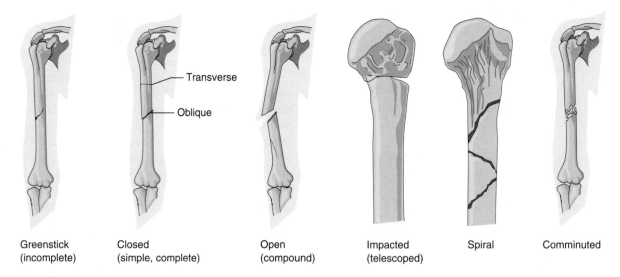

| Greenstick (incomplete) | Closed (simple, complete) | Open (compound) | Impacted (telescoped) | Spiral | Comminuted |

FIGURE 26-6 Types of bone fractures.

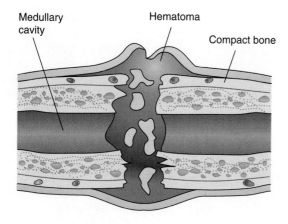

(A) A hematoma forms from blood from ruptured vessels.

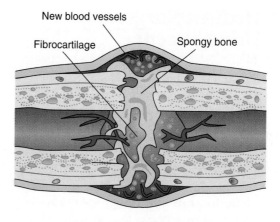

(B) Spongy bone forms close to developing blood vessels; fibrocartilage forms away from new blood vessels.

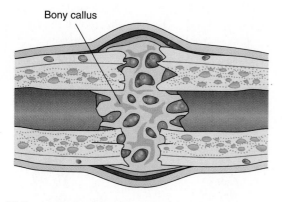

(C) Bony callus replaces fibrocartilage.

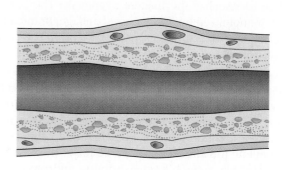

(D) Excess bony tissue is removed by osteoclasts.

FIGURE 26-7   The steps in bone repair.

and outline of the fractured bone is reestablished. Figure 26-7 outlines the healing sequence.

Complications of a fracture include infection, fat embolism, and compartment syndrome. Complications may delay healing or be life threatening.

Infections may result from an open fracture in which the bone extends through the skin allowing contamination from the outside. It may also occur following surgical repair of a fracture using an internal fixation device. Any infection may lead to a delayed union of the bone.

A fat embolism occurs when a particle of fat from the marrow of a broken bone travels in the bloodstream toward the heart and lungs. It is usually associated with fractures of the long bones, multiple fractures, or crushing injuries. An embolus may occur within twenty-four hours following a fracture. When a small area of the lungs is involved the symptoms are pain, tachycardia, and dyspnea. Larger areas of lung involvement produce more pronounced symptoms. These include severe pain, dyspnea, cyanosis, restlessness, and shock. Petechiae may appear over the neck, upper arms, chest, or abdomen. Treatment consists of bed rest, gentle handling, oxygen, and IV fluids.

▶ COMPARTMENT SYNDROME

Compartment syndrome is a form of neurovascular impairment that may lead to permanent injury of an affected limb caused by the progressive constriction of blood vessels and nerves. It can occur with any orthopedic injury as a result of bleeding into the tissue, tissue edema, or pressure from a cast or tight dressing. If untreated, in four to six hours it may lead to irreversible damage to nerves and muscles and within twenty-four to forty-eight hours permanent loss of normal limb function. A neurovascular assessment that reveals pain which is not relieved by narcotic analgesics, diminished capillary refill, weak or unequal pulses, **paresthesia**, (numbness or tingling) and paralysis are indicative of this orthopedic emergency. Treatment consists of relieving pressure by removing the cast or dressing or by performing a fasciotomy. A surgical fasciotomy is an incision into the fascia to relieve pressure on the nerves and blood vessels.

▶ *Medical/Surgical Management*

▶ *Medical*

The treatment of a fracture requires immediate attention. The most important objectives are to: (1) realign the fracture, (2) maintain the alignment, and (3) regain the function of the injured part. The method of treatment will depend on the first aid given, the site, severity, and type of the fracture, and the age and condition of the client.

Closed Reduction In closed reduction, the fracture is reduced by external manipulation. A surgical procedure is not performed. This manipulation requires three maneuvers: traction and countertraction, angulation, and rotation. Following the reduction, x-rays are taken to visualize the fracture alignment. The part is then immobilized by using a cast, bandage, or traction. A local or general anesthesia may be used to make the reduction easier and less painful to the client.

Casts A well-made and applied cast is as perfect a fixation apparatus as can be devised for the human body. Casts are made from plaster bandages or synthetic materials such as fiberglass and can be applied almost anywhere on the body. It should include the joint above and below the affected part. Three major purposes of casts include: immobilization, support and protection of the affected part, prevention of deformities which may be the result of conditions such as arthritis, and the correction of deformities like scoliosis.

Since casts dry from the inside out they should not be covered or dried with a hairdryer or heat lamp. Moisture and heat from the drying cast should be allowed to evaporate naturally. Clients should be informed that the heat they feel during the application, drying, and setting process is normal and should subside after ten to fifteen minutes. To avoid indentation, a drying cast should be placed on pillows and not on a hard surface. For the same reason, when handling the cast, only the palms of the hands should be used. A dry cast should be odorless, white and shiny in appearance, resonant when percussed, and have a temperature similar to the room air. Moisture occurring from any underlying drainage will give the cast a musty smell, dullness on percussion, a grey lusterless color, and will be cool to the touch.

Types of casts include long and short arm, which allow the fingers to be visible; long and short leg, which allow the toes to be visible; a spica, which is applied in a figure eight or spiral, and is used for hip, shoulder, and thumb dislocations or injuries. The hip spica has an abduction bar which keeps the cast in the correct position and should never be used as a turning or lifting bar. Body casts are used to immobilize the spine following surgical spinal fusions, unstable spinal injuries, or for degenerative disorders. Figure 26-8 shows different types of casts.

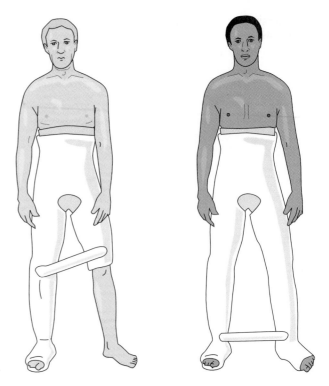

Hip spica casts

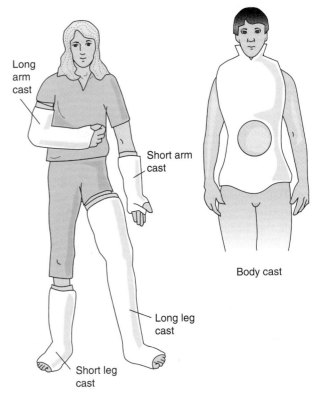

FIGURE 26-8 Casts used to correct musculoskeletal disorders.

After the application and drying of a cast, it may be necessary for the doctor to order a cast cut allowing visualization of a body area or to relieve pressure. This procedure is known as **windowing**. An arm cast may be cut in order to take a radial pulse or to dress a wound. Abdominal distention may be a reason to window a hip spica.

When a cast is removed, the client may become conscious of aches and discomforts caused by the constricted joint structures and immobilized muscles. The client's discomfort may be minimized by supporting the joint and maintaining the part in the same position as it was in the cast. The skin will be cool and pale with mottling and edema present. A yellow exudate, which is part dead skin and part secretions from oil sacs, will be on the skin. This exudate should not be rubbed or forced off.

Traction The principle of traction is to have two forces pulling in opposite directions. Traction consists of weights and counterweights. Countertraction forces can be provided by the weight of the client's body or other weight such as elevating the foot of the bed. Traction may be used to reduce a fracture, immobilize an extremity, lessen muscle spasms, or correct or prevent a deformity.

Types of traction are skeletal, skin, and manual. Skeletal traction requires the surgical insertion of pins (Steinmann) or wires (Kirschner) through the bones. Skeletal traction is continuous and is used most frequently for fractures of the femur, tibia, and cervical spine. Head tongs (e.g., Gardner-Wells tongs) are fixed in the skull to apply traction that immobilizes cervical fractures (Smeltzer & Bare 1992). Figure 26-9 shows examples of traction devices.

Skin traction is a nonsurgical method of providing necessary pull for shorter periods of time. Materials used include tapes, traction strips, cervical halters, and pelvic belts. Skin traction is frequently used to temporarily immobilize a part or stabilize a fracture. The disadvantage of skin traction for adult use is that it does not adequately control rotation and cannot be maintained for the length of time necessary for adult healing. Tapes and bandages should be applied smoothly to prevent any pressure areas.

A nurse caring for a client in traction should know the purpose of the traction, how it accomplishes its purpose, and any complications associated with the use of the traction. It is also important to know the extent of the injury and the movements and positions allowed. Care of the client should include maintenance of the injured part, general body alignment, the alignment of the traction apparatus, and range of motion in as many joints as possible.

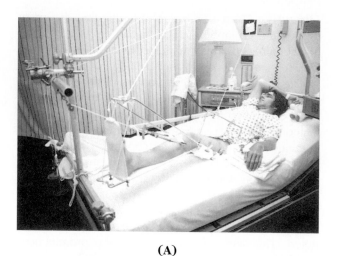

(A)

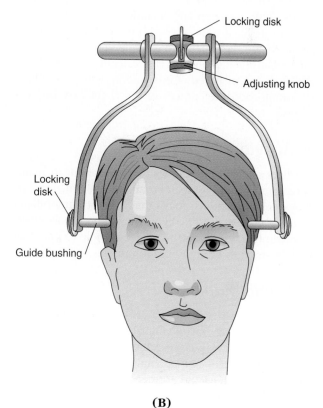

(B)

FIGURE 26-9 Types of traction devices: **(A)** Skeletal traction; **(B)** Head tongs.

▶ Surgical

Open reduction is a surgical procedure that enables the surgeon to reduce the fracture under direct visualization. When an open reduction internal fixation (ORIF) is done, orthopedic devices are used to maintain the reduction. Some of the devices used include pins, screws, nails, plates, wires, and rods. These internal fixation devices may be inserted through bone fragments or fixed to the sides of the bones.

The major disadvantage of the open reduction is the possibility of introducing infection into the bone. Other disadvantages include impaired circulation and accidental injury to major nerves, blood vessels, and bone caused by the fixation devices. X-rays may be taken during and after the open reduction to evaluate the alignment of the fracture.

▶ Pharmacological

Analgesics may be given to relieve pain. Muscle relaxants, such as cyclobenzaprine hydrochloride (Flexeril), may also be prescribed for muscle spasms. Severe or continued pain may indicate complications and should be given immediate attention. Stool softeners, such as docusate sodium (Colace), may be given to prevent constipation in the immobilized client.

▶ Diet

The client should be encouraged to eat regular meals. The meals should include foods that provide fiber, protein, calcium, phosphorus, and fluids. For the client whose dietary intake is inadequate, vitamin and mineral supplements especially calcium and phosphorus may be included. Consultation with a dietitian regarding food preferences of the client may be necessary.

▶ Activity

Client activity and exercise are important in maintaining muscle strength and tone, and minimizing cardiovascular problems. Joints that are not immobilized should be exercised either actively or passively to maintain function. Isometric exercises help to maintain muscle strength of immobilized muscles.

▶ Rehabilitation

The physician will determine when the bone has healed sufficiently for rehabilitation. Healing is monitored by periodic x-rays and physical examinations. The major objective of rehabilitation is to assist the client to return to the former level of functioning. Rehabilitation programs vary depending on the injury and the client.

Physical therapy may be started with the use of parallel bars or other exercise equipment before the client is allowed to exercise independently. The nurse has a major role in client education reinforcing the directions of both the physician and the physical therapist. Patience and encouragement are extremely important in assisting the client to feel comfortable in learning self-care techniques. The client should be taught to report any unusual signs or symptoms to the physician.

The client will also need to learn the proper use of equipment such as crutches, canes, or walkers. Crutches allow ambulation with limited weight bearing on the affected extremity. Walkers allow limited weight bearing and provide stability while the client ambulates. Canes allow the client to walk with balance and support.

The tripod position is the basic stance for crutch walking. Tips of the crutches are placed approximately 8 to 10 inches in front of and beside the client's feet. Teach the client to place his weight on the handpiece of the crutches and not on the axilla. Crutch gaits depend on the client's disability and are prescribed by the physician. See Figure 26-10 for basic crutch walking stance.

Canes are held in the hand opposite to the affected extremity. In normal walking, the opposite arm and leg move together. This same action should be done when walking with a cane. Walkers provide more support than canes or crutches. They are especially useful for clients who have poor balance. Teach the client to lift and place the walker 12 to 18 inches in front and walk toward the walker holding onto the hand grips.

▶ Nursing Process

Assessment

Subjective Data   The neurovascular assessment of a client with a fracture may reveal subjective data of pain, especially on movement, muscle spasms, and paresthesia.

Objective Data   Edema, shortening and deformity of the affected limb, and pallor may be found. Pulses in the affected and unaffected extremity must be checked and compared.

The client who has a cast applied must also have all cast edges checked for smoothness. The cast should also be checked for spots indicating wound drainage including the color and amount. Extremities including fingers, toes, hands, and feet should be assessed for changes in skin color, pulse, or temperature.

All traction wires, pulleys, and weights should be checked. Weights should hang free. The client's vital signs should be taken routinely and the general physical and mental condition of the client should be noted. The skin especially over bony prominences should be checked for color and temperature.

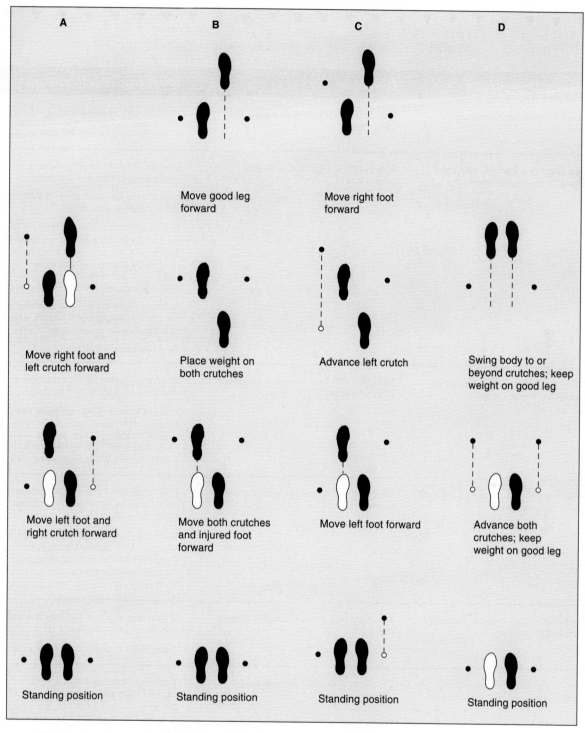

FIGURE 26-10 Crutch gaits. **(A)** Two-point; **(B)** Three-point; **(C)** Four-point; **(D)** Swing-through.

▼ ▼

Possible nursing diagnoses for a client with musculoskeletal trauma may include:

Nursing Diagnoses	Goals	Nursing Interventions
▶ *Pain (acute) related to fracture.*	The client will have relief of pain with medication.	Provide comfort measures. Administer medications for pain as ordered.
▶ *Skin integrity, impaired, high risk for related to prolonged immobility.*	The client will experience no skin breakdown.	Change client position, if allowed, maintaining correct body alignment. Check bony prominences and keep the client's skin clean and dry. For the client in a cast, check the edges of the cast for rough edges, keep the exposed skin next to the cast clean and dry, inspect of all body pressure points including the head, ears, and heels, turn the client as orders direct, and check for friction rubs. Instruct clients not to poke anything under the cast or use objects to scratch, causing skin breakdown or infections. Avoid getting the cast wet.
▶ *Tissue perfusion, altered peripheral, related to immobilizing device.*	The client will have adequate circulation to all extremities.	Perform circulatory and neurological checks at least every two hours. Perform frequent CMS checks (circulation, movement, sensation) and neurovascular checks, including pulses, edema, blanching, temperature and color of the exposed skin, and movement of the fingers and toes.
▶ *Health maintenance, altered, related to loss of independence.*	The client will regain independence in performing self-care.	Encourage the client to participate in as many self-care activities, i.e., personal hygiene, as allowed. Refer the client to a rehabilitative program which may be initiated through the combined efforts of the physical and occupational therapy departments and nursing.
▶ *Physical mobility, impaired, related to immobilizing device.*	The client will perform range of motion exercises.	If the client in a cast is allowed to turn, use an overhead trapeze. Assist client in performing ROM exercises.
▶ *Body image disturbance, related to impact of musculoskeletal condition.*	The client will adjust to body image changes.	Encourage the client with a fracture to express fears and concerns about care and recovery.

▶ *Evaluation*

Each goal must be evaluated to determine how it has been met by the client.

▲ ▲

▶ INFLAMMATORY DISORDERS

Inflammatory disorders involve the inflammation of the joints and include conditions such as rheumatoid arthritis, bursitis, polymyositis, and osteomyelitis as discussed in this section.

▶ RHEUMATOID ARTHRITIS

Rheumatoid arthritis is a chronic systemic disease of unknown etiology, with recurring inflammation involving the synovium or lining of the joints. It can also affect the lungs, heart, blood vessels, muscles, eyes, and skin. Rheumatoid arthritis is a potentially destructive and disabling disease. The course is variable with either slow or rapid progress and/or periods of remissions. Women are affected more often than men. Rheumatoid arthritis can occur at any age; however, it most commonly affects young adults. In children it occurs in a form known as juvenile rheumatoid arthritis (Still's disease). See chapter 24 for more information on rheumatoid arthritis.

▶ BURSITIS

Bursitis is inflammation of the bursa, a sac filled with synovial fluid that facilitates joint movement. Major bursae are found in the shoulder, knee, hip, and elbow. The inflammation is usually the result of trauma or repetitive movements. The client experiences painful joint movement. Diagnosis is made from the client's symptoms and x-ray which shows a calcified bursa. Treatment includes rest of the joint and the administration of anti-inflammatory drugs including salicylates and NSAIDs. For some clients, corticosteroids may be injected into the bursa.

▶ POLYMYOSITIS

Polymyositis is an inflammatory disease involving striated muscle. The etiology of this disease is unknown, but probably is an autoimmune mechanism.

It is primarily a disease of skeletal muscle; however, the heart, gastrointestinal tract, and lungs are also frequently involved. Symptoms include muscle weakness with activities like climbing the stairs, getting out of a chair, or combing the hair. The muscles of swallowing may also become involved. This weakness is the result of degeneration and necrosis of parts or entire groups of muscle fibers. Some individuals have arthralgia and Raynaud's phenomenon.

▶ Medical/Surgical Management

▶ Pharmacological

Treatment is symptomatic and begins initially with high doses of corticosteroid therapy. The doses are then modified in response to muscle enzymes. Reduction of the muscle enzymes may take several months, thus requiring long-term maintenance treatment.

▶ Diet

If the neck flexor muscles are involved, the client may need frequent small meals, antacids for reflux esophagitis, and complete bed rest with the head of the bed elevated.

▶ Activity

Physical therapy is begun to preserve muscle strength and prevent contractures.

▶ Nursing Process

Assessment

Subjective Data Ask the client questions regarding muscle or joint pain, appetite, dyspnea, and gastrointestinal symptoms.

Objective Data Objective data is gathered from observations of the client's ability to complete activities of daily living and any evidence of respiratory difficulty. Muscles and joints should be palpated for tenderness or pain.

▼ ▼

Possible nursing diagnoses for a client with polymyositis may include:

Nursing Diagnoses	Goals	Nursing Interventions
▶ *Physical mobility, impaired, related to muscle weakness.*	The client will increase physical activity as tolerated.	Assist client and encourage physical mobility, provide rest periods before and after.
▶ *Self-care deficit related to muscle weakness.*	The client will perform ADLs with minimal assistance.	Assist the client in activities whenever necessary and provide frequent position change to prevent contractures.
▶ *Nutrition, altered, less than body requirements, related to difficulty in swallowing.*	The client will maintain adequate nutritional status.	Provide small, frequent, high caloric feedings.
▶ *Knowledge deficit related to disease process, treatment, and home care management.*	The client will discuss disease process, treatment, and plans for home care.	Teach the client and family about the disease process and medications, especially management of corticosteroid therapy. Elicit plans for home care and provide referral to resources as required.

▶ Evaluation

Each goal must be evaluated to determine how it has been met by the client.

▲ ▲

▶ OSTEOMYELITIS

Osteomyelitis is the inflammation of the bone and bone marrow. The most common cause of osteomyelitis is the introduction of pathogenic bacteria into a penetrating injury such as an open fracture. Bone infections may also result from the spread of infection from another site such as infected teeth, tonsils, or an upper respiratory infection. The most common pathogen causing osteomyelitis is *Staphylococcus aureus*. Other organisms found in osteomyelitis are *Pseudomonas* and *Escherichia coli*. Osteomyelitis may become a chronic disabling problem affecting the quality of life. The affected bone may have spontaneous fractures.

Local symptoms of an acute infection are sudden pain and tenderness of the affected bone, warmth, redness, edema, and pain on movement. General symptoms with acute severe bone infections may include chills, elevated temperature, rapid pulse, and marked leukocytosis.

▶ Medical/Surgical Management

▶ Medical

The infected bone is kept at rest with the use of sandbags or casts, and the client is placed on bed rest. Antibiotics are given as soon as osteomyelitis is suspected. Unless the infective process is controlled early, a bone abscess forms. Cultures of the abscess may indicate a need for change in the antibiotic therapy. The abscess may drain naturally; however, it usually requires an incision allowing it to drain. The abscess cavity of dead bone tissue does not liquefy easily, drain, and heal as in soft tissue abscesses. A sequestrectomy to remove the dead bone tissue may need to be performed. A bone sheath forms around the sequestrum giving the appearance of healing. However, chronically infected sequestrum has the tendency to produce recurrent abscesses throughout the life of the individual.

Strict aseptic technique must be maintained when changing any dressings. Because infected bone may be extremely painful, unnecessary movement should be avoided and the affected extremity should be handled very gently.

▶ Pharmacological

Vigorous antibiotic therapy and analgesics are the medications used for the treatment of osteomyelitis. Wound irrigations with antiseptics or antibiotics are often prescribed by the physician. Specific drugs given are determined by the causative organism.

▶ Diet

A high caloric and high protein diet is generally ordered for the client with osteomyelitis. Dietary supplements of vitamins and calcium should also be given. Fluids should be increased as tolerated.

▶ Activity

There should be absolute rest of the affected extremity. Excessive handling of the extremity is very painful and should be avoided. The extremity should be handled in a smooth unhurried manner supporting the joints above and below the affected area.

▶ Nursing Process

Assessment

Subjective Data Inquire about pain and tenderness in the bone. Ask about any traumas in the area.

Objective Data Observe the client for signs of infection, including chills, elevated temperature, pain, redness, and edema of the affected extremity. The client may also experience headaches, restlessness, and irritability.

▼ ▼

Possible nursing diagnoses for a client with osteomyelitis may include:

Nursing Diagnoses	Goals	Nursing Interventions
▶ Physical mobility, impaired, related to pain.	The client will maintain full movement of unaffected extremities.	Encourage and assist client to maintain active ROM or perform passive ROM to unaffected extremities.
▶ Skin integrity, impaired, high risk for related to immobility.	The client will maintain skin integrity.	Handle the affected extremity gently, protect it from injury, keep it in good body alignment and level with the body. Irrigate wound as ordered. Use aseptic technique when irrigating the affected area and when changing the dressing. Assess skin and bony prominences for reddened areas. Encourage adequate fluid intake.
▶ Knowledge deficit related to home care management.	The client will have a plan for care at home.	Teach client the kind of care required at home. Assist client in analyzing home situation and how care requirements can be accomplished.
▶ Pain related to inflammation.	The client will verbalize absence of pain.	Protect client from jerky movements and falls. Assess wound appearance and new sites of pain. Provide diet high in protein and vitamin C. Administer pain medications as ordered.

(continued)

Nursing Diagnoses	Goals	Nursing Interventions
▶ *Knowledge deficit related to the treatment program.*	The client will be able to explain how to care for the wound using aseptic technique.	Teach client proper handwashing and strict aseptic technique. Teach wound irrigation, dressing change, medications, and activity restrictions.

▶ *Evaluation*

Each goal must be evaluated to determine how it has been met by the client.

▲ ▲

DEGENERATIVE DISORDERS

▶ OSTEOPOROSIS

Osteoporosis is an increase in the porosity of bone. It is a common disorder in bone metabolism in which both mineral and protein matrix components are diminished and the bone becomes brittle and fragile. This diminished density occurs in approximately one-fourth of all elderly persons, but more frequently in females. It is most common in women who are fair-skinned and small-framed. The reduction of bone mass in females is related to the decrease in estrogen after menopause. Other causes of osteoporosis are Cushing's syndrome, prolonged use of high doses of corticosteroids, prolonged periods of immobility, diets deficient in vitamin D and calcium, smoking, and excessive coffee and protein intake.

Symptoms are few, however, individuals especially postmenopausal women, experience pain in the lumbar spine vertebrae. Because the bone tissue loses its density, fractures and kyphosis may occur. Very slight trauma may fracture the brittle bones. With multiple vertebral fractures, the individual may experience a loss of height.

Diagnosis is made by x-ray. Laboratory tests specifically calcium, phosphorus, and phosphatase are usually normal. A CT scan provides information on bone mass.

▶ Medical/Surgical Management

There is no direct treatment for osteoporosis. Physical activity is encouraged to strengthen muscles, increase bone density, and to prevent disuse atrophy.

▶ Pharmacological

Nonnarcotic analgesics may be prescribed for relief of pain. The client may also be advised to take supplemental calcium. Postmenopausal women may be treated with estrogen therapy.

▶ Diet

The client is encouraged to maintain an adequate balanced diet rich in calcium and vitamin D. Dietary calcium and vitamin D must be adequate to maintain bone remodeling. A reduction in the consumption of caffeine, alcohol, excess protein, and the use of cigarettes is recommended.

▶ Activity

The client is encouraged to practice good body mechanics and posture. Walking, preferably outdoors for the benefits of sunshine (vitamin D), is also encouraged. This has been effective in preventing further bone loss and stimulating new bone formation.

▶ Nursing Process

Assessment

Subjective Data This includes the client's sex, age, and family health history. Any symptoms the client expresses regarding altered body image or back or neck pain that worsens when coughing, sneezing, straining, or standing should be noted. A nutritional history should be taken. Lifestyle patterns such as smoking, inactivity, or immobilization should be noted. A medical history regarding any medications is also important.

Objective Data This includes a dowager's hump, gait impairment, and posture.

▼ ▼

Possible nursing diagnoses for a client with osteoporosis may include:

Nursing Diagnoses	Goals	Nursing Interventions
▶ Pain, chronic, related to disease process.	The client will express minimal discomfort.	Administer analgesics as ordered; teach the client about the medications.
		Handle the client carefully; instruct the client to avoid any twisting movements.
		The bed should have a firm mattress or bed board for support.
▶ Injury, high risk for, related to disease process.	The client will practice correct body mechanics.	Teach client good posture and correct body mechanics.
▶ Physical mobility, impaired, related to disease process.	The client will increase physical activity.	Teach client about types of exercises and physical activities that will help maintain bone mass and isometric exercises to strengthen muscles.
		Encourage ambulation with the client using a walker or cane if necessary.
▶ Knowledge deficit related to home care management.	The client will demonstrate an understanding of home care management.	Assist client to identify potential hazards at home, such as scatter rugs.
		Allow the client to verbalize any concerns or feelings about the disease.

▶ *Evaluation*

Each goal must be evaluated to determine how it has been met by the client.

▲ ▲

▶ *OSTEOARTHRITIS*

Osteoarthritis is considered a "wear and tear" disease and is characterized by the slow and steady progressive destructive changes of the joint. It is a nonsystemic, noninflammatory disorder causing bones and joints to degenerate. It is the most common type of arthritis. The etiology of osteoarthritis is unknown. Predisposing factors include obesity, an injury to a joint, poor posture, or occupations that put strain on joints. The weight bearing joints of the lower extremities as well as the hands and cervical and lumbar vertebrae are the joints most frequently affected. The cartilage covering the bone becomes thin and then wears off. The synovial membrane thickens and fibrous tissue around the joint ossifies. The effects of degenerative changes on the knee joint is shown in Figure 26-11.

The onset of osteoarthritis begins during middleage and by age seventy most people have some degeneration. Symptoms include early morning stiffness and pain after exercise. There is joint enlargement and characteristic hypertrophic spurs, called Heberden's nodes, in the terminal interphalangeal finger joints.

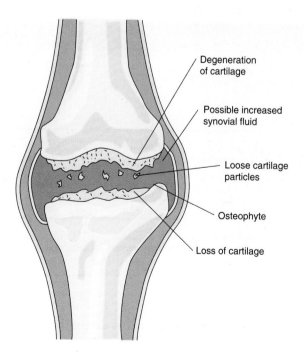

FIGURE 26-11 Degenerative changes in the cartilage of the knee.

Diagnosis is made from the client's symptoms and examination of the joints that are enlarged and tender. X-ray shows a narrowing of joint spaces and gross irregularities of joint structure.

► Medical/Surgical Management

► Medical

No treatment exists to stop the degenerative process, therefore, treatment focuses on the relief of the client's discomfort. Medical management includes local heat and rest for the affected joint, weight reduction for obese clients to relieve strain on affected joints, and orthotic devices (braces, canes, crutches) to support the inflamed joints. Physical therapy can provide exercises to strengthen muscles and teach self-management skills.

► Surgical

Surgical procedures such as total hip or knee replacement may be recommended for clients with severe osteoarthritis. Osteotomy may help correct malalignment situations. Refer to the section on total joint arthroplasty in this chapter.

► Pharmacological

Pharmacological treatment includes the use of aspirin or NSAIDs. Narcotics should be avoided because of the chronic nature of the disease.

► Nursing Process

Assessment

Subjective Data The client may describe nonspecific symptoms such as malaise, fatigue, general musculoskeletal pain, joint stiffness especially on rising, and joint pain or tenderness. Inquire about any conditions or situations that may exacerbate the client's joint pain. Some of these situations may include cold weather, overexercising, or extreme fatigue. Assess the client's understanding of the disease and its effect on his lifestyle and ability to perform activities of daily and social living.

Objective Data This includes edema around the joints and bony enlargements of distal interphalangeal joints (Heberden's nodes).

▼ ▼

Possible nursing diagnoses for a client with osteoarthritis may include:

Nursing Diagnoses	Goals	Nursing Interventions
► Pain, chronic, related to joint tenderness and edema.	The client will express minimal discomfort.	Handle the affected extremity gently and apply heat as ordered. Administer prescribed analgesic and evaluate its effectiveness.
► Physical mobility, impaired, related to joint deterioration.	The client will have increased mobility within the parameters of the disease process.	Coordinate with physical therapy and assist in a planned exercise program as ordered. Advise the client to plan rest periods during the day.
► Knowledge deficit related to disease process and home care management.	The client will verbalize understanding of self-care.	Provide information to the client about the nature of the disease and the purpose of any prescribed treatments.

► Evaluation

Each goal must be evaluated to determine how it has been met by the client.

▲ ▲

▶ TOTAL JOINT ARTHROPLASTY

Joint replacement or **arthroplasty** is the replacement of both articular surfaces within a joint capsule. The hip, knee, shoulder, and fingers are the joints most frequently replaced in this procedure. Most replacements consist of metal and polyethylene and may be cemented in the prepared bone with methyl methacrylate which has properties similar to bone. See Figure 26-12 for knee and hip replacement components.

Newer techniques use porous-coated cementless artificial joint components. These allow bone to grow into the joint component and securely fix the prosthesis. This reduces the incidence of prosthesis failure. Joint replacement is usually an elective procedure and clients are encouraged to pre-donate their own blood in case a blood transfusion is needed.

▶ *Total Hip Replacement*

Total hip replacement is the replacement of a severely damaged hip with an artificial joint. This procedure is usually reserved for clients over sixty with severe pain or irreversibly damaged hip joints. However, with improved prosthetic materials and operative techniques, younger clients with severely damaged hips are being considered for total hip replacement surgery. Potential problems with the hip replacement include dislocation of the prosthesis, excessive wound drainage, and infection.

Following a total hip replacement the client's hip and leg should be kept in a position of abduction and extension. The knees are kept apart by using foam wedges, several pillows, or an abductor pillow. The client may lie on the unoperative side. When the client turns from his back to a side-lying position, the entire leg should be supported with pillows keeping the hip abducted. The client should be instructed to avoid acute flexion of the hip. The legs should not be crossed or the hips flexed to pull up a blanket or sheet. A fracture bedpan should be used until the client can ambulate to the bathroom. In the bathroom a raised toilet seat should be used. Any specific client turning, movement, and positioning will be ordered by the physician. Vital signs and circulation, movement and sensation (CMS) checks should be done routinely.

Dressings should be inspected frequently. If the

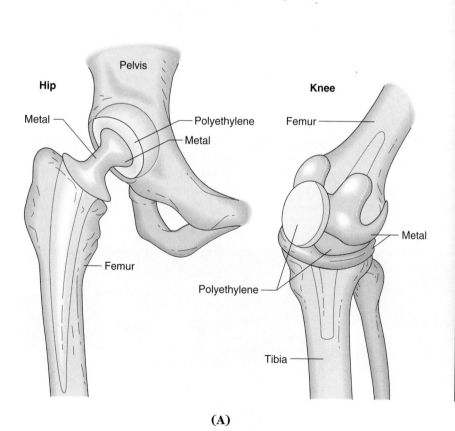

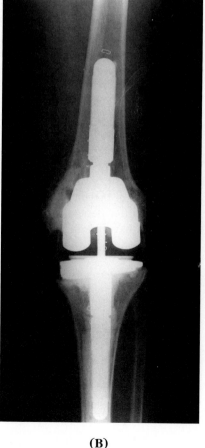

(A)   **(B)**

FIGURE 26-12 **(A)** Total hip and total knee replacement; **(B)** Radiograph of a total knee replacement (anterior-posterior view). Because the patella is plastic, it is not visible here.

surgical site is drained with a portable suction device, it should be monitored for patency, and the type and amount of drainage. Initially drainage might be 200 to 500 cc. Within forty-eight hours the drainage should decrease to 30 cc or less and the suction device can be removed.

The goal for clients who have total hip or knee joint replacement is to ambulate independently. Ambulatory activity progresses rapidly for clients with joint replacement. Clients who have total hip replacement are usually out of bed in two to three days. Gait training may begin with the use of a walker and progresses to the use of crutches or a cane. The client should avoid hip flexion of more than 90 degrees. Stair climbing should be avoided for at least three months.

▶ Total Knee Replacement

Total knee replacement, like the hip replacement, is considered for clients experiencing severe pain and functional disability related to joint destruction. The prosthesis chosen for the replacement provides the client with a painless, stable, and functional joint. Following total knee replacement surgery, clients may use a continuous passive motion machine (CPM) as shown in Figure 26-13. This machine helps to increase circulation to the operative area and promotes flexibility within the knee joint. The surgeon orders the frequency of use and the amount of tension, flexion, and extension produced by the machine.

Following knee arthroplasty, the client's knee may be immobilized with a firm compression dressing and an adjustable soft knee immobilizer. The client may transfer out of bed to a wheelchair with the immobilizer in place. No weight bearing is allowed on the knee until it is prescribed by the surgeon. If ordered, antiembolism stockings are worn to minimize the development of thrombophlebitis.

Rehabilitation generally starts the second day for clients who have total knee arthroplasty. The knee is

protected with a knee immobilizer and there should be no weight bearing on the operated knee. When the client sits in a chair, the knee should be elevated. Ambulation with assistive aids and weight bearing limits is usually started one to two days after surgery.

▶ Nursing Process

Assessment

Subjective Data This involves assessing for irritability, restlessness, orientation, and neurovascular assessment of the affected extremity for pain, numbness, tingling, and paresthesia.

Objective Data This involves assessing the incision for approximation, redness, and drainage. Assessment of skin over all bony prominences should also be made, as well as assessment for tachypnea, dyspnea, hypoxemia, and crackles and wheezes in the lungs (signs of fat embolism). Vital signs, pedal pulses, and I & O are also assessed.

The client with a total hip replacement should be assessed for position of the affected hip. The hip should be maintained in a position of abduction and extension. A complication of a total hip replacement is dislocation. The most prominent symptom of a dislocation is a clicking, popping sound. Other symptoms are a sudden sharp pain which is unrelieved by narcotic analgesics, loss of leg motion, and edema of the affected hip. The client should not be moved and the physician should be notified immediately. Surgical replacement is the only treatment for a dislocation.

Assessment of the client with a total knee replacement includes the neurovascular status of the leg, the dressing and drainage device, keeping the knee elevated, and monitoring the CPM machine. Vital signs, intake and output, and the color and temperature of the extremity are also assessed.

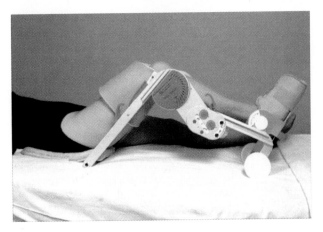 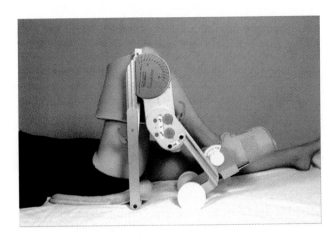

FIGURE 26-13 Continuous passive motion machine. (*Photos courtesy of US Ortho, Aurora, CO*)

▼ ▼

Possible nursing diagnoses for the client undergoing arthroplasty surgery may include:

Nursing Diagnoses	Goals	Nursing Interventions
▶ Pain, acute, related to surgery.	The client will experience pain relief.	Administer pain medications as prescribed and evaluate and document their effectiveness.
▶ Skin integrity, impaired, related to immobility and surgical incision.	The client's skin will remain free from redness or any other signs of breakdown.	Maintain a clean and dry dressing. If a drainage device is used, measure the output. Assess bony prominences for redness. Provide high protein diet with dairy products and vitamin C.
▶ Physical mobility, impaired, related to surgery.	The client will ambulate following physician's direction.	Keep client in a position of abduction. Use an abductor pillow or wedge to maintain the position when turning the client. Assist the client in accomplishing activities of daily living. Encourage client to use the trapeze to raise hips off the bed to use the bedpan.
▶ Injury, high risk for, related to unsteady gait.	The client will avoid injury by using appropriate assistive aids.	Work with physical therapy to teach ambulation skills with assistive devices. Assist or be present when client ambulates.
▶ Tissue perfusion, altered peripheral, related to surgery and immobility.	The client will have adequate circulation of lower extremity.	Encourage the client to cough and deep breathe. Monitor vital signs until stable. Assess pedal pulses and capillary refill in both extremities.

▶ Evaluation

Each goal must be evaluated to determine how it has been met by the client.

▲ ▲

MUSCULOSKELETAL DISORDERS

▶ AMPUTATIONS

An amputation is the surgical removal of all or part of an extremity. Amputations are done as a result of injuries resulting in extensive laceration of arteries or nerves or as the result of disease such as malignant tumors, infections, and peripheral vascular disorders. Other disease conditions that may require amputation include extensive osteomyelitis, or congenital disor-

ders. In severe trauma situations an amputation may be done to save the client's life. Recent advances in microsurgical techniques have allowed replantation (limb reattachment) in some injuries. These procedures involve the use of microscopes and highly specialized instruments to reconnect severed nerves and blood vessels. Amputations involving the hand or wrist are more likely to be considered for replantation rather than an injury involving a large muscle mass because of extensive tissue, bone, and muscle damage. Any amputation creates a major physical and psychological adjustment for the client.

▶ Medical/Surgical Management

▶ Surgical

Before surgery the surgeon must evaluate the client and make several decisions. These decisions include: necessity of an amputation, type of amputation (open or closed), level of amputation, potential for rehabilitation, and type of prosthesis and rehabilitation program.

The surgeon will try to save as much of the limb as possible. A closed amputation is done by using skin flaps to cover the bone end of the extremity. This type of amputation is done when there is no evidence of infection. Sometimes a Guillotine (open) amputation is necessary. This amputation requires a straight cut and allows for free drainage of infectious material. Tissue, bone, and vessels are severed at the same level without skin flaps. The major indication for doing an open amputation is infection.

The level of an amputation is determined by the vascular supply and never higher than absolutely necessary. If the blood flow at the sight of the incision is normal, the amputation is performed at that level. If the bleeding is scant a higher level of amputation is performed to ensure adequate postoperative healing.

▶ Pharmacological

Narcotic analgesics may be required immediately following surgery. After several days pain may be controlled with nonnarcotic analgesics. If a client has experienced chronic pain prior to the amputation, pain may seem mild following the surgery and an analgesic may be the only medication needed. Severe pain may indicate a hematoma or excessive pressure from a cast or elastic bandage on a bony prominence. The client may confuse **phantom limb pain** with the incisional pain. Phantom limb pain is the sensation that there is pain, soreness, and stiffness in the amputated limb. Phantom pain will decrease as inflammation subsides at the incisional site. If infection exists, a culture should be taken of the drainage to determine the appropriate antibiotic therapy.

▶ Diet

A balanced diet with adequate vitamins and protein is essential for adequate wound healing. Many elderly clients are poorly nourished or require special diets. Nutritional care plans should be discussed with the physician and a dietitian.

▶ Activity

Postoperative positioning of the stump will be determined by the surgeon. The stump may be placed in an extended position or elevated on pillows for short periods. The client should also be encouraged to spend some time in the prone position. This position helps to stretch the flexor muscles and to prevent contractions of the hip. One to two days following surgery the client may begin bed exercises. These exercises, taught by the physical therapist, are done to prevent contractures and increase muscle strength. Ambulation begins in physical therapy after transfer techniques are learned by the client. Ambulation progresses according to whether the client is to be fitted with a prosthesis immediately or at a later time.

▶ Rehabilitation

Rehabilitation for the client with an amputation requires the effort of the entire rehabilitation team. The client's physical and psychological responses to the amputation should be monitored by all members of the team. If appropriate, counseling and job training will enable many clients to return to their jobs.

▶ Nursing Process

Assessment

Subjective Data   This should include pain, sensations felt on extremity to be amputated, and the emotional status of the client.

Objective Data   This includes the color and temperature of the skin, pulse, and responses to limb movement. The unaffected extremity should also be assessed for function and circulation.

▼ ▼

Possible nursing diagnoses for the client who has an amputation may include:

Nursing Diagnoses	Goals	Nursing Interventions
► Pain, acute, related to surgery.	The client will verbalize relief from surgical pain.	Assess pain by having client identify pain on a scale of 1 to 10. Provide comfort measures, give back rub, assist client to turn. Administer analgesics as ordered for surgical pain. Refer client to counselor or clergy if the pain is associated with grief and the loss of a body part.
► Skin integrity, impaired, related to amputation.	The client will remain free from infection.	Inspect the incision for any inflammation, excessive drainage, edema, increased pain, and hypersensitivity to touch. Use aseptic technique for all dressing changes. Monitor vital signs.
► Body image disturbance related to loss of limb.	The client will participate in the care of the residual limb.	Handle the residual limb gently and treat it as though a prosthesis will be worn. Encourage client to watch dressing change and eventually assist with and do the dressing changes. Encourage the client to express feelings and concerns about the amputation.
► Physical mobility, impaired, related to loss of limb.	The client will demonstrate improved physical mobility.	Encourage the client to participate in physical therapy. Assist the client when ambulating with assistive devices. Encourage client to perform ROM exercises.
► Knowledge deficit related to lifestyle limitations.	The client will identify lifestyle limitations.	Assist client to analyze lifestyle and what changes may have to be made.

► Evaluation

Each goal must be evaluated to determine how it has been met by the client.

▲ ▲

Sample Nursing Care Plan: The Client with a Below the Knee Amputation

Mrs. Spencer is a seventy-six-year-old resident in a retirement home. She has remained active since her retirement from the secretarial job she held for twenty years. Her health history indicates she has had circulatory problems with inadequate peripheral circulation resulting from atherosclerosis. Her physician has hospitalized her for a planned below the knee amputation and has ordered an arteriogram to assist in determining the site of the amputation. The arteriogram will help determine the circulatory status of her leg necessary to promote wound healing.

The nurse's assessment of Mrs. Spencer's vital signs were B/P 120/68, pulse 72, and respirations 18. Femoral pulses were present in both extremities; however, the pedal pulse in her left foot was barely palpable, and the skin was cool and pale. She stated that lately her left foot is always cold and is a "bluish-black" color. Mrs. Spencer has expressed concern for her ability to take care of herself after she loses her foot.

Nursing Diagnosis 1 Pain, acute, related to surgical incision as evidenced by having surgery.

Goals	Nursing Interventions	Rationale	Evaluation
Mrs. Spencer will express relief from pain after taking her prescribed pain medication.	Assess symptoms of pain and administer medications as prescribed. Perform comfort measures such as position change, massage.	Documents client complaints and allows for medication adjustment. Measures reduce muscle tension, change pressure on body parts.	Mrs. Spencer states pain is less after pain medication is given.

Nursing Diagnosis 2 Infection, high risk for, related to impaired healing as evidenced by inadequate peripheral circulation.

Goals	Nursing Interventions	Rationale	Evaluation
Mrs. Spencer's skin will remain warm and will not become reddened, discolored, or edematous.	Use sterile technique when changing dressing. Administer antibiotics as ordered.	Avoids contamination of incision. Decreases incidence of infection.	Incision remains free from signs and symptoms of infection.

Nursing Diagnosis 3 Injury, high risk, for related to motor deficit as evidenced by amputation.

Goals	Nursing Interventions	Rationale	Evaluation
Mrs. Spencer will identify safety measures to prevent injuries.	Keep the environment uncluttered. Support the use of appropriate adaptive devices such as crutches, walkers, wheelchairs.	Safety factor when Mrs. Spencer begins ambulation. Decreases potential for injury.	Mrs. Spencer did not fall while using assistive devices.

Nursing Diagnosis 4 Body image disturbance, related to amputation as evidenced by statement of losing foot.

Goals	Nursing Interventions	Rationales	Evaluations
Mrs. Spencer will communicate her concerns and feelings about the changes in her body image.	Involve Mrs. Spencer in participating in her daily care. Encourage Mrs. Spencer to voice her concerns. Provide positive reinforcement when Mrs. Spencer attempts to adapt to body changes.	Gives sense of independence. Helps resolve concerns. Encourages her to continue adapting.	Mrs. Spencer has demonstrated beginning acceptance of body changes by taking an active interest in her appearance.

Nursing Diagnosis 5 Self-esteem, situational low, related to loss of body part as evidenced by express concern for ability to care for self.

Goals	Nursing Interventions	Rationales	Evaluations
Mrs. Spencer will identify at least two positive qualities about herself.	Encourage Mrs. Spencer to express her feelings about herself. Involve Mrs. Spencer in the decision-making process regarding her care. Provide Mrs. Spencer with positive feedback.	Listening helps Mrs. Spencer identify positive qualities. Helps Mrs. Spencer maintain a sense of control over her life. Gives Mrs. Spencer a feeling of approval.	Mrs. Spencer has voiced two positive qualities about herself.

Nursing Diagnosis 6 Grieving, anticipatory, related to loss associated with amputation as evidenced by her expression of concern.

Goals	Nursing Interventions	Rationales	Evaluations
Mrs. Spencer will express her feelings about the loss of her foot.	Encourage Mrs. Spencer to express her feelings by talking, crying, writing. Spend a specific amount of nonnursing time each shift with Mrs. Spencer to allow for uninterrupted conversation. Inform Mrs. Spencer and her family about support groups and organizations in the community.	Some people are uncomfortable expressing their feelings, give several options for expression. Allows expression of feelings and shows concern and understanding. May help Mrs. Spencer find new ways of adapting to loss.	Mrs. Spencer expresses feelings about her potential loss.

Nursing Diagnosis 7 Knowledge deficit related to postoperative care and activity as evidenced by concern of ability to care for self.

Goals	Nursing Interventions	Rationales	Evaluations
Mrs. Spencer will perform stump wrapping correctly.	Encourage Mrs. Spencer to participate in the care of the residual limb.	Encouraging participation helps client adjust to body changes.	Mrs. Spencer demonstrated the ability to care for the residual limb by wrapping the stump correctly.
	Instruct Mrs. Spencer on the importance of adhering to a scheduled exercise plan.	Helps Mrs. Spencer regain as much physical independence as possible.	
	Encourage Mrs. Spencer to eat well-balanced nutritious meals.	Maintains nutritional status.	
	Demonstrate how to wrap her stump, then allow her to do it several times.	Discharge instructions help clients to know how to take care of themselves.	

▶ TEMPOROMANDIBULAR JOINT DYSFUNCTION SYNDROME (TMJ)

The temporomandibular joint is the articular surface between the mandible and temporal bone of the skull. It is a combined hinge and gliding joint. Normally, the mandible moves smoothly, appears symmetrical, and is without deformity. Causes for TMJ include: uneven closure of the teeth, trauma, stress, teeth clenching or grinding (**bruxism**), and joint diseases such as rheumatoid arthritis or osteoarthritis. It is more common in women than in men. Common symptoms of TMJ include limited jaw movement, clicking or crepitus when the jaw moves, popping when chewing or talking, and pain around the ears. The clicking is caused by displaced cartilage. The jaw may lock as a result of muscle spasms.

Diagnosis of TMJ will include an x-ray to evaluate the bony structure, a CT scan to evaluate any degenerative changes, and an evaluation of the teeth and jaw in a bite position. Nursing assessment of the joint includes movement and appearance. If the mandible protrudes it may indicate a mandibular dislocation.

Medical management consists of moist heat or ultrasound to promote muscle relaxation; cold therapy, which helps to reduce muscle spasms; and analgesics or nonsteroidal anti-inflammatory drugs. Clients may be fitted with a dental retainer or bite plate to prevent teeth clenching or grinding, or splints to help realign malocclusions. Procedures such as arthroscopy or surgery to reshape the joint may be done in some cases that do not respond to medical treatment.

▶ CARPAL TUNNEL SYNDROME

Carpal tunnel syndrome occurs when the median nerve in the wrist is compressed by an inflamed, edematous flexor tendon sheath. Symptoms include pain, paresthesia (tingling, prickling, or numbness), and weakness of the thumb, index, and middle fingers. Persons working in occupations requiring repetitive movement of hands and fingers, such as computers, typing, intense quilting, or crocheting have a higher incidence of this syndrome. Diagnosis is based on a physical examination and the subjective symptoms of the client and confirmed by motor nerve velocity studies.

▶ Medical/Surgical Management

Treatment consists of rest for the hands. Splints to immobilize the hand and wrist may also be used to help relieve some of the discomfort. Hydrocortisone acetate (Cortifoam) may be injected into the carpal tunnel to relieve symptoms. If conservative medical treatment is not successful, surgery may be necessary to relieve the pressure on the nerve.

▶ Nursing Process

Assessment

Subjective Data This consists of the client's description of tingling in the hands, and numbness in the thumb, index, and middle fingers. The client may also state that there is a feeling of "puffiness" in the affected hand and is unable to grasp or hold small objects.

Objective Data This may include atrophy of the padded area at the base of the thumb.

▼ ▼

Possible nursing diagnoses for a client with carpal tunnel syndrome may include:

Nursing Diagnoses	Goals	Nursing Interventions
▶ Pain acute related to inflammation and swelling causing pressure on the median nerve.	The client will have less discomfort.	Administer analgesics as ordered and teach client about use, side effects, and dosage. Encourage client to refrain from repetitive hand movements.
▶ Disuse syndrome, hand, high risk for, related to tingling and numbness of hand.	The client will be able to use fingers and hand.	Teach client to do ROM exercises, and to prevent twisting and turning of wrist.
▶ Knowledge deficit related to lack of information about condition.	The client will be able to discuss actions needed to reduce discomfort in hand and fingers.	Teach client how to apply splint and to elevate hand for relief of edema. Teach client causes of the condition.

▶ Evaluation

Each goal must be evaluated to determine how it has been met by the client.

▲ ▲

▶ SYSTEMIC DISORDERS WITH MUSCULOSKELE-TAL MANIFESTATIONS

▶ GOUT

Gout is a hereditary metabolic disease of ineffective purine metabolism, resulting in abnormal amounts of urates in the body. Uric acid is found in blood and urine specimens. The etiology of gout may also be of unknown origin or could be secondary to the use of certain drugs. It usually attacks men between the ages of twenty and sixty. The attack generally begins abruptly with severe constant pain. The joint becomes swollen, red, and tender. The great toe is the joint most frequently involved; however, any joint may be affected. The course of gout is variable with one to two attacks being severe. If the disease is untreated the attacks may occur with increasing frequency. Clients with symptoms of gout may develop **tophi** which are nodular deposits of sodium urate crystals appearing in various parts of the body including the rim of the ears, the knuckles, and great toe. Diagnosis is made from the client's health history and an examination of the affected joint. Aspiration of the joint synovial fluid will show urate crystals. The client should be instructed to avoid foods high in purine. These foods include liver, sardines, sweetbreads, anchovies, meat gravies, and asparagus. Oral fluid intake should be increased to reduce the possibility of urate stone formation in the kidneys. Medications prescribed include colchicine and probenecid (Benemid).

▶ LYME DISEASE

Lyme disease is caused by a spirochete carried by deer ticks. In the United States it is endemic along the East Coast from Massachusetts to Virginia, and in Wisconsin, Minnesota, California, and Oregon (Smeltzer & Bare, 1992).

These ticks should be removed by using a tweezers rather than the traditional method of applying heat to the body or turpentine to the head of the tick. Early manifestations occur from spring through late fall. People living in states with a high incidence of Lyme disease should wear protective clothing and check for ticks frequently. Insect repellent containing DEET should be applied to exposed parts of the body and to clothing. Household pets should wear a flea and tick collar and also be checked frequently for ticks.

For about 30 percent of individuals, early symptoms include a red macule or papule at the site of the tick bite, a rash with round rings, headache, neck stiffness and pain. For others, symptoms may not occur until

weeks or months later as arthritis (joint swelling and pain), fatigue, and neurological abnormalities like facial palsy, meningitis, and encephalitis become evident. A polymerase chain reaction test that identifies specific spirochetes and other general blood tests are used to diagnose Lyme disease. Early treatment with antibiotics such as tetracycline (Achromycin), erythromycin (Erythrocin), and phenoxymethyl penicillin (Pen Vee) may shorten the duration of the disease. Antibiotics can also be used when symptoms develop later.

▶ CASE STUDY

George Ellis, a forty-year-old truck driver, was getting ready to help unload his cargo. He was climbing into the truck when he lost his balance and fell to the ground twisting his left leg. He stated he was in severe pain and was unable to stand. His coworkers called the emergency ambulance service to transport him to the hospital. Upon arrival in the emergency room, the nurse immediately took Mr. Ellis' vital signs. His vital signs were temperature 98.6, pulse 92, respirations 24, and blood pressure 158/90. The nurse also noted that Mr. Ellis' face was flushed and his left leg was shorter than his right.

The following questions will guide your development of a Nursing Care Plan for the case study.

1. List five types of fractures.
2. Based on the action of the fall, what type of fracture do you think Mr. Ellis received?
3. What diagnostic measures will determine whether or not Mr. Ellis has a fracture of his left leg?
4. What immediate care should have been given to Mr. Ellis?
5. List four nursing interventions for clients in traction.
6. What options may be considered for treatment of Mr. Ellis' injury?
7. List objective and subjective information the nurse would obtain regarding Mr. Ellis' injury.

SUMMARY

• When assessing the client with a musculoskeletal disorder the nurse should evaluate any changes in appearance including alignment, loss of motion, and any signs of circulatory impairment.
• Treatment of a fracture may include any one or more of the following methods: closed reduction, open reduction that may include internal fixation, casts, and traction.

• Complications of a fracture include infection, fat embolism, and compartment syndrome.
• Casts are applied using plaster bandages or synthetic materials. The cast should include the joint above and below the affected part.
• Compartment syndrome is a serious form of neurovascular impairment. Symptoms include severe pain that is not relieved with narcotic analgesics, sluggish capillary refill, weak pulses, numbness, and paralysis.

- When a client is in traction it is important to remember to preserve body alignment, maintain continuous pull and countertraction, keep the ropes moving freely through the pulleys, use the prescribed amount of weights, and keep the weights hanging freely.
- Rheumatoid arthritis is a chronic progressive inflammatory disease involving the synovium or lining of the joints. It is a potentially disabling disease.
- Osteoarthritis is characterized by slow progressive degeneration of joint articular cartilage.
- Hips, knees, and fingers are the joints most frequently considered for replacement.
- Following total hip replacement, the hip should be kept in a position of abduction and extension.
- Following total knee replacement surgery some clients may use a CPM machine that promotes knee joint flexibility and increased circulation to the operative area.
- Individuals at greatest risk for developing osteoporosis are postmenopausal women and older adults who are generally inactive.
- Carpal tunnel syndrome occurs in individuals who perform jobs requiring repetitive wrist and hand movements. The resulting trauma causes inflammation and edema which compresses the median nerve causing numbness, pain and impaired mobility to the hand and fingers.

Review Questions

1. Upon admission to the hospital the client expresses concerns for his job. This information will become which part of his nursing care plan?

    a. nursing diagnosis
    b. goal
    c. validating factor
    d. evaluation

2. A fracture caused by forceful twisting is known as what kind of a fracture?

    a. Comminuted
    b. Spiral
    c. Transverse
    d. Greenstick

3. The primary goal in the treatment of a fracture is to:

    a. aid in the formation of osteoclasts.
    b. aid in the formation of granulation tissue.
    c. establish a callus between the broken ends of bone.
    d. prevent further injury to the fractured limb.

4. A closed reduction of a fracture:

    a. always requires surgery.
    b. is completed by manual manipulation.
    c. never requires a cast.
    d. requires the use of immobilizing plates.

5. Poor body positioning and alignment of an immobilized client may result in deformities. One of the deformities that may develop is:

    a. scoliosis.
    b. lordosis.
    c. contracture.
    d. atony.

6. One of the first symptoms a client with arthritis may complain of is:

    a. nausea after each meal.
    b. joint stiffness especially on arising.
    c. an increased appetite.
    d. muscle spasms after exercising.

7. Areas of the body most often affected by arthritis are:

    a. knees, hips, fingers.
    b. shoulders, hips, ankles.
    c. back, knees, ankles.
    d. shoulders, elbows, fingers.

8. Braces, casts, or splints may be applied to joints that are painful or in spasm. This is done to prevent:

    a. deformities.
    b. edema.
    c. inflammation.
    d. fractures.

9. Traction is frequently used to treat clients with a musculoskeletal problem. One of the primary reasons for traction is to:

    a. heal a fracture.
    b. maintain a corrected position.
    c. stop muscle spasms.
    d. prevent infection.

10. Osteomyelitis:

    a. affects mainly the hip bone.
    b. is a bacterial infection of the bone.
    c. occurs most often in adults.
    d. causes a great deal of deformity.

Critical Thinking Questions

1 Prepare a teaching plan for a client to learn how to use crutches.

2. How would you explain "phantom limb pain" to a client?

Medical Terminology

arthro-	pertaining to joints
arthritis	inflammation of a joint
amph-	around; on both sides
amphiarthrosis	slightly movable joints, in all directions
amput/a-	pruning
amputation	pruning or removal of diseased or damaged body limb
osteo-	a bone
osteoporosis	abnormal condition of holes or pores in the bone
rheumat/o-	painful change
rheumatoid arthritis	chronic, painful inflammation of the lining of joints
scoli/o-	crookedness
scoliosis	crookedness or curvature of the spine

News Flash

A new technique developed in Sweden for treating damaged joints, called Autologous Chondrocyte Implantation (ACI), may offer a new therapy for the many people who injure the cartilage in their knees. Since cartilage does not have the properties to heal on its own, even minor injuries may be disabling.

The cartilage growing technique is currently controlled by an East Coast biotech company. The company offers training seminars to surgeons interested in learning about the procedure.

The new technique involves a three-step process: arthroscopy for the extraction of healthy cartilage, growth of new cells in a laboratory setting, and implantation of the new cartilage into the area of the wound. Additional arthroscopy is needed to evaluate the results.

Since full healing may take up to a year or more, at present, the best candidates are individuals under fifty who have had recent injuries to the cartilage in the area of the knee (Kalb & Cowley 1996).

27
Nervous System Disorders

Martha Ann Rust

▶ KEY TERMS

agnosia
anosognosia
aphasia
areflexia
ataxia
aura
automatism
autonomic nervous system
bradykinesia
central nervous system
cephalalgia
chorea
dysarthria

emotional lability
fasciculations
functional area
Glasgow Coma Scale
hemiparesis
hemiplegia
homonymous hemianopia
Kernig's sign
mentation
neuralgia
neurogenic shock
neurotransmitters
nuchal rigidity

nystagmus
paraplegia
peripheral nervous system (PNS)
quadriplegia
sclerotic
somatic nervous system
spinal shock
status epilepticus
stereognosis
unilateral neglect
vertigo

LIST OF DISORDERS

▶ Head Injury
▶ Brain Tumor
▶ Cerebrovascular Accident (CVA) / Transient Ischemic Attacks (TIA)
▶ Epilepsy
▶ Herniated Intervertebral Disk
▶ Spinal Cord Injury
▶ Parkinson's Disease

▶ Multiple Sclerosis
▶ Amyotrophic Lateral Sclerosis (Lou Gehrig's Disease)
▶ Alzheimer's Disease
▶ Guillain-Barre Syndrome (Polyradiculoneuropathy)
▶ Headache
▶ Trigeminal Neuralgia (tic douloureux)
▶ Encephalitis, Meningitis
▶ Huntington's Disease or Chorea
▶ Tourette Syndrome

LEARNING OBJECTIVES

Upon completion of this chapter the learner should be able to:
- Define key terms.
- Identify basic functional areas of the human nervous system.
- Perform a neurological screening and a basic neurological examination.
- Prepare a client for common neurological diagnostic examinations.
- Determine a Glasgow Coma Scale score for a client.
- Recognize common symptoms of neurological disorders.
- Plan interventions for a client with a neurological disorder.

▶ *MAKING THE CONNECTION*

INTRODUCTION

The human nervous system is a highly complex structure that controls and integrates all body systems. The purpose of the nervous system is to control motor, sensory, and autonomic functions of the body. This is done by coordinating and initiating cellular activity through the transmission of electrical impulses and various hormones. The nervous system is divided into the central nervous system, consisting of the brain and spinal cord; the peripheral nervous system, consisting of the cranial nerves and spinal nerves; and the autonomic nervous system, consisting of the sympathetic and parasympathetic systems.

ANATOMY AND PHYSIOLOGY REVIEW

Central Nervous System

The central nervous system is comprised of the brain and the spinal cord (see Figures 27-1A and 27-1B).

The Brain

The brain, composed of gray matter and white matter, controls, initiates, and integrates body functions through the use of electrical impulses and complex molecules. The gray matter on the outer part of the brain contains billions of neurons.

Neurons, the basic cells of the nervous system, have three major components, the cell body, the axon, and the dendrites (see Figure 27-2). The axon carries impulses away from the cell body, and the dendrites carry impulses toward the cell body. The cell body controls the function of the neuron. Functions include conduction of impulses and release of chemical regulators called neurotransmitters. Neurotransmitters are chemical substances that excite, inhibit, or modify the response of another neuron (Hickey, 1992).

The white matter of the inner structures of the brain contain association and projection pathways that transmit nerve impulses to communicate information to the different areas of the brain. These communication pathways are necessary for integration of brain activity (Hickey, 1992).

The brain is contained within the skull or cranium, which is a bony, rigid box that provides protection to

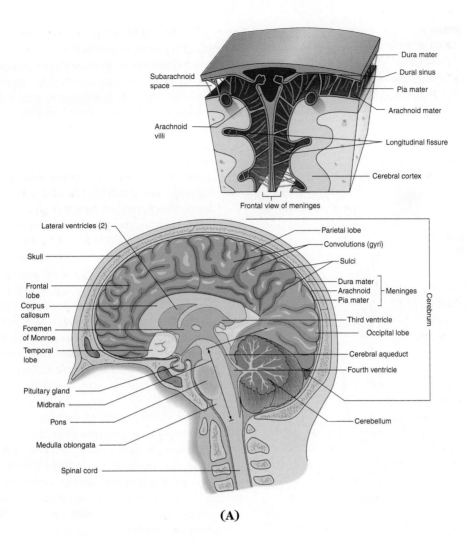

Dura mater
Dural sinus
Pia mater
Arachnoid mater
Longitudinal fissure
Cerebral cortex
Subarachnoid space
Arachnoid villi
Frontal view of meninges

Lateral ventricles (2)
Skull
Frontal lobe
Corpus callosum
Foremen of Monroe
Temporal lobe
Pituitary gland
Midbrain
Pons
Medulla oblongata
Spinal cord

Parietal lobe
Convolutions (gyri)
Sulci
Dura mater
Arachnoid — Meninges
Pia mater
Third ventricle
Occipital lobe
Cerebral aqueduct
Fourth ventricle
Cerebellum
Cerebrum

(A)

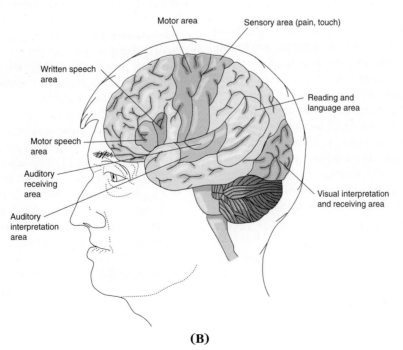

Motor area
Sensory area (pain, touch)
Written speech area
Reading and language area
Motor speech area
Auditory receiving area
Auditory interpretation area
Visual interpretation and receiving area

(B)

FIGURE 27-1 The central nervous system includes the brain, spinal cord, and meninges. **(A)** Structure of brain and **(B)** Functional areas of brain.

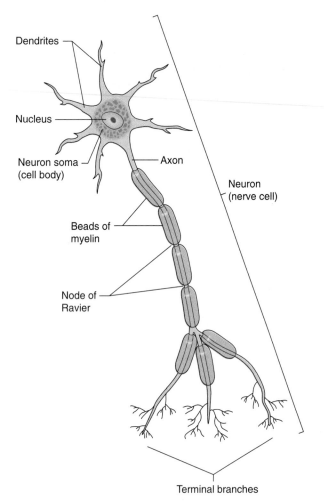

Dendrites

Nucleus

Neuron soma
(cell body)

Axon

Beads of
myelin

Neuron
(nerve cell)

Node of
Ravier

Terminal branches

FIGURE 27-2 Neuron structure.

the brain tissue. There are three coverings of the brain called meninges. They are the dura mater, arachnoid, and pia mater. The purpose of the coverings is to provide protection, support, and small amounts of nourishment. The meninges are separated by spaces.

The brain uses 20 percent of the oxygen consumed by the body (Hickey, 1992). Glucose is used for metabolism within nerve cells. The vertebral arteries and internal carotid arteries provide the blood supply to the brain (Hickey, 1992). Venous drainage is through cerebral veins emptying into dural sinuses between the dural spaces that flow into the jugular veins.

Functional Areas of the Brain Areas of the brain have specialized functions or **functional areas**. The largest amount of central nervous system tissue is in the cerebrum. The cerebrum has four lobes: the frontal, parietal, temporal, and occipital. The brain is divided into two hemispheres. The right side of the brain receives information from the left side of the body and controls the left side of the body. The left hemisphere receives information from and controls the right side of the body. Both hemispheres of the brain communicate through nerve fibers in the corpus callo-

sum. A predominate hemisphere exists for special tasks so that confusion does not occur. The right side specializes in the perception of physical environment, art, nonverbal communication, music, and spiritual aspects. The left hemisphere generally specializes in analysis, calculation, problem solving, verbal communication, interpretation, language, reading, and writing.

The hemispheres are separated by the longitudinal fissure. The lateral fissure of Sylvius separates the temporal lobe from the frontal lobe and the fissure of Rolando separates the frontal lobe from the parietal lobe. The parieto-occipital fissure separates the occipital lobe from the parietal and temporal lobes.

The frontal lobe is the largest area of the cerebrum. Emotional attitudes and responses, formation of thought processes, motor function, judgment, personality, and inhibitions are controlled by neurons in the frontal lobe. Broca's area or the motor speech area is in the frontal lobe. The left motor speech area is predominant in 95 percent of individuals. Formation of words or speech is accomplished, under the influence of the brain, by the simultaneous excitement of the muscles of the larynx, respiratory system, and the mouth.

The parietal lobe of the cerebrum is a purely sensory region for interpretation of all senses except smell (Smeltzer & Bare, 1992; Hickey, 1992). The parietal lobe also receives input from the thalamus. The purpose of the primary sensory cortex in the parietal lobe is to analyze sensations, including pain, touch, and temperature from cutaneous receptors as well as deeper receptors. Interpretations of sensations are sent to the thalamus and other cerebral areas for action to be taken by the brain (Hickey, 1992). Interpretation of position and spatial relationship of the body within the environment is another function of the parietal lobe (Beare & Myers, 1994). This allows the brain to recognize body parts, determine where the body parts are in space, determine right from left, and to identify sizes, shapes, and distance.

The temporal lobe houses the primary auditory association area, Wernicke's area, for interpretation of words that are heard. The sensations of taste, smell, and hearing are also received in this area for interpretation of meaning (Smeltzer & Bare, 1992). A specialized interpretive area called the interpretive area, located at the junction of the temporal, parietal, and occipital lobes integrates somatic, auditory, and visual sensory interpretations. Memory is also a function of the temporal lobe, especially memories that include multiple sensations or greatly detailed thoughts.

The occipital lobe is responsible for visual interpretation and visual association. Without visual interpretation and association, a person can see, but not recognize visual sensations.

The cerebellum, located below and behind the cerebrum, controls and coordinates muscles and equilibrium by coordinating sensory information relating to the positions of various body parts. Sensory interpretations, including messages from the semicircular canals in the inner ear, are continuously monitored by the cerebellum to maintain position of the body in space. Fine motor and gross motor movements are coordinated by the cerebellum.

The diencephalon is the area of the brain that houses the thalamus, hypothalamus, and the pituitary gland. The thalamus is the primary relay station for all sensations except smell. All memory, pain, and sensory impulses except smell pass through the thalamus before being relayed to the cerebrum.

The hypothalamus controls numerous functions including the autonomic nervous system, part of the peripheral nervous system consisting of the sympathetic and parasympathetic nervous systems. Fluid balance, body temperature, blood pressure, heart rate, sleep, hunger, weight control, and production of neurosecretions that cause the pituitary gland to secrete hormones are all hypothalamic functions. Responses to emotions such as blushing, clammy hands, rage, panic, and fear are regulated by the hypothalamus.

The pituitary gland, formerly referred to as the master gland of the body, is controlled by the hypothalamus. Six hormones controlling metabolic functions are secreted by the pituitary. They are growth hormone, adrenal-stimulating hormone, thyroid stimulating hormone, prolactin, follicle-stimulating hormone, and luteinizing hormone. Water regulation hormone, adrenal stimulating hormone (ADH), and oxytocin are also secreted by the pituitary gland.

The brain stem contains the midbrain, pons, and medulla. The midbrain is a nerve pathway between the cerebral hemispheres and the lower brain and is a center for auditory and visual reflexes. Cranial nerves III and IV come from the midbrain. The midbrain connects the pons and cerebellum with the cerebral hemispheres

The pons bridges the two halves of the cerebellum and the medulla with the cerebrum to provide communication pathways. The medulla transmits motor fibers from the brain to the spinal cord and sensory fibers from the spinal cord to the brain. The pons regulates respiration and the medulla regulates heart rate and blood pressure. Cranial nerves V through VIII are in the pons. Cranial nerves IX through XII pass through the medulla.

The Spinal Cord

The spinal cord is a continuation of the brain stem that exits the skull through the foramen magnum, an opening in the base of the skull. The size of the spinal cord is approximately 45 centimeters or 18 inches long and the thickness of one finger. The cord is divided into right and left halves with a shallow groove on the

dorsal side called the posterior median sulcus and a deep groove on the ventral side called the anterior median fissure. The cord tapers to a thin tip, called the conus medullaris, at the first lumbar vertebrae and terminates as a thin cord of connective tissue called the filum terminale which continues as far as the second sacral vertebrae. It provides vertical support for the cord. The meninges cover the spinal cord to provide protection. Impulses are conducted along pathways to and from higher centers in the brain and spinal cord. Reflex activity is performed within the spinal cord.

There are thirty-one pairs of spinal nerves originating from the spinal cord. Each pair contains a dorsal or posterior nerve root and a ventral or anterior nerve root. The dorsal nerve roots carry sensory impulses from the body to the brain. The ventral nerve roots carry motor impulses from the spinal cord to the body. The spinal cord has an H-shaped appearance of gray matter within the white matter. These horns forming the H shape are referred to as the anterior (ventral) horns, the posterior (dorsal) horns, and the lateral horns. These horns contain the cell bodies of neurons that innervate the skeletal muscles.

Cerebrospinal Fluid

Cerebrospinal fluid is produced primarily in the choroid plexus. Five hundred milliliters of cerebrospinal fluid are produced daily with excess reabsorbed by the arachnoid villi in the subarachnoid space. The circulation of cerebrospinal fluid is from the lateral ventricles to the third and fourth ventricles. From there it enters into the subarachnoid space to flow around the spinal cord and the brain.

The purpose of cerebrospinal fluid is to provide shock absorption and to bathe the brain and spinal cord. It contains glucose, protein, urea, and salts. The nutritive substances are delivered to the central nervous system cells and the waste and toxic substances are removed.

Cerebrospinal fluid is clear, colorless, and odorless with specific gravity of 1.007. The average amount circulating is 125 to 150 mL. Cerebrospinal fluid pressure is 60 to 180 mm of water pressure. The high glucose content of cerebrospinal fluid can differentiate it from other body fluids.

Peripheral Nervous System

The peripheral nervous system consists of the cranial nerves and the spinal nerves. All of the nerve tissue outside of the central nervous system is part of the peripheral nervous system. It has both sensory and motor components. The peripheral nervous system can be divided into the **somatic nervous system** and the autonomic nervous system. The somatic portion connects the central nervous system to the skin and skeletal muscles. It is concerned with conscious activities. The autonomic portion connects the central nervous system with visceral organs such as the heart, stomach, intestines, and various glands. It is concerned with unconscious activities.

Cranial Nerves   The twelve pairs of cranial nerves have sensory, motor, or mixed functions. See Table 27-1 for functions and assessment of cranial nerves. The cranial nerves originate from the brain or brain stem, with most originating from the brain stem. They are always identified with Roman numerals, but also have names.

Spinal Nerves

There are thirty-one pairs of spinal nerves that exit from the spinal cord through the vertebral column. The dorsal or posterior nerve roots carry sensory impulses to the brain. The ventral or anterior nerve roots carry motor impulses from the spinal cord and brain to the muscles. Motor and sensory impulses are transmitted from the body and internal organs.

Reflex activity is a stereotypical response to a stimulus that is initiated by the nervous system (Hickey, 1992). The three classifications of reflexes are muscle

Table 27-1

CRANIAL NERVES			
Cranial Nerve	**Function**	**Assessment**	**Expected Findings**
Olfactory (I)	Sensory-Smell	Have client identify smells such as coffee or alcohol, with one nostril occluded with your finger, repeat for opposite nostril.	Correct identification of smell or ability to choose smell from a list of choices.
Optic (II)	Sensory-Vision	Ask client to read printed material, identify number of fingers held in front of client, or test vision with Snellen eye chart. Test visual fields by having client identify when your finger enters visual field.	Vision intact or correctable with lenses. Visual field intact.
Oculomotor (III)	Motor-Pupil Constriction	Cranial Nerves III, IV, and VI are tested together. Inspect for ptosis or drooping of eyelid; Assess extraocular eye muscles by having client follow your finger to each quadrant of the visual field; assess for accommodation by asking the client to look at your finger held four to six inches from the client's nose, then follow your finger to 18 inches from the nose.	Pupils are equal, round, and react equally to light. No ptosis or double vision. Eyes move smoothly and consensually inward and downward. As you move your finger away from the client, the pupil will accommodate by dilating; as you move your finger closer, the pupil will normally constrict.
Trochlear (IV)	Motor-Upper eyelid elevation-Extraocular eye movement	See Oculomotor (III)	Eyes should move smoothly and consensually upward and outward without nystagmus or diplopia.
Trigeminal (V)	Sensory-Cornea, nose, and oral mucosa; Motor-Mastication	Test corneal reflex by lightly touching cornea with a small piece of cotton; check sensation of face by touching lightly with a cotton ball while client has eyes closed, asking client if sensation is present; Check motor function by having client clench jaws shut and opening to resistance of examiner's hand or have client make chewing motions.	Corneal reflex present evidenced by rapid blinking when cotton wisped across cornea. Feeling cotton ball on face indicates that facial sensation is intact. Movement of jaws symmetrical and able to overcome resistance.

Abducens (VI)	Motor-Extraocular eye movement	See Occulomotor (III)	Eyes move outward.
Facial (VII)	Motor-Facial muscles; Sensory-Taste anterior two-thirds of tongue	Ask client to smile, show teeth, wrinkle forehead or whistle; have client identify salt and sugar when dabbed on tongue.	Facial movement symmetrical; sense of taste intact.
Acoustic (VIII)	Sensory-hearing, equilibrium	Assess ability to hear ticking watch or whispered voice. Observe gait for swaying. Perform Romberg test (refer to assessment of motor function).	Sense of hearing intact, no swaying or loss of balance.
Glossopharyngeal (IX)	Sensory-sensation to throat and taste back one-third of tongue; Motor-swallowing	Identify taste of salt and sugar on back of tongue; have client say "ah" and assess for symmetrical position of uvula; test gag reflex by touching back of pharynx with tongue depressor; observe swallowing ability and speech patterns.	Taste sensation intact; uvula raises symmetrically; gag reflex intact; swallowing and speech intact.
Vagus (X)	Motor and sensory	Test along with Glossopharyngeal nerve.	
Spinal accessory (XI)	Motor-movement of uvula, soft palate, sternocleidomastoid muscle, trapezius muscle	Have client turn head against resistance by placing examiner's hand on side of client's face and asking client to turn head against resistance; have client shrug shoulders against resistance of the examiner's hand.	Ability to move shoulder and head against resistance.
Hypoglossal (XII)	Motor-Tongue movement	Ask client to stick out tongue and observe for symmetry, deviation to side, have client push tongue against tongue depressor, and move tongue from side to side.	Tongue should be centrally aligned, able to push against resistance of tongue depressor; no fasciculations (and involuntary twitching of muscle fibers) should be present.

stretch or deep tendon, superficial or cutaneous, and pathological. See section on assessment of reflexes. Reflex activity requires the function of five areas in the nervous system: the sensory fibers, the neuron relaying the impulse, the association center in the brain, the neuron relaying the motor impulse from the brain to the body, and the specific organ involved. Disease processes at any of these areas can cause an abnormal reflex response.

Autonomic Nervous System

The autonomic nervous system is part of the peripheral nervous system. The main function is to maintain internal homeostasis. There are two subdivisions, the sympathetic system and the parasympathetic system. The sympathetic system, activated by stress,

prepares the body for the "fight or flight" response. The activity of the sympathetic system causes increased heart rate, increased blood pressure, vasoconstriction, decreased peristalsis, dilated pupils, increased secretions of epinephrine and sweat, decreased digestive juices and saliva (see Figure 27-3).

The parasympathetic system conserves, restores, and maintains vital body functions (Hickey, 1992). The heart rate is slowed, gastrointestinal activity is increased, and bowel and bladder evacuation is activated by the parasympathetic system.

The sympathetic and parasympathetic systems work antagonistically to regulate smooth muscles, the heart, and glands of the body. When one system increases an action, the other system decreases the action. For example, when one stimulates, the other inhibits; when one dilates, the other one constricts. The purpose is to maintain a stable internal environment (Hickey, 1992). Both systems function simultaneously, but one can dominate the other as the need arises.

BASIC NEUROLOGICAL NURSING ASSESSMENT

A complete health history and a neurological screening assessment allow the nurse to identify areas of dysfunction in order to focus the neurological assessment. The neurological assessment utilizes all nursing assessment skills. Observation (inspection) is

necessary for the majority of the assessment. Palpation, auscultation, and percussion are also used.

Importance of Nursing History and Assessment

The complexity of the nervous system functions require the nurse to perform a thorough health history to identify data to establish nursing diagnoses. A baseline assessment is essential to determine changes in neurological functioning. Any change from the baseline assessment needs to be identified and early intervention initiated.

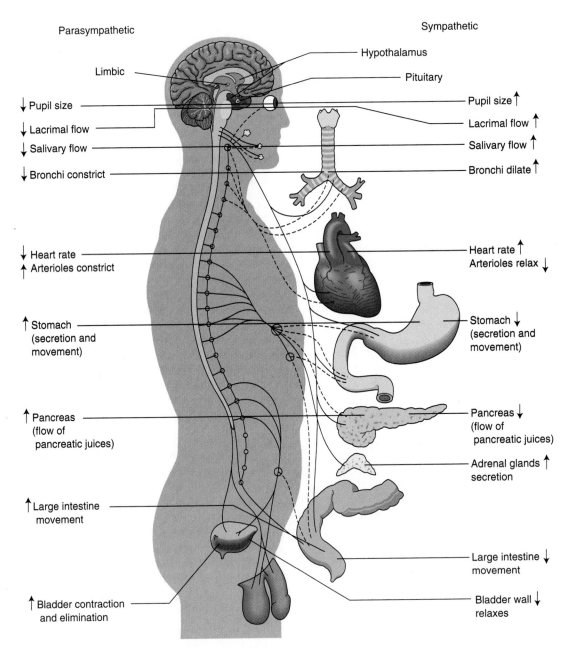

FIGURE 27-3 The autonomic nervous system (ANS)

A thorough health history includes asking the client about headaches, clumsiness, loss of function of an extremity, seizure activity, numbness or tingling, change in vision, pain, extreme fatigue, personality changes, or mood swings.

Components of a Neurological Assessment

The neurological screening includes level of consciousness and verbal responses to specific questions, selected cranial nerve assessment for eye movement and visual acuity, muscle strength, movement, gait for motor function, and tactile and pain sensation of extremities for sensory screening (Fitzgerald, 1994).

A complete nursing assessment of neurological function includes assessment of the following areas: cerebral function, cranial nerve function, motor function, sensory function, and deep tendon reflexes. The neurological nursing assessment follows in more detail.

Cerebral Function

The assessment of cerebral function includes level of consciousness, mental status, intellectual function, emotional status, pupil reaction, and communication.

Level of Consciousness Level of consciousness is assessed by determining the client's responsiveness and orientation. Responsiveness is the person's ability to perceive environmental stimuli and body reactions and then respond with thought and action. The client's responsiveness state can be described in terms of con-

Table 27-2

LEVELS OF CONSCIOUSNESS

Alert	Oriented, opens eyes spontaneously, responds appropriately.
Lethargic	Sleepy, slow to respond, but responds appropriately; oriented; opens eyes to verbal stimuli.
Stuporous	Aroused only with painful stimuli; never fully awake; conversation, if present, is confused or unclear; opens eyes to painful stimuli.
Semicomatous	May move in response to painful stimuli; does not converse; protective blink, swallowing, and pupil reflexes are present.
Comatose	Unresponsive except to severe pain; protective reflexes are absent; pupils are fixed; no voluntary movement.

Table 27-3

GLASGOW COMA SCALE

Behavior	Response	Score
Eye Opening Response	Spontaneous	4
	To Verbal Command	3
	To Pain	2
	No Response	1
Best Verbal Response	Oriented, Conversing	5
	Disoriented, Conversing	4
	Use of Inappropriate Words	3
	Incomprehensible Sounds	2
	No Response	1
Best Motor Response	Obeys Verbal Commands	6
	Moves to Localized Pain	5
	Flexion Withdrawal to Pain	4
	Abnormal Posturing—Decorticate	3
	Abnormal Posturing—Decerebrate	2
	No Response	1
Total		3–15

sciousness, such as alert, lethargic, stuporous, semicomatose, or deep coma (see Table 27-2).

A more objective assessment is done using the **Glasgow Coma Scale**, an objective, measurable tool for assessing consciousness in clients. With the Glasgow Coma Scale, eye opening, verbal response, and motor response are scored using measurable criteria (see Table 27-3). The scores are summed to indicate severity of coma and predict outcome, especially for head injuries. A score of 15 indicates a fully oriented person. A score of 3 is the lowest possible score and indicates deep coma. A score of 7 or less is considered a state of coma.

Changes in the Glasgow Coma Scale indicate changes in client condition. The nurse must quickly act upon decreasing scores to prevent further damage to the brain. Immediate measures must be taken to decrease intracranial pressure and the physician must be notified. See section on increased intracranial pressure.

Orientation is the person's awareness of self in relation to person, place, and time. In some instances awareness of situation is also a necessary measure. Using open-ended communication techniques, the nurse instructs the client to "tell me who you are", "what day of the week is it?", "where are you?", and so on in order to determine orientation of the client. It is important for the nurse to know the correct responses to the questions in order to interpret the client's orientation.

Mental Status   Assessment of mental status requires observation of the client's appearance, behavior, posture, gestures, movements, and facial expressions. The nurse compares these behaviors with expected behaviors based upon the client's age, health status, educational level, and social position. Mood is assessed by observation and by asking the client about moods and feelings. Mental assessment tools have been developed to assess cognitive ability, such as the Mini Mental Exam (see Figure 27-4).

Intellectual Function   Intellectual function is the ability of the brain to perform thought processes. Ability to concentrate, memory function both long-term and short-term, recall, calculation activities, and abstract reasoning contribute to the intellectual function.

Nursing assessment of intellectual function is performed by asking individuals to perform some tasks such as the following:

- Repeat a series of numbers such as 1, 3, 7, 1
- Tell what they ate for breakfast
- Add a couple of numbers, for example, 2 + 6
- Explain a proverb such as "a stitch in time is worth nine"

The nurse determines the status of the client's ability to process thoughts by evaluating the responses to questions such as these. The client's ability to perform these tasks prior to assessment should be known to provide comparison. For example, if the client was math illiterate prior to the nursing assessment, the client will still not be able to add or subtract.

Emotional Status   Emotional status is assessed by observation of the client's affect. Is affect appropriate for the situation? Is affect labile? Is affect consistent with verbal communication?

Pupil Reaction   Size, equality, and roundness of pupils are assessed. Size is measured in millimeters. Pupils are evaluated for symmetry in size and reaction to light. Briefly shine a penlight into the client's eye by passing the light from the outer edge of the eye toward the center of the eye. Assess reaction as brisk, sluggish, or nonreactive as well as for consensual reaction, the opposite pupil responding at the same time. Assess accommodation as in Table 27-1.

PERRLA is the abbreviation for documenting pupils equal, round, and reactive to light, and accommodation. This can be used if the pupil reaction is normal. If any part of the assessment is abnormal in one or both eyes, the assessment findings must be written out for clarity.

Communication   Communication includes both written and oral aspects. Various specialized areas of the nervous system are involved in communication. The inability to communicate, termed aphasia, can be caused by inability to form words or the inability to understand written or spoken words. To assess communication function, various approaches are necessary. Ask the client to follow a simple command such as "Close your eyes." Use a written card instructing the client to complete a simple task such as "Touch your nose." Observe client's speech for the ability to form words, appropriate use of words, and speech patterns such as clarity, rate, flow, and voice modulation. Assess client's ability for verbal and written expression of self. This can be accomplished during the health history by asking the client about expectations of hospitalization. Have the client write his name and address on paper to evaluate the ability to write.

Assessment of Cranial Nerves

Cranial nerve assessment essentially reflects brain stem activity. A complete cranial nerve examination, if required, is usually performed by the physician or advanced practice nurse. Refer to Table 27-1.

Assessment of Motor Function

The neurological screening includes assessment of muscle strength, arm and leg movement, and gait (Fitzgerald, 1994). A complete motor function assessment is performed if a deficit is identified. A complete motor function assessment includes muscle size and symmetry, muscle tone, muscle strength, coordination, and posturing.

Muscle Size and Symmetry   Assess muscle size and symmetry by palpating major muscle groups of the arms and legs and comparing with the opposite side of the body. Unilateral atrophy may indicate a nervous system problem.

Muscle Tone   Assess muscle tone as major muscle groups are palpated for size and symmetry while at rest and during passive movement. Muscles are described as flaccid, spastic, or rigid. Flaccid muscles are hypotonic or soft; assessment reveals muscles that are soft and flabby. Spastic muscles are resistant to passive movement, assessment reveals muscle that are resistant to movement, followed by release of resistance. Rigid muscles may have tremors or be constantly rigid. Rigidity is a more constant state of spasticity, with fewer periods of release of resistance.

Muscle Strength   Place each extremity through passive movement, then ask the client to move the extremity across the bed. Ask the client to move against gravity by lifting the extremity off the bed, then

Patient_____
Examiner_____
Date _____

"MINI-MENTAL STATE"

Maximum score	Score	
		ORIENTATION
5	( )	What is the (year) (season) (date) (day) (month)?
5	( )	Where are we: (state) (county) (town) (hospital) (floor)
		REGISTRATION
3	( )	Name 3 objects : 1 second to say each. Then ask the patient all 3 after you have said them. Give 1 point for each correct answer. Then repeat them until the patient learns all 3. Count trials and record.
		ATTENTION AND CALCULATION
5	( )	Serial 7's. 1 point for each correct. Stop after 5 answers. Alternatively spell "world" backwards.
		RECALL
3	( )	Ask for the 3 objects repeated above. Give 1 point for each correct.
		LANGUAGE
9	( )	Name a pencil, and watch (2 points)
		Repeat the following "No ifs, ands or buts" (1 point)
		Follow a 3-stage command:
		"Take a paper in your right hand, fold it in half, and put it on the floor" (3 points)
		Read and obey the following:
		CLOSE YOUR EYES (1 point)
		Write a sentence (1 point)
		Copy design (1 point)

_____ Total score

Assess level of consciousness along a continuum _____

| Alert | Drowsy | Stupor | Coma |

INSTRUCTIONS FOR ADMINISTRATION OF MINI-MENTAL STATE EXAMINATION

ORIENTATION
(1) Ask for the date. Then ask specifically for parts omitted, e.g., "Can you also tell me what season it is?". One point for each correct.
(2) Ask in turn "Can you tell me the name of this hospital?" (town, county, etc.). One point for each correct.

REGISTRATION
Ask the patient if you may test his or her memory. Then say the name of 3 unrelated objects, clealy and slowly, about one second for each. After you have said 3, ask patient to repeat them. The first repetition determines the score (0-3) but keep saying them until patient can repeat all 3, up to 6 trials. If the patient does not eventually learn all 3, recall cannot be meaningfully tested.

ATTENTION AND CALCULATION
Ask the patient to begin with 100 and count backwards by 7. Stop after 5 subtractions (93,86,79,72,65).
Score the total number of correct answers.
If the patient cannot or will not perform this task, ask him or her to spell the word "world" backwards. The score is the number of letters in correct order (e.g. dlrow=5, dlorw=3).

RECALL
Ask the patient if he or she can recall the 3 words you previously asked patient to remember. Score 0-3.

LANGUAGE
Naming: Show the patient a wrist watch and ask what it is. Repeat for pencil. Score 0-2
Repetition: Ask the patient to repeat the sentence after you. Allow only one trial. Score 0-1.
3-Stage command: Give the patient a piece of plain blank paper and repeat the command. Score 1 point for each part correctly executed.
Reading: On a blank piece of paper print the sentence "Close your eyes", in letters large enough for the patient to see clearly. Ask patient to read it and do what it says. Score 1 point only if patient actually closes eyes.
Writing: Give the patient a blank piece of paper and ask patient to write a sentence for you. Do not dictate a sentence, it is to be written spontaneously. It must contain a subject and verb to be sensible. Correct grammar and punctuation are not necessary.
Copying: On a clean piece of paper, draw intersecting pentagons, each side about 1 in. and ask to copy it exactly as it is. All 10 angles must be present and 2 must intersect to score 1 point. Tremor and rotation are ignored.
Estimate the patient's level of sensorium along a continuum, from alert on the left to coma on the right.

FIGURE 27-4 Mini mental exam. (*From Folstein et al.,* Journal of Psychiatric Research, *Vol 12, pp. 189, 1975, "Mini-mental state." Reproduced with permission*)

Table 27-4

MUSCLE STRENGTH	
Score	Definition
5/5	Full power of contraction
4/5	Fair or moderate power of contraction
3/5	Just able to overcome force of gravity
2/5	Can move, but not overcome power of gravity
1/5	Minimal contractile power
0/5	No movement

against resistance by placing your hand on the extremity and exerting slight resistance. Strength is graded on a scale of 0 to 5 (see Table 27-4).

Coordination   Coordination, a function of the cerebellum, is assessed by asking the client to perform repetitious movement. Ask the client to repeatedly touch his/her own nose then your fingertip. Lower extremity coordination is assessed by asking the client to run the heel of one foot down the opposite shin, then repeat with the other heel. Inability to perform these movements is termed **ataxia**, incoordination of voluntary muscle action.

Balance   Evaluate balance by using the Romberg test. Have the client stand with the feet together, arms extended in front, and eyes closed. Observe balance; a slight swaying is normal. Always stand in front of the client anticipating that the client might fall.

Posturing   Abnormal posturing occurs with injury to the motor tract. Two postures to observe for are decorticate and decerebrate posturing. Decorticate posture is characterized by flexion of the arms, adduction of the upper extremities, and extension of the lower extremities. Lesions of the cerebral hemispheres or internal structures of the brain cause decorticate posturing. Decerebrate posturing is caused by brain stem injury. It is an arcing of the back with backward flexion of the head, adduction and hyperpronation of the arms, and extension of the feet.

Abnormal posturing may be present at all times, or in response to stimuli such as loud noises, bright lights, or painful stimuli. Assess if bilateral or unilateral posturing is present and the cause of posturing if intermittent. The presence of either posture should be reported at once, because this is an ominous sign of cerebral dysfunction. Decerebrate posturing represents greater dysfunction than decorticate posturing, and any change from decorticate to decerebrate posturing indicates a worsening condition.

Assessment of Sensory Function

A subjective examination is performed with the client's eyes closed. Different pathways are used to transmit different sensory impulses. To evaluate all pathways, the examiner must test tactile, pain and temperature, vibration, proprioception, stereognosis, and integration of sensations.

Tactile Sensation   Tactile sensation is tested by using a cotton ball to lightly touch the client's arms, hands, upper legs, and feet. Comparison is done side to side. The client with eyes closed indicates whether the cotton ball is felt or not.

Pain and Temperature   Pain and temperature are transmitted along the same pathways and are evaluated using a sharp and dull touch. A paper clip or cotton-tipped applicator is used. Do not use a safety pin because skin integrity will be compromised. Touch the client with the rounded end of paper clip or cotton-tipped end of applicator to test for dull sensation and the pointed end of paper clip or uncovered end of applicator to test for sharp. Evaluate the client's ability to determine sharp and dull, again comparing both sides of the body. Test upper and lower extremities, working from upper arms to hands and from thighs to feet.

Vibration   Vibration is tested using a tuning fork. Strike the tuning fork on your palm, holding only the handle; place the end of the handle on the client's wrists and then the ankles, ask if the vibrations are felt.

Proprioception   Proprioception is the sense of joint position in space. With the client's eyes remaining closed, move a joint of the client's finger or extremity up or down in space, and ask the client to determine the position of digit or extremity. Is it up or down?

Stereognosis   Stereognosis is the ability to recognize an object by feel. Place a familiar object such as a coin or key in the client's hand and ask that the object be identified. This sensation is a function of the brain, not of the spinal pathways.

Integration of Sensation   Integration of sensation is a higher cortical function. A two-point discrimination test is performed by touching the client simultaneously on opposite sides of the body with a sharp object. Ask the client to determine the number of objects felt. The normal response is two. If only one is felt, the brain function of integration is abnormal.

Assessment of Reflexes

Reflexes are involuntary contractions of muscles or muscle groups responding to brisk stretching near the insertion site (Smeltzer & Bare, 1992). Testing of reflexes is generally the responsibility of the physician or registered nurse. Abnormal reflex responses may be an early indicator of motor or sensory dysfunction.

Examination A reflex hammer held loosely between the thumb and index finger is used to examine reflexes. The insertion site of the muscle is directly struck with the hammer or indirectly struck by placing the thumb of the examiner over the insertion site and striking the thumb. The muscle must be relaxed and the joint in midposition. Deep tendon reflexes commonly tested are the Achilles or ankle jerk, quadriceps or knee jerk, biceps, and triceps.

Description or Grading of Response Reflexes are generally described as present, absent, or diminished. If a grading scale is used, it is important to note whether a four-point or five-point scale is used. The description of each number varies between agencies, but a typical scale is presented in Table 27-5.

Abnormal Reflexes The absence of deep tendon reflexes in clients is considered as an abnormal reflex except for the absence of the ankle jerk in geriatric clients. The Babinski phenomena is the most important abnormal superficial reflex. The bottom of the foot is stroked with a key, or other object, starting at the heel and moving along the lateral side of the sole,

Table 27-5

REFLEX GRADING SCALE	
Grade	**Definition**
4	Hyperactive with clonus
3	Hyperactive
2	Normal
1	Hypoactive
0	Absent

then moving toward the big toe. The normal adult response is a slight plantar flexion or curling under of the toes. An abnormal response is dorsal flexion and fanning of the toes. This phenomena, normally present in the immature central nervous systems of children under the age of two, indicates corticospinal disease in people with mature central nervous systems.

COMMON DIAGNOSTIC TESTS

The following is a table of the commonly used diagnostic tests for clients with symptoms of nervous system disorders.

Test	Explanation /Normal Values	Nursing Responsibilities
Electroencephalogram (EEG)	Record of electrical activity generated in the brain and obtained through electrodes applied to the scalp or microelectrodes placed in brain tissue during surgery.	Omit caffeine due to stimulant effect. Give meal so blood sugar will not be altered. Client teaching—test takes approximately 45 minutes to 2 hours; electrical shock will not occur. The procedure is painless; no after-effects; client may be asked to open / close eyes during the test; there may be flashing lights or small electrical stimulations.
Lumbar Puncture (LP)	A needle is inserted into the subarachnoid space to measure CSF pressure and/or to obtain a specimen. Normal pressure — 60–180 mm water pressure. Normal Specific Gravity — 1.007. Normal Glucose — 60–80 mg/100 ml. Normal CBC — 0. Normal WBC — 0–5 cells / mm³	Obtain informed consent. Have client empty bowel and bladder prior to procedure. Position client in dorsal recumbent position on the side of bed of physician's choice. Place the hips at the edge of the bed with client's back to the physician. Assist in setting up sterile field and pouring solutions if not included in tray. Assist client to maintain position. Postprocedure: keep client flat in bed for 3 to 24 hours or as ordered by physician; encourage fluid intake to replace fluids lost; deliver specimen to the lab for diagnostic tests. Monitor vital and neurological signs.

(continued)

Test	Explanation /Normal Values	Nursing Responsibilities
		Potential complications include trauma at the puncture site, causing blood in the first sample, headache, malaise. nausea/ vomiting/ hematoma, and leg pain. Observe for backache, nuchal rigidity, elevated temperature, and difficulty voiding.
Myelogram	X-ray of spinal subarachnoid space following injection of opaque medium.	Follow nursing responsibilities for lumbar puncture. Inform client that table may be tilted during the procedure. Obtain informed consent according to facility guidelines. Omit meal prior to procedure. Administer light sedative if ordered. Post-procedure care is determined by the type of medium used, follow physician's orders for activity and fluids.
Imaging Procedures - Computerized tomography (CT), Positron Emission Tomography (PET), Single photon emission computed tomography (SPECT), Magnetic Resonance Imaging (MRI)	All imaging relies on magnets and computers to produce images. Anatomical organs, perfusion, and actual functions such as the production of dopamine can be "pictured" by the computer image.	Prepare client for the actual procedure according to facility guidelines and technology used. Administer light sedatives as ordered. Obtain informed consent according to facility guidelines.
Cerebral Angiography	Opaque dye is injected into the circulatory system for visualization of the circulation in the brain for identification of vascular abnormalities.	The test takes approximately 2 hours. Obtain informed consent according to facility guidelines. Explain that client may experience a hot feeling when dye is injected, be sure to ask about allergies especially to iodine products or shellfish. Administer a light sedative if ordered.
Brain Scan	A radioactive agent is injected into a vein and allowed to circulate to the brain; the brain is then scanned in successive layers and a picture composite of the structures developed. This is useful in identifying structural lesions whether vascular or tumors.	Same as Cerebral Angiogram
Electromyogram (EMG)	Needle electrodes are placed in the muscle to determine electrical activity to and from the muscle. It is used to differentiate between neural and muscular involvement.	Instruct the client that the procedure is not usually painful, however, some discomfort may occur. The procedure takes approximately 1 hour.

KEY ABBREVIATIONS

The following abbreviations and acronyms are used in this chapter:

ALS	amyotrophic lateral sclerosis
CSF	cerebrospinal fluid
CVA	cerebrovascular accident
DIA	diffuse axonal injury
MS	multiple sclerosis
PERRLA	pupils, equal, round, reactive to light and accommodation
RIND	reversible ischemic neurological deficit
SCI	spinal cord injury
TIA	transient ischemic attack

▶ HEAD INJURY

Head injuries involve trauma to the scalp, skull, or brain.

▶ Scalp

Scalp injuries bleed profusely because of the abundance of blood vessels. As with any break in skin integrity, infection is of major concern. The wound is cleansed and irrigated to remove foreign matter before closing the wound with sutures or butterfly dressings.

▶ Skull

Skull injuries and fractures of the skull, may be with or without brain injury. A fracture is usually caused by extreme force. Skull fractures are considered closed if the dura mater is intact or open if the dura mater is torn. Clinical manifestation of skull fracture is localized pain. If the brain is injured, other symptoms may appear.

Types of skull fractures are linear fracture, comminuted fracture, depressed fracture, and basilar fracture. Linear fractures are nondisplaced cracks in the bone. Comminuted fractures are when the bone is broken into fragments. Depressed fractures have bone fragments pressing into the intracranial cavity. Basilar skull fractures are of the bones in the base of the skull.

Basilar fractures are of particular concern because of close proximity of the fragile sinus bones and the adhesion of the dura mater to this area. The dura mater can easily tear and cerebrospinal fluid can leak from the ears or nose. The internal carotid artery and cranial nerves can also be damaged easily with a basilar skull fracture.

▶ Brain

Brain injuries are caused by primary injuries of acceleration-deceleration force, rotational force, or penetrating missile. Acceleration injuries are caused by moving objects striking the head. Deceleration injuries are when the head is moving and strikes a solid object. Rotational injuries are hyperextension, hyperflexion, or lateral flexion of the head which causes twisting of the cerebrum on the brain stem. Penetrating missile injuries are a direct penetration of an object into brain tissue (Thelan, Davie, & Urden, 1990).

▶ Open

Brain injury from skull fractures and penetrating injuries are referred to as open head injuries. Hemorrhaging from the nose, pharynx, or ears; ecchymosis over mastoid area (Battle's sign); or blood in the conjunctiva may occur in open head injuries. Cerebrospinal fluid may leak from the ears or nose. A CT scan or MRI is performed for determining the extent of injury. Neurological deficits depend upon the extent and area of injury.

▶ Closed

Closed head injuries are caused by blunt force to the head. Coup injuries are caused by the impact of the head against an object. Contrecoup injuries are caused by the impact of the brain against the opposite side of the skull (see Figure 27-5).

Types of closed head injuries are concussion, contusion, and lacerations. Concussions are transient neurological deficits caused by the shaking of the brain. Clinical manifestations may include immediate loss of consciousness lasting from minutes to hours, momentary loss of reflexes, respiratory arrest for several seconds, amnesia for the period immediately prior to and following the event. Headaches, drowsiness, confusion, dizziness, irritability, visual disturbances, and unsteady gait may also occur (Hickey, 1992).

Post-concussion syndrome may develop following the injury. This is manifested by headache and dizziness. Nervousness, irritability, emotional lability, fatigue, insomnia, loss of **mentation** (ability to concentrate, remember, or think abstractly), and sometimes other neurological deficits occur. This syndrome may last from several weeks up to a year (Hickey, 1992).

Contusions are surface bruises of the brain. Symptoms are dependent upon the area of injury. Frequently the client is unconscious for a longer period of time than with a concussion. The client may be aroused then drift back into unconsciousness. Pulse, blood pressure, and respiration are below normal. Skin is cool and pale. Cerebral edema may occur with widespread injury. See section on cerebral edema.

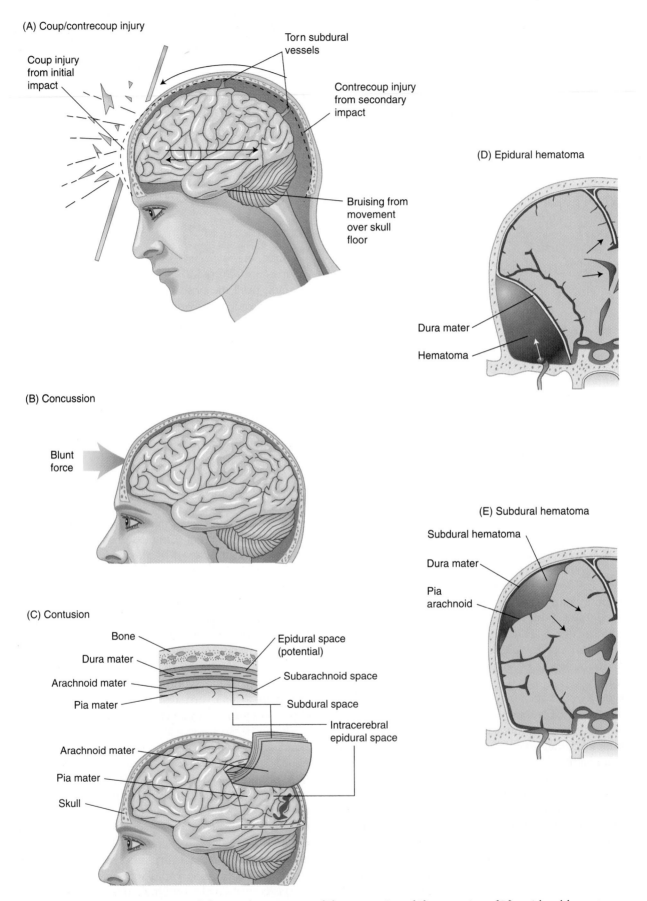

FIGURE 27-5 Brain injuries. **(A)** coup/contrecoup; **(B)** concussion; **(C)** contusion; **(D)** epidural hematoma; **(E)** subdural hematoma.

Return of consciousness may be followed with cerebral irritability to stimuli. Headache and dizziness may be present for an indefinite period. Permanent damage may cause changes in mental function or seizure disorders. Prognosis ranges from full recovery to death.

Cerebral laceration is the tearing of cortical tissue. Symptoms of brain stem injury include deep coma from time of impact, decerebrate posturing, autonomic dysfunction, nonreactive pupils, and respiratory difficulty. There is a loss of ability to relay nerve impulses from high levels in the brain. Brain stem injuries usually occur along with diffuse axonal injury (DAI). This widespread damage to nerve cells in the white matter of the brain causes immediate coma, decerebration, and increased intracranial pressure.

Hemorrhage Intracranial hemorrhage is a common complication of head injury. Bleeding may occur in the epidural space, subdural space, subarachnoid space, ventricles, or intracerebrally. Neurological change is caused by pressure on the brain from the space occupying hemorrhage. With epidural hematoma, momentary unconsciousness is followed by a conscious state of a few hours to a week depending on how rapid the bleeding is occurring. As the bleeding continues, the neurological status begins to deteriorate with decreasing level of consciousness, headache, seizures, hemiparesis, decerebration, and a dilated, fixed pupil. Treatment is surgical to evacuate the hematoma, stop the bleeding, and relieve pressure on the brain.

Subdural hematomas cause immediate pressure on the brain because of the close proximity of the arachnoid and pia mater to the brain. Classification of subdural hematomas are acute, within forty-eight hours of injury; subacute, from two to fourteen days of injury; chronic, from two weeks to months following injury. Common symptoms are headache, drowsiness, slow mentation, and confusion. The symptoms slowly progress as the size of the subdural clot increases causing increased pressure on the brain. Small hematomas are usual reabsorbed. Large hematomas require surgical removal.

Intracranial hematomas usually occur in the temporal or frontal lobes from contusions or deep in the brain from shearing forces. The hematoma usually expands rapidly. Unconsciousness may occur immediately from the injury. Headache, deteriorating level of consciousness, hemiplegia, and dilated pupil are initial signs of internal hematomas. As intracranial pressure increases herniation of the brain stem occurs causing changes in pupils, respirations, and vital signs. Craniotomy with evacuation and control of bleeding may be performed depending on the condition of the client, extent of cerebral contusion, and accessibility of the bleeding site.

Subarachnoid and intraventricular hemorrhage are common in severe head injury. The symptoms include those listed for hematoma, as well as **nuchal rigidity**, pain and rigidity in the neck. Blood in the subarachnoid space interferes with the reabsorption of cerebrospinal fluid, and thus adds to the increased intracranial pressure.

Signs and symptoms of increased intracranial pressure include a decrease in level of consciousness, initially restlessness, confusion, or difficulty in arousing. Other signs and symptoms are changes in pupil size or reaction to light. The pupil gradually dilates and becomes less responsive to light. Muscle weakness progressing to **hemiplegia**, paralysis of one side of the body, or **paraplegia**, paralysis of lower extremities, and abnormal posturing may occur. Headache and vomiting are experienced by some clients. Vital sign changes generally do not occur until the increased intracranial pressure progresses to involve the brain stem. An increase in systolic blood pressure and a widening pulse pressure accompanied by a slowing pulse are the effects of pressure on the brain stem.

Cerebral Edema and Increased Intracranial Pressure The brain is contained in a rigid container, the skull. The only normal opening to the adult skull is the foramen magnum at the base of the skull. Intracranial pressure is a result of the pressure from the contents of the skull, which are the brain, blood, and cerebrospinal fluid.

Regulatory mechanisms maintain intracranial pressure between 0 to 15 mmHg. When the intracranial pressure is measured at the level of the foramen of Monroe, which is located at midhead level, the normal pressure is 10 or below. The Monroe-Kellie hypothesis is that when there is an increase in volume of one component, there is a decrease in the volume of the others in order to compensate and maintain intracranial pressure between 0 to 15 mmHg. As long as the ability to compensate is effective, there are no neurological changes.

The decompensation phase is when the increase in volume is so excessive that decreasing the volume of remaining components cannot maintain intracranial pressure below 15 mm Hg. Neurological changes are exhibited because of cellular hypoxia and displacement of the brain which compresses neurons, especially in the brain stem. The changes are a decreasing level of consciousness, decreased motor response to commands, fixed, dilated pupils, and vital sign changes known as Cushing's triad or reflex. Cushing's triad is bradycardia, widening pulse pressure, with increasing systolic pressure, and respiratory irregularities. Respiratory changes include periods of apnea, decreased respiratory rate and depth, and irregular respirations.

Causes of increased intracranial pressure are

increased blood volume from vascular vasodilatation, increased volume of brain tissue from edema, infection, tumor, or hemorrhage, increased volume of cerebrospinal fluid, from overproduction, decreased reabsorption, or interruption of cerebrospinal fluid circulation. If intracranial pressure continues to increase, brain herniation will occur at the tentorial notch or through the foramen magnum resulting in death.

▶ Medical/Surgical Management

Management of head injury is focused toward early recognition and treatment of increasing intracranial pressure and maintenance of normal body functions. Suctioning may be necessary, but is never through the nose on a head injury client. Oxygen is given to maintain cerebral perfusion. Arterial blood gases are checked.

▶ Surgical

Decompression is performed surgically by removing a bone flap from the skull to allow room for the expansion of the brain. A space-occupying lesion such as a tumor, hematoma, or abscess may be surgically removed. Excess CSF may be drained from the ventricles (see Figure 27-6).

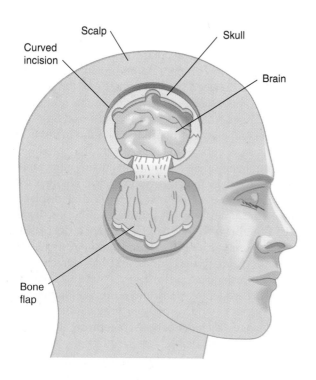

FIGURE 27-6 Bone flap—craniotomy.

▶ Pharmacological

Corticosteroids such as dexamethasone (Decadron) are given to reduce cerebral edema. Antacids such as Mylanta or Maalox, or histamine receptor antagonists such as cimetidine (Tagamet) are given to decrease the side effects of corticosteroids and stress-induced gastric acidity. Osmotic diuretics, mannitol (Osmitrol), are administered to rapidly reduce fluid in the brain tissue; muscle relaxants, sedatives, barbiturates, or muscle paralyzing agents are administered to decrease activity and reduce oxygen needs of the brain.

Antipyretic drugs are used to decrease body temperature, to decrease metabolic needs of the brain, and thereby reduce volume of blood sent to the brain to supply oxygen and glucose. Anticonvulsants are given to prevent or treat seizure activity.

▶ Activity

Activity is depressed to keep the metabolic needs of the brain at a minimum. Increased metabolic needs require more oxygen and glucose supplied by increases in blood volume in the cranium. This further increases intracranial pressure.

▶ Other

With an endotracheal tube in place, the PCO_2 can be lowered below normal. This causes a slightly alkalotic pH which decreases vasodilation and thus decreases intracranial pressure.

▶ Nursing Process

Assessment

Nursing assessment is focused on neurological status for any head injury.

Subjective Data The initial assessment includes subjective data (if the client is conscious), a history of what happened including type of trauma (acceleration, deceleration, or missile), site of blow, loss of consciousness, including when, how long, and whether able to arouse.

Objective Data This includes a neurological screening to obtain a basic neurological status, then, a more in-depth neurological exam is performed for early identification of signs of increasing intracranial pressure.

Frequent assessment of neurological status including level of consciousness, motor function, eye movement, pupil size and reaction, protective reflexes, and vital signs allow for early recognition and intervention for increasing intracranial pressure. Nursing observations also include assessing for double vision, headache, nausea, and bleeding from any orifice. Ipsilateral pupil reaction, the pupil on the same side as the injury or lesion, may occur as the result of pressure on the oculomotor nerve from the increased intracranial pressure or cerebral edema. Recognition of factors that cause increased intracranial pressure is a necessary aspect of assessment.

For the client undergoing intracranial surgery, an assessment of teaching needs of the client and family must be performed. Emotional and psychosocial needs and support systems are assessed. Client teaching includes that the head will be shaved in the area of the incision and what to expect postoperatively.

Longer term care includes assessment of bowel elimination status to prevent need for straining, skin assessment for prevention of skin breakdown, and assessment for complications of immobility.

▼ ▼

Possible nursing diagnoses for a client with a head injury may include:

Nursing Diagnoses	Goals	Nursing Interventions
► Tissue perfusion, altered, cerebral, related to disruption in cerebral blood flow.	The client will demonstrate improvement or maintenance on Glasgow Coma Scale.	Assess neurological status of client every fifteen to sixty minutes. Note finding on Glasgow Coma Scale. Compare findings with previous assessments to note changes in condition. Administer oxygen as ordered to supply a high concentration of oxygen to the brain. Position client with head of the bed up 30 to 40 degrees with head kept at midline to promote venous drainage from the head. Prevent coughing, sneezing, or valsalva maneuver to prevent increased intracranial pressure. Minimize physical activity to prevent increasing metabolic demands. Maintain blood $PCaO_2$ between 25 to 30 mmHg to prevent vasodilatation.
► Breathing patterns, ineffective, related to neurological impairment of respiratory status or mechanical ventilation.	The client will have effective breathing patterns.	Assess respiratory status every fifteen to sixty minutes. Provide mechanical ventilation if necessary. Assess ongoing arterial blood gases or pulse oximeter readings to identify need to assist respirations to prevent vasodilatation in the brain, further increasing intracranial pressure. Administer oxygen as ordered to maintain blood oxygen concentration.
► Family processes, altered, related to sudden crisis.	The client and/or family will demonstrate effective coping mechanisms.	Assess family's coping mechanisms. Provide information about the client in an ongoing fashion. Provide teaching about the injury and pathophysiology involved. Prepare family for possible outcomes of the injury. Collaborate with clergy, social support, mental health counselors, and support groups. Involve the family in client care as appropriate. Teach the family to report increased drowsiness, weakness in arm/leg, muscle twitching, nausea or vomiting, visual or hearing disturbances, and so on. Inform the family that the client may not be aware of the symptoms, that signs and symptoms of the head injury may not be apparent immediately, and that the client should rest for twenty-four hours.

▶ *Evaluation*

Each goal must be evaluated to determine how it has been met by the client.

▲ ▲

▶ *BRAIN TUMOR*

Brain tumors are space-occupying intracranial lesions, either benign or malignant. Classification of brain tumors is by location or type of tissue. Intracranial lesions may be primary lesions that begin development in brain tissue; extensions of tumors of the meninges, cranial nerves, or pituitary gland; or metastatic lesions from tumors originating in other body systems.

Pathophysiology of brain tumors is based on the increase in volume of brain tissue. The etiology is unknown. Clinical manifestations differ by the area of the lesion and the rate of growth. Intracranial pressure increases as compensatory mechanisms are unable to balance for tumor growth. Clinical manifestations commonly include alterations in consciousness, decreased mental functioning, headaches, seizures, or vomiting (sometimes sudden and projectile). Other signs and symptoms are relative to the functions of areas involved such as visual problems with occipital lobe tumors.

Diagnostic evaluation is by computerized tomography (CT) scan, magnetic resonance imaging (MRI), or electroencephalogram (EEG). Total body scans, chest x-rays, and needle biopsies of the tumor may be performed to identify the type of tumor for a basis of medical treatment.

▶ *Medical/Surgical Management*

▶ *Medical*

Medical management is based on the type of tissue, growth rate, and assessment of the client. Chemotherapy, radiation therapy, and/or surgical intervention may be used.

▶ *Surgical*

Surgical intervention, conventional or laser, includes resection of tumors (benign or malignant) to decrease the space occupied by the lesion or for obtaining tissue for biopsy. Cerebrospinal fluid may be shunted out of the brain to relieve increased pressure.

▶ *Pharmacological*

Pharmacological interventions are based on presenting symptoms. Dexamethasone (Decadron) is administered to decrease cerebral edema. Phenytoin (Dilantin) is given to prevent seizure activity. Antacids and H_2 blockers such as cimetidine (Tagamet) are given to prevent gastric irritation. Analgesics, NSAIDs or codeine are used for headaches, and stool softeners are administered to prevent straining. Antineoplastic agents may be administered based upon tumor type and whether the client meets the drug protocol.

▶ *Radiation*

Radiation therapy may be administered for treatment of specific tumor types or inoperable tumors. The goal is to destroy the tumor cells that are more susceptible to radiation than the normal cells. A typical treatment schedule is one treatment daily five days per week for four to six weeks. Radiation is also used in conjunction with surgery and chemotherapy.

▶ *Nursing Process*

Assessment

Subjective Data This includes asking the client about fatigue, pain, headache, weakness, and ability to perform daily activities. Assess for sensory changes such as hearing, visual, or olfactory changes. Pain assessment and effectiveness of interventions is necessary. A thorough psychosocial assessment, including changes in personality or judgment is the basis for providing emotional support.

Objective Data This includes assessment of functional ability, mobility, and mental status, including motor strength, gait, ability to perform activities of daily living and level of consciousness. Observe for signs of neurological changes, deficits or increased intracranial pressure such as restlessness, changes in logic, changes in vital signs, pupil responses, speech abnormalities, seizure activity, or changes in respiratory patterns.

▼ ▼

Possible nursing diagnoses for a client with a brain tumor may include:

Nursing Diagnoses	Goals	Nursing Interventions
▶ Anxiety related to fear of unknown and treatment plans.	The client will demonstrate effective use of coping mechanisms.	Allow client to verbalize feeling of anxiety and discuss coping patterns previously used. Observe for verbal and nonverbal cues of presence of anxiety. Provide emotional support by listening, guiding client to explore feeling of helplessness, fear of the unknown, and potential impending death. Teach client and family about diagnostic tests, treatments, and expected outcomes. Collaborate with pastoral care, physician, social services, and family to provide emotional support. Maintain a calm manner. Teach relaxation exercises and techniques. Administer tranquilizers and sedatives as ordered.
▶ Pain, related to pressure on the brain.	The client will state increased comfort, effective pain relief.	Assess client's level of pain. Teach client and the family about medication therapy and the use of medications to control discomfort. Administer analgesics as ordered and assess effectiveness within thirty minutes of administration. Change client's position every two to four hours. Provide planned rest periods following administration of analgesics. Provide back rubs and skin care.
▶ Fatigue related to effects of treatment.	The client will verbalize less fatigue with frequent rest periods.	Allow client to discuss feelings of fatigue. Involve client in planning daily schedule with frequent rest periods. Assess client's ability to perform activities of daily living and need for assistance to conserve energy. Cluster care activities to provide frequent rest periods that coincide with peak effectiveness of analgesics.
▶ Nutrition, altered, less than body requirement related to side effects of treatment and disease process.	The client will maintain weight within 5 pounds of initial weight.	Assess client's weight every other day. Provide frequent small feedings of high calorie and high protein foods. Offer foods of client's choice. Use nutritional supplements to maintain weight and offer fluids frequently.

▶ Evaluation

Each goal must be evaluated to determine how it has been met by the client.

▲ ▲

▶ *CEREBROVASCULAR ACCIDENT (CVA)/ TRANSIENT ISCHEMIC ATTACKS (TIA)*

Cerebrovascular accident (CVA) or stroke is a sudden loss of brain function with neurological deficit. CVA is the third highest cause of death in the United States. Death rates from stroke have steadily declined from 120/100,000 in 1970 to 60/100,000 in 1985 (Hickey, 1992). The first rise in death rates in thirty-five years, a one percent rise in stroke deaths, was recorded between 1992 and 1993, the most current available data. The rise in deaths in two groups among this population is noteworthy, African American women ages forty-five to sixty increased by 15 percent and African American men over age sixty-five increased by 10 percent (National Stroke Association, 1995). Reasons for this sharp rise have not been determined. A proposed cause is decreased mortality from other diseases such as heart disease.

Strokes are caused by ischemia from a thrombus, embolus, severe vasospasm, or a cerebral hemorrhage. Blood supply to the brain is interrupted causing neurological deficits of sensation, movement, thought, memory, or speech. The loss of function can be temporary or permanent.

The major risk factor for stroke is hypertension. Other risk factors are diabetes mellitus, atherosclerosis, aneurysm, cardiac disease, high blood cholesterol, obesity, sedentary lifestyle, smoking, stress, drug abuse, especially cocaine use, and use of oral contraceptives. People with more than one risk factor are at even higher risk.

Transient ischemic attacks, (TIAs) frequently precede a CVA. A TIA is a temporary or transient episode of neurological dysfunction caused by temporary impairment of blood flow to the brain. The loss of motor or sensory function may last from a few seconds to minutes to twenty-four hours. A classic symptom is fleeting blindness in one eye. A reversible ischemic neurological deficit (RIND) is a TIA that lasts twenty-four to forty-eight hours.

Clinical manifestations vary with the location of interrupted blood supply in the brain. As with head injury, the specific functions of the involved area of the brain are interrupted causing the symptoms. Common neurological deficits are motor deficits of hemiplegia (paralysis of one side of the body on the side opposite of the brain lesion), **hemiparesis** (weakness of one side of the body), **dysarthria** (impairment of speech muscles), and dysphagia (impairment of swallowing muscles). **Emotional lability**, loss of emotional control, inability to control behavior, and inability to process multiple pieces of information are also common manifestations of stroke.

Sensory deficits include visual deficits of double vision, decreased visual acuity, and **homonymous hemianopia**, the loss of vision in half of the visual field with the loss of vision on the same side of both eyes. There may be decreased sensation to touch, pressure, pain, heat, and cold. The client may be confused and disoriented.

Intellectual deficits include memory impairments, poor judgment, short attention span, difficulty organizing thoughts, and inability to reason or calculate. Emotional deficits include depression and decreased tolerance to stressors.

Most clients experience initial bowel and bladder dysfunction. With early recognition of the problem and use of bowel and bladder retraining programs, most clients regain continence of bowel and bladder.

Differences in the affected side of the brain have been identified. Clients with a left side CVA tend to have communication deficits of **aphasia**, inability to communicate. The three types of aphasia are expressive aphasia, receptive aphasia, or global aphasia. Expressive aphasia is difficulty transforming sound into speech. Receptive aphasia is impairment of comprehension of spoken word, that is the client can physically speak, but incorrectly uses words. Global aphasia is a combination of expressive and receptive aphasia. People with left side CVAs tend to be slow and cautious in behavior and have intellectual impairments such as memory deficits or loss of problem solving skills. Defects in the right visual field occur. If the lesion is on the left side, hemiplegia occurs on the right side.

Clients with right side CVA have left-sided paralysis and defects in the left visual fields. Spatial-perceptual defects, called **agnosia**, cause the inability to recognize familiar objects such as a hairbrush. They demonstrate poor judgment and impulsive behavior with unawareness of deficits. This is called **anosognosia**, which is gross denial of the stroke or neurological deficit. Furthermore, they are easily distracted and usually show **unilateral neglect**. Unilateral neglect is the failure to recognize or care for the affected side of the body. The right hemisphere of the brain is usually dominant in directing attention mechanisms, the function of paying attention to all stimuli affecting the body. The loss of this causes neglect of visual, auditory, and/or tactile sensations. The sensation may be intact, but the brain has difficulty directing away from stimuli in the nonneglected hemisphere to pay attention to stimuli in the neglected hemisphere (Kalbach, 1991).

Cerebral edema and increased intracranial pressure may further complicate neurological status. Cerebral edema maximizes in three to five days following the CVA. Neurological deficits begin to resolve within two days. Gradual progression from proximal to distal can occur for one to two years.

▶ Medical/Surgical Management

▶ Medical

Medical management of the client with a CVA is directed toward maintenance of airway and supportive therapy during the first twenty-four to forty-eight hours. Early diagnosis of the cause and type of stroke is necessary to determine the appropriate treatment. Maintaining adequate cerebral perfusion and preventing cerebral edema will reduce the neurological deficit. Respiratory failure will be treated with mechanical ventilation; temperature will be regulated with a hypothermia blanket if necessary. See increased intracranial pressure for prevention and treatment.

To prevent further loss of function, a focus on rehabilitation must begin on admission. Self-care and mobility that remain must be maintained.

▶ Surgical

Surgical removal of the thrombus or embolus may be necessary to relieve pressure on the brain.

▶ Pharmacological

Antihypertensive agents are used to control blood pressure. Anticoagulants, aspirin, heparin, or coumadin are used in the treatment of strokes caused by thrombi to prevent further clot formation. Thrombolytic agents such as alteplase (Activase), anistreplase (Eminase), streptokinase (Streptase), and urokinase (Abbokinase) may be ordered for strokes caused by a thrombus to dissolve the clot. A stroke caused by bleeding would not be treated with thrombolytic agents. Dexamethasone (Decadron) may be used to reduce intracranial pressure. Anticonvulsants such as phenytoin (Dilantin) may be used if convulsions are present. Calcium channel blockers should not be used as they dilate blood vessels and increase cerebral perfusion.

▶ Diet

Fluids may be restricted for a few days following a CVA. The client will however be given intravenous fluids or tube feedings.

▶ Activity

The client's bed is kept flat to increase cerebral perfusion in cases of an embolic or thrombolic stroke, and the head of the bed is elevated to decrease cerebral perfusion in the event of a hemorrhagic stroke. The type of CVA and the physician's judgment determines how long the client will stay in bed. Some physicians want the client up in a few days and others prescribe a long period of bed rest.

▶ Other Therapies

Following the initial acute phase and during rehabilitation, physical, occupational, and speech therapy are vital for the client to reach the optimal functional level of recovery.

▶ Nursing Process

Assessment

Subjective Data   This includes statements of how the client is feeling, frustration level with limitations, and feelings of pain, numbness, tingling, and sensory deficits of vision or hearing

Objective Data   Specific attention must be paid to objective findings of assessment of level of consciousness, respiratory status, hemiparesis, hemiplegia, mobility, cognitive perceptual function including inability to think clearly, ability to understand the condition, skin condition, elimination, and safety.

▼ ▼

Possible nursing diagnoses for a client with a CVA may include:

Nursing Diagnoses	Goals	Nursing Interventions
▶ *Knowledge deficit related to home care.*	The client and/or family will verbalize or demonstrate home health care management.	Assess client's and family's needs for discharge teaching and knowledge level about necessary home care.
		Develop a multidisciplinary plan for client and family teaching.
		Provide education in verbal, written, and picture form to provide different strategies for possible impairments from the stroke.

(continued)

Nursing Diagnoses	Goals	Nursing Interventions
		Teach small segments of information at a time, reinforce teaching, then have client and family return demonstration or verbalize knowledge to determine effectiveness of teaching. Primary areas of teaching are medication administration, dosages, actions, and side effects to report to the physician, mobility needs, self-care needs, safety factors, communication, swallowing, elimination, and skin care.
▶ *Communication, impaired, verbal, related to neuromuscular impairment.*	The client will communicate needs to caregiver.	Assess communication deficits and consult speech therapist for determining a method of communication if deficits are apparent.
		Allow time for the client to attempt to communicate needs, also anticipate needs to prevent client frustration in trying to communicate.
		Use gestures, pictures, and closed question for yes and no answers. Provide paper and pencil if dominant side is unaffected.
		Assign the same caregivers to provide consistency in understanding the client's needs.
▶ *Self-care deficit related to immobility.*	The client will perform optimum activities of daily living within limitations of neuromuscular impairments.	Consult occupational therapist to assist in dressing with one hand.
		Arrange items needed by the client for daily care so that they may be easily used and allow adequate time for the client to complete care.
		Consult with family and evaluate home for safety and ability to perform self-care.
		Teach client and family to place small bites of food on unaffected side, and to check for pocketed food after meals.
		Provide good oral hygiene following all meals and snacks to prevent tooth decay and oral infections.
▶ *Unilateral neglect related to neuromuscular impairment.*	The client will move paralyzed extremities with assistance from functioning extremities.	Adapt environment to prevent injury of the client with unilateral neglect by positioning water, call light, personal items on the unaffected or unneglected side. Approach the client from the unneglected side.
		Gradually cue client to remind to tend to the neglected side.
		Remind client of safety factors, such as arm trailing over edge of wheelchair or close proximity of a wall on the neglected side.
		Instruct client to scan environment for safety factors at all times.
		Teach client how to dress and tend to neglected side.
		Place arm in sling if ambulatory or on a wheelchair tray.

▶ *Evaluation*

Each goal must be evaluated to determine how it has been met by the client.

▲ ▲

▶ EPILEPSY

Epilepsy is a disorder of cerebral function with sudden attacks of altered consciousness, motor activity, or sensory phenomenon. Convulsive seizures are the most common type of attack. Most recurrent seizure patterns are due to epilepsy. Most clinicians and authors use the term "seizure disorder" for epilepsy or seizures (Hickey, 1992).

A seizure is initiated by an electrical disturbance in the neurons which causes an aberrant discharge of electrical activity from any part of the cerebral cortex, and possibly from other areas of the brain (Samuels, 1995). This electrical discharge may cause involuntary episodes of loss of consciousness, excessive muscular movement or loss of muscle tone, and changes in behavior, mood, sensation, and/or perception (Smeltzer & Bare, 1992).

The etiology of the electrical disturbance may be from birth trauma, hypoxia, infection, tumor, alcohol toxicity, drugs, drug withdrawal, carbon monoxide or lead poisoning, vascular abnormalities such as cerebral vascular accident, hypoglycemia electrolyte imbalance, or fever. Often the cause is idiopathic, or unknown.

Seizures are classified as generalized or partial. In generalized seizures, the entire brain is affected simultaneously causing bilateral, symmetrical reactions. Generalized seizures include tonic and/or clonic, absence, and myoclonic types.

Absence seizures involve loss of conscious activity without the muscular involvement of tonic-clonic seizures. Tonic-clonic seizures involve rigid tonic contractions of muscles and loss of postural control followed by a clonic stage of intermittent contraction and relaxation. Loss of continence of stool or urine is common.

Partial seizures initiate in a focal point in the brain and involve the function of those specific neurons. Two types of partial seizures are simple and complex. In simple partial seizures, the area affected may be a hand, finger, ability to talk, or a sense such as smell. Consciousness is not lost.

Complex partial seizures generally involve loss of consciousness and may produce cognitive, affective, psychosensory, or psychomotor symptoms (Chipps, Clanin, & Campbell, 1992). The client may perform inappropriate purposive behaviors, called **automatism,** like lip-smacking or walking. The seizure is not generally remembered. Automatisms are mechanical, repetitive motor behaviors performed unconsciously. **Auras,** a peculiar sensation preceding the seizure, may be of taste, smell, sight, hearing, dizziness, or just a 'funny feeling'.

Diagnostic testing to determine the type of seizure activity includes the electroencephalogram (EEG) to identify abnormal electrical activity and/or the focal point. Sleep and video electroencephalograms are performed to document activity with changes in electrical activity of the brain. Computerized tomography (CT) scans are used to identify or rule out lesion, degenerative changes, or vascular abnormalities.

▶ Medical/Surgical Management

▶ Surgical

Surgical intervention may be indicated for a very small percentage of clients. Microsurgery may be utilized to irradiate focal points of abnormal electrical discharge caused by tumor, vascular abnormality, or abscess.

▶ Pharmacological

The primary method of controlling seizure activity is pharmacological. Seizure activity in 75 percent of clients is controlled with an anticonvulsant agent or a combination of anticonvulsants (Hickey, 1992). Phenytoin (Dilantin), phenobarbital, carbamazepine (Tegretol), valproic acid (Depakene), and primidone (Mysoline) are often used. Anticonvulsant agents are started one at a time in gradually increasing doses. The client's blood levels are monitored for therapeutic range; and the client is assessed for side effects and toxicity of the drug, such as drowsiness, dizziness, gastric distress, rash, blood dyscrasias, and ataxia. Long-term use of Dilantin requires good oral hygiene because of hyperplasia in which the gums become edematous and enlarged.

The goal is to obtain seizure control with minimal side effects. Any anticonvulsant should be gradually discontinued. Abrupt withdrawal can cause **status epilepticus,** an acute prolonged episode of seizure activity lasting at least thirty minutes with or without loss of consciousness (Smeltzer & Bare, 1992). Status epilepticus is a medical emergency that can result in respiratory arrest and irreversible brain damage.

▶ Diet

Nutritionally balanced meals are required. The client should not consume alcohol.

▶ Activity

Adequate rest is required. No driving or operating machinery and no swimming is allowed until seizures are controlled.

▶ *Nursing Process*

Assessment

Subjective Data   This includes client statements of experiences prior to the seizure. What activity was the client performing? Determine whether an aura was experienced and the sensations that were manifested. Ascertain if the client has a prior history of seizure disorder.

Objective Data   Assessment of the nature of the seizure and sequencing of events is important in determining cause and management of seizure activity. During the seizure, the nurse assesses the client's respiratory status and observes for muscular stiffness or flaccidity, the position of the eyes and head, the size

and equality of the pupils, automatism, any cry or sounds made, and incontinence of urine or stool. The duration of the phases of the seizure, total duration, and whether unconsciousness occurred are noted. Also note if the onset of seizure activity was observed and what the client was doing.

Following the seizure observe the client for postictal signs of paralysis of arms or legs, inability to speak, sleep following seizure, difficulty in awakening from sleep, confusion, or general dazed effect (Smeltzer & Bare, 1992; Hickey, 1992). The postictal phase can last from several minutes to hours. Assess the client for signs of injury and obtain vital signs. Clients on anticonvulsant therapy need a thorough nursing assessment because of the wide variety of side effects involving multiple body systems.

▼ ▼

Possible nursing diagnoses for a client with a seizure may include:

Nursing Diagnoses	Goals	Nursing Interventions
▶ *Airway clearance, ineffective, related to mucus accumulation during the seizure and uncontrollable tonic-clonic muscle contractions involving the respiratory muscles.*	The client will maintain an effective airway during seizure activity.	Turn client to the side, following tonic/clonic activity to allow secretions to drain from the airway. Prepare to suction oropharynx if necessary to clear the airway. Assess skin color and respiratory rate, depth during and following seizure. Administer oxygen as needed. Insert oral airway or epistick if client's jaw is not clenched. Never insert an object if the jaw is already clenched. Do not place fingers between client's teeth. Loosen restrictive clothing.
▶ *Injury, high risk for, related to uncontrollable movements during seizure activity.*	The client will be free of injury related to seizure activity.	During seizures in bed, pad the side rails with blankets or protective pads. If the client is standing or sitting, ease the client to the floor when seizure activity begins and place client supine on floor, but do not physically restrain the client. Remove objects from around the client so that he or she will not hit them. Maintain patent airway for the client. Following the seizure, turn the client to the side to allow secretions to drain from the mouth. Assess neurological status and vital signs. Maintain a low stimulus environment to prevent further seizure activity. Observe client for injuries, i.e., tongue lacerations; broken bones; body lacerations or bruising. Inform the client that a seizure occurred and reorient if necessary.

Nursing Diagnoses	Goals	Nursing Interventions
		Teach client to maintain a safe environment including: driving restrictions; lying down in a safe area if an aura is experienced; showering instead of tub bathing; no swimming or swimming with a partner if the physician allows; and wearing a medical identification tag.
▶ *Coping, ineffective individual, related to anxiety secondary to seizure disorder and altered self-concept.*	The client will verbalize fears and concerns about seizure activity; the client will use effective coping methods.	Allow client to verbalize fears and concerns. Explore coping mechanisms with the client. Collaborate with mental health counselor or pastor to assist client with development of coping mechanisms.
▶ *Knowledge deficit related to seizure activity, medications, and safety factors.*	The client will verbalize knowledge of the pathophysiology of seizure activity; medication name, dosage, actions, side effects, and toxicity; and safety factors to prevent injury.	Develop a teaching plan for the client that covers seizure pathophysiology; medication name, action, dosage, side effects, and toxicity; safety factors and community resources. Explain the importance of maintaining therapeutic drug levels, that is, always take medications when ordered, no skipping doses. Keep all appointments with the physician.

▶ Evaluation

Each goal must be evaluated to determine how it has been met by the client.

▲ ▲

▶ HERNIATED INTERVERTEBRAL DISK

Herniated intervertebral disks are a major cause of chronic back pain. Most clients with herniated disks are thirty to fifty years of age. The majority of herniated disks occur in the lumbar or cervical spine because of the flexibility of these regions (Hickey, 1992). This can occur suddenly from trauma, lifting or twisting, or gradually because of aging, osteoporosis, or degenerative changes. Most herniated disks are caused by trauma, such as falls, accidents, or repeated lifting. Degenerative changes of arthritis, aging, or repeated minor injuries predispose the client to herniated intervertebral disks.

The intervertebral disk is a cartilaginous cushion between vertebral bodies (see Figure 27-7). In herniation or rupture of the disk, the nucleus pulposus protrudes into the fibrous ring, the annulus fibrosus. This protrusion presses upon the spinal cord and nerve roots causing pain, motor changes, sensory changes, and alterations in reflexes.

The nerve root affected and the degree of compression lead to specific symptoms. Ninety to ninety-five percent of lumbar herniations occur at the L-4 to L-5 and S-1 levels (Hickey, 1992). Low back pain that radiates across the buttock, and down the leg following the sciatic nerve is the most common symptom. The affected leg has tingling and numbness. Sneezing, straining, stooping, standing, sitting, blowing the nose, and jarring movements aggravate the pain. Positions of comfort are lying on back with knees flexed and a small pillow under the head or lying on the unaffected side with affected knee flexed.

Motor weakness may be experienced. Paresthesia and numbness of the leg and foot occur. Knee and ankle reflexes are diminished or absent. Lasegue's sign, gentle raising of the fully extended leg of the client in a supine position, causes pain at 20° to 60° because of stretching of the inflamed sciatic nerve. There may also be a positive **Kernig's sign**, which is a test for inflammation in the nerve roots. Kernig's sign is tested by placing the client in a dorsal recumbent position and having the client attempt to flex the hip and knee, then extend the knee. Normally, the client should extend the knee to 90 degrees. With a low back herniated disk, the client will not be able to extend the knee because of severe pain radiating down the hip and leg. Symptoms vary with the area and degree of nerve root compression.

Cervical herniation commonly occurs at levels C-5 to C-6 or C-6 to C-7. Symptoms of lateral herniation include pain and paresthesia in the neck, arms, and shoulders. Loss of muscle strength and reflexes may occur. Muscle mass may atrophy.

Because of anatomical positioning, cervical disks may herniate centrally more frequently than lumbar disks and compress the spinal cord. Symptoms are weakness of the lower extremities and unsteady gait. Spasticity and hyperactive reflexes may develop in the lower extremities. Difficulty voiding and sexual dysfunction may occur.

Degenerative spinal cord disease can follow compression from a herniated disk. Spinal cord tumors and herniated lumbar disk are differential diagnoses that are ruled out through the use of MRI or CT scans.

▶ Medical/Surgical Management

▶ Medical

Conservative medical treatment providing rest, stress reduction and immobility of the spine, and pain relief is often tried for several weeks.

▶ Surgical

Surgery to remove the herniated disk is done when neurological deficit or pain are not responsive to conservative treatment or when symptoms require immediate surgical intervention. Surgical interventions include the following:

- Diskectomy—removal of herniated nuclear fragments of intervertebral disk.
- Laminectomy—removal of lamina to relieve compression of the spinal cord or the nerve root, or to remove the herniated disk.
- Hemilaminectomy—removal of part of the laminal arch.
- Diskectomy with fusion—removal of herniated material with bone grafting to stabilize the spine.
- Chemonucleolysis—done if there is no nerve involvement. Local anesthesia is given. A needle is guided into the nucleus palposus and chymopapin (Discase) is injected. This dissolves the nucleus palposus.

▶ Pharmacological

Narcotic analgesics such as hydrocodone bitartrate with acetaminophen (Vicodin) and nonnarcotic analgesics such as tramadol hydrochloride (Ultram) are

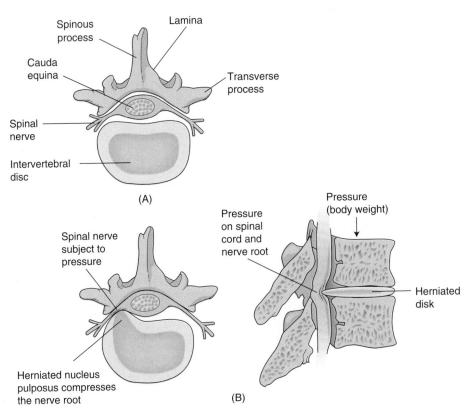

FIGURE 27-7 (**A**) Normal intervertebral disc; (**B**) Two views of a herniated disc.

ordered for pain control. Antiinflammatory drugs, steroids, or nonsteroidal antiinflammatory agents (NSAIDs) such as ibuprofen (Motrin) or naproxen (Anaprox) are prescribed to reduce the inflammatory response. Muscle relaxants such as methocarbamol (Robaxin) are given to reduce spasms of surrounding muscles which decreases the pain. Antianxiety medications such as diazepam (Valium) are given to decrease muscle tension and promote rest and immobility.

▶ Diet

Weight reduction is advocated if the client is overweight. This decreases the workload for the involved muscles. A high protein diet with calcium, vitamin D, and phosphorus is necessary for bone repair and prevention of osteoporosis. Fiber is necessary for bowel function because constipation is a common side effect of analgesics.

▶ Activity

Bed rest, support garment (back brace) or cervical collar, a firm mattress, and traction may be used to decrease stress on the affected vertebrae. Postoperatively, log roll turning is used to prevent injury to the vertebrae and spine. Turn the body as a unit without twisting the back. Place the bed in flat position, position a pillow between the legs; at least two nurses roll the client to the side as a unit. One nurse turns head and shoulders, the other turns hips and legs.

The client may not lift or carry more than 5 pounds for at least eight weeks. Twisting movements are to be avoided. The client cannot drive a car until the surgeon permits. Sitting should be limited during the early postoperative period; the client should either stand or lie down.

▶ Other Therapies

Physical therapy is focused on muscle strengthening and client comfort. Heat therapy, ultrasound, and exercises are often used to promote comfort and healing.

▶ Nursing Process

Assessment

Subjective Data Assessment includes the client's statements about motor and sensory function, pain, and effectiveness of comfort measures.

Objective Data Assessment entails a neurological evaluation of motor and sensory function of the extremities innervated below the herniated area. Reflex testing may be a part of the nursing assessment in some facilities. Assess the range of motion of the affected extremity. Assess the client's knowledge about the disease process; the planned treatment including pain management and surgery and the postsurgical care. Assess status of bowel and bladder elimination for potential nerve involvement or effects of immobility. Assess for gait alteration and limited bending.

▼ ▼

Possible nursing diagnoses for a client with herniated intervertebral disk may include:

Nursing Diagnoses	Goals	Nursing Interventions
▶ *Pain related to nerve compression or surgical intervention.*	The client will experience increase in comfort.	Assess pain intensity, location, and activities or position when pain began. Have the client rate pain on a scale of 1 to 10.
		Maintain activity level as ordered by physician.
		Place client in position of comfort, usually on back with knees slightly flexed and small pillow beneath head or on unaffected side with affected extremity flexed and a pillow between the legs.
		Maintain immobility of vertebrae with corset, brace, or traction.
		Apply moist heat as prescribed and administer medications to relieve pain, relax muscles, and to relieve inflammation and anxiety as ordered. Document effectiveness.
		Provide diversional activities.

(continued)

Nursing Diagnoses	*Goals*	*Nursing Interventions*
▶ *Physical mobility, impaired, related to nerve compression or surgical intervention.*	The client will not have complications of immobility.	Assess for complications of immobility.
		Turn client every one to two hours. The client will tend to limit position to one of comfort.
		Assist the client to logroll, that is move the body as a unit without twisting the back by placing the bed in a flat position, position a pillow between the client's legs; then at least two nurses roll the client to the side as a unit; one nurse turns head and shoulders, the other turns hips and legs.
		Ambulate as ordered by the physician.
▶ *Knowledge deficit related to disease process, treatment regimen, and postoperative care.*	The client will verbalize knowledge of treatment regimen, self-care, and disease process.	Teach the client about the disease process by reviewing the anatomy and physiology of intervertebral disk, vertebrae, spinal cord, and spinal nerves.
		Discuss goals of the treatment plan, desired effects of immobility, and the use of supportive devices.
		Teach the client about medication, actions, and side effects. Teach the log-rolling technique. Provide preoperative teaching to clients scheduled for surgery.
		Since the postoperative stay is usually twenty-four to forty-eight hours, teach home care prior to surgery.
		Teach the client to use good body mechanics and to maintain a weight reduction program if indicated, in order to reduce the chance of recurrence of a herniated disk.
		Provide the client with dietary instruction in a diet high in protein, calcium, vitamin D, and phosphorus, if the underlying disease is osteoporosis.

▶ *Evaluation*

Each goal must be evaluated to determine how it has been met by the client.

▲ ▲

▶ SPINAL CORD INJURY

Spinal cord injury (SCI) occurs from trauma to the spinal cord or from compression of the spinal cord due to injury to the supporting structures. Each year almost 8,000 new spinal cord injuries occur. Most of the victims are males between the ages of sixteen and thirty. Leading causes of the injury are motor vehicle accidents, falls, acts of violence, and sports accidents (National Spinal Cord Injury Statistical Center, 1990; Beare & Meyers, 1994; Hickey, 1992).

Numerous classification systems exist for spinal cord injuries. SCI may be classified by level of injury, mechanism of injury, or by neurological or functional level (see Figure 27-8). The injury may be considered complete or incomplete. No impulses are carried below the level of injury when injury is complete. There is complete disruption of the spinal cord functions including motor (voluntary movement), sensation, and reflexes to areas innervated by the spinal nerves at and below the level of the injury.

In an incomplete injury some of the spinal cord tracts are affected while others are able to carry impulses normally. There are four identified syndromes of incomplete spinal cord injury: anterior cord syndrome, posterior cord syndrome, central cord syndrome, and Brown-Sequard syndrome (Beare & Meyers, 1994; Buchanan & Nawoczenski, 1987; Hickey,

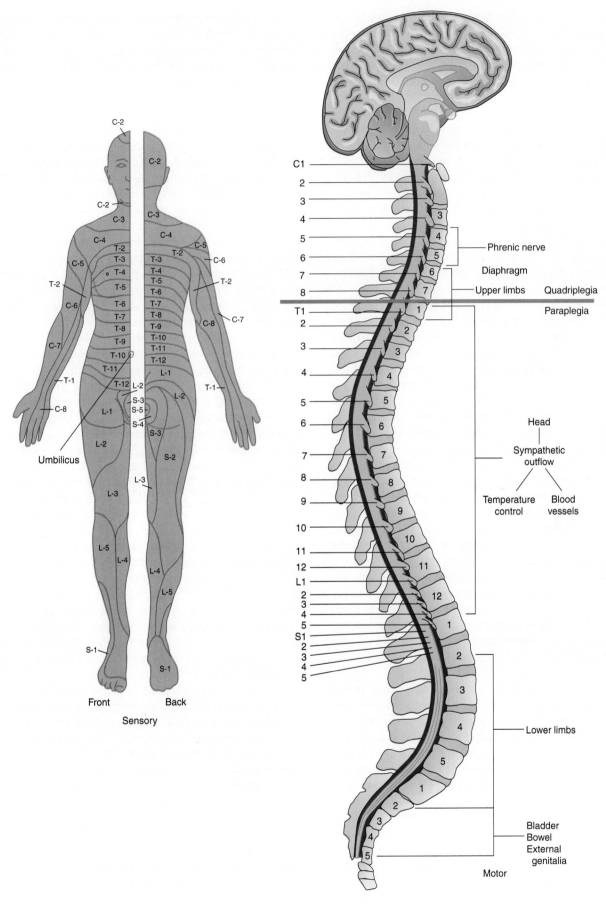

FIGURE 27-8 Spinal cord injury—levels of injury.

1992). Clinical manifestations of anterior cord syndrome are a loss of voluntary motor activity below the level of injury and loss of some sensation to light touch and pressure. Posterior cord syndrome results in loss of sensation including proprioception, discrimination, and vibration below the level of injury. Motor tracts are not usually affected. In central cord syndrome the upper extremities and respiratory system are impaired, and the lower extremities may be somewhat affected.

In Brown-Sequard syndrome, half of the spinal cord is involved causing both motor and sensory deficits. Motor function, deep touch, proprioception, and vibration are lost on the same side as the lesion. Pain, temperature, light touch, and pressure sensations are lost on the side opposite the lesion. The incomplete lesion may also include combinations of these four syndromes depending upon the nerve tracts that are involved.

The mechanism of injury is usually an acceleration-deceleration event that causes hyperflexion, hyperextension, axial loading, or excessive rotation injury (Hickey, 1992). Hyperflexion is the extreme forward movement of the head that causes compression of the vertebral bodies and damage to the posterior ligaments and intervertebral disks. Hyperextension is the extreme backward movement of the head causing injury to the posterior vertebral structures and the anterior ligaments. Axial loading or compression occurs when extreme pressure is placed upon the spinal column such as in diving accidents or falls when landing on feet or buttocks. Compression of the vertebrae causes shattering of the vertebral body. Compression fractures and posterior ligament injury can also be caused by excessive rotation or turning the head beyond the normal range.

Classification of injury by cause includes concussion, contusion, laceration, transection, hemorrhage, or damage to blood vessels supplying the spinal cord. Immediately following injury to the spinal cord, an autodestructive process begins with chemical and vascular changes that lead to ischemia and necrosis of the spinal cord.

Spinal shock (shock associated with acute spinal cord injury) and areflexia (the absence of reflexes) occur immediately upon transection of the spinal cord or upon injury to the spinal cord. There is flaccid paralysis of all skeletal muscles, loss of spinal reflexes, loss of sensation, and absence of autonomic function below the level of injury. The diaphragm is innervated at levels C3 through C5. Injuries in this area will cause partial or complete disruption of respiratory function. The client does not perspire below the level of the injury. Bowel and bladder function may be lost for a few days to months, or may be permanent. It generally lasts from one to six weeks.

As spinal shock resolves, reflex activity returns below the level of injury. The client with a lower motor neuron injury continues to have flaccid paralysis, areflexia, hypotonic bowel and bladder function, and sexual dysfunction. Lower motor neuron injury causes paraplegia, paralysis of lower extremities.

Neurogenic shock, a hypotensive situation resulting from the loss of sympathetic control of vital functions from the brain, may occur during spinal shock. This happens in clients with injury above the sixth thoracic vertebrae. The client develops orthostatic hypotension, bradycardia, decreased cardiac output, loss of ability to sweat below the level of injury, and subnormal temperature.

An upper motor neuron injury develops a spastic paralysis, loss of voluntary skeletal muscle movement, and reflexive bowel, bladder, and sexual responses. Complete upper motor neuron injury results in quadriplegia, dysfunction or paralysis of both arms, both legs, bowel, and bladder. Injuries above C5 affect respiratory function because of innervation of the diaphragm and accessory respiratory muscles. Mechanical ventilation is required to keep the client alive. Fractures below the cervical vertebrae result in diaphragmatic breathing if the phrenic nerve is functioning.

The client with an injury above the sixth thoracic vertebrae is at risk for developing autonomic dysreflexia or autonomic hyperreflexia. Autonomic dysreflexia is an emergency situation that causes a hypertensive crisis that can result in stroke or seizure activity. The cause is noxious stimuli such as a full bladder, a fecal impaction, a wrinkle in clothing, menstrual cramps, an erection, an ingrown toenail, a bladder infection, or sitting on catheter tubing. Autonomic reflexes below the level of the injury cause vasoconstriction below the level of the injury. The controlling impulses from the higher cortical levels do not transmit past the level of injury, but cause bradycardia and vasodilatation above the level of injury. Skin above the level of injury is warm and moist, but skin below the level of injury is cold with goose flesh (Beare & Meyers, 1994; Hickey, 1992; Latham, 1994).

The noxious stimuli must be removed, if possible, and the client placed in a sitting position immediately. The blood pressure must be assessed immediately and monitored every few minutes until within normal limits (Huston & Boelman, 1995). The drug of choice, nitroprusside sodium (Nipride), may be given if the conservative measure does not work. Autonomic dysreflexia must be prevented when possible, recognized when it develops, and treated immediately. Once the autonomic dysreflexia situation is relieved, the client may develop hypotension from the decreased sympathetic response and the residual effects of medication and positioning changes. A pattern of individual response to stimuli and sympathetic response is soon identified for the client. However, a client with an upper motor neuron injury above T-6 is always at risk for developing autonomic dysreflexia. Sometimes a client may have the first episode even years after the injury.

The extent of permanent injury cannot be determined immediately because of necrosis, edema, and spinal shock. Functional loss is dependent upon the level, degree, and type of injury.

▶ Medical/Surgical Management

▶ Medical

Medical management of the client with spinal cord injury begins prior to reaching the hospital. Further damage to the spinal cord is prevented by immobilizing the head, neck, and vertebral column. All trauma clients are treated as potential spinal cord injuries. When the client reaches the emergency room, x-rays of the spine are taken prior to removing the immobilizing devices such as rigid cervical collars and splinting backboards.

Respiratory function is continuously assessed and ventilatory support provided as necessary. This client may have multiple injuries that necessitate astute diagnostic skills by the emergency room physician. Assessment of the trauma client must include internal hemorrhaging, cardiac contusion, head injury, hemorrhagic shock, as well as spinal shock from the spinal cord injury. A thorough assessment is done to specifically evaluate the degree of deficit and to establish the level or degree of injury.

Immobilization of the spinal cord continues as the focus of care during the early medical management of the client. Traction may be used to maintain alignment of the spinal column. Cervical tongs and halo devices are used to apply traction and to immobilize the cervical spine. Cervical tongs and halo rings are applied under local anesthesia with spring loaded pins that are embedded into the scalp. Antiseptic solution is used to cleanse the scalp and a local anesthetic is injected into the insertion sites. Traction weights are applied to the cervical tongs or halo rings once the insertion pins are firmly embedded (see Figure 27-9). Body casts, jackets, or braces are used to immobilize thoracic and lumbar fractures.

▶ Surgical

Surgical interventions are performed for decompression, realignment, and stabilization of the vertebral

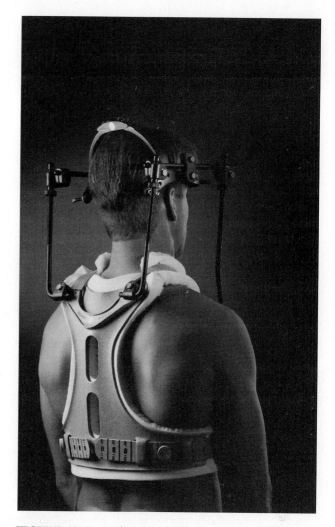

FIGURE 27-9   Halo vest. (*Courtesy of AcroMed*)

column depending upon the nature of the injury. A laminectomy may be performed to decompress the spinal cord with fusion or placement of Harrington rods to stabilize the vertebral column. Realignment is maintained by surgical manipulation of the vertebral column.

If the client has respiratory involvement, an endotracheal tube will be placed to provide mechanical ventilatory support. A tracheostomy will be performed following urgent treatment to continue ventilation.

▶ Pharmacological

Steroid therapy, dexamethasone (Decadron), is administered to prevent and reduce edema in the injured spinal cord (Ducker & Zeidman, 1994). High loading doses of steroids, methylprednisolone sodium succinate (Solu-Medrol), are given immediately with tapering dosages over the next one to two weeks to decrease and prevent edema and to improve blood flow. Mannitol, an osmotic diuretic, may be administered to decrease and prevent cord edema (Laskowski-Jones, 1993). Hydralazine hydrochloride (Apresoline) or nifedipine (Procardia) are frequently ordered to reduce blood pressure in autonomic dysreflexia.

▶ Activity

Initially, immobilization of the spinal column is necessary. In the acute phase, range of motion to all joints is performed to prevent loss of mobility and contracture of muscles. As the spine is stabilized the client progresses in activities to sitting up in a chair, performing strengthening exercises, and increasing endurance. The nurse must observe for the complication of orthostatic hypotension.

Orthostatic hypotension is caused by the venous pooling of blood in the lower body and extremities because of impairment of the sympathetic nervous system. The client becomes hypotensive, develops bradycardia, and syncope. Asystole may even occur (Laskowski-Jones, 1993). During acute phase vasopressor agents such as dopamine hydrochloride (Intropin) are given to maintain mean arterial pressure (MAP) between 80 to 90 mmHg to improve spinal cord perfusion. Prevention of orthostatic hypotension includes application of full leg support stockings, pneumatic boots, and gradually lowering the lower extremities. The client's vital signs are monitored throughout the mobilization process to determine tolerance to the procedure.

Once spinal shock has subsided, active rehabilitation begins with the interdisciplinary team optimizing the functional capabilities of the client. The physical therapist plays a major role in the activity levels. The occupational therapist is involved in activities of daily living, and the speech therapist is concerned with swallowing ability and communications. Neurological function can be regained for up to one year.

▶ Rehabilitation

An interdisciplinary approach is used for rehabilitation. Rehabilitation begins immediately with a focus on preventing disabilities and on maximizing and strengthening remaining functional ability. Refer to Chapter 17 for in-depth approach to rehabilitation.

▶ Nursing Process

Assessment

Subjective Data   This includes any input the client has concerning sensation, pain, and history of the accident. How is the client coping with the injury and resulting disability? Major lifestyle changes have occurred. How is the family or support system coping with the changes?

Objective Data   In the acute phase of care of the client with a spinal cord injury, the nursing assessment is focused upon the critical factors of airway, breathing, circulation, disability, and exposure (Laskowski-Jones, 1993).

Assessment of circulatory status involves monitoring of vital signs, observing for complications of neurogenic shock, orthostatic hypotension, hypertensive episodes of autonomic dysreflexia, and for other causes of hemorrhaging.

Disability is assessed by performing a baseline neurological assessment as described in the assessment section of this chapter.

Exposure refers to removing clothing for a thorough assessment of the client's body for condition of skin and for entrance and exit wounds. Body temperature must be monitored because of the neurological deficit in temperature regulation caused by dysfunction of the autonomic nervous system.

Subacute assessment is based upon the level of injury and neurological functioning of the client. With upper motor neuron injuries, the client is at higher risk for developing autonomic dysreflexia, so assessment includes monitoring for these signs.

All clients with spinal cord injury are assessed for condition of skin, bowel and bladder function, and respiratory status and signs and symptoms of complications of immobility. Psychosocial assessment is also very important to the well-being of the client.

▼ ▼

Possible nursing diagnoses for the client with an upper motor neuron injury in the subacute phase of care may include:

Nursing Diagnoses	Goals	Nursing Interventions
▶ *Injury, high risk for, related to motor and sensory deficits secondary to spinal fractures.*	The client will not have additional injury.	Assess the client's risk factors for additional injury.
		Monitor condition of skin for pressure areas or shearing injuries from sliding across sheets or the mats in physical therapy.
		Turn client frequently to prevent pressure areas.
		Have enough personnel available to turn client correctly to maintain alignment of spinal column.
		Provide call light that client can operate and teach to call nurse for assistance as necessary.
		Reinforce wheelchair safety factors and observe client for use of wheelchair safety.
		Prevent falls when transferring to wheelchair.
		Prevent foot drop.
		Provide passive and active range of motion exercises.
		Maintain adequate fluid intake and nutrition.
		Provide routine care for halo device by opening vest on one side to cleanse skin under vest at least daily and assess for skin breakdown. Repeat procedure on the other side.
		Monitor pin sites of halo device every shift for placement.
		Perform pin site care using facility protocol.
▶ *Powerlessness related to changes in motor and sensory function and changes in lifestyle.*	The client will make decisions regarding care, treatment, and future.	Explain all procedures and care options.
		Establish an open trusting relationship with the client to foster therapeutic communication.
		Allow time for client to express concerns, anger, and fears.
		Foster a positive environment for client to explore feelings and to accept disability.
		Allow client to participate in care decisions.
		Assess for signs and symptoms of depression.
		Collaborate with mental health professional to provide assistance in coping with lifestyle changes.
		Collaborate with family and support people to include them in the plan of care.

(continued)

Nursing Diagnoses	Goals	Nursing Interventions
▶ Dysreflexia, high risk for, related to noxious stimulation secondary to overstimulation of autonomic nervous system.	The client will state factors that cause autonomic dysreflexia, describe treatment, and notify the nurse if experiencing symptoms of dysreflexia.	Teach client causes and symptoms of autonomic dysreflexia, increased blood pressure, sudden throbbing headache, chills, pallor, goose flesh, nausea, and/or metallic taste.
		Prevent bladder distention and fecal impaction by implementing a bowel and bladder training program.
		Observe for bradycardia, vasodilatation, flushing, and diaphoresis above the level of spinal cord injury. If these symptoms occur, immediately administer medications as ordered to decrease blood pressure and notify the physician. Raise head of bed and lower legs to reduce blood pressure. Then, remove the noxious stimuli, which may be constrictive clothing, shoes, splints, or linens.
		Assess the client for a distended bladder and empty bladder if distended.
		Observe urine for signs of infection and obtain a urine specimen for culture if needed to identify the cause of the reaction.
		Check for fecal impaction using xylocaine viscous per physician's order to decrease stimulation.
		Monitor blood pressure every few minutes.

▶ Evaluation

Each goal must be evaluated to determine how it has been met by the client.

▲ ▲

▶ PARKINSON'S DISEASE

Parkinson's disease is a chronic, progressive, degenerative disease affecting the area of the brain controlling movement. The substantia nigra, an area of the basal ganglia, normally stores large amounts of dopamine. Dopamine, a neurotransmitter, controls or inhibits movement. In Parkinson's disease, the cells of the substantia nigra degenerate and are depleted of dopamine. The cause is unknown in most cases, but toxicity, hypoxia, or encephalitis may precede the onset of Parkinson's disease. Vascular and genetic factors have been implicated. Drugs such as cocaine, reserpine (Serpasil), haloperidol (Haldol), and chlorpromazine (Thorazine) may cause a parkinsonian syndrome. The theory is that these drugs interfere with the synthesis or storage of dopamine.

Typical signs and symptoms are muscular rigidity, **bradykinesia** (slowness of voluntary movement and speech), resting tremor, muscular weakness, and loss of postural reflexes. Muscular rigidity along with bradykinesia impairs the person's ability to perform daily activities and speech.

Resting tremors, usually in the upper extremities, are present when the hand is motionless. The hand moves in a "pill-rolling motion." When the person is moving or sleeping, the tremors are usually absent. Tremors also occur in other areas including the feet, lip, tongue, or jaw. The tremors usually begin unilaterally in one area and progress to other areas and to the opposite side of the body. Anxiety and concentration tend to increase the degree of tremors.

Rigidity is noted with increased muscle tone when the client is at rest. Stiffness of the trunk, head, and shoulders is present. The rigidity causes loss of arm swing, when walking. A cogwheel phenomenon is present from the muscle contractions breaking through the muscular rigidity. Cogwheel movement caused by the alternating rigidity and rhythmic contractions is a jerking-like movement. Motor impairment progressively affects facial expressions, eye blink, and the voice causing a typical presentation of a mask-like face and a monotone voice.

The posture and shuffling gait of people with Parkinson's disease is characterized by bowed head, trunk bent forward, shoulders drooped, and arms flexed. The gait is a shuffling movement with small steps. Balance is affected with a tendency to fall forward or backward. See Figure 27-10 for classic posture of a client with Parkinson's disease.

Autonomic dysfunction includes drooling, dysphagia, excessive sweating, hyperactivity of oil glands, and constipation. Orthostatic hypotension may occur from loss of the peripheral autonomic response. Urinary incontinence and frequency occur.

Mental changes may also occur. Intelligence is not impaired but problems with judgment and emotional stability may occur. Dementia is present 10 to 15 percent of the time. Depression frequently accompanies Parkinson's disease. The depression may be from the chemical changes in dopamine level or in reaction to the disorder. Cognitive, perceptual, or memory deficits may occur. Major cause of death is from the complications of immobility or injury. Fatigue increases all signs and symptoms. There is no diagnostic test specific for Parkinson's disease.

▶ Medical/Surgical Management

▶ Medical

The goals of medical management are to control the symptoms, provide supportive therapy and maintenance, maintain function with physiotherapy, and provide psychotherapy as necessary.

▶ Surgical

See News Flash for experimental treatments. Stereotactic thalamotomy, a surgical procedure to disrupt the transmission of motor impulses, is occasionally used to treat the tremors and muscular rigidity. This invasive procedure does not treat the disease, but only alleviates the tremors.

▶ Pharmacological

Drug therapy is used to control the symptoms of Parkinson's disease. L-dihydroxyphenylalanine (L-Dopa) is converted into dopamine in the basal ganglia to replace the deficit of dopamine. Dopamine is not given orally because it is metabolized before reaching the brain. L-Dopa, a precursor to dopamine, is given orally and reaches the brain to be converted into dopamine.

Dopadecarboxylase inhibitors such as carbidopa-levodopa (Sinemet) prevent the conversion of L-Dopa to dopamine in peripheral tissue. Dopamine in the peripheral tissue can cause numerous side effects as

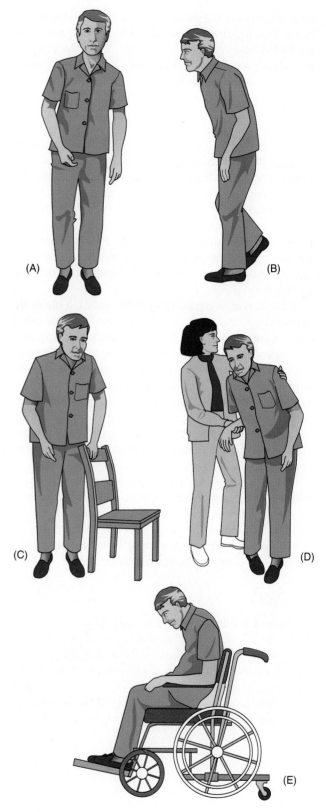

FIGURE 27-10 The stages of Parkinson's disease. **(A)** Flexion of affected arm. **(B)** Shuffling gate. **(C)** Looks for sources of support to prevent falling. **(D)** Progression of weakness, needs assistance for ambulation. **(E)** Profound weakness.

well as decrease the amount of L-dopa available to the brain. Dopadecarboxylase inhibitors that do not cross the blood-brain barrier are used to inhibit the enzyme that changes L-dopa to dopamine so that the conversion in the brain is not inhibited.

Anticholinergic drugs such as trihexyphenidyl hydrochloride (Artane), cycrimine hydrochloride (Pagitane hydrochloride), and benztropine mesylate (Cogentin), are administered to control tremors and rigidity. Anticholinergics are used alone for mild symptoms or if L-dopa is contraindicated. In other instances, it may be administered in conjunction with L-dopa.

Amantadine Hydrochloride (Symmetrel), an antiviral agent, is effective in treating Parkinsonian symptoms. The mechanism by which the drug works is not known, but the theory is that it releases dopamine storage areas or that the reuptake of dopamine is delayed by the drug.

Ethopropazine hydrochloride (Parsidol), a phenothiazine derivative, is used in combination with other anti-Parkinson drugs to alleviate symptoms. Dopamine agonist-ergot derivatives, pergolide mesylate (Permax), directly stimulates the dopamine receptors to improve the use of available dopamine. MAO inhibitor selegiline hydrochloride, (Elderpryl), inhibits dopamine breakdown. Tricyclic antidepressants amitriptyline hydrochloride (Elavil) and imipramine hydrochloride (Tofranil) alleviate depression as well as other symptoms.

Drug therapy has many side effects and dosage requirements vary greatly between individuals. Control of symptoms may vary in the same individual from day to day. A Sinemet solution may be ordered hourly while awake to maintain a more constant therapeutic level in the client for better symptom control.

▶ Diet

Pureed foods or tube feedings may be required because of dysphagia. Maintenance of weight may require high or low calorie diets. A diet that discourages formation of free radicals is being researched as a deterrent to progression of the disease. Free radical formation is thought to be discouraged by diets high in complex carbohydrates such as whole grain breads and lentils, low in fat, and high in vitamins A and E. Large doses of supplemental vitamins A and E are also given. A high-fiber diet is necessary to prevent constipation.

▶ Activity

Ambulation with assistance is necessary to maintain joint mobility. Do not hurry the client; the bradykinesia becomes worse when the client is attempting to hurry.

▶ Other Therapies

Physical therapy is directed toward the maintenance of joint mobility, posture, and gait. Occupational therapy focuses on maintaining optimal functioning in achieving activities of daily living. Speech therapy is used to promote communication and maintain swallowing function. Psychotherapy addresses the client's living with a chronic disease, depression, and psychiatric side effects of the medication regimen that may occur.

▶ Nursing Process

Assessment

Subjective Data Nursing assessment focuses on functional ability and activities. Subjective data includes client statements about control of symptoms and emotional status. Bowel and bladder elimination patterns are elicited.

Objective Data This includes evaluation of tremors, muscular rigidity, movement, posture, and gait for degree of impairment. Assessment of swallowing ability is necessary to maintain adequate nutrition and to prevent aspiration. Mental/emotional status is evaluated for signs and symptoms of depression or dementia.

Skin is assessed for diaphoresis or excessive oil production, skin integrity, and signs of injury from falls. Supine, sitting, and standing blood pressures are obtained to observe for orthostatic hypotension.

▼ ▼

Possible nursing diagnoses for a client with Parkinson's disease may include:

Nursing Diagnoses	Goals	Nursing Interventions
▶ *Physical mobility, impaired, related to muscle rigidity, gait disturbance, and bradykinesia.*	The client will maintain optimal mobility.	Assess degree of muscle involvement by testing range of motion, muscular rigidity, tremors, and gait. Administer medications within the time window that provides a constant therapeutic level for symptom control. Perform passive and active range of motion to maintain function. Ambulate client as able to tolerate. Turn client frequently while in bed.
▶ *Injury, high risk for, related to muscle rigidity, tremors, loss of postural reflexes, dysphagia, and orthostatic hypotension.*	The client will not experience injury.	Assess functional level with particular attention to postural reflexes, gait, and swallowing ability. Protect client from falls by use of assistive devices, no crepe- or rubber-soled shoes that may drag on carpet, removal of throw rugs or other obstacles to trip over, and provide assistance with ambulating and transferring as needed. Place client in upright position for eating. Provide small bites of food or pureed foods to prevent the client from choking. Have suction equipment available during meals.
▶ *Self-care deficit, related to immobility, tremors, and bradykinesia.*	The client will maintain optimal independence in self-care.	Assess client's ability to perform self-care. Encourage client to perform as much self-care as able. Consult with occupational therapy for methods to increase the ability to perform self-care. Provide daily activities the client is unable to perform. Teach the client and family to adapt home to prevent injuries by removing throw rugs, placing hand rails at steps and in the bathroom, keeping small objects off the floor, and assisting the client as needed.
▶ *Constipation, related to neuromuscular impairment.*	The client will have regular bowel movements.	Provide diet high in fiber. Encourage oral fluid intake including prune juice. Administer stool softeners or laxatives as ordered. Document bowel movements.
▶ *Swallowing, impaired, related to neuromuscular impairment.*	The client will swallow with minimal choking and coughing and no aspiration.	Position client sitting upright when eating. Have head slightly forward never extended. Encourage client to take small bites.

▶ Evaluation

Each goal must be evaluated to determine how it has been met by the client.

▲ ▲

▶ MULTIPLE SCLEROSIS

Multiple sclerosis (MS) is a chronic, progressive, degenerative disease in which scattered nerve cells of the brain and spinal cord are demyelinated. The cause of multiple sclerosis is not known. Theories suggest that viral infection before the age of fifteen, exposure to toxins, genetic factors, and immunological deficits are possible contributing factors. The disease is most prevalent in colder climates and in people who lived in colder climates before the age of fifteen. In 75 percent of the cases, onset of symptoms is in adults between the ages of twenty and forty (Chipps, Clanin, & Campbell, 1992). Women are affected slightly more often than men.

The white matter of the brain and spinal cord consists of axons covered by a white, lipid substance called myelin. This myelin sheath is an insulator that is involved in the conduction of impulses.

Multiple sclerosis is a central nervous system disease in which there is a loss of myelin in the brain or spinal cord or both and the occurrence of sclerotic patches. This interferes with the conduction of impulses. The neurological deficit that occurs is dependent upon which nerve cells are affected (Hickey, 1992).

As **sclerotic**, hardened, tissue replaces the myelin, neurological function returns. Nerve fibers begin to degenerate as periods of exacerbation become more frequent. Degeneration of the nerve fibers leads to permanent neurological deficits.

Signs and symptoms of multiple sclerosis vary with the areas of demyelination. The client may have one symptom or a combination of symptoms. Periods of exacerbation and remission also make diagnosis difficult. Symptoms may vary from hour-to-hour or day-to-day. Medical diagnosis is generally based upon history and elimination of other possible diagnoses. Magnetic resonance imaging (MRI) can be used to identify lesions of sclerotic tissue as the disease progresses. Cerebrospinal fluid (CSF) has increased white blood cells, protein, and gamma globulin (IgG).

Hickey (1992) classifies symptoms as sensory, motor, cerebellar, and other. Sensory symptoms include: visual disturbances, numbness, paresthesia (burning, prickling, tingling), pain, and decreased sense of temperature. Motor symptoms include decreased muscle strength, spasticity, paralysis, or bowel and bladder incontinence or retention.

Ataxia (loss of balance or coordination), **nystag-**mus (constant, involuntary eye movements in any direction), speech disturbances, tremors, and **vertigo** (dizziness) are cerebellar symptoms. Miscellaneous symptoms may be mood changes from depression to euphoria, overwhelming fatigue, or sexual dysfunction (Hickey, 1992).

Exacerbations are frequently precipitated by periods of emotional or physical stress, such as infections, pregnancy, trauma, or fatigue. Hot baths or strenuous exercise may aggravate motor symptoms. Periods of exacerbation may last hours to months. Commonly, the periods of exacerbation become more frequent as the disease progresses. Complications of urinary tract infection, pneumonia, pressure ulcers, contractures, and depression frequently occur. As the disease progresses and permanent neurological deficits occur, the client may become bedridden, have difficulty speaking and handling oral secretions, and/or develop emotional and intellectual disturbances.

▶ Medical/Surgical Management

There is no cure or specific treatment for multiple sclerosis. Treatment goals are to limit exacerbations, prevent complications, and maintain functional level.

▶ Pharmacological

Steroids, adrenocorticotropic hormone (ACTH) or prednisone (Delasone) are used to decrease periods of exacerbation. Muscle relaxants such as dantrolene sodium (Dantrium) or baclofen (Lioresal) are used for muscle spasticity.

Immunosuppressive agents azathioprine (Imuran), cyclophosphamide (Cytoxan), or cyclosporine (Sandimmune) are administered to decrease the immune response. Propantheline bromide (ProBanthine) is often used for urinary frequency and urgency. Bethanechol chloride (Urecholine) may be helpful for the client with a neurogenic bladder. Trimethoprim sulfamethoxazole (Bactrim or Septra) or nitrofurantoin macrocrystals (Macrodantin) is given prophylactically when urinary tract infections are a problem.

▶ Diet

A well-balanced diet with roughage is necessary to promote bowel elimination. Plenty of fluids are also necessary. If the client is obese, a dietitian should be consulted for a restricted calorie diet to help the client lose weight, yet maintain adequate nutrition.

▶ Activity

The goal of maintaining the highest possible functional level must be individualized to each client. Adequate daily exercise is necessary for clients with limited motor involvement. Physical therapy may be necessary to prevent contractures, maintain muscle strength, prevent loss of function from spasticity, or for gait training. Passive/active range of motion should be done several times per day. Occupational therapy may be used to maintain or attain self-care. Daily skills of cooking, doing laundry, or maintaining a job may also be encouraged.

▶ Nursing Process

Assessment

Subjective Data   This includes the client's listing of symptoms and an historical accounting of exacerbations and remissions. Subjective data should address incidence of visual disturbances, hazy vision, loss of central vision, or diplopia. Symptoms of weakness, numbness, fatigue, bowel or bladder problems, sexual dysfunction, emotional instability, vertigo, changes in gait, urinary incontinence or retention, constipation, or difficulty swallowing. Pain is not common.

Objective Data   Nursing assessment includes observations of gait for spastic or ataxic gait and a complete neurological examination as discussed in the section on neurological assessment.

▼ ▼

Possible nursing diagnoses for a client with multiple sclerosis may include:

Nursing Diagnoses	Goals	Nursing Interventions
▶ *Physical mobility, impaired, related to muscle weakness, ataxia, spasticity, or perceptual impairment.*	The client will maintain optimal mobility within physical limitations.	Assess motor status every four to twenty-four hours and observe for signs and symptoms of complications of immobility every eight hours: thrombophlebitis, pressure areas, diminished breath sounds, and decreased range of motion.

Provide active/passive range of motion every eight hours.

Turn bedridden clients every two hours.

Maintain proper body alignment with pillows, splints, high-topped shoes.

Encourage client to perform daily activities as able within the limitations of the disease.

Ambulate four times daily with use of assistive devices as necessary.

Provide pulmonary hygiene every two to four hours. |
| ▶ *Injury, high risk for, related to sensory deficits (paresis, visual disturbances), muscular weakness, ataxia.* | The client will be free of injury. | Assess for deficits in motor, sensory, coordination, or thought process.

Provide a safe environment.

Teach client about potential risk factors and prevention of injury: decreased temperature sensation, fall risk, use of assistive devices, and to watch feet while walking. |
| ▶ *Activity intolerance related to easily fatigued and general weakness.* | The client will experience less fatigue. | Assess client's activity tolerance and schedule activities to allow for rest periods to conserve energy. |

(continued)

Nursing Diagnoses	Goals	Nursing Interventions
		Avoid exposure to extreme temperatures, such as hot showers, use of hot tubs and saunas, going outdoors in very hot or very cold temperatures.
		Minimize stressful situations.
		Maintain well-balanced diet.
► *Urinary elimination, altered, related to changes in innervation of the bladder.*	The client will have adequate bladder elimination with minimal post-void residuals, no urinary tract infections, and no episodes of incontinence.	Assess for bladder retention or incontinence.
		Maintain fluid intake 1000 cc/day.
		Catheterize as necessary for retention or post-void residuals.
		Develop bladder program to meet individual needs of client.
		Assess for signs and symptoms of urinary tract infection.
► *Self-care deficits bathing, hygiene, dressing, grooming, and / or toileting related to neuromuscular impairment.*	The client will perform self-care as allowed within limitations of disease process.	Assess ability to perform self-care and encourage client to provide self-care as much as possible.
		Use adaptive devices to assist client in self-care: raised toilet seat, long-handled combs, and modified clothing.
		Provide the care that the client is unable to perform.
		Collaborate with occupational therapy/ physical therapy.
► *Self-esteem disturbance, related to neuromuscular and perceptual impairment.*	The client will verbalize positive statements of self-esteem.	Assess client's concept of self in relationship to changes by the disease process.
		Allow client to verbalize feelings.
		Assist client in methods of adapting to change.
		Collaborate with other health care providers, such as mental health counselors, physicians.
		Teach client about the disease process.
		Refer client to local support groups (see Resources at the end of the chapter).
► *Sexual dysfunction related to changes in sensation, genitalia and psychological response to diagnosis.*	The client will seek counseling concerning sexual dysfunction.	Assess for alterations in sexual patterns or sexual dysfunction.
		Suggest adaptations: planning time for sexual contact to conserve energy, alternatives to sexual intercourse such as touching or holding.
		Allow client to verbalize concerns.
		Refer client to appropriate health care providers.

► Evaluation

Each goal must be evaluated to determine how it has been met by the client.

▲ ▲ ▲ ▲ ▲ ▲ ▲ ▲ ▲ ▲ ▲ ▲ ▲ ▲ ▲ ▲ ▲ ▲ ▲ ▲

Sample Care Plan: The Client with Multiple Sclerosis

Mrs. Donna Jones, a thirty-seven-year-old wife and mother of two children, ages three and five, was diagnosed with multiple sclerosis two days ago. She presents with decreased sensation (paresthesia) in lower extremities and muscle weakness of the right lower extremity. She has also experienced episodes of loss of central vision. Fatigue has affected her ability to care for the children and perform household tasks. She states "I do not know what is going to happen to me." She is crying and states, "I do not know about multiple sclerosis or how I am going to take care of my children" and "I cannot keep my housework done, my children need more from me than I can give right now."

The employer where she works is concerned about her ability to perform her teaching responsibilities, but because he values her excellence as a teacher he is willing to give her a few weeks off. She has bruises on her thigh, face, and arm from a fall that she experienced several days ago. The client presents in an outpatient clinic for follow-up care with the nurse practitioner who specializes in neurological clients.

Nursing Diagnosis 1 Knowledge deficit related to disease process, lifestyle changes as evidenced by client statements, "I do not know what is going to happen to me, I do not know about multiple sclerosis or how I am going to take care of my children."

Goals	Nursing Interventions	Rationale	Evaluation
Mrs. Jones will verbalize knowledge of the disease process, pathophysiology, prognosis, and treatment; including need to reduce stressors in her life, eat a balanced diet, drink adequate fluids, and rest.	Assess Mrs. Jones's knowledge of diagnosis, treatment regimen, and lifestyle changes. Ask specific questions.	Building on the knowledge base that Mrs. Jones already has provides a frame of reference for Mrs. Jones, and helps her relate new information and integrate into her behavior.	Mrs. Jones verbalizes accurate information regarding the disease process, prognosis, and treatment. She states that by reducing stressors, maintaining a balanced diet, taking in adequate fluids, and obtaining plenty of rest that she can prevent exacerbations of multiple sclerosis.
	Begin teaching information about the pathophysiology and signs and symptoms of multiple sclerosis.	By keeping a diary of symptoms, activities, and overall feelings, the client can identify activities that exacerbate the symptoms.	
	Share lifestyle changes that need to be made, such as planning rest periods, avoiding stressors, eating a balanced diet, and drinking plenty of fluids.	Written material and a national organization provide more resources to strengthen her knowledge base.	
	Stress the importance of keeping a diary of symptoms, activities, and overall feelings in order to identify stressors that exacerbate symptoms.	Having an individual or support group to discuss similar concerns can provide a great deal of emotional support as well as offer practical solutions to problems.	

(continued)

| | Provide information about the Multiple Sclerosis Society and pamphlets that are available.

Provide the name and telephone number of a contact from the local Multiple Sclerosis Support Group or another client who is willing to share. | | |

Nursing Diagnosis 2 Home maintenance management, impaired, related to fatigue, neuromuscular impairment, and difficulty in performing child care and household tasks as evidenced by client statements, "I cannot keep my housework done, my children need more from me than I can give right now." Objective data includes decreased sensation in lower extremities, muscle weakness, and fatigue.

Goals	Nursing Interventions	Rationale	Evaluation
Mrs. Jones will identify concerns and solutions to accomplishing home maintenance management.	Allow Mrs. Jones to verbalize concerns about home maintenance management.	By allowing Mrs. Jones to verbalize fears and concerns, she can begin to plan to organize tasks and responsibilities within her ability to perform home maintenance management.	Mrs. Jones identifies that she is able to care for her children with the assistance of her husband and her mother, but that she does not have the strength to maintain the housekeeping responsibilities. Following further discussion of family commitments and availability of social supports, Mrs. Jones agrees to request weekly assistance from the women's group at her church.
	Assist Mrs. Jones in identifying areas of concern, items that can be delegated, and possible solutions.	Mrs. Jones can investigate methods of solving her home maintenance problems once she identifies concerns and explores possible solutions.	
	Assess the extended family's ability to assist with home maintenance management.	Assisting Mrs. Jones in assessment of extended family's ability to assist with home maintenance management may open opportunities that she had not considered.	
	Ask Mrs. Jones to start identifying how to decrease workload and to set priorities in expending energy.	Helps Mrs. Jones focus on needed changes.	

	Collaborate with Social Services to identify social agencies that can be of assistance.	Exploration of available resources gives Mrs. Jones other possible solutions to achieving home maintenance management.	
	Plan activities around rest periods.	Planned rest periods can conserve her strength and prevent fatigue.	
	Identify peak energy times and plan activities with peak energy in mind.	She can accomplish more by using peak energy times to perform responsibilities.	
	Explain the effects of stress, poor diet, lack of sleep, and lack of exercise on energy level.	Helps Mrs. Jones understand her condition.	

Nursing Diagnosis 3 Injury, high risk for, related to muscle weakness, decreased sensory perceptual deficits: vision, tactile, kinesthetic, and fatigue as evidenced by recent falls.

Goals	Nursing Interventions	Rationale	Evaluation
Mrs. Jones will remain free of injury.	Teach Mrs. Jones to identify risk factors in the environment.	Mrs. Jones can avoid injury by recognizing and preventing environmental risk factors.	Injuries have been prevented by increasing awareness of the risks involved with the disease process.
	Teach Mrs. Jones to identify risk factors of the disease process.	Mrs. Jones can avoid injury by identifying risk factors associated with the disease process, such as decreased sensation, weakness in legs, and visual deficits.	
	Teach Mrs. Jones to avoid hot baths, hot tubs, saunas, and so on because the muscle weakness and paraesthesia can be exacerbated with the heat.	By avoiding hot baths, hot tubs, saunas, and so on, she can prevent exacerbation of weakness and decreased sensation which increase the risk of injury.	
	Teach safety factors of wearing well-fitting, oxford style shoes.	Wearing of good fitting tie shoes decreases risk of falling.	

▶ AMYOTROPHIC LATERAL SCLEROSIS (LOU GEHRIG'S DISEASE) (ALS)

Amyotrophic lateral sclerosis is a progressive, fatal disease due to the degeneration of motor neurons in the cortex, medulla, and spinal cord. The cause of the disease is not known, but a viral-immune response is suggested by current research. A genetic defect is also being researched. Age at onset is forty to seventy years; men are affected two to three times more often than women. Average time from onset to death is three years, but some have remained active ten to twenty years after diagnosis.

The upper and lower motor neurons degenerate and deteriorate causing atrophy of the muscles innervated by those neurons. The involved motor neurons are in the anterior horns of the spinal cord and lower brain stem. The muscles of the hands, forearms, and legs usually atrophy first. As the disease progresses most body muscles are affected. Muscle spasticity and reduced muscle strength result when upper motor neurons are involved. Lower motor neuron involvement causes muscle flaccidity, paralysis, and muscle atrophy. Sensory and intellectual function are not affected. Respiratory function, ability to communicate, and emotional lability are affected as the disease progresses. Drooling, inability to handle oral secretions, and impaired swallowing occur.

▶ Medical/Surgical Management

There is no known cure for ALS. The focus of medical management is to treat the symptoms and to promote independence as long as possible.

▶ Pharmacological

Muscle relaxants including diazepam (Valium), baclofen (Lioresal), and dantrolene sodium (Dantrium) are used to reduce spasticity. Quinidine is prescribed for muscle cramping. Increased salivation is treated with trihexyphenidyl hydrochloride (Artane), clonidine hydrochloride (Catapres) or amitriptyline hydrochloride (Elavil).

▶ Diet

Regular diet with food preparation adapted to provide soft, easily chewed food is maintained as long as the client can swallow. Tube feeding may be required to provide nutrition and prevent aspiration as chewing and swallowing difficulties arise.

▶ Activity

Ambulation and other activities are encouraged as long as possible.

▶ Other Therapies

Physical and occupational therapy are used to maintain range of motion and continue independence as much as possible. Speech therapy promotes maintenance of communication skills. Mental health counseling assists with individual and family coping with a fatal disease.

▶ Nursing Process

Assessment

Subjective Data   This includes assessment of the client's and family's emotional status and knowledge status. The client may also indicate chewing or swallowing difficulties as well as dyspnea and fatigue.

Objective Data   This includes assessment of muscle weakness, muscle atrophy, fatigue and spasticity of upper extremities, flaccid paralysis, difficulty chewing and swallowing, and respiratory status.

▼ ▼

Possible diagnoses for a client with ALS may include:

Nursing Diagnoses	Goals	Nursing Interventions
▶ Physical mobility, impaired, related to muscle atrophy, weakness, and spasticity.	The client will maintain highest possible functional ability within limitations of the disease.	Provide active and passive range of motion at least twice daily. Use assistive devices to prevent contractures, for ambulation, and for muscle strengthening. Turn every two hours; assess breath sounds for presence of congestion, skin for pressure areas, and legs for thrombophlebitis.
▶ Nutrition, altered, less than body requirements, related to impaired chewing and swallowing.	The client's body weight will be maintained within ideal body weight range.	Weigh client weekly and provide oral foods and supplements that the client can swallow.
▶ Communication, impaired verbal, related to weakness of muscles used for speech.	The client will communicate verbally or through an alternative communication method as speech muscles deteriorate.	Prolong verbal communication by speech therapy interventions consisting of voice projection and speech devices. Develop alternative methods of communicating prior to the loss of verbal skills. Eye blinking for yes and no; communication boards if any arm movement remains; and computer programs can be used.
▶ Breathing pattern, ineffective, related to weakness of respiratory muscles and fatigue.	The client will maintain adequate PaO_2 levels.	Assess breathing patterns frequently and observe for aspiration and the loss of the swallow reflex. Assess breath sounds every four to eight hours depending on the progress of the disease. Provide good pulmonary hygiene to prevent aspiration and pneumonia. Turn from side to side to allow oral secretion to drain from mouth and suction oral pharynx as necessary. Provide ventilation support as ordered.
▶ Powerlessness, related to loss of control over life, physical dependence, and presence of fatal disease.	The client will communicate wishes to significant others while still able to communicate so that some control over decisions remains.	Explore client and family emotional status and coping abilities. Allow client to verbalize feelings while still able to communicate and make decisions in daily care. Promote discussion of client's wishes with family, health care team, and legal representative while still able to speak. Provide client education about the disease process, support groups, and counseling to provide support.

▶ Evaluation

Each goal must be evaluated to determine how it has been met by the client.

▲ ▲

▶ ALZHEIMER'S DISEASE (AD)

Alzheimer's disease (AD) is a progressive, degenerative neurological disease in which brain cells are destroyed. The cerebral cortex atrophies, there is a loss of neurons, and changes occur within the brain cells. Risk factors have been identified as increased age, female sex, following head injuries, a history of thyroid disorders, and chromosome abnormalities.

The cause of Alzheimer's disease is unknown. Some hypothesized causes are genetic, viral, toxic, immunological, traumatic, biochemical, or nutritional reasons. The neurons of the frontal and medial temporal lobes are affected with biochemical and structural changes. Characteristic physiologic changes are neurofibrillary tangles and neuritic plaques (deposits of protein) that interfere with the cells' ability to transmit impulses (see Figure 27-11). These changes are found in the association areas and scattered throughout the cortex. The hippocampus, a part of the limbic system which is responsible for learning, memory, and emotions is affected (Selkoe, 1992). The cells most affected are neurons that use acetylcholine as the neurotransmitter. There is a decrease in the size of the brain and in the amount of acetylcholine. There is also an increase in aluminum found in the brain tissue on autopsy. (Hickey, 1992; Smeltzer & Bare, 1992).

Diagnosis of the disease is difficult because of the variety of clinical manifestations and there is no test specific to Alzheimer's disease. Diagnosis is based upon the clinical picture and the exclusion of other conditions that can cause similar clinical patterns, such as overmedication, metabolic disorders, depression, thyroid imbalance, or brain tumors. Computerized tomography (CT) or magnetic resonance images (MRI) indicate brain atrophy, and rule out other conditions.

In late stages of the disease, the electroencephalogram (EEG) may indicate general slowing of brain waves. Diagnosis is usually done in the middle stage. Definitive diagnosis is determined on autopsy with a brain biopsy. Alzheimer's disease is generally a disease of older people, but does occur in people ages forty to fifty. The older the person, the higher the incidence of the disease. Clients usually recognize their own name into the later stages of the disease process.

The stages of Alzheimer's disease are scaled from early to late. Different authors identify from three to six stages of the disease. The time frame for each stage varies from person to person. See Table 27-6 for clinical manifestations of early, middle, and late stages of Alzheimer's Disease.

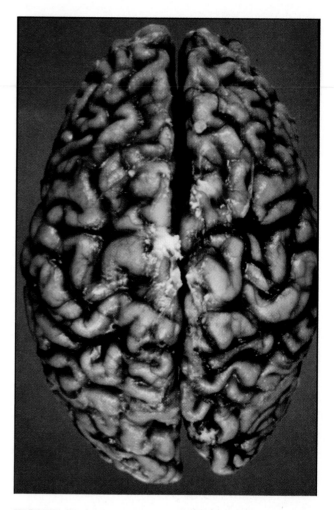

FIGURE 27-11 At autopsy, this brain shows changes in the cerebral cortex caused by Alzheimer's disease. (*Courtesy of National Institute of Neurological Disorders and Stroke, Bethesda, MD*)

▶ Medical/Surgical Management

There is no curative treatment for Alzheimer's disease. Management of the client with the disease is aimed at controlling undesirable symptoms. Other conditions such as drug reaction, depression, brain tumors, pernicious anemia, or hormonal imbalances must be ruled out.

▶ Pharmacological

Antipsychotics, sedatives, antianxiety agents and antidepressants may be used to treat behavioral symptoms. Medications often make symptoms worse. Several medications that affect transmission of chemicals

Table 27-6

STAGES OF ALZHEIMER'S DISEASE

Stage 1 Early	Forgetfulness, often subtle, masked by client
	Indecisiveness
	Increased self-centeredness, decreased interest in others, environment, social activities
	Difficulty learning new information
	Slowed reaction time
	Performance at home and at work is beginning to fail
Stage 2 Middle	Forgetfulness progresses. Unable to remember names of family members or close friends. Loses things
	Confusion
	Fearful
	Easily frustrated and irritable. Sometimes outbursts of anger
	Repeats stories
	Communication problems begin, unable to remember words, appears to be aphasic
	Unable to follow simple directions
	Difficulty calculating numbers
	Begins to get lost in familiar places
	Evasive or anxious interactions with others
	Becomes physically active, paces, wanders
	Sleep-rest cycle changes, frequently active at night
	Eating patterns change. May be hungry all the time or not eat at all
	Neglects activities of daily living, personal hygiene, changes in bowel and bladder continence, and dressing
	Needs supervision to maintain safety
	Loses social behaviors
	Paranoid
Stage 3 Late	Unable to communicate
	Unable to eat
	Incontinent of urine and freces
	Does not recognize family or friends
	Bedridden
	Totally dependent for care

across synapses are under study. Tacrine hydrochloride (Cognex), an anticholinesterase, has demonstrated effectiveness in increasing cognitive function of Alzheimer's clients. There is a high incidence of liver toxicity, nausea, and vomiting with the drug. A recent study by Stewart as cited in a newspaper article ("Anti-inflammatories," 1996) suggests that use of nonsteroidal anti-inflammatory drugs may decrease the formation of the protein deposits linked to Alzheimer's. More research is needed to determine the merit of this study.

▶ *Diet*

A high-fiber diet is used to prevent constipation. A high-caloric diet is needed for hyperactive clients. Frequent feedings of high nutritive value are preferable to three meals a day.

▶ Nursing Process

Assessment

Subjective Data Data about sleeping and eating habits is necessary. Each client must be assessed for individual signs and symptoms.

Objective Data An objective neurological examination with particular attention to memory loss and gradual loss of thought processes and impaired judgment is important. Observe eating patterns, bowel and bladder control, aggressiveness, depression, ambulation, agitation, restlessness, sleep patterns, vision, and hearing. The client is an expert at hiding these deficits in the early stages of the disease. A family interview may be helpful in ascertaining health and personal history. The client's ability to provide self-care, manage finances, drive, prepare meals, use the telephone, and perform housekeeping, communicate needs, and perceive the environment also need to be assessed. Attention must be directed to assess the support system, the family caregiver, support groups, availability of respite care for the caregiver. The care of the caregiver is often the focus of nursing care of the client with Alzheimer's disease.

▼ ▼

Possible nursing diagnoses for the client with Alzheimer's may include:

Nursing Diagnoses	Goals	Nursing Interventions
▶ *Injury, high risk for, related to inability to perceive danger in the environment, confusion, impaired judgment, and weakness.*	The client will not experience injury.	Assess client's ability to perceive environmental hazards. Maintain a safe environment: uncluttered, position furniture/equipment in same place, monitor hot water and food temperature, maintain monitoring system to prevent wandering into adverse climate or into traffic; provide adequate lighting, orient client and family to surroundings, and reorient as necessary. Teach family to provide a safe home environment, including precautions for the following: sharp items, such as knives, forks, razors; hot items, such as coffee and heaters; poisonous solutions, such as cleaning supplies, paints, medications, insecticides; hazardous items, such as power tools, guns, electric fans; and use of stairs without railings. Ensure that the client wears well-fitting tie shoes to prevent fall injury.
▶ *Thought processes, altered, related to neuron degeneration, sleep deprivation.*	The client will maintain optimal cognitive ability.	Assess for cognitive, memory, and communication deficits. Develop memory aids and cues to help client remember. Maintain a consistent environment and daily schedule. Approach the client in a quiet, nonthreatening manner. Do not confront the client with reality if it will only upset and agitate him. For example, do not tell a ninety-year-old client who wants his mother that she is dead. Listen to nonverbal cues for unmet needs, i.e., pacing, grimacing, crying, agitation. The client may be hungry, have a full bladder, or be unable to ask to be repositioned. Get a picture of the client that can be recognized by the client. A current photo of the client may appear as a stranger to the client, but a picture of the client at age 20 or 30 may be remembered. Give simple, single instructions.
▶ *Self-care deficit: feeding, dressing/grooming, bathing/ hygiene related to cognitive impairment and decreased motor function.*	The client will maintain independent activities of daily living as long as possible.	Assess the client's ability to perform self-care. Promote independence in performing self-care; by cuing client through self-care, for example, demonstrate use of washcloth which may not be recognized by the client. Provide range of motion active or passive at least twice daily to all extremities.

Nursing Diagnoses	Goals	Nursing Interventions
		Listen to nonverbal cues for care needs, i.e., toileting.
		Anticipate client's needs.
		Provide for care as needed.
		Do not hurry the client.
		Allow a few choices (i.e., the choice of clothes).
▶ *Sleep pattern disturbance, related to disorientation, irritability, or poor judgment.*	The client will sleep six hours each night.	Advise the client to avoid caffeine.
		Maintain a quiet environment.
		Provide a night light.
		Increase activities to tolerance.
		Use exercise to tire the client.
		Provide comfort measures.

▶ Evaluation

Each goal must be evaluated to determine how it has been met by the client.

▲ ▲

▶ GUILLAIN-BARRE SYNDROME (POLYRADICULO-NEUROPATHY)

Guillain-Barre syndrome is an acute inflammatory process primarily involving the motor neurons of the peripheral nervous system.

The cause of Guillain-Barre syndrome is not identified, but most cases are preceded by a nonspecific infection. There may be an autoimmune basis for this syndrome or a viral agent. Both spinal and cranial motor nerves may be involved. Sensory neurons may also be affected. The demyelination process begins in distal nerves and ascends symmetrically. Remyelination occurs from proximal to distal (Hickey, 1992).

Clinical manifestation occurs in differing patterns, but include motor weakness and areflexia, absence of reflexes. Characteristically, motor weakness begins in the legs and progresses up the body. Respiratory failure results from loss of respiratory muscle function. Cranial nerve involvement results in facial muscle deficits, difficulty swallowing, and autonomic dysfunctions. Autonomic functions affected may be cardiac rhythm, blood pressure regulation, gastrointestinal mobility, or urine elimination.

Sensory involvement causes paresthesia and pain to hands and feet. The pain progresses up the body and can interfere with sleep.

The three stages of Guillain-Barre are acute onset, lasting one to three weeks, the plateau period lasting several days to two weeks, and the recovery phase involving remyelination which may last up to two years.

Diagnosis is based upon the clinical picture of a recent viral infection, motor and possibly sensory deficits, along with characteristic diagnostic results. Diagnostic results include an elevated protein level in cerebrospinal fluid without elevation of red blood cells or white blood cells and electromyelogram (EMG) showing slowed nerve conduction velocity of paralyzed muscles.

▶ Medical/Surgical Management

▶ Medical

The goal of medical management is prevention and treatment of complications, immobility, infection, and respiratory failure.

Plasma exchanges have been found to decrease the severity and duration of symptoms. Plasmapheresis is performed in severe cases. A complete plasma exchange removes the antibodies affecting the myelin sheath. Three to four exchanges one to two days apart are initiated within the first two weeks of onset of Guillain-Barre. Plasmapheresis may also be used late in the disease process for continued demyelination or lack of progress in remyelination. Mechanical ventilatory support will be initiated for decreased or lost respiratory function. Blood gas monitoring is used to assess respiratory function.

▶ Surgical

Those who develop respiratory failure may require a tracheostomy along with mechanical ventilation.

▶ Pharmacological

Steroids, adrenocorticotrophic hormone (ACTH) and prednisone (Detasone), immunosuppressive agents azathioprine (Imuran) or cyclophosphamide (Cytoxan) are prescribed to slow the demyelination process. Low doses of anticoagulants such as heparin are ordered to prevent thrombophlebitis.

▶ Diet

A balanced diet is necessary to prevent tissue and muscle breakdown and to promote healing. If there is severe paralysis, a gastrostomy tube may be used to provide adequate nutrition.

▶ Activity

Range of motion and muscle strength are maintained through physical therapy. Occupational therapy activities teach the client to maintain optional self-care within the limitation of the disease process. Pool therapy is often used to maintain and gain strength of muscles.

▶ Nursing Process

Assessment

Subjective Data   This includes client statements about return of sensation, pain, respiratory function, and knowledge.

Objective Data   Assessment includes the status of motor and sensory function which is monitored continuously in the acute phase of the illness. Progression of loss of function from distal to proximal is monitored with particular assessment of respiratory status. Decreased depth and quality of respirations and diminished breath sounds may be found. Status of autonomic functions is monitored by assessment of blood pressure, cardiac rhythm, urinary elimination, and bowel sounds. Assessment for complications of immobility includes breath sounds, signs of thrombophlebitis, loss of range of motion, skin condition, and temperature.

▼ ▼

Possible nursing diagnoses for a client with Guillain-Barre syndrome may include:

Nursing Diagnoses	Goals	Nursing Interventions
▶ Breathing pattern, ineffective, high risk for, related to loss of respiratory muscle function.	The client will be adequately ventilated.	Monitor respiratory status of the client by assessing breath sounds, respiratory rate, and respiratory quality. Position the client to allow for maximal expansion of the chest wall for optimal breathing. Monitor oxygenation by assessing skin color, mental status, pulse oximeter readings and blood gas values. Administer oxygen as ordered. Report decreasing respiratory status to the physician. Provide mechanical ventilation for respiratory failure.
▶ Physical mobility, impaired, related to progressive loss of motor function.	The client will avoid complications of immobility (pneumonia, thrombophlebitis, pressure areas, and loss of range of motion).	Monitor status of motor and sensory function in an ongoing fashion. Have client turn, deep breathe, and cough. Suction client as necessary.

Nursing Diagnoses	Goals	Nursing Interventions
		Perform respiratory assessment for diminished breath sounds or congestion.
		Monitor vital signs, blood pressure, pulse, respiration, and temperature every four to eight hours.
		Assess for calf tenderness, redness, or increased warmth.
		Monitor for positive Homan's sign indicating deep vein thrombosis.
		Perform range of motion to lower extremities every two to four hours.
		Use plexipulse boots, intermittent pumping boots that promote return blood flow from lower extremities.
		See Vascular Disorders Chapter 21 for information about Homan's sign and Plexipulse boots.
		Administer low doses of heparin or other anticoagulants as prescribed.
		Apply antiembolism stockings.
		Assess condition of skin for pressure areas.
		Turn to relieve pressure on pressure points every two hours.
		Apply specialty mattress.
		Massage back and pressure points with lotion three times a day.
		Assist client to sitting positions in wheelchair two to three times daily.
		Progress to ambulation as motor function returns.
		Apply high-topped shoes to prevent footdrop.
▶ *Powerlessness related to inability to communicate, inability to perform self-care, and long-term effects of the disease process.*	The client will participate in decision making regarding care and treatment.	Teach client about disease process and expected body changes.
		Allow time for client to express needs and wishes verbally or through alternative communication methods.
		If possible discuss wishes for care early in the disease process before communication skills are affected.
		Provide opportunity for client to make decisions in daily care.
		Prepare written plan of client's daily care choices.
		Promote normalcy in activities such as hairstyle, permanent wave, nail care, and so forth.
		Encourage client that there will be progress with increase of function as remyelination occurs.
		Encourage rehabilitation throughout the course of the disease.

(continued)

Nursing Diagnoses	Goals	Nursing Interventions
▶ *Self-care deficit related to decreased motor function.*	The client will have self-care needs met.	Encourage self-care within the limitations of the neurological deficits.
		Maintain muscle strength and range of motion with physical therapy.
		Provide range of motion to all extremities three to four times daily.
		Provide daily care needs that client is unable to perform.
		Initiate rehabilitation following acute phase of illness with strengthening exercises, occupational therapy, getting client out of bed several times per day to build strength and endurance.

▶ Evaluation

Each goal must be evaluated to determine how it has been met by the client.

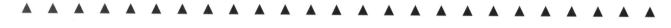

▶ HEADACHE

Headache, or **cephalalgia**, the condition of pain in the head, is caused by stimulation of pain sensitive structures in the cranium, head, or neck. Headaches are classified as symptoms rather than a disease.

The pain sensitive areas of the intracranial structure include peripheral nerves, cerebral vasculature, and parts of the dura mater. The external supporting structures skin, muscles, and nasal passages are also sensitive to pain. The skull, brain tissue, and most of the meninges are insensitive to pain.

Clinical manifestations vary with the type and cause of the headache. The Headache Classification Committee of the International Headache Society (1988) presented twelve classifications of headaches.

1. Migraine with or without aura
2. Tension type headaches
3. Cluster headaches and paroxysmal hemicrania
4. Miscellaneous headaches associated with structural lesion
5. Headache associated with head trauma
6. Headache associated with vascular disorder such as subarachnoid hemorrhage
7. Headache associated with nonvascular intracranial disorders such as brain tumor
8. Headache associated with use of chemical substances or their withdrawal
9. Headache associated with noncephalic infection
10. Headache associated with metabolic disorder such as hypoglycemia
11. Headache or facial pain associated with disorders of the head or neck, such as acute glaucoma

12. Cranial neuralgia, persistent pain originating from a cranial nerve

▶ Primary Headaches

Primary headaches have no known cause. They include classic migraine, common migraine, and cluster headaches.

▶ Migraine Headaches

Migraine headaches are vascular and recurrent. The initial vasoconstriction can cause neurological symptoms or an aura prior to the vasodilatation which causes the headache. Serotonin levels are increased in the initial phase prior to the onset of the headache. This indicates involvement of neurotransmitters in the pathophysiology.

Some migraine type headaches may be triggered by certain foods or chemicals. Alcohol, cured meats containing nitrates; aged cheeses, monosodium glutamate (MSG), citrus fruits, chocolate, and red wines can precipitate a migraine type headache in susceptible people. Tension and stress also precipitate headaches (see Table 27-7).

▶ Secondary Headaches

Secondary headaches are the result of pathological conditions such as aneurysm, brain tumor, or inflammation of cranial nerves. The headache is caused by compression, inflammation, or hypoxia of pain-sensitive structures.

Table 27-7

PRIMARY HEADACHE PATTERNS

Type	Aura	Pain	Typical Pattern	Duration
Classic Migraine	15 to 30 minutes; sensory, usually visual, bright spots, zigzag lines; unilateral or bilateral numbness or tingling in lips, face, or hand; difficulty thinking; confusion or drowsiness; some people experience premonition 24 hours before.	Throbbing, intense; begins unilaterally, may progress to bilateral headache; tenderness in scalp; muscle contractions in neck and scalp followed by feelings of exhaustion.	Periodic, recurrent; usually begins on awakening; begins in childhood or early adolescence. Tends to be familial; nausea and vomiting are typical.	Hours to days
Common Migraine	None, but may experience premonitions of coming headache.	Throbbing, intense; progresses to nonthrobbing generalized head pain.	Usually begins gradually frontal or temporal areas; Slight to no nausea or vomiting; begins at any age; hereditary correlation; increases with life crisis and with premenstrual fluid retention.	Hours to days
Cluster	None	Intense throbbing; unilateral pain in orbitotemporal area.	Awaken 2 to 3 times during the night with headache; accompanied by watering eyes, nasal congestion, runny nose, facial flushing over the throbbing area; after this cluster of headaches may be free of symptoms for weeks to months; same side of head is usually involved; usually older men.	30 minutes to 2 hours

▸ Medical/Surgical Management

▸ Medical

Medical management is based upon the underlying cause of the headache. A thorough history of headache pattern, dietary pattern, and coping patterns is essential. Underlying pathology of brain tumor, aneurysm, and infection must be ruled out. If pathology is identified, treatment will be based upon findings. If no cause is found, management of secondary headaches will be based upon symptoms.

▸ Surgical

Surgical management may include clipping of an aneurysm or resection of a brain tumor.

▸ Pharmacological

Management is either abortive to stop the headache or prophylactic to prevent the occurrence or decrease the frequency of headaches. Abortive therapy for vas-

cular headaches includes: ergotamine tartrate (Ergostat), administered orally, sublingually, rectally, intramuscularly, or subcutaneously at the beginning of a migraine headache. Cafergot, containing ergotamine and caffeine, is also used for abortive therapy. A pregnant woman cannot take ergotamine because it causes the uterus to contract. The action is to cause vasoconstriction and to block serotonin uptake. Promethazine hydrochloride (Phenergan) is often used to control nausea and vomiting. Narcotic or nonnarcotic analgesics are administered for pain relief.

Prophylactic treatment includes beta blockers, propranolol hydrochloride (Inderal) and methysergide maleate (Sansert), to prevent dilation of the blood vessels and interrupt the serotonin mechanism. Clonidine hydrochloride (Catapres) directly affects the ability of the blood vessels to constrict or dilate. Tricyclic antidepressants, amitriptyline hydrochloride (Elavil), block the uptake of serotonin.

▸ Diet

A strict diet history should be kept to identify precipitating foods. Once all suspect foods are eliminated, skin testing for allergies may be performed. Introduction of potentially precipitating foods may be added one at a time to identify triggering foods. Alcohol, cured meats containing nitrates, aged cheeses containing monamine oxidaze, citrus fruits, chocolates, and red wines are common precipitating foods.

▶ Activity

Activities that precipitate headaches need to be identified and eliminated if possible. Stressful situations are frequently precipitating agents. Biofeedback, relaxation techniques, stress reduction, and development of more effective coping mechanisms are useful in reducing the occurrence of headaches caused by stress and tension.

▶ Nursing Interventions

Nursing interventions focus on the relief of pain and assisting the client in managing the pain. Identify methods of decreasing pain, such as effective use of medications, managing the environment to decrease stimulation such as decreasing light, noise, activity.

Assist the client in developing a plan for accomplishing daily activities when incapacitated by a headache. Teach the client to keep a diary of headache history, to determine patterns in headache development. Assist the client in changing lifestyle to decrease incidence of headaches, such as decreasing stress, avoiding certain foods, reducing salt intake during premenstrual period, and use of relaxation techniques to better handle stress.

▶ TRIGEMINAL NEURALGIA (TIC DOULOUREUX)

Trigeminal neuralgia is a condition of cranial nerve V which is characterized by abrupt paroxysms of pain and facial muscle contractions. **Neuralgia** is nerve pain. The pain follows one of the three branches of the trigeminal nerve, the ophthalmic, maxillary, or mandibular. The last two branches are most commonly affected.

The etiology of trigeminal neuralgia is not known but injury, dental caries, dental work, and anatomical position of the nerves have been identified as possible causes. Pain is precipitated when trigger points are stimulated causing periods of intense pain and facial twitching lasting from seconds to minutes. These periods may last several weeks to months. Periods of remission interspersed with exacerbations occur with increasing frequency with aging (Hickey, 1992).

▶ Medical/Surgical Management

Drug therapy, nerve blocks, and surgery are treatment modalities for trigeminal neuralgia.

▶ Surgical

Surgical approaches to relieve pain include percutaneous electrocoagulation with radio frequency. This affects the pain sensory fibers with little damage to touch, proprioception or motor fibers. Longer-term relief or permanent relief may be obtained.

▶ Pharmacological

Phenytoin (Dilantin) and carbamazepine (Tegretol) are used to shorten the length of the paroxysmal pain. Nerve blocks using alcohol and phenol injections into the nerve provide temporary relief for eight to sixteen months.

▶ Nursing Interventions

Goals of nursing interventions are for relief of pain, prevention of injury, prevention of self-care deficits, and promotion of social interaction. The client experiencing trigeminal neuralgia frequently experiences such severe pain, that grooming, talking, and eating are avoided. It is especially important to provide good oral hygiene if the client is on phenytoin (Dilantin) because of the hyperplasia of the gums caused by the medication. Teach the client to identify trigger points that stimulate the pain, and how to avoid those areas without neglecting daily needs.

The client who has had surgery may have lost the protective mechanisms that protect the eye from injury. Teach the client not to touch his or her eye and to observe for redness of the eye and conjunctiva. The client may not feel pain from dental caries following surgery, so it is important to routinely visit the dentist for an oral examination.

▶ ENCEPHALITIS, MENINGITIS

Encephalitis is inflammation of the brain. Meningitis is inflammation of the meninges. The most common cause of encephalitis or meningitis is a virus. Bacteria, fungi, or parasites can also be causative factors. The virus or other causative agent enters the brain through the bloodstream by direct extension from trauma, or via nerve pathways.

The inflammatory process causes demyelination of white matter and degeneration of neurons. Cerebral edema, hemorrhage, and necrosis of brain tissue can occur (Chipps, et al., 1992). Clinical manifestations vary, depending upon the causative agent, area of involvement, and degree of damage to nerve tissue. Fever, headache, nuchal rigidity, photophobia, irritability, lethargy, nausea, and vomiting are typical signs and symptoms. As the disease progresses the level of consciousness may decrease and other neurological dysfunctions occur including motor weakness, aphasia, seizures, behavioral changes, or even death. A lumbar puncture is performed to test cerebrospinal fluid for causative agent, presence of white blood cells or red blood cells, and elevated protein levels. A complete blood count is done to identify the presence of viral or bacterial infection.

▶ *Medical/Surgical Management*

Treatment is supportive based upon presenting symptoms. The aim of treatment is to prevent or decrease intracranial pressure and to minimize neurological deficits. Intravenous fluids will be given to rehydrate the client.

▶ *Pharmacological*

Antibiotics or antiinfectives will be administered in massive doses as appropriate for the causative agent. They may be given intravenously or intrathecally into the spinal canal. Most viral agents do not respond to antibiotics or antiinfectives. Glucocorticosteroids will be administered to prevent cerebral edema. Osmotic diuretics may be used to decrease cerebral edema. To prevent seizures, anticonvulsants are often ordered. Antipyretics are often given to reduce fever.

▶ *Diet*

Nutritional status must be maintained to promote response to the infection.

▶ *Activity*

A quiet environment with minimal stimulation of noise, light, client activity is maintained. Routine turning, range of motion, pulmonary hygiene, and skin care are required to prevent the complications of immobility.

▶ *Nursing Interventions*

In the acute stages, the client must be monitored for changes in neurological status, especially changes in level of consciousness and for signs of increasing intracranial pressure. Provide a quiet environment to decrease external stimulation. Observe the client for seizure activity and protect from injury. Provide comfort measures such as oral hygiene, tepid baths, and administration of analgesics for relief of headaches.

▶ *HUNTINGTON'S DISEASE OR CHOREA*

Huntington's disease is a chronic, progressive hereditary disease of the nervous system. It is characterized by a progressive involuntary choreiform movement and progressive dementia.

The cells of the basal ganglia which control movement die prematurely. Cells in the cerebral cortex also die which interferes with thought processes, memory, perception, and judgment. Age of onset is usually thirty-five to forty-five years with death occurring in ten to fifteen years (Smeltzer & Bare, 1992). The theory of cause is the lack of γ-aminobutyric acid (GABA), a neurotransmitter. There is a 50 percent chance of developing Huntington's disease for each child of a person with Huntington's disease. A genetic marker has been discovered that indicates if the person will develop the disease. However, there is no cure for this devastating progressive disease.

Clinical manifestations are **chorea**, abnormal involuntary, purposeless movements of all musculature of the body. Facial tic, grimacing, difficulty chewing and swallowing, speech impairments, disorganized gait, and bowel and bladder incontinence all occur. Mental or intellectual impairment progresses to dementia. The client may experience paranoia, hallucinations, or delusions. Emotions are labile from outbursts of anger to profound depression, apathy, or euphoria. A ravenous appetite is usually present, but because of the constant movement, the client is often emaciated and exhausted. Death usually results from heart failure, pneumonia, infection, or an accident (Smeltzer & Bare, 1992).

The entire family experiences this disease in an emotional, physical, social, and financial way. Supportive care is required as the family progresses through life with a loved one with Huntington's disease. Because of the hereditary factor, genetic counseling is necessary.

▶ *Medical/Surgical Management*

The goal of treatment is to control the symptoms.

▶ *Pharmacological*

Medications used to decrease choreiform movement are dopamine receptor blockers, chlorpromazine (Thorazine), haloperidol (Haldol), and thiothixene

(Navane), and reserpine (Serpasil) which depletes presynaptic dopamine. Antidepressants, such as desipramine hydrochloride (Norpramin) and fluoxetine hydrochloride (Prozac) and antipsycotics, such as fluphenazine hydrochloride (Prolixin) are used for emotional disturbances.

▶ Diet

The diet must be high in calories to provide for the high energy needs caused by the continuous movement. Chewing and swallowing difficulties require foods that are easy to chew or foods cut into small pieces to prevent choking hazards.

▶ Activity

Ambulation is maintained as long as possible. A safe environment needs to be maintained to prevent injury from falls or from sharp objects. Driving is usually restricted when choreiform movement or impaired judgment interferes with the ability to drive safely.

▶ Nursing Interventions

Nursing interventions include a holistic approach to the client's care. Collaboration with the social worker, the chaplain, the physician, and the mental health worker are necessary.

Teach the client and his or her family about the disease process, the progress of the disease, and the genetic factors involved. Safety factors need to be considered. Fall prevention, such as removing throw rugs and small objects from the floor, and injury prevention by removing sharp or dangerous objects such as guns and knives from the home are implemented. The hazard of choking also needs to be addressed, by teaching the family to cut the client's food in small pieces, serve soft foods, and teaching the Heimlich maneuver.

▶ TOURETTE SYNDROME

Tourette syndrome is a neurological movement disorder that also has prominent behavioral manifestations. Clinical manifestations include motor tics, involuntary repetitive movements of mouth, face, head, or neck muscles. The trunk and extremities may also be included. Motor tics may be forceful eye blinking or toe touching. Vocal tics, repetitive involuntary

vocalizations may be sniffing, grunting, or throat clearing or may be coprolalia (involuntary and inappropriate swearing). Other complex motor and vocal tics may also be present; these include copropraxia, involuntary and affectively appropriate use of obscene gestures; echolalia, involuntary repetition of the speech of others; and palilia, involuntary repetition of the person's own speech. (Hyde & Weinberger, 1995). Obsessive-compulsive symptoms of repetitive handwashing or checking rituals may be exhibited.

Structural abnormalities in the basal ganglia and prefrontal cortex have been identified in research as the possible site of pathology of Tourette syndrome (Hyde & Weinberger, 1995). Genetic tendencies have been documented. Depression and obsessive compulsive disorders may also exist.

▶ Medical/Surgical Management

Medical management is focused on manifestations of the disease.

▶ Pharmacological

Primozide (Orap) blocks dopamine receptors in the brain. Methylphenidate hydrochloride (Ritalin) combined with haloperidol (Haldol) may help control behavior. Acetaminophen (Tylenol) may help muscle spasms discomfort.

▶ Other Therapies

Clients, as they get older, learn to suppress tics in social situations. Psychotherapy and family counseling are beneficial in coping with social stigma and adjustment problems.

▶ Nursing Interventions

The client and the family with Tourette's syndrome need a lot of emotion support. Teach them about the availability of support groups for clients with Tourette's syndrome. Also teach about the disease process and expectations for the client. Behavioral modification techniques are generally effective, so the nurse needs to know what modification is being performed and follow through with consistent responses.

▶ CASE STUDY

Mr. George Mason, a seventy-six-year-old retired farmer, was admitted to the emergency room with a left-sided hemiplegia, difficulty swallowing, and inability to speak. He was awake and watching the staff upon admission. He moved his right arm to indicate that Mrs. Mason was his wife, but was unable to speak or form sounds. Mrs. Mason stated that he was working in the garden picking tomatoes and cucumbers when he fell to the ground thirty minutes before admission. The emergency room nurse administered oxygen per nasal cannula at 2 liters per minute and obtained vital signs. The blood pressure was 182/98, pulse was 88, respirations were 20, and temperature was 100.5. The emergency room physician ordered a MRI scan of the head STAT, a complete blood count, and prothrombin time. The MRI indicated that Mr. Mason experienced a cerebrovascular accident caused by a bleeding into the brain.

The following questions will guide your development of a Nursing Care Plan for the case study.

1. List clinical manifestations other than the ones Mr. Mason experienced that can occur when having a cerebrovascular accident.

2. List subjective and objective data a nurse would want to obtain.

3. Identify three individualized nursing diagnoses and goals for Mr. Mason.

4. Mr. Mason is transferred to a general medical unit for three days, then is transferred to a rehabilitation center for intensive therapy. What pertinent nursing actions should a nurse perform in caring for Mr. Mason in the acute setting and the rehabilitation setting related to:

    Mobility
    Safety
    Elimination
    Skin Integrity
    Comfort/Rest

5. What teaching will Mr. Mason need before discharge from the rehabilitation facility?

6. List at least three client outcomes for Mr. Mason.

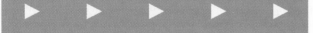

SUMMARY

- The nervous system controls all bodily functions, from movement, to thinking, to processing information, to autonomic responses.
- Functional areas of the brain specialize in specific tasks.
- The frontal lobe of the cerebrum specializes in emotional attitudes and responses, formation of thought processes, motor function, judgment, personality, and inhibitions.
- The parietal lobe of the cerebrum is a purely sensory region for interpretation of senses except smell, the purpose is to analyze sensations, includ-

ing pain, touch, and temperature from receptors in the skin.
- The temporal lobe of the cerebrum houses the primary auditory association area, Wernicke's area, for interpretation of words that are heard. Memory is also a function of the temporal lobe, especially memories that include multiple sensations or greatly detailed thoughts.
- A special interpretive area located at the junction of the temporal, parietal, and occipital lobes integrates somatic, auditory, and visual sensory interpretations.
- The occipital lobe of the cerebrum is responsible for visual interpretation and visual association.

- The cerebellum is responsible for visual interpretation and visual association.
- Disorders of the nervous system cause complex dysfunctions in which the nurse must use assessment skills and quickly recognize changes in condition.
- The plan of care must be modified based upon reassessment of client status.
- Teaching to prevent injury and to understand the effects and prognosis of the disorder are required to meet physical and psychosocial needs of the client and family.
- Many neurological disorders cause a potential for injury. Nursing care must provide the client and the family with necessary safety information.
- Rehabilitation is initiated from the first contact with the client in order to maintain and restore functional ability.

Review Questions

1. The most important indicator of neurological status is:

    a. level of consciousness.
    b. pupil reaction.
    c. vital signs.
    d. motor function.

2. Cranial nerves III, IV, and VI all have functions affecting:

    a. special senses.
    b. facial movement.
    c. eye movement.
    d. gag reflex.

3. Assessment of intellectual function requires that the nurse:

    a. have knowledge of the client's prior ability to function.
    b. administer a written test to determine the client's IQ level.
    c. utilize auscultation, percussion, and palpation skills.
    d. observe the client's behavior, posture, and facial expression.

4. Contusion of the brain is a (an):

    a. shaking of the brain.
    b. bleeding into the brain tissue.
    c. open head injury.
    d. bruising of the brain.

5. Benign brain tumors can be:

    a. less anxiety producing than malignant tumors.
    b. less life threatening than malignant tumors.
    c. treated with radiation therapy.
    d. the cause of increased intracranial pressure.

6. Miss Webster, a 24-year-old client with Guillain-Barre Syndrome can be told which of the following:

    a. the nerve degeneration slowing continues to progress in this chronic degenerative nerve disease.
    b. the disease is an acute inflammatory process with most clients regaining complete function.
    c. respiratory failure may occur requiring chronic ventilatory support.
    d. motor function deficit will occur, but sensation will remain.

Critical Thinking Questions

1. What lifestyle changes would be necessary for a person with hemiplegia or paraplegia?

2. How would you feel if a grandparent had Alzheimer's disease?

News Flash 1

A recent study by Dr. Reiman, et al. (1996) suggests using a blood test for identification of a gene, apolipoprotein ε, and a PET scan to identify potential clients with Alzheimer's disease. The gene has three varieties: ε-2, ε-3, and ε-4. Apolipoprotein ε-2 is suspected of protecting people from getting Alzheimer's, ε-4 causes Alzheimer's to start at a younger age, and ε-3 falls in between. People who inherit two ε-4 genes, about two to three percent of the population of the United States develop Alzheimer's disease at an average age of seventy. Next, the researchers performed a PET scan on Alzheimer's victims and people with two ε-4 genes. Deficits showing decreased metabolism were identified in specific locations in the brain of both groups. More research is necessary to determine the usefulness and replicability of these findings.

Medical Terminology

a/an-	prefix for without
aphasia	inability to communicate
cerebr/o-	main brain mass
cerebral palsy	
encephal/o-	pertaining to brain
encephalitis	inflammation of the brain
hemi-	half
hemiplegia	total paralysis of one side of the body
mening/o-	membrane
meningocele	protrusion of the membranes of the brain or spinal cord
neuro-	pertaining to or affecting a nerve or the nervous system
neuropathy	any disease of the nervous system
para-	lower extremities
paraplegia	paralysis of both legs and the lower part of the body
-paresis	weakness
hemiparesis	paralysis affecting only one side of the body
-phas/o	speech
dysphasia	impairment of speech due to a brain lesion
-plegia	paralysis of
cardioplegia	paralysis of the muscles of the heart
quad-	four
quadriplegia	paralysis of all four extremities

News Flash 2

Strokes claimed 145,000 American lives in 1996. The National Institute of Neurological Disorders and Strokes is developing guidelines for new treatments for stroke victims. One of these treatments is the administration of tPA within 3 hours of the onset of stroke symptoms. This drug dissolves clots and restores blood to the tissues in the effected area of the brain, thus preventing the permanent symptoms often suffered by stroke clients. tPA must be administered within 3 hours of the symptoms or it can make the stroke worse (*The Journal Gazette* 1997).

28

Sensory Disorders

Robin Theresa McKenzie
Raymond Phillips

▶ KEY TERMS

astigmatism
cerumen
conductive
cycloplegic
hyperopia
mydriatic
myopia
nystagmus
presbyopia
sensorineural
strabismus
tinnitus
uveitis
vertigo

LIST OF DISORDERS

Disorders of the Ear
- ▶ Impaired Hearing
- ▶ Meniere's Disease
- ▶ Otosclerosis
- ▶ Acoustic Neuroma
- ▶ Otitis Media
- ▶ Otitis Externa
- ▶ Mastoiditis

Disorders of the Eye
- ▶ Cataracts
- ▶ Glaucoma
- ▶ Retinal Detachment
- ▶ Infections of the Eye
  - • Keratitis
  - • Stye
  - • Chalazion
  - • Conjunctivitis (Pink-eye)
- ▶ Refractive Errors
- ▶ Eye Injuries
- ▶ Impaired Vision
- ▶ Macular Degeneration

LEARNING OBJECTIVES

Upon completion of this chapter the learner should be able to:
- Define key terms.
- Compare and differentiate common disorders of the special senses.
- Identify the structure and function of the major parts of the eye and ear.

- Explain the purpose of the common diagnostic tests for sensory problems.
- List the nursing assessments and common nursing diagnoses related to sensory impairment.

- Assist in planning nursing care for clients with sensory disorders.
- List some of the common sensory aids for the visual and hearing impaired.

▶ *MAKING THE CONNECTION*

Refer to the topics in the following chapters to increase your understanding of sensory disorders:

- **Chapter 5, Communication:** Nonverbal Communication, p. 70; Therapeutic Communication, p. 71; Psychosocial Aspects of Communication, p. 73; Nurse/Client Communication, p. 75
- **Chapter 8, Health Maintenance:** Cataracts, p. 131; Glaucoma, p. 131
- **Chapter 10, Nursing Assessment:** Head-to-Toe Assessment, p. 176
- **Chapter 12, Pain Management:** Therapeutic Approaches to Pain, p. 214

- **Chapter 13, Perioperative Nursing:** Elderly Clients Undergoing Surgery, p. 259
- **Chapter 16, Caring for the Older Adult:** Common Disorders Related to Aging/Vision, p. 339; Common Disorders Related to Aging/Hearing, p. 339
- **Chapter 18, The Dying Process/Hospice:** Care of the Mouth, Eyes, and Nose, p. 375
- **Chapter 27, Nervous System Disorders:** Anatomy and Physiology Review, p. 680; Table 27-1, Cranial Nerves, p. 684; Basic Neurological Nursing Assessment, p. 686

INTRODUCTION

From the moment we wake in the morning until we fall asleep at night, we are inundated with information from the outside world through our special senses. It is difficult to imagine not being able to hear children laughing, birds singing, or music playing. We savor the aroma and taste of freshly brewed coffee, enjoy reading the morning paper, and love hugging our family before heading off to school or work. Although most of us do not consider our special senses as organs of protection, we depend on visual and auditory alarms to keep us from harm. This chapter reviews the structure and function, identifies appropriate nursing diagnoses and presents the medical and nursing management of the five special senses: vision, hearing, taste, smell, and touch.

ANATOMY AND PHYSIOLOGY REVIEW OF THE EAR

The human ear can be divided into three main anatomical components: the outer ear, middle ear, and inner ear (see Figure 28-1). Each part plays a major role in hearing. Similar to other paired organs in the body, dysfunction of part or all of one ear does not affect the function of the other.

Outer Ear

The outer ear is composed of the auricle (pinna), a cartilaginous flap on the temporal sides of the head, and the external ear canal or external auditory meatus. The outer ear is responsible for collecting, conducting, and amplifying sound waves. The auricle directs sounds through the external ear canal to the tympanic membrane (eardrum). This canal is lined with ceruminous glands that secrete **cerumen** (ear wax), a yellowish brown protective substance that guards against certain bacteria, small insects, and traps dust and debris that may damage the inner ear. There are two kinds of cerumen, waxy and dry. Normally, the cerumen works its way out of the ear as we eat, chew, or speak. However, cerumen can build up and actually cause significant hearing loss in the affected ear.

The tympanic membrane (TM) serves as a boundary between the outer and middle ear. As sound waves vibrate against the membrane, the motion is transmitted to the bones of the inner ear. In an acute ear infection,

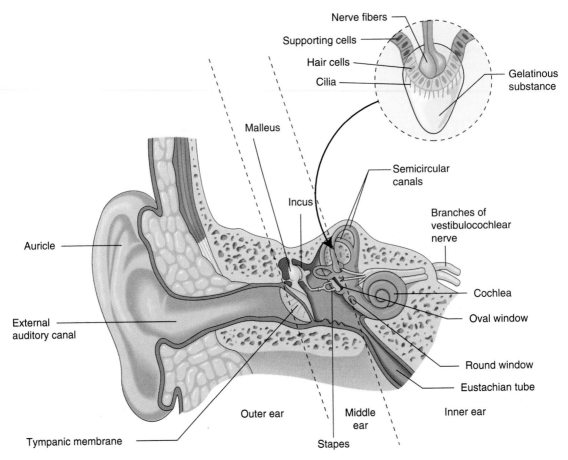

FIGURE 28-1 Structures of the ear: internal and external.

fluid fills the middle ear, creating significant pressure on the tympanic membrane. The TM is normally concave on otoscopic exam, so a convex or bulging TM is an important sign of an acute infectious process.

Middle Ear

The three bones of the middle ear are collectively referred to as the ossicles and include: the malleus (hammer), incus (anvil), and stapes (stirrup), so named because they resemble the tools of a blacksmith's trade. The malleus is attached to the upper, inner portion of the tympanic membrane. The head of the malleus connects with the next ossicle, the incus which joins the third ossicle, the stapes. The flat oval bone of the stapes, called the footplate, rests on the oval window (part of the inner ear). The vibration created by sound waves passes through the outer ear canal to the tympanic membrane and then transmitted to these three bones (see Figure 28-2).

The eustachian tube opens into the pharynx from the middle ear. It is approximately 3 to 4 cm long, and

its primary function is to equalize pressure on both sides of the eardrum by providing a path (via the nasal passages) to relieve the pressure. In addition to pressure equalization, the functions of the middle ear include amplification of the sound waves and stimulation of the oval window to move the fluids of the inner ear.

Inner Ear

The inner ear has two main functions: hearing and equilibrium. It consists of a complex series of interconnected, fluid-filled chambers and tubes called the labyrinth. It can be divided into three main parts: the semicircular canals, the vestibule, and the cochlea all located in the temporal bone. The semicircular canals, which function in providing the sense of balance, open into the vestibule. The vestibule is the central chamber of the inner ear and on one side of it a membranous structure called the oval window is connected to the footplate of the stapes (in the middle ear). The cochlea is a snail-shaped structure that contains the auditory organ for the sense of hearing. It consists of a long coiled tube and is partially divided through its length by a thin spiral shelf of bone called the osseous spiral lamina. The basilar membrane across this shelf divides the canal into two passages. The lower passage is known as the scala tympani and has an opening called the round window. The upper passage is the scala vestibuli. The scala vestibuli and scala tympani contain perilymph. The central duct, located between the scala tympani and the scala vestibuli is called the scali media and it is filled with endolymph. The Organ of Corti lies on the upper surface of the basilar membrane which forms the floor of the scala medi and extends from the base to the apex of the cochlea. Multiple rows of hair cells, also known as cilia, line the surface of the Organ of Corti. Above the Organ of Corti, is a rooflike membrane, the tectorial membrane, that makes contact with the tips of the hair cells.

The mechanical vibration of the stapes on the oval window creates pressure and causes the perilymph to vibrate. Different frequencies from different sounds cause a different portion of the basilar membrane to move, which in turn causes the cilia of the specific hair cells to bend. As they brush against the tectorial membrane, this bending causes the nerves at the base of the hair cells to respond to different sounds and initiate neural responses that are sent along the auditory nerve (VIII cranial nerve) to the brain. Thus, mechanical information is translated into nerve impulses and sent to the brain which translates the sound into meaningful impressions and language.

ANATOMY AND PHYSIOLOGY REVIEW OF THE EYE

The eyes are a pair of spherical organs located in bony orbital cavities in the front of the skull. They are the sensory receptor organs of the visual system that transduce light from the environment into electrical impulses, which the optic nerve then transmits to the brain where they are interpreted as the sensation of vision (see Figure 28-3). The adult eyeball measures about 1 inch in diameter. Of its total surface area, only the anterior one-sixth is exposed. The remainder is recessed and protected by the bony orbit into which it fits. Anatomically, the eye can be divided into three separate coats or "tunics": the outer fibrous tunic, the middle vascular tunic, and the inner nervous tunic.

Fibrous Tunic

The fibrous tunic is the outer coat of the eyeball and is composed posteriorly of the sclera and anteriorly of the transparent cornea. The sclera is leathery, white, and relatively thick, i.e., "the white of the eye," and is composed of connective tissue. The cornea, or "window of the eye" is a continuation of the sclera and forms a transparent rounded bulge through which light passes.

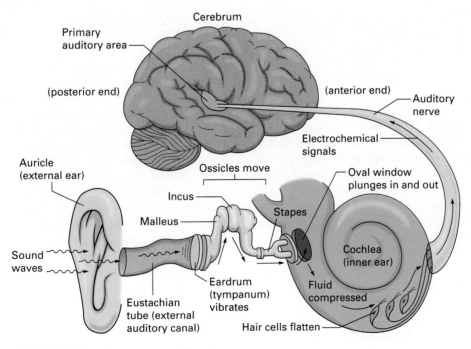

FIGURE 28-2 The process of hearing.

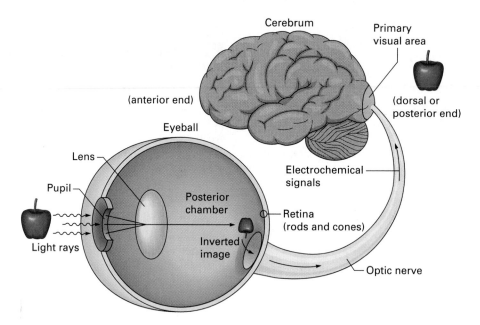

FIGURE 28-3 The process of vision.

Vascular Tunic

The vascular tunic is the eye's middle layer and is composed of three portions: the posterior choroid, the anterior ciliary body, and the iris. Collectively, these three structures are called the uveal tract. The choroid carries the blood vessels for the eyeball and contains a large amount of pigment, thus preventing internal reflection of light. Around the edge of the cornea the choroid forms the ciliary body, a thickened structure containing smooth muscle. A thin diaphragm of mostly connective tissue and smooth muscle fibers with an opening in the center is attached around the anterior margin of the ciliary body. The muscles of the ciliary body serve to change the shape of the lens, allowing changes in the focal distance of the eye. The third portion of the vascular tunic is known as the iris, and contains the pigment responsible for the color of the eye. The hole in the iris is the pupil, which permits light to enter the eye. Some of the smooth muscle fibers in the iris encircle the pupil and others radiate from it. Contraction of the radial muscle dilates the pupil and contraction of the circular muscle constricts the pupil. By their control of pupil diameter these muscles regulate the amount of light entering the eye.

Nervous Tunic

The third and innermost tunic of the eye, the retina, translates light waves into neural impulses. An extremely complex structure, the retina contains several layers of nerve cells and their processes, including two types of receptors, the rods for vision in dim light and the cones for daytime or color vision. Cones are stimulated only by bright light. This is why we cannot see color by moonlight. Cones are most densely concentrated in the central fovea, a small depression in the center of the macula lutea. The macula lutea, or yellow spot, is in the central part of the retina. The fovea is the area of sharpest vision because the highest concentration of cones are located there. Rods are absent from the fovea and macula, but they increase in density toward the periphery of the retina. The optic disk, where the optic nerve exits the eye, is a weak spot in the fundus (posterior wall) of the eye because it is not reinforced by the sclera. The optic disk is also called the blind spot, because it lacks photoreceptors and light focused on it will not be detected.

The interior of the eyeball contains an anterior and posterior chamber separated by the lens. The anterior chamber is filled with a watery fluid called the aqueous humor, which maintains intraocular pressure, provides nourishment, and helps maintain the shape of the eye ball. The posterior chamber is filled with a jellylike substance called the vitreous humor, which maintains the spherical shape of the eye and supports the inner structures. Both substances are transparent, thus allowing light to pass through the eye to the retina (see Figure 28-4).

The lens, located in the anterior chamber of the eye, is a transparent biconvex crystalline body enclosed in an elastic capsule suspended by suspensory ligaments. The shape of the lens changes to focus the image.

At the junction of the sclera and cornea is a venous sinus known as the canal of Schlemm. It is a small canal that serves to return the aqueous humor to the venous system of the eye.

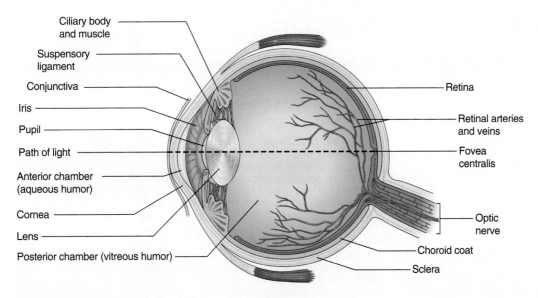

FIGURE 28-4 Lateral view of the interior eyeball.

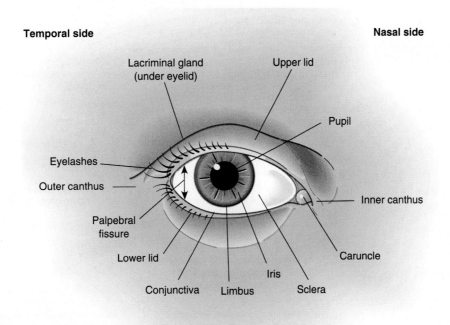

FIGURE 28-5 External view of the eye.

The eyeball is protected from the external world by the eyelid, which contains a thin protective layer of epithelium, the conjunctiva. The conjunctiva covers the anterior portion of the eyeball and lines the eyelid. Projecting from the border of each eyelid is a row of short, thick hairs, the eyelashes. In the upper lid, the hairs are long and turn upward; in the lower lid, they are short and turn downward.

The lacrimal gland produces a secretion called tears which contain a lysozyme, muramidase, to destroy pathogens. The constant flow of tears is from the upper outer lid diagonally across the eye lubricating the eye and washing off foreign particles (see Figure 28-5).

COMMON DIAGNOSTIC TESTS

The following is a table of commonly used diagnostic tests for clients with problems in hearing and vision:

Test	Explanation/Normal Values	Nursing Responsibilities
Weber test (tuning fork)	Detects loss of hearing in one ear or both. Tuning fork is struck and the handle is placed in the middle of the forehead. Clients with normal hearing or bilateral deafness will hear or not hear the sound equally in both ears. Clients with unilateral hearing loss will only hear the sound in the unaffected ear.	Explain purpose and procedure to the client.
Rinne test (tuning fork)	Detects loss of hearing in one or both ears. Tuning fork is struck and placed against the mastoid bone to measure sound conduction through bone. Then the tuning fork is placed beside and parallel to the ear to test conduction through the air. If the sound is louder when the tines are placed beside the ear, then hearing is normal or the hearing loss is sensorineural. If the sound is louder when conducted through bone, then the hearing loss is conductive.	Explain the purpose and procedure to the client.
Audiometric testing	Evaluates both bone and air conduction and determines the degree of hearing loss. The client wears headphones and signals to the audiologist when the tone is audible. A series of tones are delivered at different frequencies through the earphones. The results are recorded on an audiogram. The client is in a sound proof booth during the test.	Explain the purpose and procedure to the client. Ensure that the client is not claustrophobic.
Speech Audiometry (Spondee Threshold)	Evaluates ability to hear and understand the spoken word. A series of two-syllable words commonly recognized by their vowel sounds (like toothbrush and baseball) are delivered through the earphones. When the client correctly repeats the word, the sound intensity is recorded in decibels. This test is normally conducted in a soundproof booth.	Explain the purpose and procedure to the client. Ensure client is not claustrophobic.
Caloric Test	Assess alteration in vestibular function. The client is placed in a supine or Fowler's position and each ear is irrigated with cold and then warm water. A normal response includes vertigo, nystagmus, nausea, vomiting, and unsteady gait. A decreased response or failure to respond within 3 minutes indicates an abnormality may be present. This test is most commonly done on comatose clients. A punctured eardrum or Meniere's disease may be a contraindication for the test.	Explain the purpose and procedure to the client. Tell the client he will experience nystagmus, vertigo, nausea, vomiting, and an unsteady gait with a normal response. Stay with the client and have an emesis basin and tissues available.
Brainstem auditory evoked response (ErA and BAER)	Detects hearing dysfunctions of the central nervous system and cochlear nerve (VIII cranial nerve). Valuable for testing comatose clients, clients with neurologic damage, and children. An altered appearance of the brainstem waveforms or delayed or loss of a waveform indicates an abnormality including a possible cochlear lesion or acoustic neuroma.	Explain the purpose and procedure to the client. The client will be in a darkened room with electrodes attached to the head and earphones in place.

Test	Explanation/Normal Values	Nursing Responsibilities
Typanometry	Measures the movement of the eardrum in response to air pressure in the ear canal. Evaluates the presence of fluid in the middle ear and is commonly used to evaluate otitis media in children or adults.	Explain the procedure to the client. A small burst of air is introduced through the otoscope and may produce an uncomfortable sensation.
Computed Tomography (CT)	Detects bony tumors, mastoid infection, and acoustic neuroma through radiographic imaging.	Explain the procedure to the client and that they will be lying on a large table with the head positioned inside a large tunnel-like machine. The client must lie very still and all metal objects, such as jewelry, must be removed. Check for claustrophobia.
Magnetic Resonance Imaging (MRI)	Detects soft tissue abnormalities such as a meningioma, brain tumor, or acoustic neuroma.	Explain the procedure to the client, and that the head will be positioned in a large donut-like machine. The client must lie very still and all metal objects such as jewelry, must be removed. Check for claustrophobia.
Romberg Test	To assess vestibular (balance) function. The client stands with eyes closed, arms extended in front, and both feet together. Slight swaying is normal.	Explain the purpose and procedure to the client. Stand close and reassure the client someone will catch him if he begins to fall.
Otoscopic Exam	Visual examination of the ear canal using an otoscope. The examiner looks for signs of inflammation, discharge, or foreign bodies. The tympanic membrane is normally pearly gray. The position and color of the membrane is noted as well as any unusual appearance.	Explain the purpose and procedure to the client. The ear should be clear of cerumen. The head is tilted away from the examiner and the earlobe is pulled up, back and out to straighten the auditory canal. In children, the earlobe is pulled down and out to straighten the canal.
Past-point Testing	Measures the ability or inability to accurately place a finger on some part of the body, usually the client's or examiner's face and fingers. For example, the examiner will instruct the client to close her eyes and touch her nose, then touch the examiner's nose; or touch the examiner's index finger.	Explain the test and procedure to the client. Explain that it is painless and a helpful measure of vestibular, (coordinated) function.
Color Vision Tests	Most common color vision tests use pseudoisochromatic (seemingly the same color) plates made up of patterns of dots of the primary colors superimposed on backgrounds of randomly mixed colors. A client with normal vision can identify the patterns; a client with a color deficiency cannot distinguish between the pattern and the background.	Explain the test and procedure to the client.
Tonometry	Used to measure intraocular pressure and to aid in the diagnosis and follow-up evaluation of glaucoma. There are two types of tonometric devices used for assessment: applanation and indentation. An applanation tonometer is the most accurate and commonly used device and measures the force (delineated by the reading on the tension dial on the tonometer) required to flatten a small, standard area of the cornea. An indentation tonometer measures the deformation of the globe in response to a standard weight placed on the cornea. Before use of either apparatus the eyes are anesthetized with a local ophthalmic	Explain the test and procedure to the client. Explain to the client that this test measures the pressure within the eyes. The test requires that the client's eyes be anesthetized, but the anesthesia will wear off shortly after the examination is complete. Reassure that the procedure is painless.

(continued)

Test	Explanation/Normal Values	Nursing Responsibilities
	solution, such as benoxinate with fluorescein or tetracaine so that the tonometer's pressure will not be felt. Normal = 12 - 22 mmHg.	
Slit Lamp Examination	The cornea is examined with the aid of a slit lamp. A slit-like beam facilitates visualization of the layers of the cornea and lens; one can thus evaluate the thickness of these structures and more accurately localize disease processes. It is useful in detecting and evaluating abnormalities of anterior segment tissues and structures. This examination may reveal disorders such as iritis, corneal abrasions, conjunctivitis, and lens opacities (cataracts).	Explain the test and procedure to client.
Perimetry	Perimetry is used to detect or monitor visual field loss. Loss of visual field is the major clinical manifestation of optic nerve damage from glaucoma and is, therefore, used both in the diagnosis of glaucoma and in the evaluation of the response to treatment. A perimeter is used to plot the topography of the island of vision and is used to recognize any variations from normal in either localized areas or the overall visual field.	Explain test and procedure to the client.
Visual Acuity	This examination is used to test distant and near visual acuity and to identify refractive errors in vision. Distant visual acuity is measured with a standardized visual acuity chart, e.g., Snellen's chart. Near visual acuity is measured with a Jaeger card (a card with print in graded sizes). Visual acuity is recorded as a fraction. The fraction's numerator represents the distance to the chart; the denominator represents the distance at which a normal eye can read the line. Thus, the larger the denominator, the poorer the client's visual acuity. For example, if the client's vision is normal, results are expressed as 20/20, which means that the smallest symbol one can identify at 20 feet is the same symbol the normal eye can identify from the same distance.	Explain the test and procedure to the client. The client must stand a specific distance from the eye chart, usually 10 feet. One eye must be alternately covered during the exam. If the client wears glasses, the test should be done with the glasses on and with glasses off.
Electroretinogram (ERG)	An electroretinogram (ERG) is a record of the changes in the retina's electric potential following stimulation by light. The ERG is clinically useful in some clients with retinal disease. An ERG is obtained by placing a contact lens electrode on the anesthetized cornea. The electrical potential recorded on the cornea is identical with the response that would be obtained if the electrodes were placed directly upon the surface of the retina.	Explain the test and procedure to the client.
Ocular ultrasonography	Ocular ultrasonography involves the transmission of high frequency sound waves through the eye and the measurement of their reflection from ocular structures. An A-scan converts the	Explain the test and procedure to the client. A small transducer (soft disk) is placed on the eyelid. It transmits high frequency sound waves that are reflected by the structures in the eye. The client may

Test	Explanation/Normal Values	Nursing Responsibilities
	resulting echoes into waveforms whose crests represent the positions of different structures, giving a linear dimensional picture. The more common B-scan converts the echoes into patterns of dots that form a two-dimensional, cross-sectional image. This test is helpful to evaluate a cataract or vitreous hemorrhage and to locate an intraocular foreign body or diagnoses retinal detachment.	be asked to move his eye or change his gaze during the procedure. The client's cooperation is paramount to ensure accurate determination of test results. Reassure the client that the test will cause only slight discomfort.
Ophthalmoscopic Examination	Examination of the fundus (posterior eye) performed with an ophthalmoscope. Magnifies vascular and nerve tissue of the fundus, including the optic disk, retinal vessels, macula, and retina. Used to diagnose diseases of the eye and aberrations in the refractive mechanism.	Explain the test and procedure to the client.
Orbital Computerized Tomography	Allows visualization of abnormalities not readily seen on standard x-rays, delineating size, position, and relationship to adjoining structures. The orbital CT is a series of images reconstructed by a computer and displayed as anatomic slices on an oscilloscope. It identifies space-occupying lesions earlier and more accurately than other x-ray techniques. It also provides three-dimensional images of orbital structures, especially the ocular muscles and optic nerve. Enhancement with a contrast agent may help define ocular tissue and circulation abnormalities.	Explain the test and procedure to client. The client is positioned on an x-ray table. The head of the table is moved into the scanner. The scanner rotates during the test and may make loud, crackling sounds. If an IV contrast agent is required, the client may feel flushed and warm or experience a transient headache. A salty taste, nausea, and vomiting may occur following injection of intravenous contrast dye. Reassure the client that the reaction is common and she may signal the technician if she is unable to tolerate the test.
Fluoresce in Angiography	Rapid sequence photographs of the fundus are taken with a special camera, following intravenous injection of sodium fluorescein. Visibility of microvascular structures of the retina and choroid are enhanced allowing evaluation of the entire retinal vascular bed.	Eye drops are instilled to dilate the pupils. The client will have an IV so the sodium fluorescein can be injected. The IV is removed following completion of the test. Skin and urine may be yellow for 24 to 48 hours

KEY ABBREVIATIONS

The following abbreviations and acronyms are used in relation to sensory disorders:

TM	tympanic membrane
IOL	intraocular lens
IOP	intraocular pressure
TDD	telecommunication device for the deaf

▶ DISORDERS OF THE EAR

▶ IMPAIRED HEARING

There are three types of specialists who care for the client with a hearing disorder: audiologists, otolaryngologists, and the hearing aid specialist. The audiologist evaluates hearing and determines the extent and type of hearing loss. The audiologist also provides nonmedical treatment such as the fitting of hearing aids, advice about assistive listening devices, and communication/aural rehabilitative training. The otolaryngologist (ear, nose, and throat physician) provides medical evaluation of hearing disorders and medical and surgical interventions. The hearing aid specialist is licensed to dispense hearing aids but does not have a medical background or training.

► *Types of Hearing Loss*

Hearing loss is generally categorized in two ways, **conductive** and **sensorineural**. Mixed hearing loss, both conductive and sensorineural, is possible, but far less likely. Either may occur at birth (congenital), develop later in life, be genetic, or caused by injury or trauma.

► *Conductive Hearing Loss*

Conductive hearing loss indicates an inability of the sound waves to reach the inner ear. This may be due to cerumen buildup or blockage, perforated tympanic membrane, or fixation of one or all of the ossicles.

► *Sensorineural Hearing Loss*

In sensorineural hearing loss, the inner ear or cochlear portion of the cranial nerve VIII may be abnormal or diseased. A tumor, infection, or temporal bone skull fracture may cause destruction of the nerve and result in sensorineural hearing loss.

► *Behaviors Indicating Hearing Loss*

A hearing impairment is a serious disorder that is often debilitating and embarrassing to the client. Hearing is a protective mechanism that alerts us to potential danger such as a car horn or smoke alarm. Hearing is part of the communication process and the inability to hear may cause the person to do or say the wrong thing in response to a question or command. Persons with hearing impairment may withdraw from conversation or seem indifferent to their surroundings or to those around them.

In infants and toddlers, speech may be severely delayed or absent. In adults, speech can deteriorate as manifested by muttering, slurring words, and dropping consonants or syllables. Individuals with hearing impairments may not notice the changes in their own speech pattern unless or until someone (often a loved one) constantly asks them to repeat themselves or to speak clearly. Indifference and withdrawal are common behaviors in response to hearing loss. If left undiagnosed and untreated, the person may truly regress, become unhappy, lonely, and possibly even paranoid. Some individuals become very loud and aggressive.

Profound bilateral hearing loss may be secondary to hereditary abnormalities, lesions in the inner ear, trauma, bilateral Meniere's disease, ototoxic drugs, syphilis, or many other disorders. Until recently, clients with profound hearing loss usually learned lip reading to cope with this severe sensory deficit.

Recognition of hearing loss by a family member, the nurse, or other health care provider can make the dif-ference between early treatment and a confident happy lifestyle and a life of seclusion, loneliness, and depression.

Research on hearing impairment has created many devices to aid speech and sound discrimination. Early diagnosis, treatment, and rehabilitation are essential to help hearing impaired persons enjoy and appreciate the world they live in.

► *Hearing Aids/ Assistive Devices*

Hearing aids today come in a variety of designs and sizes. Some are quite small and tinted to a person's skin color so as to be virtually unnoticeable. Some are worn in the ear, behind the ear, or are part of eyeglasses frames. Persons with bilateral hearing loss may need binaural (worn in both ears) hearing aids.

A hearing aid converts environmental sound and speech into electronic signals that are amplified and converted to acoustic signals. It makes speech and sound louder, but not necessarily clearer. Depending on the extent of hearing impairment and preference, the client may need to experiment with several different types of hearing aids. In addition, speech therapy, lip reading, and auditory training may be necessary to help discriminate speech and develop better listening skills.

Special instruction in the use and care of a hearing aid is necessary. The health care provider who assists with the choice of a hearing device is required to provide the following information to the client.

1. A medical evaluation should be performed prior to purchasing a hearing aid. Certain medical conditions such as an acute infection or sudden hearing loss require more thorough evaluation.
2. Written and verbal instructions in the use and care of the device. This should include proper cleansing and battery changes.
3. Repair service availability.
4. Avoidable things that could damage the hearing aid in daily use.
5. Reportable conditions resulting from irritation or improper use of the hearing aid.

Many other assistive hearing devices are available for the hearing impaired. Numerous television programs are closed-caption. Advanced technology allows telecommunication through a device called Telecommunication Device for the Deaf (TDD) (also called TTY Typewriter) which sends a printed message onto a small screen. Both sender and receiver must have the typewriter/telephone device. Many businesses offer this option to conduct transactions.

Alarm clocks offer strobe lights or vibrators to awaken clients. State of the art receivers give instant access to radio, television, computer, and stereos to enhance receiving and listening systems. For travelers, complete kits are available to provide ready access for smoke alarm, clock, TDD, and door knock alert in hotels or inns.

Hearing guide dogs are also available. The animals are specially trained to meet the needs of their owner. At home, the dog responds to alarms, knocking on doors, and babies crying. In public, the dog takes a position between owner and a potential threat. Special identifiers, such as a collar for the dog and ID card for the owner are available. The dogs are trained to go wherever their master goes including restaurants, grocery stores, and on public transportation.

▶ Medical/Surgical Management

▶ Medical

It is important to identify the type of hearing loss and underlying etiology to determine the best medical or surgical management. The client should undergo a complete physical examination as well as thorough diagnostic hearing tests. Once the etiology is determined, the client and doctor can determine the best course of therapy.

▶ Surgical

Silverstein (1992) offers a very recent technological advancement called the cochlear implant as a possible treatment for persons with profound deafness. Studies thus far indicate better success with the implant in children than in adults. In this procedure, a receiver/ stimulator is implanted in the skull and a group of electrodes are planted in front of the round window in the inner ear. The client wears a microphone near the ear that picks up and translates sound into electrical signals. These signals are then transmitted to the brain via the cochlear implant and cranial nerve VIII.

▶ Pharmacological

There are no pharmacologic agents for the treatment of hearing loss.

▶ Nursing Process

Assessment

Subjective Data Subjective data may be obtained by asking the client to describe the initial onset of symptoms and possible familial traits. Ask the client about recent infections of the ears, nose, or upper respiratory system. Inquire about recent trauma and past surgery as well as medical history such as diabetes, heart disease, or cancer. Note allergies to food, drugs, or environmental factors. Ask the client about their work history which may reveal exposure to loud noises. Ask the client about associated symptoms such as **tinnitus** (ringing in the ear), **vertigo** (dizziness), nausea, and vomiting.

Objective Data Objective data may be obtained by listening closely to the client and noting any deterioration of speech, slurring, or dropping of word endings. Note current and recent medication use.

Inspect the outer ear for abnormalities, lesions, or cerumen. Palpate the mastoid process, neck, jaw, and temporal regions of the head for swelling or tenderness to touch. Note the degree of hearing loss as reported by the client and compare it to the diagnostic tests such as the speech audiogram. The client's perception of hearing loss may be significantly different from the diagnostic findings.

▼ ▼

Possible nursing diagnoses for a client with impaired hearing may include:

Nursing Diagnoses	Goals	Nursing Interventions
▶ Anxiety, related to potential difficulty in communicating with hearing people.	The client will develop effective means of communication and maximize ability to hear and/or understand the spoken word.	Encourage client to express anxieties about communication difficulties.
		Speak slowly and distinctly after getting the client's attention.
		Face the client and sit or stand to be at eye level with the client.
		Use short simple sentences and give the client time to respond. Repeat or rephrase if necessary.
		Use written materials when possible to communicate information.

(continued)

Nursing Diagnoses	Goals	Nursing Interventions
		Keep a notepad and pen or pencil available to write down new or unfamiliar words and concepts.
		If sign language is the client's preferred method of communication, locate a person who understands sign language.
		If the client wears a hearing aid, make sure that the battery is functional, it is turned on, and adjusted to a comfortable level.
▶ *Social isolation, related to hearing impairment.*	The client will participate in conversations and other social situations.	Take time to engage client in conversation.
		Speak slowly and distinctly.
		Make sure you have the client's attention and be at eye level.
		Give the client time to respond.
		Advise client to seek audiological testing to determine etiology of hearing impairment.
		Provide the client and family members written information regarding the availability, variety, and quality of assistive hearing devices.
		Encourage client to participate in social situations.

▶ Evaluation

Each goal must be evaluated to determine how it has been met by the client.

▲ ▲

▶ MENIERE'S DISEASE

Meniere's disease is also known as endolymphatic hydrops. Although the exact cause is unknown, it is postulated that the cause is an excessive accumulation of endolymph in the cochlear duct and possible leakage of endolymph into the perilymph due to increased capillary permeability. Mixing of the two fluids chemically alters the homeostasis of the perilymph and endolymph and can be responsible for the symptoms associated with Meniere's disease.

The major symptoms are the classic triad of vertigo, tinnitus, and unilateral fluctuating hearing loss. The vertigo is often associated with nausea and vomiting. Tinnitus may either be a preceding aura or occur simultaneously with the vertigo. Initially, tinnitus is intermittent, but as the disease progresses, it may be a constant, low-pitched roaring sound.

The third classic symptom is a fluctuating, unilateral hearing loss. With each attack, the hearing deficit becomes more profound.

The symptoms are frequently at their worst during the first attack which may last a few minutes or three to six hours. **Nystagmus**, repetitive and involuntary movement of the eyeballs, and diaphoresis may occur during an attack. Subsequent attacks are less severe, but over time may involve both ears and cause permanent bilateral hearing loss. Clients report many different precipitating events such as stress, weather changes, menstruation, pregnancy, and various dietary influences such as caffeine, alcohol, and salt. Smoking has also been implicated.

▶ Medical/Surgical Management

▶ Medical

Medical management is the preferred treatment and most helpful to about 80 to 85 percent of persons affected with this disease. Diagnosis is not difficult and is usually made on the client's symptoms. Diagnosis may also be confirmed with caloric stimulation (though this test is primarily conducted on comatose clients) and an MRI to rule out a tumor. Medical management is symptomatic.

► Surgical

Surgical intervention is usually needed only when the attacks are frequent and debilitating, or when the disease severely impacts the quality of life and the ability for self-care. Surgical treatment includes endolymphatic, subarachnoid shunt placement to drain excessive endolymph. With this procedure, hearing is preserved in 60 to 70 percent of the clients. With a vestibular neurectomy, the vestibular portion of cranial nerve VIII is severed, yet preserves hearing in 90 percent of the clients. In surgical destruction of the labyrinth, hearing is destroyed but the incapacitating vertigo is completely relieved.

► Pharmacological

A number of medications are useful to help control the symptoms such as antihistamines, antiemetics, benzodiazepines, diuretics, tranquilizers, vasoactive agents, and oral niacin. The medications may be prescribed for long-term use or at the onset of symptoms. Since the cause is unknown, there is no cure.

► Diet

Dietary interventions include strict salt restriction and avoidance of those foods or beverages that precipitate or aggravate an attack. Examples are beer, wine, soda, salty food or snacks, chocolate, and coffee and tea that have caffeine.

► Activity

Activity is not limited in a normal daily routine. However, during or after an attack, clients may require prolonged bed rest and restriction of activities that may be unsafe, such as driving or operating heavy equipment.

► Nursing Process

Assessment

Subjective Data   Identify significant contributory data by starting with an in-depth history. Subjective data may be obtained by asking the client to describe the initial onset of symptoms including, but not limited to the classic triad of tinnitus, vertigo, and fluctuating unilateral hearing loss.

Include questions related to recent viral illness, upper respiratory infections, past medical, surgical, and dental history and any problems related to the neck and face. Ask the client about food, drug, or environmental allergies. Record any current or recent long-term medications. Identify the client's occupation and hobbies that may contribute to hearing loss.

Objective Data   Objective data may be obtained with a thorough physical examination that includes looking at the ear for abnormalities, lesions and cerumen blockage, or unusual drainage. Palpate the neck, jaw, and mastoid process for possible lymph node enlargement and tenderness. Assist with the otologic examination as needed. Audiological testing determines unilateral or bilateral hearing loss.

▼ ▼

Possible nursing diagnoses for a client with Meniere's disease may include:

Nursing Diagnoses	Goals	Nursing Interventions
► Activity intolerance, related to severe vertigo.	The client will be able to tolerate activities of daily living.	Provide adequate periods of bed rest.
		Keep the room dim and quiet when possible.
		Keep side rails up and explain safety precautions to client.
		Avoid jarring the bed and caution client to avoid sudden movements.
		Administer antiemetic before symptoms become too severe.
		Offer food and fluids as tolerated.
		Provide assistance with ambulation and encourage increased activity as tolerated.

(continued)

Nursing Diagnoses	*Goals*	*Nursing Interventions*
▶ *Anxiety, related to abrupt onset and unknown progression of the disease.*	The client will verbalize understanding of the disease process and potential precipitating factors and how to manage or control the symptoms.	Assess the client's current knowledge of the disease process.
		Review the disease process and underlying etiology of Meniere's disease.
		Ask the client to identify possible precipitating factors such as stress or dietary habits.
		Discuss health promotion programs for stress management and healthy cooking classes.
		Suggest consultations with dietary and social services.
		Review follow-up appointments, medications, dietary management, activity, and rest parameters.
		Evaluate client's readiness to discuss progressive hearing loss and current assistive hearing devices available.
▶ *Adjustment, impaired, related to progressive hearing loss and possible bilateral deafness.*	The client will verbalize feelings related to adjustment and potential hearing loss.	Examine the client's feelings regarding progressive hearing loss and changes in activities of daily living, employment, and quality of life issues.
		Discuss common modalities for assisted hearing devices and consult social services as needed.
		Speak directly to the client in comfortable tones.
		If possible and agreeable, arrange a meeting with a support person whose disease process closely correlates to client's.
		Provide written materials that identify community resources and support groups to help client avoid social isolation and withdrawal.
▶ *Communication, impaired, verbal, related to unilateral or bilateral hearing loss.*	The client will develop an effective means of communication and maximize the ability to hear and/or understand the spoken word.	Identify hospital and community resources for the hearing impaired.
		Collaborate with family members or significant other to learn lip reading.
		Teach the client acoustic strategies such as sitting where the conversation can best be heard, usually in the corner of a room.
		Demonstrate that cupping the ear or turning toward the sound or conversation is often helpful.
		Describe benefits of a hearing aid with assistance from a well-trained audiologist.
		Discuss long-term speech and auditory training.
		Recommend that the client engage in quiet activities to avoid a noisy environment.

Nursing Diagnoses	Goals	Nursing Interventions
▶ *Injury, high risk for, related to vertigo.*	The client will not fall or be injured because of vertigo.	Keep side rails up. Teach client to move or turn slowly. Reiterate need to call for assistance when ambulating. Keep call bell within client's reach. Administer medications for vertigo prior to worsening of symptoms. Avoid glaring, bright lights. Instruct client to sit or lie down when vertigo occurs.
▶ *Sensory/perceptual, alterations, vestibular, auditory, related to disease process.*	The client will be able to verbalize ways to deal with sudden episodes of vertigo and hearing loss.	Teach the client to sit or lie down when vertigo occurs. If driving or operating complex machinery, the client must stop the activity and seek help. Identify contributing factors such as stress, changes in weather, and diet that may contribute to onset of symptoms. Discuss options to reduce stress and avoid those foods that may potentiate an attack. If medications are ordered, review the prescribed instructions for use. As hearing loss worsens, the client should be instructed in assistive hearing devices and community resources for the hearing impaired.

▶ Evaluation

Each goal must be evaluated to determine how it has been met by the client.

▲ ▲

▶ OTOSCLEROSIS

Otosclerosis is a conductive hearing loss secondary to a pathologic change of the bones in the middle ear. The exact cause is unknown. The ossicles are normally hard, but over time and without warning, the bone becomes softened, spongy, highly vascular, and partially or totally fixed. This fixation reduces or prevents transmission of source waves to inner ear fluids. Although all three bones may be affected, the stapes, which must vibrate on the oval window in order to transmit sound waves, is most commonly afflicted.

Otosclerosis is more common in adults, women are affected more often than men, and it is familial in some cases. It is the most common cause of conductive hearing loss.

The primary clinical manifestations are subtle changes in hearing and low-pitched tinnitus. It becomes more difficult to distinguish a whisper, or to hear in crowded places or understand conversation. Individuals affected by otosclerosis often blame others for speaking too softly or mumbling. Frequently, rather than asking others to speak up or to repeat themselves, the person will be irritable and withdrawn.

Diagnostic testing begins with the Weber and Rinne tuning fork tests. In addition, audiometric testing should be performed. Schwartz's sign, a pink blush, is seen on otoscopic examination. Tympanometry shows stiffness in the sound conduction system.

▶ Medical/Surgical Management

▶ Medical

Treatment for otosclerosis is limited to three options. The individual may choose to do nothing and obtain periodic audiometry to evaluate progression of the disease. The second choice is to use a hearing aid and the third choice is surgical management with a procedure known as a stapedectomy.

▶ *Surgical*

A stapedectomy is the preferred surgical technique for improving hearing loss due to otosclerosis. A stapedectomy may be done under local or general anesthesia and routinely requires a surgical incision in the posterior ear canal, removal of the stapes, and implantation of a plastic prosthesis. A new technique, laser stapedectomy, may be performed through the ear canal without an incision. The stapes tendon is vaporized, chards are removed with delicate micro instruments and an opening is made allowing the surgeon to implant a prosthetic piston. This restores normal vibration against the inner ear.

▶ *Pharmacological, Diet, Activity*

Pharmacologic intervention is not useful in this disease process. No changes are required in diet or activity.

▶ *Nursing Process*

Assessment

Subjective Data   Subjective data will include a careful history to discover possible hereditary traits or acquired disease. Ask the client about recent infections of the ears, nose, or upper respiratory system. Inquire about past surgery, trauma, or other illnesses such as diabetes, heart disease, or cancer. Ask the client about associated symptoms such as dizziness, tinnitus, vertigo, and nausea.

Note allergies to foods, drugs, or any environmental factors. Ask about the client's work history that may reveal exposure to loud noises. Record current and recent medications especially those known to be ototoxic.

Objective Data   Objective data includes a thorough physical examination. Inspect the outer ear for abnormalities, lesions, or impacted ear wax. Palpate the mastoid process, neck, jaw, and temporal regions of the head for pain or swelling. Note the degree of hearing loss. The client may be vomiting.

▼ ▼

Possible nursing diagnoses for the client with otosclerosis may include:

Nursing Diagnoses	*Goals*	*Nursing Interventions*
▶ *Anxiety, related to decrease or loss in hearing.*	The client will show evidence of reduced anxiety and verbalize understanding of the disease process and treatment regimen.	Encourage the client to explore feelings of anxiety and to ask questions to clarify concerns.
		Provide honest and realistic feedback.
		Collaborate with the physician to provide thorough and clear explanations of the disease process, treatment options, and anticipated results.
▶ *Knowledge deficit, related to preoperative preparations and postoperative care.*	The client will verbalize understanding of preoperative preparations and of postoperative care.	Provide written and verbal information on the procedure, risks, and expected results and what not to do postoperatively.
		Answer questions knowledgeably and in terms the client understands.
		Clarify NPO status.
		Suggest bringing an overnight bag in case it is needed.
		Instruct client to wear hair up to avoid betadine prep solution from getting into hair.
		Discuss postoperative care related to pain control, antiemetic, antibiotics, bed rest, and activity restrictions such as avoiding sudden movements, blowing nose, and sneezing.

Nursing Diagnoses	Goals	Nursing Interventions
▶ Injury, high risk for, related to vertigo.	The client will not fall or be injured because of vertigo.	Keep side rails up. Instruct the client to move or turn slowly. Reiterate need to call for assistance when ambulating and keep call bell within client's reach. Administer medications for vertigo prior to worsening of symptoms. Keep room well lit when client is ambulating.
▶ Trauma, high risk for, related to increased middle ear pressure with displacement of prosthesis.	The client will minimize risks for prosthesis displacement.	Maintain bed rest for twenty-four to forty-eight hours, or as ordered. Remind client to avoid sudden movement, sneezing, or blowing the nose. Monitor vital signs q4h. Be particularly attentive to temperature for evidence of infection, excessive clear or bloody drainage, and pain not controlled with prescribed analgesics. Administer analgesics and/or sedatives to reduce discomfort and promote rest.
▶ Knowledge deficit, related to activities after surgery.	The client will demonstrate the ability to change dressing correctly and verbalize knowledge of self-care and follow-up.	Teach client how and when to perform dressing change and have client demonstrate the procedure. Instruct client to avoid pressure changes (such as flying in an unpressurized aircraft), avoid heavy lifting (60 lbs) for one month, avoid nose blowing for ten days and if sneezing occurs, keep mouth open. Advise client to keep water out of the ear and keep the ear exposed to air as much as possible for one month. There will be some drainage which is initially red, then pink, and then brownish as the dissolvable pack works its way out of the ear. Tell client to report any greenish, yellowish, or foul smelling drainage. Instruct client to take all antibiotics as prescribed and complete the full course of treatment. Advise client there should be very little pain or discomfort but if there is, take prescribed analgesics and notify doctor if pain is prolonged or intense. Warn client that hearing may be decreased for three to four weeks after surgery until gel-foam packing dissolves. Inform client that audiometric testing will be conducted one month after surgery. Instruct client to schedule an appointment with the physician in one month but call physician if uncontrolled pain is experienced or a malodorous, greenish discharge comes from the ear.

▶ Evaluation

Each goal must be evaluated to determine how it has been met by the client.

▲ ▲

▶ *ACOUSTIC NEUROMA*

Acoustic neuroma is a slow-growing and usually benign tumor of the vestibular portion of the inner ear (cranial nerve VIII). Detection at the onset of symptoms is essential and may be accomplished with an MRI. Presenting symptoms of dizziness, tinnitus, and hearing loss are common to many dysfunctions of the ear and the possibility of acoustic neuroma must not be overlooked.

Clients who present with dizziness, tinnitus, and hearing loss should have a complete workup for auditory and vestibular (balance) function. Facial weakness may be caused by compression of the tumor on cranial nerve VIII. The Vth cranial nerve may also be affected as the tumor grows causing paresthesia of the face and loss of the corneal reflex. Large neuromas can cause increased intracranial pressure, papilledema, vomiting, and headache.

▶ *Medical/Surgical Management*

Treatment is almost always surgical excision of the tumor. Although antihistamines may reduce the dizziness, the pharmacologic treatment is only temporary until diagnostic tests are completed and surgery is planned.

▶ *Nursing Process*

Assessment

Subjective Data   Subjective data may be obtained through the client history of the chief complaint, reported signs and symptoms, and all contributing data.

Objective Data   Objective data will be obtained with the physical examination and should include a complete cranial nerve evaluation performed by the physician or audiologist to determine the extent of cranial nerve involvement.

▼ ▼

Possible nursing diagnoses, already covered in this chapter, for a client with acoustic neuroma may include:

- Anxiety, related to decrease or loss of hearing.
- Knowledge deficit, related to preoperative preparations and postoperative care.
- Injury, high risk for, related to dizziness.
- Knowledge deficit, related to activities after surgery.
- Adjustment, impaired, related to hearing loss and possible deafness.

An additional, possible nursing diagnosis for a client with acoustic neuroma may include:

Nursing Diagnoses	Goals	Nursing Interventions
▶ *Grieving, anticipatory, related to diminished quality of life, loss of ability for self-care, or possible loss of life.*	The client will express feelings of grief and demonstrate adaptive coping mechanisms.	Assist the client to express feelings about progressive hearing loss and changes in activities of daily living, employment, and quality of life issues.
		Collaborate with physician and other members of the health care team to provide thorough and clear explanations of the disease process, treatment options, and anticipated results.
		Observe the client's coping styles. Support those that the client finds helpful and explore other coping mechanisms that may prove useful in time (e.g., hobbies and other diversional activities, prayer, reading, and so on).
		Include the family in all interventions that the client desires.

Nursing Diagnoses	Goals	Nursing Interventions
		Examine the family's feelings and ability to cope.
		Consult social services, pastoral care, or other hospital and community resources when appropriate.

▶ Evaluation

Each goal must be evaluated to determine how it has been met by the client.

▲ ▲

▶ OTITIS MEDIA

Otitis media is an inflammation of the external auditory meatus and/or the middle ear and a common cause of conductive hearing loss, though usually temporary. Presenting symptoms include ear pain, fever, redness of auricle and ear canal, and sometimes enlarged lymph nodes over the mastoid process, parotids, and upper neck. Otitis media occurs more frequently in children than in adults.

Fluid accumulates behind the eardrum due to blockage of the eustachian tube (see Figure 28-6). This may be secondary to an upper respiratory infection, allergies, or acute bacterial infection. On physical examination the tympanic membrane may be retracted, normal, or bulging. A pneumatic otoscope allows the doctor to blow soft puffs of air against the tympanic membrane to assess movement. A stiff, nonmoving, or bulging TM may indicate inflammation, or fluid accumulation in the middle ear. Visualization of the normal landmarks may be obscured. The Rinne tuning fork test and audiometry confirm a conductive hearing loss.

▶ Medical/Surgical Management

▶ Medical

Topical heat and systemic analgesics may be used to control pain.

▶ Surgical

Surgical management may be necessary for diagnostic or therapeutic reasons. A myringotomy may be performed. An incision is made in the eardrum and fluid is aspirated. A polyethylene tube may be placed in the eardrum to equalize the air pressure and allow drainage of fluid.

A tympanoplasty may be needed if the tympanic membrane is ruptured. If there is a large tympanic membrane perforation, the malleus, which is connected to the tympanic membrane, or other ossicles may be damaged. Ossicular chain reconstruction typically refers to the removal of the actual bones or some of them and replacement with a plastic prosthesis. Often the prosthesis and the tympanic membrane reconstruction result in a significant improvement in hearing.

A–SEROUS OTITIS MEDIA

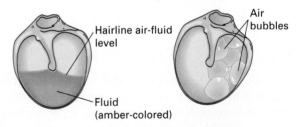

B–ACUTE PURULENT OTITIS MEDIA

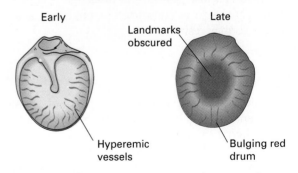

FIGURE 28-6 The tympanic membrane in the presence of otitis media. **(A)** Serous Otitis media; **(B)** Acute purulent otitis media. Hyperemic means there is increased blood within the vessels.

▶ *Pharmacological*

Medications used include the use of decongestants such as pseudoephedrine hydrochloride (Sudafed), antihistamines such as diphenhydramine hydrochloride (Benadryl), and systemic antibiotics such as ampicillin (Omnipen).

▶ *Diet and Activity*

Diet and activity are not restricted unless surgical management is indicated. The information and nursing diagnoses for otosclerosis may be used to guide nursing management.

▼ ▼

Possible nursing diagnoses for a client with otitis media may include:

Nursing Diagnoses	Goals	Nursing Interventions
▶ Pain, acute, related to inflammation in the middle ear.	The client will experience pain relief.	Administer antibiotics as ordered.
		Teach client and family the importance of administering medications as ordered and to complete full course of prescription.
		Administer analgesics as ordered.
		Apply heating pad, set on low, for twenty minutes every two hours. Do not use on small children.
		Teach client if pain is unrelieved in forty-eight hours, to contact physician.

▶ *Evaluation*

Each goal must be evaluated to determine how it has been met by the client.

▲ ▲

▶ *OTITIS EXTERNA*

Otitis externa or "swimmer's ear" typically involves a bacterial infection of the external ear canal skin. The canal skin becomes red and edematous. If the swelling is severe enough, it will block the ear passage and cause a mild conductive hearing loss. Also, in most cases there is a discharge. If the discharge is copious and the canal size is constricted, a mild conductive hearing loss may result.

▶ *MASTOIDITIS*

Mastoiditis is most often the direct result of chronic or recurrent bacterial otitis media. The recurrent infection may find its way into the bone and structures surrounding the middle ear which, if left untreated, can cause severe damage, sensorineural deafness, facial weakness, brain abscess, and meningitis. Other symptoms include earache, fever, headache, and malaise. Antibiotics are given for a trial period. If symptoms do not resolve, surgical intervention such as mastoidectomy or meatoplasty may be necessary.

▶ *DISORDERS OF THE EYE*

Eye disorders may be treated by either an ophthalmologist or an optometrist. An ophthalmologist is a medical doctor who specializes in the diagnosis and treatment, both medical and surgical, of diseases of the eye, visual disorders, and eye injuries. An optometrist is a doctor of optometry and is licensed to examine, diagnose, manage and treat vision problems, diseases, and other abnormalities of the eyes and related structures.

▶ *CATARACTS*

A cataract is a disorder that causes the lens or its capsule to lose its transparency and/or become opaque (see Figure 28-7). The lens is normally clear and transparent and allows light to pass through to the retina. As clouding develops, visual impairment occurs. Cataracts usually affect both eyes; however the degree of visual impairment is often different in each eye.

Cataracts are usually associated with aging; how-

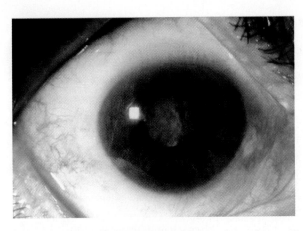

FIGURE 28-7 A cataract results in the loss of transparency of the lens of the eye. (*Courtesy of National Eye Institute, Bethesda, MD*)

ever, they may be congenital, caused by severe eye injury, or secondary to certain systemic diseases characterized by metabolic problems (diabetes mellitus) and chronic eye disease (uveitis). Ophthalmoscopic examination is the primary method of evaluation.

▶ Medical/Surgical Management

▶ Surgical

The only treatment for a cataract is surgical removal of the lens. However, the mere finding of a cataract is not an indication for surgery. Surgery is indicated when significant vision loss has occurred. The lens may be removed by the intracapsular or extracapsular approach. During the intracapsular cataract extraction, the ophthalmologist removes the lens within its capsule. Extracapsular cataract extraction is the procedure most commonly used (see Figure 28-8). The ophthalmologist removes the anterior portion of the capsule and then expresses, or removes, the lens. An intraocular lens (IOL) is generally implanted. Glasses or special contact lenses may also be used.

Most eye surgery is done on an outpatient basis under local anesthesia. General anesthesia can be used at the client's request and for clients who are extremely anxious, deaf, or mentally retarded. A tranquilizer such as diazepam (Valium) is often given to reduce anxiety when receiving injections on the face and around the eye.

Preoperatively, the client can receive several types of eye medications to prepare the eye for surgery: mydriatic (makes pupil dilate) and cycloplegic (paralyzes ciliary muscle) eye drops, antibiotic eye drops as a prophylaxis against infection, and an intravenous infusion of an agent to lower intraocular pressure (mannitol or a carbonic anhydrase inhibitor).

The client is instructed to have a driver available to provide transportation postoperatively because driving is restricted for a few days. After the anesthesia wears off, the client is discharged.

Postoperatively, the client has a patch over the eye. The patch is removed and reapplied on the first postoperative day when miotic (makes pupil contract) eye drops are begun. Mild discomfort and scratchiness are expected. Atropine sulfate eye drops and cold compresses may be ordered to relieve these discomforts.

▶ Nursing Process

Assessment

Subjective Data Obtain a general medical history as well as a history of symptoms. Symptoms may include: haziness, cloudiness, blurred vision, double vision, altered color perception, and glare when looking at lights, especially with night driving. Fear of losing one's eyesight can be very devastating. There is often a great deal of anxiety when the client seeks an eye examination.

Objective Data Upon inspection of the eye the usual black pupil appears clouded, progressing to a milky white appearance which is a characteristic finding of a mature cataract indicating significant vision loss.

Lens Implant Surgery for Cataracts

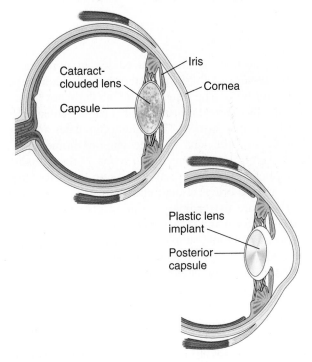

FIGURE 28-8 In extracapsular extraction, the lens is removed, the posterior lens capsule is left intact, and the intraocular lens (IOL) is placed.

▼ ▼

Possible nursing diagnoses for a client with cataracts may include:

Nursing Diagnoses	Goals	Nursing Interventions
▶ *Sensory/perceptual alterations, visual, related to ocular lens opacity.*	The client will demonstrate improved ability to process visual stimuli and communicate visual limitations.	Assess and document baseline visual acuity. Elicit functional description of what the client can and cannot see.
▶ *Injury, high risk for, related to difficulty in processing visual images and altered depth perception.*	The client will avoid activities associated with increased potential for injury.	Teach the client to change position slowly. Teach the client to avoid reaching for objects to maintain stability when ambulating.
▶ *Home maintenance management, impaired, related to age, limited vision or activity restrictions imposed by surgery.*	The client will perform self-care activities in home environment.	Discuss the client's desired location for home recovery following surgery. Discuss the client's ability to meet self-care needs and activities of daily living. Evaluate how the client's current functional ability will be affected by activity restrictions and postoperative care needs. Help the client decide on a realistic site for postoperative care needs.

▶ *Evaluation*

Each goal must be evaluated to determine how it has been met by the client.

▲ ▲

▶ GLAUCOMA

This disorder is characterized by an abnormally high pressure of fluid inside the eyeball (intraocular pressure, IOP). The aqueous humor does not return into the bloodstream through the canal of Schlemm as quickly as it is formed. The fluid accumulates and, by compressing the lens into the vitreous humor, puts pressure on the neurons of the retina. If the pressure continues over a long period of time, it destroys the neurons and brings about blindness.

There are two primary forms of glaucoma: open-angle glaucoma and closed-angle glaucoma. Open-angle glaucoma (chronic simple glaucoma) is characterized by a gradual rise in intraocular pressure and absence of symptoms causing slowly progressive loss of peripheral vision and, when controlled, a late loss of central vision and ultimate blindness. This is the most prevalent form of glaucoma and is usually bilateral. Closed-angle glaucoma (acute glaucoma) is characterized by attacks of suddenly increased intraocular pressure, exhibited clinically by a bulging iris, which is an emer-gency situation. Closed-angle glaucoma is usually unilateral with severe pain and loss of vision caused by acute obstruction of aqueous humor drainage within the eye.

Secondary glaucoma results from ocular or systemic disorders that are responsible for the elevation in IOP. These disorders or conditions indirectly disrupt the activity of the structures involved in circulation and/or reabsorption of aqueous humor. This can happen suddenly and without warning.

▶ *Medical/Surgical Management*

▶ *Medical*

Medical management for glaucoma is focused on drug therapy and the main objective is to reduce intraocular pressure. Two mechanisms for reducing this pressure include: (1) physically constricting the pupil so that the ciliary muscle is contracted, which allows better circulation of the aqueous humor to the site of absorption, and (2) inhibiting the production of aqueous humor.

▶ Surgical

Surgical intervention to facilitate drainage of the aqueous humor is called an iridectomy. A surgical incision is made through the cornea to remove a portion of the iris to facilitate aqueous drainage.

A laser may also be used to treat various eye disorders. In open-angle glaucoma a laser is used to create multiple scars around the trabecular meshwork (a supporting or anchoring strand that allows increased outflow of aqueous humor) thereby reducing intraocular pressure. In closed-angle glaucoma laser energy is used to create a hole in the periphery of the iris, creating an opening between the anterior and posterior chambers for aqueous drainage.

▶ Pharmacological

Drugs that enhance pupillary constriction are commonly used to treat glaucoma. Miotics and cholinesterase inhibitors such as pilocarpine hydrochloride (Isopto Carpine), carbachol (Carbacel) and demecarium bromide (Humorsol) are frequently used.

Beta-adrenergics such as timolol maleate (Timoptic Solution) are the drugs of choice for decreasing IOP. When used as eye drops, beta-adrenergics reduce aqueous humor production without pupil constriction and are used only for clients who have heart conditions.

Carbonic anhydrase inhibitors, such as acetazolamide (Diamox), reduce production of aqueous humor to help maintain a lowered IOP. Side effects reported are numbness, weakness, tingling of extremities, and rashes. Adrenergics such as epinephrine bitartrate (Epitrate) also reduce aqueous humor production. Osmotic agents such as mannitol and glycerin (Osmoglyn) may be administered systemically to the client with closed-angle glaucoma in an emergency as an effort to decrease IOP. The high osmolarity of these agents is used to draw fluid into the intravascular space, which lowers the IOP.

It is important to continue the use of eye medications as ordered. The client needs continued medical supervision for observation of intraocular pressure to ensure control of the disorder. The client should avoid exertion, stooping, heavy lifting, or wearing constrictive clothing as these increase intraocular pressure.

▶ Nursing Process

Assessment

Subjective Data Obtain a history or presence of risk factors: positive family history (believed to be linked in open-angle glaucoma), eye tumor, intraocular hemorrhage, intraocular inflammation (uveitis), or contusion of the eye from trauma during cataract surgery.

Symptoms of open-angle glaucoma include gradual loss of peripheral vision, eye pain, difficulty adjusting to darkness, halos around lights and an inability to detect color. For closed-angle glaucoma symptoms include sudden onset of severe pain in the eye often accompanied by headache, nausea, vomiting, malaise, rainbow halos around lights and blurred vision.

Objective Data Acute increased intraocular pressure (21 to 32 mmHg) as measured with a tonometer. Normal = 12 to 22 mmHg.

▼ ▼

A possible nursing diagnosis for a client with glaucoma may include:

Nursing Diagnoses	Goals	Nursing Interventions
▶ Pain, acute, related to closed-angle glaucoma.	The client will verbalize relief from discomfort.	Administer prescribed ophthalmic agent for glaucoma.
		Notify physician of the following: hypotension, urinary output less than 240 mL for eight hours, no relief in eye pain within thirty minutes of drug therapy, and continual diminishing visual acuity.
		Monitor blood pressure, pulse, and respiration every four hours if not receiving osmotic agent intravenously and every two hours if receiving intravenous osmotic agent.

(continued)

Nursing Diagnoses	Goals	Nursing Interventions
		Monitor degree of eye pain every thirty minutes during the acute phase.
		Monitor intake and output every eight hours while receiving intravenous osmotic agent.
		Monitor visual acuity prior to each instillation of prescribed ophthalmic agent by asking if objects are clear or blurred and if the client can read printed material held at arm's length.
		Remind the client that miotics may cause blurred vision for one to two hours after use and that adaptation to dark environments is difficult because of the pupillary constriction.

▶ Evaluation

Each goal must be evaluated to determine how it has been met by the client.

▲ ▲

▶ RETINAL DETACHMENT

In retinal detachment, there is an actual separation of the retina from the choroid. Partial separation becomes complete, if untreated, with the subsequent total loss of vision. A tear or hole in the retina can extend the separation as vitreous humor seeps through the opening and separates the retina from the choroid. The cause of retinal detachment may be from severe trauma to the eye or from intraocular disorders such as cataract extraction, perforating injuries, or severe **myopia** (nearsightedness). This condition is painless since there are no pain receptors in the retina.

▶ Medical/Surgical Management

▶ Medical

Early corrective intervention to reattach the retina may use one of several techniques. Three procedures can be used to create an inflammatory reaction that when healing and scarring occur the retina is reattached to the choroid. One such technique is electrodiathermy (heat therapy) which uses an ultrasonic probe to burn (seal) the scleral surface directly over the retinal break. Another technique is cryotherapy which uses an intensely cold probe applied to the scleral surface directly over the hole in the retina. Laser photocoagulation is also used to seal tears or holes in the retina.

▶ Surgical

A surgical procedure called scleral buckling is sometimes used. This operation reduces the scleral surface and allows contact between the choroid and retina.

▶ Pharmacological

Cycloplegic-mydriatic and antiinfective eyedrops are often ordered following the attachment procedure.

▶ Activity

Bed rest and patches on one or both eyes restricts activity. If air is injected into the vitreous humor, the client either lies prone or sits forward with the unaffected eye upward.

▶ Nursing Process

Assessment

Subjective Data   Obtain a medical history of presence of causative factors: trauma, recent cataract surgery, eye tumor, severe myopia, uveitis. The client may describe sudden flashes of light (photopsia), floating spots (caused by bleeding into the vitreous cavity), blurred vision that becomes progressively worse, or complaints of a sensation of a veil in the line of sight.

Objective Data   Ophthalmoscopic examination visualizes the detachment.

▼ ▼

Possible nursing diagnoses for a client with retinal detachment may include:

Nursing Diagnoses	Goals	Nursing Interventions
▶ *Anxiety, related to sensory visual impairment and lack of understanding about treatment.*	The client will demonstrate reduction of emotional stress, fear, and depression; and acceptance of surgery.	Assess degree and duration of visual impairment.
		Encourage conversation to determine client's concerns, feelings, and level of understanding.
		Answer questions, offer support, assist client to devise methods for coping.
		Orient client to new surroundings.
		Explain perioperative routine. Preoperative: Level of activity-ocular rest which includes bilateral eye patching and bed rest to facilitate settling of the retina and prevent detachment from worsening. The client will be NPO after midnight. The affected eye is maximally dilated before surgery to permit adequate visualization of the fundus. Intraoperative: Client must lie still during surgery or give surgeon warning if needs to cough or change position. Face covered with drapes. Air and oxygen provided. Unfamiliar noises from equipment. Monitoring, including frequent blood pressure measurements. Postoperative: Positioning (supine with a small pillow under the head), bilateral eye patches, activity restrictions, and need to call for assistance with ambulation until stable and vision is adequate.
		Explain interventions clearly.
		Announce yourself with each interaction; interpret unfamiliar sounds; use touch to assist with verbal communication.
		Encourage to carry out ADL as ability allows.
		Order finger foods for those who cannot see well enough or do not have the coping skills to use implements.
		Encourage participation of family or significant others in client care.
		Encourage participation in social and diversional activities as allowed (visitor, radio, audio tapes, television, crafts, games).
▶ *Injury, high risk for, related to visual impairment or knowledge deficit.*	The client will not have injury caused by visual impairment.	Assist client when able to ambulate postoperatively until stable and has adequate vision or coping skills (remember that clients with bilateral eye patches are unable to see).
		Assist client in arranging environment and do not rearrange furnishings without reorienting client.
		Discuss importance of wearing metal shield or glasses as ordered.
		Apply no pressure to the affected eye.
		Use proper procedure to administer eye medications.

(continued)

Nursing Diagnoses	Goals	Nursing Interventions
▶ *Pain, related to trauma, increased IOP, surgical intervention, or instillation of dilating drops.*	The client will report reduction of pain.	Administer medications for pain and IOP control as prescribed.
		Apply cold compresses as ordered for blunt trauma.
		Reduce light levels; light dimmed, shades/drapes drawn.
		Encourage use of dark glasses in strong light.

▶ *Evaluation*

Each goal must be evaluated to determine how it has been met by the client.

▲ ▲

▶ *INFECTIONS OF THE EYE*

▶ *Keratitis*

Keratitis is inflammation of the cornea that may be caused by infection, irritation, injury, or allergies. Symptoms associated with keratitis include severe eye pain, red watering eye, photophobia, sometimes reduced vision, and sometimes rash, e.g., herpes simplex, herpes zoster, or rosacea.

Treatment of keratitis includes optical anesthetics to relieve pain and mydriatics to dilate the pupil. Dark glasses should be worn to relieve the photophobia. Antibiotic solutions are prescribed for the specific type of infection, since the microorganism may be bacterial, viral, or fungal.

▶ *Stye*

A stye is also referred to as a hordeolum. It is a pustular inflammation of an eyelash follicle or sebaceous gland on the lid margin commonly caused by staphylococcal organisms. Symptoms include pain, redness, and swelling of a specific area of the eyelid. Treatment consists of warm compresses and topical antibiotic ointments. More severe cases may require incision and drainage. Once the pus drains, the pain is relieved and healing begins.

▶ *Chalazion*

A chalazion is a cyst of the meibomian glands, which are sebaceous glands located at the junction of the conjunctiva and inner eyelid margins. The hard cyst is filled with fatty material from the chronically obstructed meibomian glands. The inherent feature of a chalazion is painless localized swelling that develops over a period of weeks. Treatment usually involves surgical excision if the cyst is large, becomes infected, or interferes with vision or closure of the eyelids. The cyst remains when the inflammation subsides.

▶ *Conjunctivitis (Pink-eye)*

Conjunctivitis is an inflammation of the conjunctiva, a membrane that lines the inside of the eyelids and covers the cornea, that results from invasion by bacterial, viral, or rickettsial organisms, allergens, or irritants. Symptoms include burning and itching of eyes, discharge, swelling, pain, and redness. Treatment consists of applying warm compresses using saline or boric acid solution and instilling antibiotic or antiviral ointments. When caused by allergens treatment includes avoiding the allergen, taking antihistamines, or being desensitized.

Conjunctivitis is contagious. Proper handwashing must be done by nurse and client. Gloves should be worn when applying compresses or instilling ointment. The client's linen should be disinfected to prevent spread of the infection.

▶ *REFRACTIVE ERRORS*

Refraction is the deflection or bending of light rays when they pass from a medium of one density to a medium of another density. In the case of the eye, light waves pass through the air, less dense, into the fluids of the eye, more dense so that they can be brought to focus on the retina. The eye has four media of refraction: cornea, aqueous humor, lens, and vitreous humor.

Refractive errors include myopia (nearsightedness), **hyperopia** (farsightedness), **astigmatism** (asymmet-

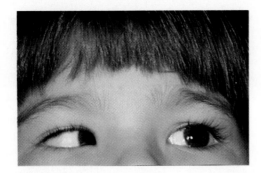

FIGURE 28-9 Strabismus.

ric focus), **presbyopia** (inability to change focus), and **strabismus** (inability of the eyes to focus in the same direction). Figure 28-9 shows a client with strabismus.

With myopia, parallel light rays come to focus in front of the retina because the refractive system is too strong, or the eyeball is elongated. Near vision is normal, but distant vision is poor.

With hyperopia, parallel light rays come to focus behind the retina because the refractive system is too weak or the eyeball is flattened. Vision beyond 20 feet is normal, but near vision is poor. Figure 28-10 illustrates the light rays focus for myopia and hyperopia.

Astigmatism is a visual defect due to unequal curvatures of the refractive surfaces of the eye. Light rays from a point do not come to focus on the retina which creates visual distortion.

Presbyopia is the loss of elasticity of the lens of the eye caused by aging that causes the near point of vision to recede. The eye loses the ability to accommodate to near objects but remains accommodated for far objects.

▶ Medical/Surgical Management

▶ Medical

Refractory errors may be corrected by prescription glasses or contact lenses. The corrective lenses bend light rays to compensate for a client's refractive error.

▶ Surgical

Radial keratotomy is a surgical procedure used to correct myopia and astigmatism. Under local anesthesia, incisions that resemble the spokes of a wheel are made in the cornea. These incisions start near the center of the cornea and extend outward to the edge. The incisions are made by a special knife that can be calibrated to cut at a predetermined depth. After the cuts are made, pressure in the anterior chamber of the eye reshapes the cornea to a normal or near-normal curvature.

▶ Nursing Process

Assessment

Subjective Data Obtain a general medical history as well as a history of symptoms. Symptoms may include blurred vision, headache, or eye fatigue.

Objective Data The client is asked to view an eye chart while lenses of different strengths are systematically placed in front of the eye. The client is asked if the lenses sharpen or blur vision. The power or strength of the lens necessary to permit focusing of the image on the retina is expressed in measurements called diopters.

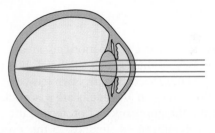

A Normal eye
Light rays focus on the retina

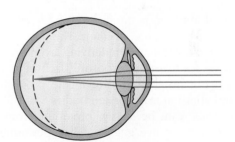

B Myopia (nearsightedness)
Light rays focus in front
of the retina

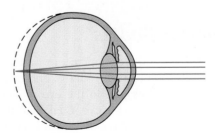

C Hyperopia (farsightedness)
Light rays focus beyond
the retina

FIGURE 28-10 Refraction. **(A)** Normal eye; **(B)** Myopia; **(C)** Hyperopia.

▼ ▼

A possible nursing diagnosis for a client with refractive errors may include:

Nursing Diagnoses	Goals	Nursing Interventions
▶ *Anxiety, related to impaired vision and having to wear glasses or contact lenses.*	The client will accept wearing glasses or contact lenses.	Allow client to discuss impact of wearing glasses or contact lenses.
		Encourage client to wear the glasses or contact lenses as prescribed.

▶ *Evaluation*

Each goal must be evaluated to determine how it has been met by the client.

▲ ▲

▶ *EYE INJURIES*

Injury to the eye or periorbital area can result from a variety of things such as chemical sprays, tree branches, slingshots, BB guns, lawn mowers, and fireworks. Both children and adults are susceptible to eye injuries and the importance of protecting the eyes cannot be overemphasized. Injuries to the eyes require immediate attention by an ophthalmologist. Even a few hours delay in treatment may lead to permanent damage.

Corneal abrasion is the disruption of cells and the loss of the superficial epithelium. The outer surface is easily separated from the underlying layers and can be injured or destroyed by exposure (lack of moisture), chemical irritants that dissolve in the protective tear film, and abrasion from foreign bodies.

The eyes can be easily protected from injury by wearing protective goggles when performing eye hazardous tasks. Those who wear contact lenses should follow the recommendations for wearing them during certain activities such as swimming or when sleeping.

▶ *Foreign Bodies*

Foreign bodies in the conjunctiva or on the cornea may cause excessive tearing, redness, and complaints of a foreign body sensation in the eye or under the eyelid, or just irritation in the eye. Conjunctival foreign bodies often become embedded in the conjunctiva under the upper eyelid. The lid must be everted and the client is instructed to look up to facilitate inspection and removal. If the particle is not located and removed, sterile fluorescein drops or strips should be instilled to visualize minute foreign bodies not readily visible with the naked eye.

▶ *Chemical Burns*

Emergency treatment of chemical burns to the conjunctiva or cornea includes immediate lavage of the eye with tap water and referral to an emergency room or ophthalmologist. In the emergency room, a specially made lid speculum is placed directly on the eyeball and connected to a minimum of one liter of isotonic saline solution for irrigation. A topical anesthetic may be instilled to minimize the pain during irrigation. Do not attempt to neutralize the chemical, since the heat generated by the chemical reaction may cause further injury. Both eyes should then be patched to allow more comfort and the client should be referred to a physician.

▶ *IMPAIRED VISION*

The term blindness evokes an image of total darkness and is used for many legal purposes when central visual acuity is 20/200 or less with corrective lenses, in the better eye. Those who have visual acuity between 20/70 and 20/200 in the better eye, with the use of glasses, are often referred to as partially sighted.

The aids that follow are designed to make the most of the available vision (those in italics can also be used by persons who are blind): magnifying glasses, hand and stand magnifiers, telescopes, large print books, newspapers, magazines, talking books, *Braille,* closed-circuit television which produces highly magnified image, *tactually marked watches and clocks, tactually modified table top games,* enlarged telephone dials, kitchen implements, tools, medication devices, talking clocks, timers, scales, calculators, computers, *text scanner which converts text to audio mode or Braille,* speech synthesizer, flashlight eye sonar devices, canes, laser canes, and seeing eye dogs.

▶ MACULAR DEGENERATION

Macular degeneration is atrophy or deterioration of the macula, the point on the retina where light rays meet as they are focused by the cornea and lens of the eye. The person loses central vision, but still has peripheral vision.

The most common form of macular degeneration is associated with the aging process and is called age-related macular degeneration. Other forms of this disorder include exudative (wet) macular degeneration (sudden growth of new blood vessels in the area of the macula) and injury, infection, or inflammation that damages the macula.

▶ Medical/Surgical Management

▶ Medical

The treatment of age-related macular degeneration is geared toward assisting the client to maximize the use of the remaining vision. The loss of central vision may interfere with the client's ability to read, write, recognize safety hazards, and drive.

Management of clients with exudative macular degeneration is geared toward halting the initiating process and identifying further changes in visual perception. Fluid and blood may resorb in a small percentage of clients with exudative degeneration. Laser therapy to seal the leaking blood vessels in or near the macula may also limit the extent of the damage.

▶ Nursing Process

Assessment

Subjective Data   Obtain a general medical history as well as a history of symptoms. Symptoms would include blurred vision, disturbance in color vision (colors become dim), difficulty in reading or doing close work, distortion of objects (especially those with lines), and an empty area within the central field of vision.

Objective Data   Assess behavior including coping mechanisms such as turning head to use peripheral vision.

▼ ▼

A possible nursing diagnosis for the client with macular degeneration may include:

Nursing Diagnoses	Goals	Nursing Interventions
▶ Sensory-perceptual alterations, visual, related to macular degeneration.	The client will discuss the impact of vision loss on lifestyle.	Allow client to express feelings about vision loss such as its impact on lifestyle. Convey a willingness to listen, but do not pressure client to talk.
		Provide a safe environment by removing excess furniture or equipment from client's surroundings.
		Orient client to surroundings and show how to use call light.
		Do not move furniture or leave objects in hallway.
		Modify the environment to maximize any vision the client may have.
		Always introduce yourself or announce your presence on entering the client's room; let client know when you are leaving.
		Provide sensory stimulation by using tactile, auditory, and gustatory stimuli to help compensate for vision loss.
		Suggest large print-books, talking books, audiotapes, or radio as preferred by client.
		Provide reality orientation if client is confused or disoriented.

(continued)

Nursing Diagnoses	Goals	Nursing Interventions
		Give clear, concise explanations of treatments and procedures but avoid information overload.
		When speaking, enunciate words clearly, slowly, and in a normal speaking voice.
		Make sure that health care personnel are aware of client's vision loss. Record information on the client's chart or post in room.
		Respond to call light quickly.
		Provide continuity by assigning same staff members to care for client when possible.
		Refer to appropriate community resources.

▶ *Evaluation*

Each goal must be evaluated to determine how it has been met by the client.

▲ ▲

Sample Nursing Care Plan: The Client with Macular Degeneration

Mr. Datal is a sixty-year-old high school Latin teacher. He describes having blurred vision in both eyes with a gradual loss of vision in only the right eye. He has trouble reading and is afraid to drive because he can no longer recognize safety hazards. He denies having pain. He also relates having fallen several times recently at home while going up and down the stairs. The family practitioner referred him to an ophthalmologist who diagnosed Mr. Datal as having macular degeneration in the right eye.

Nursing Diagnosis 1 Sensory-perceptual alterations, visual, related to macular degeneration as evidenced by his inability to recognize safety hazards when driving.

Goals	Nursing Interventions	Rationale	Evaluation
Mr. Datal will discuss impact of vision loss on lifestyle.	Encourage Mr. Datal to express feelings about vision loss, such as the impact on lifestyle.	Allowing Mr. Datal to discuss the impact of vision loss aids in the acceptance of it.	Mr. Datal discussed the effects of vision loss on his lifestyle and contacted a local agency that provides assistance to the visually impaired.
	Convey a willingness to listen, but do not pressure Mr. Datal to talk. Discuss Mr. Datal's current ability to meet self-care needs and activities of daily living.	Discussion can determine needs for assistance which will, in part, be based on current functional level and determines Mr. Datal's awareness of his limitations.	
	Educate Mr. Datal in alternative ways of coping with vision loss; care of such adaptive devices as eyeglasses, magnifying glass, and contact lenses.	A knowledgeable client will be better able to cope with vision loss.	
	Refer to appropriate community resources to help Mr. Datal and his family adapt to his vision loss.	Support from outside resources will help Mr. Datal and his family cope better with his vision loss.	

Nursing Diagnosis 2 Injury, high risk for, related to difficulty in processing visual images and altered depth perception as evidenced by recent falls.

Goals	Nursing Interventions	Rationale	Evaluation
Mr. Datal will not experience injury or visual compromise resulting from a fall.	Advise Mr. Datal that depth perception is changed with macular degeneration.	Information promotes understanding.	Mr. Datal has not fallen in two weeks.
	Teach Mr. Datal to avoid reaching for objects for stability when ambulating.	Objects may not be located where they are perceived. Excessive reaching alters the center of gravity which can precipitate a fall.	

(continued)

| | Advise Mr. Datal to go up and down steps one at a time. | Going up and down steps one at a time enhances the sense of balance. | |

Nursing Diagnosis 3 Home maintenance management, impaired, related to limited vision, as evidenced by recent falls at home.

Goals	Nursing Interventions	Rationale	Evaluation
Mr. Datal will develop a plan for self-care in the desired living environment.	Inform Mr. Datal about required self-care activities: personal care, eyedrop instillation, activities permitted, activity restrictions, medications, and how to monitor for complications.	Knowing what self-care activities are needed will help Mr. Datal plan for his care at home.	Mr. Datal is working on a plan so he can care for himself at home.
	Assist Mr. Datal to determine which activities will require assistance: personal care, meal preparation, eyedrop instillation, or shopping.	Helps Mr. Datal to plan for his care at home.	
	Evaluate sources of assistance: friends/family, home health care (skilled nursing care), or home care aids.	Determines availability of assistance.	
	Critique the safety of Mr. Datal's home: location of telephone, emergency plan, presence of loose rugs or carpets.	Changes can then be made to make Mr. Datal's home safer.	

SENSE OF TASTE

The special sense of taste (gustation) serves as a protector from rotten or putrid food and provides delightful sensations of creamy chocolate, crunchy chips, chewy taffy, and fruitful pies. Taste sensors are most efficient at room temperature and respond only to substances in solution. The taste buds are located in four areas of the tongue that sense sweet, salt, bitter, and sour as shown in Figure 28-11.

The tongue is not only an important organ of taste, but also aids in swallowing and speech. Motor movement is controlled by the hypoglossal (XII) nerve and temperature and position are controlled by the trigeminal (V) nerve and glossopharyngeal (IX) nerve.

Taste sensations can be altered secondary to neurological disorders or trauma. Clients who complain of food not "tasting good" should be evaluated for possible causes including dietary habits, medication use, smoking and caffeine use, as well as olfactory disturbances. The sense of taste works very closely with the sense of smell for identification of the taste sensations.

SENSE OF SMELL

The sense of smell (olfaction) also serves as a guardian from danger. Our nose warns us of impending danger from gas leaks, smoke, fires, rancid meat or fish, and sour dairy products. Body odors and halitosis are obvious clues regarding the need to maintain personal hygiene and dental care.

Disorders of the olfactory sense often go unnoticed. Sexual function and emotional changes can be associated with a loss of smell. New tests such as the University of Pennsylvania Smell Identification Test (UPSIT) allow self-testing of smelling deficiencies. Early identification of the loss of the sense of smell may offer clues to alterations in dietary habits, weight loss or gain, anorexia, malnourishment, and changes in daily habits such as bathing and brushing teeth. The receptors for the sense of smell are located in the roof of the nasal cavity. If these cells are damaged, the sense of smell is impaired. The body cannot regenerate the olfactory cells.

SENSE OF TOUCH

The sense of touch (tactile) includes sensations pertaining to the skin. The tactile receptors are located throughout the integumentary system. Cutaneous sensations of touch, pressure, vibration, cold, heat, and pain are examples. Clients who are unable to sense temperature variations should be taught cautionary measures when applying heat or cold therapies, preparing bath water, cooking or exposing self to hot or cold climates and environmental temperatures.

Clients with reduced or loss of tactile sensation risk injury when their condition confines them to bed. They are unable to sense pressure on bony prominences or the need to change position. The nurse's role to reduce or prevent impairment of skin integrity is important and crucial. Timely positioning, securing tubes or devices away from the client's body, and using products to minimize skin breakdown are a few of the interventions vital to excellent client care.

▶ Proprioception

Proprioception is the awareness of precise position and movement of parts of the body such as the head, arms, or legs. Sensory nerve endings in muscles, tendons, and joints work with the inner ear to maintain proper position and movement.

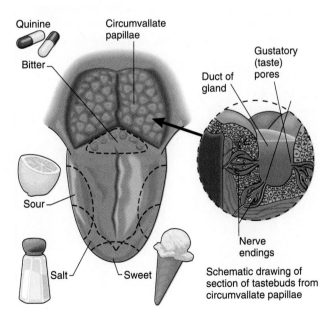

FIGURE 28-11 Taste regions of the tongue.

► *CASE STUDY*

Katie Rollins is a thirty-four-year-old nurse who was diagnosed with a right ear hearing impairment during a routine physical examination. She admitted to her doctor that she noticed she would only use her left ear to talk on the phone and that she had particular difficulty hearing her family or friends in a crowded restaurant or other public settings. She also noted that her husband asked her why she played the television so loud, yet if he turned it down to his normal hearing level, she could not hear it clearly. Her physician ordered an audiogram which showed a conductive hearing loss of 40 percent secondary to otosclerosis. Hearing in her left ear was normal.

Katie's doctor gave her three medical treatment options.

1. Do nothing and monitor her hearing impairment by audiogram every six months. If it were to worsen, other options would be considered.
2. Be fitted with a hearing aid.
3. Have a surgical procedure to correct the hearing loss.

Katie agreed to have surgery. She thought she would be too self-conscious to wear a hearing aid, after all she was only thirty-four, but she simply could not ignore the problem by doing nothing. Katie was scheduled for same-day surgery.

The following questions will guide your development of a Nursing Care Plan for the case study.

1. What diagnostic tests were done on the initial examination to diagnose a conductive hearing loss? List other diagnostic tests that may have been ordered for Katie.

2. How is a conductive hearing loss differentiated from a sensorineural hearing loss?

3. What does an audiogram tell you? What special things should Katie know before she has the audiogram.

4. Describe the surgical procedure that will most likely be used to correct the conductive hearing loss.

5. What will you teach Katie prior to her surgery about the procedure and expected postoperative course?

6. List four individualized nursing diagnoses and expected outcomes for Katie and nursing interventions for each diagnosis.

7. How might Katie's pain be controlled?

8. Describe the expected discharge instructions that Katie must know related to diet, medications, activity restrictions, and follow-up care.

Summary

- Hearing loss may be conductive, sensorineural, or a combination of the two. It may also be congenital.
- Meniere's disease is a result of excessive accumulation of endolymph causing severe vertigo, dizziness, and hearing loss. Treatment is primarily symptomatic.
- Otosclerosis is a conductive hearing loss resulting from fixation of the stapes and may be treated medically with the use of a hearing aid or surgically with a stapedectomy.
- Acoustic neuroma is a slow-growing, often benign tumor that may cause a hearing loss from impinging on the eighth cranial nerve. Surgical treatment is recommended.
- Otitis media is inflammation of the middle ear. Treatment usually includes antibiotics, decongestants, and possibly a myringotomy.
- Many resources are available for the hearing impaired through community and national agencies.
- The special senses of taste, smell, and touch are essential to our enjoyment of life and serve to protect us from danger or harm.

Review Questions

1. The three bones of the middle ear are:
   a. hammer, nail, and stirrup.
   b. malleus, incus, and cochlea.
   c. malleus, humorous, and stapes.
   d. malleus, incus, and stapes.

2. In a conductive hearing loss:
   a. the endolymph may cross the capillary membrane and mix with the perilymph resulting in severe vertigo.
   b. the ossicles of the middle ear fracture resulting in a tear of the eighth cranial nerve.
   c. sound waves are not transmitted through the ear canal to inner ear fluid.
   d. a tumor in the inner ear blocks the flow of fluid through the bony and membranous labyrinths.

3. A possible nursing diagnosis for a client with Meniere's disease is:
   a. activity intolerance related to impaired hearing.
   b. knowledge deficit related to surgical shunt placement to drain excessive endolymph.
   c. communication, impaired, verbal, related to tinnitus.
   d. injury, high risk, related to Menier's disease.

4. Persons with hearing impairment or loss may benefit from:
   a. sitting in the middle of a crowded room so as to listen to all conversations at once.
   b. learning to lip read with family members.
   c. using a poorly fitted hearing aid with proper amplification.
   d. cupping the ear and turning the head toward the person speaking to them.

5. Chemical burns of the eye are treated with:
   a. local anesthetics and antibacterial drops for twenty-four to thirty-six hours.
   b. hot compresses applied at fifteen-minute intervals.
   c. flushing of the lids, conjunctiva, and cornea with water.
   d. cleansing of the conjunctiva with a small cotton-tipped applicator.

6. Postoperatively, the client who has cataract surgery should be placed:
   a. flat on their back with pillows supporting both sides of the head to prevent unnecessary movement.
   b. in high-Fowler's position with the neck supported with a neck collar to prevent unnecessary jarring and to minimize eye movement.
   c. on the side opposite the surgery to eliminate pressure near the surgical area.
   d. supine with a small pillow under the head.

7. Increased ocular pressure is indicated by a reading of:
   a. 0 to 5 mmHg.
   b. 6 to 10 mmHg.
   c. 11 to 20 mmHg.
   d. 23 to 30 mmHg.

8. A clinical symptom(s) of a detached retina is (are):
   a. a sensation of floating particles.
   b. an area of vague vision.
   c. momentary flashes of light.
   d. pain in the eye.

9. Macular degeneration is characterized by:
   a. purulent periorbital drainage.
   b. pupil dilation.
   c. loss of central vision.
   d. ptosis (droopy lid).

Critical Thinking Questions

1 What would have to change in your life if you suddenly could not see?

2. What would change in your life if you suddenly could not hear?

Medical Terminology

audio-	pertaining to hearing
audiogram	record of hearing test
cochlea-	pertaining to a snail
cochlea	spiral-shaped bony portion of the inner ear
endo-	within
endolymph	fluid within the cochlear duct
lymph	colorless fluid
ocular	pertaining to or affecting the eye
oculo-	a combining form denoting relationship to the eye
oculus	the organ of vision
optic	pertaining to the eye
optical	pertaining to or subserving vision
ophthalmic	pertaining to the eye
ophthalmology	branch of medicine dealing with the eye, its anatomy, physiology, and pathology
oto-	pertaining to the ear
otitis	inflammation of the ear
peri-	around, within
perilymph	fluid within the inner ear
tympan-	pertaining to a drum
tympanic membrane	the eardrum that separates the outer and inner ear
vestibule	a space or cavity that serves as an entrance or passageway
vestibular apparatus	sends messages between the inner ear and the brain related to the position and movement of the head.

News Flash: Photorefractive Keratectomy

Photorefractive keratectomy (PRK) is a new procedure that will correct refractive errors such as myopia (nearsightedness) and hyperopia (farsightedness). It was recently approved by the FDA for the general public.

An excimer laser is used to shape the cornea by removing tenths of microns of cells from the cornea. The excimer laser breaks the molecular bonds of the corneal stroma while inflicting no underlying thermal trauma. The laser is pulsed (5 or 10 pulses per second) and the shaping is computer controlled. The ablation of the cells from the cornea is only a fraction of the true depth of the cornea and does not weaken the cornea.

The client undergoes routine preoperative procedures such as an extensive eye exam. The operation is done under local anesthetic and takes less than ten minutes to complete. The client may experience mild pain within the first twelve to twenty-four hours and have complete vision restored in as few as seven days postoperatively. Trials thus far have proven highly successful. Side effects are reportedly few and may include glare or halos at night, loss of corrected vision and scar formation. (*Maquen, et al., 1994*).

UNIT
9

System Regulation

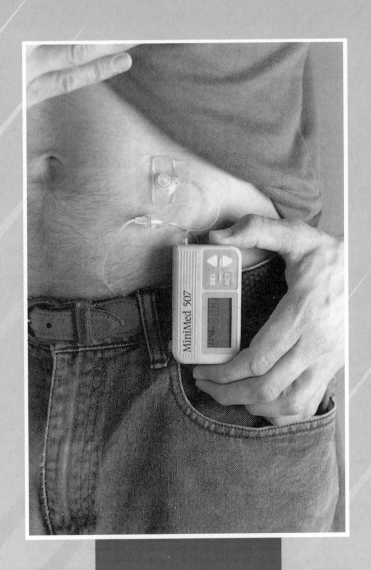

CHAPTER 29

Endocrine Disorders

Russlyn A. St. John

▶ *KEY TERMS*

agranulocytosis
alopecia
autosomal
Chvostek's sign
endocrine
exophthalmos
goiter
gynecomastia
hormone
hypovolemia
iatrogenic
idiopathic
paroxysmal
prognathism
tetany
Trousseau's sign

LIST OF DISORDERS

Pituitary Disorders

- Hyperpituitarism
- Hypopituitarism
- Simmonds' Disease
- Pituitary Tumors
- Diabetes Insipidus

Thyroid Disorders

- Hyperthyroidism
- Hypothyroidism
- Thyroid Tumors
- Cancer of the Thyroid
- Goiter
- Hashimoto's Thyroiditis

Parathyroid Disorders

- Hyperparathyroidism
- Hypoparathyroidism

Adrenal Disorders

- Cushing's Syndrome (Adrenal Hyperfunction)
- Addison's Disease (Adrenal Hypofunction)
- Pheochromocytoma

LEARNING OBJECTIVES

Upon completion of this chapter the learner should be able to:

- Define key terms.
- Identify and locate the endocrine glands and list function(s) and hormone(s) secreted by each.

- Discuss rationale for the pituitary gland being traditionally called the "master" gland.
- Compare symptoms of the disease process resulting from a hyper- or hyposecretion of an endocrine gland.

- Discuss assessment techniques for a client suspected of having an endocrine disorder.
- Formulate a nursing care plan for the client with an endocrine disorder.

▶ *MAKING THE CONNECTION*

Refer to the topics in the following chapters to increase your understanding of endocrine disorders:

- **Chapter 10, Nursing Assessment:** Head-to-Toe Assessment, p. 176
- **Chapter 14, Fluid, Electrolyte, and Acid-Base Balances:** Basic Physiology of Body Fluids and Electrolytes, p. 268; Hypokalemia, p. 277; Sample Nursing Care Plan: The Client with Cushing Syndrome Due to Long-Term Use of Corticosteroids, p. 280; Hypercalcemia, p. 282; Hypomagnesemia, p. 283; Hypermagnesemia, p. 285
- **Chapter 15, Oncology Nursing:** Lymphomas, p. 313
- **Chapter 16, Caring for the Older Adult:** Exercise, p. xx; Common Disorders Related to Aging/Endocrine System, p. 345

- **Chapter 20, Cardiac Disorders:** Cardiac Dysrhythmias, p. 455
- **Chapter 24, Allergies, Immune, and Autoimmune Disorders:** Myasthenia Gravis, p. 609
- **Chapter 26, Musculoskeletal Disorders:** Common Diagnostic Tests, p. 650; Musculoskeletal Assessment, p. 650
- **Chapter 27, Nervous System Disorders:** Basic Neurological Assessment, p. 686
- **Chapter 31, Female Reproductive Disorders:** Anatomy and Physiology Review, p. 857; Common Diagnostic Tests, p. 859
- **Chapter 32, Male Reproductive Disorders:** Anatomy and Physiology Review, p. 915; Common Diagnostic Tests, p. 917

INTRODUCTION

The endocrine system is unique in that the components are not in direct physical contact but scattered throughout the body. The endocrine system provides the same general functions as the nervous system: communication and control. The endocrine system is generally slower and has longer lasting control over the various body activities and functions. It exerts this control through the secretion of hormones that circulate through the blood. A malfunction of any part of the endocrine system can result in a shift of homeostasis with far-reaching systemic reactions.

Assessment of the endocrine system is difficult. Not only are the components not in direct contact, but only the thyroid gland is close enough to the body surface for direct physical assessment. Still the nurse needs to be familiar with the normal functioning of the endocrine system. In assessing the client for endocrine dysfunction, the nurse must take note of negative findings as well as positive ones. The nurse's assessment must also include results of diagnostic tests as well as any precipitating or aggravating factors. The nurse

must detect the connecting link between the signs and symptoms exhibited by the client with the involved gland of the endocrine system.

ANATOMY AND PHYSIOLOGY REVIEW

The endocrine system is composed of a group of various glands scattered throughout the body. The term **endocrine** (endo-within, crin-secrete) indicates that the secretions formed by these glands directly enter the blood or lymph circulation, rather than being transported via tubes or ducts. These secretions, called **hormones**, are chemical substances that initiate or regulate activity of another organ, system, or gland in another part of the body. The level of hormone in the blood is regulated by the homeostasis mechanism called negative feedback. If the blood level for a specific hormone falls below normal, negative feedback causes the specific endocrine gland to produce more of the hormone to increase the hormone to the normal level.

The glands discussed in this chapter that comprise

the endocrine system are: the hypothalamus, pituitary, thyroid, parathyroid, and adrenals (see Figure 29-1). Several endocrine glands such as the pineal, thymus, pancreas, ovaries, and testes are of great importance; however, they will be discussed in other chapters in connection with the organ system in which they function.

The pituitary gland consists of an anterior and a posterior lobe. It has traditionally been called the "master" gland because so many of its secretions influence other endocrine glands and body systems. It is attached to the hypothalamus by a stalk called the infundibulum. The hypothalamus is located in the lower portion of the brain and produces secretions influencing the production and release of the anterior pituitary hormones as well as the production of the posterior pituitary hormones. Both the pituitary and hypothalamus are located in the head. The pituitary, about the size of a pea, is located in the sella turcica, a small depression in the sphenoid bone. The anterior pituitary, or adenohypophysis, produces and secretes the following seven hormones:

- Thyroid-stimulating hormone (TSH)
- Adrenocorticotropic hormone (ACTH)
- Follicle-stimulating hormone (FSH)
- Luteinizing hormone (LH)
- Melanocyte-stimulating hormone (MSH)
- Growth hormone (GH)
- Prolactin or lactogenic hormone.

The posterior pituitary, or neurohypophysis, releases two hormones—antidiuretic hormone (ADH) and oxytocin. The pituitary hormones have a variety of functions. Refer to Table 29-1 for specific endocrine hormones and functions.

The thyroid gland is butterfly-shaped and lies in the neck. It consists of two lobes—one on each side of the trachea connected by an isthmus. The gland sits saddlelike starting on the anterior surface of the trachea just below the larynx and surrounds it partway. The thyroid gland stores iodine. The thyroid gland produces thyroid hormones including thyroxine which is the most abundant and triiodothyronine. It regulates the metabolic rate for carbohydrates, protein, and fats.

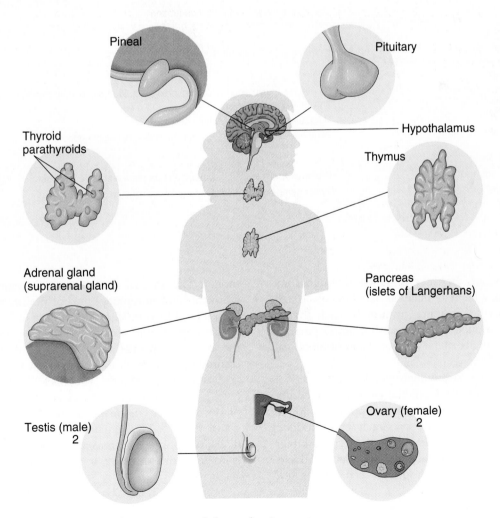

FIGURE 29-1 The structures of the endocrine system.

Table 29-1

ENDOCRINE GLAND HORMONES

Hormone	Function
Anterior Pituitary	
Thyroid-stimulating hormone (TSH)	Stimulates thyroid growth and secretion of the thyroid hormone
Adrenocorticotropic hormone (ACTH)	Stimulates adrenal cortex growth and secretion of glucocorticoids
Follicle-stimulating hormone (FSH)	Stimulates ovarian follicle to mature and produce estrogen; in the male, stimulates sperm production
Luteinizing hormone (LH)	Acts with FSH to stimulate estrogen production; causes ovulation; stimulates progesterone production by corpus luteum; in male, stimulates testes to produce testosterone
Melanocyte-stimulating hormone (MSH)	Causes increase in synthesis and spread of melanin (pigment) in skin
Growth hormone (GH)	Stimulates growth
Prolacting or Lactogenic hormone	Stimulates breast development during pregnancy and milk secretion after delivery of baby
Posterior Pituitary	
Antidiuretic hormone (ADH)	Stimulates water retention by kidneys to decrease urine secretion
Oxytocin	Stimulates uterine contractions; causes breast to release milk into ducts
Thyroid Gland	
Thyroid hormone (thyroxine T_4 and triiodothyronine T_3	Increases metabolic rate
Calcitonin	Decreases blood calcium concentration
Parathyroid Gland	
Parathyroid hormone	Increases blood calcium concentration
Adrenal Cortex	
Glucocorticoids (cortisol, hydrocortisone)	Stimulates gluconeogenesis and increases blood glucose; antiinflammatory; antiimmunity; antiallergy
Mineralocorticoids	Regulates electrolyte and fluid homeostasis
Sex hormones (androgen)	Stimulate sexual drive in females; in males, negligible effect
Adrenal Medulla	
Epinephrine (adrenalin)	Prolongs and intensifies sympathetic nervous response to stress
Norepinephrine	Prolongs and intensifies sympathetic nervous response to stress

There are four parathyroid glands although some individuals may have as many as six. Two glands are embedded in the posterior portion of each thyroid lobe. They produce parathyroid hormone, parahormone, which regulates the concentration of blood calcium and phosphorus.

The adrenal, or suprarenal, glands are located on top of each kidney. Each adrenal gland is divided into two parts, the cortex, or the outer portion, and the medulla, or the inner portion. Each part produces its own secretions. The adrenal cortex secretes mineralocorticoids including aldosterone, glucocorticoids including cortisol, and androgens which are sex hor-

mones. The adrenal medulla secretes epinephrine or adrenalin and norepinephrine or noradrenalin which help the body to function under stress.

It is important to understand the normal function of the endocrine glands and hormones. Most endocrine disorders are a result of either overactivity or underactivity of these glands. Feedback of the hormonal level in the blood indicates a need for either increased or decreased hormone production by the endocrine gland. If the endocrine gland is unable to produce sufficient hormone or produces excessive hormone, there is an endocrine disorder.

COMMON DIAGNOSTIC TESTS

The following is a table of commonly used diagnostic tests for clients with endocrine disorders.

Test	Explanation/Normal Values	Nursing Responsibilities
PITUITARY GLAND DIAGNOSTIC TESTS		
Adrenocorticotropic Hormone (ACTH), Corticotropin	This blood test determines the function of the anterior pituitary. Since there is diurnal variation, specimens should be drawn in both morning and evening. Normal = AM = 15–100 pg/mL or 10–80 ng/L PM = < 50 pg/mL or < 50 ng/L	Emotional or physical stress, or recent radioisotope scans can interfere with test results. Drugs that may increase ACTH levels include: corticosteroids, estrogens, ethanol, and spironolactone. Explain procedure. This is especially important to decrease client stress levels. Evaluate client for increased stress levels. Nothing by mouth after midnight. This venous blood specimen must be drawn with a heparinized syringe and chilled by placing the specimen on ice for immediate transport to lab.
Antidiuretic Hormone (ADH), Vasopressin	This blood test determines the production of ADH from the posterior pituitary. Normal = 1–5 pg/mL or < 1.5 ng/L	Explain procedure to client. Blood specimen should be collected in plastic, not glass, container. Note any drugs that could interfere with test results. Drugs that elevate ADH levels include: acetaminophen, barbiturates, cholinergic agents, estrogen, nicotine, oral hypoglycemic agents, some diuretics such as thiazides, and tricyclic antidepressants. Drugs that decrease ADH levels include: alcohol, beta-adrenergic agents, morphine antagonists, and phenytoin (Dilantin). Client should fast for 12 hours before test. Evaluate client for high levels of physical or emotional stress.
Follicle-Stimulating Hormone (FSH)	This blood test determines anterior pituitary function. Usually measured with luteinizing hormone level. Normal = varies with phase of menstrual cycle. Follicular = 5–20 mU/mL Midcycle peak = 15–30 mU/mL Luteal = 5–15 mU/mL Males = 5–20 mU/mL Postmenopause = 50–100 mU/mL	Recent use of radioisotopes can interfere with test results. Estrogen and progesterone may decrease FSH levels. Explain procedure to client. Indicate the date of the last menstrual period (LMP) or if postmenopausal on laboratory requisition. Indicate use of estrogen or progesterone on laboratory requisition. Client should be relaxed and recumbent for 30 minutes before test.

(continued)

Test	Explanation/Normal Values	Nursing Responsibilities
Growth Hormone (GH), Human GH, HGH, Somatotropin Hormone, SH	Although this blood test determines the function of the anterior pituitary, other tests such as the growth stimulation test are more accurate. Normal = Females = < 10 ng/mL or < 10 μg/L Males = < 5 ng/mL or < 5 μg/L	Random measurements of growth hormone is not adequate because it is not secreted constantly. A radioactive scan within the week, stress, exercise, or decreased blood glucose levels can interfere with test results. Drugs that may increase GH levels include: amphetamines, arginine, dopamine, estrogens, glucagon, histamine, insulin, levodopa, methyldopa, and nicotinic acid. Drugs that may decrease GH levels include: corticosteroids and phenothiazines. Explain procedure to the client. Client should be well rested and not emotionally or physically stressed. Client should fast but may have water. Additional blood specimens should be obtained during sleeping hours. Additional information for the laboratory requisition includes fasting time, time specimen collected, and client's recent activity. Since GH half-life is only 20 to 25 minutes, the specimen should be taken to the laboratory immediately.
Growth Hormone Stimulation test, GH Provocation test, Insulin tolerance test, ITT, Arginine Test	This blood test indicates growth hormone deficiency. Normal = > 10 ng/mL or 10 μg/L	This test is not to be done on a client with epilepsy, cerebrovascular disease, myocardial infarction, or decreased basal plasma cortisol levels. Explain procedure to the client and parents. Nothing by mouth after midnight except water. To prevent multiple puncture, a heparin lock should be inserted. Baseline growth hormone, cortisol, and glucose levels are done. An injection of insulin or arginine is given. Blood specimens for growth hormone are drawn at 0, 60, and 90 minutes after injection. Blood glucose levels are monitored every 15 to 30 minutes. Blood glucose needs to drop to 40 mg/dL for effectiveness. Monitor client for signs and symptoms of hypoglycemia. This test takes about 2 hours. Although the test can be performed by a nurse, a physician should be readily available. If vigorous exercise is used instead of medication, this should be running or stair-climbing for 20 minutes. Blood specimens are drawn at 0, 20, and 40 minute intervals. At the conclusion of the test, the client is given cookies and punch or IV glucose. Blood specimens should be taken to the laboratory immediately after being drawn. Test results take about a week.

Test	Explanation/Normal Values	Nursing Responsibilities
Luteinizing Hormone Assay (LH) Assay	This blood test determines anterior pituitary function. It can be used to determine if ovulation has occurred. It can also determine if gonadal insufficiency is primary or secondary. Normal = Females = > 6–30 mU/mL Males = 7–24 mU/mL	Recent use of radioisotopes can interfere with test results. Estrogen and progesterone may decrease LH levels. Explain procedure to client. Indicate the date of the last menstrual period or if postmenopausal on laboratory requisition.
Prolactin Levels (PRL)	This blood test determines anterior pituitary secretion. Among the problems indicated by an elevated level are pituitary tumors or primary hypothyroidism. Normal = Females or Males = 0–20 ng/mL Pregnant = 20–400 ng/mL	Drugs that may increase prolactin levels include: phenothiazines, oral contraceptives, reserpine, opiates, verapamil, histamine antagonists, monoamine oxidase inhibitors, and antihistamines. Drugs that may decrease prolactin levels include: ergot alkaloid derivatives, clonidine, levodopa, and dopamine. Explain procedure to client. Blood specimen should be obtained in the morning. It should be placed on ice if not taken immediately to the laboratory.
Thyrotropin-Releasing Hormone test, TRH test, Thyrotropin-Releasing Factor test, TRF test	This blood test assesses the responsiveness of the anterior pituitary by its secretion of TSH in response to an IV injection of TRH. It also tests the function of the thyroid gland. Normal = undetectable to 15 μIU/mL	Pregnancy may increase the TSH response to TRH. Drugs that may modify the TSH response include: antithyroid drugs, aspirin, corticosteroids, estrogens, levodopa, and T_4. Explain procedure to client. Any thyroid preparations should be discontinued for 3 to 4 weeks before the test.
Urine Specific Gravity	This measures the concentration of particles in the urine. Normal = 1.005–1.030	Recent radiographic dyes can interfere with test results. Explain procedure to client. The first voided morning specimen is best. Label container with client's name, date, and time. Transport to the laboratory as soon as possible but within 2 hours. Refrigerate specimen if test is not run immediately.
Long Bone X-rays	Serial x-rays of the long bones determine bone growth.	Explain procedure to client. Client will need to keep extremities still while x-ray taken. Shield ovaries, testes, or pregnant uterus. Remove all metallic objects from area being x-rayed.
Sella Turcica X-ray	A radiographic skull film that shows erosion and destruction of the normal sella turcica indicates pituitary tumors.	Explain procedure to client. Client must remove all objects above the neck.

(continued)

Test	Explanation/Normal Values	Nursing Responsibilities
Computed Tomography of Head (CT Scan of Head), Computerized Axial Transverse Tomography (CATT)	A noninvasive x-ray to detect abnormalities of the head displayed on a television screen and recorded on Polaroid or x-ray film. This image can be enhanced by repeating CT scan after administration of an iodinated contrast dye.	This test cannot be done on client allergic to iodinated dye or shellfish, pregnant, unstable vital signs, very obese over 300 lbs, or claustrophobic. Explain procedure to client showing picture of machine. Encourage verbalization of concerns. Obtain informed consent if required. Assess allergies. Premedicate if needed. Nothing by mouth for 4 hours before test. Wigs, hairpins, clips, or partial dental plate cannot be worn during test. The client will have head resting on snug-fitting rubber cap inside a water-filled box. The head is enclosed only to the hair line with face uncovered. Sponges are placed on each side of the head to prevent movement. There may be a clicking noise during the test. If a dye is used, the client may experience salty taste, flushing, or warmth.

THYROID GLAND DIAGNOSTIC TESTS

Test	Explanation/Normal Values	Nursing Responsibilities
Antithyroid Microsomal Antibody, Antimicrosomal Antibody, Microsomal Antibody, Thyroid Autoantibody, Thyroid Antimicrosomal Antibody	This blood test is used to detect thyroid microsomal antibodies found in clients with Hashimoto's thyroiditis. Normal = titer < 1:100	Explain procedure to client.
Calcitonin, HCT, Thyrocalcitonin	This blood test determines thyroid and parathyroid activity. It is also used as a tumor marker to detect thyroid cancer and several other cancers. Normal = basal Females = ≤ 14 pg/mL or ≤ 14 ng/L Males = ≤ 19 pg/mL or ≤ 19 ng/L	Drugs that may increase calcitonin levels include: calcium, cholecystokinin, epinephrine, glucagon, pentagastrin, and oral contraceptives. Explain procedure to client. The client should fast overnight but may have water.
Serum Free Triiodothyronine (T_3)	This blood test measures the amount of free T_3 that actually enters the cells and is active in metabolism. It is a true indicator of thyroid activity and can be used to diagnose thyroid status in pregnant females or clients on drugs that can interfere with results of other tests. Normal = 0.2–0.6 ng/dL	Explain procedure to client. Blood specimens for T_3 and T_4 uptake must be obtained to calculate T_3.
Thyroid-Stimulating Hormone (TSH), Thyrotropin	This blood test determines thyroid function as well as monitors exogenous thyroid replacement. Normal = 2–10 µU/mL or 2–10 mU/L	Recent radiographic administration may affect test results. Severe illness may decrease TSH levels. Drugs that may increase TSH levels include: antithyroid drugs, lithium, potassium iodide, and TSH injection. Drugs that may decrease TSH levels include: aspirin, dopamine, heparin, steroids, and T_3. Explain procedure to client. The client should be relaxed and recumbent for 30 minutes before the test.

Test	Explanation/Normal Values	Nursing Responsibilities
Thyroid-Stimulating Hormone Stimulation test, TSH Stimulation test	This blood test differentiates between primary and secondary hypothyroidism. Normal = none given	Explain procedure to client. Obtain baseline levels of radioactive iodine intake or serum T_4. Administer 5–10 units of TSH intramuscularly for 3 days. Repeat radioactive iodine intake or T_4 as indicated for comparison studies.
Thyroxine Index Free, FTI, FT_4 Index	This blood test measures the amount of free T_4 that actually enters the cells and is active in metabolism. It is a true indicator of thyroid activity and can be used to diagnose thyroid status in pregnant females or clients on drugs that can interfere with results of other tests. Normal = 0.8–2.4 ng/dL or 10–31 pmol/L	Recent radionuclear scans can interfere with test results. Explain procedure to client. Blood specimens for T_4 and T_3 uptake must be obtained to calculate T_4.
Thyroxine, T_4, Thyroxine Screen	This blood test directly measures the amount of T_4 present. Normal = radioimmunoassay = 5–12 µg/dL or 65–155 nmol/L	X-ray iodinated contrast studies may increase T_4 levels. Pregnancy will increase T_4 levels. Drugs that may increase T_4 levels include: clofibrate, estrogens, heroin, methadone, and oral contraceptives. Drugs that may decrease T_4 levels include: anabolic steroids, androgens, antithyroid drugs, lithium, phenytoin (Dilantin), and propranolol (Inderal). Explain procedure to client. Evaluate client drug history. If needed, instruct client to stop exogenous T_4 medications for a month prior to test.
Triiodothyronine, T_3 radioimmunoassay, T_3 by RIA	This blood test determines thyroid gland function. Normal = 110–230 ng/dL or 1.2–1.5 nmol/L	Radioisotope administration may interfere with test results. Pregnancy increases T_3 results. Drugs that may increase T_3 levels include: estrogen, methadone, and oral contraceptives. Drugs that may decrease T_3 levels include: anabolic steroids, androgens, phenytoin (Dilantin), propranolol (Inderal), reserpine, and salicylates (high dose). Explain procedure to client. Determine if exogenous T_3 is being taken. Withhold drugs with physician's approval that would interfere with test results.
Radioactive Iodine Uptake, (RAIU), Iodine Uptake test, ^{131}I Uptake	This nuclear scan uses oral radioactive iodine to determine thyroid function by its ability to trap and retain iodine. Normal = 2 hours = 4–12% absorbed 6 hours = 6–15% absorbed 24 hours = 8–30% absorbed	The client who is allergic to iodine or shellfish or pregnant should not have the test done. Exogenous iodine preparations or recent x-ray studies using iodinated contrast material will decrease thyroid gland uptake. Drugs that may increase RAIU levels include: barbiturates, estrogen, lithium, phenothiazines, and TSH. Drugs that may decrease RAIU levels include: ACTH, antihistamines, saturated solution of potassium iodine, thyroid drugs, antithyroid drugs, and tolbutamide.

(continued)

Test	Explanation/Normal Values	Nursing Responsibilities
		Explain procedure to client. Assess allergies. Some laboratories prefer nothing by mouth after midnight. Restrict iodine and thyroid preparations a week before test.
		Radioactive iodine may be given orally or IV. Client may eat 45 to 60 minutes after iodine is given. A list of times to report to radiology will be given. The client will lie supine for test which takes about 30 minutes. Isolation or specific urine precautions are not necessary.
Thyroid Scan, Thyroid Scintiscan	This nuclear scan uses a radioactive substance to visualize the size, shape, position, and function of the thyroid gland. Normal = no growth or enlargement.	Client allergic to iodine or shellfish or pregnant should not have this test. Iodine-containing foods or recent administration of x-ray iodinated contrast agents can interfere with test results. Drugs that can interfere with test results include: cough medicines, multiple vitamins, some oral contraceptives, and thyroid drugs. Explain procedure to client. Assess allergies. Certain drugs may have to be restricted for weeks before the test. Obtain a history concerning previous contrast x-ray studies, nuclear scans, or intake of thyroid-suppressive or antithyroid drugs. Fasting is usually not required. The scan may be taken 2 hours or 24 hours after oral ingestion of radioactive substance. The client should remove all jewelry, metal objects, and dentures before scan. The scan takes about 30 minutes. Isolation or specific urine precautions are not necessary.
Thyroid Ultrasound, Thyroid Echogram, Thyroid Sonogram	This ultrasound detects the size, shape, and position of the thyroid gland. Normal = no growth or enlargement	Explain procedure to client. The client will lie supine with the neck hyperextended. Breathing or swallowing will not be affected by the sound transducer. A liberal amount of lubricating gel will be placed on the neck for the transducer. A series of photos will be taken over a 15 minute period. Assist the client in removing lubricant.
Thyroid Biopsy	This is the excision of thyroid tissue for histologic examination after noninvasive tests are abnormal or inconclusive. The tissue can be obtained through needle biopsy or open surgical biopsy under general anesthesia.	Explain procedure to client. Client must give informed consent. Assess allergies. Have coagulation blood studies done. Client must be assessed for bleeding, respiratory or swallowing difficulty after the test. To prevent undue strain on biopsy site, client should be instructed to put both hands behind neck when sitting up. Client should be warned that a sore throat is possible after the biopsy.

PARATHYROID GLAND DIAGNOSTIC TESTS

Test	Explanation/Normal Values	Nursing Responsibilities
Parathyroid Hormone (PTH), Parathormone	This blood test measures the quantity of PTH to determine hyperparathyroidism or to distinguish if hypercalcemia is caused by parathyroid glands. Normal = < 2000 pg/mL	Recent radioisotope injections can interfere with test results. Explain procedure to client. Nothing by mouth after midnight except water. Obtain morning blood specimen indicating time of collection.

Test	Explanation/Normal Values	Nursing Responsibilities
Calcium, total/ionized Ca⁺⁺	Total blood calcium indicates parathyroid gland function and calcium metabolism. Since ionized calcium is unaffected by serum albumin, it can give more accurate results; however, most laboratories do not have the equipment to perform the test. Normal = Total = 9–10.5 mg/dL or 2.25–2.75 nmol/L Ionized = 4.5–5.6 ng/dL or 1.05–1.30 nmol/L	Vitamin D and excessive milk ingestion can interfere with test results. Drugs that may increase serum calcium levels include: calcium salts, hydralazine, lithium, thiazide diuretics, parathyroid hormone (PTH), thyroid hormone, and vitamin D. Drugs that may decrease serum calcium levels include: acetazolamide, anticonvulsants, asparaginase, aspirin, calcitonin, cisplatin, corticosteroids, heparin, laxatives, loop diuretics, magnesium salts, and oral contraceptives. Explain procedure to client. Fasting is not required for serum calcium but might be required if drawn with other blood chemistry tests.
Phosphorus	This blood test determines the level of phosphorus in blood. Normal = 3.0–4.5 ng/dL or 0.97–1.45 nmol/L	Laxatives or enemas containing sodium phosphate can increase serum phosphorus levels. Drugs that may increase serum phosphorus levels include: methicillin and excessive vitamin D. Recent carbohydrate ingestion including IV administration cause decreased serum phosphorus levels. Drugs that may decrease serum phosphorus levels include: antacids and mannitol. Explain procedure to client. Nothing by mouth after midnight. Discontinue IV fluids with glucose for several hours before test if possible.

ADRENAL GLANDS DIAGNOSTIC TESTS

Test	Explanation/Normal Values	Nursing Responsibilities
Adrenocorticotropic Hormone Stimulation test, ACTH Stimulation test, Cortisol Stimulation test, Cosyntropin test	This blood test monitors plasma cortisol levels to indicate adrenal gland response to ACTH. Normal = Rapid = ↑ 7 µg/dL above baseline 24 hours = > 40 µg/dL 3 days = > 40 µg/dL	Drugs that may increase plasma cortisol levels include: cortisone, estrogens, hydrocortisone, and spironolactone. Explain procedure to client. Nothing by mouth after midnight. For all tests, obtain baseline serum cortisol level. Rapid Test: Administer IV injection of cosyntropin over 2 minutes. Draw blood specimen at 30 and 60 minutes after injection. 24-Hour Test: Start an IV infusion of cosyntropin in 1 liter normal saline and run at 2 units/hour for 24 hours. Draw plasma cortisol level after 24 hours. 3-Day Test: Administer 25 units cosyntropin IV over 8 hours for 2 or 3 days. At the end of 3 days, draw plasma cortisol level.
Cortisol, Hydrocortisone	This blood test determines adrenal cortex function. There is normally a diurnal variation with higher levels around 6 to 8 A.M. and falling to lowest levels around midnight.	Physical or emotional stress can artificially elevate plasma cortisol levels. Recent use of radioisotopes can interfere with test results.

(continued)

Test	Explanation/Normal Values	Nursing Responsibilities
	Normals = 8 A.M. = 6–28 µg/dL or 170–625 nmol/L 4 P.M. = 2–12 µg/dL or 80–413 nmol/L	Drugs that may increase plasma cortisol levels include: estrogen, oral contraceptives, and spironolactone. Drugs that may decrease plasma cortisol levels include: androgens and phenytoin (Dilantin). Explain procedure to client. There will be 2 specimens drawn—one at 8 A.M. and another at 4 P.M. Assess client for physical or emotional stress and report to physician. Indicate times of collection on laboratory requisitions.
Dexamethasone Suppression test (DST), Prolonged/Rapid DST, Cortisol Suppression test, ACTH Suppression test	This blood test monitors plasma cortisol levels to indicate adrenal gland function. Normal = nearly 0 cortisol level	Stress can interfere with test results. Drugs that can interfere with test results include: barbiturates, estrogens, oral contraceptives, phenytoin (Dilantin), spironolactone, steroids, and tetracyclines. Explain procedure to client. Weigh client for baseline weight. Rapid Test: Administer dexamethasone 1 mg orally at 11 P.M. Give with milk or antacid. Administer sedative if ordered. At 8 A.M. before client rises, draw plasma cortisol level. Overnight 8 mg Dexamethasone Suppression Test: If no cortisol suppression, repeat test using 8 mg dexamethasone. If there is still no cortisol suppression, a prolonged test over 6 days involving six 24-hour urine collections should be done.
Plasma Renin Assay, Plasma Renin Activity, PRA	This blood test measures the amount of renin and is used as a screening procedure to detect essential or renal hypertension. When combined with plasma aldosterone level, it determines adrenal cortex activity. Normal = Upright position, sodium depleted or restricted diet: 20–39 years: 2.9–24 ng/mL/h > 40 years: 2.9–10.8 ng/mL/h Upright position, sodium repleted or Normal diet: 20–39 years: 0.1–4.3 ng/mL/h > 40 years: 0.1–3.0 ng/mL/h	Pregnancy, salt intake, or licorice ingestion can interfere with test results. Time of day (early in the day), client on low-salt diet, or client in upright position increase renin values. Drugs that may interfere with test results include: antihypertensives, diuretics, estrogens, oral contraceptives, and vasodilators. Explain procedure to client. The client should maintain a normal diet with sodium restricted to 3 grams per day for 3 days before test. Drugs and licorice should be discontinued for 2 to 4 weeks before test. The client should stand or sit upright for 2 hours before blood drawn. Client position, dietary status, time of day, and drugs should be recorded on laboratory requisition. Blood specimen should be placed in ice and taken immediately to laboratory. After blood specimen is obtained, client may resume a normal diet and restart medications.
Progesterone Assay	This blood test determines ovulation and function of corpus luteum. Adrenal tumors can elevate levels. Normal = Midcycle: 300–2400 ng/dL	Recent use of radioisotopes or hemolysis resulting from rough-handling of blood specimen can interfere with test results. Drugs that may interfere with test results include: estrogen and progesterone. Explain procedure to client. Indicate date of last menstrual period on laboratory requisition.

Test	Explanation/Normal Values	Nursing Responsibilities
Aldosterone Assay	This can be a blood test or 24-hour urine collection to evaluate adrenal cortex, especially for tumors. The 24-hour urine is more reliable, but the blood specimen is more convenient. Normal = Blood: Supine: 3–10 ng/dL or 0.08–0.30 nmol/L Upright: Female: 5–30 ng/dL or 0.14–0.80 nmol/L Male: 6–22 ng/dL or 0.17–0.61 nmol/L Urine: 2–80 µg/24h or 5.5–72 nmol/24h	Strenuous exercise and stress can increase aldosterone levels. Excessive licorice ingestion can decrease aldosterone levels. Posture, diet sodium, and pregnancy can interfere with test results. Drugs that may increase aldosterone levels include: diazoxide, hydralazine, and nitroprusside. Drugs that may decrease aldosterone levels include: fludrocortisone and propranolol (Inderal). Explain procedure to client. Client should have a normal diet with 3 grams of sodium/day and no licorice for at least 2 weeks before test. Medications should be stopped for at least 2 weeks before test if possible. Blood: Blood should be drawn before client gets out of bed. A second blood specimen might be obtained 4 hours later. Indicate time and client position on laboratory requisition. Transport blood specimen on ice to laboratory. 24-Hour Urine: Collect 24-hour urine after discarding first specimen. Post signs with times of collection. Each voiding does not have to be measured. Instruct client not to contaminate urine with feces or toilet tissue. Force fluids unless medically contraindicated. Collection needs a preservative and refrigeration. Indicate times of collection and any drugs that could interfere with results on laboratory requisition. Send collection immediately upon conclusion.
17-Hydroxycorticosteroids (17-OHCS)	This 24-hour urine measures adrenal cortex function. Normal = Female: 2.5–10 mg/24h Male: 4.5–10 mg/24h	Emotional or physical stress or licorice ingestion may increase adrenal activity. Drugs that may increase 17-OHCS levels include: acetazolamide, chloral hydrate, chlorpromazine, colchicine, erythromycin, meprobamate, paraldehyde, quinidine, quinine, and spironolactone. Drugs that may decrease 17-OHCS levels include: estrogens, oral contraceptives, phenothiazines, and reserpine. Explain procedure to client. Collect 24-hour urine after discarding first specimen. Post signs with times of collection. Each voiding does not have to be measured. Instruct client not to contaminate urine with feces or toilet tissue. Force fluids unless medically contraindicated. Collection needs refrigeration. Indicate times of collection and any drugs that could interfere with results on laboratory requisition. Send collection immediately upon conclusion.
17-Ketosteroids (17-KS)	This 24-hour urine measures adrenal cortex function. Normal: Female: 4–15 mg/24h or 14–52 µmol/d Male: 7–25 mg/24h or 24–88 µmol/d	Stress may increase adrenal activity. Drugs that increase 17-KS levels include: antibiotics, chloramphenicol, chlorpromazine, dexamethasone, meprobamate, phenothiazines, quinidine, secobarbital, and spironolactone.

(continued)

Test	Explanation/Normal Values	Nursing Responsibilities
		Drugs that may decrease 17-KS levels include: estrogen, oral contraceptives, probenecid, promazine, reserpine, salicylates (prolonged use), and thiazide diuretics.
		Explain procedure to client. Withhold all drugs with physician's approval for several days before test. Monitor client for stress and report to physician.
		Collect 24-hour urine after discarding first specimen. Post signs with times of collection. Each voiding does not have to be measured. Instruct client not to contaminate urine with feces or toilet tissue. Force fluids unless medically contraindicated. Collection needs a preservative and refrigeration. Indicate times of collection and any drugs that could interfere with results on laboratory requisition. Send collection immediately upon conclusion.
Urine Cortisol, Hydrocortisone	This 24-hour urine measures adrenal cortex function. Normal: 10–100 µg/24h or 27–276 nmol/d	Pregnancy or stress increases cortisol levels.
		Recent radioisotope scans can interfere with test results.
		Drugs that may interfere with test results include: oral contraceptives and spironolactone.
		Explain procedure to client. Assess for stress and report to physician.
		Collect 24-hour urine after discarding first specimen. Post signs with times of collection. Each voiding does not have to be measured. Instruct client not to contaminate urine with feces or toilet tissue. Force fluids unless medically contraindicated. Collection needs a preservative and refrigeration. Indicate times of collection and any drugs that could interfere with results on laboratory requisition. Send collection immediately upon conclusion.
Vanillylmandelic Acid & Catecholamines, VMA & Epinephrine, Norepinephrine, Metanephrine, Normetanephrine, Dopamine	This 24-hour urine diagnoses pheochromocytoma and other adrenal tumors. Normal = VMA: 2–7 mg/24h or 10–35 µmol/24h Epinephrine: 0.5–20 µg/24h or <275 nmol/24h Norepinephrine: 15–80 µg/24h Metanephrine: 24–96 µg/24h Normetanephrine: 75–375 µg/24h Dopamine: 65–400 µg/24h	Certain foods (tea, coffee, cocoa, vanilla, chocolate, etc.), vigorous exercise, stress, or starvation may increase VMA levels.
		Uremia, alkaline urine, or iodinated contrast dyes may falsely decrease VMA levels.
		Drugs that may increase VMA levels include: caffeine, epinephrine, levodopa, lithium, and nitroglycerine.
		Drugs that may decrease VMA levels include: clonidine, disulfiram (Antabuse), guanethidine, imipramine, monoamine oxidase inhibitors, phenothiazines, and reserpine.
		Drugs that may increase catecholamine levels include: ethyl alcohol, aminophylline, caffeine, chloral hydrate, clonidine (chronic therapy), contrast media (iodine containing), disulfiram (Antabuse), epinephrine, erythromycin, insulin, methenamine, methyldopa, nicotinic acid (large doses), nitroglycerin, quinidine, riboflavin, and tetracyclines.
		Drugs that may decrease catecholamine levels include: guanethidine, reserpine, and salicylates.
		Explain procedure to client. Client should be on a VMA restricted diet for 2 to 3 days

Test	Explanation/Normal Values	Nursing Responsibilities
		before test. Items restricted include: coffee, tea, bananas, chocolate, cocoa, licorice, citrus fruit, anything with vanilla, and aspirin. Client should not take antihypertensive drugs before test. Collect 24-hour urine after discarding first specimen. Post signs with times of collection. Each voiding does not have to be measured. Instruct client not to contaminate urine with feces or toilet tissue. Collection may need a preservative (see lab) and is to be refrigerated. Indicate times of collection and any drugs which could interfere with results.
Adrenal Angiography, Adrenal Arteriogram	Radiologic study of adrenal glands and arterial system after injection of radiopaque dye to detect benign or malignant tumors or hyperplasia of the adrenal glands. Normal = no growth or enlargement	Contradicted for allergies to shellfish or iodinated dyes, client with arteriosclerosis, pregnancy, or client with blood disorders. Explain procedure to client. Assess allergies. Informed and written consent must be obtained before procedure. Note if client has been taking anticoagulants. Nothing by mouth after midnight. Mark peripheral pulses with pen before procedure. Inform client a warm flush may be felt when dye is injected. Observe puncture site. Monitor vital signs. Monitor peripheral pulses, color, and temperature of extremities. Bed rest for 12 to 24 hours. Cold compresses to puncture site if needed. Force fluids to prevent possible dehydration from dye.
Adrenal Venography	This test involves insertion of catheter through femoral vein into adrenal vein to withdraw blood specimen to detect function of each adrenal gland. A contrast dye is injected to visualize size and position of adrenal glands. Normal = no growth or enlargement	Explain procedure to client. Assess allergies. Obtain informed and written consent. Inform client that a burning sensation may be experienced when dye is injected. Although this study involves the venous system, monitor vital signs, injection site, and pulses, temperature, and color of extremities.
Computed Tomography of Adrenals, CAT Scan of Adrenals, CT Scan of Adrenals	A noninvasive x-ray to detect abnormalities of the adrenals is displayed on a television screen and recorded on Polaroid or x-ray film. The image can be enhanced by repeating CT scan after administration of iodinated contrast dye. Normal = no growth or enlargement	Test cannot be done on client allergic to iodinated dye or shellfish, pregnancy, unstable vital signs, very obese over 300 lbs, or claustrophobic. Presence of metallic objects, retained barium, or large amount of fecal material or gas in bowel can interfere with test results. Explain procedure to client showing picture of machine. Encourage verbalization of concerns. Obtain informed consent if required. Assess allergies. Premedicate if needed. Nothing by mouth for 4 hours before test. Client must lie motionless. Test takes 30 minutes unless contrast dye is used then takes 1 hour. There may be a clicking noise during the test. If a dye is used, the client may experience salty taste, flushing, or warmth. Evaluate for delayed reaction to dye if used. Force fluids to promote excretion of dye.

KEY ABBREVIATIONS

The following abbreviations and acronyms are used in this chapter:

ACTH	adrenocorticotropic hormone
ADH	antidiuretic hormone
FSH	follicle-stimulating hormone
GH	growth hormone
LH	luteinizing hormone
MSH	melanocyte-stimulating hormone
PBI	protein-bound iodine
PTH	parathyroid hormone
PTU	propylthiouracil
RAI	radioactive iodine
TSH	thyroid-stimulating hormone

▶ *PITUITARY DISORDERS*

▶ *HYPERPITUITARISM*

Hyperpituitarism is a chronic progressive disease marked by hormonal dysfunction and startling skeletal growth. It generally results from a tumor of the anterior pituitary gland. Since it may affect members of a family, there may be genetic factors involved. Hyperpituitarism is most commonly diagnosed between the second and fourth decade of life but can appear in infancy and childhood. Although other pituitary hormones may be affected, the most common one is the growth hormone. As a result, either gigantism or acromegaly occurs.

Gigantism begins before the epiphyseal closure in bones. This causes proportional overgrowth of all body tissues. Since the disease is progressive, there can be a loss of various trophic hormones (thyroid-stimulating hormone, luteinizing hormone, follicle-stimulating hormone, or adrenocorticotropic hormone) leading to various metabolic dysfunctions (Norris, 1994). Gigantism affects infants and children causing them to increase the growth rate. By the time they are adults, they may reach more than 8 feet tall.

Since acromegaly occurs after epiphyseal closure of bones, there is bone thickening with transverse growth and tissue enlargement. This occurs between thirty and fifty years of age. Photographs over years will reveal a progressive enlargement of the face (See Figure 29-2).

Acromegaly involves a gradual onset of clinical manifestations including: visual defects from pressure of the pituitary tumor on the optic nerve, soft tissue swelling, or hypertrophy of the face and extremities. The cartilaginous and connective tissue overgrowths result in a characteristic hulking appearance with thickened ears and nose, and marked **prognathism** (projection of jaw). The jaw can appear enlarged and the tongue may also thicken. The paranasal sinuses can become enlarged. Also laryngeal hypertrophy can occur. The client has thick fingers with tips that appear "tufted" (shaped like arrowheads on x-rays). Because of the changes in appearance, the client may be irritable or hostile. The client exhibits a characteristic moist, weak, doughy handshake. The heart, liver, and spleen may enlarge. Some other characteristics are: diaphoresis (profuse perspiration), oily or leathery skin, fatigue, heat intolerance, weight gain, headache, joint pain, hirsutism (excessive hairiness especially in females), and sleep disturbance. The client may experience decreased libido or impotence, oligomenorrhea (scanty or infrequent menstruation), and infertility.

The client's history and clinical manifestations along with cranial x-rays and a CT scan make a diagnosis of acromegaly. Serum growth hormone levels are elevated.

Prognosis depends upon the causative factor; however, there is generally a reduced life span. Diabetes mellitus is a possible complication of hyperpituitarism because of glucose intolerance caused by the insulin-antagonistic character of the growth hormone.

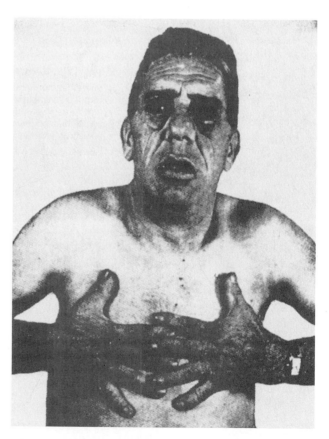

FIGURE 29-2 Acromegaly. (*From Chaffee & Lytle,* Basic Physiology and Anatomy, *4th ed., Philadelphia, PA: J. B. Lippincott Co., 1980*)

▶ *Medical/ Surgical Management*

▶ *Medical*

Medical treatment consists of either medication that affects the growth hormone or irradiation of the pituitary gland. Irradiation would be considered if the cause is the result of a tumor. Proton beam therapy is used to destroy GH secreting tumors. It uses a very low dose of radiation and is much less destructive to nearby tissue than conventional radiation therapy.

▶ *Surgical*

Surgical treatment for hyperpituitarism is to remove the pituitary gland. Two surgical approaches to remove the pituitary are transfrontal or transsphenoid hypophysectomy. The transfrontal approach is rarely used because it has a high risk of mortality as well as permanent loss of smell and taste and causes severe diabetes insipidus. The transsphenoid approach involves an incision in the superior maxillary gingiva. Surgery may be the treatment of choice or used after attempting medical treatment.

The preoperative care is similar to any client undergoing surgery. Regardless of approach, postoperative care will be the same. The nurse will monitor the client for vital signs, neurological check, and intake and output. If the client has nasal packing, it should be checked for clear colorless drainage. If it occurs, the drainage must be documented and reported to the physician. If this drainage is suspected of being cerebrospinal fluid, it should be checked for glucose which is found in cerebrospinal fluid. The nurse should observe for infection which includes elevated leukocytes, sudden temperature elevation, or complaints of headache or nuchal rigidity. Analgesics are administered as needed. The client should avoid activities such as coughing, straining, vomiting, or sneezing. The client should be encouraged to use an incentive spirometer instead of coughing. The client should not brush teeth for two weeks to avoid problems with the incision. Mouthwash can be used. The client should be instructed to avoid lifting and bending at the waist for two to three months after surgery.

▶ *Pharmacological*

Two drugs may be prescribed for hyperpituitarism. Bromocriptine mesylate (Parlodel) is a nonhormonal drug which activates dopamine receptors to inhibit the release of the growth hormone and prolactin. Bromocriptine mesylate (Parlodel) should be given with food to decrease gastric upset. Since it can cause drowsiness or dizziness, the client should be instructed to avoid activities that require mental alertness. If the client is on oral contraceptives, alternate contraceptive measures should also be used because bromocriptine can be used to stimulate ovulation.

The other drug is octreotide acetate (Sandostatin) which inhibits the growth hormone. Although octreotide is given by injection, it can still cause gastric distress. The injections should be given between meals and at bedtime. Clients with diabetes mellitus should closely monitor blood sugar levels.

Octreotide acetate (Sandostatin) can interfere with the production of other pituitary hormones. If the client exhibits clinical manifestations of hypothyroidism, decreased adrenal function, or decreased gonadal function, the appropriate hormone may have to be replaced. Some of the replacements may be thyroid, cortisone, or gonadal hormones. If the client has surgery, replacement therapy will be indicated.

▶ *Nursing Process*

Assessment

Subjective Data Obtain a thorough nursing history and ask about vision impairment, headache, muscular weakness and psychological disturbances.

Objective Data Objective data includes gait changes, vital sign changes (tachycardia or hypotension which may indicate congestive heart failure), and dyspnea. The jaw is enlarged and projected, so the client may have difficulty in chewing.

▼ ▼

Possible nursing diagnoses for a client with hyperpituitarism may include:

Nursing Diagnoses	Goals	Nursing Interventions
▶ *Growth and development, altered, related to increased levels in growth hormone.*	The client will comply with treatment to minimize hyperpituitarism and stop excessive growth with treatment.	Assist client with activities of daily living. Provide meticulous skin care using alcohol-free skin cleansers and emollient lotion. Administer medications as ordered. Assist client with range of motion exercises. Remind client to carry medications on person.
▶ *Body image disturbance, related to irreversible physical changes.*	The client will acknowledge changed body image, express positive feelings about self, and exhibit ability to cope with altered body image.	Encourage client to verbalize feelings. Offer emotional support and help client to develop coping strategies. Show respect and acceptance of the client as a person. Refer to professional counseling as needed. Refer to community resources as needed. Provide a positive but realistic assessment of the situation.
▶ *Injury, high risk for, related to long-term effects of excessive growth hormone (muscle weakness, gait changes).*	The client will comply with medical or surgical treatment to decrease growth hormone; and avoid complications of hyperpituitarism.	Remind client to wear medical alert bracelet or identification. Place objects within the client's visual field. Assist the client to identify environmental hazards so ambulation can be maintained.

▶ *Evaluation*

Each goal must be evaluated to determine how it has been met by the client.

▲ ▲

▶ HYPOPITUITARISM

Hypopituitarism is a complex syndrome marked by metabolic dysfunction, sexual immaturity, and growth retardation when it occurs in childhood. Panhypopituitarism occurs when there is partial or complete failure by the pituitary gland to produce all six vital hormones. Each hormone produced must be evaluated. Deficiency of the growth hormone results in dwarfism.

The most common cause of hypopituitarism is a tumor. Other causes are: congenital defects (hypoplasia or aplasia), pituitary infarction (from postpartum hemorrhage), pituitary surgery or irradiation, or chemical agents. A rare cause is from granulomatous disease such as tuberculosis. Hypopituitarism can be primary meaning there is no known cause or secondary. Secondary hypopituitarism can be a result of a deficiency of hypothalamic releasing hormones. This deficiency can be **idiopathic** (without a known cause) or a result of infection, trauma, or tumor.

Clinical manifestations develop slowly and generally are not apparent until 75 percent of the pituitary is destroyed. Specific manifestations will vary with the specific hormone that is deficient.

Deficiency of the growth hormone becomes apparent by about six months of age as the infant exhibits growth retardation, with chubbiness in the lower trunk and a short stature. As it progresses, secondary tooth eruption is delayed and later there is a delay in puberty. Growth continues at about half the normal rate until the child reaches about 4 feet in height. Body proportions are normal as is mental development. Frequently in adulthood, sex organs may not develop normally unless treated with hormones. Clients experience an accelerated pattern of aging, resulting in the lifespan being shortened by as much as twenty years. If the deficiency occurs in adults, manifestations are not as apparent. There are subtle signs such as wrinkles near the mouth and eyes.

Deficiencies of follicle-stimulating hormone (FSH) and luteinizing hormone (LH) cause differences in clinical manifestations between female and male clients. In the female, symptoms include: amenorrhea, dyspareunia, infertility, decreased libido, breast atrophy, sparse or absent axillary and pubic hair, and dry skin. In the male, symptoms include: weakness, impotence, decreased libido, decreased muscle strength, testicular softening and shrinkage, and retarded secondary sexual hair growth.

In a child a deficiency of thyroid-stimulating hormone (TSH) will result in severe growth retardation even with treatment. Other deficiency manifestations include: cold intolerance, constipation, increased or decreased menstrual flow, lethargy, dry pale puffy skin, and bradycardia. Thought processes may also be slowed.

A deficiency of adrenocorticotrophic hormone (ACTH) results in fatigue, nausea, vomiting, anorexia, weight loss, and depigmentation of the skin and nipples. Vital signs taken during periods of stress would show fever and hypotension.

Prolactin deficiency results in absent postpartum lactation, amenorrhea, and sparse or absent axillary and pubic hair. There may also be manifestations of thyroid or adrenal cortex failure.

Findings of hypopituitarism depend upon the specific hormone, client's age, and severity of condition when detected. Diagnosis depends on finding decreased levels of plasma GH. X-rays of the wrist determine bone age and a skull series will rule out a pituitary tumor. Total failure of the pituitary without treatment is fatal; however, prognosis is good with treatment by the appropriate hormone(s). Complications of hypopituitarism include a deficiency of the various hormones. Pituitary apoplexy, caused by abrupt hemorrhaging from the rupture of thin-walled vessels into the pituitary, is life threatening. This is a treatable medical emergency. Another complication of hypopituitarism is an inability to cope with minor stressors resulting in high fever, shock, coma, and death. In secondary hypopituitarism, the posterior pituitary can be damaged resulting in diabetes insipidus.

Medical/Surgical Management

Medical

Medical management consists primarily of replacement therapy for the deficient hormone(s). Treatments of the causative factor can vary. If the causative factor is a tumor, surgery is a choice for treatment. Refer to hypophysectomy with the previous discussion of hyperpituitarism.

Pharmacological

The replacement of hormones could include: hydrocortisone (Cortef) (the most important), levothyroxine sodium (Levothroid) and testosterone (Andro 100) or conjugated estrogens (Premarin) on a cyclic basis. In an attempt to boost fertility, menotropins (Pergonal) and human chorionic gonadotropin HCG (Pregnyl) would be administered. Somatotropin (Humatrope) stimulates growth in children with dwarfism. It can cause an increase of 4 to 6 inches the first year, but growth will taper after that. Before administering somatotropin, the physician must assess the child to ascertain that there is no epiphyseal closure. This treatment involves a series of injections. During this time, the child's height and weight must be monitored.

Nursing Process

Assessment

Subjective Data Obtain a thorough nursing history. Ask about growth pattern, menstrual periods, weakness, decreased libido, cold intolerance, lethargy and infertility.

Objective Data Assess height and weight, breast atrophy, sparse or absent axillary and pubic hair, bradycardia, testicular softening and dry skin.

▼ ▼

Possible nursing diagnoses for a client with hypopituitarism may include:

Nursing Diagnoses	Goals	Nursing Interventions
▶ Protection, altered, related to lack of anterior pituitary hormones.	The client will take medications as ordered, use stress reduction techniques, and seek medical help as needed.	Teach client medication schedule and importance of maintaining that schedule. Teach client techniques to reduce stress. If the client has cold intolerance, provide extra blanket and adjust the room temperature as needed. Teach measures to conserve energy and manage stress. Advise to keep follow-up appointments and seek medical help as needed.
▶ Infection, high risk for, related to chronic steroid therapy.	The client will wash hands frequently especially before preparing food, stay away from people who have infections and use precautions in activities of daily living to reduce or prevent infections.	Use good handwashing technique. Teach the client proper handwashing technique. Advise client to stay away from people with infections (cold, flu). Teach measures to prevent infection (avoid fatigue, adequate rest, balanced diet with adequate fluids and calories, and good personal hygiene).
▶ Body image disturbance, related to physical changes.	The client will accept body image changes.	Encourage the client to verbalize feelings about body appearance and rejection by others. Assist the client to develop a realistic assessment of the situation. Encourage development of interests supporting a positive self-image and decrease emphasis on appearance.

▶ Evaluation

Each goal must be evaluated to determine how it has been met by the client.

▲ ▲

▶ SIMMONDS' DISEASE

Simmonds' disease is defined as a total absence of all pituitary secretions. This is also called panhypopituitarism. This disease results from surgery, infection, injury, or tumor. It may also occur after a difficult labor in childbirth due to thrombosis formation during or after delivery.

Clinical manifestations which vary in intensity include: extreme weight loss, general debility, lethargy, pallor, and dry yellowish skin.

There is a loss of libido, amenorrhea, and intolerance to cold. It leads to loss of axillary and pubic hair and atrophy of genitalia and breasts. It progresses to bradycardia (slow pulse), hypotension, premature wrinkling of the skin, and atrophy of the thyroid and adrenal glands.

Treatment consists of administration of ACTH, TSH, or thyroid, adrenal, and sex hormones for a lifetime.

▶ PITUITARY TUMORS

Pituitary tumors more often affect the anterior pituitary rather than the posterior portion. They account for 6 to 15 percent of intracranial neoplasms. Adenomas of the pituitary, which are rarely malignant, replace glandular tissue and enlarge the sella turcica. The cause is unknown, but there may be a predisposition toward tumor formation from an inherited **auto-**

somal dominant trait, which means it is a dominant characteristic carried on any chromosome other than the one determining sex.

Clinical manifestations frequently start with a headache unrelated to stress or other factors. The next obvious manifestation is visual problems caused by the tumor putting pressure on the optic nerve. Others include personality changes, dementia, amenorrhea, impotence, lethargy, and weakness. The client may complain of cold intolerance, increased fatigue, and constipation. The client may have seizures. Although the tumor is not malignant, damage is done by tumor invasion of normal tissue.

Treatment is removal of the tumor. Complications of pituitary tumors are endocrine abnormalities if there is no replacement therapy after removal of the tumor. If the hypothalamus is compressed, diabetes insipidus can result. If the tumor has eroded the base of the skull, the client may have rhinorrhea (thin watery nasal discharge). Prognosis depends upon the extent of invasion. In most cases, the tumor causes excessive secretion of the anterior pituitary hormones.

▶ Medical/Surgical Management

▶ Medical

Medical treatment of a pituitary tumor would be radiation therapy. This can be used for small tumors or if the client is a poor surgical risk. Radiation can also be used after surgery to shrink tissue remaining after surgical excision. Another alternative to surgery is cryohypophysectomy. This involves freezing the area with a probe inserted via the transsphenoidal approach.

▶ Surgical

Large tumors, especially those impinging on the optic nerve, are generally removed by using the transfrontal approach. Smaller tumors can be resected via the transsphenoidal approach with a 70 to 90 percent success rate.

▶ Pharmacological

After surgery, the client will need hormone replacement therapy. These can include corticosteroids, thyroid hormone, sex hormones, or insulin.

Ergonovine maleate (Ergotrate) may be administered to decrease prolactin and growth hormone secreting tumors.

▶ Nursing Process

Assessment

Subjective Data Obtain a thorough nursing history and assess for manifestations of a tumor such as visual problems, headache, impotence, lethargy, cold intolerance, fatigue, or constipation. Speak with the family to determine any personality changes.

Objective Data Assess for tilting of the head to compensate for visual disturbances, axillary and pubic hair loss, a waxy appearance to the skin, and few wrinkles.

▼ ▼

Possible nursing diagnoses for a client with a pituitary tumor may include:

Nursing Diagnoses	Goals	Nursing Interventions
▶ Fatigue, related to decreased ACTH and TSH levels.	The client will communicate an understanding of the relationship between fatigue, the disease, and activity level, understand measures to decrease fatigue in activities of daily living, and express feeling of increasing energy as treatment progresses.	Explain relationship between pituitary tumor, fatigue, and activity level. Suggest alternating periods of activity with periods of rest. Encourage completion of all treatments.
▶ Sensory/perceptual alterations (vision), related to pressure on optic nerve by the pituitary tumor.	The client will use adaptive devices and appropriate resources to compensate for visual changes, express feelings of comfort, safety, and security, and regain normal vision with treatment.	Provide information about adaptive devices and resources for visual changes. Provide a safe clutter-free environment. Make certain that the bed is in the low position and the call signal in reach of the client. Use side rails as needed. Explain treatment and encourage completing it.

(continued)

Nursing Diagnoses	Goals	Nursing Interventions
▶ *Sexual dysfunction, related to hormone imbalance.*	The client will acknowledge changes in sexual function, communicate understanding of cause for sexual changes, and reestablish sexual function with treatment.	Provide opportunity for client to discuss change in sexual function. Explain causes for sexual changes. Encourage following treatment plan.

▶ *Evaluation*

Each goal must be evaluated to determine how it has been met by the client.

▲ ▲

▶ *DIABETES INSIPIDUS*

Diabetes insipidus is a deficiency of vasopressin or antidiuretic hormone (ADH) causing a metabolic disorder characterized by severe polyuria and polydipsia. Diabetes insipidus generally starts in childhood or early adulthood with a median onset of twenty-one years. It affects males more often than females. Although a deficiency of vasopressin or antidiuretic hormone is the most common cause, diabetes insipidus can also be caused by failure of the kidneys to respond to ADH. About half the cases are primary, either familial or idiopathic in origin. Diabetes insipidus can occur in neonates as a result of central nervous system congenital malformations, infection, trauma, or tumor. Diabetes insipidus can be secondary to intracranial tumors, hypophysectomy, neurosurgery, skull fracture, head trauma, infection, vascular lesion, or granulomatous disease such as tuberculosis. ADH secretion can be inhibited by alcohol, phenytoin (Dilantin), some anesthetics, lithium carbonate (Lithotabs), and mannitol.

Clinical manifestations have an abrupt onset. The client experiences extreme polyuria of 4 to 16 liters of dilute urine daily. In some cases, there can be up to 30 liters of urine per day. The client also has extreme thirst, preferring cold beverages. Even though there is an extraordinary volume of fluid intake, weight is lost. Other manifestations include dizziness, weakness, constipation, slight to moderate nocturia, and fatigue which could be a result of inadequate rest due to frequent voiding and excess thirst.

Complications of untreated diabetes insipidus are **hypovolemia** (decreased circulatory blood volume), circulatory collapse, unconsciousness, and central nervous system damage. Prolonged urine flow can cause chronic urinary system conditions such as bladder distension, enlarged calyces, and hydronephrosis.

Prognosis is generally good with fluid replacement in uncomplicated cases. Prognosis also depends upon the underlying cause of diabetes insipidus.

▶ *Medical/Surgical Management*

▶ *Pharmacological*

In addition to intravenous fluids, several medications can be used to treat diabetes insipidus. Desmopressin acetate (Stimate), a synthetic antidiuretic hormone which can be given parenterally or nasally, is the drug of choice. Lypressin (Diapid), another synthetic antidiuretic hormone, is given nasally. The nurse needs to make certain that the nasal passage is clear before administering the medication. Monitor intake and output and assess for hypovolemia and electrolyte imbalance.

▶ *Nursing Process*

Assessment

Subjective Data   Obtain a thorough nursing history. Ask about severity of thirst, weakness, fatigue, and lethargy.

Objective Data   Assess for weight loss, constipation, and signs of fluid volume deficit such as dry skin and mucous membranes, fever, dyspnea, and poor skin turgor. Check urine for color, amount, and specific gravity. Assess weight daily.

▼ ▼

Possible nursing diagnoses for a client with diabetes insipidus may include:

Nursing Diagnoses	Goals	Nursing Interventions
▶ Urine elimination, altered, related to polyuria.	The client will express understanding of polyuria and how medications control it, recover and maintain normal output with treatment.	Check the client's urine specific gravity. Teach client how to check the urine specific gravity. Explain action of medication and how to use it.
▶ Fluid volume deficit, high risk for, related to polyuria.	The client will have sufficient fluid intake to prevent dehydration, recover and maintain normal intake and output (equal), and have no complications from fluid volume deficit.	Provide easy access to bedpan/bathroom. Answer call signal promptly. Monitor the client for dizziness and weakness. Monitor client intake and output. Provide fluids as ordered to cover output. Teach client and family how to monitor intake and output. Monitor weight daily. If the client is on replacement hormones, instruct the client to taper off the medication and not to stop abruptly. Provide oral care. Use a soft toothbrush, mild mouthwash, and petroleum jelly for the lips. Assess condition of oral mucous membranes.
▶ Knowledge deficit related to diabetes insipidus and treatment.	The client will express desire to learn about diabetes insipidus and treatment, communicate understanding of how the treatment controls symptoms, and correctly administer medications.	Assess client's knowledge of diabetes insipidus and its treatment. Provide information about treatment. Teach client how to administer the medication.
▶ Skin integrity, impaired, high risk for, related to altered hydration.	The client will maintain skin integrity.	Assess skin, especially pressure points, three times a day. Prevent pressure on skin by turning or ambulating client. Use eggcrate mattress or sheepskin. Encourage adequate intake of fluids, protein, vitamin C, and calories.

▶ Evaluation

Each goal must be evaluated to determine how it has been met by the client.

▲ ▲

▶ THYROID DISORDERS

▶ HYPERTHYROIDISM

Hyperthyroidism is a collective term for a condition marked by increased thyroid activity and overproduction of thyroid hormones thyroxine (T_4) and triiodothyronine (T_3). The thyroid gland itself may be enlarged. Variations of hyperthyroidism are Grave's disease, Basedow's disease, Parry's disease, or thyrotoxicosis. Although these are different forms of hyperthyroidism, Grave's disease is the most common. It generally affects females seven to ten times more often than males; however, it tends to affect males more severely. The highest incidence is in the thirty- to forty-year-old group, especially if there is a family history of thyroid abnormality. It affects about 5 percent of persons under the age of fifteen.

The origin of hyperthyroidism is not clear. There may not be a single cause, but a combination of several factors. There may be a genetic influence since there is an increased incidence in identical twins.

There also may be immunologic factors. Hyperthyroidism sometimes coexists with an abnormal iodine metabolism or other endocrine problems such as diabetes mellitus, thyroiditis, or hyperparathyroidism. It may be associated with the production of autoantibodies (immunoglobulins that react against normal cells in the body). Attacks can be triggered by severe emotional or physical stress.

Clinical manifestations include two obvious physical changes. The thyroid can be palpated for asymmetry and size. It may enlarge three to four times its normal size. The enlargement of the thyroid gland is called **goiter**. This is generally a result of overactivity of the thyroid gland. If there is an accumulation of orbital fluid behind the eyeball forcing it to protrude, this is called **exophthalmos** (see Figure 29-3). This occurs in about half the cases of hyperthyroidism. It produces a characteristic stare.

As a result of increased thyroid hormone production, the client has an increased metabolic rate. This leads to weight loss despite increased appetite, fatigue, poor tolerance to heat, and profuse perspiration. The client is very nervous leading to restlessness, irritability, difficulty concentrating, emotional lability, mood swings, possible personality changes, and sleep disturbances. The client may have fine tremors of the fingers and tongue, shaky handwriting, clumsiness, trouble climbing stairs, or dyspnea on exertion and possibly at rest. The skin is warm and moist with a velvety texture as well as flushed with increased areas of pigmentation clearly different from normal pigmentation. The skin may be a characteristic salmon color. The hair is fine and soft with premature graying and increased hair loss. The nails appear fragile with distal nail separation from the nail bed (onycholysis). There may be general or local muscle atrophy and acropachy (soft tissue swelling with underlying bone changes where new bone forms). There is a tachycardia with bounding pulse up to 160 beats per minute and down to 80 beats per minute during sleep. Pulse pressure is widened.

Diagnostic tests generally include T_3, T_4, radioactive iodine uptake, and a thyroid scan.

There are some complications since this condition affects almost all body tissues. The older client particularly develops cardiovascular problems such as arrhythmias (atrial fibrillation), cardiac insufficiency leading to cardiac decompensation, and resistance to the usual dose of digoxin. There can be muscular weakness and atrophy, osteoporosis, and paralysis. There may be vitiligo which is characterized by milky-white patches on the skin surrounded by areas of normal pigmentation. There is decreased libido, impaired fertility, and **gynecomastia** (abnormal enlargement of one or both breasts in males).

One major complication is thyrotoxic crisis, also called thyroid storm. This is a medical emergency that can lead to cardiac, hepatic, or renal failure. Thyroid storm can be precipitated by stressful situations such as surgery, infection, or trauma. Less common causes are cerebrovascular accident (CVA), myocardial infarction, sudden discontinuing of antithyroid medications, subtotal thyroidectomy with excess intake of synthetic thyroid hormone, toxemia, or diabetic ketoacidosis. Any of these events can lead to overproduction of thyroid hormone which, in turn, causes an increase in systemic adrenergic activity. This causes an overproduction of epinephrine and severe hypermetabolism leading to rapid cardiac, gastrointestinal, and sympathetic nervous system decompensation. The client will exhibit severe and rapid clinical manifestations of hyperthyroidism.

If the nurse suspects that the client is experiencing thyrotoxic crisis, the physician must be informed immediately. The client will be transferred to intensive care for closer monitoring of vital signs, EKG pattern, and cardiopulmonary status. Antithyroid therapy will be initiated immediately. The client's temperature is monitored and cooling measures initiated as needed. Acetaminophen may be administered to lower the temperature, but aspirin will not be given since it could cause a further increase in the client's metabolic rate. Supportive care would be given until the client is out of the thyrotoxic crisis.

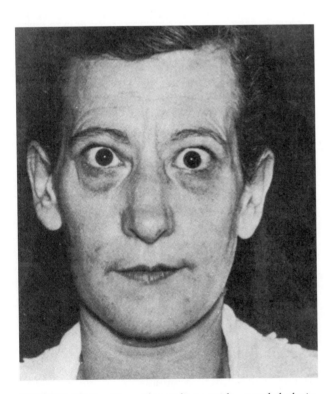

FIGURE 29-3 Hyperthyroidism with exophthalmia. (*From DeGroot, The Thyroid and Its Diseases, 4th ed. New York: John Wiley & Sons, Inc., 1975*)

▶ Medical/Surgical Management

▶ Medical

The goal of managing hyperthyroidism is to decrease excessive thyroid hormone production. With treatment to decrease the thyroid production of its hormone, the prognosis is good. The client can live a normal life. There can be a combination of treatment methods. The first method is to administer antithyroid medications. If this is not effective, the thyroid gland can be irradiated. Surgical removal of part or all of the thyroid gland may be necessary.

Radiation therapy of the thyroid gland could consist of external radiation to the neck; however, the more accepted method is the oral administration of a radioactive iodine that targets the thyroid tissue. This is the treatment of choice for the client who is a poor surgical risk and does not respond to antithyroid medications. It is most commonly used for the woman past the reproductive years or clients who do not plan to have children. If the client is of reproductive age, the client must sign an informed consent form since small amounts of the radioactive iodine could lodge in the gonads. Pregnant females should not have this method of treatment since the radioactive iodine crosses the placenta to the fetus. The method should be used with caution in children and adolescents because of the potential to develop cancer or leukemia in later years.

The client should stop taking antithyroid medications four to seven days prior to injection. The physician needs to be informed if the client is receiving amiodarone hydrochloride (Cordarone), an antiarrhythmic because it contains large amounts of iodine. The oral ^{131}I should not be given to the client with severe vomiting or diarrhea.

This method involves a single dose of ^{131}I orally. It will destroy some iodine concentrating cells that produce the thyroxine. Clinical manifestations decrease in about three weeks with the full effect in about three months. Some clients may require a second or third dose.

If the client is to be hospitalized because this method is to be used, there are several precautions that should be initiated. No pregnant nurse should care for the client. The client should expectorate carefully for the first day since the saliva is radioactive. The client should drink plenty of fluids for two days to help circulate and eliminate the radioactive iodine. The toilet should be flushed twice after each use for at least two days or throughout the hospitalization. Disposable eating utensils should be used by the client. Close contact with children or pregnant females should be avoided for a week after the administration.

Diversional activities should be planned for the client during this time. If the client is treated on an outpatient basis, the same precautions should be followed.

The client usually resumes the thyroid hormone antagonist three to five days after ^{131}I therapy until the physician determines the thyroid to be atrophic (decreased in size). The physician may have the client continue to take propranolol hydrochloride (Inderal) for tachycardia, tremor, and diaphoresis. The client requires continued monitoring of thyroid hormone blood levels and physical condition.

The most common complication is hypothyroidism, which occurs about two to four months after treatment. If the hypothyroidism is severe, the client may be placed on thyroid replacement therapy. If the hypothyroidism persists for six to nine months, the client may need to have replacement therapy for a lifetime.

If there is an exacerbation of hyperthyroidism within three to fourteen days after treatment, the physician must be notified. Females should not get pregnant for six months after treatment.

▶ Surgical

A subtotal or partial thyroidectomy is the choice for the client over forty with a large goiter not resolving with medications. Generally just a portion of the thyroid gland is removed, but a total thyroidectomy may be performed. A thyroidectomy may also be done for respiratory obstruction by a goiter or thyroid cancer. If a partial thyroidectomy is done, the remaining thyroid tissue should provide adequate amounts of thyroid hormones. If a complete thyroidectomy is done, the client will require thyroid hormone replacement for a lifetime.

Preoperatively, the client should be given explanations concerning activities after surgery. There will be a neck incision generally with some type of drain. The client may experience a sore throat and hoarseness. The client probably has taken propylthiouracil PTU for four to six weeks prior to surgery. Iodine preparations may have been prescribed ten to fourteen days before surgery to decrease thyroid vascularity and decrease bleeding. Depending upon the symptoms of hyperthyroidism, the client may also be taking propranolol hydrochloride (Inderal). Thyroid function tests and an EKG would be performed before surgery to provide baseline information. Informed consent must be obtained.

After surgery, the client is placed in high-Fowler's position to promote venous drainage. The client should support the head with a hand when moving the head to prevent strain on the incision. Observe for respiratory problems. Respiratory obstruction can be a result of tracheal collapse, tracheal mucous accumulation, laryngeal or local tissue edema. A tracheotomy tray or endotracheal tubes and insertion tray must be kept readily available at the client's bedside in case of a respiratory emergency. Since the thyroid is so vascular, the dressing must be checked frequently for drainage. Check at the back of the neck for bleeding. If there is a drain, approximately 50 cc of drainage is expected the first day. If there is no drainage, the drain must be checked for kinks or obstruction of the tubing. The nurse should encourage voice rest for forty-eight hours with voice checks every two to four hours as ordered to make certain there is no laryngeal nerve damage. Because the parathyroid glands could be accidentally removed during the thyroidectomy, the client's blood calcium level must be monitored. Check for **Chvostek's sign** or **Trousseau's sign**. (These will be discussed more fully in hypoparathyroidism.) Analgesics are administered as needed.

Complications of thyroidectomy are respiratory distress and hemorrhage. There can be damage to the laryngeal nerves affecting the voice. Manipulation of the thyroid gland during surgery can cause a release of large amounts of thyroid hormone causing thyroid storm which is rare but may occur. The client must be advised that **tetany** can occur up to ten days after surgery. Tetany is sharp flexion of the wrist and ankle joints, muscle twitchings, or cramps caused by decreased blood calcium levels.

► *Pharmacological*

Antithyroid therapy is used for children, younger adults, pregnant females, the client who refuses surgery, or clients following surgery. There are several drugs that can be used for antithyroid therapy. Propylthiouracil (PTU) is used frequently, especially in cases of thyroid storm. It reduces the production of the thyroid hormones. It should be given with food. The client must be instructed to avoid foods high in iodine such as shellfish and iodized salt. Over-the-counter preparations must be checked to see if they contain iodine. This drug requires several weeks to exert the full effect and it may be administered up to two years. This drug can cause **agranulocytosis** (a decreased number of granulocytes, types of white blood cells) so it is important to report signs and symptoms of infection immediately to the physician. If the drug is administered to a pregnant female, the minimum dosage should be prescribed to avoid fetal hypothyroidism. The drug should not be given to a lactating mother.

Methimazole (Tapazole) is another antithyroid preparation that interferes with thyroid hormone synthesis. It has a more rapid onset than PTU; however, it does not have as much consistency in effect. It should be administered at evenly spaced intervals with food to prevent gastric upset. This drug can also cause agranulocytosis, particularly in the client over the age of forty.

Iodide preparations may be given to the client with hyperthyroidism. Because iodides inhibit the release of thyroid hormones rather than the synthesis, they take effect in two days. Two common preparations are potassium iodide saturated solution, SSKI and a solution of 5% iodine and 10% potassium iodide which is called Lugol's solution. When iodide preparations are administered orally, they should be mixed with milk, juice, or water to decrease gastric upset. Drinking the preparations through a straw will decrease discoloration of the teeth. These drugs are contraindicated in the client with acute bronchitis or a known hypersensitivity to iodine.

Clients may be prescribed propranolol hydrochloride (Inderal) to counteract tachycardia and peripheral effects of hyperthyroidism. Clients should not smoke while taking this medication. Abrupt withdrawal of the drug can cause hypertension, myocardial ischemia, or cardiac arrhythmias. Clients should rise slowly from a sitting or lying position in order to prevent orthostatic hypotension.

Topical medications such as isotonic eye drops may be ordered to protect the eyes of the client with exophthalmos. Care must be taken that the eyes are not injured or infected. Some physicians may order high doses of corticosteroids to help reduce exophthalmos.

During a thyrotoxic crisis, antithyroid drugs are given. Other medications that may be used are propranolol, corticosteroids, and iodine preparations. Individual client needs could indicate a need for vitamins, nutrients, fluids, or sedation.

► *Diet*

Since the client has a greatly increased metabolic rate as well as weight loss, diet is a consideration. The client may require between 4,000 to 5,000 calories per day. There is a need for increased protein, vitamins (especially vitamins B and C), and minerals. In addition to three meals a day, the client may need additional meals or snacks to meet the increased dietary needs. Fluids should be encouraged, but caffeine should be avoided.

► **Nursing Process**

Assessment

Subjective Data   Obtain a thorough nursing history and ask about the ability to concentrate, nervousness, insomnia, jitteriness, excitability, or emotional lability.

Objective Data   Assess for dysphagia, insomnia, rapid pulse, elevated blood pressure, warm skin, elevated temperature, diaphoresis, or hand tremors.

▼ ▼

Possible nursing diagnoses for a client with hyperthyroidism may include:

Nursing Diagnoses	Goals	Nursing Interventions
▶ *Nutrition, altered, less than body requirements related to inability to ingest adequate nutrients for the increased metabolic rate.*	The client will eat a nutritionally balanced diet with enough calories to prevent weight loss and have no nutritional deficiency.	Arrange a consultation with the dietitian to assist in determining the client's increased nutritional needs. Encourage client to eat a well-balanced diet.
▶ *Thought processes, altered, related to emotional lability.*	The client will regain emotional stability and normal thought processes with treatment.	Reassure the client and family that mood swings, altered thought processes, and nervous problems will decrease with treatments. Be nonjudgmental in caring for clients. Schedule periods of rest with the room quiet and the lights dimmed.
▶ *Cardiac output, decreased, high risk for, related to tachycardia from uncontrolled hypermetabolic state.*	The client will regain and maintain normal heart rate as measured by an EKG with treatment, and maintain adequate cardiac output as indicated by normal vital signs and be alert and oriented in all three spheres.	Administer medications as ordered. Monitor the client's vital signs, intake and output, weight, serum electrolytes, orientation, and EKG. Avoid excessive palpation of the thyroid; it could cause thyrotoxic crisis. Signs could be posted to caution about excessive palpation.
▶ *Injury, high risk for, related to exophthalmos.*	The client's eyes will not be injured from exophthalmos.	Administer isotonic solutions or eye lubricants to keep the eye moist. At night, elevate head of the bed which may assist in keeping the eyelids closed or the eyes may be taped shut to prevent drying. Suggest to client that dark or tinted wraparound glasses may conceal the condition and protect the eyes from wind and airborne particles.
▶ *Body image disturbance related to neck scar.*	The client will accept the presence of the neck scar.	Keep the incision clean and dry. Suggest wearing loosely buttoned collars, high-necked tops, jewelry, or scarves. Suggest that a mild body lotion may soften the scar tissue. If the neck appears to be enlarging, measure the neck circumference daily and note any increase.
▶ *Knowledge deficit related to thyroidectomy complications of hypothyroidism and hypoparathyroidism.*	The client will describe clinical manifestation of hypothyroidism and hypoparathyroidism.	Describe clinical manifestations of hypothyroidism and hypoparathyroidism.

▶ *Evaluation*

Each goal must be evaluated to determine how it has been met by the client.

▲ ▲

Sample Nursing Care Plan: The Client with Hyperthyroidism

Janey Jackson, thirty-three years old, has returned to her physician's office to find out results of her tests for hyperthyroidism. She continues to have multiple complaints. "I have lost fifteen pounds in the last month despite eating everything all the time. I am restless and can't sleep. I feel jittery and irritable. My family says my moods change so rapidly they don't know what to expect from me. I feel so hot most of the time and sweat a lot."

The office nurse notes Mrs. Jackson appears flushed and her eyes protrude slightly. Her vital signs, T.-100.6 orally, P.-120, R.-26, and B/P.-140/88, are slightly elevated from her previous office visit. Her test results confirm that she has hyperthyroidism.

Nursing Diagnosis 1 Nutrition, altered, less than body requirements related to increased metabolism as evidenced by weight loss despite eating.

Goals	Nursing Interventions	Rationale	Evaluation
Mrs. Jackson will eat a nutritionally balanced diet with enough calories to prevent weight loss.	Monitor amount of food ingested and caloric intake.	Provides data to determine if diet adequate to prevent weight loss.	Mrs. Jackson gained or maintained weight.
	Monitor weight daily.	Determines weight gains or losses.	
	Provide a diet high in calories, protein, and carbohydrates.	Maintains or increases weight while preventing muscle mass breakdown yet providing adequate energy.	
	Advise Mrs. Jackson to avoid highly seasoned or fibrous foods or foods causing flatulence.	Gas accumulation is common and could cause increased peristalsis resulting in diarrhea.	
	Provide small frequent meals spread over waking hours.	Provides adequate calories over the waking hours without extremely large meals.	
	Obtain nutritional consult as needed.	Assists with meal planning to ensure nutritional status while considering personal food preferences.	

Nursing Diagnosis 2 Thought processes, altered, related to emotional lability as evidenced by restlessness, irritability, feeling jittery, and mood swings.

Goals	Nursing Interventions	Rationale	Evaluation
Mrs. Jackson will have a safe and protected environment and receive emotional support and understanding.	Reassure Mrs. Jackson and family that mood swings will decrease with treatment.	Mood swings are manifestations of untreated hyperthyroidism.	Mrs. Jackson expressed her feelings and experienced fewer mood swings.

	Allow Mrs. Jackson to verbalize feelings.	Good listening skills can assist the nurse to assist Mrs. Jackson in understanding these feelings.	
	Assist Mrs. Jackson in identifying and developing coping strategies.	Mrs. Jackson may not be able to identify coping strategies.	
	Refer to mental health professional as needed.	Mrs. Jackson may require more emotional support than the nurse can supply.	

Nursing Diagnosis 3 Hyperthermia related to increased metabolic rate as evidenced by complaints of feeling hot, flushing, and elevated temperature.

Goals	Nursing Interventions	Rationale	Evaluation
Mrs. Jackson's body temperature will be within normal range.	Assess for elevated temperature, heat intolerance, and diaphoresis.	Indicates increased heat production from increased metabolic rate.	Mrs. Jackson maintained her temperature in a normal range.
	Provide a well-ventilated room with temperature controlled to coolness for comfort.	Promotes comfort if heat intolerant.	
	Suggest wearing cool loose-fitting lightweight clothing.	Provides comfort and prevents overheating.	
	Provide frequent bathing and changes in linens or clothing.	Promotes comfort if diaphoretic.	
	Provide fluids up to 3 liters per day.	Replaces fluid if diaphoretic.	

Nursing Diagnosis 4 Skin integrity, impaired, high risk for, related to diaphoresis as evidenced by excessive sweating.

Goals	Nursing Interventions	Rationale	Evaluation
Mrs. Jackson's skin will remain intact and free of injury.	Assess skin for flushing and moisture.	Indicates heat intolerance.	Mrs. Jackson maintained an intact skin without impairment.
	Monitor skin for redness or breakdown, especially bony prominences.	Indicates potential for breakdown.	
	Keep Mrs. Jackson clean and dry.	Prevents skin breakdown.	

(continued)

Nursing Diagnosis 5 Injury, high risk for, related to increased metabolic rate and exophthalmos as evidenced by restlessness, irritability, and eyes slightly protruding.

Goals	Nursing Interventions	Rationale	Evaluation
Mrs. Jackson will not suffer any injury to her eyes.	Provide adequate eye care such as isotonic eye drops or lubricants, taping eyes shut at night, and wearing dark or tinted glasses.	Prevents injury to the eyes from dryness, injury, or wind.	Mrs. Jackson did not suffer any eye injury.
	Provide adequate rest alternated with activity.	Overactivity can result in injury.	
	Monitor state of anxiety and agitation.	Anxiety and agitation can result in injury.	

▶ HYPOTHYROIDISM

Hypothyroidism is a condition in which the metabolic processes are decreased because of a deficiency of the thyroid hormone. It is termed primary if the problem arises from a dysfunction solely of the thyroid. It is secondary if the thyroid gland is not stimulated to produce normally or if the target cells fail to respond to normal thyroid functioning. This condition is five times more common in females than males. There is a significant increase in incidence between the ages of forty to fifty.

A congenital condition due to a lack of thyroid hormones causes defective physical development and mental retardation. This is called cretinism. This occurs in about 1 of 4,000 live births. The child generally has a large head, short limbs, puffy eyes, thick and protruding tongue, excessively dry skin, and a lack of coordination. If untreated, the child will be permanently dwarfed, mentally retarded, and sterile. This condition is rare in the United States and is tested by the T_4.

Myxedema is the term for severe hypothyroidism in adults (see Figure 29-4).

There are a variety of abnormalities that lead to decreased thyroid hormone production. The obvious ones are thyroid gland surgery such as thyroidectomy or irradiation of the thyroid gland. Some other causes are chronic autoimmune Hashimoto's thyroiditis, inflammatory conditions (sarcoidosis), pituitary failure to produce TSH, or hypothalamus failure to produce thyrotropin-releasing hormone. There may be an inability to synthesize thyroid hormones related to iodine deficiency (rarely from general diet deficiency) or resulting from taking antithyroid medications.

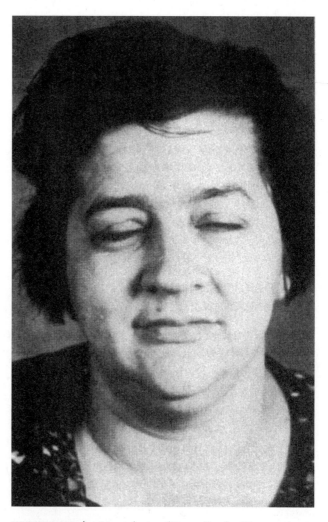

FIGURE 29-4 Myxedema. (*From Burke,* Human Anatomy and Physiology for the Health Sciences, *3rd ed. Copyright 1992, Delmar Publishers Inc.*)

Clinical manifestations are vague and varied, developing slowly over a period of time. These include an energy loss, fatigue, forgetfulness, sensitivity to cold, unexplained weight gain, and constipation. As the condition progresses, manifestations include reduced libido, menorrhagia, paresthesias, joint stiffness, and muscle cramping. There is a characteristic alteration in overall appearance and behavior including decreased mental stability and a thick and dry tongue, causing hoarseness and slow, slurred speech. The skin is flaky and inelastic, feels cool, dry, rough, and doughy. There is edema of the face, hands, and feet. The hair is dry and sparse, with patchy hair loss including loss of outer third of the eyebrow. The nails are thick and brittle with visible transverse and longitudinal grooves. The pulse is weak and bradycardic. There is muscle weakness and delayed reflex relaxation time especially the Achilles tendon (Norris, 1994). The thyroid gland may be so small that it may not be palpated unless there is a goiter. The blood pressure is generally lower than normal for the client.

Diagnostic tests generally include: TSH, T_3, T_4, radioactive iodine uptake, and a thyroid scan.

Complications affect almost every system. Cardiovascular complications include ischemic heart disease, poor peripheral circulation, enlarged heart, or pleural or pericardial effusion. Gastrointestinal complications include adynamic colon (decreased functioning of the colon), megacolon (massive and abnormal dilation of the colon), or intestinal obstruction. Other complications include conductive or sensorineural deafness, psychiatric disorders, carpal tunnel syndrome, or impotence or infertility. Prognosis depends upon the organs involved, duration, and severity of condition.

Myxedema coma or hypothyroid crisis is a serious complication of extreme or prolonged hypothyroidism. It is life threatening. It is characterized by severe metabolic disorders, hypothermia, and cardiovascular collapse leading to coma. It has a gradual onset but is triggered by severe stress such as infection, exposure to cold, or trauma. Abrupt withdrawal of thyroid medication or the use of narcotics, sedatives, or anesthetics can also cause myxedema coma. If myxedema coma occurs, it must be reported to the physician immediately. The client would be moved to the intensive care unit. The client will be monitored closely for vital signs, EKG changes, and cardiopulmonary status. Wrapping the client in blankets will warm the client, but a warming blanket should not be used as it could cause peripheral vasodilation and shock. Thyroid medications and possibly corticosteroids would be administered. Supportive care would be given until the client comes out of the myxedema coma. Myxedema coma is often fatal.

▶ Medical/Surgical Management

▶ Pharmacological

Thyroid replacement therapy lasts a lifetime. Thyroid (Armour Thyroid) is a natural form while levothyroxine sodium (Levothroid, Synthroid) is a synthetic. The physician will order thyroid hormone to begin slowly and increase dosage every two to three weeks until the desired response is achieved. The medication should be given in one dose in the morning to prevent insomnia. It should be stored in a cool, dark place away from moisture and light. Since there may be differences between brands, brand change is not recommended without consulting a physician or pharmacist. Certain foods such as cabbage, turnips, pears, and peaches can alter the requirements for thyroid hormone. The thyroid hormones increase the client's toxicity to iodine so the client should avoid foods high in iodine (dried kelp, shellfish, iodized salt, saltwater fish), multivitamins, dentifrices, and nonprescription medications containing iodine. A dietary consultation for meal planning and a list of foods to avoid should be provided to the client.

If the client has diabetes mellitus, insulin or oral hypoglycemic dosage might have to be adjusted. The client should monitor blood sugar levels closely. If the client is on anticoagulant therapy, thyroid hormones potentiate the anticoagulant action. The client needs to be informed to watch for excessive bleeding or bruising. Digitalis preparations are also potentiated by thyroid hormone.

Because hypothyroidism impairs the metabolic rate, the client may have difficulty metabolizing medications. The client may have an increased sensitivity to hypnotics, sedatives, or opiates. Dosage may have to be adjusted appropriately. Synthesis of the thyroid hormone can be impaired by drugs such as lithium carbonate (Lithotabs), or aminoglutethimide (Cytadren).

▶ Diet

The client should be instructed to avoid foods high in iodine and foods that interfere with thyroid hormone replacement. The diet is designed to increase weight loss and combat constipation. The diet should be high in bulk or fiber and low in calories. Sodium should be decreased to prevent fluid retention. The diet should be increased in protein, carbohydrates, vitamins B complex and C, and iron.

▶ *Nursing Process*

Assessment

Subjective Data Obtain a thorough nursing history and ask about lethargy, depression, irritability, impaired memory, and slowing of thought processes. Also assess psychosocial manifestations.

Objective Data Assess for hearing and speech deficits, anorexia, constipation, decreased libido, thin hair, skin dry and thickened, enlarged facial features, masklike expression, voice low and hoarse, bradycardia, decreased blood pressure and respirations, and exercise intolerance. If the client is a child, the nurse must assess the family as well as the client for understanding of the disease process and proposed treatment.

▼ ▼

Possible nursing diagnoses for the client with hypothyroidism may include:

Nursing Diagnoses	*Goals*	*Nursing Interventions*
▶ *Activity intolerance related to decreased metabolic and energy level.*	The client will express understanding for the need to increase activity level gradually.	Assist the client to gradually increase activity level but rest between activities to avoid fatigue and decrease cardiac oxygen demands.
	The client will maintain blood pressure, pulse, and respirations within normal limits when active.	Measure the client's legs correctly so antiembolic hose, which help venous return, will fit properly when worn.
	The client will regain and maintain normal activity levels.	Reposition client every two hours and encourage client to continue activity when normal activity level is achieved.
▶ *Tissue perfusion, altered, cardiopulmonary related to decreased cardiac output caused by bradycardia.*	The client will not have chest pain at rest.	Assess for chest pain and advise client to report any episodes of angina immediately.
	The client will have a normal heart rate and rhythm.	Monitor the client's vital signs.
	The client will avoid ischemic EKG changes.	Monitor cardiac status through EKG and assessment of heart and lung sounds plus checking for edema.
	The client will maintain adequate cardiopulmonary perfusion.	Restrict fluid and sodium during the time of cardiac decompensation as ordered and monitor intake and output and weight.
▶ *Body image disturbance related to changes in weight, skin, and hair.*	The client will express feelings about body image changes.	Provide client an opportunity to express feelings about body image.
	The client will comply with treatment to improve body image; and regain a positive self-image and express positive feelings about self.	Encourage treatment compliance. Assist client to develop interests to enhance a positive self-image and de-emphasize appearance.

▶ *Evaluation*

Each goal must be evaluated to determine how it has been met by the client.

▲ ▲

▶ THYROID TUMORS

There are several neoplasms of the thyroid gland. The benign thyroid cyst and adenoma are firm, encapsulated, noninvasive, slowly growing neoplasms of unknown etiology. Diagnosis of benign neoplasms is done by needle biopsy. These growths tend to be nonfunctioning (not affecting the functioning of the thyroid gland) so there is no treatment other than continued monitoring. If the adenoma is functioning (increasing the functioning of the thyroid gland), then it is treated by radioactive iodine or surgery.

▶ CANCER OF THE THYROID

Cancer of the thyroid occurs in all age groups, but individuals who have had radiation therapy to the neck are more susceptible. There are four major types of thyroid cancer.

- Papillary carcinoma is the most common type affecting 60 percent of the cases. It can affect any age but is more common in females of childbearing age. It is multifocal and bilateral. It slowly metastasizes to the neck nodes, mediastinum, and lungs. It is the least virulent form.
- Follicular carcinoma affects 20 percent of the cases. It is likely to recur. It metastasizes to the regional lymph nodes and spreads through the blood vessels to the bone, liver, and lungs.
- Medullary carcinoma is a solid carcinoma. There may be a familial tendency possibly through the autosomal dominant gene. It is associated with pheochromocytoma. This form is fairly rare affecting only 5 percent of the cases. It affects females over the age of forty. It is curable if detected before signs and symptoms occur. Without treatment, it grows rapidly metastasizing to the bones, liver, and kidneys.
- Anaplastic or undifferentiated carcinoma resists radiation. It is almost never curable by resection. It metastasizes rapidly generally causing death by invasion of the trachea and adjacent structures. It occurs in 10 to 15 percent of the cases, generally affecting individuals over the age of sixty.

Since there is no known cause of cancer, there are several risk factors. They are radiation exposure, prolonged secretion of TSH resulting from radiation or heredity, familial disposition, or chronic goiter.

The first clinical manifestation is a painless lump. As it enlarges, it destroys the thyroid which leads to clinical manifestations of hypothyroidism. Although rare, the tumor could trigger excessive thyroid hormone production causing the client to display the clinical manifestations of hyperthyroidism. There can be dysphagia, hoarseness, and vocal stridor. There may be a detectable, disfiguring thyroid mass with a firm nodule on palpation.

The thyroid scan shows a "cold" nodule (decreased uptake of ^{131}I) for papillary carcinoma. Follicular carcinoma and benign adenomas show a "hot" nodule. Thyroid function tests are usually normal. A needle biopsy may be done to confirm diagnosis.

▶ Medical/Surgical Management

▶ Surgical

All carcinomas can be treated with surgery (discussed previously). Radioactive iodine or external radiation therapy may also be used. Response of the tumor will depend upon early diagnosis and treatment. These methods of treatment may be used individually or in combination. Client care is the same as for hyperthyroidism.

▶ Pharmacological

Exogenous thyroid hormone may suppress thyroid activity. To increase tolerance to surgery or radiation therapy, the physician may prescribe simultaneous exogenous thyroid hormone and adrenergic blocker such as propranolol hydrochloride (Inderal). If there is widespread metastasis, the cancers will be treated with neoplastic chemotherapy.

▶ Nursing Process

Assessment

Subjective Data Obtain a thorough nursing history and ask about difficulty eating, breathing, or swallowing. Assess client for clinical psychological effects of cancer.

Objective Data Palpate client's neck and nearby lymph nodes for tumor formation. Assess respirations and breath sounds.

▼ ▼

Possible nursing diagnoses for the client with a thyroid tumor may include:

Nursing Diagnoses	Goals	Nursing Interventions
▶ Nutrition, altered, less than body requirements related to dysphagia.	The client will maintain weight and consume an adequate amount of a nutritionally balanced diet daily.	Monitor intake and output and weight. Monitor the client's nutritional intake and provide a nutritionally balanced diet in six or more small meals daily.
▶ Swallowing, impaired, related to presence of the tumor.	The client will adjust eating habits to compensate for impairment and not develop complications of aspiration pneumonia or malnutrition; and regain normal swallowing with treatment.	Provide soft or pureed diet for ease in swallowing. Encourage client to sit up straight when eating; provide nutritional snacks between meals. If the client is to have thyroid surgery, explanations must be given.
▶ Communication, impaired verbal, related to presence of the tumor.	The client will communicate needs and desires by alternate means without undue frustration and regain normal speaking ability with treatment.	Warn client about a temporary voice loss or hoarseness for several days after surgery. Provide paper and pencils. Ask questions that can be answered by yes or no. Encourage client to comply with selected treatment. Refer client to the American Cancer Society.

▶ *Evaluation*

Each goal must be evaluated to determine how it has been met by the client.

▲ ▲

▶ *GOITER*

A goiter is an enlargement of the thyroid unrelated to inflammation or neoplasm. There are three types of goiter. One type is a diffuse toxic goiter found in hyperthyroidism. This type of goiter may be moderate to massively enlarged. The consistency varies from soft to firm and rubbery. It generally feels smooth. Frequently it is associated with exophthalmos.

Another type of goiter is a simple nontoxic goiter. It develops when the thyroid is unable to utilize iodine properly or in response to low iodine levels in the blood. These goiters are more common in females. They develop during times of great metabolic demands such as adolescence or pregnancy. A deficiency of iodine can cause goiter formation. Goiters found in specific geographic regions away from the seacoast are referred to as endemic goiters. Clinical manifestations depend upon the size of the goiter. There is an obvious enlargement of the thyroid gland. A large goiter can compress the esophagus or trachea causing dysphagia, a choking sensation, or respiratory difficulty. If the goiter impairs venous return from the head and neck, the client may experience dizziness and syncope. Diagnosis is based on history, clinical manifestations, and results of thyroid function tests. T_3 is generally very low. Treatment concentrates on the underlying cause. This may involve thyroid hormone replacement therapy or prescribing iodine supplements or increasing dietary iodine sources. Surgery is done when respiration or swallowing is impaired or for cosmetic effect.

The third type of goiter is the nodular goiter. It is similar to the simple goiter except that palpation reveals multiple nodules causing the enlargement. It is found frequently in females over forty. It usually is asymptomatic. Treatment varies with the client's age and clinical manifestations.

▶ *HASHIMOTO'S THYROIDITIS*

Hashimoto's thyroiditis is an autoimmune disease characterized by the production of antibodies in response to thyroid antigens and the replacement of normal thyroid structures by lymphocytes and lymphoid germinal centers. The disease occurs twenty times more often in females than in males. It occurs more frequently between the ages of thirty and fifty and shows a marked hereditary pattern. There is an increased incidence of Hashimoto's thyroiditis in clients with Down's syndrome and Turner's syndrome.

Clinical manifestations include a thyroid that is enlarged and has a lumpy surface. Generally the goiter is asymptomatic, but it could cause dysphagia and feeling of local pressure. The thymus gland is also enlarged. Other clinical manifestations are similar to hypothyroidism.

Treatment of Hashimoto's thyroiditis is also similar to that of hypothyroidism. Thyroid hormone replacement is used. This is a chronic disorder that can be treated, but not cured. The client will be on lifetime thyroid hormone replacement.

▶ PARATHYROID DISORDERS

▶ HYPERPARATHYROIDISM

Hyperparathyroidism is a condition resulting from overactivity of one or more of the parathyroid glands. It results in increased secretion of parathyroid hormone (PTH), which causes calcium to leave the bones and accumulate in the blood. This cannot be compensated by renal excretion or uptake into the soft tissues. It occurs twice as often in postmenopausal females than males. It occurs frequently between the ages of thirty-five and sixty-five. Hypercalcemia may also be caused by excessive intake of thiazide diuretics, vitamin D, or calcium supplements.

X-rays will show skeletal decalcification. Blood PTH and alkaline phosphate levels are increased. Serum calcium level is elevated.

It is termed primary if there is an enlargement of one or more of the parathyroid glands increasing secretion of PTH and thus increasing blood calcium levels. The most common cause is adenoma, but other primary causes include genetics or multiple endocrine neoplasms.

The condition is termed secondary if there is excess compensatory production of PTH stemming from a hypocalcemia-producing abnormality other than the parathyroid gland. Some of these abnormalities are rickets, chronic renal failure, vitamin D deficiency, or osteomalacia due to laxative abuse or phenytoin (Dilantin).

Many clients are asymptomatic; however, there are several clinical manifestations. The client may have polyuria, chronic low back pain, bone tenderness, or renal calculi. The client may also experience nausea, vomiting, anorexia, constipation, lethargy, or drowsiness. There can be changes in level of consciousness,

disorientation, stupor, coma, or personality changes with a loss of initiative and memory. There may be marked muscle weakness and atrophy especially of the legs, joint hyperextensibility, long bone skeletal deformity, or hyporeflexia.

Without treatment, there can be permanent damage to the skeleton or kidneys. There can be bone and articular problems including pathologic fracture. Renal complications include calculi, colic, nephrolithiasis, urinary tract infection, and renal insufficiency leading to chronic renal failure. Other complications may be stone formation in various organs, cardiac or vascular problems, or central nervous system changes.

▶ Medical/Surgical Management

▶ Medical

Medical management is aimed at decreasing overactivity of the parathyroid glands. This may be accomplished by medication therapy or surgery. If there is severe renal involvement, the client may require dialysis.

▶ Surgical

Primary hyperparathyroidism can be treated by surgical removal of three and one half of the four parathyroid glands. Surgery can relieve bone pain in three days but may not reverse renal damage.

Preoperative care includes explanations, encourage fluids, limiting calcium intake, and administering medications to lower blood calcium levels.

Postoperative care involves administration of magnesium or phosphate. The client may receive calcium supplements for several days. The nursing care is similar to that provided to the client with thyroidectomy (refer to hyperthyroidism). A major complication is airway obstruction.

▶ Pharmacological

Pharmacological treatment is aimed toward correcting secondary hyperparathyroidism. This involves treating the underlying cause. Since hypercalcemia is a major manifestation, medications are geared to decrease the calcium level in the blood. This includes the use of diuretics such as furosemide (Lasix) and ethacrynic acid (Edecrin).

Other drugs that decrease the calcium levels of the blood are calcitonin-human (Cibacalcin), plicamycin (Mithracin), and magnesium- or phosphate-based drugs. Magnesium and calcium are antagonists (Monahan et al., 1994). Phosphate-based drugs lower calcium levels based on the inverse relationship between phosphorus and calcium.

▶ *Nursing Process*

Assessment

Subjective Data   The nurse should obtain a thorough nursing history and ask about muscle weakness, apathy, nausea, mental status, and pain (low back or renal). Assess for increased calcium intake either dietary or supplements.

Objective Data   Assess for fatigue, drowsiness, anorexia, constipation, personality changes, renal colic, skeletal deformity, output, hematuria, vomiting, weight loss, hypertension, bradycardia, or dysrhythmias.

▼ ▼

Possible nursing diagnoses for the client with hyperparathyroidism may include:

Nursing Diagnoses	*Goals*	*Nursing Interventions*
▶ *Activity intolerance related to neuromuscular symptoms.*	The client will regain and maintain normal muscle mass and strength, maintain maximum joint range of motion, and perform self-care activity as tolerated.	Alternate rest and activity periods. Assist client with moderate, weight bearing activities. Assist client with ROM exercises. Encourage client to perform self-care.
▶ *Injury, high risk for, related to effects of elevated serum calcium level.*	The client will express understanding of how elevated serum calcium levels affect the body, comply with treatment, and suffer no injury from elevated serum calcium level.	To prevent renal problems, encourage fluids to a minimum of 3 liters a day, include cranberry and prune juices. Monitor the client's intake and output and weight. Strain urine to detect any renal calculi.
▶ *Pain related to musculoskeletal changes resulting from persistently increased serum calcium level.*	The client will express relief after analgesics, use comfort measures to decrease pain, and be pain-free when serum calcium level reaches normal.	Administer analgesics as ordered. Provide comfort measures for bone pain, and include turning and repositioning every two hours and supporting affected extremity with pillows. Assess pain level and compare to serum calcium level. Assess environment for hazards and eliminate them. Assist the client to ambulate. Maintain the bed in a low position with siderails up and call light in reach. Lift and move the client gently to prevent pathologic fractures. If the client is on digoxin, monitor level since an elevated serum calcium level can interfere with it. Inform client to avoid calcium antacids.

▶ *Evaluation*

Each goal must be evaluated to determine how it has been met by the client.

▲ ▲

▶ *HYPOPARATHYROIDISM*

Hypoparathyroidism is a condition resulting from a deficiency of parathyroid hormone (PTH) secretion by the parathyroids or the decreased action of peripheral PTH. Since the parathyroids normally regulate the serum calcium level, hypoparathyroidism will result in a decreased serum calcium level. PTH normally maintains the serum calcium level by increasing bone resorption and gastric reabsorption. It also maintains the inverse relationship between calcium and phosphorus levels. Hypoparathyroidism can be acute or chronic.

If hypoparathyroidism is idiopathic, it may be the result of an autoimmune disorder or congenital absence of parathyroid glands. Acquired hypoparathyroidism is generally irreversible. The most common cause is accidental removal during thyroid or other neck surgery. It could also be a result of ischemic infarction during surgery, sarcoidosis, tuberculosis, neoplasms, trauma, or massive thyroid irradiation. Reversible hypoparathyroidism can result from hypomagnesemia-induced impairment of hormone synthesis, suppression of normal gland function because of hypercalcemia, or delayed maturation of the parathyroid glands.

The characteristic sign of hypoparathyroidism is tetany, which is muscle spasms and tremors caused by a lack of calcium. Other clinical manifestations include dry skin, brittle hair, **alopecia** (loss of hair or baldness), and loss of eyelashes and fingernails. The teeth are stained, cracked, and decayed due to weak enamel. The client may have altered neuromuscular irritability, tingling and twitching of the face and hands, and increased deep tendon reflexes. There may be personality changes or EKG changes.

There are two diagnostic assessment tests that can be performed. One is the Chvostek's sign which is an abnormal spasm of the facial muscles in response to a light tapping of the facial nerve. The other test is Trousseau's sign which is a carpal spasm caused by inflating a blood pressure cuff above the client's systolic pressure and leaving it in place for three minutes (see Figure 29-5).

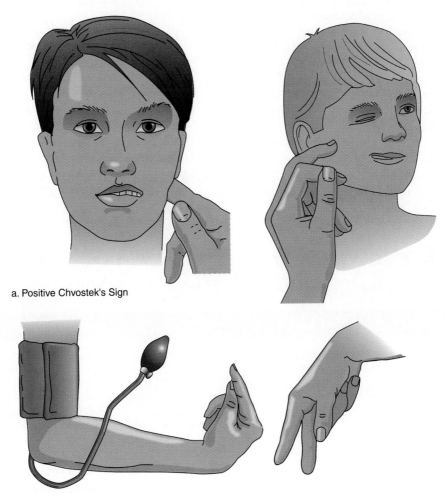

a. Positive Chvostek's Sign

b. Positive Trousseau's Sign

FIGURE 29-5 Signs of hypocalcemia and hypoparathyroidism: **(A)** Chvostek's sign; **(B)** Trousseau's sign.

Expected test results include: decreased serum calcium, increased urinary calcium, increased serum phosphorus, and decreased urinary phosphorus.

Complications are related to longstanding hypocalcemia. This leads to decreased heart contractility leading to cardiac failure. There can be cataract formation or papillary edema from increased intracranial pressure. There may be bone deformity. In cases of severe tetany, the client can experience laryngospasm, respiratory stridor, anoxia, paralysis of vocal cords, and death. A child with hypoparathyroidism may have mental retardation, stunted growth, and malformed teeth.

▶ Medical/Surgical Management

▶ Pharmacological

Calcium gluconate or calcium chloride may be given intravenously. Give calcium chloride very slowly since it is very irritating to the vessel wall. Too rapid IV calcium infusion can cause cardiac arrest. After initial IV dose, then calcium may be given orally.

Unless the hypoparathyroidism is reversible, the client will require lifelong replacement. There are a large number of calcium supplements available. The client should not just take vitamin and mineral supplements because they do not contain sufficient amounts of calcium. Vitamin D may also be given to assist in the absorption of calcium. The calcium supplements should be given one to one-and-one-half hours after meals to increase absorption. The client may take the supplements orally. If the client cannot swallow the large tablets, they could be dissolved in hot water and the suspension cooled before administering to the client. The best sources of calcium are from the diet. The client needs to take calcium as ordered and not abruptly stop taking the drug. Since calcium potentiates digitalis actions, the physician needs to be advised if the client is also taking a digitalis preparation. The client must be advised that calcium may cause digitalis toxicity. Cimetidine (Tagamet) interferes with normal parathyroid functioning.

▶ Diet

The diet should be high in calcium and low in phosphorus containing foods. Since many foods that are high in calcium are also high in phosphorus, the client should be given a list of foods that are high in calcium but lower in phosphorus. Foods on this list include vegetables such as asparagus, broccoli, collards, and tomatoes; fruits such as apricots, bananas, cantaloupe, and many berries, and other foods such as kidney beans, lima beans, and brown sugar. Foods that have a high phosphorus content and should be avoided include: most legumes, nuts, cheeses, and seafood.

▶ Nursing Process

Assessment

Subjective Data   Obtain a thorough nursing history and ask the client about recent surgery or irradiation, use of alcohol, numbness or tingling of the skin, anxiety, headache, irritability, depression, or nausea.

Objective Data   Assess for dysphagia, laryngeal spasm, stridor, cyanosis, or dysrhythmias. Check Chvostek's sign and Trousseau's sign.

▼ ▼

Possible nursing diagnoses for the client with hypoparathyroidism may include:

Nursing Diagnoses	Goals	Nursing Interventions
▶ *Thought processes, altered, related to hypocalcemia-induced neurologic dysfunction.*	The client will regain and maintain normal thought processes.	Maintain a patent IV line and administer calcium gluconate or calcium chloride as ordered.
▶ *Injury, high risk for, related to calcium deficiency.*	The client will not exhibit signs and symptoms of tetany, and prevent injury from hypocalcemia.	Monitor Chvostek's and Trousseau's signs, serum calcium and phosphorus levels, as well as EKG changes.
		Keep tracheotomy tray readily available and maintain seizure precautions.
		Support the client while walking to prevent injury.
		Monitor the client taking digoxin for toxicity.

Nursing Diagnoses	Goals	Nursing Interventions
▶ Nutrition, altered, less than body requirements, related to calcium intake.	The client will have adequate calcium intake.	Provide diet with calcium-rich foods. Give calcium replacement as ordered. The client who is taking digoxin must be monitored for toxicity.

▶ Evaluation

Each goal must be evaluated to determine how it has been met by the client.

▲ ▲

▶ ADRENAL DISORDERS

▶ CUSHING'S SYNDROME (ADRENAL HYPERFUNCTION)

Cushing's syndrome is a condition resulting from overactivity of the adrenal cortex causing excess production of the hormone cortisol. It is fairly rare with only ten cases per one million of the population in the United States yearly. It occurs in females eight times more than males, generally between the third and fourth decades of life.

Excess production of androgens is called adrenogenital syndrome. When aldosterone is produced in excess, it is termed primary aldosteronism.

Cushing's syndrome can be classified into three types according to etiology: primary, secondary, and **iatrogenic** (caused by treatment or diagnostic procedures). About 70 percent of the cases stem from hyperplasia of the adrenal cortex with excess production of corticotropin. It can also be a result of increased pituitary secretion of ACTH. Corticotropin-producing tumors in another organ such as oat cell carcinoma of the lungs, occur more in males. Between 25 percent and 30 percent of the cases are a result of cortisol-secreting adrenal tumors which are generally benign. Administration of synthetic glucocorticoids or corticotropin can occasionally cause Cushing's syndrome.

Classic clinical manifestations are adiposity of the face, neck, and trunk which give rise to the moon-shaped face and buffalo hump. Others include purple striae on the abdomen, hirsutism, and thin extremities due to muscle wasting. Boys will exhibit an early onset of puberty while girls exhibit development of masculine characteristics. The client may complain of fatigue, muscle weakness, sleep disturbances, water retention, amenorrhea, decreased libido, irritability, and emotional lability. There could be petechiae, ecchymoses, decreased wound healing, or swollen ankles (see Figure 29-6).

There are multiple complications of Cushing's syndrome most of which are produced by the stimulating and catabolic effects of cortisol. There can be increased calcium resorption from the bone leading to osteoporosis and pathologic fractures. It can cause increased hepatic gluconeogenesis and insulin resis-

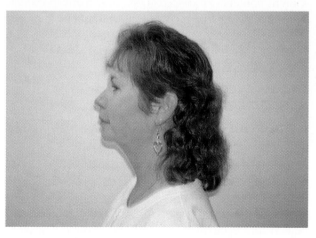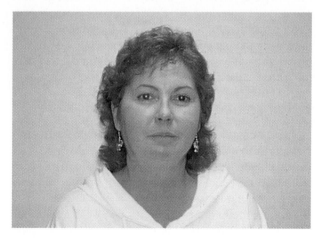

FIGURE 29-6 A client with Cushing's syndrome: Untreated. (*Photos courtesy of Dr. Matthew Leinung, Acting Head, Division of Endocrinology, Albany Medical College, Albany, NY*)

tance causing glucose intolerance and diabetes mellitus. The client may have frequent infections and slowed wound healing. There is a suppressed inflammatory response that can mask severe infections. The client may have decreased ability to handle stress which could lead to psychological problems from mood swings to psychosis. Other complications include hypertension, ischemic heart disease, congestive heart failure, menstrual disturbances, and sexual dysfunction.

Plasma cortisol level is elevated. Plasma ACTH level may be elevated or low. Adrenalangiography is done for adrenal tumor. Twenty-four-hour urines for seventeen ketosteroids and seventeen hydroxysteroids are elevated.

Prognosis depends upon early diagnosis, identifying the underlying cause, and effective treatment. Without treatment, about half will die within five years.

▶ Medical/Surgical Management

▶ Medical

The major goal is to restore hormone balance. Treatment is based on the causative factor. This is accomplished primarily by medications. If there is adrenal cancer, the client may either have radiation therapy to the adrenal gland or surgery on either the pituitary gland or the adrenal glands, or all three treatments.

▶ Surgical

If the underlying cause of Cushing's syndrome is related to the pituitary gland, the client may have a hypophysectomy done. Refer to hypophysectomy in section on hyperpituitarism.

For an adrenal tumor, an adrenalectomy is performed. This could be unilateral or bilateral. During the first twenty-four to forty-eight hours after surgery, the client is observed closely for hemorrhage and shock. Vital signs and urine output must be monitored. Glucocorticoids are administered with changing dosage until a maintenance dose is established. The client's blood glucose level needs to be monitored especially for hypoglycemia.

▶ Pharmacological

Cyproheptadine hydrochloride (Periactin) is an antihistamine that also decreases cortisol levels. It can cause drowsiness or dizziness so the client must be instructed to avoid activities that require mental alertness or manual dexterity.

Aminoglutethimide (Cytaden) also decreases cortisol levels. It can cause dizziness or drowsiness. The client should be instructed to avoid activities requiring mental alertness or manual dexterity. It may be given

in combination with metyrapone to treat metastatic adrenal carcinoma.

Mitotane (Lysodren) directly suppresses the activity of the adrenal cortex. This cytotoxic agent is generally used for inoperable adrenal cortex cancer. It is given for at least three months. The client should avoid situations that cause injury or exposure to infections.

If the client had pituitary or adrenal surgery, cortisol therapy may be given before and after surgery to decrease physical stress. Steroid therapy could be a lifetime situation. The client should take the drug with food or antacids to decrease gastric distress. Two-thirds dose of the steroids should be taken in the morning with the remaining one-third in the early evening to mimic the body's diurnal schedule. Steroids can lead to osteoporosis and the possibility of pathologic fractures. Females should be warned that steroid use can interfere with oral contraceptive effectiveness. There may be an adverse effect on the male's sperm production and count. The client with diabetes mellitus may have to adjust insulin dosage because the steroids can affect the glucose levels. Steroids can mask severe infections and cause some immunosuppression. Wounds are slower to heal. The client should be instructed to contact a physician before using over-the-counter preparations. The client should not abruptly discontinue the steroid drug. Dosage should be tapered before discontinuing.

▶ Diet

The diet should be high in protein and potassium but low in sodium. Foods high in protein include: eggs, milk, whole grains, legumes, and meat; however, milk, cheeses, and whole grains depending upon processing are also high in sodium. Many foods high in potassium are also low in sodium. These foods are: legumes; fruits, such as figs, oranges, bananas, prunes, and raisins; and vegetables, such as avocado, potato, and spinach. The client should be advised to read labels for sodium content. Processed foods and many preservatives have high sodium content and should be avoided.

▶ Nursing Process

Assessment

Subjective Data Obtain a thorough nursing history and ask about the use of steroids, stress, methods of coping with stress, irritability, depression, mood swings, loss of libido, and the possibility of suicide. Ask about the use of steroids.

Objective Data Assess for thin and fragile skin, petechiae, ecchymoses, delayed wound healing, weight gain, increased abdominal girth, purple striae, hyperglycemia, and hypokalemia.

▼ ▼

Possible nursing diagnoses for the client with Cushing's syndrome may include:

Nursing Diagnoses	Goals	Nursing Interventions
▶ *Body image disturbance related to changes in physical appearance.*	The client will verbalize feelings about changed appearance.	Encourage the client to verbalize feelings about changed body image and sexual dysfunction. Offer emotional support and a positive realistic assessment of the condition.
▶ *Infection, high risk for, related to suppressed inflammatory response from excessive corticosteroid production and skin and capillary fragility.*	The client will take precautions to avoid or decrease exposure to infection and maintain normal temperature, leukocyte count, and differential.	Advise client to avoid people with infections. Provide a private room with reverse or protective isolation as indicated. Monitor the client's vital signs, intake and output, and weight.
▶ *Injury, high risk for, related to stimulating and catabolic effects of excessive corticosteroid production on body tissues.*	The client will identify early signs and symptoms of complications and importance to seek medical attention quickly and, express understanding of measures to prevent complications such as adequate rest, well-balanced diet, compliance with treatment.	Teach early signs and symptoms of complications. Instruct client how to recognize stressful situations and methods to reduce stress. Teach relaxation techniques and diversional activities. Provide alternating rest and activity periods. Monitor the client's activity tolerance and increase activity gradually. Assure safety precautions, including the client wearing shoes when out of bed. Keep bed in low position with the siderails up as needed and the call signal in reach. Assist the client to ambulate. Handle client with extreme caution to minimize skin trauma and bone stress.

▶ *Evaluation*

Each goal must be evaluated to determine how it has been met by the client.

▲ ▲

▶ ADDISON'S DISEASE (ADRENAL HYPOFUNCTION)

Addison's disease, the chronic form of adrenal hypofunctioning, involves decreased functioning of the adrenal cortex and its secretions—mineralocorticoids, glucocorticoids, and androgens. It can also be called adrenal hypofunction or insufficiency. It is fairly uncommon occurring in one per 100,000 people in the United States. Although it affects all ages and both sexes, it is less common among the elderly. There is an increased incidence if there is a history of autoimmune disease or chronic steroid therapy.

Addison's disease occurs when more than 90 percent of the adrenal gland is destroyed. It may be primary such as an autoimmune disease. It can be caused by bilateral adrenalectomy or hemorrhage into the adrenal gland related to anticoagulant therapy. Some infections such as tuberculosis, histoplasmosis, HIV, and meningococcal pneumonia can cause Addison's disease. It can also be caused by cancer of the adrenal gland. It is termed secondary if it resulted from decreased pituitary function, abrupt withdrawal of long-term steroid therapy, or tumor of the pituitary gland.

A classical clinical manifestation of Addison's disease is a bronze coloration of the skin resembling a deep suntan especially in the creases on the hands, elbows, and knees. There may be some areas of pigmentation loss and other areas more darkly pigmented. The client may complain of fatigue, muscle weakness, becoming lightheaded when rising, weight loss, and craving for salty foods. The client may have decreased tolerance even to minor stress. The client is anxious, irritable, and may become confused. The pulse may be weak and irregular. There may be hypotension. There can be a variety of GI complaints.

The acute form is called adrenal crisis. It may occur when there is trauma, surgery, other physiologic stress, or abrupt withdrawal of steroids. The clinical manifestations are the same only more severe with a rapid onset. The crisis requires immediate treatment. The client will be placed on intravenous therapy and IV administration of hydrocortisone (Cortef, Hydrocortone). Measures to maintain a stable blood pressure and normal water and sodium levels are instituted. After the crisis, the client will be placed on a maintenance dose of hydrocortisone.

Expected test results include: low serum sodium, high serum potassium, low serum glucose, low cortisol and aldosterone serum levels, and decreased urinary 17-ketosteroid and 17-hydroxysteroid levels.

► Medical/Surgical Management

► Medical

Treatment is geared toward prompt restoration of fluid and electrolyte balance and replacement of deficient adrenal hormones.

► Pharmacological

The client will require lifetime maintenance of steroids. Refer to Cushing's syndrome for steroid therapy. Administration of glucocorticoids should be in late afternoon or evening in order to prevent insomnia. Mineralocorticoids may be given in the afternoon or evening. Fludrocortisone acetate (Florinef) may be given to decrease dangerous dehydration and hypotension.

If the female has muscular weakness and decreased libido, testosterone may be given. Depending upon the dosage, it may cause the female to develop more masculine characteristics.

► Diet

The diet should be high in sodium and low in potassium. It should contain adequate calories and protein. If the client is anorexic, six small meals may increase caloric intake. A late afternoon or evening snack should be available if there is a drop in the client's blood glucose level.

► Nursing Process

Assessment

Subjective Data The nurse should obtain a thorough nursing history and ask about recent synthetic steroid use, adrenal surgery, recent infection, craving salt, nausea, weakness, vertigo, headache, disorientation, emotional status, anxiety, and apprehension.

Objective Data Assess for postural hypotension, inability to perform normal activities, syncope, dark pigmented areas on skin and mucous membrane, weight loss, vomiting, diarrhea, and very low or very high temperature.

Possible nursing diagnoses for the client with Addison's disease may include:

Nursing Diagnoses	Goals	Nursing Interventions
► Fluid volume deficit, related to low sodium level, vomiting, diarrhea, and increased renal losses.	The client will have normal fluid and electrolyte balance.	Monitor the client's vital signs, level of consciousness, intake and output, and weight. Administer IV fluids as ordered and encourage fluid intake.
► Infection, high risk for, related to suppressed inflammatory response.	The client will maintain normal temperature and leukocyte count and differential and use precautions to avoid or reduce risks of infection.	Monitor temperature every four hours unless elevated then every two hours. Provide a private room with reverse or protective isolation as needed.

Nursing Diagnoses	Goals	Nursing Interventions
		Teach proper handwashing.
		Limit visitors.
		Monitor laboratory test results for WBC and differential.
▶ *Knowledge deficit related to inadequate understanding of decreased adrenal function and steroid therapy.*	The client will express need to know about decreased adrenal function and steroid therapy, and describe adrenal insufficiency and steroid therapy.	Assess client's current knowledge of decreased adrenal function and steroid therapy.
		Teach client about decreased adrenal function and steroid therapy.

▶ Evaluation

Each goal must be evaluated to determine how it has been met by the client.

▲ ▲

▶ PHEOCHROMOCYTOMA

Pheochromocytoma, sometimes known as chromaffin cell tumor, is a rare disease characterized by **paroxysmal** (a symptom that begins and ends abruptly) or sustained hypertension due to excessive secretion of epinephrine and norepinephrine. Some medical experts estimate that about one-half percent of newly diagnosed clients with hypertension have pheochromocytoma. Although the tumor is generally benign, it can be malignant in 5 to 10 percent of the cases. It affects all races and both sexes. It is most common in females ages thirty to fifty years.

It is caused by a chromaffin cell tumor of the adrenal medulla (more commonly on the right side). Extraadrenal pheochromocytomas can occur in the abdomen, thorax, urinary bladder, neck, or associated with cranial nerves IX (glossopharyngeal) and X (vagus) (Norris, 1994). Epinephrine overproduction occurs with the adrenal pheochromocytoma; however, norepinephrine overproduction is associated with both adrenal and extraadrenal pheochromocytoma. It is associated with a familial history of pheochromocytoma or endocrine gland cancer. It is considered to be inherited on the autosomal dominant gene in about 5 percent of the cases.

The major clinical manifestation is hypertension. The client may have episodes of malignant hypertension with blood pressure readings of 300/180 or more. These episodes can last from a few minutes to several hours. Most episodes last about forty minutes. The client may have had previous unpredictable episodes of hypertensive crisis. Paroxysmal symptoms could be a result of a seizure disorder or anxiety. The hypertension responds poorly to conventional treatment. Other clinical manifestations include headache, palpitations, visual disturbances, nausea, or vomiting. The client may have severe diaphoresis, feelings of impending doom, or precordial or abdominal pain. These attacks may be triggered by activities or conditions that displace the abdominal contents such as heavy lifting, exercise, bladder distention, or pregnancy. Severe attacks can be precipitated by administration of opiates, histamine, glucagon, and corticotropin. Some attacks may have no precipitating factor. Some other clinical manifestations are mild to moderate weight loss due to increased metabolism or orthostatic hypotension when arising to an upright position. The client will have tachycardia. The actual tumor is rarely palpable; however, palpation could trigger a hypertensive attack.

The complications are similar to those of severe and persistent hypertension. These complications are stroke, retinopathy, heart disease, or irreversible kidney disease. Pheochromocytoma is frequently diagnosed during pregnancy when the enlarged uterus puts pressure on the tumor causing more frequent attacks. The attacks could prove fatal to both mother and fetus. Although there is an increased risk of spontaneous abortion, most fetal deaths occur during labor or immediately after delivery. The client with pheochromocytoma has an increased risk of severe complications or death during invasive diagnostic tests or surgery.

Although pheochromocytoma can be potentially fatal, the prognosis is good with treatment. About 90 percent of the clients are cured with treatment.

▶ Medical/Surgical Management

▶ Surgical

The treatment of choice is surgical removal of the tumor. Sometimes the adrenal gland is removed, too.

The blood pressure is monitored closely during the immediate postoperative period. The client may have hypotension, but hypertension is more common. About 10 percent of the cases are not surgical candidates. These would be treated with medications to lower the blood pressure. Some may be given neoplastic chemotherapy. Refer to adrenalectomy in section on Cushing's syndrome.

▶ *Pharmacological*

During acute hypertensive attacks, the drugs of choice are phentolamine mesylate (Regitine) or nitroprusside sodium (Nipride). Phentolamine mesylate (Regitine) and phenoxybenzamine HCl (Dibenzyline) are alpha-adrenergic blocking agents. They are used to control hypertension before surgery or when surgery is contraindicated. The client's blood pressure and pulse should be monitored. The client should be warned about orthostatic hypotension and rise slowly from a supine position to an upright position. The client should not take over-the-counter drugs or alcohol.

Nitroprusside sodium (Nipride, Nitropress) acts on the vascular smooth muscle to cause peripheral vasodilation. The drug is given in an intravenous infusion. It should be protected from heat, light, and moisture. During the intravenous infusion, the fluid bag and tubing should be wrapped with an opaque covering such as aluminum foil. An electronic infusion device must be used to monitor the infusion rate. The client's blood pressure is used to titrate the infusion rate per the physician's orders.

Metyrosine (Demser) is used to block catecholamine synthesis. This drug must be continued for life if the tumor is inoperable. Ongoing medications include adrenergic blockers such as propranolol hydrochloride (Inderal), atenolol (Tenormin), prazosin HCl (Minipress), labetalol HCl (Normodyne) or nifedipine (Procardia), a calcium channel blocker. The client's blood pressure must be monitored frequently to determine the effectiveness of the medication.

Propranolol hydrochloride (Inderal) should not be stopped abruptly. The client should not smoke while taking this medication. Atenolol (Tenormin) may enhance the client's sensitivity to cold. Prazosin HCl (Minipress) should be taken on an empty stomach. The initial dose should be given at bedtime. The client should not use cough, cold, or allergy medications without the physician's knowledge. If the client is given parenteral labetalol HCl (Normodyne, Trandate), the client should remain supine for three hours to decrease the possibility of orthostatic hypotension. Nifedipine (Adalat, Procardia) should be protected from light and moisture and stored at room temperature. Over-the-counter medications should not be taken.

▶ *Diet*

The diet should be high in protein with adequate calories. Stimulating foods such as aged cheeses and yogurt, and caffeine containing beverages such as coffee, tea and soft drinks; beer, and red wine should also be avoided (Smeltzer & Bare, 1996).

▶ **Nursing Process**

Assessment

Subjective Data   Obtain a thorough nursing history and ask about heat intolerance, severe headaches during hypertensive crisis, anxiety, trouble sleeping, palpitations, nervousness, dizziness, paresthesias, and nausea.

Objective Data   Assess for dyspnea, tremors, diaphoresis, glycosuria, hyperglycemia, or dilated pupils. Frequently assess blood pressure, pulse, and respirations for elevations. Observe for signs of anxiety to prevent it from triggering a hypertensive crisis.

▼ ▼

Possible nursing diagnoses for the client with pheochromocytoma may include:

Nursing Diagnoses	*Goals*	*Nursing Interventions*
▶ *Tissue perfusion, altered, renal, related to adverse effects of hypertension.*	The client will maintain adequate renal function and have normal renal function studies.	Monitor the blood pressure and pulse of the client. Monitor and record intake and output.
		Monitor cardiac function through telemetry and renal function through laboratory tests.
▶ *Anxiety related to potential seriousness and associated complications of pheochromocytoma.*	The client will identify and express feelings about diagnosis and perform activities to decrease anxiety.	Assist client to identify and express feelings about diagnosis.
		Teach client relaxation techniques.

Nursing Diagnoses	Goals	Nursing Interventions
▶ *Injury, high risk for, related to potential for hypertensive crisis.*	The client will identify signs and symptoms of hypertensive crisis and seek help immediately and avoid factors known to precipitate hypertensive crisis.	Teach client to seek medical help if headache, palpitations, visual distrubances, nausea, and vomiting are present. Teach client to avoid heavy lifting, exercise, or bladder distention.

▶ Evaluation

Each goal must be evaluated to determine how it has been met by the client.

▲ ▲

▶ CASE STUDY

Mary Jane Trudell, forty-three years of age, was diagnosed with Addison's disease when she was thirty-four years old and placed on long-term steroid therapy. Due to sudden financial problems, she was unable to refill her prescription for steroids. She came to the emergency room with a rapid onset of fatigue, muscle weakness, lightheadedness upon rising, weight loss, and a craving for salty foods. She is anxious, irritable, and slightly confused. She is diagnosed as being in addisonian crisis and admitted to the hospital. Her orders include: vital signs q4h, IV of D-5-RL @ 125 cc/hr continuous, Solu-Cortef 100 mg IVP now, then IVPB q8h, regular diet, bedrest with bathroom privileges.

The following questions will guide your development of a Nursing Care Plan for this case study.

1. Discuss the difference in clinical manifestations between Addison's disease and adrenal crisis.
2. Discuss vital signs the nurse should expect to find when assessing Ms. Trudell.
3. List three nursing diagnoses and goals for Ms. Trudell.
4. List teaching that Ms. Trudell will need concerning long term steroid use.
5. List three successful outcomes for Ms. Trudell.

SUMMARY

• The endocrine system is composed of glands at various body locations producing secretions (hormones) that directly enter the blood or lymph circulation.

• The endocrine system provides slower and longer lasting control over various body activities and functions.
• A malfunction of any part of the endocrine system can result in a shift of homeostasis with far-reaching systemic reactions.

- Assessment of the endocrine system can be difficult since the glands are scattered. Negative findings are as important as positive findings.
- Hyperthyroidism causes an increase in the metabolic rate that can make it difficult for the body to meet its own metabolic needs.
- Goiter formation can occur with either hyperthyroidism or hypothyroidism.
- The two major complications of thyroidectomy are respiratory distress and hemorrhage.
- Regardless of disorder, the client should wear a medic alert bracelet and be aware that the treatment generally lasts a lifetime.

Review Questions

1. Explanations prior to diagnostic tests for an endocrine disorder are most important to
   a. enable the client to collect a twenty-four-hour urine specimen.
   b. ensure client compliance for test instructions.
   c. prevent taking medications that interfere with test results.
   d. reduce stress that can interfere with test results.

2. Which of the following nursing diagnoses would be most appropriate for the client with diabetes insipidus?
   a. Alteration in growth and development related to increased growth hormone production
   b. Alteration in thought processes related to decreased neurologic function
   c. Fluid volume deficit related to polyuria
   d. Hypothermia related to decreased metabolic rate

3. Meticulous skin care is especially important for the client with hyperthyroidism because of:
   a. diaphoresis from heat intolerance.
   b. edema from sodium and water retention.
   c. poor nutrition due to nausea and vomiting.
   d. pressure from immobility due to paralysis.

4. The nurse would assess for which of the following clinical manifestations in the client with hypothyroidism?
   a. hypertension, diaphoresis, nausea, and vomiting
   b. tetany, irritability, dry skin, and brittle nails
   c. unexplained weight gain, energy loss, and cold intolerance
   d. water retention, moon-faced, hirsutism, and purple striae

5. The client with hyperparathyroidism should have extremities handled gently because:
   a. decreased calcium bone deposits can lead to pathologic fractures.
   b. edema causes stretched tissue to tear easily.
   c. hypertension can lead to a stroke with residual paralysis.
   d. polyuria leads to dry skin and mucous membranes that can breakdown.

6. Which of the following assessments would the nurse expect to observe in the client with pheochromocytoma?
   a. bradycardia and tetany
   b. nausea, vomiting, and diarrhea
   c. personality changes
   d. systolic pressure up to 300 mmHg

Critical Thinking Questions

1. Discuss lifestyle changes necessary for each endocrine disorder.

2. How could a person cope with the physical changes and body image disturbance of the endocrine disorders?

Medical Terminology

cortic-	pertaining to the cortex
endo-	within, inward
endocrine	a group of cells secreting substances directly into the blood or lymph circulation
exo-	outside, outward
exocrine	external secretion of a gland
horm-	an impulse, to urge or stimulate
hormone	a substance produced by an endocrine gland that stimulates activity in another part of the body
thyro-	pertaining to the thyroid
hyperthyroidism	a condition marked by increased thyroid activity

News Flash:
Do Growth Hormone Injections Work?

Although there are about 7,000 children in the United States suffering from growth hormone deficiency, an estimated 20,000 to 25,000 children receive growth hormone injections. The cost per child for the injections ranges from $15,000 to $20,000 per year. Studies show that the child with a growth hormone deficiency receiving injections for five to ten years can increase adult height up to 6 inches. Children without an endocrine or metabolic disorder who receive growth hormone injections show little to no change in adult height projections. The difference is that these children have an increase in the speed of growth rather than increase in height itself. A pharmaceutical spokesman responded that healthy, short children might gain psychological benefits from reaching adult height sooner even if there is no actual increase in height.

Rick Weiss, a reporter for the *Washington Post,* reported that the results of a new study indicate that growth hormone injections on healthy, short children have little to no effect. The National Institutes for Health is conducting the biggest trial study; however, these results will not be complete for several years (*Weiss, 1994*).

CHAPTER
30
Diabetes Mellitus

Mary Kay Schultz

▶ KEY TERMS

dawn phenomenon
glucagon
glucose
glycosuria
hyperglycemia
hypoglycemia
insulin
ketone
ketonuria
lipodystrophy
polydipsia
polyphagia
polyuria
Somogyi phenomenon

LIST OF DISORDERS

▶ Diabetes Mellitus
  • Insulin Dependent Diabetes Mellitus (IDDM)
  • Non-insulin Dependent Diabetes Mellitus (NIDDM)

LEARNING OBJECTIVES

Upon completion of this chapter the learner should be able to:
• Define key terms.
• Differentiate between insulin dependent and noninsulin dependent diabetes in terms of pathophysiology, presenting symptoms and treatment.
• Describe the role of diagnostic testing in the diagnosis, treatment, and self-management of diabetes mellitus.
• Discuss the action, side effects, and routes of administration of insulin.
• Describe the role of oral antidiabetic agents in the treatment of the noninsulin diabetic client.
• Discuss the roles of diet and exercise in the management of diabetes mellitus.
• Utilize the nursing process in developing a plan of care for the diabetic client.
• Develop teaching plans for the diabetic client that focus on the importance of self-management and metabolic control in the prevention of short- and long-term complications.
• Identify signs, causes, and treatment of complications of hypoglycemia, diabetic ketoacidosis, and hyperosmolar hyperglycemic nonketotic syndrome.
• Relate the major long-term complications of diabetes.
• Describe nursing care of the diabetic client experiencing infection, illness, surgery.

...

▶ MAKING THE CONNECTION

Refer to the topics in the following chapters to increase your understanding of diabetes mellitus.

INTRODUCTION

Diabetes mellitus is a group of disorders characterized by chronic **hyperglycemia** (elevated blood **glucose**, sugar) and other disorders of carbohydrate, fat, and glucose metabolism. It is a systemic disease caused by an imbalance between insulin supply and insulin demand. Insulin dependent diabetes mellitus (IDDM) and noninsulin dependent diabetes mellitus (NIDDM) are the two most common forms and are discussed in detail in this chapter.

Diabetes mellitus is an endocrine disorder of the pancreas of major importance in the United States. According to the Centers for Disease Control and Prevention (CDC), it is estimated that 12 to 14 million Americans have diabetes mellitus. Because of the insidious nature of symptoms associated with NIDDM, approximately one-half of these diabetics remain undiagnosed and, hence, untreated. Diabetes is the third leading cause of death in the United States and is associated with many serious complications. Diabetes is the leading cause of new blindness among adults, the leading cause of new cases of renal failure, and is present in more than half of persons experiencing nontraumatic lower extremity amputations. Diabetes and its complications shorten a person's life span, create disability, and impose an economic burden on persons who have the disease (Geiss et al., 1993).

Diabetes is seen in all age groups and races (Figure

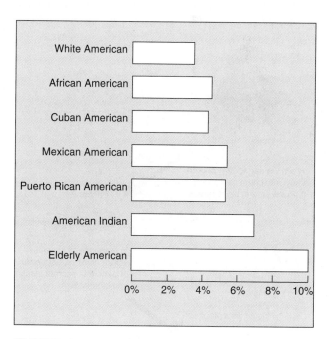

FIGURE 30-1 Americans with diagnosed diabetes. (*From U.S. Department of Health and Human Services. Public Health Service:* Diabetes in the United States: A strategy for prevention *[map reference]. National Center for Chronic Disease Control and Prevention. Division of Diabetes Translation. Washington, DC, 1992, U.S. Government Printing Office*).

30-1). One-third of the clients with diabetes are over the age of sixty. African American, Hispanic, and some Native American populations have a higher incidence of noninsulin dependent diabetes than the white population. The incidence of insulin dependent diabetes is slightly higher in white persons than nonwhite.

The goal of diabetes management is controlling the blood glucose level within acceptable levels, thereby minimizing the long-term complications associated with diabetes. Management of diabetes mellitus requires individual planning that impacts all areas of the client's life including diet, exercise, and medications. By understanding the disease process, its treatments, and complications, the nurse can assist and support the client in controlling this disorder and achieve optimal outcomes.

ANATOMY AND PHYSIOLOGY REVIEW

Diabetes mellitus is a disorder of metabolism. When we eat, most of the food we eat is broken down by digestive juices into chemicals, including a simple sugar called glucose. Of the food we eat, 100 percent of carbohydrate and approximately 58 percent of protein and 10 percent of fat is broken down to glucose. For the glucose to get into the cells, insulin must be present (see Figure 30-2).

Insulin is a hormone produced and secreted by the beta cells in the islets of Langerhans of the pancreas.

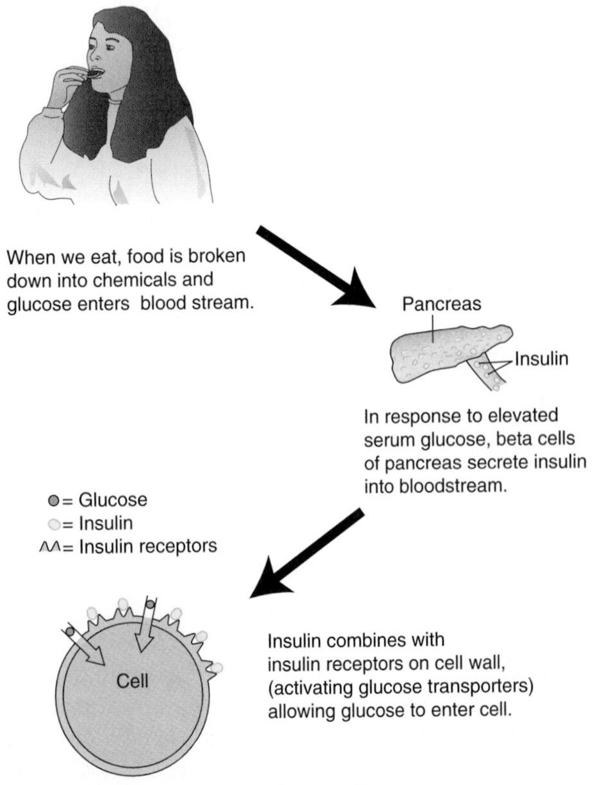

When we eat, food is broken down into chemicals and glucose enters blood stream.

Pancreas

Insulin

In response to elevated serum glucose, beta cells of pancreas secrete insulin into bloodstream.

● = Glucose
◌ = Insulin
ᴧᴧ = Insulin receptors

Insulin combines with insulin receptors on cell wall, (activating glucose transporters) allowing glucose to enter cell.

Cell

FIGURE 30-2   How insulin works.

Insulin stimulates the active transport of glucose into muscle and adipose tissue cells, making it available for cell use. For glucose to cross the cell membrane, insulin must connect with a receptor on the cell membrane. Some clients with diabetes mellitus have enough insulin, but too few functioning receptor sites. Others have inadequate or no insulin production. Blood glucose can always be used by the brain and kidneys. Insulin is not needed for glucose to enter brain cells or cells of the glomeruli.

The amount of glucose in the blood regulates the rate of insulin secretion. When a meal is eaten, the blood glucose elevates and the beta cells of the islets of Langerhans release insulin. As the blood glucose level drops, insulin secretion diminishes. It is important to note that during times of fasting (overnight or between meals) a low level of insulin continues to be secreted along with **glucagon**. Glucagon, another pancreatic hormone, stimulates release of glucose by the liver. The balance and interactions of insulin and glucagon serve to maintain a constant serum glucose level.

Other functions of insulin include:

- Promoting conversion of glucose to glycogen for storage in the liver and inhibiting conversion of glycogen to glucose
- Promoting the conversion of fatty acids into fat that can be stored as adipose tissue and preventing breakdown of adipose tissue and conversion of fat to ketone bodies
- Stimulating protein synthesis within tissues and inhibiting the breakdown of protein into amino acids

In summary, insulin actively promotes those processes that lower the blood glucose level and inhibits those processes that raise the blood glucose level. Insulin deficiency results in hyperglycemia. Excess insulin results in **hypoglycemia** (low blood glucose).

ASSESSMENT OF THE CLIENT WITH DIABETES MELLITUS

Assessment of the client with diabetes mellitus requires a holistic approach. Complaints related to pancreas dysfunction cause problems in several other body systems because the endocrine system functions interdependently with other body systems. Keep in mind that diabetes mellitus can greatly alter a person's lifestyle. The nurse needs to be aware of how this disease is affecting the individual both physically and psychosocially.

Begin the assessment by asking questions regarding the main area of concern. Common complaints associated with diabetes are fatigue, weakness, weight changes, mental status changes, polyuria, and polyphagia, polydipsia. It is also helpful to determine if others in the client's family have diabetes mellitus. When performing an assessment the following aspects should be investigated.

Ask about the client's overall health status. Determine if they are feeling tired or lethargic. Decreased energy level may occur with changes in the blood glucose level. Ask if the client feels any numbness or tingling of the arms or legs. This may be an indication of peripheral neuropathy that occurs with diabetes mellitus. Ask if she is experiencing any vision problems especially blurred vision as this can be an early sign of hyperglycemia. Assess how her appetite has been as increased appetite is an indication of diabetes mellitus. Assess the vascularity of the extremities for dependent redness or cyanosis and the absence of hair on the lower extremities may indicate arterial insufficiency related to diabetes mellitus. Look for any manifestation related to arteriosclerosis as the client with diabetes is especially prone to the accelerated effects of this disease.

COMMON DIAGNOSTIC TESTS

The following is a table of commonly used diagnostic tests for clients with diabetes mellitus.

Test	Explanation/Normal Values	Nursing Responsibilities
Blood glucose, Fasting Blood Sugar, (FBS)	Measure of blood level of glucose (serum values). Depends on method used by laboratory. Normal = 70–115 mg/dL Diabetic ≥ 140 mg/dL Critical values: > 400 mg/dL < 50 mg/dL	Client must fast (except for water) 6–8 hrs. Withhold insulin or oral antidiabetic meds until blood drawn. Be certain client receives meds and meal after fasting specimen drawn. Cortisone, thiazide and loop diuretics cause increase.
2 hour post prandial glucose, (2h PPG) or 2 hour post prandial blood sugar (2h PPBS)	Measure of blood glucose 2 hours after a meal. Normal = 70–140 mg/dL Diabetic > 140 mg/dL	Instruct client to eat entire meal, and then not eat anything else until blood drawn. Notify lab of time meal is completed.
Glucose Tolerance Test (GTT)	Evaluates blood and urine glucose 30 min. before, and 1, 2, 3 & 4 hours after a standard glucose load. Normal = blood glucose ≤ 140 mg/dL within 2 hrs.; urine negative Diabetic: > 140 for more than 2 hrs., possibly never returns to normal; urine positive for glucose	Client must fast (except for water) 6–8 hrs. Withhold drugs that interfere with results. After administration of glucose load, client may not eat anything else until test completed. Should drink water. Collect urine specimens at hourly periods. Administer meal and meds after test completed.
Glycosylated Hemoglobin (GHb)	Serum measure of glycohemoglobin, evaluating average blood glucose level over 120 days Normal = 4–8% Good control = 7.5% or less Fair control = 7.6–8.9% Poor control ≥ 9% or more	Fasting not indicated. Blood can be drawn any time.

Random and Fasting Serum Glucose Levels

Elevated serum (blood) glucose levels are the criteria upon which the diagnosis of diabetes mellitus is determined. A fasting glucose level greater than 140 mg/dL, or nonfasting (random) level greater than 200 mg/dL, on two separate occasions suggests a diagnosis of diabetes (American Diabetes Association, 1995).

Self-Monitoring Blood Glucose (SMBG)

The availability and use of home glucose monitoring equipment to evaluate serum (blood) glucose has revolutionized self-care for the diabetic client (see Figure 30-3). Also called "finger stick blood glucose" (FSBG), self-monitoring of blood glucose can be done quickly using capillary blood that provides an accurate reading of the current blood glucose. Most often, the glucose level is checked before meals and at bedtime, thus allowing the client to adjust the treatment plan accordingly. Self-monitoring of blood glucose is recommended for all clients requiring insulin and for clients with widely fluctuating glucose levels. Symptoms of hypoglycemia at any time warrant immediate evaluation of the blood glucose level.

Urine Testing

Since the advent of home glucose monitoring devices, urine testing for glucose is rarely used for the estimation of serum glucose levels in the management of diabetes. Testing urine for **ketone** (product of fatty acid oxidation) production, however, continues to be recommended when the blood glucose level is consistently ≥ 240 mg/dL or when any symptoms of ketoacidosis are present.

KEY ABBREVIATIONS

The following abbreviations and acronyms are used in this chapter:

DKA	diabetic ketoacidosis
FBS	fasting blood sugar
FSBG	finger stick blood glucose
GDM	gestational diabetes mellitus
GHb	glycosylated hemoglobin
GTT	glucose tolerance test
HHNK	hyperosmolar hyperglycemic nonketotic syndrome
IGT	impaired glucose tolerance
IDDM	insulin dependent diabetes mellitus
NIDDM	non-insulin dependent diabetes mellitus
PPBS	post prandial blood sugar
PPG	post prandial glucose
PVD	peripheral vascular disease
SMBG	self-monitor blood glucose
U-100	100 units insulin per cc

DIABETES MELLITUS

Diabetes mellitus is actually a group of disorders with glucose intolerance in common. Diabetes results from an imbalance between insulin availability and insulin need. The major classifications of diabetes are:

- *Insulin dependent diabetes mellitus (IDDM),* or Type I, was previously called juvenile-onset diabetes. About 5 to 10 percent of diabetics have insulin dependent

FIGURE 30-3 Diabetic blood testing equipment: glucose meter, cotton balls, lancet, alcohol, blood testing strips, gloves, and watch.

or Type I diabetes. IDDM is characterized by an absolute insulin deficiency and always requires management with insulin injections. Onset of IDDM peaks at age eleven to thirteen and rarely occurs before age 1 or after age 30. IDDM has an abrupt onset and because of the acute nature of its symptoms, IDDM does not go undetected for very long.

- *Non-insulin dependent diabetes mellitus (NIDDM),* or Type II, was previously called adult-onset diabetes. The majority, approximately 85 to 90 percent of diabetics, have non-insulin dependent, or Type II, diabetes. This type rarely occurs before the age of forty, has a gradual onset, and is frequently associated with obesity and aging. Diabetics with NIDDM retain the ability to produce some insulin and may or may not require insulin therapy. Because there is some insulin production, the onset and progression of symptoms can be slow, and the disease can go undetected for years.

- *Gestational diabetes mellitus (GDM)* develops during pregnancy. Most gestational diabetes mellitus clients return to normal glucose tolerance when the pregnancy is over, but 40 to 60 percent of women who have had GDM will develop NIDDM later in their lives.

- *Impaired Glucose Tolerance (IGT),* is sometimes referred to as "borderline diabetes." Persons with IGT have hyperglycemia, but at lower levels than that which qualifies as a diagnosis of diabetes. Symptoms of diabetes are absent. IGT is thought to be a forerunner of NIDDM and 15 to 25 percent of people with IGT will progress to diabetes later in life. Persons with IGT should be supported in attaining their ideal body weight and screened periodically for diabetes.

- Diabetes mellitus may be associated with other conditions or syndromes such as malnutrition, hormone disorders, or drug therapy.

Insulin Dependent Diabetes Mellitus

IDDM is thought to be the result of a gradual autoimmune destruction of the islet cells of the pancreas. The presence of islet cell antibodies in 85 percent of persons with IDDM provides strong evidence for an autoimmune pathology. Current theories of causation hold that islet-cell destruction occurs predominantly in genetically susceptible people. Approximately 10 percent of individuals with IDDM have a first degree relative (parent or sibling) with IDDM.

Environmental agents have been implicated as "triggers" to the autoimmune process. Environmental agents that have been associated with altered pancreatic function are chemical toxins and viruses, including mumps and the coxsackievirus B.

It appears that the immune system attacks and destroys the insulin-producing beta cells of the islet of Langerhans. Before hyperglycemia occurs, 80 to 90 percent of the insulin-secreting cells must be destroyed.

In the absence of insulin, glucose from food eaten cannot be used or stored and remains in the bloodstream, resulting in hyperglycemia. In addition, glucose production from the liver goes unchecked, further elevating the blood glucose level.

As the serum glucose rises, the kidney begins to excrete excess glucose in the urine (**glycosuria**). Glucose eliminated in the urine pulls excessive amounts of water with it (osmotic diuresis), resulting in fluid volume deficit and producing symptoms of thirst (**polydipsia**) and increased urination (**polyuria**).

Insulin deficiency also results in impaired metabolism of fats and proteins. Because of the impaired glucose, fat, and protein metabolism and the inability to store glucose, clients with IDDM frequently experience protein wasting, weight loss, and increased hunger (**polyphagia**).

Metabolism of fat stores for energy leads to production of acid byproducts called ketones, which can be detected in the urine (**ketonuria**). As ketones accumulate, the associated decrease in pH leads to metabolic acidosis, or more specifically a condition known as diabetic ketoacidosis, discussed later in this chapter.

Non-Insulin Dependent Diabetes

The cause of NIDDM is unknown although it is thought to be autosomal recessive. NIDDM may be caused by some combination of gene-environmental interaction although the contribution of each component is not clearly understood. Heredity, aging, and obesity play major roles in the development of NIDDM.

In NIDDM, hyperglycemia results when the pancreas cannot match the body's need for insulin and/or when the number of insulin receptor sites are decreased or altered. Although available insulin may be insufficient to meet the body's metabolic needs and prevent hyperglycemia, there is a sufficient amount of insulin to prevent fat breakdown for energy and the resulting ketoacidosis associated with IDDM. Extremely elevated glucose in the non-insulin dependent diabetics will result in development of hyperosmolar hyperglycemic nonketotic syndrome (HHNK), discussed later in this chapter.

Obesity has been implicated as a major contributor to the development of NIDDM. Approximately 80 percent of all clients with NIDDM are 20 percent or more over their ideal body weight. It is possible that the pancreas of an overweight person may not be able to meet the increased need for insulin production. Some persons with NIDDM, however, have an increased insulin level (hyperinsulinism). Current theories suggest that the cells of obese individuals may have defective or a decreased number of insulin receptors, leading to insulin resistance.

Contributing Factors

Persons with a family history of diabetes are at greater risk for developing diabetes. The incidence of diabetes in first degree relatives (parent or sibling) of persons with NIDDM is increased 10 to 15 percent, and the incidence is increased 5 to 10 percent for first degree relatives of persons with IDDM. It is believed that people do not inherit the disease diabetes, but rather they inherit the ability to develop diabetes.

At present, development of diabetes cannot be predicted or prevented. In persons susceptible to develop IDDM, it is believed that exposure to certain environmental factors, such as chemical toxins or viruses, trigger diabetes to develop. Prevention of the disease may someday be possible if the environmental triggers can be identified and exposure prevented, vaccines can be developed, or methods are refined to suppress the autoimmune destruction of the islet cell in the pancreas.

In addition to family history, factors associated with NIDDM include obesity, aging, and ethnic group. The most powerful risk factor for NIDDM is obesity, increasing a person's risk for developing NIDDM ten times. In persons with a family history of NIDDM, maintenance of an ideal body weight may delay or prevent the onset of diabetes.

Aging can also be considered a contributing factor. Incidence of NIDDM occurs almost ten times more often in persons over age sixty-five, possibly related to decreased immune function associated with aging.

It is known that members of certain racial groups are more likely to develop diabetes. In the United States, there is a greater chance of developing NIDDM for Hispanics, certain Native American populations, and African Americans.

Other groups at risk for development of diabetes include those with a history of gestational diabetes or impaired glucose tolerance (IGT). Approximately 10 to 15 percent of persons with IGT and 40 to 60 percent of persons with a history of gestational diabetes will develop diabetes.

Clinical Manifestations

Table 30-1 compares and contrasts the clinical manifestations of IDDM and NIDDM.

Insulin Dependent Diabetes Mellitus

Initial symptoms of IDDM usually have an acute onset and develop rapidly. The untreated diabetic appears thin and emaciated. Classic symptoms include weight loss, polyuria, polydipsia, and polyphagia. Ketoacidosis, caused by increased amounts of circulating ketones, may also be present.

Noninsulin Dependent Diabetes

NIDDM is associated with a gradual onset of symptoms and may go undetected for years. Although clients with NIDDM may present the classic symptoms of diabetes (polyuria, polydipsia, polyphagia), they are more likely to experience fatigue, visual changes, paresthesias, and recurrent infections. The client is frequently overweight. NIDDM is often diagnosed while the client is being evaluated or treated for another disorder.

Medical/Surgical Management

There is no known cure for diabetes to date. The goal of therapeutic management is aimed at the control of blood sugar, and the prevention and early

Table 30-1

A COMPARISON OF THE CLINICAL MANIFESTATIONS OF IDDM AND NIDDM

	Types of Diabetes Mellitus	
Synonyms	*IDDM* Type I, Juvenile, Brittle/labile	*NIDDM* Type II, Adult Onset
Etiology	Autoimmune, probably due to genetic and environmental factors with risk factors	Genetic susceptibility associated. Usually associated with long duration obesity
Age of Onset	Rare before age 1 or after age 30	Rare before age 40. Incidence increases with age
Percent of diabetics	5–10%	85–90%
Onset	Abrupt, rapid	Gradual, over years
Body weight at onset	Normal or thin	80% are overweight
Insulin production	None	Less than normal, normal, or greater than normal
Insulin injection	Always	Necessary for approximately 30%
Ketosis	May occur	Unlikely
Management	Insulin, diet, exercise	Diet and weight loss, exercise, possibly oral hypoglycemics or insulin

detection of the complications associated with diabetes. Diabetes is considered under control if the client maintains ideal body weight and enjoys good health, pre-prandial glucose levels are less than 140 mg/dL, postprandial glucose levels do not rise above 180 mg/dL, and glycosylated hemoglobin is within normal limits (4 to 8 percent).

Treatment plans vary and are individualized for each client. Control of blood glucose generally involves a balance of a dietary prescription, an exercise plan, and medications. Ultimately, the client is the manager of the treatment plan and, therefore, must be very well informed about diabetes and involved in all aspects of care planning and decision making.

The client with insulin-dependent diabetes will always require administration of insulin to lower the glucose level and prevent complications of diabetes. Diet and exercise regimens are also important for the control of the glucose level and maintenance of health.

Dietary management is the cornerstone of treatment for the person with non-insulin dependent diabetes (NIDDM). As the obese person loses weight, the body's insulin requirements decrease, resulting in improved glucose tolerance. Exercise can also play a valuable role in losing weight and lowering the blood glucose level. NIDDM not controlled by diet and exercise may necessitate administration of medications. Oral hypoglycemic agents or parenteral administration of insulin may be required for optimal control.

Diet

Nutritional therapy continues to be considered the cornerstone of diabetic management. There is no one diabetic or ADA (American Diabetic Association) diet. The recommended diet is a dietary prescription based on nutritional assessment and treatment goals of the client.

Dietary prescriptions are individualized to meet client and family needs. Consideration must be given to usual eating habits and other lifestyle factors such as dietary likes and dislikes, cultural influences, who prepares the meals, and family finances. It is important that meals remain a social experience, and the diabetic person does not feel isolated or different.

The goals of nutrition are to maintain as near-normal blood glucose level as possible, achieve optimal serum lipid levels, provide adequate energy for maintaining or attaining a reasonable weight, prevent complications of diabetes, and improve overall health. Because of the complexity of nutrition issues, it is recommended that clients be referred early to a registered dietician for nutritional education. Table 30-2 summarizes the dietary recommendations of the American Diabetes Association.

Diabetes is a strong risk factor for atherosclerosis

Table 30-2

ADA DIETARY RECOMMENDATIONS

Calories: Sufficient to achieve and maintain ideal body weight.

Protein: Same recommendation as for general population. 10–12% of total calories 80–90% of calories remain to be distributed between dietary fat and carbohydrates, and can vary based on nutritional assessment and treatment goals.

Fat: ≤ 30% total calories, including < 10% saturated fats < 10% polyunsaturated fats

Carbohydrates: 50–70% total calories Sucrose, fructose and other nutritive sweeteners may be included in modest amounts, depending on glycemic control. Recommendations for fiber are same as general population (20–35 grams/day).

Sodium: Same as general population (≤ 3000 mg/day)

Alcohol: ≤ 2 alcoholic beverages (1 beverage = 12 oz beer, 5 oz wine, or 1.5 oz distilled liquor) When calculating intake as part of dietary exchange, 1 alcoholic beverage = 2 fat exchanges. Alcohol may increase the risk for hypoglycemia in people treated with insulin or sulfonyureas, and therefore should be ingested with a meal.

Vitamins and Minerals: When dietary intake is adequate, there is no need for additional vitamin and mineral supplement.

(*From* Nutrition recommendations and principles for people with diabetes, *American Diabetes Association: Clinical Practice Recommendations 1995.*)

and cardiovascular disease. Therefore, reducing serum lipid levels is a goal of diabetic nutrition therapy. To reduce the risk of cardiovascular disease, the ADA recommendations incorporate a reduction in saturated fat and cholesterol consumption.

It is recommended that individuals taking insulin or oral hypoglycemic agents eat at consistent times synchronized with the actions of the medications used. Distribution of calories over twenty-four hours, with regular meals and snacks helps to prevent extreme highs and lows in blood glucose.

Exchange System The diabetic exchange system, developed by the American Diabetes Association and the American Dietetic Association, is the most frequently used system for ensuring that the diabetic integrates all aspects of the dietary prescription. This system divides food into six categories according to the amount of protein, carbohydrate, fat, and calories supplied by the food. The six groups, and examples of exchanges are listed in Table 30-3. Clients are given meal plans or prescriptions, specifying the number of exchanges from each list that should be eaten at each meal. With the exchange group system, any food in the proper amount may be substituted for another food in the same exchange list. Table 30-4 shows a sample menu based on the exchange system. The diabetic exchange system continues to be widely used. Once it is learned, it is simple, flexible, and provides wide variety.

Other Diet Systems   Many tools and plans for dietary compliance are available to diabetics. Another system gaining more popularity is one that monitors the amount of carbohydrate available in each meal. Insulin doses are then regulated according to total available carbohydrate.

Position Statement: American Diabetes Association   According to *Nutrition Recommendations and Principles for People with Diabetes Mellitus, 1996,* there are five goals of nutrition therapy besides improved metabolic control. They are:

1. Maintain as near-normal blood glucose level.
2. Achieve optimal serum lipid levels.
3. Provide adequate calories to maintain or attain a reasonable weight (reasonable weight is determined by client and health care provider).
4. Prevent and treat acute complications of insulin-treated diabetes.
5. Improve overall health through optimal nutrition (Dietary Guidelines for Americans and Food Guide Pyramid are examples to follow).

Protein intake of both animal and vegetable sources should make up 10 to 20 percent of the daily calorie intake. If nephropathy is present, protein should be 10 percent of the daily calorie intake.

Total fat intake depends on the goals set by the client and health care provider for desired levels of glucose, lipid, and weight. If lipid levels are normal, 30 percent or less of calories should come from fat with less than 10 percent from saturated fat. If weight loss is a primary issue, reduction in fat intake is an efficient way to reduce calorie intake. When lipid levels are a problem, decrease saturated fat intake to < 7 percent of the total calories, total fat to < 30 percent of total calories and cholesterol to < 200 mg/day.

The remainder of the calorie intake comes from carbohydrates. The amount consumed is more important than the source of the carbohydrate.

Persons with diabetes should follow the same precautions regarding the use of alcohol as applied to the general public. Alcohol may increase the risk for hypoglycemia in people treated with insulin or sul-

Table 30-3

ADA EXCHANGE LISTS—SAMPLE FOOD SERVINGS

Starch/bread (80 cal): 15 g CHO, 3 g pro, trace fat

oatmeal, ½ c	corn, ⅓ c
bread, 1 slice	peas, ½ c
bran muffin, 1	bagel, ½
crackers, 5	tortilla, 1
brown rice, 1 c	cooked pasta, ½ c
dinner roll, 1 small	hamburger bun, ½
popcorn (plain), 2 c	potato, ½ small

Meats

Lean (55 cal): 7 g pro, 3 g fat
   fish, 2 oz
   tuna fish, ¼ c
   meat, 1 oz lean pork, veal poultry without skin
   cottage cheese, ¼ c
Medium (75 cal): 7 g pro, 5 g fat
   boiled ham, 1 oz
   liver, 1 oz
   egg, 1
High fat (100 cal): 7 g pro, 8 g fat
   peanut butter, 1 tbsp
   lunchmeat, 1 oz

Vegetables (25 cal): 5 g CHO, 2 g pro
   lettuce, as desired
   vegetable soup, ½ c
   tomato, 1 medium
   carrots, green beans, eggplant, brussels sprouts, onion, cabbage, ½ c cooked or 1 c raw

Fruits (60 cal): 15 g CHO
   cantaloupe, ⅛
   applesauce, ½ c
   grapes, 15
   banana, ½
   peach, pear, apple, orange, 1 small

Milks (80 cal): 12 g CHO, 8 g pro, trace fat (if skim)
   skim milk, 1 c
   nonfat yogurt 1 c

Fat (45 cal): 5 g fat

mayonnaise, 1 tsp	avocado, ⅛
salad dressing, 1 tbsp	bacon, 1 strip
margarine, 1 tsp	cream cheese, 1 tbsp

Free exchanges (0 cal)

calorie-free beverages	coffee, tea
unsweetened gelatin	boullion

(*Adapted from:* Exchange lists for meal planning, *American Diabetes Association and American Dietetic Association, 1986.*)

Table 30-4

SAMPLE ADA DIET, USING EXCHANGE SYSTEM (2,200 CAL)						
Food Group	Total Exchanges	Breakfast	Lunch	Dinner	Snacks P.M.	HS
Milk	2	1				1
Vegetable	4		2	2		
Fruit	3	1	1		1	
Bread	12.5	3	3	3	2	1.5
Meat	8	1	2	4		1
Fat	7	2	2	3		

Breakfast
1 medium peach
½ c oatmeal
1 poached egg on slice wheat toast
1 bran muffin
2 tsp margarine
1 c skim milk
coffee

Lunch
vegetable soup
5 wheat crackers
tuna sandwich (2 breads, ½ c tuna, 2 tsp mayo)
1 medium pear
Diet soda

P.M. Snack
10 crackers
2 tbsp peanut butter
1 orange

Dinner
4 oz pork chop
1 c brown rice
½ c green beans
Tossed green salad with Italian dressing (3 tbsp)
½ c applesauce
1 dinner roll

HS Snack
3 c popcorn, plain
1 oz cheese
1 c skim milk

(*Adapted from:* Essential of Nutrition and Diet Therapy, *Williams, S.R., 1994*).

fonylureas such as acetohexamide (Dymelor), chlorpropamide (Diabinese), or tolazamide (Tolinase).

Pharmacological

Various pharmacological treatments that are used in the management of IDDM and NIDDM are discussed as follows.

Insulin Persons with IDDM always require insulin administration. Persons with NIDDM often do not require insulin when initially diagnosed, but insulin therapy may become necessary over time, as endogenous insulin production decreases. The client with NIDDM may also require insulin during times of stress or illness.

Historically, insulin has been obtained from beef or pork pancreas. Today, biosynthetic human insulin is used almost exclusively, but there are some clients still using pork or beef insulin. Human insulin is purer, more effective, and has a much lower incidence of causing insulin allergies and resistance. Insulin is available in short-, intermediate-, and long-acting forms that can be injected separately or mixed in the same syringe. Premixed insulins are also available. See Table 30-5 for descriptions of types of insulins and their

actions. Insulin is routinely administered subcutaneously. Regular insulin (short-acting) may be administered intravenously when immediate response is desired, as in treatment of greatly elevated glucose levels occurring with diabetic ketoacidosis (DKA) or hyperosmolar hyperglycemic nonketotic syndrome (HHNK). Regular insulin, which is the only clear insulin, is the *only* insulin that can be given intravenously (IV).

The strength of insulin correlates to the number of units of insulin per cubic centimeter. The most common concentration of insulin used today is U-100 insulin (100 units of insulin per 1 cc). U-500 insulin is also available for clients who have developed insulin resistance and require very high doses.

Insulin should always be measured in an insulin syringe which is marked in units. When mixing two types of insulin in the same syringe, it is important that the Regular (clear, short-acting) insulin be drawn up first. The policy of many health care institutions requires that two nurses check insulin dosages prior to administration. Even if the facility does not have such a policy, checking the insulin dosage with another nurse will help protect against an adverse reaction due to error.

Insulin dosages are individually determined, usually requiring two or more injections per day and involving

Table 30-5

TYPES OF INSULIN AND THEIR ACTIONS

Types of Insulin	Appearance	Action in Hours		
		Onset	Peak	Duration
Short-acting				
Humulin R	clear	½–1	2–4	6–8
Intermediate				
Humulin N	cloudy	1–2	4–12	10–14
Humulin L	cloudy	2	8–12	12–16
Long				
Humulin U	cloudy	8	18	24–36
Premixed				
Reg/Humulin N				
Humulin 70/30	cloudy	1/2	2–12	18–24
Humulin 50/50				

a combination of a short-acting and a longer-acting insulin. Various regimens of insulin administration can be used, each with its own advantages and disadvantages. In general, the more complex the regimen, the more normal the blood glucose levels throughout the day. Clients can be taught to use the results of their self monitoring blood glucose to adjust their insulin doses, allowing more flexibility in their meals and schedules. Recent studies strongly support the theory that intensive insulin regimens that tightly control the blood glucose level delays the onset and progression of complications of diabetic retinopathy, nephropathy, and neuropathy.

Sliding Insulin Scale   During times of surgery, illness, or stress, clients with IDDM and NIDDM may have their glucose level managed with an insulin sliding scale in lieu of their regular regimen of insulin or oral hypoglycemics. A sliding scale determines insulin dosage based on fingerstick blood glucose level. Regular (short-acting) insulin is used and a dose is administered every four or six hours based on the blood glucose level. The sliding scale allows for much flexibility and ensures frequent monitoring of and response to changes in the client's glucose level. An example sliding scale might be:

- 4u Humulin R Insulin for glucose 151–200 mg/dL
- 6u Humulin R Insulin for glucose 201–250 mg/dL
- 8u Humulin R Insulin for glucose 251–300 mg/dL
- 10u Humulin R Insulin for glucose 301–350 mg/dL
- Call physician for glucose > 350 mg/dL

Insulin Injections   Insulin injections are administered into the subcutaneous tissue. If an inch can be pinched, inject needle at a ninety degree angle, otherwise, at a forty-five degree angle. The four main areas for injection are the abdomen, arms, thighs, and hips (see Figure 30-4). Factors affecting absorption should be considered when selecting an injection site. Absorption occurs most quickly in the abdomen, followed by the arms, thighs, and hips.

Rotation of sites for injection has traditionally been recommended to prevent **lipodystrophies** (local changes in the subcutaneous fat). More recently, some authorities are recommending that the abdomen, which provides the most predictable absorption of insulin, be used exclusively for insulin administration.

If sites other than the abdomen are used, site rotation needs to be done in a systematic manner to prevent erratic absorption. One system of rotation is to always use the same area of injection the same time each day, for example, always using the abdomen in the morning and the thigh in the afternoon. Another system of rotation is to use all available injection sites in one area before moving to another.

Areas of lipodystrophy should not be used for injection, as absorption may be diminished. Exercise will increase the rate of absorption, so diabetics planning to exercise should not inject insulin into the areas to be exercised.

Vials of insulin not being used should be refrigerated to prevent loss of potency. Vials in use may be kept at room temperature to decrease local irritation at the injection site, which can occur when cold insulin is used. When mixing a short-acting (Humulin) and a longer-acting (Humulin N, Humulin L, Humulin U) insulin in the same syringe, the Regular (clear) should always be drawn up into the syringe first, followed by the longer-acting (cloudy) insulin. Figure 30-5 illustrates mixing and administering insulin.

It is recommended that insulin syringes be used

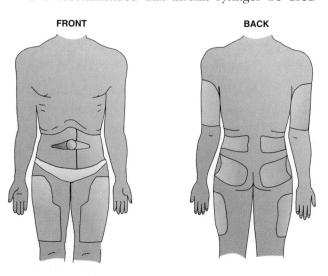

FIGURE 30-4   Suggested sites for insulin administration.

only once and then discarded. In the home, however, some clients are able to safely reuse insulin syringes to decrease expense. The syringe should be discarded when the needle becomes dull, has been bent, or has come into contact with any surface other than the skin. If syringes are reused by the client, the needle must be recapped after each use. Syringe reuse is not advisable for clients with poor hygiene, open wounds, or decreased resistance to infection.

The visually and/or neurologically impaired diabetic may benefit from assistive devices available to facilitate drawing up the insulin and administering it. Diabetics dependent on others for drawing up their insulin may benefit from prefilled syringes, which are considered stable for up to three weeks when stored in the refrigerator.

The nurse should keep in mind that the most important factor in the administration of insulin is consistency in technique. Also, simplification of the pro-cedure may have a major impact on a clients ability to comply and to maintain independence. It is important that the nurse understand the basic principles of insulin administration and thereby remain flexible when teaching new clients or assessing the skills of experienced clients.

Insulin Pumps A portable insulin infusion pump delivers insulin continuously through a subcutaneous needle, usually anchored in the abdomen (see Figure 30-6). A continuous, or basal rate, of regular (rapid-acting) insulin is programmed and delivered to closely imitate the body's natural insulin secretion. Additional boluses can be manually administered to coordinate with meal times. The injection site is changed every twenty-four to forty-eight hours. The use of the insulin pump prevents multiple injections and allows flexibility in meal size and time. Use of the pump requires a motivated and educated client, because intensive self-monitoring of blood glucose is essential.

Mixing insulins

The client may withdraw two different types of insulin into the same syringe. In this series of diagrams, a rapid-acting insulin (R vial) is combined with an intermediate-acting insulin (N vial).

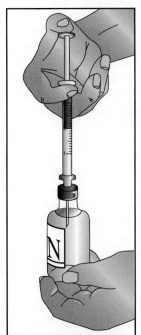

1 After cleaning the rubber stopper on both vials with an alcohol wipe, inject the amount of air equal to the dose of the intermediate-acting insulin into the N vial.

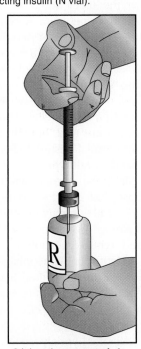

2 Inject the amount of air equal to the dose of the rapid-acting insulin into the R vial.

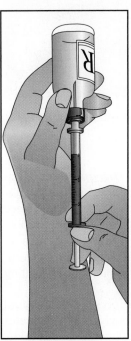

3 Withdraw the correct amount of rapid-acting insulin.

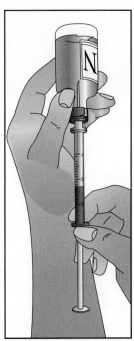

4 Withdraw the correct amount of intermediate acting insulin. (Note: pull the plunger down to the unit mark that equals the dose of rapid-acting insulin plus the dose of intermediate-acting insulin. The insulins will mix immediately in the syringe. If too large an amount of intermediate acting insulin is withdrawn, the entire contents of the syringe must be discarded.)

FIGURE 30-5 How to mix insulin. (*Adapted from Baer, C.L. & Williams, B.R. (1996),* Clinical Pharmacology and Nursing, *3rd edition. Springhouse, PA: Springhouse Corporation.*)

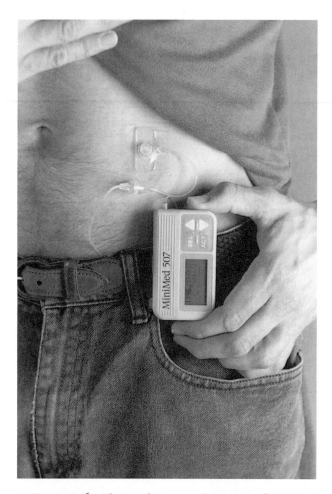

FIGURE 30-6 The insulin pump. (*Courtesy of MiniMed*)

Complications of Insulin Therapy Complications of insulin therapy include hypoglycemia (discussed later in this chapter), insulin resistance (requiring more than 200 units/day), lipodystrophy, Somogyi phenomenon and the dawn phenomenon. Lipodystrophy can be minimized by using human insulin, using room temperature insulin, and by rotating sites of insulin injection.

The **Somogyi phenomenon** occurs when a rapid decrease in blood glucose (hypoglycemia) generates the release of glucose-elevating hormones (epinephrine, cortisol, glucagon). The hypoglycemia usually occurs during the night, but manifests as an elevated glucose in the morning and may be inadvertently treated with an increase in insulin dosage. The Somogyi phenomenon can be diagnosed by checking the blood glucose during the night at about 3 A.M. Adjusting the insulin regimen to avoid the peaking of insulin during the night will correct this effect.

The **dawn phenomenon** is an early morning glucose elevation produced by the release of growth hormone. Administering the evening insulin dose at a later time will coordinate the insulin peak with the hormone release.

Oral Hypoglycemic Agents Oral hypoglycemic agents are used in the treatment of persons with NIDDM who are not controlled with exercise and diet. About 35 percent of diabetics are treated with oral medications. Oral hypoglycemics are not insulin and work by other mechanisms.

Sulfonylurea is the class of oral hypoglycemic medications most commonly used for diabetes therapy. The sulfonylureas work primarily by increasing the ability of the islet cells of the pancreas to excrete insulin. It is also believed that they have some effect by increasing the cells' sensitivity to insulin and decreasing glucose production by the liver.

Most sulfonylureas should be administered half an hour before meals, except for glipizide (Glucotrol) which can be administered on a more flexible schedule. Hypoglycemia can occur in any client taking a sulfonyluric oral hypoglycemic, but hypoglycemia is more common and more dangerous in the elderly. Recognition of hypoglycemia may be more difficult for the older adult because aging decreases the adrenergic mediated hypoglycemic responses of shaking, sweating, and nervousness. Older adults are also more likely to be taking medications for other chronic illnesses that may interact with the oral hypoglycemic. Various medications have the potential to interfere with or enhance the action of oral hypoglycemics.

Other side effects of sulfonyluric oral hypoglycemic agents are rare, but can include skin rashes and gastrointestinal disturbances. Clients should be warned that the oral hypoglycemics, especially chlorpropamide (Diabinese), are known to produce a disulfiram (Antabuse)-like effect in some clients when ingesting alcohol. Reaction may be severe and include symptoms of flushing, sweating, nausea and vomiting, palpitations, and hyperventilation.

Metformin (Glucophage), a biguanide, was approved for use in the United States in 1995. Metformin does not increase insulin release but works by making existing insulin more effective at the cellular level. Metformin may be given alone or in combination with other oral hypoglycemics. In some clients, Glucophage works more effectively if given with some dose of Diabeta. Because it does not stimulate increased insulin release, metformin is not associated with episodes of hypoglycemia. The major side effects of metformin are gastrointestinal and include anorexia, nausea, abdominal discomfort, and diarrhea.

Oral hypoglycemics require some production of insulin by the pancreas and, therefore, are not useful in the treatment of IDDM. See Table 30-6 for a description of oral hypoglycemic agents available in the United States.

Pancreas Transplants

Pancreas transplantations have been performed and have successfully eliminated the need for exogenous insulin in some clients. At present pancreas transplants are being performed primarily on clients with IDDM who also need kidney or other organ transplants. This is because the serious side effects of the antirejection medications do not justify a pancreas transplant alone. Pancreatic islet cell transplants are also being done experimentally with limited success, but hold much promise for the future.

Activity

The beneficial effects of regular exercise for the diabetic are multiple. Exercise decreases the blood glucose by increasing the uptake of glucose by body muscles and improving insulin usage. Exercise also increases circulation, improves cardiovascular status, decreases stress, and assists with weight loss.

Before starting an exercise program, the diabetic individual should have a complete physical and review the exercise plan with the physician or primary health care provider. Regular daily exercise rather than sporadic exercise should be encouraged.

Diabetics need to correlate exercise with their blood glucose, taking care to avoid periods of hypoglycemia or exercising when blood glucose is too high. Exercise potentiates the action of insulin, resulting in lower insulin requirements and an increased risk of hypoglycemia during and after exercise. On the other hand, in the diabetic who is insulin deficient, exercise may cause a further rise in blood glucose and rapid development of ketosis. Diabetics must know they should not exercise at the peak of insulin activity, when blood glucose is greater than 250 mg/dL, or if they have ketones in their urine. See Table 30-7, Guidelines for Exercising.

Discharge Planning

Self-Monitoring Blood Glucose (SMBG) The development of monitors, whereby diabetics can evaluate and thus more easily regulate their own glucose level, are considered a major breakthrough in diabetes management. Monitors allow for detection of hypo- and hyperglycemia. They play a major role in keeping the blood glucose level in the normal range and possibly reducing long-term complications associated with diabetes. SMBG is a useful procedure for all diabetics and is considered essential for all intensive insulin regimens. Most clients check their blood glucose two times a day, but may test prior to each meal, during episodes of hypo- or hyperglycemia, or PRN during illness.

The monitors used for finger-stick glucose are technique dependent and because treatment and insulin

Table 30-6

ORAL HYPOGLYCEMICS

Generic (Brand)	Usual Dose	Onset Time (hours)	Duration (hours)
tobutamide (Orinase)	500–2,000 mg divided dose	1	6–12
acetohexamide (Dymelor)	250–1500 mg single or divided dose	1	12–24
tolazamide (Tolinase)	100–1,000 mg single or divided dose	4–6	12–24
chlorpropamide (Diabanese)	100–750 mg single dose	1	60
glipizide (Glucatrol)	2.5–40 mg single or divided dose	1	10–24
glyburide (Diabeta, Micronase)	1.25–20 mg single or divided dose	2–4	24
metformin (Glucophage)	1–2.5 gm two or three divided doses		

doses are often based on results, accuracy is a major concern. Client teaching regarding monitor use and maintenance is a primary concern for the diabetic educator.

Sick Day Management It is important that diabetics have a plan for managing their diabetes in the event of illness. They should know that it is important that they continue to receive their insulin or oral hypoglycemic medication when they are experiencing illness, as illness and fever can increase blood glucose and the need for insulin. Some diabetics who do not normally take short-acting insulin may require insulin coverage during times of fever or illness. Blood glucose should be monitored four to six times per day and urine should be checked for ketones. Blood glucose greater than 300 mg/dL or ketones in the urine should be reported to the physician.

If the client cannot ingest the planned meal, carbohydrates in the form of soft foods and liquids can be substituted. Extreme nausea and vomiting or diarrhea should be reported to the physician because extreme fluid loss can be dangerous. Clients with IDDM who are unable to retain fluids may need to be hospitalized to avoid ketoacidosis.

Table 30-7

GUIDELINES FOR EXERCISING

- Try to exercise at the same time and in the same amount each day.
- Test blood glucose levels before, during, and after exercise.
- Do not inject your insulin into a limb that you will be exercising.
- Do not exercise at the peak of your insulin activity.
- Do not exercise before meals unless you are trying to lower your serum glucose level.
- Do not exercise with blood glucose levels over 250 mg/dL or if you have ketones in your urine. This indicates severe insulin deficiency and may predispose client to hyperglycemia.
- Do eat a snack (15 gm carbohydrate) prior to or during exercise if appropriate, based on blood glucose.
- Always carry a source of carbohydrates and emergency cash, if away from home, in case you become hypoglycemic while exercising.
- Always carry personal and medical alert identification.
- Watch for post-exercise hypoglycemia. Individuals who have more than usual exercise during the day should increase their carbohydrate intake and test their glucose during the night to detect nocturnal hypoglycemia. (Hypoglycemia can occur 8 to 15 hours following exercise.)

Acute Complications of Diabetes

There are three major acute complications of diabetes related to blood glucose imbalance: hypoglycemia, diabetic ketoacidosis (DKA), and hyperosmolar hyperglycemic nonketotic syndrome (HHNK).

Hypoglycemia (Insulin Reaction)

Hypoglycemia (low blood glucose) occurs when a client's glucose level drops below 70 mg/dL with the most severe reactions occurring when it drops below 50 mg/dL. Hypoglycemia can occur anytime of the day, but most often will occur before meals or when insulin action is peaking. Factors that can contribute to the development of a hypoglycemic reaction are skipping meals or eating late, unplanned exercise, and administration of excess insulin.

Hypoglycemic symptoms can occur suddenly and unexpectedly, and vary from client to client (see Table 30-8). *Always believe clients who tell you they are having an insulin reaction.* Most diabetics have had hypoglycemic reactions before, so they know the symptoms that precede an insulin reaction.

When a hypoglycemic reaction is suspected, the nurse must respond immediately according to the institution's protocol. Treatment involves assessing the client, checking blood glucose level, and administering glucose in the most appropriate form. Always

remember, hypoglycemic reactions can be fatal. *Leaving the client untreated is more dangerous than causing mild hyperglycemia with overtreatment.* Figure 30-7 provides a sample hypoglycemic protocol.

Diabetics and their families must be instructed about the symptoms and treatment for hypoglycemia. Hypoglycemic episodes can be prevented by following a regular pattern of eating, exercise, and insulin administration. Between meals and bedtime snacks can be used to cover times of peak insulin action. Additional food should be eaten when engaging in greater than usual exercise. Blood glucose level should be checked at the first suspicion of hypoglycemia. All diabetics should wear an identification bracelet or tag indicating that they have diabetes, as hypoglycemic reactions can occur unexpectedly.

Table 30-8

SYMPTOMS OF ACUTE COMPLICATIONS OF DIABETES

Symptoms of Hypoglycemia (Insulin Reaction)

Mild hypoglycemia
- Diaphoresis
- Pallor
- Palpitations
- Hunger
- Paresthesias
- Tremors
- Anxiety

Moderate to severe hypoglycemia
- Confusion, disorientation, loss of consciousness
- Slurred speech
- Behavior changes
- Seizures

*Nursing Alert: Severe hypoglycemia is a medical emergency. Administer some form of glucose immediately.

Symptoms of Hyperosmolar Hyperglycemic Nonketotic Coma (HHNK)

- Polyuria
- Polydipsia
- Skin hot, dry, decreased turgor
- Dehydration—hypotension, increased pulse
- Blurred vision
- Weakness
- Mental status changes, confusion to coma

Symptoms of Diabetic Ketoacidosis (DKA)

Same as HHNK plus symptoms of acidosis:
- "fruity" odor to breath
- Kussmaul's respirations (deep, non-labored)

Diabetic Ketoacidosis (DKA)

Diabetic ketoacidosis (DKA) is one of the most serious complications of hyperglycemia. Glucose is a hyperosmolar substance drawing fluid out of the cell and into the circulation where it is excreted by the kidneys. This oncotic diuresis results in polyuria (increased urine output), dehydration, and electrolyte imbalances. Increased fat metabolism results in accumulation of ketones, resulting in metabolic acidosis. Surgery, stress, or illness may trigger DKA which usually develops in clients with IDDM, although it can occur in clients with NIDDM. The client with undiagnosed IDDM may also present with DKA.

The onset of DKA may be gradual or sudden. Classic symptoms of hyperglycemia (polyuria, polyphagia, polydipsia) usually precede DKA. Other symptoms include nausea and vomiting, abdominal pain from acidosis, headache, weakness, fatigue, and blurred vision. Assessment may reveal hot, flushed skin and signs of hypovolemia or shock. Acidosis will produce signs of hyperpnea (Kussmaul's breathing), fruity odor to breath from respiratory elimination of acetone, and decreased level of consciousness ranging from lethargy to coma.

Laboratory values will reveal blood glucose from 300 to 800 mg/dL and metabolic acidosis. Urine will be positive for glucose and ketones.

Hyperosmolar Hyperglycemic Nonketotic (HHNK) Syndrome

Hyperosmolar hyperglycemic nonketotic (HHNK) syndrome occurs when there is insufficient insulin to

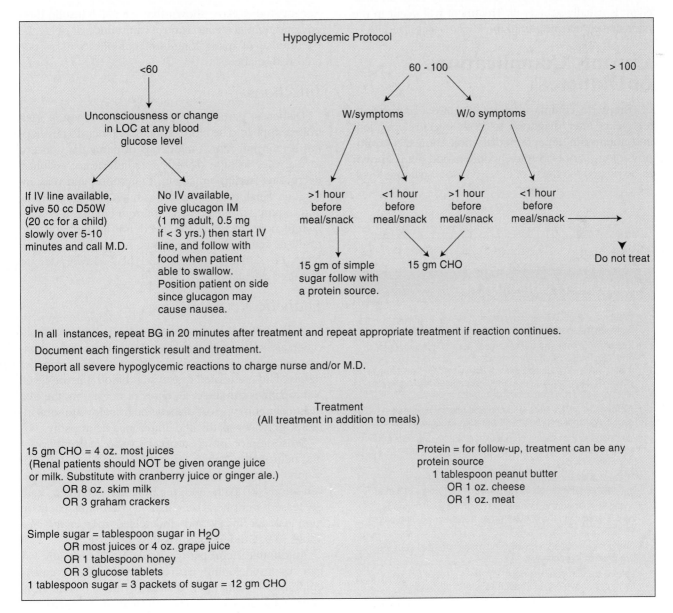

FIGURE 30-7 Hypoglycemic protocol.

prevent hyperglycemia, but enough insulin to prevent ketoacidosis. HHNK occurs in persons with NIDDM. Because symptoms of acidosis do not occur, hyperglycemia and oncotic diuresis can be much more severe.

HHNK occurs most often in the elderly client with undiagnosed NIDDM. HHNK can also occur in the poorly controlled client and is usually precipitated by illness or other stressor.

Clinical manifestations of HHNK reflect dehydration and shock. Hyperosmolality eventually results in lethargy, seizures, and coma (Table 30-8). Blood glucose level ranges from 600 to 2000 mg/dL and serum osmolality > 350 mOsm/L.

Medical Management of DKA and HHNK
Management involves fluid and electrolyte replacement (particularly potassium), insulin therapy, and treatment of any precipitating factors. DKA and HHNK are associated with significant mortality rates and the client is usually acutely ill. Treatment will occur in the intensive care setting until the client is stabilized.

Chronic Complications of Diabetes

Long-term complications of diabetes occur five to ten years after diagnosis in both insulin-dependent and noninsulin-dependent diabetics. The exact pathophysiology is not completely understood but is known to be related to effects of elevated blood glucose level.

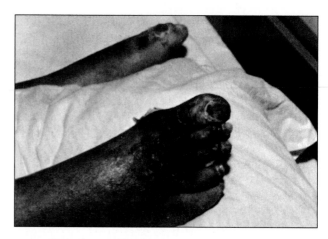

FIGURE 30-8 Gangrene of the toes and foot as a result of an infection often means eventual amputation.

Recent studies have shown that intensive insulin therapy and tight glycemic control can reduce or delay the occurrence of many long-term complications associated with diabetes.

Infections

Diabetics, particularly clients who are poorly controlled, appear to be more prone than others to developing certain infections. Infections of particular concern to diabetics include diabetic foot infections, cellulitis, necrotizing fasciitis, urinary tract infections, and yeast infections. Small cuts on the feet can become gangrenous and require amputation as shown in Figure 30-8.

Infections increase the need for insulin and can result in ketoacidosis. Infections, once they occur can often be difficult to treat and heal slowly due to impaired circulation.

Diabetic Neuropathies

Neuropathies are the most common chronic complication associated with diabetes. The incidence of peripheral neuropathies increases with age and duration of disease and are related to elevated blood glucose level. Neuropathies can affect all types of nerves but the two most common types of diabetic neuropathy are sensorimotor polyneuropathy and autonomic neuropathy.

Sensorimotor polyneuropathy, also called peripheral neuropathy, causes paresthesias and burning sensations, primarily in the lower extremities. Decreased sensations of pain and temperature, coupled with decreased peripheral circulation place the client at high risk for injury and undetected foot injury. See Table 30-9, Guidelines to Healthy Feet.

Autonomic neuropathy can affect almost any organ system including: gastrointestinal (delayed gastric emptying, constipation, diarrhea), urinary (retention, neurogenic bladder) and sexual (male impotence) dysfunction.

Table 30-9

GUIDELINES TO HEALTHY FEET

- Wash your feet daily and dry them carefully, especially between the toes.
- Inspect your feet and between your toes for blisters, cuts, and infections. Use a mirror to see the bottoms of your feet. If your vision is impaired, have a family member examine your feet. Remember, because of decreased feeling in your feet, you may have an infection and not know it.
- Avoid activities that will restrict blood flow to your feet, especially smoking. Do not sit with legs crossed.
- Wear shoes that are comfortable, well-fitting, and closed toed. Wear new shoes for short intervals until broken in. Do not walk barefoot.
- Prevent cuts and irritations. Always wear stockings. Look inside shoes for rough edges, nail points, foreign objects.
- Avoid temperature extremes. Test bath water with hands before getting in. Do not use water bottles or heating pads on feet.
- See your physician regularly and make sure that your feet are examined each visit.
- When you trim your toe nails, cut them straight across. When you have corns of calluses, see a physician or prodiatrist. Do not cut them yourself.

Sample Nursing Care Plan: The Diabetic Client with a Foot Ulcer

Mr. Kucharski is a seventy-year-old insulin dependent diabetic with an infected ulcer on the heel of his left foot. He is admitted to a skilled care facility for wound care and IV antibiotic therapy. Mr. Kucharski stated the ulcer developed after he stepped on a sharp stone while walking barefoot in his yard. He has decreased sensation in his feet and did not realize it had not healed until sero-purulent drainage developed several days later. He tried treating it at home for two weeks with little success and now has a Stage III ulcer of the foot. The tissue is red, with yellow purulent drainage. VS are BP146/90, P 100, R 20, T 101.4°F. Mr. Kucharski has been giving himself two injections of insulin each day: 20U NPH and 5U Regular each AM, and 8U NPH each afternoon. SMBG (Self-monitoring blood glucose) which he checks each AM, usually ranges 100–130 mg/dL. Since development of his foot ulcer and infection, his glucose has usually been over 200 mg/dL. Mr. Kucharski is a widower and lives alone in his own home.

Upon admission, the physician ordered blood glucose monitoring per SMBG to be done q.i.d. with Regular insulin to be given on a sliding scale. Mr. Kucharski is somewhat anxious. When talking with him he states "I didn't think a little sore like that could turn so ugly, or I'd have watched it more closely. I walk barefoot all the time and nothing like this has ever happened. You don't think they'll have to cut it off, do you? My father was a bad diabetic and he ended up with both his feet amputated."

Nursing Diagnosis 1 Tissue integrity, impaired, related to injury decreased circulation, decreased sensation and impaired healing associated with diabetes mellitus as evidenced by foot ulcer.

Goals	Nursing Interventions	Rationale	Evaluation
Mr. Kucharski's ulcer will show signs of healing: absence of further breakdown, decrease in size, pink tissue, and absence of exudate.	Provide local wound care as prescribed.	Begins the healing process.	Mr. Kucharski is able to correctly demonstrate wound care. Tissue is pink, exudate is absent. Wound continues to be Stage III with no decrease in size at time of discharge.
	Teach Mr. Kucharski wound care and allow opportunity for return demonstration.	Gives Mr. Kucharski control of his health care.	
	Arrange for a home health agency to evaluate wound care and assist as necessary after Mr. Kucharski's discharge.	Diabetic foot ulcers may take weeks to months to heal; Clients are not hospitalized until ulcer has healed and need for wound care may continue for weeks to months at home.	

Nursing Diagnosis 2 Nutrition altered, less than body requirements, related to diabetes mellitus and metabolic alterations associated with stress and infection as evidenced by elevated glucose levels.

Goals	Nursing Interventions	Rationale	Evaluation
Mr. Kucharski's blood glucose level will remain within a controlled range (80–140 mg/dL) during his illness.	Monitor urine for ketones when glucose level remains elevated or is unstable.	Changes in insulin regime also place Mr. Kucharski at risk for complication of hypoglycemia.	Mr. Kucharski experienced no episodes of hypoglycemia. He was able to demonstrate
	Monitor blood glucose q.i.d. and prn as	Maintaining glucose levels within a	*(continued)*

Mr. Kucharski will verbalize understanding of the effects of illness on blood glucose level and of appropriate interventions to monitor glucose and diabetes during times of illness.

symptoms dictate. Administer insulin per sliding scale as ordered.

Review with Mr. Kucharski procedures for SMBG and checking urine for ketones.

Monitor Mr. Kucharski for signs of hyper- and hypoglycemia and review with him symptoms and self-management of hyper- and hypoglycemia.

Explain to him how illness influences glucose levels.

controlled range will facilitate tissue healing.

Regular SMBG may help minimize severe fluctuations in blood glucose levels.

Early detection of hyper- and hypoglycemia enables prompt intervention and may prevent serious complications.

Illness and fever can increase blood glucose causing symptoms of hyperglycemia and increasing need for insulin.

Anticipating the effects of illness on the glucose level may alert client to symptoms of complications.

Early detection of ketones can prevent development of ketoacidosis.

correct techniques for SMBG and check urine for ketones, and describe when it would be appropriate to do so. His glucose initially ranged from 80–250 but stabilized after several days as his temperature and signs of infections decreased. At time of discharge, Mr. Kucharski was able to return to his b.i.d. insulin regime, but was still checking SMBG q.i.d.

Nursing Diagnosis 3 Knowledge deficit, foot care, related to not appreciating importance of as evidenced by walking barefoot, not visually inspecting feet, and developing a foot ulcer.

Goals	Nursing Interventions	Rationale	Evaluation
Mr. Kucharski will demonstrate appropriate diabetic foot care and verbalize intent to perform on a daily basis.	Explain to Mr. Kucharski that persons with diabetes are at high risk for foot problems. Teach him measures to prevent foot problems (see Table 30-9, Guidelines to Healthy Feet), the importance of maintaining normal blood glucose level, daily inspection of feet, and contacting health care provider at first sign of problem or infection.	The feet of diabetic persons are more prone to injury because of decreased circulation and impaired healing. Because of decreased sensation, Mr. Kucharski may be unaware of injury if visual inspection is not done on a daily basis. Early detection and prompt treatment can prevent infection and more severe complications.	At time of discharge, Mr. Kucharski was able to demonstrate correct foot care and verbalized intent to perform on a daily basis.

Nursing Diagnosis 4 Fear related to complications of foot ulcer as evidenced by anxiety and verbalizations.

Goals	Nursing Interventions	Rationale	Evaluation
Mr. Kucharski will effectively communicate feelings regarding diagnoses and complications, implement positive coping mechanisms, and verbalize a reduction or absence of fear.	Acknowledge awareness of Mr. Kucharski's fear and concerns. Encourage him to talk about his fears and feelings and establish a working relationship through continuity of care. Assist Mr. Kucharski in assessing the situation realistically, but avoid false reassurances. Assist him in identifying and practicing strategies used to deal with fear (exercises in relaxation, meditation, guided imagery, calming self-talk, and so on).	Acknowledgment of Mr. Kucharski's feelings validates the feelings and communicates acceptance. The presence of a trusted person assures him of security and safety. Accurate information and feedback are important as fears may be based on unrealistic or unlikely outcomes. Provides Mr. Kucharski with additional coping methods.	Mr. Kucharski appears less anxious but continues to express some concerns and fear of amputation as ulcer is healing so slowly.

Nephropathy (Chronic Renal Failure)

Diabetic nephropathy develops slowly over many years, progressing eventually to kidney failure. Persons with diabetes have a 20 to 40 percent chance of developing renal disease and renal failure. Controlling hypertension and blood glucose level may decrease or delay renal damage. There is now firm evidence that ACE-inhibitors (antihypertensive drugs) may prevent or delay kidney failure in persons with diabetes. Refer to Chapter 35 for discussion of renal failure.

Retinopathy

Changes in the small vessels of the retina result in diabetic retinopathy, which is a major cause of blindness among diabetics. Fifty percent of persons with diabetes develop retinopathy within ten years of diagnosis and 80 percent within fifteen years. Because of the insidious onset of NIDDM, retinopathy is often present at diagnosis. The severity and progression of retinopathy appear to be closely related to glucose control. Blindness/loss of vision can be reduced by 50 percent with timely laser photocoagulation available today. Diabetics also develop cataracts at an earlier age. Although the majority of clients develop some degree of retinopathy, most do not develop visual impairment. To facilitate early detection, diabetics should have ophthalmologic evaluations every six to twelve months.

Vascular Changes

Diabetes is an independent risk factor for atherosclerotic vessel disease. Atherosclerotic changes that occur in diabetics are similar to those that occur in nondiabetics, but occur at earlier ages and progress at a more rapid rate.

Cardiovascular Hypertension is twice as common in diabetics and is an important factor in the progression of retinopathy, nephropathy, and vascular (large vessel) disease. The incidence of coronary artery disease, angina, and myocardial infarction is two times higher for diabetic men and three times higher for diabetic women compared to the nondiabetic population. Cerebral vascular disease and cerebral vascular accident are also more common in persons with diabetes.

Therapies aimed at lowering risk factors and effects of atherosclerosis are recommended for the diabetic client. These management techniques include weight control, low-fat diet, treatment of hypertension and hyperlipidemia, regular exercise, and control of blood glucose levels.

Peripheral Vascular Disease (PVD) PVD occurs most commonly in diabetics with hypertension or hyperlipidemia and in diabetics who smoke. Diabetics have two to three times the incidence of occlusive peripheral arterial disease when compared to the nondiabetic population. Diabetes is present in more than half of persons experiencing nontraumatic lower extremity amputations.

▶ *Nursing Process*

Diabetes management is ultimately dependent on the client. Client education and involvement in decision making and planning are essential for effective self-care.

Assessment

Assessment of the diabetic client has several foci, depending on the stage of illness and the current situation.

Subjective Data This includes assessment of the health history, diet, activity regimen, and the understanding of the disease and medical therapies.

Objective Data Objective data should focus on the symptoms of diabetes, the common acute and chronic complications, and the results of diagnostic tests.

▼ ▼

Nursing diagnoses, based on the assessment findings, may be varied and extensive due to the multiple problems and complications caused by diabetes mellitus. Possible nursing diagnoses may include:

Nursing Diagnoses	*Goals*	*Nursing Interventions*
▶ *Knowledge deficit, diabetes, medical regimen, diet, exercise, self-care management skills (insulin injection, SMBG) related to new diagnosis or changes in treatment.*	The client will relate basic understanding of pathophysiology of diabetes, and relationship between insulin and hyper-/hypoglycemia.	Teach client about diabetes and the use of insulin to prevent hyper- hypoglycemia or assist client to enroll in a formal diabetic education program.
	The client will verbalize how/when to take oral hypoglycemics and the side effects to report or will demonstrate correctly how to administer insulin and rotate sites.	Teach client about oral hypoglycemics or insulin, whichever the client will be using.
	The client will relate importance of an exercise program.	Discuss how exercise is related to diabetes management.
	The client will describe the relationship between dietary management and glycemic control; choose foods that comply with diet prescription.	Discuss how dietary management is related to the control of blood glucose and provide an exchange list of foods.
	The client will correctly demonstrate how to use SMBG to determine blood glucose level.	Teach client how to perform SMBG and have client return demonstration.
	The client will verbalize symptoms and treatment of hypoglycemia.	Provide client with a list of symptoms and treatment for hypoglycemia.
▶ *Fluid volume deficit, high risk for, related to hyperglycemia, polyuria, and dehydration.*	The client will exhibit normal skin turgor, moist mucous membranes, and maintain oral fluid intake of 2500–3000 mL/day.	Measure client's intake and output, administer intravenous fluids as ordered and encourage oral fluids.
	The client will have vital signs within normal limits.	Monitor vital signs and serum electrolytes.
▶ *Nutrition, altered, less than body requirements, related to imbalance between insulin, diet and activity.*	The client will have weight within normal range for height and age.	Assist client to adjust dietary intake in order to maintain weight in normal range.

▶ *Evaluation*

Each goal must be evaluated to determine how it has been met by the client.

▲ ▲

GERONTOLOGIC CONSIDERATIONS

- The number of older adults with diabetes is predicted to increase, the result of both increased incidence of the disease with aging, and increase in the numbers of persons over age sixty-five. Diabetes occurs in 18 percent of persons between the ages of sixty-five and seventy, and in 40 percent of persons eighty years or older.
- Responses of older adults to diabetes are often different than those of young or middle-age adults. The symptoms of diabetes reported by older persons may be the usual symptoms, or may be loss of energy, blurred or decreased vision, pain or cramps in legs, feet, or fingers, slow healing of cuts, and frequent infections of the skin, gums, or genitalia.
- The older adult may be asymptomatic, or ignore manifestations of the disease.

- Polyuria may cause incontinence. Increased voiding may interfere with sleep and contribute to falls. Increased voiding may be blamed on urinary tract infections, enlarged prostate, or diuretics. Dehydration may cause malaise. Changes in mentation due to hyperglycemia or hypoglycemia may be attributed to aging, dementia, or TIAs.
- Anorexia, common in the elderly, due to disease, decreased sensation of taste, medication, poverty, or depression, can result in hypoglycemia.
- The elderly may lack the dexterity to monitor their glucose or administer insulin. Compliance may be further impaired by cognitive dysfunction, decreased short-term memory or poor vision. Written instructions (large print) and assistive devices may be of some assistance to the elderly.

▶ *CASE STUDY*

Mr. Carnes, a forty-four year-old black male, is admitted to the medical unit from his physician's office. He reports that he has lost 18 pounds over the last month and has been very tired. He also reports symptoms of thirst, frequent urination, and blurred vision. His vital signs are: BP 166/92, P 88, R 16, T 99.2°. Physical assessment reveals hot, dry flushed skin. Laboratory exams reveal a blood glucose 490 mg/dL and urine negative for ketones. Mr. Carnes is a truck driver and leads a fairly sedentary lifestyle. History reveals that he is usually 30 to 35 pounds overweight, but has otherwise been in good health. He reports that his mother died from diabetes and renal failure, and an older brother was diagnosed as having NIDDM three years ago.

The following questions will guide your development of a Nursing Care Plan for this case study:

1. List physical symptoms that Mr. Carnes is experiencing that are suggestive of diabetes.

2. Based on history and laboratory values, would you expect Mr. Carnes to be diagnosed with IDDM or NIDDM?

3. Which nursing diagnoses would you identify as priority for Mr. Carnes right now? List two.

4. Mr. Carnes is treated with IV fluids and insulin sliding scale until his blood glucose is stabilized. Describe what an insulin sliding scale is, and when it is used.

5. A 2,000 calorie ADA diet is ordered for Mr. Carnes. Mr. Carnes does not care to eat the apple that came on his breakfast tray and asks if he can exchange it for another serving of scrambled eggs. How would you respond to Mr. Carnes?

6. Mr. Carnes is being discharged and will continue to attend diabetic education classes at a local diabetic treatment center. Assuming Mr. Carnes is to continue on a diabetic diet and will be receiving mixed insulin injections, list the pertinent information Mr. Carnes will need to know about his disease and therapies related to:

    *   Diabetes and symptoms of hyperglycemia
    *   Role of exercise
    *   Effects of diet
    *   Self-monitoring blood glucose
    *   Insulin injections/technique
    *   Symptoms of hypoglycemia
    *   Sick day care
    *   Long-term complications

SUMMARY

- Diabetes is a complex chronic disease with multiple acute and chronic complications. It is a systemic disease caused by an imbalance between insulin supply and demand. There are two primary types of diabetes: insulin dependent diabetes mellitus (IDDM) and non-insulin dependent diabetes (NIDDM).
- Approximately 5 to 10 percent of diabetics have IDDM. IDDM occurs before the age of 30 and is characterized by an absolute deficiency of insulin.
- NIDDM is much more common, rarely occurs before the age of forty, and has a much higher incidence in the obese. In NIDDM there may be a deficiency of insulin, or insulin levels may be adequate but body cells are resistant to the insulin that is produced.
- A coordinated program of exercise, diet, and medications is used to achieve diabetic control. Persons with NIDDM are managed through diet and exercise, and may or may not require oral hypoglycemic agents or insulin. Persons with IDDM always require insulin therapy in addition to dietary control and an exercise program.
- Acute complications of diabetes include hypoglycemia, diabetic ketoacidosis, and hyperosmolar hyperglycemic nonketotic syndrome.
- Chronic complications include increased incidence of infections, neuropathies, nephropathy, retinopathy, coronary artery disease, and peripheral vascular disease.
- Initial and ongoing education are extremely important regarding: the disease and its complications; effects and management of diet; insulin administration; self-monitoring blood glucose; and self-care skills for prevention and early detection of complications.
- The goal of diabetes management is enabling the diabetic to manage the disease by maintaining a blood glucose level within an acceptable range and thereby minimizing the incidence of acute and chronic complications.

Review Questions

1. Mrs. Gavin tells the nurse that she is surprised that she developed diabetes at forty years of age. The nurse knows that the development of diabetes in middle-aged people is most directly the result of:
   a. atherosclerosis.
   b. eating too much sugar.
   c. obesity.
   d. viral infection.

2. Glycosylated hemoglobin is:
   a. a blood test that shows the pattern of blood glucose levels over several months.
   b. a form of anemia that occurs in diabetic clients.
   c. a type of insulin reaction in which hemoglobin is hemolyzed.
   d. a type of blood glucose monitor used to check daily glucose levels at home.

3. When teaching the diabetic client about mixing short- and longer-acting (NPH) insulin in the same syringe, the nurse should teach that:
   a. regular insulin should be drawn up first.
   b. the NPH insulin should be drawn up first.
   c. it does not matter which insulin is drawn up first since they will be mixed anyway.
   d. the two insulins do not mix and should be drawn up and administered separately.

4. Which of the following principles is used when planning for a diabetic who is to undergo surgery?
   a. All insulin is withheld until surgery is over and the client is eating.
   b. Insulin or oral hypoglycemics are given as usual.
   c. Sliding scale insulin is used to regulate glucose levels during the operative period.
   d. Hyperglycemia poses the most serious danger to the client during surgery.

5. Mr. Schultz and the nurse collaborate to establish a meal plan for his 1,800 calorie ADA diet. The principle used in the exchange system is based on the fact that Mr. Schultz:
   a. may eat any food as long as he has three meals and limits his calories to 1,800 calories.
   b. may substitute any food in the correct amount for another on the same exchange list.
   c. can eat any food any time as long as it is on an exchange list.
   d. must weigh all food before determining serving size.

6. JoAnne is a twenty-one-year-old college student who has been diagnosed with IDDM for seven years. In reviewing principles of insulin administration with JoAnne, the nurse knows that she understands the relationship of her food intake and action of regular insulin when she tells the nurse she eats:
   a. within thirty minutes after her insulin injection.
   b. a bedtime snack.
   c. between meal snacks.
   d. when she is hungry.

7. Ms. Perez, who has IDDM, complains of weakness and shakiness. She is pale, diaphoretic, and her pulse rate is increased. The nurse should recognize these symptoms as indications of:

    a. hyperglycemia.
    b. hypoglycemia.
    c. ketoacidosis.
    d. potassium excess.

8. Mrs. Lally, age twenty-four, is a newly diagnosed insulin-dependent diabetic. If Mrs. Lally's husband comes home and finds her unconscious, what is the first thing he should do?

    a. Place some easily absorbed glucose under her tongue (e.g., monogel) or give glucagon SC or IM.
    b. Call the doctor.
    c. Administer 20U Regular insulin.
    d. Add sugar to orange juice and administer orally.

9. You have been teaching Mr. Morales to give himself insulin injections. Which of the following statements indicates that he understands what you've taught him?

    a. "Before drawing up the insulin, I'll shake the bottle really good to mix it up."
    b. "I'll clean the injection site carefully before administering."
    c. "I'll make sure I inject the insulin deep into the muscle."
    d. "After injecting the insulin, I'll exercise that area to increase absorption."

10. To which one of the following diseases is the diabetic most predisposed?

    a. Anemia
    b. Arthritis
    c. Atherosclerosis
    d. Osteoporosis

Critical Thinking Questions

1. How would you react if you were diagnosed with IDDM?

2. If a friend related symptoms of diabetes, what should he be encouraged to do?

3. Prepare a teaching plan for a client just diagnosed with NIDDN.

Medical Terminology

diabet/o-	siphon
diabetes	condition characterized by excessive urination
insul/in	little island; a substance
insulin	a substance secreted from "little islands" within the pancreas
glyc-	sweet, sugar
glycogen	a stored form of sugar
-emia	a blood condition of
hyper-	excessive
hyperglycemia	condition of excessive blood sugar
hypo-	deficient
hypoglycemia	deficiency of blood sugar
mellit/us	presence of honey
diabetes mellitus	the most common type of diabetes
-pathy	disease
neuropathy	disease of nerves
retinopathy	disease of retina
nephropathy	disease of kidneys
poly-	much or many
polydypsia	much (excessive) thirst
polyphagia	eating an abnormally large amount of food
polyuria	much urine

News Flash

Genetic Markers

The fact that IDDM is thought to be the result of genetic and environmental factors has led to research on methods of identifying those at risk for development of IDDM, prevention, and early control. Scientists are searching for genes that may be involved in NIDDM and IDDM. Some genetic markers for IDDM have been identified, and it may soon be possible to screen relatives of people with diabetes to see if they are at risk for developing diabetes. (Diabetes Overview, 1994)

Immune Therapy for Prevention

Studies are now underway using drugs that stop the immune system from attacking the beta cells to try to prevent IDDM from developing in people who are at high risk for the disorder. One substance currently under study as a preventive is glutamic acid decarboxylase, also called GAD.

In other studies, researchers are using a method similar to the desensitization process used to ward off allergic reactions. Researchers are investigating the possibility of administering agents to those at risk for IDDM that might induce the immune system to tolerate the presence of insulin and delay or prevent the onset of diabetes.

Other methods under study include encapsulating the beta cells in a semipermeable membrane to protect them from immune attack and implanting the cells in the thymus as a way of inducing tolerance by the immune system. (Diabetes Overview, 1994)

Transplantation

Transplantation of the pancreas or insulin-producing cells offers the best hope of cure for people with IDDM. Although some success with pancreatic transplants has been achieved, the cost and serious side effect associated with the necessary antirejection drugs continues to prohibit many transplants from being performed. Scientists are working to develop less harmful drugs and better methods of pancreatic tissue transplantation. (Budingar & Donnelly, 1994)

Blood Glucose Monitors

Several companies are working on the development of devices that measure blood glucose by passing a beam of light through a client's fingertips, thus eliminating the need for a finger stick. Implantable glucose sensors that provide constant blood glucose readings are also being researched and developed (Robinsons, 1992).

Insulin

Experiments are being done to develop a new faster-acting analog of human insulin (insulin lispro). This faster-acting insulin will act immediately and peak in less than an hour—twice as fast as rapid-acting (Regular) insulin. This insulin will allow clients to take the insulin right at mealtime, rather than having to time an injection for half an hour before they eat.

Other studies are working on the development of insulin that can be taken nasally or orally and bioengineering to create artificial beta cells that secrete insulin in response to glucose (Betz, 1995).

UNIT
10

Reproductive and Sexual Disorders

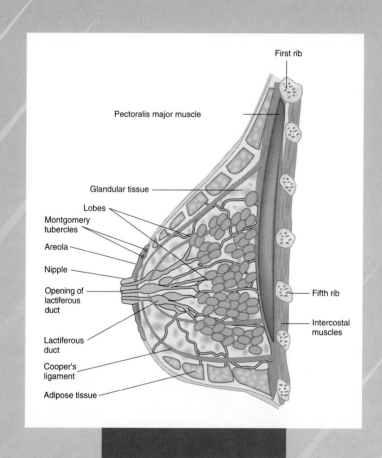

First rib

Pectoralis major muscle

Glandular tissue

Lobes

Montgomery tubercles

Areola

Nipple

Opening of lactiferous duct

Fifth rib

Intercostal muscles

Lactiferous duct

Cooper's ligament

Adipose tissue

CHAPTER
31
Female Reproductive Disorders

Mary Elias

KEY TERMS

abortion
amenorrhea
contraception
cystocele
dysmenorrhea
dyspareunia
gynecology
infertility
menopause
menorrhagia
metrorrhagia
oligomenorrhea
polymenorrhea
rectocele
tenesmus
urethrocele

LIST OF DISORDERS

▶ Pelvic Inflammatory Disease
Neoplasms
   ▶ Fibrocystic Breast Disease
   ▶ Breast Cancer
   ▶ Cervical Cancer
   ▶ Fibroid Tumors (Leiomyoma)
   ▶ Uterine Cancer
   ▶ Ovarian Cancer
▶ Endometriosis
▶ Vaginitis
Menstrual Disorders
   ▶ Dysmenorrhea
   ▶ Amenorrhea
   ▶ Premenstrual Syndrome (PMS)
▶ Cystocele/Urethrocele/Rectocele/Prolapsed Uterus
▶ Complications of Menopause
▶ Infertility
▶ Contraception
▶ Abortion
▶ Toxic Shock Syndrome (TSS)

LEARNING OBJECTIVES

Upon completion of this chapter the learner should be able to:
- Define key terms.
- Describe the role and responsibilities of the nurse in caring for the female client with a disorder of the reproductive system in a variety of health care environments.

- Discuss normal and abnormal anatomy and physiology of the female reproductive system, including the menstrual cycle.
- Discuss pertinent nursing assessment factors for the initial and ongoing care of the female client.
- Describe the signs and symptoms of infections, inflammations, and abnormal function of female reproductive organs.
- Describe diagnostic tests for disorders of the female reproductive system.

- Discuss common medical and surgical interventions.
- Discuss contraceptive methods including actions, side effects, and client teaching.
- Utilize the nursing process in caring for the female client, to develop a care plan for medical and surgical gynecological disorders.
- Demonstrate the ability to teach clients with gynecological disorders.

▶ *MAKING THE CONNECTION*

INTRODUCTION

The branch of medicine dealing with the female reproductive system is **gynecology**. The physician who specializes in this field is the gynecologist. Registered nurses with advanced degrees and specialized education in obstetrics and gynecology are nurse practitioners (OB-GYN NP) and practice in gynecologists' offices, clinics, or hospitals. Care provided by the physician or the nurse practitioner includes routine annual health examinations, Pap smears, breast examinations, prenatal and postpartum examinations, and treatment for disorders of the reproductive system. A member of a holistic health care team in many health care settings, the nurse actively participates in prevention, maintenance, and restoration for women experiencing reproductive system disorders.

For the majority of women, the reproductive system functions without problems throughout the life span from puberty through **menopause** (cessation of menses). For others, minor and major gynecological disorders may be treated by physicians or nurse practitioners. Some of the problems are related to alterations in structure, while others are related more to altered physiology of the reproductive system. This chapter discusses disorders of the female reproductive system by applying the steps of the nursing process.

ANATOMY AND PHYSIOLOGY REVIEW

External Female Structures

The area known as the vulva includes the external female structures, such as the mons pubis, the labia majora, labia minora, and clitoris. The Bartholin glands and Skene's glands, located proximal to the vaginal opening, produce and secrete lubricating fluids. The labia majora and minora serve as protective barriers for the softer internal structures. The clitoris, located proximal to the mons pubis, and superior to the urinary meatus, plays a role in sexual arousal in the female, and is considered analogous to the male penis. During foreplay, the clitoris engorges and stimulates orgasm or climax in the female. It is covered by a small hood called the prepuce. The perineum is the distal portion of the vulva, located below the vaginal opening and superior to the anus. This is the area that is cut to perform an episiotomy at the time of delivery.

The breasts are also a part of the external female reproductive system (see Figure 31-1). Their external structures include the nipple, areola, and Montgomery tubercles. The nipples have several openings or ducts that lead from the lactiferous glands inside the breast. Milk is ejected through the ducts when the infant sucks on the breast. The areola, or the darker area around the nipple, becomes darker in response to the in-creased hormone levels during pregnancy. Small, mole-like, raised areas around the areola are the Montgomery tubercles. These glands produce a lubricant that keeps the nipple soft and supple.

Internally, the breasts each contain approximately twenty lobules made of many acini, or alveoli, which produce the breast milk. The alveoli respond to an elevated level of the anterior pituitary hormone, prolactin, which stimulates the production of the milk. The milk travels from the alveoli through the lactiferous ducts to the lactiferous sinuses. The tiny muscles in the walls of the sinuses are stimulated to contract and eject the milk when the baby sucks at the breast. Oxytocin, a posterior pituitary hormone is responsible for this letdown reflex, which ejects the milk.

Internal Structures

The vagina is an elastic, tube-like structure leading from the outside of the female body to the cervix. Approximately 2 to 3 inches long, it contains many rugae that allow it to stretch during intercourse and also permit the passage of the baby during delivery. The pH environment of the vagina is normally acidic, providing protection from microorganisms that could cause infections.

The uterus is a 3-inch long, 2-inch wide, 1-inch thick hollow, muscular structure as seen in Figure 31-2. The top is the fundus, the middle is the body (corpus), and the lower portion is the cervix, which extends down into the upper part of the vagina. Four sets of ligaments hold the uterus in its normal anteverted (forward) position, and permit it the freedom to grow and move during pregnancy. The uterus has three distinct layers: the innermost layer is the endometrium, which sloughs with menstruation each month. The myometrium is the middle layer, which is constructed of many muscle fibers that are interwoven for strength, stretch and contractility. The outer layer is the perimetrium, which is an external serous membrane covering. The uterus is capable of expanding 17 to 20 times its normal size during pregnancy. The muscle fibers of the myometrium must function efficiently during the labor process to expel the fetus or the woman will experience dysfunctional labor or dystocia.

The fallopian tubes are connected to the uterus on either side. They are continuous with the mucous membrane lining of the endometrium on the inside. Billions of cilia line each fallopian tube and make a sweeping motion toward the uterus, especially at the time of ovulation. This sweeping action moves the ovum along the path toward the uterus. The movement may also impede the progress of the sperm that must swim upstream against the downward current produced by the cilia.

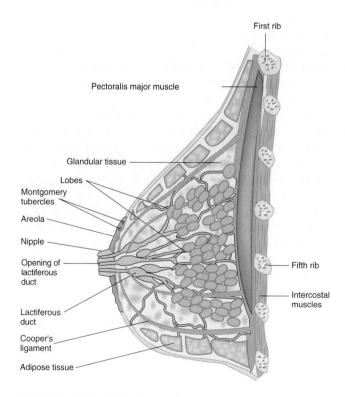

First rib

Pectoralis major muscle

Glandular tissue

Lobes

Montgomery tubercles

Areola

Nipple

Opening of lactiferous duct

Lactiferous duct

Cooper's ligament

Adipose tissue

Fifth rib

Intercostal muscles

FIGURE 31-1 The female breast.

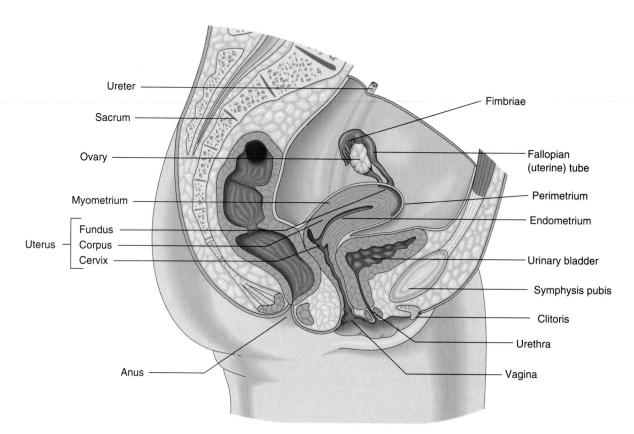

FIGURE 31-2 The female reproductive system.

The cervix is the lower portion of the uterus and extends into the vaginal vault (see Figure 31-2). Like the vagina, the cervix has muscle layers that allow it to stretch to a diameter of at least 10 centimeters during delivery. The cervix in the non-pregnant woman feels like gristle, or like the tip of the nose. In a pregnant woman, hormones cause the cervix to soften significantly so that it feels very soft and almost pudding-like in consistency by the end of pregnancy.

An almond-shaped ovary, about 2 inches long and 1 inch wide, is located within the broad ligament on either side of the uterus, just below the fimbriae, the fingerlike projections at the distal end of the fallopian tubes. The ovaries contain all of the ova (eggs) that a woman will have from puberty until menopause. Each month, the ovary responds to hormonal signals from the anterior pituitary gland to ripen one or more ova. In this negative feedback system, follicle-stimulating hormone (FSH) is released by the anterior pituitary and sends a message to the ovary that it is time to develop the ovum. Once the ovary has received the initial signal from the pituitary gland, it begins to release estrogen, which causes the ovum to ripen and

become larger. The ovum, now surrounded by a liquid-filled sac, is called the graafian follicle. As the level of estrogen rises, another signal is sent back to the pituitary letting it know that the graafian follicle is ready to be released. The entire first part of the cycle is known as the proliferative phase. Once the message from the ovary is received by the pituitary, luteinizing hormone (LH) is released. LH triggers a chain of events that stimulates the ovary to release the ovum. This point in the menstrual cycle is called ovulation. The area on the ovary where the ovum had been growing and developing now becomes the corpus luteum or "yellow body." Its function is to produce another hormone called progesterone, which causes the glands and blood vessels of the endometrial lining to grow and thicken as they prepare for the implantation of a fertilized ovum. If fertilization does not occur, the progesterone level will decrease, the endometrium will be sloughed off, and the woman experiences menstruation. If fertilization does occur, the progesterone level remains elevated to ensure the optimal environment for implantation of the zygote in about six to eight days following fertilization. Figure 31-3 illustrates the menstrual cycle.

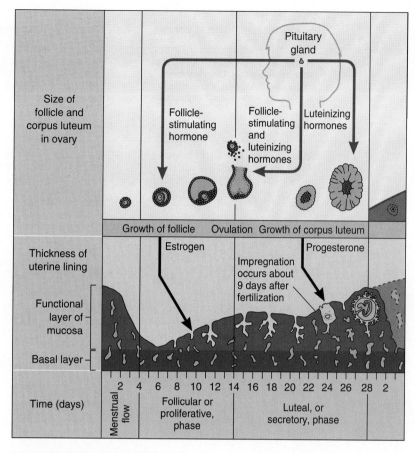

FIGURE 31-3 Approximate time and sequence of events in the menstrual cycle.

COMMON DIAGNOSTIC TESTS

The following is a table of the commonly used diagnostic tests for clients with disorders of the female reproductive system.

Test	Explanation/Normal Values	Nursing Responsibilities
Pelvic exam recommended annually for women over 18 through menopause.	Performed by Doctor or NP to visualize the external and internal pelvic structures, a bi-manual exam to palpate pelvic organs and a speculum exam of the cervix. A Pap smear and rectovaginal exam are included. Cultures and wet smears may be obtained.	Explain procedures, prepare the client by having her void and undress, position the client on the exam table in a dorsal lithotomy position; help the client with relaxation during the exam, prepare slides and culture medium, obtain other supplies; assist with the procedure.
Pap Smear (Papanicolaou)	Cells obtained from the external and internal cervical canal. Diagnostic for cervical dysplasia or cancer.	Prepare the client as above. Prepare microscopic slides for pathology. Instruct the client on the importance of annual pap smear.
Cultures	Discharge obtained by swab from the vagina and cervix. Diagnostic for STDs and other microorganisms.	Prepare the client as above. Prepare the culture medium and send to the lab. Instruct the client in measures to prevent sexually transmitted infections and other types of infections. Teach the proper use of vaginal or oral medication to treat infections, and good health hygiene practices.

(continued)

Test	Explanation/Normal Values	Nursing Responsibilities
Endometrial Biopsy	Tissue sample obtained with special biopsy instruments. Diagnostic for endometrial tissue abnormalities.	Prepare the client as above. Explain the procedure. Prepare tissue preservation agent, label and send to pathology. Assist the client in relaxation during the procedure due to the discomfort/cramping she may experience.
Mammography	Special radiologic exam to diagnose benign and malignant disorders.	Explain the procedure. The breast will be compressed and may be uncomfortable for several seconds. Explain that it is important to have a baseline mammogram done between the ages of 35 to 40 and a breast exam done by a doctor or NP every 3 to 4 years. For the woman 40 to 49, a mammogram every 1 to 2 years, and for those over 50, an annual mammogram is recommended along with an annual breast exam by doctor or NP.
Breast Biopsy	Performed with or without local or general anesthesia by aspiration, needle biopsy, excision, or incision. Tissue or fluid is obtained and sent to pathology for examination and identification of abnormal cells. New method of obtaining breast biopsies may be done with the stereotactic mammography studies.	Explain the procedure. Have the client undress down to the waist. Cleanse the biopsy region and shave the area if needed. Drape the breast and adjacent skin. Provide emotional support prior to, during, and following the procedure. Monitor vital signs. Apply a sterile dressing or bandage. Instruct the client in post-biopsy wound care.

SURGICAL TESTS

Test	Explanation/Normal Values	Nursing Responsibilities
Dilatation and Curettage (D & C)	Surgical scraping of the endometrial lining, performed under general, epidural, or paracervical anesthesia as an outpatient. Diagnostic or therapeutic for uterine bleeding disorders.	Explain the procedure. Pre- and postoperative assessment and care. Provide discharge instructions related to activities and follow-up appointments.
Hysterosalpingogram	Radiopaque dye instilled through the cervix during the radiologic exam. Diagnostic for uterine cavity and tubal abnormalities. Performed as a part of an infertility workup.	Explain the procedure and prepare the client in lithotomy position. Test is done in radiology department. Inquire about allergies to iodine or other dyes. Assist the doctor.
Huhner Test (Post Coital Test)	Performed in the office. The couple has intercourse 2 hours before the appointment. A sample of secretions is removed from the vagina and placed on a microscopic slide. The sperm are observed for the number present and their motility in the cervical mucous. A minimum of 20 sperm per field should be visible with good motility.	Explain the procedure and schedule near client's normal ovulation. Prepare the client in lithotomy position. Assist the doctor or NP with the procedure. Perform microscopic observations as directed.
Colposcopy	Direct visualization of the vagina and cervix through a high-powered microscope. Acetic acid or other solution is applied to the tissue to dehydrate the cells for improved visualization. Diagnostic for cervical dysplasia or carcinoma *in situ* of the cervix. Biopsies may be obtained as needed.	Explain the procedure and prepare the client in dorsal lithotomy position. Assist with procedure. Prepare biopsy specimens for pathologic exam.

Test	Explanation/Normal Values	Nursing Responsibilities
Schiller Test	Performed during colposcopy. An iodine solution is applied to the cells of the cervix. Healthy, normal cells turn brown. Abnormal cells turn white or yellow. This aids in visualization of the abnormal tissue and indicates areas for biopsy.	Explain the reason for the application of the solution. Assist with the biopsy procedure as necessary. Label tissue specimens and send to histology.
Laparoscopy	Examination of the internal pelvic structures by direct visualization with a laparoscope. Usually performed under general anesthesia. Diagnostic for pelvic disorders or infertility problems.	Explain the procedure. Prepare the client. Pre- and postoperative assessment and interventions. Provide discharge instructions in activity and follow-up.
Ultrasound	Diagnostic test that utilizes sound waves bounced off of internal structures. Diagnostic for cysts, tumors, pregnancy, fetal gestational age, and multiple gestation.	Explain the procedure. Instruct the client to drink enough fluid to fill her bladder prior to the procedure.

KEY ABBREVIATIONS

The following abbreviations and acronyms are used in this chapter:

AID	artificial insemination by donor
AIH	artificial insemination by husband
CIS	carcinoma *in situ*
CPAP	continuous positive airway pressure
CSM	circulation, sensation, movement
DES	diethylstilbestrol
FBD	fibrocystic breast disease
GIFT	gamete-intra-fallopian transfer
HCG	human chorionic gonadotropin
HPV	human papillomavirus
IUD	intrauterine device
IVF-ER	*in vitro* fertilization and embryo replacement
PCA	patient-controlled analgesic
PID	pelvic inflammatory disease
PMS	premenstrual syndrome
TRAM	transplantation of the rectus abdominous muscle
TSS	toxic shock syndrome
WNL	within normal limits
ZIFT	zygote-intra-fallopian transfer

ASSESSMENT

The purpose of the physical assessment is to provide information regarding the status of the reproductive organs. The physical assessment includes a breast examination, genital and pelvic assessment. A nurse will usually assist the physician or nurse practitioner when a gynecological examination or pelvic assessment of the client is performed. However, a nurse must be prepared to assess the breasts and external genitalia of clients.

Breasts

Examination of the breast is accomplished using inspection and palpation. Important questions to ask the client include: "Are you experiencing any pain?" "Have you noticed any lumps or thickening?" "Are you experiencing any discharge?" "Do you have any rash or swelling of the breast?" "Is there a history of breast disease or cancer in your family?" "Have you ever had a mammogram?" "When was your last mammogram?"

Have the client seated with both arms at the side. The breasts should be completely exposed for inspection. Note the symmetry, size, shape, skin color, texture, vascular pattern, and presence of any lesions. Determine the symmetry of nipples and any discharge. Next, ask the client to raise her arms above her head. This allows the nurse to note any signs of skin retraction. Both breasts should move symmetrically. Ask the client to push her hands into her hips to contract the pectoralis muscles and note any dimpling or puckering, which is an indication of skin retraction.

Examine the axilla for signs of any rash or infection. Palpation of the axilla is important to detect any enlarged nodes. This is accomplished by lifting the woman's arm and supporting it to promote relaxation. Reach high into the axilla with your fingers and move them down the chest wall at the mid-axillary line, then palpate along the anterior and posterior borders of the axilla and along the inner aspect of the upper arm.

Repeat this on the opposite axilla. Usually nodes are not palpable, however, the client may experience some tenderness as you palpate high in the axilla.

Next, place the client in the supine position. Place a small pad under the side to be examined and raise the client's arm over her head. The nurse uses the pads of the first three fingers to palpate the breast in concentric circles toward the periphery. Move in a clockwise fashion palpating all areas of the breast. It is important to palpate the tail of Spence of the breast that extends into the axilla. Next palpate the areola for any masses or discharge. Note the color, consistency, and odor of any discharge.

Developmental considerations should be kept in mind. The newborn's breasts may be enlarged and may have a clear or white discharge referred to as "witch's milk." As an adolescent develops, there may be asymmetry of breast growth, in both sexes. Breast development usually occurs between the ages of ten and thirteen years of age. A pregnant individual often has enlarged breasts with nipples that darken and enlarge. The elderly client's breasts tend to be pendulous and less firm. The elderly woman often develops cartilage below the breast, which is referred to as the inframammary ridge. Reinforcement of the importance of breast self-examination needs to occur throughout the life cycle.

Genitalia

It is important for the nurse to allay any anxiety the client may have about an internal examination and prepare the client. Ask the client to empty her bladder and ask any pertinent historical questions before having the client disrobe. Pertinent historical questions include determination of the client's menstrual and obstetric history, such as the date of the last menstrual period and the usual pattern of her menstrual flow, number of pregnancies, and how many babies delivered. Determine if the client is menopausal and if she is experiencing any symptoms related to menopause. It is important to determine if she has any unusual vaginal discharge and have her describe the character of the secretion. Sexual activity and contraceptive use may also be pertinent to the client's condition.

Position the client in the lithotomy position for an internal pelvic examination. The upper body should be covered with a gown or street clothes.

In many cases, a complete gynecological examination is not required, but inspection is indicated. In the acute care facility or long-term care facility, this is best accomplished during the bath.

Begin the assessment by inspecting the pubic area for distribution of pubic hair. In an adult, pubic hair is thick and appears on the mons pubis and inner aspects of the superior thighs. In early adolescence, pubic hair growth is sparse, fine, and found along the labia. The elderly client's labia will be thin and the pubic hair is often sparse, thin, gray, and straight.

With a gloved hand, gently spread the labia majora and inspect the labia minora, clitoris, urinary meatus, and vaginal opening, which should be pink, moist, and free of any lesions. Note any skin lesions, masses, infestations, or discharge. Odorless vaginal secretions are normal; however, the discharge changes in character throughout the menstrual cycle. After menstruation, there may be a scant, white discharge. As ovulation approaches, the discharge is clear and thin; after ovulation the discharge may return to a white, thickened consistency. Examples of abnormal discharge would include a frothy, malodorous, greenish gray watery discharge, which may indicate a *Trichomonas* or *Haemophilus* infection. If the client has an inflamed vulva and thick, white discharge it may indicate candidiasis.

Developmental considerations need to be kept in mind during inspection of the genitalia. A newborn's genitalia is often engorged as a consequence of the mother's hormones. Vaginal secretions may be blood-tinged during the first week. In a child of any age, inflammation of the vulva with any lesions or open irritated areas could indicate sexual abuse. If sexual abuse is suspected, follow the agency's procedure for reporting such incidents.

▶ PELVIC INFLAMMATORY DISEASE

Pelvic inflammatory disease (PID) is an inflammatory process involving pathogenic invasion of the fallopian tubes (salpingitis) and/or ovaries (oophoritis), as well as any vascular or supporting structures within the pelvis, except the uterus. Pathogenic microorganisms such as gonococcus, streptococcus, and staphylococcus are frequently causes of PID. Infections are usually ascending by nature, that is, the pathogens are introduced into the reproductive system from outside and travel upward from the vagina to the fallopian tubes and then out into the pelvis. Risk factors associated with the incidence of PID include multiple sexual partners, frequent intercourse, IUDs (intrauterine contraceptive device), and childbirth. The use of barrier contraceptives has been shown to reduce the risk factors of PID in some high risk groups.

The symptoms of PID include a low grade fever, pelvic pain, abdominal pain, a "bearing down" backache, a foul-smelling vaginal discharge, nausea and vomiting, **dysmenorrhea** (painful menstruation), **dyspareunia** (painful intercourse), and intense pelvic tenderness upon examination. Peritonitis or pelvic abscesses may develop as complications of PID if the pathogens spread into the pelvic cavity. Future **infertility** (inability or diminished ability to produce offspring) problems can be related to scarring and strictures of the fallopian tubes, which have developed as a result of a chronic inflammatory process within the pelvis. These problems have been associated with ectopic pregnancies because the fertilized ovum becomes trapped inside the fallopian tube before it can complete its trip to the uterus.

The condition is often diagnosed during a pelvic examination. The nurse usually obtains a history of the client's symptoms and documents it in the client's chart. Frequently, vaginal and cervical cultures are obtained at the time of the exam to determine the causative agent. A pelvic ultrasound may be ordered to rule out other causes of pelvic pain. The nurse needs to instruct the client in the purpose of these procedures and any special preparations that may be required, such as having a full bladder.

▶ Medical/Surgical Management

▶ Surgical

If the inflammation is extensive, the client may require a hysterectomy. Medical treatment is preferred initially; however, it is not always successful and the client may develop chronic PID.

▶ Pharmacological

The client who is not acutely ill from PID may be treated as an outpatient at home with oral antibiotics and bed rest, unless the infection is herpes simplex virus II. Clients with herpes simplex II infections may require more intensive care in the hospital with IV antibiotic therapy. The physician may also order medicated vaginal suppositories for the vaginal discharge.

However, the acutely ill client may require hospitalization for IV antibiotic therapy such as doxycycline monohydrate (Vibramycin) or metronidazole (Flagyl). IV fluids are frequently administered to promote adequate hydration. A 5 percent dextrose in lactated Ringer's solution or plain lactated ringers solution are often used.

▶ Activity

During hospitalization, the client is placed on bed rest with bathroom privileges. A semi-Fowler's position is preferred because it will facilitate drainage of the pelvis. If vaginal suppositories are used, the client should lie in a supine position for thirty minutes.

▶ Nursing Process

Assessment

Subjective Data On the initial assessment, the nurse should inquire about the client's sexual activity, including contraceptive methods and number of partners. Unprotected intercourse is the most frequent method of entry for the microorganisms that cause PID. The nurse should also include the client's history of **contraception** (prevention of pregnancy), sexual activity, previous vaginal infections and treatments, obstetrical history, and normal hygiene practices such as douching and tampon use. Complaints of nagging pelvic pain and a low grade fever should alert the nurse to notify the physician for follow-up treatment.

Objective Data The nurse may also note an elevated temperature, flushed, dry skin, the presence of a malodorous vaginal discharge, and positive vaginal or cervical cultures.

▼ ▼

Possible nursing diagnoses for a client with PID may include:

Nursing Diagnoses	Goals	Nursing Interventions
▶ Pain related to inflammation of the pelvic structures caused by invasion of pathogens.	Using a pain rating scale of 0 to 10, the client will report that her pain has decreased to two or less within forty-eight hours after the initiation of treatment.	Assess client's pain level every four hours, noting the location, duration, sensation, intensity, and factors that increase or decrease the pain. Administer analegesics as ordered.
▶ Knowledge deficit related to the etiology of the pelvic inflammatory process, treatment regimen, self-care, and preventive measures.	The client will follow prescribed treatment regimen, self-care, and preventive measures.	If suppositories are ordered, the nurse should instruct the client in the proper method of insertion (see Teaching Tip). Provide instructions to the client and partner about the causes of PID and ways to prevent the inflammation. Teach proper pericare and hygiene, especially

(continued)

Nursing Diagnoses	Goals	Nursing Interventions
		handwashing before and after changing sanitary pads. Change sanitary pads every three to four hours. Encourage client to make time for rest periods during the acute phase of the inflammation. Instruct client about pelvic rest, which includes no douching, tampons, or intercourse. Teach client to avoid strenuous activities like straining or heavy lifting. Advise client to wear underpants with a cotton crotch. Teach client to cleanse the perineal area from front to back after each voiding or bowel movement. Provide a written copy of discharge instructions to help her recall specific information after she has gone home. Discuss and encourage the use of safe sexual practices and the use of barrier contraceptives to prevent recurrence of PID symptoms.
	The client will contact her health care provider if her symptoms persist, worsen, or return.	Encourage client to notify the NP or physician at the first sign of PID symptoms. Advise client to monitor her own temperature, upon discharge, twice daily for two weeks and notify the physician or NP if the temperature remains elevated or increases.
▶ *Hyperthermia related to physiologic responses to the inflammatory or infectious process.*	The client's temperature will return to normal range within twenty-four hours after the initiation of therapy.	Monitor client's vital signs every four hours. Administer antipyretic and antibiotic as ordered by the physician. Give sponge baths with tepid water to help decrease the fever.
▶ *Anxiety related to hospitalization, discomfort, and multiple psychosocial factors.*	The client will demonstrate a decreased level of anxiety.	Encourage client to discuss fears and concerns that cause anxiety.
▶ *Infection, high risk for, related to the spread of the inflammation within the pelvic cavity or the transmission of the inflammation to sexual partners.*	The client will perform measures to prevent the transmission of inflammation or infection and follow the activity restrictions prescribed while at home or in the hospital and after discharge.	Follow standard precautions and teach to client. Explain the importance of completing the entire course of antibiotics and other medications to ensure eradication of the pathogens from the pelvic organs. Maintain the semi-Fowler's position and help reposition the client every two hours. Use pillows to support body parts and increase rest.

▶ Evaluation

Each goal must be evaluated to determine how it has been met by the client.

▲ ▲

▶ Teaching Tip: Teaching the Client to Insert Vaginal Suppositories

First, have the client wash her hands, then cleanse the vulva with a mild soap and warm water to remove any external discharge. Next, she should lie down in a supine position with her knees flexed. With one hand, the client can separate the labia and gently insert the suppository high inside the vagina. Once the suppository is in place, the client should remain supine for a minimum of thirty minutes to ensure adequate absorption of the medication through the vaginal mucosa.

▶ NEOPLASMS

▶ FIBROCYSTIC BREAST DISEASE

Fibrocystic breast disease (FBD) is also called chronic cystic mastitis or lumpy breast syndrome. It is the most common breast lesion in females and usually occurs between thirty-five and fifty years of age. Many cases will subside after menopause. The incidence of the potential for developing breast cancer is increased three to four times with fibrocystic breast disease. There appears to be a familial tendency toward the development of breast cancer.

Lumps may occur as single or multiple cysts which are frequently fluid filled. It is difficult to differentiate fibrocystic tissue changes from other breast lesions because the dense fibrocystic areas may mask areas of breast cancer. Figure 31-4 shows the differences among cysts, fibroids, and carcinomas of the breast.

The pathophysiology of fibrocystic breast disease is found in the formation of fibrous tissue caused by hyperplasia of the epithelial cells in the breast lobules and ducts. The proliferation of the fibrous tissue deviates from the expected normal cyclic response to female hormone shifts during the menstrual cycle. Research on fibrocystic breast disease has indicated that there may be a link between caffeine intake and the growth of the abnormal tissue. The caffeine may keep the hormonal triggers in an "on" position and they foster the hyperplasia.

Routine mammograms may be ordered to provide baseline information and to differentiate the palpable breast lumps between benign and malignant types. With the stereotactic mammogram, a computer-directed biopsy may be performed during the procedure. The client will experience a pinching sensation as the biopsies are taken and the areas are covered with a Band-Aid® afterward. This method of biopsy is more specific because the lesion can be pinpointed by the computer and guessing the location is eliminated.

Women should be taught breast self-examination (BSE) as adolescents and encouraged to practice the procedure on a monthly basis at the end of each menstrual cycle when it is easier to palpate the breast tis-

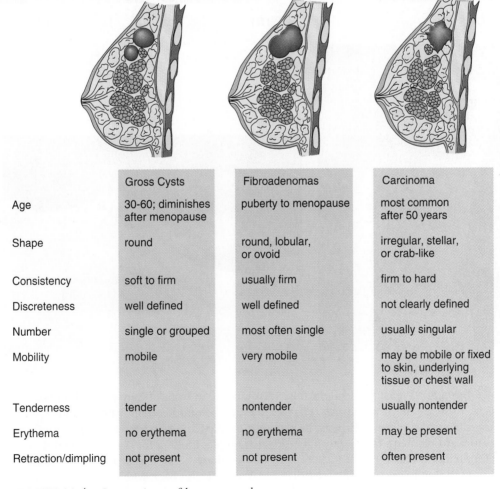

	Gross Cysts	Fibroadenomas	Carcinoma
Age	30-60; diminishes after menopause	puberty to menopause	most common after 50 years
Shape	round	round, lobular, or ovoid	irregular, stellar, or crab-like
Consistency	soft to firm	usually firm	firm to hard
Discreteness	well defined	well defined	not clearly defined
Number	single or grouped	most often single	usually singular
Mobility	mobile	very mobile	may be mobile or fixed to skin, underlying tissue or chest wall
Tenderness	tender	nontender	usually nontender
Erythema	no erythema	no erythema	may be present
Retraction/dimpling	not present	not present	often present

FIGURE 31-4 Comparison of breast neoplasms.

sue. Figure 31-5 provides specific information on how to perform a breast self examination.

A yellow-greenish, sticky discharge is occasionally present with fibrocystic breast disease. A Pap smear may be done on the discharge to rule out the presence of malignant cells. The presence of any breast discharge should be noted and reported to the health care provider as soon as possible. The physician or NP may recommend a biopsy or aspiration of the abnormal areas. Aspiration may be performed in the office

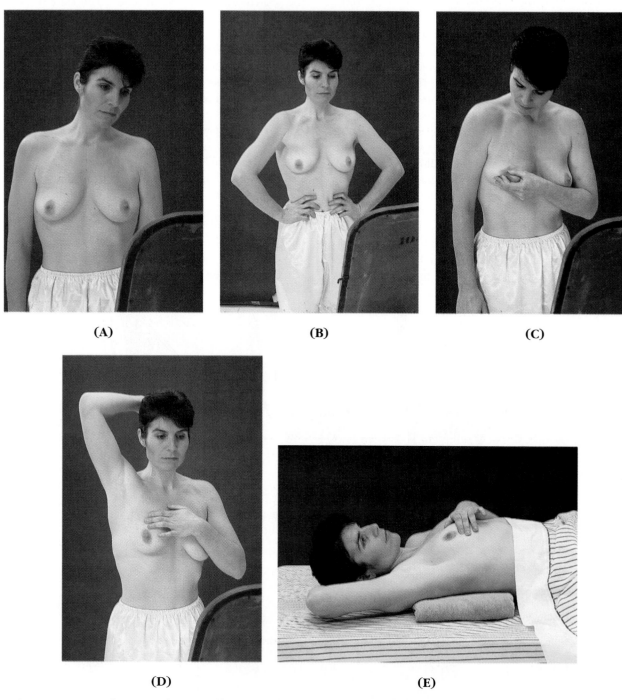

(A) **(B)** **(C)**

(D) **(E)**

FIGURE 31-5 Performing a breast self-examination. **(A)** Standing in front of mirror, check breasts for puckering, dimpling, scaliness, or discharge from nipples. **(B)** Clasp hands behind head and press hands forward, watching for changes in the shape or contour of breasts. Press hands on hips and bend toward mirror while pulling shoulders and elbows forward (shown). **(C)** Gently squeeze each nipple, looking for discharge. **(D)** Raise one arm and use fingers of other hand to check breast for lumps or masses under skin. Use a pattern of motion (circular, up-and-down, etc.) to cover entire breast. **(E)** Repeat "D" while lying flat on back with one arm over head and a towel under the shoulder.

with a syringe and a 23-gauge needle. If fluid is obtained from the area, it should be sent to pathology for examination. If no fluid is obtained, it may be a solid cyst or tumor, and biopsy may be required.

In the office, a breast biopsy may be performed with a local anesthetic. If there is any question of malignancy, or if the physician suspects that the lesion will be malignant based upon the mammography report, the biopsy may be performed in the hospital under general anesthetic so that additional tissue may be removed if necessary. A frozen section may be obtained and sent to the laboratory for a preliminary examination to rule out a malignant lesion. The client usually signs a surgical consent form giving the surgeon permission to remove the affected tissue if it appears to be cancerous.

► Medical/Surgical Management

► Surgical

Aspiration or surgical excision may be indicated for diagnostic or therapeutic reasons. The cystic tissue may be aspirated with a small gauge needle and syringe. The nurse prepares the client for the procedure and assists the doctor or NP with the procedure. Assist the client into a supine position on the examination table. Set up the equipment and instruments needed for the procedure. Cleanse the area to be biopsied and assist with the procedure as directed by the doctor or NP. Upon completion of the aspiration or biopsy, label the specimen and send it to the pathology department.

If the areas of fibrocystic tissue are extensive and have not responded to conservative treatments and methods, or if the risk of cancer is high, the tissue may be excised completely. Removal of fibrocystic tissue does not guarantee that the client will not develop

breast cancer in the remaining tissue, and she must continue to perform monthly BSE.

► Pharmacological

Some physicians recommend up to 600 units of vitamin E daily. It is believed that the vitamin supplement helps to breakdown the fibrocystic tissue because it reacts with the polyunsaturated fats in the membrane of the cell. It may also have some effect on the balance of female hormones.

► Diet

Most health care providers recommend limiting or completely eliminating caffeine-containing products from the woman's diet. This would include teas, colas, coffee, and chocolate. These products are all available in caffeine-free forms.

► Nursing Process

Assessment

Subjective Data The client may report that the lumps are more tender as she approaches her menstrual period and that there is a greenish, sticky discharge from one or both breasts. The nurse should inquire about the client's dietary habits, especially caffeine intake, frequency of BSE, and the date of the most recent mammogram, if applicable. Since FBD lumps are more tender near the menses, the client should be seen for an exam the week following her period. The tissue contains less fluid during that time and palpation is easier.

Objective Data When examined, single or multiple lumps may be palpated in both breasts. The lumps are not always discrete, but should be freely movable.

▼ ▼

Possible nursing diagnoses for a client with FBD may include:

Nursing Diagnoses	Goals	Nursing Interventions
► Pain related to tender cysts in the breasts.	The client will have decreased breast discomfort.	Advise the client to wear a well-fitting brassiere day and night when the breasts are the most tender to help lessen the client's discomfort.
► Knowledge deficit related to the cause and treatment of fibrocystic breast disease.	The client will verbalize and demonstrate her understanding of the cause of FBD and her role in treatment.	Demonstrate BSE for the client either in person or by video with a follow-up return demonstration by the client. Observe the client as she performs the BSE so that immediate feedback can be given. Explain the best timing for the BSE and the rationale for performing the procedure after the menses.

(continued)

Nursing Diagnoses	Goals	Nursing Interventions
		Schedule the mammogram and encourage follow-up mammography at regular intervals dependent upon the client's age and risk factors.
		Teach the client about dietary modifications, such as limiting caffeine.
▶ *Anxiety related to the underlying potential and risk of breast cancer.*	The client will display behaviors of decreased anxiety related to the potential for breast cancer.	Clarify for the client the differences between malignant breast lesions and FBD to help alleviate the client's anxiety.

▶ Evaluation

Each goal must be evaluated to determine how it has been met by the client.

▲ ▲

▶ BREAST CANCER

Cancer of the female reproductive system will affect the lives of one in every nine women annually. The number one fatal cancer in females is lung cancer (22 percent), followed by breast cancer (19 percent) (Knobf & Morra, 1993). Many cancers could be prevented by wise lifestyle choices and simple changes in habits known to increase the potential for certain types of cancers. Nursing plays an important role in educating women on the value of routine physical examinations, including mammograms, breast self-examination, and Pap smears. The National Cancer Society and The American Cancer Society are two referral resources that provide free information about cancer prevention, screening, and treatment.

The American Cancer Society recommends that women under forty have a general physical examination every three years, and annually after forty years of age. BSE is highly recommended on a monthly basis. Women who are sexually active or who have multiple sexual partners should have an annual Pap smear done. An increased number of sexual partners has been associated with an increased risk of cervical cancer. Postmenopausal women also need to continue annual breast and pelvic examinations by a health care professional, especially if they are currently taking hormonal replacement therapy.

Breast cancer is the most common cancer in females in the United States. Two of the most common types of breast cancer are ductal and lobular, which means they originate within the breast tissue. Two-thirds of breast cancer cases occur in women over fifty years of age. Women at greatest risk for developing breast cancer are those who:

- Had a mother or sibling with breast cancer
- Never had children or had their first child after the age of thirty

- Never breast fed
- Have a history of fibrocystic breast disease
- Started menstruating before age ten
- Are obese
- Consume a high fat diet and a moderate amount of alcohol
- Smoke
- Experienced a late menopause

A woman generally presents herself at the physician or NP's office after the discovery of a tender or non-tender lump in her breast. If she has been performing BSE routinely each month, she is more likely to be familiar with even minute changes in the breast tissue. Breast cancers often occur in the upper, outer quadrant of the breast and may extend into the tail of the breast, which spread upward into the axilla. It is important to teach women to examine the axillary region as well as the breast during BSE (refer to Figure 31-5 for BSE).

Women also seek medical advice because they notice a discharge from the breast, dimpling of the skin, retraction of the nipple, pain, a unilateral change in breast size, or a puckering (orange peel appearance) of the skin. Dimpling and puckering are usually associated with the breast tissue or tumor attaching to the skin or the underlying muscle mass which does not permit movement. The nurse should not be misled by the client's report of a tender lump or mass and assume it is FBD. All new or enlarged lumps or masses in the breast require medical assessment.

Baron & Walsh (1995) reported that an estimated 182,000 women would develop breast cancer that year. Approximately 96 percent of women know about the importance of performing BSE monthly, however, only 33 percent actually perform it on a regular basis (Barton & Walsh, 1995). Frequently, (an estimated 95 percent), the earliest detection of a breast lump is when it is discovered by the woman or her partner. Sometimes, careful physical examination of the breast performed by an experienced health care provider may be the time of initial discovery. The presence of tiny clusters of calcium, or "microclusters," may be an early sign of breast cancer. These should be followed closely with mammography every six to twelve months to detect subtle changes in shape or size. The American Cancer Society recommends that women ages twenty to forty perform BSE each month and have a clinical breast examination every three to four years. For women forty-one to forty-nine years of age, BSE should also be performed monthly, a clinical examination every one to two years, and a mammogram every one to two years. Women fifty and older should follow the monthly routine for BSE and have a clinical examination and mammogram every year (Baron & Walsh, 1995). Figure 31-6 shows the staging of breast cancer.

A mammogram is a radiologic examination of the breast that may be ordered for baseline data or to confirm a tentative diagnosis of benign or malignant breast conditions. The procedure involves placing the breast on a radiologic surface and compressing the tissue as flat as possible prior to taking the x-ray. The procedure produces moderate discomfort, but it does not take too long. The nurse should advise the client to take a mild analgesic like acetaminophen or ibuprophen thirty to sixty minutes before the test to minimize the pain. Some women will experience minor bruising of the tissue following the test. The client should limit caffeine consumption for at least one week prior to the mammogram. The client should avoid wearing deodorant or talcum powder at the time of the test. Figure 31-7 illustrates a normal and abnormal mammogram.

Another type of mammography is performed by the

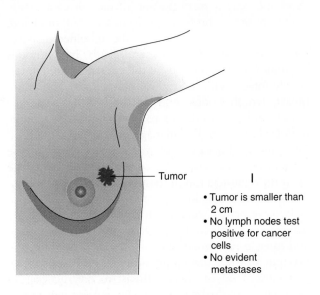

I
• Tumor is smaller than 2 cm
• No lymph nodes test positive for cancer cells
• No evident metastases

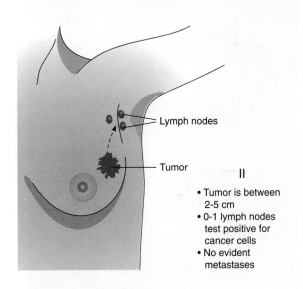

II
• Tumor is between 2-5 cm
• 0-1 lymph nodes test positive for cancer cells
• No evident metastases

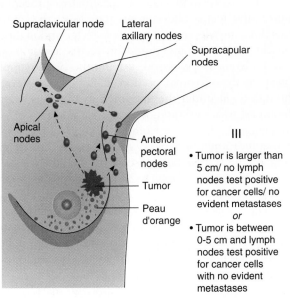

III
• Tumor is larger than 5 cm/ no lymph nodes test positive for cancer cells/ no evident metastases
  or
• Tumor is between 0-5 cm and lymph nodes test positive for cancer cells with no evident metastases

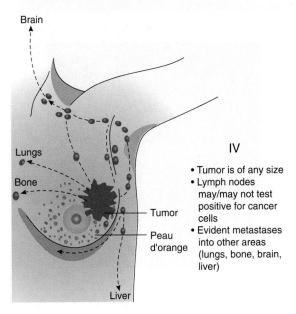

IV
• Tumor is of any size
• Lymph nodes may/may not test positive for cancer cells
• Evident metastases into other areas (lungs, bone, brain, liver)

FIGURE 31-6 Breast cancer staging.

stereotactic computer guided technique. This advanced method allows needle biopsies to be taken at the same time if necessary. Often, the physician or NP will recommend this method after an initial mammogram has shown suspicious areas. This technique is less costly than excisional biopsy and can be performed with little discomfort to the client. The client is placed in a prone position on the special examination table with her breast hanging down through the opening in the table. The operator can move the position of the table and visualize the entire breast area via computerized guidance.

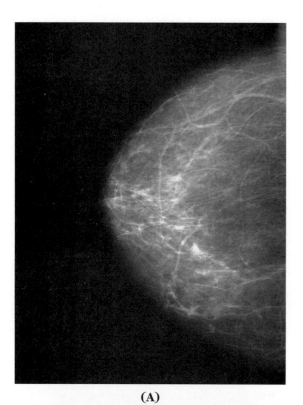

(A)

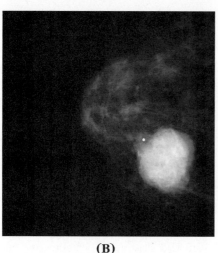

(B)

FIGURE 31-7 Mammograms. **(A)** A normal mammogram. **(B)** A large mass is visible in breast.

After the breast has been biopsied and the tissue has been examined by the pathologist, if a malignancy is confirmed, the client may be advised to proceed with surgical removal of the affected tissue. This procedure is referred to as a lumpectomy or mastectomy.

▶ Medical/Surgical Management

▶ Surgical

There is an abundance of lymphatic vessels proximal to the breast. Malignant cells can thus escape into the general lymphatic system and be spread throughout the body. Some surgeons prefer a conservative approach to mastectomy and perform the lumpectomy procedure. A simple mastectomy removes the tumor mass and only a small portion of the adjacent tissue. Some physicians prefer to perform a partial, modified, or total radical procedure. In the modified mastectomy, the entire breast tissue and nearby lymph nodes are removed. The muscles of the chest wall are left relatively intact. With the radical mastectomy, the entire breast, lymph nodes, and the underlying pectoralis muscle are removed. Figure 31-8 shows the various options in the surgical management of breast cancer. The greater the extent of the surgical removal, the longer the client's recovery process and the greater the need for rehabilitation in the use of the upper extremity on the affected side.

Reconstructive surgery following a mastectomy may be determined by the amount of breast tissue and muscle remaining after the initial procedure, the position of the mastectomy scar, and the probability of recurrent breast cancer. Breast reconstruction can help the client deal with the disfigurement that results from the mastectomy. One reconstructive procedure utilizes the rectus abdominous muscle or the latissimus dorsi muscle. In the transverse rectus abdominous muscle or TRAM procedure, the rectus abdominous is freed from its distal end, leaving the blood supply intact on the proximal portion. It is then transferred through a slit under the abdomen to the area where the breast tissue was removed and sutured into place. Subcutaneous fat tissue from the abdomen is cut and shaped to form a new breast and placed on top of the muscle. The skin is then closed over the newly reconstructed breast and a new areola may be made.

The client's desire for reconstruction and her psychological status play an important role in determining the personal value of additional surgery. In the United States particularly, the breast is associated with childbearing and female sexuality. It may be difficult for the client to express her concerns regarding her sexuality and desirability to her partner after the mastectomy. She may have difficulty facing the physical alteration

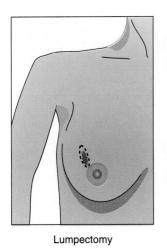

Lumpectomy

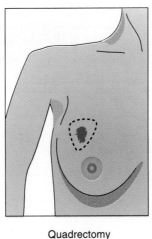

Quadrectomy

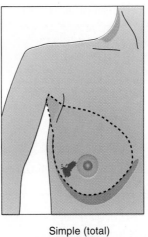

Simple (total)
Mastectomy

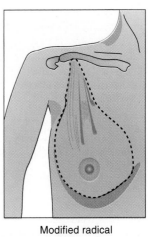

Modified radical
Mastectomy

FIGURE 31-8 Surgical options for breast cancer.

immediately after surgery and for some time in the future. The caring nurse with good interpersonal communication skills can help the client identify and verbalize her feelings of loss and thus promote the psychological healing process and acceptance of the altered body image.

Breast prostheses constructed to look and feel like real breast tissue, are available. The prosthesis fits into a special pocket inside the brassiere. Some types are available for swim suits and strapless tops. The construction of the prosthesis varies from sponge rubber to fluid- or air-filled. They are washable and should be protected from excessive heat.

Volunteers from the local cancer society often visit new mastectomy clients to assist them in the physical and psychological transition and adjustment following breast surgery. The American Cancer Society publishes a pamphlet entitled *Help Yourself to Recovery,* which includes simple postmastectomy exercises to perform as a part of the rehabilitation process.

▶ Pharmacological

Some of the agents used in the treatment of breast cancer include antineoplastic drugs like antiestrogens: megestrol acetate (Megace), medroxyprogesterone acetate (Depo-Provera), tamoxifen citrate (Nolvadex), and aminoglutethamide (Cytadren). Androgens for postmenopausal clients include testolactone (Teslac); methyltestosterone (Testred), and/or rotating combinations of chemotherapy agents such as cyclophosphamide (Cytoxan), an alkalating agent, doxorubicin hydrochloride (Adriamycin), an antitumor antibiotic; 5-fluorouracil (Adrucil) and methotrexate sodium (Rheumatrex), antimetabolites; and prednisone (Orasone), a glucocorticoid via intravenous or oral routes. These drugs may be initiated prior to or following surgery. These anti-

neoplastic agents act in several ways to either inhibit cellular growth or interfere with DNA replication. A laboratory test called tissue assay determines if estrogen or progesterone stimulates the cancer cells to grow. If the cancerous growth is stimulated by estrogen, antiestrogen drugs are used to treat the breast cancer. When the tumors are not estrogen dependent, estrogen is used as a chemotherapy agent to treat breast cancers. Examples of two estrogen medications are diethylstilbestrol diphosphate (Stilphostrol) and ethinyl estradiol (Estinyl).

Paclitaxel (Taxol), a drug made from the bark of the Pacific yew, has demonstrated positive results in clinical trials with breast cancer therapies. It acts by prohibiting cell replication. One of the benefits of this agent is that it causes milder nausea than many of the other chemotherapy agents that are used. It has the potential to cause severe anaphylactic reactions when it is administered due to a histamine release. To avoid this problem, the client should be medicated with the following medications prior to Taxol infusion therapy: a corticosteroid like dexamethasone (Decadron), a histamine blocker like cimetidine (Tagamet), and an antihistamine diphenhydramine hydrochloride (Benadryl).

▶ Radiation Therapy

Breast tissue and lymphatic regions may be radiated before or after surgical excision of the tumor. This treatment may be done prophylactically to prevent the metastasis of malignant cells to other areas, or it may be done as a palliative measure to maintain the client's comfort. Figure 31-9 illustrates brachytherapy, one form of radiation therapy used in the treatment of breast cancer. Metastasis of breast cancer often progresses to the lymph system, then bone, and finally to the lung.

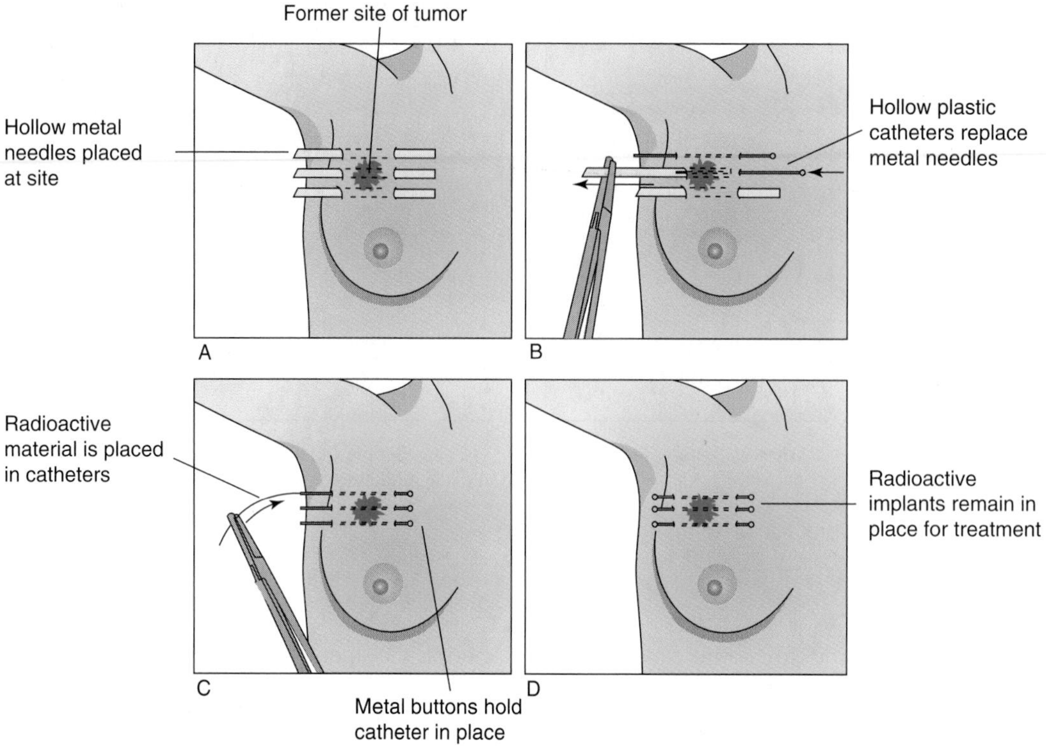

Former site of tumor

Hollow metal
needles placed
at site

Hollow plastic
catheters replace
metal needles

A

B

Radioactive
material is placed
in catheters

Radioactive
implants remain in
place for treatment

C

D

Metal buttons hold
catheter in place

FIGURE 31-9   Brachytherapy for treatment of breast cancer.

▶ *Nursing Process*

Assessment

Subjective Data   The client may come to the office concerned about a newly discovered breast lump and other changes in the breast, such as dimpling, pucker-

ing, or discharge. Ask how long the lump has been present, whether or not it is movable, whether it is tender or not, the frequency that BSE is performed, and the date of the most recent mammogram and current medications being taken. Other questions should include the risk factors also discussed in this section.

Objective Data   Assess vital signs and weight. Review report of the last mammogram.

▼ ▼

Possible nursing diagnoses for a client with breast cancer may include:

Nursing Diagnoses	*Goals*	*Nursing Interventions*
▶ *Anxiety related to possible metastasis, surgery, and disfigurement.*	The client will express feelings of decreased anxiety related to hospitalization and surgical interventions or procedures.	Encourage client to express feelings of anxiety.
		Take extra time to clarify or explain instructions.
		Provide written back-up instructions along with verbal instructions.
		Encourage family members to remain with the client before and after surgery.
		Suggest a preoperative visit by a member of the cancer society to facilitate the client's acceptance of the surgery.
▶ *Knowledge deficit related to diagnostic tests, BSE, and signs of breast cancer.*	The client will verbalize or demonstrate her understanding of diagnostic tests, BSE, and preoperative/postoperative teaching.	Assess the client's understanding and knowledge of BSE, cancer risk factors, diagnostic tests/procedures, medications, and the medical plan of treatment.

Nursing Diagnoses	Goals	Nursing Interventions
		Encourage the client to ask questions.
		Provide her with the American Cancer Society's booklets about breast cancer and literature pertaining to BSE and mammography.
		Provide the client with information regarding surgical and medical treatment options for breast cancer.
▶ *Coping, individual, ineffective, related to medical or surgical interventions to treat the breast cancer.*	The client will demonstrate effective coping strategies during the pre- and postoperative periods.	Assess the client's previous coping patterns with major life stressors.
		Spend time with client to answer questions.
		Provide client with time alone to allow her to adjust and vent her feelings.
▶ *Body image disturbance, related to psychological reactions to removal of the breast.*	The client will discuss her feelings related to the loss of her breast and demonstrate acceptance of the change in physical appearance.	Remain attentive to signals from the client indicating her readiness to look at the surgical site and encourage her to do so when she displays readiness.
		Be alert for client's comments regarding her body changes.
		Encourage client recommended for chemotherapy to obtain a wig before therapy begins. Approximately 80 percent of clients undergoing chemotherapy will experience hair loss and, if the client becomes accustomed to wearing a wig before her hair begins to fall out, she may feel more comfortable in it later.
		Anticipate the client's need to grieve the loss of her breast.
		Refer her to a breast cancer support group.
		Inform client that she may have decreased sensation and lymphatic fluid retention in the arm on the affected side.
		Teach her to keep this arm elevated above the level of the heart to promote lymph drainage.
		Encourage client to wear a properly fitting elastic compression sleeve on the affected arm that will help reduce the lymphedema.
▶ *Skin integrity, impaired, related to surgical intervention or radiation effects.*	The client's surgical incision will heal without signs or symptoms of infection or complication.	Instruct the client in proper postoperative skin care.
		Teach client to avoid soaps, creams, and deodorants near the surgical site.
		Teach client signs and symptoms of complications such as elevated temperature, redness, warmth, swelling near the surgical incision, an increase in wound drainage or change in the color or odor of the drainage, or breakdown of sutures around the incision.
		Explain to client that she may notice areas of pin point hemorrhage (petechiae) or larger areas (ecchymosis) on her skin, or bleeding from her gums.
▶ *Pain, related to surgery or radiation implants and exposed tissue.*	The client's pain will be controlled at a level tolerable for the client to continue activities of daily living during the postoperative period.	Assess pain on 1 to 10 scale.
		Administer analgesics as ordered.
		Advise client to use warm saline rinses several times a day to ease mouth discomforts.

(continued)

Nursing Diagnoses	Goals	Nursing Interventions
		Inform the client that she may experience "phantom pain or sensations" after the surgery. This phenomena appear to be more common in women over fifty years of age.
▶ Breathing pattern, ineffective, related to the proximity of the surgical incision to respiratory muscles and pain with respiratory effort.	The client's breath sounds will remain clear to auscultation and she will effectively cough and deep breathe every two hours.	Preoperatively, teach the client to how to turn, cough, and deep breathe. Postoperatively, assess the client's breath sounds, rate, and quality of respirations every four to eight hours. Encourage deep breathing or the use of incentive spirometry every two hours. Medicate the client or encourage her to use the PCA pump prior to performing exercises or deep breathing.
▶ Infection, high risk for, related to surgical wound and wound drainage.	The client will be free of infection, and vital signs will remain within normal limits.	Monitor CBC reports for RBC and WBC levels since bone marrow depression is also a side effect of chemotherapy drugs. Instruct the client to contact her health care provider at the first signs of an infection or if she develops a fever above 101 degrees. Teach client to protect herself from contact with others who have infections, colds, or the flu. Postoperatively, observe the wound, and assess for lymphedema. Assess the surgical wound for redness, edema, warmth, and drainage at least every 4 hours once the dressing has been removed. Monitor the drainage for type, amount, color, and odor. Anticipate the presence of one or two drainage tubes in the wound and use caution when removing the old dressing so that the drains do not become dislodged. Administer antibiotics as ordered. Elevate the affected arm on pillows to reduce edema. Monitor and record vital signs every four to eight hours. Check for adequate circulation, sensation, and movement (CSM) of the hand and fingers on the affected side.
▶ Self-care deficit, related to limited use and range of motion on the affected side and post-operative discomforts.	The client will gradually regain ROM and provide self-care.	Begin passive range of motion exercises on the first or second postop day as ordered. Demonstrate postoperative exercises for the affected arm or request a consult from the physical therapy department. Observe the client as she performs the exercises and reinforce correct performance. Encourage active ROM as soon as ordered by the physician to strengthen the operative side. This may be difficult at first due to tissue soreness from surgery.

▶ Evaluation

Each goal must be evaluated to determine how it has been met by the client.

▲ ▲

Sample Nursing Care Plan: The Client with Breast Cancer

Claire Wilder, age fifty-seven, is married, with two children ages twenty-four and twenty-two. During a bath, she noted a small, movable lump in her right breast, grew concerned, and went to see her health care provider. Family history is significant for fibrocystic breast disease and breast cancer on the maternal side (mother, aunt, sister). Personal history: onset of menses at age ten with regular twenty-eight day cycle, five day flow. She is 5' 5" tall and weighs 175 pounds. Her history is negative for alcohol use, but she smokes one to one-and-one-half packs of cigarettes daily. She did not breast-feed the children. Her last mammogram was fifteen years ago. BSE is not practiced routinely. States: "I'm not sure just how to do the exam anyway."

Physical examination reveals a pea-sized lump in the URQ of the R breast and multiple clusters of lumps throughout each breast. Dimpling is present superior to the nipple. No nipple discharge noted. The remainder of the exam was unremarkable. Vital signs were WNL. A mammogram revealed a suspicious mass and a biopsy performed using stereotactic visualization, was positive for cancer cells. A modified mastectomy was performed the next day with biopsies of adjacent lymph nodes. Six of ten nodes were also positive. Hormone assay reveals that the tumor had estrogen-positive receptors.

The morning after surgery, Claire displayed behaviors which the nurse interpreted as anxiety. She confided in the nurse that she was afraid she was going to die like her mother did from the cancer. Claire had a large chest pressure dressing with two Jackson-Pratt drains in place. She stated that she was glad she had the PCA pump to take care of the pain.

Nursing Diagnosis 1 Self-care deficit, bathing/dressing, related to temporary altered function of arm as evidenced by large chest pressure dressing and two drains in place.

Goals	Nursing Interventions	Rationale	Evaluation
Claire will meet her daily hygiene needs.	Assess Claire's ability to use affected arm to perform ADLs.	Assessment provides the nurse with baseline information related to Claire's abilities and limitations.	Claire's hygiene needs were met.
	Provide assistance as needed to complete hygiene tasks, such as bathing and grooming.	Assisting with tasks and encouraging Claire to participate, will facilitate the return of function and self-esteem.	
	Encourage gradual resumption of activities as Claire indicates readiness.	By gradually increasing the use of the affected arm, Claire will regain strength and maintain the mobility of the extremity. Claire is empowered to help perform her own care which validates her self-image and worth.	
	Instruct Claire in arm exercise to maintain range of motion.	Maintaining ROM will facilitate the use of her arm.	
	Provide a sling for support of affected arm.	A sling will provide support for the arm.	
	Elevate the affected arm above the level of the heart when in bed or sitting to reduce lymph edema.	Arm elevation will assist in fluid draining from arm.	

(continued)

Nursing Diagnosis 2. Fear, related to removal of the breast as evidenced by her fear of dying like her mother.

Goals	Nursing Interventions	Rationale	Evaluation
Claire will have less fear about breast removal.	Encourage Claire and family to verbalize their feelings and concerns related to the diagnosis and treatment.	Sharing feelings and concerns often relieves fear. Claire and family perceptions may differ from health care worker's and should be identified.	Claire verbalized having less fear about her surgery.
	Assess Claire's normal or previously used coping behaviors	Identification of previous coping patterns enables the nurse to help the client use or change coping behaviors.	
	Involve Claire and her family in care planning.	By involving the client and the family in the planning of the care, they are more likely to feel a part of the team rather than simply accepting a passive "client role."	

Nursing Diagnosis 3. Pain related to surgical manipulation of tissues and excision of tissue as evidenced by client statement that she was glad she had the PCA pump to take care of the pain.

Goals	Nursing Interventions	Rationale	Evaluation
Claire will verbalize that pain is controlled.	Assess Claire's pain level and response to analgesia every two hours.	The nurse must be alert to increasing pain and how the client is tolerating the pain medication.	Claire reports pain is controlled at less than 2 on a one to ten scale.
	Instruct Claire how to use the PCA pump to administer Demerol 10 mg q 10 minutes.	Use of the PCA pump allows the client greater control over analgesia and provides consistent relief from pain.	
	Evaluate the effectiveness of analgesia q 2 hours.	Evaluating the client's response to medication allows the nurse to identify any untoward effects and effectiveness of the medication. The nurse may need to contact the physician for different analgesia	

		orders if the current medication is ineffective in controlling her pain at the desired level of comfort.	
Reposition Claire q 2 hours.		Changing positions helps to improve vascular flow and relieves pressure on bony prominences.	
Elevate the arm on the right side on pillows to facilitate venous flow and decrease edema.		Increased venous flow decreases edema and discomfort due to pressure on nerves in the area.	

Teaching Tips: Post-surgery

There are important instructions for the client prior to discharge from the hospital for her on-going recovery and restoration of function. Advise the client to avoid carrying items in the affected arm, or wearing purse straps over the affected shoulder. Vaccinations and lab tests or blood draws should be done on the unaffected side only. Minor injuries and infections of the affected side require immediate medical attention to prevent complications.

▶ CERVICAL CANCER

An abnormal condition of the cervix known as dysplasia may be an early sign of developing cervical cancer. Dysplasia is a change in the size and shape of the cervical cells, and it is classified as mild, moderate, or severe. An abnormal Pap smear may be the first indication of a problem. Pap smears are classified from 1 through 5. A "1" is considered a normal cervix and a "5" would indicate a malignant condition.

Cancer of the cervix is more prevalent in women with multiple sexual partners than in women in monogamous relationships. Recent research has indicated that there is a link between the human papilloma virus (HPV), which causes venereal warts (condyloma acuminatum) and the incidence of cervical cancer. Other associated etiologies include chronic infections and exposure to viruses, like herpes simplex II. A higher incidence of cervical cancer has been observed in women from lower socioeconomic populations, African Americans, and diethylstilbestrol (DES) daughters. There is also an increased incidence of cervical cancer in women who had their first intercourse at an early age.

Although cervical cancer can occur at any age, it occurs more frequently in women between thirty-five and fifty-five years of age. It is usually insidious in its onset because it is asymptomatic. Cervical cancer has a high cure rate in the early stages, and it is easily detected by the routine annual Pap smear.

The nurse should immediately bring any abnormal Pap smear results to the attention of the physician or NP so the client can be notified and the appropriate follow-up treatment initiated. A repeat Pap smear may be indicated after treatment with a vaginal antibiotic cream or colposcopy may be performed.

Staging of the cancer progresses from 0 to IV (see Figure 31-10). Carcinoma *in situ* (CIS) means that the cancerous cells remain within the cervix and have not yet spread to adjacent areas. The higher the number on the staging table, the more the cancer has metastasized to other structures. Stage II through IV would indicate that the cancer cells have invaded the bladder, vagina, or other pelvic organs.

▶ Medical/Surgical Management

▶ Surgical

Treatment modalities may include conization, a surgical excision of a cone-shaped section of the abnormal cervical tissues. This procedure is desirable if the client is of childbearing age and wants to bear children in the future. However, a problem known as incompetent cervix is associated with conization and may affect the client's future pregnancies. With this condition the cervix begins to open or dilate prior to the full term of the pregnancy as the fetal weight increases and the fetus may be delivered preterm. The end result of the conization may be success in removing the cancer, but may interfere with the client's childbearing abilities. Laser surgery, cryosurgery (freezing of the cells with liquid nitrogen), or cauterization (burning) may be performed as alternative methods of treatment if the cervical lesions are easily visible for the procedure. A total hysterectomy or radical pelvic surgery may be required to eradicate the cancer. If the spread of the disease has become too extensive, treatment will be directed toward palliative measures and focused on maintaining the client's comfort as long as possible.

STAGING SYSTEM FOR CANCER OF THE CERVIX		
Stage	Characteristics	
I IA IA1 IA2 IB	• Carcinoma is strictly confined to cervix (extension to corpus should be disregarded) • Preclinical carcinoma • Minimal microscopically evident stromal invasion • Microscopic lesions no more than 5 mm depth measured from base of epithelium surface or glandular from which it originates, and horizontal spread not to exceed 7 mm • All other cases of stage I; occult cancer should be marked "occ"	
II IIA IIB	• Carcinoma extends beyond cervix but has not extended to pelvic wall; it involves vagina, but not as far as lower third • No obvious parametrical involvement • Obvious parametrical involvement	
III IIIA IIIB	• Carcinoma has extended to pelvic wall; on rectal examination, there is no cancer-free space between tumor and pelvic wall; tumor involves lower third of vagina; all cases with hydronephrosis or nonfunctioning kidney should be included, unless they are known to be due to another cause • No extension to pelvic wall, but involvement of lower third of vagina • Extension to pelvic wall, or hydronephrosis or nonfunctioning kidney due to tumor	
IV IVA IVB	• Carcinoma has extended beyond true pelvis or has clinically involved mucosa of bladder or rectum • Spread of growth to adjacent pelvic organs • Spread to distant organs	

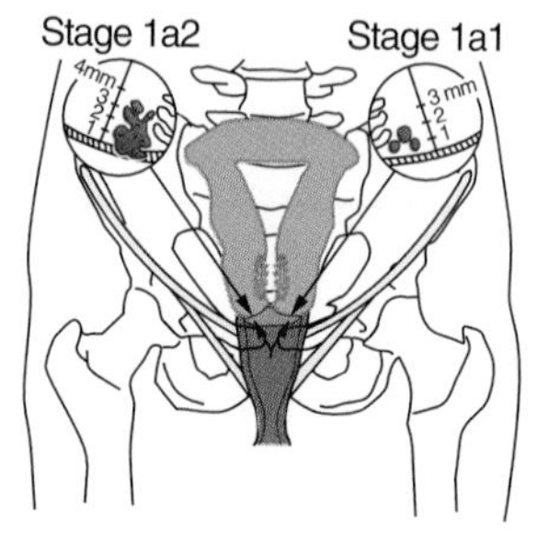

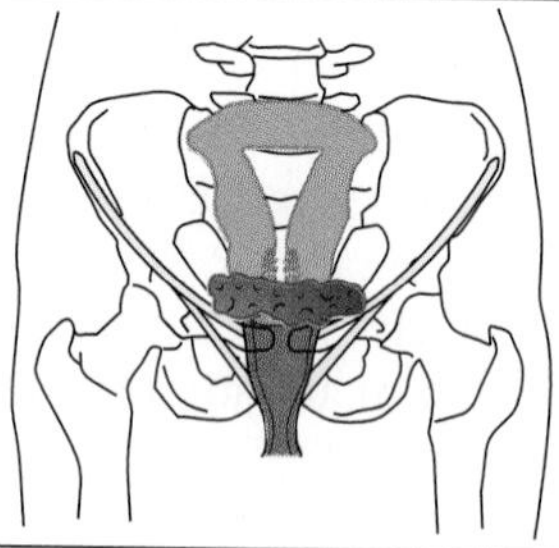

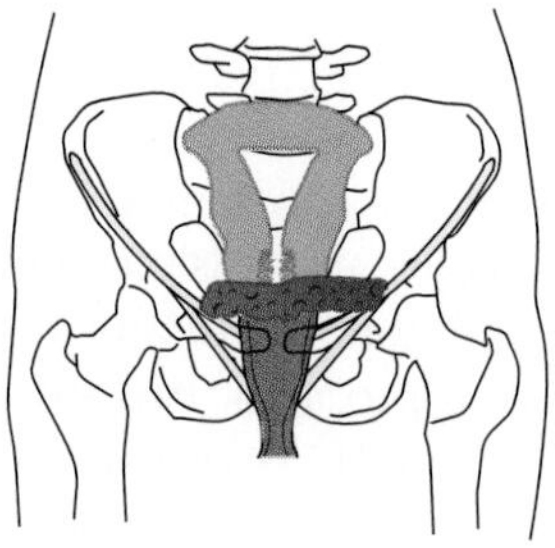

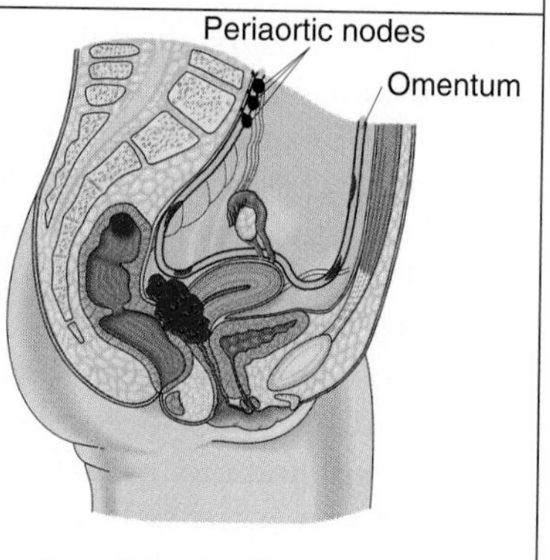

FIGURE 31-10 Cervical cancer staging.

▶ Radiation Therapy

The physician may recommend the use of radium implants or radiation therapy prior to the surgical excision of the cervix. In addition, chemotherapy may be utilized as an adjunct therapy to help shrink the tumor or slow its growth. The nurse must be cautious in providing nursing care for the client with radium implants. Pregnant nurses or female nurses of childbearing age should not care for this client or spend extended periods of time at the bedside. Direct client care should be organized to optimize time spent at the bedside. A sign should be hung on the door to indicate that radiation is being used in the room and provide a warning for visitors to limit their visit time. With the implants in place, the client will remain on complete bed rest.

▶ Nursing Process

Assessment

Subjective Data   The client may complain of postcoital bleeding (bleeding after intercourse), or spotting between menstrual periods or after menopause, and occasionally a foul smelling vaginal discharge. Later, as the disease progresses, she may complain of increased or bloody discharge, and pain that radiates down the lower back and legs.

Objective Data   Objective data may include the presence and appearance of a vaginal discharge. The cervix may appear eroded or raw and may bleed easily when touched with a cotton tipped applicator or Pap scraper. Necrotic tissue may be present and cause the foul odor. Pap smear results will probably indicate dysplasia or Class II through Class IV cell changes. Tissue samples obtained through colposcopic examination will also demonstrate cellular changes. In advanced disease, weight loss and anemia may be present. Laparotomy may be performed to stage the disease along with other laboratory and diagnostic testing to identify metastases. Areas most likely to be investigated will be proximal to the cervix, including the rectum, vagina, bladder, and pelvis.

▼ ▼

Possible nursing diagnoses for a client with cervical cancer may include:

Nursing Diagnoses	Goals	Nursing Interventions
▶ *Sexuality patterns, altered, related to vaginal bleeding and discomfort and procedures.*	The client will return to normal sexual functioning following recovery from treatment for cervical cancer.	Inform client that she may experience dyspareunia related to vaginal dryness following radiation therapy. Instruct client to use a water soluble lubricant during intercourse or to use lubricated condoms to decrease irritation.
▶ *Anxiety related to unknown outcome and possible treatments.*	The client will verbalize having less anxiety about treatment and possible outcome.	Be aware of the client's emotional state throughout the course of care and use effective interpersonal communication to facilitate the client's acceptance of her condition and the treatments. Explain diagnostic tests and procedures to client to decrease her anxiety. Provide therapeutic emotional support to client to help her cope with feelings of guilt, alteration of body image, or self-concept.
▶ *Knowledge deficit, related to cause and prevention, treatment, and ongoing therapy.*	The client will verbalize her understanding of the condition and treatment alternatives.	Inform the client of what she should expect both physically and psychologically prior to surgery and follow-up treatments. Teach the client how to turn, cough, and deep breathe in preparation for postoperative care. Inform the client about the placement of the intracavity radiation device that will be performed during surgery and remain in place for twenty-four to seventy-two hours.

(continued)

Nursing Diagnoses	*Goals*	*Nursing Interventions*
		Teach the client the importance of keeping follow-up appointments after dismissal from the hospital.
► *Infection, high risk for, related to open internal areas of the cervix and exposure to external factors.*	The client will be free of signs and symptoms of infection before and after surgery.	Administer preoperative cleansing enemas and vaginal douches as ordered.
		Assess client each shift for vaginal discharge, bleeding, pain, and other signs indicative of radiation sickness.
		Following intracavity radiation therapy, administer cleansing enema and vaginal douche as ordered.
► *Pain, related to surgical procedures, chemotherapy, and radiation therapy.*	The client will identify pain at a level of less than 3 on a 1 to 10 scale.	Provide client with an egg crate mattress postoperatively to aid in comfort.
		Inform client that a Foley catheter will probably be inserted to prevent pressure on the radiation device and promote her comfort during period of bed rest.
		Administer analgesic as ordered.
► *Body image disturbance, related to effects of the disease, chemotherapy, and radiation.*	The client will maintain a positive body image.	Refer the client to the American Cancer Society or one of its members for support.
► *Self-care deficit, related to required bed rest during intracavitary radiation therapy.*	The client will participate in activities of daily living as permitted by bed rest.	Encourage client to perform as much of her daily hygiene as she can, then complete the remainder for her.
► *Urinary elimination, altered and incontinence, bowel, related to potential damage from radiation effects on the bowel and bladder.*	The client will maintain normal patterns of elimination, and will be maintained throughout therapy.	Assess the function of the Foley catheter to assure patency.
		Maintain client's adherence to a low residue diet, as ordered by physician, to keep the bowel quiet and nonactive.
		Encourage the client to drink many fluids to flush the kidneys and decrease risk of UTI.
► *Skin integrity altered, high risk for, related to effects of intracavity radiation implants.*	The client will maintain skin integrity throughout therapy.	Assess client for development of petechiae and eccyhmosis.
		Prior to discharge, teach client proper skin care, including patting skin instead of rubbing it dry and avoiding irritating soaps, powders, and sprays.

► Evaluation

Each goal must be evaluated to determine how it has been met by the client.

▲ ▲

► Nursing Alert

Remember, due to the risk of radiation exposure to the caregiver, from the radiation implant device, procedures that require exposure to the client's perineal area should be kept at a minimum.

▶ FIBROID TUMORS (LEIOMYOMA)

Fibroids (leiomyomas) are benign tumors that grow in or on the uterus. A higher incidence is seen with nulliparous women and those who are over thirty years old. These benign tumors are also more prevalent in certain ethnic groups such as African Americans and Mediterraneans with darker skin. The fibroids may appear below the serosal membrane or the mucosa. An early symptom is often **menorrhagia**, an excessively heavy menstrual flow. Later, the client may experience increasing pelvic pressure as the tumors grow, along with dysmenorrhea, abdominal enlargement, and constipation. Growth of the fibroids is usually slow, but can be stimulated by estrogen. During pregnancy, when the estrogen level and progesterone level dramatically increase, the tumors grow much faster. Concern arises for the fetus when the fibroids begin to enlarge and crowd the uterus. Overcrowding may compress the fetus or initiate the onset of preterm labor. With either situation, the pregnancy must be monitored more carefully.

A medical diagnosis of uterine fibroids may initially be based upon the client's symptoms and the findings of the pelvic examination. If on palpation the uterus feels like an irregular mass or several masses, a pelvic ultrasound would be ordered to confirm the diagnosis.

▶ Medical/Surgical Management

▶ Medical

The physician may opt to wait and observe the growth pattern of the fibroids before advising the client to have surgery. This "wait and see" attitude may be swayed by the significance of the client's symptoms, size of the fibroids, amount of discomfort the client is experiencing, and the amount of menorrhagia and/or **metrorrhagia**, vaginal bleeding between menstrual periods. Reexamination should be encouraged at least every six months.

▶ Surgical

If the menorrhagia is significant with each menstrual cycle, a dilatation and curettage (D & C) may be performed to determine the exact etiology of the bleeding. A myomectomy, a surgical procedure to remove the tumor, may be performed if the client desires future pregnancies. In the case of severe menorrhagia, with a dropping hemoglobin level or multiple tumors, the physician may recommend a hysterectomy as the option of choice.

▶ Nursing Process

Assessment

Subjective Data   This would include the client's description of excessive menstrual flow, dysmenorrhea, and/or pelvic pain and pressure. She may also have difficulty fitting into clothes because her abdomen has enlarged.

Objective Data   This would include counting the number of sanitary pads the client saturates in an hour; observing the presence or absence of clots in the blood, and a hemoglobin level of less than 12 mg/dL. The nurse may observe that the client's skin color is pale. Her blood pressure may be slightly lower than normal and her pulse may be increased as a compensatory mechanism. When the pelvic examination is performed, the physician or NP may palpate irregularities in or on the uterus.

▼ ▼

Possible nursing diagnoses for a client with fibroids may include:

Nursing Diagnoses	Goals	Nursing Interventions
▶ *Fluid volume deficit, high risk for, related to excessive blood losses.*	The client will have a hemoglobin above 12mg /dL and will maintain fluid balance.	Assess client's blood loss for amount, color, and clots.
		Provide an accurate count of the saturated sanitary pads, along with the length of time taken to saturate a pad.
		Monitor vital signs at least every 4 hours, or more frequently if the client is having active blood loss.

(continued)

Nursing Diagnoses	*Goals*	*Nursing Interventions*
		Monitor client after initiation of blood transfusion postoperatively, if required. This would include observing for any reaction and monitoring the client's vital signs every fifteen to thirty minutes.
▶ *Pain, related to pressure on pelvic structures caused by growing tumors and cramping during the menses.*	The client will verbalize less discomfort and pelvic pressure.	Administer analgesics as ordered. Provide discharge instructions pertaining to pain management, activity restrictions, and follow-up appointments with the physician or nurse practitioner.
▶ *Knowledge deficit, related to the source of the bleeding and possible treatments.*	The client will verbalize an understanding of the causes of the bleeding and treatment alternatives.	Educate the client about the cause of the bleeding, explaining what fibroids are and how they cause the symptoms she is experiencing. Discuss tentative treatments. If surgery is required, prepare the client by discussing preoperative and postoperative care and expectations.
▶ *Anxiety, related to active blood loss and possible hospitalization or transfusion.*	The client will verbalize a decrease in anxiety.	Provide time for the client to ask questions. Actively listen to the client. Explain all treatments and procedures.

▶ Evaluation

Each goal must be evaluated to determine how it has been met by the client.

▲ ▲

▶ UTERINE CANCER

Postmenopausal women are at the greatest risk for uterine cancer, especially if they have taken estrogen replacement therapy for several years (usually more than five years). Research has shown that unopposed estrogen stimulation of the endometrial lining has a strong relationship with the development of uterine cancer. During the normal menstrual cycle, estrogen and progesterone rise and fall. These hormonal fluctuations affect the stimulation of the endometrial tissue to grow or to be sloughed off, in a sense, in opposition to each other. Without the progesterone effects, the endometrial tissue is not sloughed off at regular intervals and may undergo cellular changes leading to a high risk for endometrial dysplasia or cancer. For this reason, many physicians and nurse practitioners recommend estrogen/progesterone therapy for clients who experience menopausal symptoms. The combination of the two hormones stimulates the normal menstrual hormonal cycle and causes monthly sloughing of the endometrium. Clients may resist this combination therapy because they are reluctant to continue having menstrual periods in their fifties and sixties.

Other risk factors associated with uterine cancer may include never having borne a child, being Caucasian, middle class, never having had sexual intercourse, or being of Jewish descent.

Cancer of the uterus usually does not produce symptoms until it becomes relatively advanced. Routine Pap smear and pelvic examinations are inadequate for early diagnosis. An endometrial biopsy, which examines the tissue from the uterine lining under a microscope, is the best diagnostic tool to identify cellular changes. This may be done on an annual basis when the client has her routine examination. The medical follow-up treatment plan is dependent upon the biopsy results. D & C has a potential for spreading the cancer cells to adjacent tissues because the malignant cells may escape into the bloodstream at the time of the procedure. This is not usually a problem with the biopsy because the amount of tissue removed is so small and blood loss is minimal. A D&C is also more expensive, higher risk, and requires some type of anesthesia.

▶ Medical/Surgical Management

Treatments for uterine cancer may range from radiation, radium implants, chemotherapy, or surgery to a combination of any of the above. The choices of treatment are related to the staging of the cancer.

▶ Medical

Intravenous fluid administration will be implemented to replace fluids lost by the excessive bleeding. A blood transfusion may also be ordered due to a low hemoglobin. A hemoglobin above 10 gm/dL is preferred prior to surgical intervention. The physician may order whole blood or packed red blood cells to increase the hemoglobin rapidly.

▶ Surgical

Surgery for uterine or cervical cancer includes hysterectomy. A total hysterectomy is the removal of the cervix and the uterus. In a subtotal hysterectomy, only the uterus is removed and the cervix remains. A radical or pan hysterectomy is the removal of the ovaries, cervix, uterus and fallopian tubes, pelvic lymph nodes, and part of the vagina. Vaginal hysterectomy procedures have been refined with the laparoscopic approach so that many clients are released from the hospital within twenty-four to thirty-six hours postoperatively. If the cancer has spread beyond the uterus into the pelvic region, an abdominal hysterectomy may be the best approach for visualization and maneuvering room during the surgical procedure. The physician may recommend a course of radiation therapy following surgery.

▶ Pharmacological

Hormonal therapy with megestrol acetate (Megace); medroxyprogesterone acetate (Depo-Provera); or hydroxyprogesterone caproate (Prodrox), may be administered to suppress tumor growth when the cancer is considered inoperable or has metastasized, especially if the tumor receptors are estrogen stimulated.

▶ Radiation Therapy

There is a tendency for uterine cancer to confine itself to the uterus which increases the client's five-year survival prognosis. Uterine cancer is also one that usually responds well to the therapies available at this time, including radiation. Radiation may be delivered to the pelvic region via external sources or it may be delivered via intracavitary devices or implants with radium or cesium. There is a potential danger for injury to adjacent pelvic structures during radiation therapy. The nurse should be alert for signs of complications, such as bleeding from the rectum, moderate to severe abdominal pain, constipation, or diarrhea. New therapies are being developed using protons that are capable of more direct application of radiation which decreases the chance of injury to other organs or structures.

Nursing care of the client receiving radiation for uterine cancer is the same as the care previously discussed for cervical cancer.

▶ Nursing Process

Assessment

Subjective Data One of the earliest symptoms reported by many clients is vaginal bleeding. If the client is postmenopausal, it is imperative that all bleeding be investigated as soon as possible unless it is from hormonally induced periods. Late in the progression of the cancer, the client may experience symptoms similar to those discussed with cervical cancer. Pain is often associated with the spread of cancer to adjacent organs and is considered a late sign.

Objective Data Objective data may be collected from the client's physical exam findings, biopsy reports, and a history of hormone replacement therapy with or without the estrogen/progesterone combination.

▶ OVARIAN CANCER

Ovarian cancer most often originates in the epithelial tissue of the ovary, and like cervical and uterine cancer, does not produce symptoms until it is in an advanced, inoperable stage and is sometimes called "the silent killer." Its symptoms are vague and may be ignored for a long time before the client seeks medical attention.

The annual death toll from ovarian cancer exceeds 12,000 women. The incidence is greater in women between forty-five to sixty-five years old. It is the number one cause of gynecological deaths and the third most frequent gynecological cancer (Brunner & Suddarth, 1995). Nulliparity (never having borne a child), smoking, alcohol, infertility, and a high fat diet are factors that place the client at higher risk for developing ovarian cancer. There is an extremely low survival rate, less than 40 percent, for women with ovarian cancer due to the advanced stage present at the time of discovery. Metastasis occurs in over 75 percent of cases prior to diagnosis, and often the cancer has spread beyond the pelvis. The colon is the most frequent site of ovarian cancer metastasis, then the stomach, and diaphragm.

Unfortunately, medical research has not yet developed an early diagnostic or screening tool to detect ovarian cancer. It is believed, however, that there is an increased risk of ovarian cancer for clients with breast cancer and vice versa. A family history of two or more female relatives with breast or ovarian cancer provides a sound rationale for more frequent breast and pelvic examinations. Often the physician or NP palpates an ovarian mass on a routine bi-manual examination. This finding is cause for further investigation by pelvic ultrasound or CT scan to determine the size, character, and consistency (solid or fluid filled) of the mass, and whether or not other pelvic structures are involved. Some experts believe that there is a link between the occurrence of ovarian cysts and the development of ovarian cancers in certain women.

General diagnostic studies, such as a lower GI series, chest x-ray, intravenous pyelogram (IVP), and laparoscopy may be useful in determining the extent of the primary and secondary lesions. A substance called CA-125 may be measured in the blood if ovarian cancer is suspected because this type of malignancy produces the CA-125. Used alone, this is not diagnostic of ovarian cancer because the CA-125 marker in the blood may be present in some benign conditions of the ovary, such as benign ovarian cysts (National Cancer Institute, 1991). If the client develops peritoneal fluid or ascites as the cancer progresses, it may be removed by abdominal paracentesis for cytologic examination.

Recurrent disease is common and may occur in two years or less. Continued medical surveillance is recommended every two months for a period of two years for the earliest possible detection of new lesions.

▶ Medical/Surgical Management

Surgical excision of the ovary is rarely successful due to the extensiveness of the disease. Most often a combination of radiation, chemotherapy, immunotherapy, and surgery produce the best results, even if they are only palliative for the client. The client must be actively involved and informed of her treatment options as well as her prognosis to enable her to make sound choices in the treatments chosen.

▶ *Pharmacological*

Chemotherapy drugs that have been used with ovarian cancer treatment include cyclophosphamide (Cytoxan), doxorubicin hydrochloride (Adriamycin), mitomycin (Mutamycin) and paclitaxel (Taxol). These may be administered by regional or intraarterial perfusion techniques. These percutaneous modes direct the drugs to the lesion's vascular supply. If the cancer has not metastasized, a regimen of chemotherapy using a single drug, such as Cytoxan, may be administered over the course of five days and repeated again at regular intervals over the course of a year. A combination of the chemotherapy agents, mentioned in the chapter, used in a rotating series, is often more effective for reproductive cancers in the advanced stages. For example, the client would receive one drug over the course of five days, then switch to another drug for five days, and then a third drug for five days. This series may be repeated over the year in a similar pattern to that used with a single agent.

▶ Nursing Process

Assessment

Subjective Data   The client may describe fatigue, malaise, diarrhea or constipation, pelvic pressure, frequency with urination, loss of appetite, nausea, weight gain or loss, vaginal bleeding or spotting with intercourse, a foul-smelling vaginal discharge, and pain in the lower back. The list of symptoms is very vague and could be related to many reproductive and nonreproductive disorders.

Objective Data   Objective data pertinent to all cancers of the pelvic reproductive organs may include information from the client's previous health history, reproductive history (onset of menses, pregnancies, contraceptives methods, infections, hormonal replacement therapy, and surgeries), the discovery of a palpable mass during a bi-manual examination, an abnormal appearance of the cervix or adjacent tissues, abnormal Pap smear results greater than Class II dysplasia, abnormal cervical or endometrial biopsies, increased abdominal girth, or the presence of ascites and pleural effusion.

Diagnostic tests and laboratory studies may include all or some of the following: Papinicolaou test (Pap smear), pelvic ultrasound, a chest x-ray, an IVP (intravenous pyelogram), a kidney/ureters/bladder x-ray (KUB), CBC with differential, blood chemistry studies, bleeding and clotting time, endometrial biopsy, cervical biopsy, D & C tissue specimens, Schiller's test and colposcopy, laparoscopy, barium enema, and a bone scan.

▼ ▼

Possible nursing diagnoses for a client with ovarian or uterine cancer may include:

Nursing Diagnoses, Preoperative	Goals, Preoperative	Nursing Interventions, Preoperative
▶ Anxiety /fear related to tentative diagnoses, pending surgical procedures, cancer treatment and its side effects, incapacitating or extended illness with resulting dependence, and or death.	The client will verbalize or demonstrate behaviors consistent with reduced anxiety or fear prior to and following surgery.	Facilitate the client's expression of anxiety or fear by encouraging the client's open discussion of her concerns. Be alert for nonverbal cues as well. Explore sources of the client's anxiety if a high level of anxiety is detected on admission. Arrange a consultation with a social worker or chaplain, if appropriate.
▶ Pain, related to the spread of cancer throughout the pelvis and adjacent structures.	The client will have pain controlled at a level which allows the client to continue to function in her activities of daily living as long as possible.	Administer analgesics as ordered. Provide comfort measures, such as changing position and back rub.
▶ Knowledge deficit, related to the disease process, treatments, preoperative and postoperative care and the disease prognosis.	The client and her family will verbalize an understanding of diagnostic test procedures, surgical and medical interventions, treatment modalities, preoperative and postoperative care and expectations.	Explain all diagnostic tests and procedures. Answer client's questions thoroughly. Prepare the client for upcoming events of surgery and postoperative care. Teach client proper coughing and deep breathing techniques. Explain abdominal splinting, medications, and other treatments. Obtain baseline vital signs and complete a preoperative check list.
▶ Coping, individual, ineffective, related to difficulty in dealing with the disease process, and changes in role or relationships, possible death.	The client will effectively cope with the physical and emotional stresses of cancer.	Assess the client's usual coping methods. Identify client's strengths and weaknesses. Assist client in identifying needs during the hospitalization and convalescence.
▶ Urinary elimination, altered, incontinence, bowel or constipation, related to pressure from tumor growth, or organ involvement/invasion, posttherapy side effects of radiation and irritation.	The client will have normal bowel and bladder function.	Obtain a baseline assessment of the client's bowel and bladder elimination patterns. Insert and anchor foley catheter and give enema as ordered. Monitor intake and output and bowel elimination.
▶ Nutrition, altered, less than body requirements, related to presence of nausea, loss of appetite, chemotherapy side effects, or dietary modifications associated with therapy.	The client will have adequate dietary intake to maintain body weight and metabolic needs.	Assess the client's dietary intake prior to therapy, including her likes and dislikes. Provide a pleasant environment for meal times. Provide nutritionally balanced meals of client's likes.

(continued)

Nursing Diagnoses, Postoperative	Goals, Postoperative	Nursing Interventions, Postoperative
▶ *Skin integrity, impaired, related to surgical interventions, radiation, and chemotherapy side effects.*	The client will recover skin integrity.	Provide the client with proper skin care instructions during and after radiation therapy that may include avoiding soaps, creams, powder, deodorants, soaps, and other substances on the skin around the incision that may irritate the skin, not washing off the radiation markings, and avoiding tight clothing around the area.
		Teach client to look for signs of reactions to radiation therapy, such as tenderness, pink color (like a sunburn), delayed wound healing, and itching.
		Perform daily cleansing of the incisional area with water only.
		If the client is on complete bed rest due to radium implant therapy, provide a complete bedbath as well as with morning and bedtime skin care.
		Organize time near the client's bedside to brief periods to avoid overexposure to radiation.
		Wear rubber gloves when disposing of soiled materials.
		Put soiled dressings in a biohazard waste container.
▶ *Self-esteem disturbance, related to radiation and chemotherapy side effects. Psychological response to changes in appearance, and declining general health with metastatic disease.*	The client will maintain self-esteem.	Encourage client to verbalize her feelings regarding her femininity as reproductive organs and childbearing capability may be strongly linked to the female role and self-esteem of some clients.
		Encourage the client to seek psychological counseling, if recommended by the physician.
▶ *Noncompliance with the medical plan of treatment related to physical and emotional effects of cancer.*	The client will be compliant with the medical plan of treatment.	Provide a clear, thorough explanation of the medical plan for follow-up care prior to the client's dismissal from the hospital.
		Determine if arrangements have been made for the client's financial needs, transportation, equipment and supplies, home health caregivers, and home maintenance activities.
		Ideally, begin discharge planning on the client's admission to effectively coordinate the multiple aspects of follow-up care.
		Obtain information about the client's home environment and support system.
		Obtain referrals to community support groups and other resources.
▶ *Sexual dysfunction, related to physical or emotional obstacles to intercourse.*	The client will resume a fulfilling sexual relationship with her partner.	Be sensitive to client cues related to her sexuality concerns.
		Listen to what the client says and does not say, but implies.
		Instruct the client not to resume sexual activity until after she has seen the physician for her postoperative check-up.
		Advise client that intercourse may be uncomfortable initially following a hysterectomy or other vaginal procedures until the tissues have completely healed, about 4 to 6 weeks.

Nursing Diagnoses, Postoperative	Goals, Postoperative	Nursing Interventions, Postoperative
		Advise the client whose ovaries have been removed and who is not taking hormone replacement that she may experience vaginal dryness.
		Recommend use of water soluble lubricants placed in the vagina prior to sexual activity.
		Encourage the client to openly discuss her feelings with her partner.
		Help the client set realistic goals during her recovery period to facilitate a new outlook on her relationship.
▶ *Pain, related to surgical procedures and incisions.*	The client will have pain controlled at a level which allows the client to continue to function in her activities of daily living.	Keep the client as comfortable as possible without significant sedation.
		Administer pain medications as ordered by physician.
▶ *Urinary elimination, altered, incontinence, bowel or constipation, related to the proximity of surgical site to bowel and bladder, spread of cancer to adjacent structures, manipulation of organs during surgery, administration of narcotic analgesics, lack of activity, and changes in dietary intake.*	The client will have adequate bowel and bladder function during the postoperative period.	Explain dietary modifications designed to reduce residue. The diet should be limited in dairy products, raw fruits, grains, and vegetables. Meats must be well cooked and possibly ground.
		If the client is not receiving radium implant therapy, weigh her daily on the same scale at the same time of the day.
		Review the client's normal elimination patterns from the baseline assessment data to help identify early changes in bowel or bladder elimination.
		Forewarn the client of radiation enteritis and cystitis, common tissue responses to radiation therapy, and instruct her to report them, such as diarrhea, cramping, frequency, urgency, and dysuria.
		Assess bowel sounds and abdominal distention at least every four to eight hours.
		Carefully monitor the client's urinary pattern and maintain an accurate intake and output record.
		Observe urine and stool for color, consistency, amount, and the presence of blood.
		Monitor the client for other gastrointestinal problems, such as nausea, vomiting, and **tenesmus** (involuntary, painful straining).
▶ *Fluid volume deficit, high risk for, related to decreased oral intake, and blood loss during surgery.*	The client will maintain fluid balance.	Be alert for the possibility of fluid and electrolyte imbalances due to excessive fluid losses and resulting metabolic alkalosis.
		Monitor intake and output.
		Monitor laboratory reports for electrolyte levels.
▶ *Infection, high risk for, related to invasive procedures.*	The client will be free of signs and symptoms of infection.	Assess client's status and monitor vital signs when she returns to room.
		Compare the postoperative vital signs with those obtained prior to surgery.
		Perform assessments every hour. When the client is stable, assessment is performed every four hours for the first twenty-four to forty-eight hours.

(continued)

Nursing Diagnoses, Postoperative	Goals, Postoperative	Nursing Interventions, Postoperative
		Be alert for even subtle changes in the client's condition.
		Assess the surgical site every four to eight hours. The incision should remain clean, dry, intact, and well approximated.
		When the dressing is removed, inspect the incision for redness, tenderness, edema, warmth, and drainage.
► Breathing pattern, ineffective, related to ineffective cough and deep breathing exercises after surgery and general anesthesia.	The client will demonstrate normal respiratory effort, quality, and rate and be free of adventitious breath sounds.	Encourage coughing and deep breathing every two hours. Assess breath sounds every four hours. Encourage use of incentive spirometer.
► Physical mobility, impaired, related to intracavity radiation.	The client will not develop deep vein thrombosis.	Accurately measure the client's legs to assure the proper fit of the hose. Apply thigh-high antiembolitic stockings (TEDS) as ordered. Assist client to ambulate when allowed.

► Evaluation

Each goal must be evaluated to determine how it has been met by the client.

▲ ▲

Teaching Tip

Some of the pain associated with reproductive cancers may be alleviated by removal of the tumor, however, if the cancer is in an advanced stage, or if it has metastasized to other organs, the client may continue to experience, severe, chronic pain. The majority of women in later stages of cancer find pain management to be a problem. Narcotic agents are frequently used to manage the pain associated with cancer. Addiction, a craving for a drug in the absence of pain, is not a common occurrence with clients who have cancer. Due to the chronic, severe nature of the pain, clients may need more frequent doses of medication or higher doses to maintain the same level of control. This is referred to as "tolerance" to the narcotic's effects.

Sometimes two or three different medications are necessary to achieve this goal. Intravenous medications are often given by a PCA pump with continuous low dose narcotics. This method seems more effective for the client than regular IV bolus doses every four hours. IV medications may also be given slow IV push (an RN procedure), orally in tablets or liquids, intramuscular injections, or by trans-

dermal patches (Duragesic). A liquid mixture of syrup, cocaine, morphine, alcohol, flavoring, and water called "Brompton's mixture or elixir" may be ordered. The client may drink up to 20 cc every three to four hours for pain relief. Most of these methods of narcotic administration are equally effective and may be used in the home care or hospice setting. Other types of medication that may be given include tranquilizers, antiemetics, and laxatives.

► ENDOMETRIOSIS

Endometriosis is the presence of endometrial tissue, the normal lining of the uterus, in the pelvic cavity. The disease occurs more frequently in women thirty years and older and tends to be familial. Personality types or characteristics occasionally associated with the disease include overachievers, perfectionists, and women with higher than average IQs. It predominantly affects Caucasian females who have not given birth and is more common among the higher socioeconomic population. Endometriosis has been called the "career woman's disorder," because it is often diagnosed in the late twenties or thirties when the working woman makes plans for childbearing.

The endometrial tissue implants itself on other pelvic structures (Figure 31-11). Two of the most common areas for endometrial implants are the pouch of Douglas and the ovaries. The tissue implants respond to the monthly hormonal changes in the same way as the endometrial tissue inside the uterus does. Bleeding of the implants during the menses results in the formation of adhesions and scar tissue. The endometriosis appears as brownish/black "powder burns" or larger lesions. If the endometriosis becomes encapsulated in an ovarian cyst it is called a "chocolate cyst." The disease appears to be progressive and has a tendency to be recurrent. Some women with minimal endometriosis experience severe monthly symptoms, such as lower backache, painful intercourse, a feeling of heaviness on the pelvis, and spotting. Other women have a more extensive disease but have minimal symptoms. Thus, the amount of endometriosis present may or may not indicate the severity of the symptoms experienced by the client. Endometriosis is one cause of female infertility. Pregnancy inhibits the growth and

bleeding of the endometrial implants because ovulation is suppressed. Often it is difficult for the client to become pregnant due to the amount of scar tissue and adhesions around the pelvic organs, ligaments, and fallopian tubes.

▶ Medical/Surgical Management

▶ Medical

Endometriosis may be tentatively diagnosed by palpation of endometrial implants within the pelvis, but this method is inconclusive for treatment. Further investigation is required to confirm the diagnosis. Laparoscopy, performed under general anesthesia, is the best method of diagnosis by direct visualization of the pelvic structures. Consideration for treatment is dependent upon the client's age and desire for future childbearing. Sometimes pregnancy relieves the symptoms even after delivery. The older multigravida who is experiencing severe, debilitating symptoms that

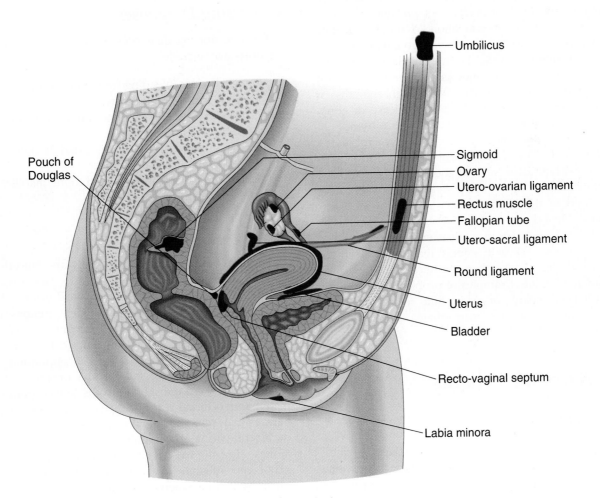

FIGURE 31-11 Common sites of endometriosis.

affect her lifestyle and normal functions, role or activity, may desire a hysterectomy.

▶ Surgical

If the lesions are large and/or extensive, a laparotomy may be performed for adequate removal. However, if the implants are small and scattered, cauterization or laser vaporization may be most desirable. Lysis of pelvic adhesion would be done at the same time.

▶ Pharmacological

The goals of pharmacological therapy are to suppress ovulation, reduce symptoms, and cause the implants to shrink. Medications used in the treatment of endometriosis must effectively suppress the monthly a hypothalamic-pituitary-ovarian hormonal stimulation of ovulation. Some medications act on the body as "pseudopregnancy" agents that produce anovulation, breast tenderness, nausea, weight gain, and hirsutism. Other hormonal therapies cause a temporary medically induced menopause state. Medications like oral contraceptives are administered cyclically or continuously. Oral contraceptives prevent ovulation, and thus inhibit menstruation. Nafarelin acetate (Synarel) is a nasally administered gonadatropin analog that inhibits cyclic hormone release. Danazol (Danocrine) is another androgen hormone that must be taken continuously for six to eight months or longer. This medication inhibits the release of gonadotropin. The resulting **amenorrhea** (absence of menstrual period) will suppress the growth of the endometrial tissue. This medication is used in moderate to severe case of endometriosis. Occasionally, Danocrine is given following surgical removal or cauterization of the endometriosis to relieve symptoms from residual disease.

All medications used to treat endometriosis cause mild to moderate side effects that may affect the client's desire to take them or her compliance with continuous usage. Examples of problems that may be experienced include oily skin, fluid retention, weight gain, acne, hot flashes, metrorrhagia, mastalgia, and depression.

▶ Nursing Process

Assessment

Subjective Data The data to be gathered include complaints of pelvic pain, which is especially worse around the time of her menstrual period. She may also voice concerns about pelvic discomfort with intercourse. The nurse should be alert to what the client

says as well as what is left unsaid. Dyspareunia may result in marital tension if the client avoids sexual intimacy to reduce her pain. Equally important to the client's pain is the occurrence of prolonged, excessive menstrual periods. The client may report that she is experiencing periods that are getting closer and closer together. Another sign, although not as significant, is pain with defecation during the menstrual period. In obtaining a client history, the nurse should note the onset of menses, regularity of cycles and any changes the client has noted in the frequency, discomfort, duration, and amount of menstrual flow. It is important to note the onset of the client's symptoms in relationship to the menstrual cycle, the severity as reported by the client, any alterations in lifestyle related to the pain or other symptoms, and the client's future plans for childbearing.

Objective Data The nurse's role in caring for this client is usually focused on collecting subjective data from the client interview. The nurse may assist the physician during actual procedures such as palpating for the presence of irregular lesions in the pelvis during the bi-manual exam.

▶ Nursing Diagnoses

Possible nursing diagnoses for a client with endometriosis may include:

1. Pain, related to bleeding from endometrial implants in the pelvic cavity.
2. Anxiety, related to treatment options, possible side effects, and infertility.
3. Sexuality patterns, altered, or sexual dysfunction, related to painful intercourse.
4. Self-esteem disturbance, related to the inability to conceive.

▶ VAGINITIS

Several common types of vaginitis are caused by bacteria, protozoa, virus, and yeast. The vaginal mucosa is normally protected by an acid mantle. The acidic pH (less than 5.0) environment inhibits the growth of many pathogenic microorganisms. Due to the proximity of the vaginal opening to the external environment, microorganisms have an opportunity to invade the reproductive tract. Some organisms that cause vaginitis are transmitted to the female from the male partner during sexual contact. Natural protective barriers may vary with the fluctuating hormonal levels during the woman's monthly cycle because the hormones affect the vaginal pH. At ovulation, the vaginal pH becomes slightly less acidic due to the high level of estrogen. Periods when the woman's system has lower estrogen levels, such as immediately following the menses and after menopause, are also times when there is a higher risk for infections because the epithelium is less active, no glycogen is present, and the pH may reach as high as 7.0.

Occasionally, superinfections may develop during or after a course of antibiotic therapy to treat another problem. These usually result from a decrease in the presence of the normal flora along with pathogens, which allows an overgrowth of yeast (fungus). *Candida albicans* is present on the human skin most of the time and is usually harmless, but if conditions permit, the yeast cells will flourish due to changes in the skin's acid mantle or a compromised immune system. Fungal infections will produce internal and external symptoms. Women with multiple sexual partners place themselves at a greater risk of sexually transmitted infections.

The physician or NP should determine the specific causative agent before prescribing treatment. Diagnosis is made after performing a vaginal examination and obtaining a sample of the vaginal discharge. When the client contacts the physician or nurse practitioner to report her symptoms of vaginitis, the nurse should instruct her to avoid douching or using tampons prior to being examined. Douching will wash away the discharge needed to be examined and tampons will absorb it.

Common types of vaginitis include candidiasis caused by the fungus *Candida albicans*, trichomoniasis caused by the protozoan *Trichomonas vaginalis*, *Gardnerella vaginalis* (a bacteria) and *Chlamydia trachomatis* (a parasite). Other causes of vaginitis symptoms may include streptococcus, staphylococcus, gonococcus, and herpes simplex II. Usually the symptoms depend upon the causative agent. The client's description of her symptoms along with the examination of the discharge help confirm the diagnosis. Most infections have a characteristic discharge, irritation, with burning and/or itching which may be internal, external or both. The nurse should obtain assessment information from the client regarding the nature of her symptoms, the onset, menstrual history, contraceptive methods, recent or current use of antibiotics or other medications, recent illness, diabetes mellitus, sexual history, pregnancy history, usual hygiene practices like douching, deodorant sprays, bubble baths, wearing panty hose, type of underwear, and use of deodorized tampons or pads.

Predisposing factors for candidiasis, also called monilia, may include obesity, diabetes, pregnancy, oral contraceptives, antibiotics, and frequent douching. Many of these factors alter the pH of the vagina. Symptoms of this yeast infection include a thick, white, cheesy or curd-like discharge with a musty, sweet odor, accompanied by vaginal and/or vulvar itching and irritation. Upon examination. the vaginal mucosa will have patches of white discharge present. If the patches are scraped off, the tissue underneath will appear reddened and may bleed. Externally, the vulva may be reddened and edematous. The client may have scratches from attempting to ease the itching.

The preferred treatment is administered with vaginal applications of antifungal creams or suppositories such as miconazole (Monistat), clotrimazole (Mycelex-G, Gyne-Lotrimin), or nystatin (Mycostatin). The length of treatment is usually seven days. Alternate therapies include douching with white vinegar solution (1 tablespoon/1 pint of water) twice a day for a week. This restores the acid balance of the vagina and washes away the *Candida albicans*. Eating cultured yogurt with active acidophilus or applying the yogurt directly to the labia help restore the normal bacteria and protective mechanisms in the vagina. Instruct the client to insert vaginal creams or suppositories at night for the most effectiveness. The applicator should be washed after each use. The nurse may instruct the client in other ways to decrease the risk of vaginitis such as wearing cotton crotch underwear, avoiding sitting in a wet bathing suit in warm weather for long periods, seeking prompt medical attention at the first signs of infections, and eating an 8 oz container of yogurt daily with active cultures while taking antibiotics.

Trichomonasis is frequently passed from partner to partner during intercourse. A copious green-yellow, foul smelling, frothy vaginal discharge is characteristic of this type of vaginal infection. It may produce itching or external burning and irritation. Metronidazole (Flagyl) is taken orally by both partners as a treatment of choice for this infection. Both partners should be instructed to take the medication at the same time to assure that the organisms are killed. This simultaneous treatment is not recommended by the Centers for Disease Control and Prevention unless the infection is recurrent.

Flagyl is normally contraindicated in the first trimester of pregnancy, so obtaining a menstrual history or a pregnancy test may be needed prior to the client starting the medication. It is also essential to inform the client and her partner to avoid any alcohol intake during therapy. Flagyl causes a strong antabuse-like effect. This effect will cause severe nausea and vomiting. Caution the client to read labels on over-the-counter medications being taken concurrently with the Flagyl because many preparations contain alcohol bases. An alternative remedy for treating trichomonas vaginitis is made by brewing a solution of chaparral chamomile with one quart of water and using it as a douche two to three times a week for two weeks (Long & Glazer, 1993).

The nurse should instruct the client and her partner to abstain from intercourse during therapy and to finish all of the medication.

Gardnerella vaginalis, often produces a gray-white vaginal discharge with a strong fishy odor or the woman may remain asymptomatic. If itching or burning are present, it may suggest another microorganism. For the treatment of *Gardnerella,* and other bacterial vaginitis, the physician may order Flagyl or an oral antibiotic like tetracycline hydrochloride (Achromycin) or ampicillin (Omnipen). Sulfa-based creams like Sultrin, Triple Sulfa, and AVC may be used vaginally in conjunction with the oral medications once or twice a day for 6 to 14 days to completely treat this type of infection. Bacterial vaginitis has been associated with the onset of preterm labor in as many as 40 percent of women who experience preterm labor.

Chlamydial vaginitis infections are often asymptomatic, but have been associated with infertility problems. A culture of vaginal secretions is necessary to specifically identify the organism. The treatment is usually oral antibiotics for at least seven days. A repeat culture is recommended following treatment to assure that the parasites have been eradicated.

Postmenopausal vaginitis (atrophic) is caused by a decreased level of estrogen in the vaginal tissue. The client may complain of painful intercourse (dyspareunia), itching, burning, or irritation. Estrogen replacement therapy often relieves the symptoms of this type of vaginitis. The medication may be administered orally, vaginally, or by transdermal patch.

▶ *Nursing Diagnoses*

Possible diagnoses for a client with vaginitis, regardless of the etiology, may include:

1. Knowledge deficit, related to the origin of the infection, prevention, and treatment options.
2. Tissue integrity, impaired, related to the presence of vaginal discharge, itching, or irritation.
3. Sexual dysfunction, related to discomfort during intercourse or fear of transmitting the infection to the sexual partner.
4. Skin integrity, high risk for, impaired, related to internal and external irritation from discharge and itching.

▶ MENSTRUAL DISORDERS

Abnormalities of menstruation may be associated with an increase or decrease in secretion from any of the following glands: hypothalamus, pituitary, ovaries, adrenals, and thyroid. The normal menstrual pattern is controlled by a series of hormonal negative feedback mechanisms. The average menstrual cycle occurs every twenty-eight to thirty days when the endometrial lining of the uterus sloughs off in the absence of a fertilized ovum.

▶ DYSMENORRHEA

Painful menstruation, dysmenorrhea, also called "menstrual cramps," is more common in nulliparous women and in women who are not having intercourse. The exact pathophysiology is unknown but it may be related to endocrine secretions like prostaglandin F which causes uterine cramping, irritation, and contractions. Other causes may include uterine anatomical anomalies, chronic illness, and/or psychological factors.

The primary symptom is pelvic pain before or at the onset of the menses that may be due to spasms of the uterus, narrowing of the cervical canal, emotional factors, endometriosis, pelvic inflammatory disease, or the presence of an intrauterine contraceptive device (IUD). The client may also state that the pain radiates across the lower back and downward into the legs.

The condition is diagnosed based upon the client's complaints and description of the timing of the onset of symptoms. The nurse should obtain information pertaining to the menstrual history and general health status of the client. A thorough physical exam will be performed by the physician which includes a bimanual exam to rule out other possible causes. A pelvic ultrasound may be ordered.

One effective preventive intervention may begin before the young woman begins menstruation. A positive parental attitude toward the onset of menstruation can aid the young girl in adjusting to the physiological and psychological changes that occur with puberty.

Certain medications have been used over the last ten to fifteen years that are effective in the treatment of dysmenorrhea. Analgesics like acetaminophen and ibuprofen are useful in relieving pain. Oral contraceptives have been used for some clients to inhibit ovulation which appears to be an associated cause. Prostaglandin inhibitors like naproxen sodium (Anaprox) and mefenamic acid (Ponstel) are useful if taken at the earliest sign of discomfort.

▶ AMENORRHEA

Amenorrhea, the absence of menstruation, may be primary or secondary. Primary amenorrhea is defined as the absence of menstruation by the age of seventeen. Possible causes are related to anatomical or genetic abnormalities (Turner's syndrome). The treatment is dependent upon the cause. Secondary amenorrhea is defined as the absence of menstruation after six months of regular periods, or after twelve months of irregular periods. Several etiologies are possible for secondary amenorrhea which include anatomical abnormalities, nutritional deficits (anorexia nervosa), excessive exercise with significant decreases in body fat, endocrine dysfunction, emotional disturbances, side effects of medications, pregnancy, and lactation.

This condition is diagnosed based upon the length of absence of menstruation. A complete physical examination should be performed including a pelvic examination to rule out many factors discussed earlier. A progesterone challenge test may be administered in an attempt to force the body to respond hormonally. Medroxyprogesterone acetate (Depo-Provera) is taken orally for five to ten days as ordered by the physician. When the medication is finished, the client should have a menstrual period within three to four days. A menstrual flow after taking the medication may be an indicator that the client has not been ovulating. If no bleeding occurs, further investigation may be necessary to uncover other causes. Hormonal imbalances, microscopic pituitary tumors, and nutritional deficits are common etiologies of secondary amenorrhea. A microscopic pituitary tumor will cause an elevation in the prolactin level and result in anovulation and amenorrhea. A serum prolactin level should be ordered, especially if the client has noticed any breast discharge. Normal prolactin level should not exceed 15 ng/dL. With pituitary tumors, the prolactin level may exceed 400 ng/dL. In these cases, the drug of choice is bromocriptine mesylate (Parlodel) which had been used in the past to suppress lactation in mothers who did not breast-feed their newborns. A careful examination of the client is needed prior to administration of Parlodel, due to an increased potential for cardiovascular problems recently associated with this medication. Because of this risk, the medication is no longer used for the postpartum client to suppress milk production. Other medical or surgical interventions will be dependent upon the source of the amenorrhea.

Other menstrual disorders include menorrhagia and metrorrhagia. Both types of abnormal bleeding can be problematic for the client and require further investigation. **Polymenorrhea** is a term used to describe short menstrual cycles of less than twenty-one days in length. The causes are similar to those of the other menstrual disorders. **Oligomenorrhea** is a diminished menstrual flow, but it is not classified as amenorrhea. It may be associated with low dose oral contraceptives that inhibit the growth of the endometrium and result in minimal tissue sloughing at the end of the cycle. Other causes may be metabolic or hormonal. Again, treatment is specific to the etiology.

For conditions associated with heavy bleeding or bleeding between periods, a dilatation and curettage (D & C) may be performed. In this case, the procedure may be diagnostic and therapeutic. Tissue removed from the uterus will be examined microscopically and

histologically to evaluate its stage in the menstrual cycle. A hysterectomy may be indicated if abnormalities are discovered or if the bleeding is so excessive that the client is significantly compromised. The client may require a blood transfusion to correct low hemoglobin and hematocrit levels prior to any other procedures. Supplemental iron generally is prescribed by the physician to also help correct the deficiency.

▶ Nursing Process

Assessment

Subjective data The nurse should ask the client about the onset of the bleeding and its relationship to the timing of her normal menstruation, the color of the bleeding, amount, pads saturated, presence of clots, and presence of pain with the bleeding. A history of current medications, contraception, and the possibility of pregnancy are additional assessment data. Any preexisting health problems that could affect bleeding and clotting times, as well as life stressors should be explored by the nurse during the data gathering process.

Objective Data Assess vital signs, may have hypertension and tachycardia. Monitor laboratory test results.

▶ Nursing Diagnoses

Possible diagnoses for a client with any of the menstrual disorders discussed in this section may include:

1. Pain related to uterine cramping or heavy bleeding.
2. Cardiac output, decreased, related to excessive blood loss.
3. Fatigue related to decreased hemoglobin and hematocrit levels.
4. Body image disturbance related to the absence of menstruation.

▶ PREMENSTRUAL SYNDROME (PMS)

One-third to one-half of women between twenty and fifty years old experience some of the symptoms known as premenstrual syndrome (PMS). Once, this condition was thought by many physicians to be a psychological problem of women; however, recent research has supported data that there are many physiologic as well as psychological factors involved. PMS often occurs during the secretory phase of the menstrual cycle following ovulation. Risk factors associated with the development of PMS include age (over thirty), multiple life stressors, inappropriate nutritional status, a previous reaction to or side effects from oral contraceptives, a sedentary lifestyle, marital status, a history of preeclampsia in pregnancy, and multiparity.

Over 150 symptoms have been reported that have been related to PMS. These include: weight gain, bloating, irritability, edema, headache, mood swings, inability to concentrate, food cravings, acne, and numerous others. For many women, the PMS symptoms are merely a monthly nuisance, but for others, the symptoms are so incapacitating that they cannot function in their normal roles or responsibilities. The onset of symptoms is usually seven to ten days before the menstrual period starts and ends after the menstrual flow begins.

Research has correlated hormonal imbalances of estrogen, progesterone, ACTH, and androgens with the symptoms of PMS. The presence of prostaglandin F in the tissue may also be a cause of some of the symptoms. Prostaglandins are associated with many inflammatory responses in the tissues.

The first step in identifying PMS is a physical examination to rule out possible other disorders of the reproductive system. The client may be asked to keep a monthly calendar of symptoms to see if there are patterns in severity, type, or onset. Blood tests may be ordered to assess estrogen and progesterone levels, as well as checking the glucose level. Low blood glucose level has been associated with irritability that sometimes accompanies PMS symptoms. The client should receive counseling, if needed, to facilitate coping with life stressors that may be complicating the complexity of the PMS symptoms.

▶ Medical/Surgical Management

▶ Pharmacological

Some physicians and NP recommend medication like acetaminophen (Tylenol), naproxen (Naprosyn), mefenamic acid (Ponstel), and ibuprofen (Advil) for the relief of minor discomforts of PMS. These are most useful for relieving dysmenorrhea. Tranquilizers and antidepressants have not proven to be effective for short term use in PMS, however, in severe cases, they may be a last resort. Several PMS symptoms are thought to be related to a low progesterone level. For some clients, the use of progesterone suppositories or oral progesterone to supplement their own production during the secretory phase of the menstrual cycle has been useful.

▶ Activity

As mentioned previously, a sedentary lifestyle and lack of exercise are associated with PMS. A regular exercise routine, coupled with the use of stress management techniques like deep breathing and relaxation exercises help the client cope with the increased sense of anxiety or irritability that may accompany the PMS. Meditation, positive affirmation, visualization, and imagery may be helpful. Other alternative therapies may include acupressure, neurolymphatic or neurovascular massage, and yoga.

▶ Diet

A thorough diet history should be included in the assessment data collected. Certain nutritional deficits and/or cravings have been linked to the worsening of PMS. Items such as sugar, salt, and caffeine and chocolate are in this category. Many studies have shown that limiting these substances may be helpful. Caffeinated beverages may increase anxiety, irritability, and deplete vitamin B stores in the body. Dairy products interfere with the absorption of magnesium which helps stabilize the mood. Chocolates have been related to increased sugar cravings, mood swings, fluid retention, and increased vitamin B demands. Oranges and other fruits or vegetables that are highly acidic may worsen PMS. Foods that are recommended are whole grains, nuts, pasta, legumes, root vegetables, fruits like apples and pears, poultry, and seafood. A good vitamin supplement rich in vitamin B-complex, calcium, magnesium, and zinc should be taken daily, especially during the PMS period. Herbal tea formulas have shown some promise as alternative methods of relieving PMS. One is a mixture of burdock root, ginger root, and sarsaparilla, and another is a mixture of dandelion, alfalfa, and burdock root.

▶ Nursing Process

Assessment

Subjective Data The client should describe her symptoms and the impact on her lifestyle. Many times, clients will seek medical attention for their PMS symptoms when the emotional impact has caused friction in the home, marriage, work, or family environment. Symptoms described may include weight gain, bloating, irritability, headache, mood swings, inability to concentrate, or food cravings. Ask client to relate symptoms to time of menstrual cycle.

Objective Data Assess for weight gain and edema. Review results of all laboratory tests ordered.

▼ ▼

Possible nursing diagnoses for a client with premenstrual syndrome may include:

Nursing Diagnoses	Goals	Nursing Interventions
▶ Fluid volume excess, related to hormonal imbalance and increased sodium or sugar intake.	The client's intake and output will be balanced and edema will be decreased.	Advise client that a certain amount of fluid retention is normal prior to the onset of the menstrual period and cannot be avoided, but by limiting sodium and sugar intake, she may be able to influence the amount of fluid retained.
▶ Coping, individual, ineffective, related to client perceptions of stressors during PMS episodes.	The client will demonstrate effective coping skills during PMS episodes.	Encourage client to practice relaxation techniques such as deep breathing or taking a short nap. Advise client to seek counseling to help cope with PMS, if appropriate.
▶ Health seeking behaviors, related to finding methods to cope with symptoms of PMS.	The client will develop effective health promotion skills to increase coping with PMS symptoms or to decrease symptom severity or frequency.	Teach client how to keep a monthly PMS calendar of events. Discuss prescribed medications with the client including the dosage, expected effects, and side effects. Discuss relationship of foods to PMS.
▶ Knowledge deficit, related to causes and self-management of PMS symptoms.	The client will verbalize her understanding of the cause and treatment of PMS and her role in symptom management.	Assess client's lifestyle, nutritional, and stress factors and discuss with client their effects on her risks for PMS.
▶ Nutrition, altered, potential for more than body requirement related to cravings for sugar, sodium, and caffeine.	The client will modify her dietary intake of sugar, sodium, and caffeine to decrease PMS symptoms.	Advise the client in ways to modify her dietary intake and limit foods and beverages associated with PMS.
▶ Self-esteem, situational, low, related to client's perception of appearance and relationship problems during PMS episodes.	The client's self-esteem will be maintained.	Encourage client to discuss her feelings about herself during PMS. Remind client that she is not alone in her condition, but that millions of other women experience similar symptoms as this may help the client accept that she is not mentally ill, but having a temporary problem associated with hormone imbalance.

▶ Evaluation

Each goal must be evaluated to determine how it has been met by the client.

▲ ▲

▶ CYSTOCELE, URETHROCELE, RECTOCELE, PROLAPSED UTERUS

These conditions are often associated with relaxation of the pelvic muscles that support the uterus, bladder, and rectum. A **cystocele** is a downward displacement of the bladder into the anterior wall of the vagina (Figure 31-12A). A **urethrocele** is a downward displacement of the urethra into the vagina and a **rectocele** is an anterior displacement of the rectum into the posterior vaginal wall (Figure 31-12B&C). Prolapsed uterus is a downward displacement of the uterus into the vagina (Figure 31-12D). Possible causes for the four conditions are multiple pregnancies, third or fourth degree perineal lacerations with childbirth, and weakening of the pelvic muscles as an aging process.

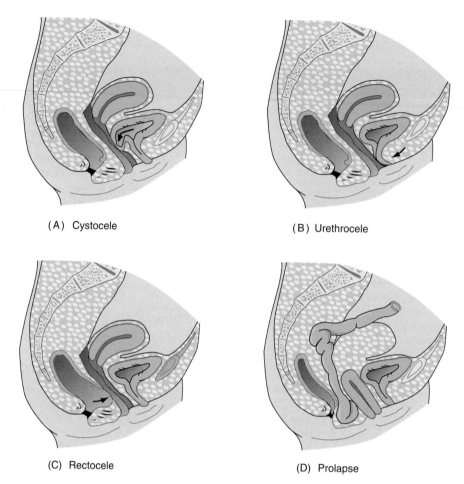

(A) Cystocele   (B) Urethrocele

(C) Rectocele   (D) Prolapse

FIGURE 31-12 **(A)** Cystocele, **(B)** urethrocele, **(C)** rectocele, **(D)** uterine prolapse.

A prolapsed uterus is often accompanied by a cystocele and/or rectocele. Variations in the severity of uterine prolapse are described as first, second, and third degree. With a first degree prolapse, the cervix is visible at the vaginal introitus or opening without straining. The cervix extends beyond the vaginal opening to the perineum with a second degree prolapse, and with a third degree, the uterus protrudes outside of the vagina. This severe condition is called *procidentia uteri*. Medical and surgical interventions for the treatment of each of these conditions are focused on relief of the discomforts and restoration of the structure and function of the pelvic organs.

▶ *Medical/Surgical Management*

▶ *Surgical*

Surgery for a prolapsed uterus may require a hysterectomy. If the prolapse is accompanied by a cystocele or rectocele, an A & P repair may also be performed.

An A & P repair (anterior/posterior colporrhaphy) may be performed vaginally to replace the bladder, urethra, or rectum in the correct anatomical position. Another procedure, the Marshall-Marchette-Krantz, may be performed to attach the bladder to the inferior surface of the pubic bone. Postoperatively, the client may be sent home with an indwelling Foley catheter due to the potential inability to void. This is a common postoperative situation that usually resolves itself spontaneously within one to two weeks after discharge.

▶ *Activity*

Clients should be taught Kegel exercises before childbearing. These exercises are performed by tightening and releasing the perineal muscles. An important muscle group called the "levators," help lift and support the organs inside the pelvis. When giving the initial instructions on Kegel performance, the nurse may suggest that the client practice them when she has a full bladder. If she can successfully start and stop the flow of urine from the bladder, she is identifying and using the correct muscle groups. The muscles should be tightened and held for five to ten seconds and then released slowly. The exercises should be repeated at least ten times. Kegel exercises can be practiced anytime and anyplace. A secondary benefit of increasing the strength and contractility of the pelvic and perineal muscles is seen in an improvement in pelvic sensations for both partners during intercourse.

▶ Assistive Devices

The pessary is a small molded plastic or rubber apparatus that fits into the vagina behind the pubic bone and in front of the rectum. Its function is to provide an artificial or mechanical support for the uterus. Pessaries are not uncomfortable and should not be felt by the client if it has been properly fitted and is in the correct position. The client should be taught how to insert and remove the pessary so it can be cleaned. The pessary may be washed in warm, soapy water once every one to two weeks. Prolonged use of a mechanical device like a pessary may result in vaginal necrosis and ulceration. Periodic examination by a health care professional is recommended, especially with weight gain or loss of greater than 10 to 15 pounds.

▶ Nursing Process

Assessment

Subjective Data The client often describes stress incontinence which is a loss of urine when she coughs, sneezes, laughs, or jumps. She may describe it as "a leaky bladder." She may notice that her panties are damp or that she dribbles urine. Many women complain of frequent urination in small quantities with a feeling of urgency but there is no burning or dysuria. The client may notice that she has been experiencing more constipation or a sense of bearing down pressure in the pelvis with a rectocele. Many of these symptoms will decrease or subside completely when she is lying down. The nurse should obtain information about the client's childbearing history, onset of current symptoms, and any other pertinent gynecological data.

Objective Data This includes the visualization of a bulging of the bladder, urethra, or rectum into the vagina. The bulging increases when the client is asked to bear down. Assess results of urinalysis.

▼ ▼

Possible nursing diagnoses for a client experiencing symptoms of uterine prolapse, cystocele, rectocele, or urethrocele may include:

Nursing Diagnoses	Goals	Nursing Interventions
▶ Incontinence, stress, related to relaxation of the pelvic muscles.	The client will not have stress incontinence.	Teach the client Kegel exercises and encourage routine practice daily. Encourage client to empty bladder frequently.
▶ Constipation, related to relaxation of the anterior rectal wall into the vagina and decreased function.	The client will not have constipation.	Encourage client to defecate at same time each day. Encourage client to eat high fiber foods.
▶ Knowledge deficit, related to the cause of symptoms and treatment.	The client will understand the causes of her condition and treatment.	Discuss procedure with client preoperatively and encourage client to discuss her concerns. Describe to client possible causes of her condition.
▶ Pain, chronic, related to fatigue and bearing down sensation from displacement of the pelvic structures and organs.	The client will have relief from pelvic pressure and discomfort.	Administer pain medication as ordered. Offer the client pain medication prior to removing the vaginal packing postoperatively.
▶ Infection, high risk for, related to exposure of internal tissues to external environmental factors.	The client will be free of signs and symptoms of infection.	Monitor the client's vital signs. Encourage client to practice proper personal hygiene and wear clean undergarments daily.

(continued)

Nursing Diagnoses	Goals	Nursing Interventions
▶ *Sexual dysfunction, related to discomforts with intercourse.*	The client will have a fulfilling sexual relationship without discomfort.	Be sensitive to client cues related to her sexual concerns.
		Encourage the client to openly discuss her feelings with her partner.
		Help the client set realistic goals during her recovery period to facilitate a new outlook on her relationship.
▶ *Anxiety, related to the potential for surgical correction of pelvic muscle relaxation.*	The client will have decreased anxiety related to surgery and hospitalization.	Encourage the client to verbalize her fears regarding surgery and pessary use.
		Describe what client should expect after surgery.

▶ Evaluation

Each goal must be evaluated to determine how it has been met by the client.

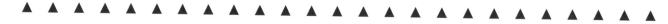

▶ COMPLICATIONS OF MENOPAUSE

Menopause or climacteric is the cessation of menstruation. It may occur as a natural hormonal decline or it may be surgically induced by removal of the uterus and ovaries. Some people may think of menopause as the "change of life." Many women will begin to experience signs and symptoms of approaching menopause around fifty years of age, however, for some it is earlier, and for others later. The range is from forty-nine to fifty-five years old. Menstrual cycles become further apart and the flow decreases. The onset is usually gradual and may take over a year before the woman has completely ceased menstruation. Reproductive capability is also lost with menopause. For some women this is a sad time perceived as the loss of womanhood, while for others it is a welcome relief from monthly blood loss.

The decreasing level of ovarian hormone production affects women in a variety of ways, more than just the end of menstruation. There may be a relaxation of the pelvic support structures, loss of skin turgor and elasticity, thinning of the hair on the head, axilla, and pubic regions. Other signs of decreasing hormones (estrogen and progesterone) are vaginal dryness, thinning of the vaginal mucosa, weight gain, dry skin, and stress incontinence. The estrogen level plays an important protective role in maintaining an adequate calcium balance in the bones, and preventing coronary artery disease. Calcium is important to bone strength and without it, the bones become brittle, and there is an increased risk of fractures and osteoporosis. The femur and spine are areas of vulnerability. A baseline bone density study may be recommended prior to menopause.

Some women experience psychological responses to menopause such as mild to moderate depression, nervousness, and insomnia. Consultation with a psychologist, minister, or counselor may be useful in facilitating the transition through this period for some women.

Women may also experience mild to moderate periods of profuse perspiration called "hot flashes." These usually move from the waist upward. They are caused by the decreased estrogen level and its effect on the hypothalamus. The sensation may last from a few seconds to two to three minutes. It appears that many different things can trigger a hot flash—from drinking hot beverages, to spicy foods, smoking, caffeine, and alcohol, or emotional swings, to red wine, chocolate, and aged cheese. The last three substances contain tyramine, an amino acid, that can trigger a release of norepinephrine and reset the body's thermostat.

▶ Medical/Surgical Management

▶ Pharmacological

For some women, estrogen replacement therapy is recommended, especially if they are experiencing moderately uncomfortable symptoms. Estrogen replacement therapy (ERT) may help decrease some symptoms like the insomnia, hot flashes, mood swings, and lack of concentration. Another positive benefit of taking estrogen is its protective nature against osteoporosis and cardiovascular disease. Estrogen elevates the high density lipoproteins (healthy ones) and lowers the low density lipoproteins (unhealthy) in the circulation. Estrogen may be administered orally or as a transdermal patch, or as a vaginal cream. The transdermal patch releases the hormone into the bloodstream percutaneously. This results in a by-pass of the stomach and liver which means less gastrointestinal tract irritation for the client. The patch is a good option of estrogen administration for clients with liver disease. Occasionally, the client may complain of a rash or skin irritation from the patch that is usually related to the adhesive. It is important to teach the client to rotate the application sites of the patch every three to four days. Holding the patch to the open air for ten to fifteen seconds before application may decrease the potential for skin irritation. There may be less protection from the estrogen patch than the client receives from oral estrogen related to the bone and heart problems. Conjugated estrogen

(Premarin), estradiol (Estrace), and estropipate (Ogen) are examples of oral estrogens available. Estrogen creams or water soluble jells like Lubrifax or K-Y, may be used to combat the vaginal dryness and resulting dyspareunia.

Many health care providers are concerned about the possible effects of unopposed estrogen causing endometrial cancer. To alleviate some of this concern, a progesterone supplement may be added to the hormone regimen if the client still has a uterus. Progesterone, along with the estrogen replacement, will cause the woman to have some amount of endometrial sloughing every month, a menstrual period. This prevents the build up of tissue inside the uterus that has the potential to undergo cellular changes or mutation into cancerous cells. Some studies have suggested that a woman should be on ERT for approximately ten to fifteen years after menopause to reach the maximum benefits of the therapy (see Table 31-1).

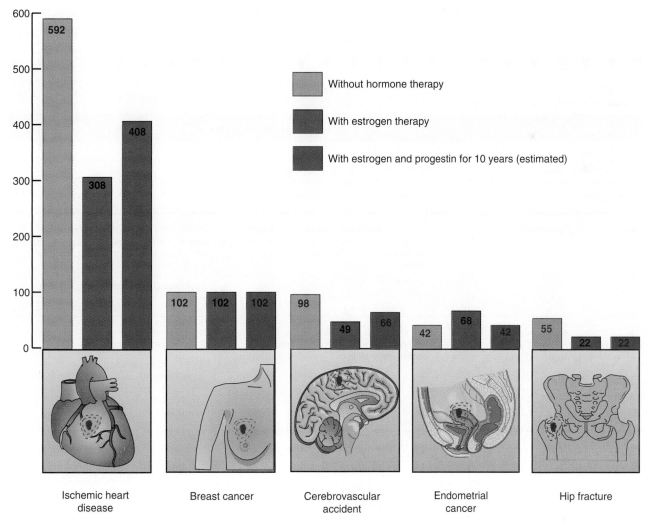

TABLE 31-1 Estrogen Replacement Therapy and Analysis of Morbidity/Mortality Rates (*Adapted from ERT: A statistical analysis,* RN Magazine, *September 1992*).

▶ Diet

The nurse should provide the client with instructions regarding the importance of an adequate daily intake of calcium rich products, such as dairy products. Many low-fat, high-calcium products are available if the client has a concern about weight gain. Calcium supplements may also be taken in a tablet form. The woman should consult her health care provider before adding a calcium supplement because too much calcium increases the risk for other health problems. Herbal teas, vitamin E, magnesium, and primrose oil have been used as alternative methods to alleviate or decrease hot flashes and promote relaxation for some women.

▶ Activity

One important way that the client can decrease the potential for calcium loss from weight bearing bones is to exercise. A planned thirty minute program, performed at least three times per week is adequate to maintain bone density. Exercises such as walking or swimming are excellent. Swimming provides good nonweight bearing activity and promotes active movement of all extremities. Biking is a good exercise to maintain joint mobility in the lower extremities, but it does not require the use of the same muscle groups as walking.

▶ Nursing Process

Assessment

Subjective Data The client may be seen in the physician's office with concerns about decreasing regularity of menstruation or hot flashes. The nurse should obtain information from the client about gynecological and obstetrical history, including menstruation. It is helpful to know when the client began experiencing symptoms in predicting the length of time they may continue.

Objective Data This includes a physical examination and Pap smear. The results of the Pap smear can indicate if there is less estrogen present in the cervical tissue than normal.

▼ ▼

Possible nursing diagnoses for a client experiencing menopausal symptoms may include:

Nursing Diagnoses	Goals	Nursing Interventions
▶ Health-seeking behaviors, related to perceived physiological and psychological impact of decreased estrogen.	The client will develop effective health promotion skills to increase coping with menopausal symptoms or to decrease symptom severity or frequency.	Encourage the client to continue to see her health care provider for annual Pap smears and breast examinations.
▶ Tissue integrity, impaired, related to vaginal dryness and dry skin.	The client will have skin integrity, vagina will not be dry, and she will continue a satisfactory sexual relationship with her partner.	Advise client to try estrogen creams or water soluble jells like Lubrifax or K-Y, to combat the vaginal dryness and resulting dyspareunia. Encourage client to use body lotion to prevent dry skin.
▶ Thermoregulation, ineffective, related to endocrine imbalance and resulting neurosensations.	The client will have minimal thermal discomfort from symptoms caused by decreasing estrogen.	Encourage client to verbalize her feelings related to physical sensations. Teach the client to avoid certain foods, especially those containing tyramine, an amino acid, that can trigger a release of norepinephrine and reset the body's thermostat.
▶ Incontinence, stress, related to relaxation of the pelvic support structures.	The client will not experience stress incontinence.	Teach client to perform Kegel exercise daily. Encourage client to keep bladder empty.

Nursing Diagnoses	Goals	Nursing Interventions
▶ *Decisional conflict, related to taking supplemental estrogen therapy.*	The client will make informed decison about taking supplemental estrogen.	Discuss the advantages and disadvantages of estrogen replacement therapy with the client.
		Remind the client that if she has a uterus and takes hormonal replacements, she will continue to have monthly menstrual cycles.
▶ *Knowledge deficit, related to factors causing symptoms and methods to prevent or relieve symptoms.*	The client will verbalize an understanding of menopause, the effects of hormones, and treatment options.	Instruct the client in the normalcy of menopause and the reasons for the physiologic changes resulting from decreased ovarian function.
		Explain nutritional requirements for vitamins and calcium that increase with menopause.
		Encourage the client to begin a regular exercise program that includes weight bearing activities such as walking to prevent loss of calcium from the bones.

▶ Evaluation

Each goal must be evaluated to determine how it has been met by the client.

▲ ▲

▶ INFERTILITY

Approximately one is every six couples experiences infertility, the inability to produce offspring. Infertility may be primary or secondary. In primary infertility, the couple have never achieved a pregnancy or have never carried a pregnancy to viability. Secondary infertility involves problems that arise after the couple has had a successful pregnancy. Many factors may be investigated as causes of infertility in both male and female clients. This chapter will focus primarily on the female infertility problems. See Chapter 32 for information on male infertility problems. Forty percent of infertility factors are female related, 40 percent are male related, and 20 percent are a combination of multiple factors that involve both partners. The more factors that are involved, the more difficult the infertility resolution. It has been estimated that about 80 percent of couples without infertility problems should be able to conceive within the first twelve months of unprotected intercourse. The average couple who seeks medical advice for infertility have been trying to conceive for at least that period of time.

The etiology of infertility may be related to anatomical or endocrine problems. The female anatomic or structural abnormalities may include blocked passages through the cervix or fallopian tubes caused by failed development or by past infections, such as PID, or STDs. Uterine and cervical abnormalities may also occur. The cervix may be too narrow or closed and sperm are unable to navigate through the passage. The uterus may have a partial or complete septum inside

that limits the internal cavity space. Immune problems involve the development of antibodies by the woman's system to the male's sperm. These antibodies may be present in the cervical mucus and kill the sperm on contact. Hyposecretion or hypersecretion of FSH, LH, estrogen, or progesterone have been associated with infertility.

A basic infertility workup may be initiated when the client has been unable to conceive after six to twelve months of unprotected intercourse. Many physicians do not see clients for infertility until after the first year of trying for a pregnancy. One simple, noninvasive procedure is the use of a basal body temperature chart. The chart is kept for a minimum of three months and then reviewed for normal ovulatory fluctuations in the basal temperature. During the first half of the menstrual cycle, the body temperature may remain below 98 degrees. At ovulation, there is often a slight decrease in the temperature for a twenty-four hour period. This is the optimal period of fertility. After ovulation, the woman's basal body temperature should go above 98 degrees and remain in that range for a period of fourteen days. The length of the luteal phase (secretory phase) of the cycle following ovulation is a critical factor in some infertility disorders. Variations in the temperature chart may indicate that the client has had an anovulatory cycle or has a shortened luteal phase. Since the fertilized ovum does not implant in the endometrium until 6 to 8 days after conception, the luteal phase is critical to maintain the blood-rich lining long enough for implantation to occur. Low progesterone levels during the luteal phase may result in spontaneous **abortion** (ending a pregnancy before the age of viability) of the fertilized ovum prior to implantation. Blood tests and endometrial biopsies may be done to detect hormone levels and tissue responses during both phases of the menstrual cycle. There is no ideal solution for this infertility problem, except by-passing the cervical mucus with artificial insemination directly into the uterus with the partner's sperm. Laparoscopy may be utilized to discover conditions like endometriosis, adhesions, or scar tissue that potentially immobilize the fimbria or polycystic ovarian disease (Stein-Leventhal syndrome).

▶ *Medical/Surgical Management*

There is no one treatment for infertility problems. The goal of treatment is successful achievement of a pregnancy that is carried to full term and produces a healthy offspring.

▶ *Medical*

Infertility treatment may include artificial insemination with either the partner's sperm or donor sperm. This method is particularly useful if the male partner has a low sperm count, abnormal sperm, or no sperm production. With the procedure, the semen is placed directly into the cervix or uterus with a small flexible catheter and a syringe. If donor sperm is used, it may be frozen from a sperm bank or fresh from a local donor. Sperm banks are located across the United States. They are responsible for screening potential donors, collecting the specimens, preparing the sperm, and verifying that the specimens are free of infectious agents. The nurse's role may involve matching the donor characteristics with those of the couple, ordering the specimens, assuring proper storage of the sperm in a liquid nitrogen tank until it is needed, and preparing it prior to the procedure. The nurse may also assist the physician or NP with the procedure. For AID (artificial insemination by donor) or AIH (artificial insemination by husband), it is essential to follow the client's hormonal cycle to assure that the procedure is performed at or very close to ovulation. If the couple are contemplating artificial insemination by donor as an infertility option, it may be recommended that they seek a qualified or board certified infertility or endocrine specialist. It is important for the couple to know how successful the health provider has been in helping couples achieve pregnancy with the AID. Frequently, couples are also advised to undergo a series of evaluations by a psychologist prior to beginning insemination by donor to assure that both partners can accept a pregnancy if and when it occurs.

▶ *Surgical*

Several methods can be used to accomplish a pregnancy, but each one is directed toward a different underlying cause of the infertility. One method is *in vitro* fertilization. This may be by GIFT (gamete-intra-fallopian transfer), or ZIFT (zygote-intra-fallopian transfer). The GIFT technique was developed in 1984 by Dr. Richado H. Asch to help couples with infertility problems who did not respond to other conventional therapies. The female partner receives monthly cyclic hormone injections which are followed with a series of pelvic or transvaginal ultrasounds to monitor the development of the graafian follicle's maturation. The hormones may cause more than one ovum to ripen during each cycle which enhances the possibility of more than one ovum being fertilized and implanted in the uterus. A semen specimen is collected from the male partner one to two hours prior to the GIFT procedure. The semen is washed and prepared in a special solution and then centrifuged. The strongest, most active sperm swim to the top of the tube and are then placed into a special catheter. The ripened ovum is obtained from the female via laparoscopy or ultrasound aspiration. After microscopic examination, the ovum is loaded into the catheter in a sequential manner with the sperm and then injected through the fimbrial end of the fallopian tube also by laparoscopy. This procedure takes approximately one hour to complete. Pregnancy is confirmed within seven to ten days with a blood hormonal test (Beta HCG) and/or an ultrasound.

The ZIFT procedure is similar to GIFT. However, several ova are obtained just prior to ovulation. After the ova are retrieved, they are placed in a special fluid for several hours while the sperm are prepared, then the ova and sperm are carefully mixed and closely observed for two to three days. The fertilized ova (now zygotes) are transferred into the fallopian tube or into the uterine cavity. The woman must return to the hospital or clinic for the transfer procedure. She may remain in the hospital for several hours following the procedure and is placed in a modified Trendelenburg position to facilitate the attachment of the embryo to the uterus. Another name for the ZIFT procedure is IVF-ER (in vitro fertilization and embryo replacement) which more clearly defines what actually occurs. The following one to two days, she should limit her physical activity, after which she can go about her normal routine. Both GIFT and ZIFT are relatively expensive infertility procedures (approximately $5,000 or more per cycle), and may or may not be covered by health insurance. For many couples, these are final efforts to conceive. If either procedure is performed by laparoscopy, the client may receive a light general anesthetic or an epidural anesthesia. No anesthesia is needed for the embryo transfer because a fine, special catheter is used to insert the embryo through the vagina, cervix, and into the uterine cavity.

Microsurgery is an alternative treatment which is required to correct some structural problems in the fallopian tubes, for lysis of adhesions, or to reverse a previous sterilization. It is also an expensive procedure and often requires an extensive hospitalization.

► Pharmacological

Several medications are used in the treatment of infertility disorders and most are focused on hormone imbalances or deficiencies. Clomiphene citrate (Clomid), stimulates release of follicle stimulating hormone and luteinizing hormone, and is used to induce ovulation. Clomid is administered orally beginning on the fifth day of the menstrual cycle. If ovulation does not occur, the dosage will be increased for five days in the next cycle. If ovulation does not occur by the time the dose has been increased four or five times, it may be considered a Clomid failure. There is some chance of multiple gestation while the client is taking Clomid and she should be informed of the potential. Most often it is a twin pregnancy, but occasionally triplets may be conceived.

Menotropins (Pergonal) mimics FSH anf LH causing follicular growth and maturation. It is administered by intramuscular injection. Although Pergonal is an expensive drug, it has been shown to increase the possibility for ovulation in clients who have not responded to other medications.

Human chorionic gonadotropin (Pregnyl) may also be administered with the Clomid or Pergonal therapy to help maintain the endometrial lining for implantation. It stimulates the production of progesterone from the ovary until the fertilized ovum implants and the placenta begins to function. Progesterone suppositories may be used vaginally two times a day to help correct a luteal phase defect by lengthening the time from ovulation until the onset of the menses or through implantation and pregnancy. Some clients continue with the progesterone suppositories throughout the first few weeks of the pregnancy to assure that the endometrium remains intact.

► Prevention

Seeking prompt medical treatment for infections that involve the reproductive system is an essential means of preventing infertility problems, especially with STDs and PID. PID causes scarring of the outside of the fallopian tubes and gonorrhea can result in scarring or strictures of the internal fallopian tube. Either cause can result in an ectopic pregnancy when the fertilized ovum cannot pass through the tube.

Other considerations may include wise choices in contraceptive methods. The use of oral contraceptives has been associated with primary and secondary infertility due to decreased pituitary function. This condition may resolve spontaneously or medications may be required to stimulate ovulation in order to conceive.

Multiple sexual partners have also been associated with an increased risk of sexually transmitted disease, infections, and cervical cancer. Condoms should be used along with a contraceptive foam when the client is involved with more than one person sexually. This measure may also prevent the formation of antisperm antibodies in some women.

► Resources

Couples may be referred to several infertility support groups that have local or national chapters. Refer to the Resources section at the end of this chapter.

When efforts, finances, and other resources invested in their infertility workup and investigation have been exhausted, the couple may come to a conclusion to remain child-free or investigate other options, like adoption. There are long waiting lists with both public and private adoption agencies. Many couples are looking for a baby with certain characteristics, while others are just looking for a baby. Some couples resort to placing advertisements in local and distant newspapers looking for birth mothers who might consider adoption. Their seeking is often unsuccessful. The infertility journey is long and tedious and sometimes takes its toll on the couple and their marriage.

► CONTRACEPTION

Contraception, or preventing pregnancy, has been accomplished by many methods over the centuries. It may be accomplished by natural means or medical interventions. This section of the chapter will discuss a basic overview of the types of contraceptive methods currently available, the advantages and disadvantages, the effectiveness of each kind, the mechanisms by which they work and client education that should accompany the methods (see Table 31-2).

► Methods

► Natural

Natural methods of contraception may include what is called the "rhythm method." During the woman's fertile period of the month, usually seven days (three days prior to ovulation and three days after) the couple should abstain from intercourse. The determination of the fertile period is made based upon the time of ovulation. Sperm can live up to seventy-two hours after ejaculation and it is possible for sperm to still be

TABLE 31-2

CONTRACEPTION METHODS, EFFECTIVENESS, AND CONCERNS.

Method	Effectiveness Rate	Risks	Side Effects	Other Advantages
Oral contraceptives	97%	Cardiovascular complications such as stroke, blood clots, high blood pressure, and heart attacks with the higher-dose combined oral contraceptive	Possible nausea, headaches, dizziness, spotting, weight gain, breast tenderness, chloasma, cramping	Protects against PID, decreases risk of ovarian and endometrial cancer, decreases menstrual blood loss and dysmenorrhea (cramps), decreases benign breast disease, regulates irregular menses, protects bone density, decreases risk of atherosclerosis, lessens the risk of rheumatoid arthritis, decreases uterine fibroids, and decreases ovarian cysts
IUD	94%	Pelvic inflammatory disease, uterine perforation, anemia	Menstrual cramping, spotting, increased bleeding	None known except progestin-releasing IUD, which may decrease menstrual pain and blood loss
Condoms	86%	None known	Decreased sensation, allergy to latex, less spontaneity in lovemaking	Protects against sexually transmitted disease, including AIDS; delays premature ejaculation
Norplant implants	N/A	Infection at implant site	Menstrual changes, weight gain, headaches	May protect against PID, may decrease menstrual cramps, and blood loss
Sterilization female male	99.6% 99.8%	Infection	Pain at surgical site, psychological reaction with subsequent regret	None known
Abstinence	100%	None known	Psychological reactions	Prevents infections including AIDS
Barriers diaphragm cervical cap spermicide	84% 73–92% 79%	Mechanical irritaton, vaginal infections, toxic shock syndrome	Pelvic pressure, cervical erosion, vaginal discharges if left in too long	Protects to some degree against sexually transmitted diseases
Depo-Provera	N/A	Pulmonary embolism	Headache, depression, hypertension, edema, nausea	Effective to treat obstructive sleep apnea

in the cervix or uterus if the couple had intercourse three days before ovulation. The couple may also decide to maintain a basal body temperature chart to more accurately pinpoint ovulation each month. Another method to determine the approaching ovulation, is to monitor the stretchiness of the cervical mucus. This is called "spinnbarkeit." As the woman nears ovulation, the hormones (estrogen) cause the cervical mucus to become clear, thin, and stretchy. This type of mucus provides a favorable environment for the sperm and helps their motility toward the ova. The cervical secretions are high in sodium chloride

and if they are removed and dried on a microscopic slide, the sodium chloride (NaCl) will appear as crystals that resemble Boston ferns. This fern pattern grows larger the closer the woman is to ovulation. Immediately following ovulation, the cervical mucus becomes hostile to sperm. It becomes thick, cloudy, and more acid. It also loses its stretchiness. Kits are available for purchase from the local drug store or pharmacy that react to chemicals in the cervical mucus and predict the time of ovulation. The kits are inexpensive and simple to use, much like home pregnancy tests.

▶ Barriers and Spermicides

Methods of barrier contraception include male and female condoms, the diaphragm, and the cervical cap. Another barrier method, the sponge, was taken off the market. These devices work by blocking the pathway of the sperm through the cervix into the uterus. Spermicides kill sperm before they can enter the cervix. This type of contraceptive requires some preplanning on the part of one or both of the partners and may reduce the spontaneity of the sex act.

Spermicides contain a chemical, nonoxynol-9, that kills sperm on contact. If used alone, spermicidal agents have a lower efficacy rate than if used with a condom. The nurse should advise the couple to use a spermicidal gel, foam suppository, or film in addition to another barrier method for the greatest effectiveness. Foam should not be used with the diaphragm because it can result in deterioration of the latex. These agents must be placed in the vagina at least fifteen minutes prior to intercourse to promote the spermicidal reaction. This method is safe and inexpensive, but requires a high level of compliance each time or the effectiveness of the method drops significantly.

▶ Hormonal

Oral Contraceptives   The "pill" has been available as a contraceptive method for many years. Since its earliest form, it has been refined and the levels of hormones needed have been reduced. Oral contraceptives work by suppressing ovulation. In a sense, the body thinks it is pregnant when the pill is used. Some oral contraceptives contain estrogen and progesterone, while others contain only progestins. Many physicians recommend starting the pill pack on a Sunday immediately following the menses for ease in remembering. Once the pack has been started, the client continues to take a pill daily for twenty-one or twenty-eight days. In the twenty-eight day pack, there are six placebo tablets. These are helpful for the client who remembers to take a pill if she has to do it everyday. It is important to instruct the client not to miss a pill. If she does, she should take the one she missed as soon as possible. The next dose should be taken at the regular time. In the event that the client forgets two pills, she should finish the pack, but also use another type of barrier contraception for the remainder of the cycle, because ovulation could occur.

In response to the pseudopregnancy state, the client may experience mild side effects and discomforts often associated with pregnancy such as, nausea, headache, breast tenderness, and/or weight gain. Major side effects from oral contraceptives may include cardiovascular accidents and/or thrombophlebitis. There is approximately a one in 200 chance of becoming pregnant while taking the oral contraceptive. If the woman thinks that she might be pregnant, she should stop the pill immediately and contact her physician. When the woman and her partner decide that it is time for a pregnancy, she should discontinue the oral contraceptive for at least two to three cycles before having unprotected intercourse. This will lessen the possibility of pill effects remaining in her system and allow her body to return to its own natural rhythm. Some women will find that they experience primary or secondary infertility problems after being on the pill for several years due to pituitary suppression. The remedy is often fertility drugs like clomiphene citrate (Clomid). Women who have never established a regular pattern of menstruation may not be good candidates for oral contraceptives, except as being used to regulate the cycle by artificial means. Other clients who should not take oral contraceptives include women with a history of preexisting hypertension, diabetes, cardiovascular disease, or thrombophlebitis. Some physicians may consider oral contraceptives in the newer low dose combinations for clients who were previously in this high risk group.

Norplant   A relatively new contraceptive, levonorgestrel (Norplant System) consists of six small progestin-filled pellets that are inserted under the skin of the upper arm under a local anesthetic. Theoretically, Norplant is effective for up to five years. Some clients will experience mild breakthrough bleeding during the first few months after the Norplant is in place. This usually subsides or lessens with time, but for some clients it is an inconvenience. This is a good option for the woman who is sure she does not desire a pregnancy for at least five years, although the pellets may be removed before the end of that time. Due to the expense of the Norplant and placement procedure, the nurse or physician should make sure the client has a clear understanding of the method before proceeding. It is important that the Norplant be inserted by a qualified physician or NP.

Depo-Provera   The medroxyprogesterone acetate (Depo-Provera) injection is administered intramuscularly every twelve weeks. It works like oral contraceptives to suppress ovulation. The client may experience breakthrough bleeding after the first injection, but this is not an indication that the hormone is not working. It usually requires about three weeks following the first injection before the contraceptive is effective, so the client should be advised to use a barrier contraceptive method during that period. The client must receive the injections at regular intervals to assure effectiveness. Norplant and Depo-Provera are good options for the client who is approaching her forties or who smokes because it only contains progestins which decrease her risk of cardiovascular problems.

▶ Intrauterine Contraceptive Devices (IUD)

The IUD has been used for many years and has undergone several changes. The Dalcon shield which was used in the 1960s and 1970s caused many problems from infection to infertility. The IUD works by causing an irritation inside the uterine cavity that results in a hostile environment for the fertilized ovum that causes it not to implant. It is then sloughed off with the menstrual flow. The intrauterine device is recommended for women who have had children because the cervix has been dilated. This allows for easier insertion of the device. The IUD is inserted or removed while the client is having her period because there is slight dilatation of the cervix at that time. A string is attached to the distal end of the device that hangs out of the cervix into the vagina. The client is instructed to check the string each month after the menstrual period to make sure the device has not been expelled. Some women experience more dysmenorrhea with the IUD in place and a heavier menstrual flow. Because there is an increased risk of infection with the IUD, a monogamous relationship is advisable for the client. The intrauterine devices that are currently available are effective for one year or seven years.

▶ Sterilization

This method of contraception is considered permanent and very effective. In a rare incident, a woman will become pregnant after a tubal ligation. The procedure interrupts the pathway through the fallopian tube. Sterilization may be performed on an outpatient basis in a surgical clinic or the outpatient department at the hospital. The tubal ligation is done under a general or epidural anesthetic with laparoscopy. The sterilization may be performed by cutting and tying the tubes, cutting and cauterizing, crushing the tubes, or by removing the fimbriated ends. Additional time is required for recovery if the client has had a general anesthetic. The procedure takes about thirty to sixty minutes. The abdomen is distended with a gas to permit better visualization of the pelvic structures during the procedure. This may result in some discomfort for the client afterward, even though most of the gas is removed before the small incisions are closed. The woman may experience some abdominal or shoulder soreness for a day or two following the procedure. The shoulder pain is usually from the small amount of gas remaining in the abdominal cavity which is gradually absorbed by the body. Acetominophen (Tylenol) or another mild analgesic is normally adequate to manage this discomfort. The female sterilization is more expensive and because it requires more anes-

thesia, it carries a slightly higher risk than the male procedure.

As mentioned, sterilization procedures are considered permanent; however, with refined microsurgical techniques, it is possible to reverse the procedures. The reversals are not always successful and the couple need to consider the odds of success before venturing into the expense of this type of surgery.

Reanastomosis of the fallopian tubes is an extensive and expensive surgery and it requires hospitalization for several days following the procedure. During the hospitalization, the physician will instill medication or air through the tubes to ensure their patency.

▶ ABORTION

Abortion is defined as the termination of a pregnancy before the age of viability. It may be spontaneous or induced. Approximately 75 percent of spontaneous abortions occur within the first twelve weeks of pregnancy. Miscarriage is the lay term that is used to describe spontaneous abortion. The exact pathophysiology is unknown. One possible cause is a blighted ovum. In this case, the ovum has been fertilized, but an embryo does not develop as it should. There are definite changes in the endometrium that appear consistent with pregnancy, but when the uterine contents is examined, there is no fetus. Other causes include placental abnormalities, implantation problems, and maternal disease (infections, diabetes, or endocrine imbalances).

▶ Spontaneous

Spontaneous abortion may be classified in the following ways. A threatened abortion is characterized by uterine cramping and brown or reddish vaginal bleeding. The cervix has not dilated. The client is usually advised to remain on bed rest until the cramping subsides or an abortion becomes inevitable. An inevitable abortion is characterized by cramping, brown to bright red vaginal bleeding and cervical dilation with eventual expulsion of the products of conception. A complete abortion is the expulsion of all of the products of conception. In an incomplete abortion, some tissue is expelled, but some remains. In this case, the client may continue to have heavy bleeding. This places the client at high risk for hemorrhage and a D & C may be required. A habitual abortion is a term used for the client who experiences three or more spontaneous abortions without an apparent cause. This may be related to an incompetent cervix or some genetic problem. In the case of the incompetent cervix, a surgical banding of the cervix may be done. This procedure is called a cerclage or Shirodkar procedure. A purse string suture is placed around the cervix to keep it tightly closed until the pregnancy has reached near term. The procedure is done as an outpatient and the client may be monitored in the labor and delivery area following her recovery to detect any signs of preterm labor.

If the suspected cause of the habitual abortion is genetic, the couple should be referred for genetic counseling. If a hormonal imbalance is diagnosed, the physician may prescribe various treatments such as those that were discussed in the infertility section.

A missed abortion means that the embryo died in the uterus, but was not expelled. The woman often experiences the usual early pregnancy signs and symptoms and then notices that the symptoms disappear. A bi-manual examination may reveal a slightly enlarged uterus and other presumptive signs of pregnancy. An ultrasound may show a sac or embryo without a heartbeat. A D & C is generally performed.

▶ Induced

Induced abortions may be either therapeutic or elective. A therapeutic abortion is performed when the mother's life is endangered by continuing the pregnancy. An elective abortion is the termination of the pregnancy by medical intervention at the client's request. Both types of induced abortion are controversial. An ethics committee may be required to review a request to perform a therapeutic abortion and grant permission before the physician may proceed. Some hospitals prohibit therapeutic abortions based upon religious beliefs.

Methods used for the induced abortion may include the instillation of prostaglandin F suppositories vaginally to induce contractions, dilatation and curettage (D & C), a dilatation and evacuation (D & E), instillation of intrauterine saline solution, or a hysterotomy. The majority of induced abortions in the United States are performed by surgical intervention depending upon the gestation of the pregnancy. Induced abortion, regardless of the method chosen, carries some risk inherent to the procedure, especially if it is performed after the first trimester.

Newer chemical methods of inducing abortion include RU-486 and a methotrexate/Cytotec combination. RU-486, known as mifepristone (Mifegyne), is a progesterone antagonist that induces sloughing of the endometrium. It has been available in Europe for several years and was introduced into the United States in 1993. It has not been approved at this time by the FDA as an abortion drug, but is being used in research against various cancers. RU-486 must be taken early in the cycle, after fertilization has occurred, and it will induce an abortion. If taken in the first days to one week of the pregnancy, it is about 85 percent effective. It is often called the "morning after pill."

A combination of methotrexate, an antimetabolite used for chemotherapy, and misoprostol (Cytotec) a medication used to treat peptic ulcer disease have been tried recently as a contraceptive method that induces abortion in the early weeks of pregnancy. Neither drug has been approved for this use at this time but can be used by the physician for other reasons.

Many times, the client who has an elective or therapeutic abortion will experience long-term emotional reactions to the loss of the pregnancy. This also occurs with the spontaneous loss of pregnancy. Abortion is a personal and emotional decision. Prior to 1970, legal abortions were not available in the United States. Roe vs. Wade and Doe vs. Bolton are two famous court cases which resulted in the Supreme Court decision to legalize abortion in this country. Issues and restrictions related to abortion provisions vary in the laws from state to state including waiting periods, informed consent, parental or spousal notification and/or permission, and the possibility of hospitalization.

Health care providers (nurses, doctors, and counselors) are obligated to provide information to the client in a nonjudgmental manner regarding pregnancy options and offer her support in discussing those options, making referral, and exploring the emotional aspect of abortion. Pro-choice advocates believe that the client should have full control and decision over what occurs to and in her body and whether she desires pregnancy at that time. Pro-life advocates believe that life begins at conception and to terminate a pregnancy is killing a human being. Because this is a controversial topic, nurses should examine their own personal values, beliefs, and feelings about abortion. Personal views may impact where the nurse chooses to seek employment and the comfort level in discussing abortion options or alternatives with the clients.

▶ Nursing Interventions

The nurse should carefully assess the client who is experiencing signs of an abortion. Essential parts of the assessment include monitoring the vital signs and bleeding. A vaginal pad count is often recommended if the client is bleeding heavily. The nurse should also observe for the passage of the uterine contents. The client may be given an analgesic medication if she is experiencing a lot of cramping and pain. If a D & C is required, the nurse will help prepare the client for surgery and monitor her status following surgery. If the client is stable after the surgery, she will be dismissed within a few hours. The nurse should advise the client to rest at home for the next day or two and to notify her physician if she has any increased vaginal bleeding or if she develops an elevated temperature or other signs of infection. Pregnancy should be avoided for a minimum of three months following an abortion to allow the body to heal and return to its normal non-pregnant state. Fertility is not affected by abortion and the client should be advised to use an effective contraceptive method as soon as she resumes sexual activity. The physician usually advises the client about sexual activity after she has been seen for a postoperative check-up. The nurse may need to instruct the client in family planning methods and assist the client in the selection of the best method for her individual needs and desire for future pregnancies.

The nurse's role in helping the client cope with her pregnancy loss is often as an active listener. Allowing the client time to grieve for the end of the pregnancy, and the child she will never know, is part of the process. There are varied reactions to an abortion, whether it is spontaneous or induced. The nurse should avoid using cliche remarks or comments as they are not therapeutic and may block communication.

▶ TOXIC SHOCK SYNDROME

Toxic shock syndrome (TSS) is a condition most often associated with *Staphylococcus aureus,* which enters the bloodstream. A strong relationship has been found between the use of tampons (especially super absorbent) during menstruation and the onset of TSS symptoms. It has been hypothesized that the fibers from the tampon lower the level of magnesium in the woman's body and, therefore, produce a favorable environment for the growth of pathogenic microorganisms. The condition was first diagnosed in the mid-seventies and the incidence increased throughout the eighties. A high percentage of women who are affected by toxic shock syndrome are under thirty. TSS can also occur in nonmenstruating women and men.

The client may present with a temperature to 102 degrees or greater, vomiting, diarrhea, and progressive hypotension. She may also experience flulike symptoms of malaise, muscle soreness, sore throat, and headache. There may be a macular erythematous (flat,

red) rash that is followed in one to two weeks by the peeling of the palms and soles. Disorientation may occur from the release of toxins and dehydration.

▶ Medical/Surgical Management

▶ Medical

Blood, urine, genitourinary, and throat cultures may be obtained and are usually negative except for *Staphylococcus aureus.* The goals of treatment are focused on the control of the falling blood pressure, fluid volume replacement, halting the infectious process, and maintaining adequate ventilation efforts. IV fluids are administered per the physician's order. The client may require mechanical ventilation and CPAP (continuous positive airway pressure).

▶ Pharmacological

Broad spectrum antibiotic therapy is recommended. Culture and sensitivity tests will indicate which type of antibiotic is best against the staphylococcus organism. Examples may include dicloxacillin sodium (Dynapen), clexacillin sodium (Tegopen), nafcillin sodium (Nafcil), and methicillin sodium (Staphcillin). The medication regimen is continued for at least two weeks to ensure control of the pathogens.

▶ Activity

Bed rest is usually prescribed.

▶ Nursing Process

Assessment

Subjective Data Data to be obtained includes recent use of tampons, length tampon is left in before changing, sore throat, headache, myalgia, and fatigue.

Objective Data Assess for erythematous rash, edema, peeling of palms and soles, hypotension, level of consciousness, nonpurulent conjunctivitis, and hyperemia of vagina and oropharynx.

▼ ▼

Possible nursing diagnoses for a client with TSS may include:

Nursing Diagnoses	Goals	Nursing Interventions
▶ Hyperthermia, related to inflammatory process.	The client will have normal range temperature within forty-eight hours.	Administer antipyretics as ordered. Give cooling sponge bath. Encourage oral fluids as tolerated.
▶ Fluid volume deficit, related to diarrhea, vomiting, fever, and decreased intake.	The client will have fluid and electrolyte balance within twenty-four hours.	Administer intravenous fluids as ordered. Encourage oral fluids if client is not vomiting. Administer antiemetic and antidiarrheal medications as ordered. Assess skin turgor and mucous membranes. Monitor I & O.
▶ Skin/tissue integrity, impaired, related to dehydration and effects of circulating toxins.	The client will have skin and tissue integrity.	Encourage or assist with position change every two hours. Provide or assist with personal hygiene. Assess bony prominences for reddened areas.
▶ Pain, related to inflammatory process.	The client will report reduction in pain within twenty-four hours.	Administer analgesics as ordered. Provide comfort measures.

▶ *Evaluation*

Each goal must be evaluated to determine how it has been met by the client.

▲ ▲

▶ *Teaching Tip*

Client education is essential to prevent a recurrence of the TSS. If the client recovers from the TSS, she should be instructed to avoid tampon use for several cycles. If she chooses to use tampons in the future, she should change them every two to three hours, especially the super-absorbent types.

▶ *CASE STUDY*

Mrs. Mary Keiver, a forty-year-old, African American school teacher, nullipara, was seen by her physician because of heavy menstrual bleeding. She stated that she had been saturating a sanitary pad every thirty minutes since early that same morning. She reported that her menstrual periods had been getting heavier for the past six months and were accompanied by severe cramping. She also noted that after her period she felt "physically drained." Other symptoms that Mary had observed included an increasing sense of heaviness in her pelvis and that her skirts and slacks were too tight around the abdomen, even though her weight had not changed significantly.

When Mary was examined by the physician, it was noted that her uterus was enlarged approximately equal to twelve weeks gestational size and it felt irregular in shape. Mary's skin was pale and cool to touch. Her mucous membranes and conjunctival sacs were pale pink. Her blood pressure was 100/60, pulse 90, temperature 98.8. The results of an H & H were as follows: Hgb-7.0 mg/dL and HCT-26. An ultrasound confirmed the findings of the pelvic exam for the presence of multiple uterine fibroids. The bleeding did not subside, and Mary was admitted for an outpatient dilatation and curettage with a diagnosis of menorrhagia secondary to uterine leiomyoma.

The following questions will guide your development of a nursing care plan for the case study.

1. List the clinical signs and symptoms manifested by this client that suggest that the heavy bleeding may be related to uterine fibroids.
2. List two reasons why a hemoglobin and hematocrit were ordered.
3. Describe what other diagnostic tests were ordered and why.
4. List the subjective and objective data the nurse should obtain during the assessment.
5. Write three individualized nursing diagnoses and goals for Mrs. Keiver.
6. Describe pertinent nursing actions/interventions to be taken in caring for this client prior to and following the D & C related to:
   - Bleeding
   - Cardiac output
   - Comfort/rest
   - Activity
   - Medications
   - Teaching
7. List a minimum of three specific topics the nurse should discuss when talking to this client regarding her condition.
8. Discuss discharge instructions or teaching necessary for this client.
9. List a minimum of three successful outcomes for this client.
10. Discuss how the nurse might evaluate the effectiveness of treatment and care for this client.

SUMMARY

- Potential complications from PID may include sterility or infertility from scarring of fallopian tubes.
- A BSE is an important method for detecting breast changes and should be practiced each month. Breast cancer is the most common female cancer in the United States.
- Cervical cancer is more common in women with multiple sexual partners.
- Uterine cancer often only produces symptoms once it is widespread. Any unusual vagina bleeding should be investigated, especially if it occurs after menopause.
- Menstrual disorders are often associated with hormonal imbalances, increased or decreased function of the endocrine glands, or neoplasms.
- Menopause is a normal, gradual decline in the ovarian production of female hormones that occurs around age fifty. Estrogen replacement therapy is recommended by many health care providers to decrease the symptoms of menopause and as a preventive measure against cardiovascular disease and osteoporosis.
- Infertility affects at least one in every four couples in the United States and is caused by hormonal imbalances, and structural or physiological abnormalities in both male and female clients.
- Clients who smoke and women over forty are at greater risk of major complications while using oral contraceptives. Major health risks include cardiovascular accidents and deep vein thrombosis.
- Toxic shock syndrome (TSS) often occurs during the menses and a strong correlation exists between the onset and use of super-absorbent tampons.

Review Questions

1. The best method of screening for cervical cancer is:
   a. genitourinary cultures.
   b. cervical biopsy.
   c. Pap smear.
   d. ultrasound.

2. The client should perform BSE (breast self-examination):
   a. just before the menstrual period.
   b. just after the menstrual period.
   c. at ovulation.
   d. any time of the month.

3. The "silent killer" of many women is:
   a. cervical cancer.
   b. uterine cancer.
   c. breast cancer.
   d. ovarian cancer.

4. If the client complains of heavy bleeding between her normal menstrual cycles it is called:
   a. amenorrhea.
   b. polymenorrhea.
   c. metrorrhagia.
   d. menorrhagia.

5. Bowel and bladder complications that may follow pelvic radiation therapy for uterine cancer are often caused by:
   a. dehydration.
   b. lack of mobility.
   c. damage to the tissue from radiation effects.
   d. damage to tissues during surgery.

6. The most common cancer of the female reproductive system is:
   a. breast.
   b. ovarian.
   c. cervical.
   d. uterine.

7. An example of an antiestrogenic drug used in the treatment of female reproductive cancers, especially in breast cancer, is:
   a. Megace.
   b. Cytoxan.
   c. 5-FU.
   d. Teslac.

8. The primary microorganism associated with the occurrence of toxic shock syndrome is:
   a. *E-coli.*
   b. *Streptococcus aureus.*
   c. *Staphylococcus aureus.*
   d. *Pseudomonas.*

9. An example of a barrier method of contraception is:
   a. condom.
   b. the "pill."
   c. an IUD.
   d. Norplant.

10. A dietary element frequently associated with fibrocystic breast disease is:
    a. fats.
    b. protein.
    c. sodium.
    d. caffeine.

11. Bright red vaginal bleeding, cramping, and cervical dilation during the first trimester of pregnancy are symptoms of which type of abortion?
    a. missed
    b. complete
    c. threatened
    d. inevitable

12. Which of the following are characteristic signs of a trichomonas vaginitis?

    a. thick, white, "cheesy" discharge with itching
    b. frothy, foul smelling, yellow discharge with itching and irritation
    c. creamy, thin, vaginal discharge with a musty/fishy odor
    d. painful intercourse due to decreased lubrication

13. The drug of choice to treat PID (pelvic inflammatory disease) is:

    a. penicillin.
    b. doxycycline.
    c. erythromycin.
    d. cyclophosphamide.

14. What degree of prolapse is described when the cervix and the uterus extend out of the body, past the vaginal opening?

    a. first degree
    b. second degree
    c. third degree
    d. fourth degree

Critical Thinking Questions

1. How would you respond to a diagnosis of breast cancer requiring surgery and chemotherapy and/or radiation? Or, how would you respond if someone close to you had this diagnosis?

2. Prepare a teaching plan for a breast self examination.

Medical Terminology

ameno-	prefix refers to "without" or absence of
amenorrhea	absence of menstruation
-cele	suffix meaning sac or pouch
cystocele	a bladder hernia that protrudes into the vagina
-ception	suffix refers to pregnancy
contra-	prefix meaning against or to prevent; example, contraception
contraception	prevention of pregnancy by natural or artificial methods
cyst-	suffix or stand alone. Refers to sac or bladder. Fluid or solid
dys-	prefix meaning difficult or painful
dysmenorrhea	painful cramping associated with menstrual period
hyster-	prefix refers to uterus
-ectomy	suffix meaning to excise surgically
hysterectomy	surgical removal or excision of the uterus, and/or the uterus, fallopian tubes, and ovaries
fibro-	meaning formation of fibrous tissue
fibrocystic	benign overgrowth of fibrous tissue
meno-	prefix refers to menstruation
menopause	that period which marks the permanent cessation of menstrual activity
metro-	prefix refers to uterus
metrorrhagia	vaginal bleeding between menstrual periods
oligo-	prefix meaning decreased or infrequent
-rrhea	suffix meaning flow of blood
oligomenorrhea	infrequent menstrual periods or decreased menstrual flow
poly-	prefix meaning increased or more frequent
polymenorrhea	menstrual periods that are abnormally frequent
recto-	refers to rectum
rectocele	relaxation of the posterior vaginal wall which allows the protrusion of the rectum into the vagina
-rrhagia	suffix meaning excessive flow of blood
menorrhagia	excessively heavy or prolonged menstrual flow
urethro-	prefix refers to urethra
urethrocele	relaxation of the anterior vaginal wall which allows the bladder and/or urethra to protrude into the vagina

News Flash

Estrogen replacement therapy was supported for postmenopausal women in a longitudinal research project at the University of Pittsburgh. A sample of 9,704 Caucasian women who were sixty-five years old or older, and were taking estrogen or an estrogen/progesterone combination therapy, experienced a 30% decrease in heart disease over a ten-year period. It appears that the benefits of estrogen replacement extend even after the woman is no longer taking the hormone. The greatest benefits were demonstrated in the women who ranged from sixty-five to seventy-four. The study concluded that women over seventy-five, or those on ERT less than ten years also experienced a significant benefit. Based on figures from the American Heart Association, heart disease affects six out of nine women. This may further support the use of estrogen replacement therapy for postmenopausal clients (Cauley, 1995).

CHAPTER

32

Male Reproductive Disorders

Sandra Liming

► KEY TERMS

androgenic
Bellevue bridge
coitus interruptus
gynecomastia
hematuria
hesitancy
Kegel exercise
nocturia
orchiectomy
post void residual
priapism
spermatogenesis
stent
tumescence
urethrostomy
vasectomy

LIST OF DISORDERS

Benign Neoplasms
► Benign Prostatic Hypertrophy
Malignant Neoplasms
► Prostate Cancer
► Testicular Cancer
► Penile Cancer
► Breast Cancer
Inflammatory Disorders
► Epididymitis
► Orchitis
► Prostatitis
Structural Disorders
► Cryptorchidism
► Hydrocele
► Hypospadias and Epispadias
► Spermatocele
► Varicocele
► Torsion of the Spermatic Cord
Impotence, Infertility and Contraception
► Impotence
► Infertility
► Contraception

LEARNING OBJECTIVES

Upon completion of this chapter, the learner should be able to:
• Define key terms.
• Identify the components of the male reproductive system.
• Describe the hormonal mechanisms that regulate male reproductive functions.

- Describe the changes in the male reproductive system that occur with aging.
- Differentiate between impotence and infertility.
- Describe disorders of the male reproductive system and related treatments.

- Describe male fertility disorders and related treatments.
- Discuss methods of contraception for a male client.
- Apply the nursing process when caring for a male client with a disorder of the reproductive system.

► MAKING THE CONNECTION

Refer to the topics in the following chapters to increase your understanding of male reproductive disorders:

- **Chapter 8, Health Maintenance:** Sexually Transmitted Diseases, p. 130
- **Chapter 10, Nursing Assessment:** Thoracic Assessment, p. 179; Abdominal Assessment, p. 181
- **Chapter 13, Perioperative Nursing:** Intraoperative, p. 240; Postoperative, p. 247
- **Chapter 14, Fluid, Electrolyte, and Acid-Base Balances:** Hormonal Control, p. 269
- **Chapter 15, Oncology Nursing:** Breast Cancer, p. 311; Prostate Cancer, p. 312; Testicular Cancer, p. 312
- **Chapter 16, Caring for the Older Adult:** Common Disorders Related to Aging/Male

Reproductive System, p. 341; Urinary System, p. 344

- **Chapter 20, Cardiac Disorders:** Arteriosclerosis, p. 472
- **Chapter 21, Vascular Disorders:** Hypertension, p. 508
- **Chapter 25, HIV Disorders:** Modes of Transmission, p. 621
- **Chapter 30, Diabetes Mellitus:** Chronic Complications of Diabetes, p. 842
- **Chapter 33, Sexually Transmitted Diseases:** Chlamydia, p. 948; Gonorrhea, p. 949; Syphilis, p. 949; Herpes Genitalis, p. 950; Human Papillomavirus, p. 954; Trichomoniasis, p. 955
- **Chapter 35, Urinary Disorders:** Changes with Aging, p. 1017; Renal Failure, p. 1039

INTRODUCTION

Because of modern technology, current medical and nursing knowledge, and health education programs, laypersons have access to much information about their bodies. However, men continue to be seriously affected by male health disorders. In some instances men may lack knowledge of how to detect signs and symptoms of these disorders. Often they simply delay routine medical examinations or avoid seeking medical treatment. In addition, males may have difficulty discussing symptoms related to their reproductive system.

Routine health care must be maintained and early diagnosis made in order to reduce the incidence and seriousness of male health disorders. These goals can be facilitated with skilled nursing assessment and client education. This chapter is designed to provide the learner with detailed descriptions of disorders of the male reproductive system along with explanations of related treatment and nursing care. The learner will

also be provided with a review of anatomy and physiology of the male reproductive system to assist in identifying key structures involved in the various disorders.

ANATOMY AND PHYSIOLOGY REVIEW

The male reproductive organs and associated structures are illustrated in Figure 32-1. The scrotum is a fleshy structure that is suspended below the perineum, anterior to the anus. It is divided into two parts, each of which contains a testis, an epididymis, and a portion of the spermatic cord (vas deferens). The left side of the scrotum is usually lower than the right because the left spermatic cord is often longer.

The testes, two smooth, oval endocrine glands, are suspended in the scrotum. This location helps to maintain proper temperature and also protects the testes from trauma. Certain cells of the epithelium lining the seminiferous tubules of the testes produce one-half

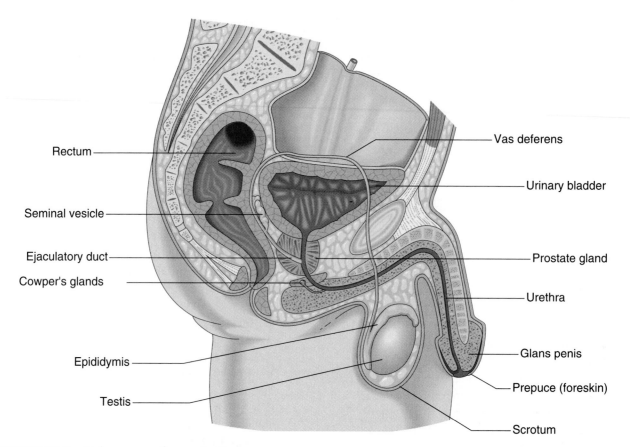

Rectum

Seminal vesicle

Ejaculatory duct

Cowper's glands

Epididymis

Testis

Vas deferens

Urinary bladder

Prostate gland

Urethra

Glans penis

Prepuce (foreskin)

Scrotum

FIGURE 32-1 Male organs of reproduction.

billion sperm daily (**spermatogenesis**). They also secrete the **androgenic** (male) hormone, testosterone. Spermatogenesis is regulated by the follicle stimulating hormone (FSH), which is produced by the anterior pituitary gland. The production of testosterone is regulated by luteinizing hormone (LH), which is also produced by the anterior pituitary gland. The sperm move through the rete testis, a network of tubules, on the way to the epididymis where they are stored for maturation. After the sperm mature, they travel through the vas (ductus) deferens, a long tube that is attached to the epididymis. The vas deferens, along with associated nerves and blood vessels, forms the spermatic cord.

The vas deferens travels up and around the bladder and carries sperm from the epididymis to the seminal vesicle. The seminal vesicle is a small pouch that produces secretions which, when mixed with sperm and prostatic fluid, forms semen. The prostate is an encapsulated gland that encircles the proximal portion of the urethra. It is divided into a median lobe and two lateral lobes. The prostatic fossa, a depression on the cranial border of the prostate, allows entry of the ejaculatory ducts. Within the prostate is a cluster of thirty to fifty tubuloalveolar glands that secrete prostatic fluid. The prostate gland is of clinical significance because as men age, it is a common site for malignant disease or benign enlargement that can cause urethral obstruction.

The penis is a cylindrical organ through which urine is passed to the outside and semen is ejaculated into the female vagina during sexual intercourse. Half of the penis is located within the body. The external half of the penis is flaccid, unless the male is sexually aroused, at which time it becomes erect due to engorgement with blood. There are three cylindrical columns of erectile tissue; two corpora cavernosa and the corpus spongiosum. A fold of skin, the prepuce, surrounds the tip of the penis in the uncircumcised male. Circumcision is performed on many Western society infants to remove the prepuce or foreskin. In 1975 the American Academy of Pediatrics (AAP) did not support any medical need for routine circumcision. In 1988 they reversed their position, based on increased evidence that circumcision reduces the incidence of urinary tract infections. Also, circumcision is performed for cultural or religious reasons.

COMMON DIAGNOSTIC TESTS

The following is a table of the commonly used diagnostic tests for male clients who present with reproductive disorders.

Test	Explanation/Normal Values	Nursing Responsibilities
Alpha-Fetoprotein	Test for tumor marker; Elevated in nonseminomatous testicular cancer. normal = 0.9 ng/mL	Apply pressure to site and watch for bleeding or hematoma.
Human Chorionic Gonadotropin (HCG)	Test for tumor marker; Elevated in germ cell testicular cancer. Normal = 0–5 U/L	Apply pressure to site and watch for bleeding or hematoma.
Prostate-specific antigen (PSA)	Serum measurement of prostate specific antigen and acid phosphate. Accuracy varies as normal values may require age-specific adjustments. Normal = 0.0–4.0 ng/mL.	Apply pressure to the site and watch for bleeding or hematoma.
Serum Acid Phosphatase (prostatic)	Serum measurement of prostatic acid phosphatase, elevated with malignancy; because it detects cancer in the later stages, no longer commonly used. Normal = 0.0–0.8 U/L	Apply pressure to site and watch for bleeding or hematoma.
Serum Alkaline Phosphatase	Serum measurement of alkaline phosphates, elevated with malignancy. Normal = 30–120 U/L	Apply pressure to site and watch for bleeding or hematoma.
Serum Calcium	Serum measurement of calcium, Normal = 8.8–10.3 mg/dL.	Apply pressure to site and watch for bleeding or hematoma.
Semen Analysis	Determine presence, number, and motility of sperm.	Client education about proper collection of sperm.
Segmented Bacteriologic Localization Cultures	Collect first 5–10 mL urine, discard next 200 mL, then collect 5–10 mL midstream. Prostate massaged until prostatic secretions collected. Next, 5–10 mL urine collected, then empty bladder. Four samples are needed in sterile culture tubes.	Make sure the client is well hydrated and has a full bladder.
Prostatic Smears	Microscopic examination of prostatic secretions obtained via rectal massage performed by a physician.	Explain that to obtain the specimen the prostate will need to be massaged via the rectum and there will be some discomfort.
Prostatic Biopsy	Removal of a small piece of tissue for microscopic examination.	Monitor and educate about signs and symptoms of hemorrhage, infection, and pain post procedure.
Testicular Biopsy	Determine presence of sperm and rule out vas deferens obstruction.	Monitor and/or educate about signs and symptoms of infection or hemorrhage.
Dynamic Infusion Cavernosometry and Cavernosography (DICC)	Group of diagnostic tests that measure neururovascular events of penile erection venous/increased pressure erection within blood vessels.	Baseline assessment, monitor during the procedure, and assess for complications postoperatively; advise client of possible discomfort related to injection.

(continued)

Test	Explanation/Normal Values	Nursing Responsibilities
Ultrasound (Transrectal Bladder)	Use of ultrasound to produce an image or photograph the prostate or bladder and surrounding tissue.	Client education about procedure.
Nocturnal Tumescence Penile Monitoring	Various devices are attached to penis at night to monitor swelling (**tumescence**) that occurs.	Explain to client that test will require application of a device to the penis, to be worn while sleeping; show client the device and explain how to apply.

KEY ABBREVIATIONS

The following abbreviations and acronyms are used in this chapter:

AAP	American Academy of Pediatrics
BPH	benign prostatic hypertrophy
BSE	breast self examination
BVI	bladder volume indicator
DES	diethylstilbestrol
FSH	follicle stimulating hormone
HIV	human immunodeficiency virus
LH	luteinizing hormone
LHRH	luteinizing hormone releasing hormone
TSE	testicular self-examination
TURP	transurethral resection of prostate
TULIP	transurethral ultrasound-guided laser induced prostatectomy
UTI	urinary tract infection
VCD	vacuum constriction device

▶ BENIGN NEOPLASMS

▶ BENIGN PROSTATIC HYPERTROPHY

Benign prostatic hypertrophy (BPH) is a progressive adenomatous enlargement of the prostate gland that occurs with aging. More than 50 percent of men over the age of fifty and 75 percent of men over the age of seventy demonstrate some increase in the size of the prostate gland (Martini, 1995). While this disorder is not harmful, the urinary outlet obstruction that may be associated with the disorder is a problem.

Because the urethra is encircled by the prostate, common early symptoms of BPH are related to partial or complete obstruction of the urethra. Early symptoms include **hesitancy** (difficulty initiating the urinary stream), decreased force of stream, urinary frequency,

and **nocturia** (awakening at night to void). However, a temporary reduction of these symptoms may occur as the bladder muscles hypertrophy in response to the increased work they must do to force the urinary stream past the obstruction.

While this bladder muscle compensatory response may temporarily reduce symptoms, eventually the muscle decompensates, becoming noncompliant and hypotonic. This leads to atony of the mucous membranes between the muscle bands that causes stagnant urine to collect in the small compartments (cellules) of the membranes. In addition, the man is unable to completely empty the bladder when voiding (**post void residual**). Because these changes in urinary function promote urinary alkalosis by increasing the urine pH, a perfect environment for bacterial growth is created. This bacterial growth can cause a urinary tract infection (UTI), which may eventually lead to kidney damage.

▶ Medical/Surgical Management

▶ Medical

The physician will perform a digital rectal examination in order to identify any enlargement of the lateral lobes or nodular lumps on the surface of the prostate gland. Diagnostic tests will be ordered to learn more about the client's condition; these may include a PSA, measuring residual urine, cystoscopy, intravenous pyelogram, and ultrasonography. The physician will also carefully monitor the client's condition to detect any exacerbation of symptoms such as increased hesitancy, urgency, hematuria, or repeated urinary tract infections and suggest appropriate treatment options.

Many alternatives to surgical treatment of BPH have been introduced over the past several years. Medical treatment methods have ranged from balloon dilation of the prostate and prostate urethral **stents**, as shown in Figure 32-2, to thermotherapy. Balloon dilation of the prostate during an endoscopic examination is done to break the prostatic capsule and facilitate

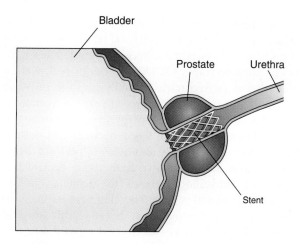

FIGURE 32-2 Urethral stent.

decompression of the prostate. A stent is material that is used to hold tissue in place or, in this instance, to provide support to the urethra which is being compressed by the prostate. Various types of thermotherapy that may be used are microwave thermotherapy and hyperthermia. While these minimally invasive treatments are safe, they do not remove the urinary obstruction.

▶ *Surgical*

The traditional surgical intervention for enlargement of the portion of the prostate that surrounds the urethra has been transurethral resection of the prostate

(TURP). This surgery is performed via a resectoscope, an instrument that includes a cutting and cauterization device (see Figure 32-3). The client receives either a general or spinal anesthetic and the resectoscope is passed through the urethra for the purpose of removing small pieces of prostate tissue while controlling bleeding. The bladder is continuously irrigated with normal saline or another solution during the procedure. This irrigation is continued during the postoperative period to reduce clot formation that would interfere with urinary drainage.

The traditional surgical alternatives to a TURP are open operations. A suprapubic resection, where the prostate is removed from around the urethra via the bladder, is performed when the prostate mass is large. When a retropubic prostatectomy is performed, the bladder is not opened but instead retracted and prostatic tissue is removed through an incision in the anterior prostatic capsule. Both of these alternatives involve an abdominal incision (see Figure 32-4). In a perineal prostatectomy, a perineal incision is made and the prostatic tissue is removed through an incision in the posterior postatic capsule.

While these traditional surgeries successfully relieve bladder obstruction, they are costly and postoperative complications can endanger or seriously affect the quality of a man's life. These complications include hemorrhage, water intoxication, infection, thrombosis, damage to surrounding structures, sexual dysfunction, and urinary incontinence.

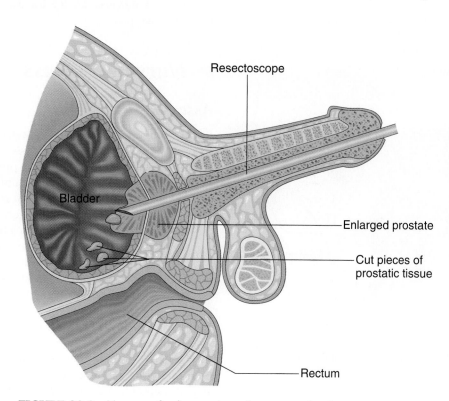

FIGURE 32-3 Transurethral resection of prostate gland via resectoscope.

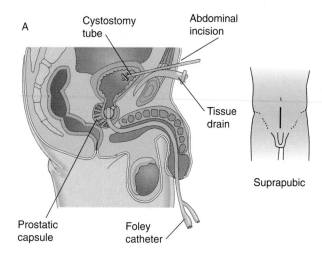

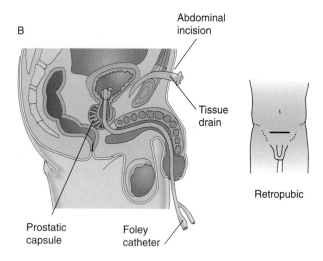

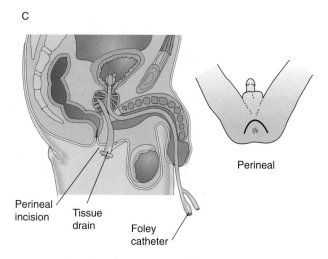

FIGURE 32-4 Three types of prostatectomies: **(A)** Suprapubic; **(B)** Retropubic; **(C)** Perineal.

Laser prostatectomy, the most recently developed surgical intervention for BPH, is based on thermal action. The transurethral ultrasound-guided laser induced prostatectomy (TULIP) is performed with a probe that is passed transurethrally into the prostatic urethra. While the adjacent prostate area is visualized via ultrasound, the laser energy is directed at the prostate tissue, resulting in tissue necrosis and sloughing. The procedure is easy and quick to perform, however, the large amount of sloughing tissue necessitates having an indwelling catheter to facilitate bladder drainage for several weeks. The client is less likely to experience water intoxication because this surgical method allows blood vessels to seal rapidly, keeping irrigant fluid from being forced into the circulation. Although this procedure is relatively new, thus far client outcomes appear to be positive.

▶ *Pharmacological*

A pharmacological intervention that has been successfully used to treat BPH is the use of alpha blockers. These drugs are thought to decrease the resistance along the urinary tract without compromising normal urinary control reflexes. Because the use of the alpha blockers terazosin hydrochloride (Hytrin) and doxazosin mesylate (Cardura) has been shown to be safe and provided men with improved urinary function, they offer a treatment alternative for BPH other than the traditional surgery. Belladonna and opium (B & O) suppositories are used to reduce postoperative bladder spasms and narcotic analgesics are used to relieve postoperative pain.

▶ *Nursing Process*

Assessment

Subjective Data Urinary patterns are the primary focus of a preoperative nursing assessment of a client with BPH. Ask the client about the presence of urinary frequency, hesitancy, dribbling, number of times he gets up at night to void, and the force of the urinary stream. In addition to a careful general medical history, any information pertaining to a history of chronic urinary tract infections needs to be noted.

Postoperative nursing assessment should include assessing for pain related to bladder spasms. This data can be objectified by incorporating the use of a pain scale, which allows the client to rate his pain by using a scale of 1 to 10. The client's emotional needs should also be assessed as he may be experiencing anticipatory grieving, body image disturbance, anxiety, or concerns about alteration in sexuality patterns or possible sexual dysfunction. Assess for any behavioral or verbal cues from the client that may indicate a need for further information or reassurance regarding his condition and related treatment.

Objective Data When assessing for hemorrhagic shock or postoperative infection, monitor vital signs, avoiding the use of a rectal thermometer. A bright red urine color persisting for more than a few hours after surgery may be a sign of hemorrhage. Hemorrhage, hyperthermia, hypotension (low blood pressure), and tachycardia should be reported to the physician immediately. (See Chapter 20 for further information on cardiac disorders.)

Following a TURP, the client will have a three-way Foley catheter and continuous bladder irrigation (see Figure 32-5) for at least twenty-four hours. After the catheter is removed, monitor for bladder distention by palpating the bladder, doing post void catheterizations, or assessing with a bladder volume indicator (BVI). A bladder volume indicator is an ultrasonic device that can be used to measure the amount of post void residual in the bladder. Intake and output will also need to be monitored to ensure that the client has adequate oral intake to promote urinary flow and reduce the infection risk. When measuring output, the amount of irrigant must be subtracted from the total output in order to determine the actual urinary output. After the catheter is removed, the client should be assessed for post void residual and incontinence. This can be accomplished by using a BVI to measure post void residual, palpating the abdomen for bladder distention, checking the bed linens and clothing for signs of incontinence, or asking the client if he is experiencing loss of urinary control.

It is important for the nurse to assess for water intoxication, which may be the result of absorbing irrigating fluid in addition to the IV fluids. The most common early symptoms of water intoxication are changes in the client's mental status. These may be manifested by agitation, confusion and later, convulsions. The client may also have a slow bounding pulse with an increase in systolic and decrease in diastolic blood pressure.

A suprapubic or retropubic prostatectomy does not require a three-way Foley. Instead the client will have a urethral catheter, a tissue drain from the prostatic

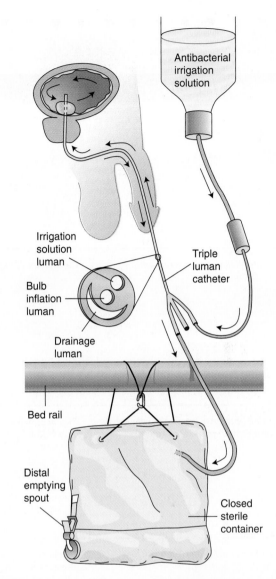

FIGURE 32-5 Continuous bladder irrigation set-up used for transurethral resection of the prostate (TURP).

fossa and an abdominal dressing (refer to Figure 32-4). The nurse needs to assess for incisional pain and do a dressing check, being careful to also check the linens underneath the client's back.

▼ ▼

Possible nursing diagnoses for a client with benign prostatic hypertrophy may include:

Nursing Diagnoses	Goals	Nursing Interventions
▶ *Urinary retention, acute, related to obstruction secondary to TURP.*	The client will avoid urinary retention.	Monitor the client's urinary output, noting the amount, color, and presence of clots. After twenty-four hours, the urine should be a light pink color. Increase rate of flow of the bladder irrigant if the urine has clots, a darker color, or decreased output. Monitor the client's intake; encourage a fluid intake of 2500 to 3000 mL/day.
▶ *Pain related to bladder spasms or incision.*	The client will experience minimal pain.	Maintain traction on the urethral catheter by anchoring the catheter to the leg with tape, taking care that accidental additional traction will not occur with leg movement. Monitor for bladder spasm pain and administer analgesics and antispasmodics as ordered. Instruct the client not to void around the catheter, even though the presence of the catheter produces a sensation of fullness.
▶ *Injury, high risk for, due to hemorrhage or infection, related to surgery.*	The client will experience minimal bleeding and avoid infection.	Monitor the client's vital signs and incisional drainage. Report hyperthermia, tachycardia, hypotension, or increased incisional drainage to the physician immediately. Maintain strict asepsis when handling urinary drainage, wound drains, and dressings.
▶ *Fluid volume excess, high risk for, related to postoperative irrigation.*	The client will not experience water intoxication.	Monitor for changes in the client's behavior, especially confusion and agitation which may be the first signs of cerebral edema. Monitor for hypertension, bradycardia, weakness, and seizures.
▶ *Incontinence, stress or urge, related to catheter removal following surgery.*	The client will achieve urinary control following removal of the catheter.	Advise the client that temporary urinary incontinence frequently occurs following surgery, and reassure him that this is normal. Teach the client perineal exercises which will help him regain urinary control. These exercises consist of tightening and relaxing gluteal muscles, such as with the **Kegel exercise.**
▶ *Knowledge deficit, related to surgery and postoperative care.*	The client will demonstrate understanding of postoperative activity restrictions and medical follow-up.	Teach the client that vigorous exercise and heavy lifting should be avoided for three to four weeks. Instruct the client to avoid straining at stool and to use stool softeners or mild cathartics as ordered. Encourage the client to maintain a fluid intake of 2500 to 3000 mL/day. Instruct the client to report any bleeding or diminished urinary stream to the physician.

Nursing Diagnoses	Goals	Nursing Interventions
▶ *Sexual dysfunction, high risk for, related to surgery.*	The client will maintain sexual function postoperatively.	Monitor client's statements to determine if he has any misunderstanding of the surgery and sexual function.
		Provide the client with opportunities to voice his feelings and ask questions.
		Reassure the client that impotency can be a complication of a radical perineal prostatectomy, but does not occur with the other types of prostatectomies.
▶ *Anxiety, high risk for, related to surgery.*	The client will experience minimal anxiety about pending surgery.	Provide the client with information about the operative procedure, postoperative and discharge care. When available, a video may be used to present this information. Be available to answer the client's questions.
▶ *Anticipatory grieving related to surgery.*	The client will maintain a positive attitude about his recovery or seek appropriate counseling if this goal is not achieved.	Monitor the client's statements and behaviors that indicate concern about loss of masculinity, anger, or sadness. Be sensitive to the client's feelings and concerns.
		Provide the client with opportunities to express these.
		Be alert for signs that the client is not resolving these issues and suggest counseling as necessary.
▶ *Sexuality patterns, altered, high risk for, related to surgery.*	The client will maintain his usual sexuality patterns.	Instruct the client to avoid sexual intercourse for three to four weeks postoperatively and that it may take time for his previous level of sexual function to return.
		Advise the client that it is normal and not harmful if his urine has a milky appearance due to retrograde ejaculation.

▶ Evaluation

Each goal must be evaluated to determine how it has been met by the client.

▲ ▲

▶ MALIGNANT NEOPLASMS

The majority of male reproductive tract tumors are malignant and involve the testes, prostate gland and penis. Usually by the time these tumors are detected they have metastasized. For early detection and improved survival rate, men must become educated about the importance of routine medical examinations.

▶ PROSTATE CANCER

Prostate cancer is the second most prevalent type of cancer in men and appears to have a familial ten-

dency. In 1994, 200,000 men were diagnosed with the disorder and 38,000 men died (Twillie, et al., 1994) Although prostate cancer is more common in males over the age of fifty, it is much more lethal in younger men. The encouraging news is that improved detection methods have greatly increased the number of individuals having positive outcomes. Diagnostic tests that may be performed are measurement of serum prostate specific antigen (PSA), transrectal ultrasonic examination, and prostatic biopsy. Studies indicate that the use of the PSA for routine screening is not necessarily useful due to the number of false positive levels reported in men with BPH and the false negative levels in men with prostate cancer. Therefore, the most useful screening method continues to be a rectal examination, which all men over the age of forty should have annually.

Changes in urinary patterns are often the earliest signs of prostate cancer. These changes include frequency, urgency, and nocturia. Later symptoms are related to complete urethral obstruction or hematuria. Blood in the urine (**hematuria**), which can lead to anemia, occurs due to the rupture of blood vessels that have been overstretched.

▶ Medical/Surgical Management

▶ Medical

Radiation is the traditional alternative to surgical removal of the malignant prostate gland. However, radiation may fail to eradicate the tumor or may lead to diarrhea, bowel obstruction, lymphocele formation, edema of the extremities, pulmonary embolism, wound infections, infection, impotence, incontinence, or radiation cystitis. An alternative successful radiation treatment option for early stage prostate cancer is transrectal assisted radioactive seed implant. With the use of ultrasound, the physician is able to precisely position the rice-sized radioactive seeds inside the malignant prostate gland. During the first five years of clinical trials, 91 percent of the men remained disease-free and their PSA level remained normal (Wolcott, 1995). In addition, the men have reported no incontinence and the impotency rate is less than half that reported with traditional surgical treatment.

▶ Surgical

Surgical treatment of prostatic cancer involves removal of the entire prostate gland, including the capsule and adjacent tissue. The urethra is then anastomosed to the bladder neck. Sometimes the retropubic approach is used, but the usual approach is perineal where the incision is made between the scrotum and the rectum. Because of the proximity of the bladder sphincters to the prostate gland, urinary incontinence may be a complication. Other complications include sexual dysfunction and the universal surgical risks of hemorrhage, infection, thrombosis, and strictures. Removal of the testes (**orchiectomy**) may also be done as a palliative measure to help eliminate the androgenic effect that promotes tumor growth.

Another surgical alternative is cryosurgical ablation. This method was used in the 1960s but abandoned due to the complications of tissue sloughing and fistula development. With the advent of the transrectal ultrasound and the transurethral warming device, cryosurgery has become a more viable alternative. The ultrasound allows the surgeon to selectively freeze prostate gland tissue while the temperature of the prostatic urethra is kept at 44°C by irrigation with heated water. This surgical approach is an option for those who cannot tolerate more extensive surgery, have a localized tumor, or do not have successful radiation treatment. It can be performed more than once, involves a shorter hospital stay, and produces fewer side effects.

▶ Pharmacological

Other treatment options include chemotherapy, hormones, and corticosteroids. Early reports indicate that adjuvant treatment with an antimetabolite, interleukin-6 may significantly reduce the morbidity and improve the quality for men treated surgically. Palliative treatments include estrogen therapy with diethylstilbestrol (DES), a female hormone, and luteinizing hormone-releasing-hormone, LHRH (Factrel), agonists. These treatments are used to eliminate or suppress the androgenic effect that promotes tumor growth. If there are metastases to the bone, corticosteroids may be used for bone pain.

▶ Nursing Process

Assessment

Subjective Data When prostate cancer is suspected, a complete medical history needs to be obtained. Providing an opportunity for the client to discuss any perceived threat of altered body or sexual function will help the nurse identify his educational and emotional needs. These assessments are important because the client's anxiety is likely to increase when he does not have adequate information concerning his condition and treatment options. He needs to describe the location and nature of his pain or any other related symptoms such as weight loss, changes in bowel or bladder function, and the color of his urine. Postoperatively the client needs to be asked about pain, using a pain scale to objectify data.

Objective Data The client needs a complete physical assessment that includes palpation of the abdomen and skin assessment. The abdomen is palpated to determine if there is any bladder distention. Skin assessment is important when incontinence or catheter patency is a problem because the client is at risk for skin breakdown. If he has a perineal prostatectomy, he will return from surgery with an indwelling urethral catheter and possibly an ostomy bag around the incisional dressing (refer to Figure 32-4). It is not unusual for the client to have a large amount of urinary drainage at the incision site for several hours postoperatively, which is the reason for an ostomy bag. Assess vital signs, the incisional site, intake and output.

Hyperthermia, hypotension, tachycardia, or increased incisional drainage should be reported to the physician immediately.

Because the catheter is used to maintain urinary drainage and as a splint for the urethral anastomosis rather than for hemostasis, there are minimal bladder spasms. However, the catheter is subject to blockage and dislodgement especially during the first hour, so it is important to maintain a patent catheter and not have tension on the catheter. Patency of the catheter can be monitored by assessing the drainage for color, amount, and presence of clots. If the tubing is not draining freely, reposition or milk the tubing. The nurse should call the physician if these measure fail to restore patency. During the first week of the postoperative period the client also needs to be monitored for fecal incontinence related to relaxation of the perineal sphincter. This is a complication that occurs when a perineal surgical approach is used because the incision is made between the scrotum and the rectum.

▼ ▼

Possible nursing diagnoses for a client with prostate cancer may include:

Nursing Diagnoses	Goals	Nursing Interventions
▶ Urinary retention, acute, high risk for, related to urethral obstruction, secondary to urethral anastomosis.	The client will not experience urinary retention.	Monitor the client's urinary output, noting the amount, color, and presence of clots. The urine should not appear bright red for more than a few hours postoperatively, after which time it should be dark red.

Reposition or milk the catheter tubing if not patent. If these interventions fail, notify the physician.

Monitor the client's intake, encouraging a fluid intake of 2500 to 3000 mL/day. |
| ▶ Pain, related to incision. | The client will experience minimal incisional pain. | Monitor for incisional pain.

Administer analgesics as ordered. |
| ▶ Injury, high risk for, due to hemorrhage or infection related to surgery. | The client will experience minimal bleeding and avoid infection. | Monitor the client's vital signs and incisional drainage. Report hyperthermia, tachycardia, hypotension, or increased incisional drainage to the physician immediately.

Avoid the use of rectal thermometers, rectal examinations, and enemas.

Advise the client to avoid the Valsalva maneuver.

Maintain strict asepsis when handling urinary drainage, wound drains, and dressings. |
| ▶ Incontinence, functional, related to bladder sphincter trauma. | The client will achieve urinary control following removal of the catheter. | Advise the client that temporary urinary incontinence frequently occurs following surgery, and reassure him that this is normal.

Teach the client perineal exercises that will help him regain urinary control. These exercises consist of tightening and relaxing perineal and gluteal muscles and can be performed in a variety of ways. One example is the Kegel exercise. |
| ▶ Incontinence, bowel, related to relaxation of the perineal musculature. | The client will achieve perineal musculature control. | Advise the client that temporary fecal incontinence frequently occurs following a perineal incision.

Teach the client perineal exercises that will help him regain bowel control. |

(continued)

Nursing Diagnoses	Goals	Nursing Interventions
▶ *Skin integrity, impaired, high risk for, related to incontinence.*	The client will not experience skin breakdown.	Keep the client clean and dry, especially if he is experiencing fecal or urinary incontinence. Monitor the ostomy bag for leakage.
▶ *Sexual dysfunction, high risk for, related to surgery.*	The client will maintain sexual function postoperatively.	Monitor statements made by the client to determine his understanding of the surgery and sexual function.
		Provide the client with opportunities to voice his feelings and ask questions.
		Reassure the client that impotency can be a complication of a radical perineal prostatectomy, but does not occur with the other types of prostatectomies.
▶ *Knowledge deficit, related to surgery and postoperative care.*	The client will demonstrate understanding of postoperative activity restrictions and medical follow-up.	Teach the client that vigorous exercise and heavy lifting should be avoided for three to four weeks.
		Instruct the client to avoid straining at stool and to use stool softeners or mild cathartics as ordered.
		Encourage the client to maintain a fluid intake of 2500 to 3000 mL/day.
		Instruct the client to report any bleeding or a diminished urinary stream to the physician.
▶ *Anxiety, high risk for, related to diagnosis.*	The client will experience minimal anxiety.	Provide the client with information about the operative procedure, postoperative and discharge care. When available, a video may be used to present this information, with the nurse being available to answer the client's questions.

▶ Evaluation

Each goal must be evaluated to determine how it has been met by the client.

▲ ▲

▶ TESTICULAR CANCER

Although testicular cancer occurs at a relatively low rate, it is the most common form of cancer in young men between the ages of fifteen and thirty-five. The incidence is higher in men with undescended testicles (cryptorchidism). The number of whites diagnosed with testicular cancer has more than doubled since the 1930s. With improved treatment methods, the cure rate has increased to over 90 percent in 1994 (Martini, 1994). The most common form of testicular cancer is seminoma.

Symptoms of testicular cancer include painless enlarged testis and **gynecomastia** (enlargement of breast tissue). Because early diagnosis of testicular cancer is so essential for a positive surgical outcome, young men need to be taught how to perform a testicular self-examination (TSE) and be encouraged to routinely perform that examination (see Figure 32-6).

TSE is performed as follows:

- Perform TSE after a bath or shower when scrotum is warm and most relaxed.
- Grasp testis with both hands and palpate gently between thumbs and forefingers.
- The testis should feel smooth, egg-shaped, and firm to the touch.
- The epididymis, located behind the testis, should feel like a soft tube.
- Any abnormal lumps or changes in the testes should be reported to a physician.

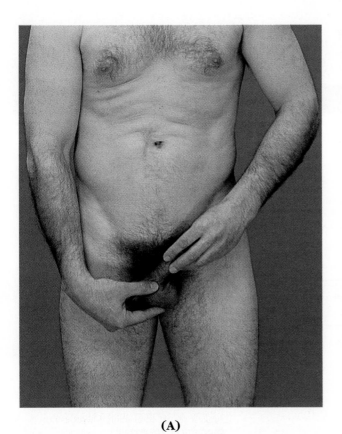
(A)

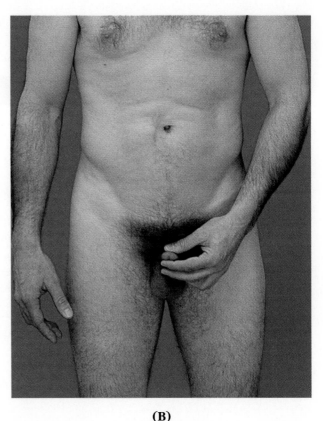
(B)

FIGURE 32-6 Performing a testicular self-exam.

▶ Medical/Surgical Management

▶ Medical

In addition to a testicular ultrasound, the client may have a serum acid or alkaline phosphatase test done. They are both elevated in malignancies. Testicular ultrasound is used to study the testes for enlargement or lesions.

▶ Surgical

Biopsy of the testis is contraindicated because of the increased potential for metastases. Removal of the testis with examination of the nodes, is indicated instead. If unilateral removal of a testis is indicated, the remaining healthy testis will continue to maintain sperm and androgen production. Surgical removal of the testis, spermatic cord, and inguinal canal contents, with examination of the nodes, is indicated for testicular cancers.

▶ Pharmacological

While chemotherapy and radiation are used as adjuvant treatments, radical inguinal orchiectomy remains the primary intervention. Combination chemotherapy with cisplatin (Platinol), vinblastine sulfate (Velban) and bleomycin sulfate (Blenoxane) is effective.

▶ Nursing Process

Assessment

Subjective Data Listen carefully as the client describes his pain. He may describe a feeling of heaviness in the scrotum. Ask about weight loss. During the postoperative phase, the client needs to be assessed for pain, using a pain scale to objectify data. He also needs to have emotional and educational needs assessed. For example, the client should be able to accurately describe his activity restrictions and how to provide scrotal support postoperatively. His behaviors and statements need to be monitored for signs of anxiety or depression.

Objective Data Physical examination should include palpation of the abdomen and assessment of the scrotum. Positive findings in the scrotum include a firm, painless mass in the testis and an enlarged scrotum. As gynecomastia is another symptom of testicular cancer, the client's breast tissue should be assessed for enlargement. Postoperative assessment includes monitoring vital signs to detect signs of hemorrhage or infection. Also, the incisional site should be monitored for excess drainage, swelling, or redness.

▼ ▼

Possible nursing diagnoses for the client with testicular cancer may include:

Nursing Diagnoses	Goals	Nursing Interventions
▶ *Injury, high risk for, due to infection and hemorrhage related to surgery.*	The client will experience minimal bleeding and avoid infection.	Monitor the client's vital signs and incisional drainage. Report hyperthermia, tachycardia, hypotension, increased incisional drainage, and swelling or redness around the incision to the physician immediately. Maintain strict asepsis when handling wound dressings.
▶ *Fluid volume excess, related to surgery.*	The client will experience minimal scrotal swelling.	Monitor for incisional pain. Administer analgesics as ordered.
▶ *Pain, related to the incision.*	The client will experience minimal incisional pain.	Apply ice to and elevate the scrotum on a towel to help reduce edema.
▶ *Body image disturbance, high risk for, related to surgery.*	The client will maintain a positive body image.	Provide the client with opportunities to voice his concerns and ask questions. Monitor the client for statements and behaviors that indicate concern about loss of masculinity. Suggest sexual counseling if he does not appear to be resolving these issues. Advise the client that unilateral removal of a testis will not cause him to be sterile or demasculinized.
▶ *Knowledge deficit, related to surgery and postoperative care.*	The client will demonstrate understanding of postoperative activity restrictions and medical follow-up.	Advise the client that he needs to be on bed rest for twelve to twenty-four hours postoperatively. Instruct the client to wear tight fitting underwear or an athletic supporter when ambulating and avoid heavy lifting for four to six weeks.
▶ *Anxiety, high risk for, related to diagnosis.*	The client will experience minimal anxiety.	Provide the client with information about the operative procedure, postoperative and discharge care. When available, a video may be used to present this information, with the nurse being available to answer the client's questions.

▶ Evaluation

Each goal must be evaluated to determine how it has been met by the client.

▲ ▲

▶ PENILE CANCER

Penile cancer is rare and has a high correlation with poor hygiene and delayed or no circumcision. The bacteria harbored in the foreskin of the uncircumcised male are irritants to the glans penis and the prepuce. The chronic nature of this irritation is thought to be carcinogenic. Males with a history of STDs are also predisposed to developing penile cancer. Symptoms of penile cancer include a painless, nodular growth on the foreskin, fatigue, and weight loss. Unfortunately, metastases are common with this form of cancer.

▶ Medical/Surgical Management

▶ Medical

The primary penile cancer treatment is surgery. Treatment with radiation alone is ineffective and chemotherapy alone is used only for palliative treatment of penile cancer with deep distant metastases. However, the client may receive adjuvant therapy with either radiation or chemotherapy.

▶ Surgical

If the tumor is not extensive and no metastases are involved, the remaining penis should be long enough for the client to void standing and avoid soiling himself. If a penectomy is necessary, the urethra will be redirected to an opening between the scrotum and the anus (**urethrostomy**).

▶ Nursing Process

Assessment

Subjective Data Although the tumor is painless, the client should be asked if he is experiencing any pain, to rule out other possible diagnoses. The client also needs to be asked if he is experiencing fatigue or weight loss. Preoperatively, the client needs an assessment of his emotional and educational needs. He needs to be asked questions that can be used to determine his understanding of the surgical procedure and the need for counseling. Postoperative assessment also includes monitoring for pain, using a pain scale to objectify data.

Objective Data The client needs a physical assessment that includes inspection of the penis for the presence of painless, nodular growths. During the postoperative phase, monitoring of his vital signs, incisional site, intake and output must be done. Hypotension, tachycardia, excessive incisional drainage, redness or swelling around the incision, bright red or low urinary output could be signs of complications.

▼ ▼

Possible nursing diagnoses for a client with penile cancer may include:

Nursing Diagnoses	Goals	Nursing Interventions
▶ *Injury, high risk for, due to infection and hemorrhage related to surgery.*	The client will experience minimal bleeding and avoid infection.	Monitor the client's vital signs and incisional drainage.
		Report hyperthermia, tachycardia, hypotension, increased incisional drainage, and swelling or redness around the incision to the physician immediately.
		Maintain strict asepsis when handling wound dressings.
▶ *Pain, related to the incision.*	The client will experience minimal incisional pain.	Monitor for incisional pain.
		Administer analgesics as ordered.
▶ *Body image disturbance, related to surgery.*	The client will maintain a positive body image.	Provide the client with opportunities to voice his concerns and ask questions.
		Keep in mind the typically young age of the client and the associated self-image and sexuality issues.

(continued)

Nursing Diagnoses	Goals	Nursing Interventions
		Monitor the client for statements and behaviors that indicate he is concerned about loss of masculinity. Suggest sexual counseling if he does not appear to be resolving these issues.
▶ Anxiety, related to surgery.	The client will experience minimal anxiety.	Provide the client with information about the operative procedure, postoperative and discharge care. When available, a video may be used to present this information, with the nurse being available to answer the client's questions.
▶ Knowledge deficit, related to surgery and postoperative care.	The client will list the postoperative activity restrictions and medical follow-up.	Advise the client that if he is able to void while standing, direct the stream and not void on himself, that sexual function will probably be retained. Advise the client with a penectomy that with stimulation of the perineal, scrotal and testicular regions, some men are able to experience orgasm and ejaculation.
▶ Sexuality patterns, altered, related to the surgery.	The client will maintain normal sexuality patterns postoperatively.	Advise the client to seek sexual counseling for both himself and his partner if he is unable to maintain normal sexuality patterns.
▶ Urinary elimination, altered patterns, related to surgery.	The client will achieve urinary control postoperatively.	Monitor the client's intake and output. Report low urinary output to the physician immediately.

▶ Evaluation

Each goal must be evaluated to determine how it has been met by the client.

▲ ▲

▶ BREAST CANCER

While males may have gynecomastia of breast tissue as a result of puberty, older age, or medications, breast cancer in the male is an uncommon disorder. Because it is so uncommon, breast cancer in men is all the more dangerous since it is not considered a threat. Late diagnosis is quite common; therefore, males need to be educated in the technique of and encouraged to do self-breast examinations (SBE). Signs and symptoms of breast cancer include breast lumps, pain, or discharge from the nipple.

▶ Medical/Surgical Management

▶ Medical

The primary form of treatment is surgery. Adjuvant therapy with radiation and chemotherapy are also indicated.

▶ Surgical

Removal of the tumor is indicated. The surgery may be limited to the tumor or more extensive based on whether there are metastases involved.

▶ Nursing Process

Assessment

Subjective Data Preoperatively, assess the client's emotional and educational needs. Preoperatively and postoperatively, assess for pain, using a pain scale to objectify data.

Objective Data Examine the breasts for lumps and discharge from the nipples. During the postoperative phase the nurse needs to assess the client's vital signs and incisional site. Also monitor the client's statements and behaviors to determine his emotional status.

▼ ▼

Possible nursing diagnoses for the male client with breast cancer may include:

Nursing Diagnoses	Goals	Nursing Interventions
▶ *Injury, high risk for, due to hemorrhage and infection related to the surgery.*	The client will experience minimal bleeding and avoid infection.	Monitor the client's vital signs and incisional drainage. Report hyperthermia, tachycardia, hypotension, increased incisional drainage, and swelling or redness around the incision to the physician immediately. Maintain strict asepsis when handling wound dressings.
▶ *Pain, related to the incision.*	The client will experience minimal incisional pain.	Monitor for incisional pain. Administer analgesics as ordered.
▶ *Knowledge deficit, related to the surgery.*	The client will demonstrate understanding of postoperative medical follow-up.	Provide the client with information concerning any follow-up treatments such as radiation or chemotherapy.

▶ Evaluation

Each goal must be evaluated to determine how it has been met by the client.

▲ ▲

▶ INFLAMMATORY DISORDERS

▶ EPIDIDYMITIS

Epididymitis can be a sterile or nonsterile inflammation of the epididymis. A sterile inflammation may be caused by direct injury or reflux of urine down the vas deferens. Urinary reflux that is related to strain exerted by a male while his bladder is full, can be caused by lifting heavy objects or doing strenuous exercises. Nonsterile inflammation may occur as a complication of gonorrhea, chlamydia, mumps, tuberculosis, prostatitis, or urethritis. Prolonged use of an indwelling catheter or an invasive procedure can also lead to nonsterile inflammation.

Signs and symptoms of epididymitis include sudden, severe pain in the scrotum, scrotal swelling, fever, dysuria, and pyuria. Treatment includes bed rest, antibiotics, scrotal support, and ice compresses to the area. Bilateral epididymitis can cause sterility. Untreated epididymitis leads quickly to testicular tissue necrosis, septicemia, and death.

▶ ORCHITIS

Orchitis is an inflammation of the testes that most often occurs as a complication of a bloodborne infection originating in the epididymis. Other causes of orchitis include gonorrhea, trauma, surgical manipulation, and tuberculosis and mumps that occur after puberty. In most instances, both testes are involved, which often results in sterility. In orchitis, unilateral involvement does not cause sterility. Orchitis signs and symptoms include sudden scrotal pain with pain radiating to the inguinal canal, scrotal edema, chills, fever, nausea, and vomiting. Treatment includes bed rest, scrotal support, and ice to the area.

▶ PROSTATITIS

Prostatitis, an inflammation of the prostate, is a common complication of urethritis caused by chlamydia or gonorrhea. Infecting organisms may reach the genital tract by direct spread through the urethra or be borne by blood or lymph. The condition may be acute or chronic with the chronic form leading to development of fibrotic tissue. This fibrotic tissue causes the prostate to harden, so prostatitis may be difficult to differentiate from prostate cancer. It may take three to six months for the granulomatous form to resolve. Signs and symptoms of prostatitis include perineal pain, fever, dysuria, and urethral discharge.

▶ Medical/Surgical Management

▶ Medical

When it is suspected that the client currently has urethritis, he should not be catheterized because the infection spreads rapidly to the genital organs. This is due to the trauma of catheterization and possible spread of bacteria from the nonsterile distal part of the urethra. The physician may order that segmented bacteriologic localization cultures be obtained.

▶ Activity

Treatment of prostatitis includes bed rest. While the client is in bed, his scrotum should be elevated and cold packs applied to the area. The client should be encouraged to drink a large amount of fluids and use sitz baths for comfort. These interventions are used to reduce inflammation, swelling, and discomfort. Periodic digital massage of the prostate by the physician increases the flow of infected prostatic secretions.

▶ Pharmacological

Pharmacological treatment of prostatitis includes antibiotics, analgesics, and stool softeners. Treatment of epididymitis and orchitis includes antibiotics and injection of procaine around the spermatic cord.

▶ Nursing Process

Assessment

Subjective Data Question the client about the presence of urethral discharge or dysuria as well as the nature and location of his pain. Complaints of pain may include arthralgia, low back pain, and myalgia. In addition, a careful medical history should be obtained. A positive history of recent bacterial or viral infection is of special significance. Ongoing nursing assessment should include monitoring for pain, using a pain scale to objectify data. Ask the client if he is experiencing nausea, as this could be a sign that his condition is deteriorating. The client also needs an assessment of his educational and emotional needs as he may be worrying needlessly about possible sterility or impotence.

Objective Data Monitor the client's vital signs, especially his temperature. An increase in temperature may be an indicator that the client's condition is worsening. Assess the client for scrotal edema and purulent urethral discharge. Intake and output need to be monitored. The client also needs to be monitored for constipation.

▼ ▼

Possible nursing diagnoses for the male client with an inflammatory disorder may include:

Nursing Diagnoses	*Goals*	*Nursing Interventions*
▶ *Injury, high risk for, related to worsening of the inflammatory process.*	The client will not experience worsening of his condition.	Monitor the client's vital signs, especially his temperature.
		Monitor the client for signs of nausea, as this could be a sign that his condition is deteriorating.
		Report hyperthermia, hypotension, nausea, and tachycardia to the physician immediately.
▶ *Fluid volume deficit, related to nausea and vomiting.*	The client will maintain fluid balance.	Monitor the client's intake and output and encourage him to drink plenty of fluids.
▶ *Pain, acute, related to inflammation.*	The client will experience minimal pain.	Monitor for pain.
		Administer analgesics as ordered.
		Encourage the client to maintain bed rest.

Nursing Diagnoses	Goals	Nursing Interventions
		Provide diversional activities to increase compliance.
		Encourage the client with prostatitis to take a sitz bath, but never the client with epididymitis or orchitis as local heat may increase destruction of sperm cells. Fill a plastic glove with crushed ice and place it under the scrotum when heat is contra-indicated. Remove the ice for short intervals every hour to prevent ice burns.
▶ Constipation, high risk for, related to bed rest and analgesics.	The client will maintain normal bowel habits.	Encourage the client to drink plenty of fluids.
		Administer stool softeners as ordered.
▶ Fluid volume excess, high risk for, related to the inflammatory process.	The client will not experience scrotal swelling.	Encourage the client to maintain bed rest and to elevate the scrotum. A folded towel can be placed under the scrotum with adhesive or strapping (**Bellevue bridge**, as seen in Figure 32-7).
▶ Knowledge deficit, related to condition and treatment regimen.	The client will be able to identify behaviors that may predispose him to these disorders.	Educate the client about behaviors that may predispose him to prostatitis. Provide information about "safe sex" and the use of condoms to reduce his risk of contracting STDs.
	The client will demonstrate understanding of the importance of finishing his antibiotics.	Advise about the importance of finishing his antibiotics.
▶ Anxiety, related to concerns about possible sterility or impotence.	The client will experience minimal anxiety.	Reassure the client that with proper treatment, sterility and impotence are not likely complications of prostatitis.

▶ Evaluation

Each goal must be evaluated to determine how it has been met by the client.

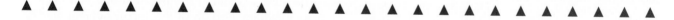

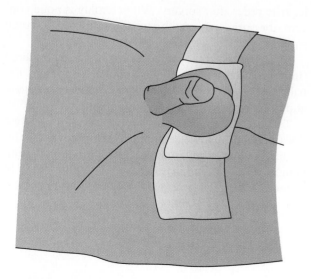

FIGURE 32-7 A Bellevue bridge.

▶ STRUCTURAL DISORDERS

▶ CRYPTORCHIDISM

Cryptorchidism is a condition where one or both testicles fail to descend into the scrotum by the time of birth. The cause is usually unknown. Decrease or loss of sperm production may occur because of the damage that occurs to the seminiferous epithelium. When the testes are within the normal path and do not descend or cannot be pulled into the scrotum, surgery (orchiopexy) is usually done between five to seven years of age. Even with the corrective surgery, as adults, these males have a ten to thirty times higher incidence of testicular cancer.

▶ *HYDROCELE*

A hydrocele is a benign, nontender collection of clear amber fluid within the space of the testes and the tunica vaginalis or along the spermatic cord. This collection of fluid may result in scrotal swelling, which can be painful if it develops suddenly. Inflammation of the epididymis or testis or a lymphatic or venous obstruction may cause this condition. Congenital hydrocele in the newborn occurs when the canal between the peritoneal cavity and the scrotum does not close completely during fetal development. Aspiration of the fluid serves only as a temporary measure and can lead to secondary infection. Therefore, treatment for the condition is surgery.

▶ *HYPOSPADIAS AND EPISPADIAS*

Hypospadias is an abnormal placement of the urethral opening on the ventral surface of the penis. Epispadias is the opening of the urethra on the dorsal surface of the penis. The treatment is determined by the position of the urethra on the penis. Infants with either condition should not be circumcised before a urology consultation is obtained, as the foreskin is used in the repair.

▶ *SPERMATOCELE*

A spermatocele is a benign nontender cyst of either the epididymis or the rete testis. It contains milky fluid and sperm. Usually this condition is painless and does not require medical treatment.

▶ *VARICOCELE*

A varicocele is dilation of the veins of the scrotum that occurs when the venous system that drains the testicle lengthens and enlarges. This dilation occurs when incompetent or absent valves in the spermatic venous system permit blood to accumulate, resulting in increased hydrostatic pressure. This condition is more commonly found on the left side because of the increased retrograde pressure of the renal vein, the length, and fewer competent valves. It is theorized that the hyperthermia that occurs with this condition decreases spermatogenesis, resulting in decreased fertility. Symptoms may include a bluish discoloration of the scrotal skin or palpation of a wormlike mass when the male bears down. These seldom require treatment.

▶ *TORSION OF THE SPERMATIC CORD*

Torsion of the spermatic cord occurs when the vascular pedicle of the testis twists, resulting in partial or complete venous occlusion. The three forms of this disorder are (1) rotation of the spermatic cord, (2) torsion of a testicular appendage, or (3) torsion of the spermatic cord and epididymis. Testicular torsion may be related to recent trauma, and the onset of symptoms often occurs quite suddenly. Symptoms of testicular torsion may include abdominal and scrotal pain, scrotal edema, nausea and vomiting and, possibly, a slight fever. The pain caused by testicular torsion is not relieved by bed rest or scrotal support.

▶ *Medical/Surgical Management*

Medical/surgical management of male structural disorders is specific to the condition. Cryptorchidism may be treated with hormonal therapy. If this is not successful, surgery should be done within the first eighteen months of life, in order to avoid possible sterility. In some newborns a hydrocele may resolve without medical intervention. Clients of all ages may have aspiration performed to reduce the swelling caused by fluid or a hematoma. However, this solution is usually only temporary, while surgical removal of the sac provides the only permanent solution to the problem. While a spermatocele usually does not require treatment, sometimes surgical aspiration or excision is necessary.

Because a common complication of a varicocele is male infertility, ligation of the spermatic vein may be performed if infertility is a concern. Sometimes this does not resolve infertility problems because varicoceles may recur after surgery. When fertility is not a concern, the varicocele may be treated simply with scrotal support.

Hypospadias and epispadias are surgically repaired (urethroplasty) before the child is one year of age. Usually, successful repair requires more than one surgery and often results in scarring of the penis.

Torsion of the spermatic cord is one disorder that does require immediate surgery to remove the infarcted testis and minimize possible reaction to antigenic sperm, which may lead to infertility. Also of concern is the high potential for hemorrhagic necrosis.

▶ Nursing Process

Assessment

Subjective Data Diagnostic assessment for all structural disorders should include asking the client about the type and location of his pain. He should also be asked about related symptoms such as alteration in urinary patterns, warmth, fatigue, nausea, or vomiting. Postoperative assessments include monitoring for pain and using a pain scale to objectify data. The client's knowledge of his condition, treatment, and follow-up care also need to be assessed. Ask about the implications of sterility and impotence to the client's life.

Objective Data Physical assessment should include inspection and palpation of the genitals to detect presence of swelling or skin changes. Assess for scrotal swelling, testicular enlargement, scrotal immobility, redness and warmth of the scrotum. Small varicoceles may be diagnosed by the presence of a wormlike mass in the scrotum when the man is asked to bear down. Large varicoceles may be visible through the scrotal skin as a bluish discoloration. Include bilateral palpation of the newborn's scrotum, to determine the bilateral presence of testes. A firm, oval-shaped mobile mass should be detected on both sides of the scrotum. If the client has surgical treatment of his disorder he will need monitoring of vital signs and the incisional site.

▼ ▼

Possible nursing diagnoses for a male client with a structural disorder of the reproductive system may include:

Nursing Diagnoses	Goals	Nursing Interventions
▶ Injury, high risk for, related to inflammation and hemorrhage.	The client will experience minimal bleeding and avoid infection.	Monitor the client's vital signs and incisional drainage. Report hyperthermia, tachycardia, hypotension, increased incisional drainage, and swelling or redness around the incision to the physician immediately. Maintain strict asepsis when handling wound dressings.
▶ Pain, related to the incision.	The client will experience minimal incisional pain.	Monitor for incisional pain. Administer analgesics and antiinflammatories as ordered.
▶ Fluid volume excess, high risk for, related to surgery.	The client will experience minimal scrotal swelling.	Elevate the scrotum on a folded towel or a Bellevue bridge. Place a plastic glove filled with ice, under the scrotum.
▶ Body image disturbance, related to the condition.	The client will maintain a positive body image.	Provide the client with opportunities to voice his concerns and ask questions.
▶ Anxiety, high risk for, related to the treatment outcome.	The client will experience minimal anxiety.	Monitor the client for statements and behaviors that indicate he is concerned about the success of the treatment.
▶ Knowledge deficit, related to the condition and possible complications.	The client will demonstrate understanding of the possible complications of his condition.	Monitor statements made by the client to determine if there is any misunderstanding about how the surgery will affect his masculinity and fertility. Provide the client with opportunities to voice his feelings and ask questions.

▶ Evaluation

Each goal must be evaluated to determine how it has been met by the client.

▲ ▲

IMPOTENCE, INFERTILITY, AND CONTRACEPTION

▶ IMPOTENCE

It is estimated that chronic impotence affects up to 20 percent of American men (Gray, 1992). Impotence is defined as the inability for an adult male to have an erection firm enough or to maintain it long enough to complete sexual intercourse. There are three types of impotence: functional, atonic, and anatomical. Psychological factors that lead to concerns about sexual performance may contribute to functional impotence. These factors include aging and difficulty with communication or relationships.

Atonic impotence may be the result of medications such as antihypertensives, sedatives, antidepressants, or tranquilizers. For example, since antihypertensives lower blood pressure in all arteries of the body, reduction of the blood pressure to penile arteries may lead to failure of the penis to fill sufficiently to achieve erection. The use of alcohol, cocaine, and nicotine can also decrease potency. Disease processes leading to atonic impotence include diabetes, vascular and neurologic disorders. Diabetic clients are at increased risk for impotence due to their tendency to develop atherosclerosis and autonomic neuropathy. Vascular and neurologic disorders include atherosclerosis, hypertension, spinal cord injuries, and multiple sclerosis. End-stage renal disease and chronic obstructive pulmonary disorders can also decrease potency.

Peyronie's disease causes development of nonelastic, fibrous tissue just beneath the penile skin, leading to anatomical impotence. The resulting loss of elasticity leads to a decreased ability of the penis to fill with and store blood during an erection. Peyronie's disease often causes the penis to bend upward, possibly lead-ing to pain and an inability to penetrate the vagina (see Figure 32-8).

As the nature of many human beings is to consider themselves as a grouping of unrelated systems, men are often surprised to learn that conditions affecting other parts of their body are related to their impotence (Clowers, 1995). When impotence is discussed with a client in a holistic fashion, he is able to recognize the relationship of medications, alcohol, nicotine, or disease processes to the potency difficulty.

▶ Medical/Surgical Management

▶ Medical

The first step in treating impotency is to determine whether the client's lifestyle is a factor. Further assessment may include nocturnal penile tumescence monitoring or DICC. Treatment will be based on the assessment findings and test results. Treatment may include changes in lifestyle to reduce the need for medications, manage stress, lose weight, and exercise. These changes often help to improve the client's physical health, self-image and attitude about his ability to function sexually.

▶ Surgical

Surgical interventions for impotency include revascularization and penile implants. For those clients with impotency related to blocked arteries, revascularization is done to bypass blocked arteries and remove veins that are causing excessive drainage. For those clients who are not candidates for revascularization, penile prostheses are another option (see Figure 32-9). One type is a semirigid implant which is a silicone cylinder that may be flexible or inflexible. Another type is a hydraulic implant that has a cylinder that can be inflated by squeezing a pump located in the scrotum or at the end of the penis. Because of its ability to fill and empty, the hydraulic implant, unlike the silicone implant which is always semirigid, most closely mimics flaccidity and erection. The disadvantages of surgical interventions are expense and postoperative complications, the most serious being postoperative infection.

▶ Pharmacological

Medications that promote erections are available. One side effect of drug therapy is prolonged erection that does not occur in response to sexual stimulation (**priapism**). While oral neurotransmitters have been used with variable success, sublingual apomorphine shows some promise as an erectogenic agent. When

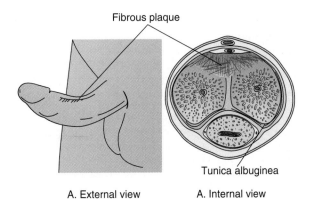

Fibrous plaque

Tunica albuginea

A. External view   A. Internal view

FIGURE 32-8 Peyronie's disease. **(A)** Plaque causes a curvature of the penis. **(B)** Cross section of the penis showing plaque.

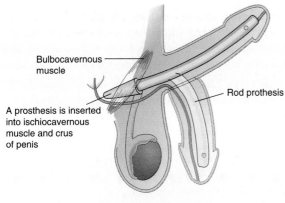

Bulbocavernous muscle

A prosthesis is inserted into ischiocavernous muscle and crus of penis

Rod prothesis

(A) Semirigid implant in place

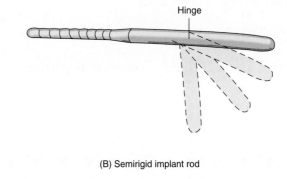

Hinge

(B) Semirigid implant rod

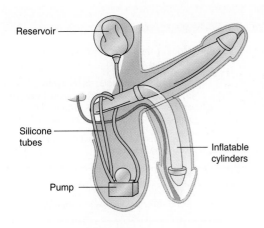

Reservoir

Silicone tubes

Pump

Inflatable cylinders

(C) Hydraulic implant, pump in scrotum

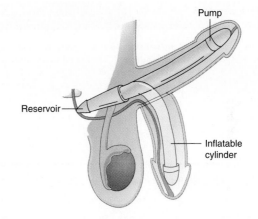

Pump

Reservoir

Inflatable cylinder

(D) Hydraulic implant, pump in end of penis

FIGURE 32-9 Penile prostheses.

administered sublingually rather than subcutaneously, as was done in the past, there are fewer side effects. Self-injections of vasodilators or other drugs may result in serious complications.

▶ External Devices

External devices can be used to promote an erection. A vacuum constriction device (VCD) may be used to increase the blood supply to the penis, causing engorgement and rigidity (Figure 32-10). The client inserts his penis into a plastic cylinder and squeezes a pump to withdraw the air from the cylinder, creating a vacuum that draws blood into the penis. Once an erection has been achieved in this manner, a rubber ring is moved from the bottom of the cylinder to the base of the penis. This permits the blood to be safely trapped in the penis for up to one-half hour. Advantages of the VCD over surgical intervention are decreased expense and complications.

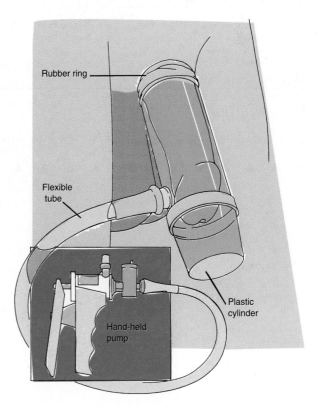

Rubber ring

Flexible tube

Hand-held pump

Plastic cylinder

FIGURE 32-10 Vacuum constriction device.

▶ *Nursing Process*

Assessment

Subjective Data Perform a complete assessment that includes a history of illicit and prescribed drug use, alcohol consumption, previous diagnoses, lifestyle, sexual functioning, and family disorders. Assess the client's emotional and educational needs to determine whether anxiety about sexual performance or lack of knowledge are contributing factors to his impotence.

Objective Data If the client has surgery, the nurse needs to monitor his vital signs, incisional site, intake and output.

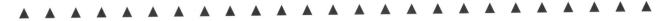

Possible nursing diagnoses for a client who is impotent may include:

Nursing Diagnoses	Goals	Nursing Interventions
▶ *Injury, high risk for, due to infection and hemorrhage related to surgery.*	The client will experience minimal bleeding and avoid infection.	Monitor the client's vital signs and incisional drainage. Report hyperthermia, tachycardia, hypotension, increased incisional drainage, and swelling or redness around the incision to the physician immediately. Maintain strict asepsis when handling wound dressings.
▶ *Pain, related to the incision.*	The client will experience minimal incisional pain.	Monitor for incisional pain. Administer analgesics as ordered.
▶ *Body image disturbance, related to the condition.*	The client will achieve a positive self-image.	Provide the client with opportunities to voice his concerns and ask questions related to body image and sexuality issues.
▶ *Knowledge deficit, related to the condition.*	The client will demonstrate understanding of how to use the penile implant.	Provide the client with information about how to use the penile implant. Emphasize the importance of seeking sexual or marital counseling, in conjunction with the surgical treatment.

▶ *Evaluation*

Each goal must be evaluated to determine how it has been met by the client.

Sample Nursing Care Plan: The Client with Impotence

Mr. Parry is a fifty-five-year-old, married male with diabetes and atherosclerosis. He recently also has been diagnosed as being impotent. He has trouble making eye contact as he discusses his condition and says he has told no one of his diagnoses, not even his wife. He tells you he doesn't understand why this is happening to him now when things have been going so well for him.

Nursing Diagnoses 1 Body image disturbance related to his condition, as evidenced by Mr. Parry's lack of eye contact and statement that he has not told his wife.

Goals	Nursing Interventions	Rationale	Evaluation
Mr. Parry will achieve a positive self-image or seek counseling to assist him with that goal.	Provide Mr. Parry with opportunities to voice his concerns and ask questions in a private, comfortable atmosphere.	The related self-image and sexuality issues are often difficult to discuss.	Mr. Parry verbalizes that he is afraid that his wife will leave him if he is not able to perform sexually. He agrees to attend professional counseling with his wife to discuss these concerns.
	Monitor Mr. Parry for statements and behaviors that indicate he is experiencing a body image disturbance.	The nurse needs to observe Mr. Parry and listen to what he is saying in order to determine his concerns and needs.	
	Suggest that Mr. Parry seek sexual or marital counseling, if indicated.	If Mr. Parry does not appear to be meeting his goal, alternative resources may help him achieve his goals.	

Nursing Diagnosis 2 Knowledge deficit, related to his condition, as evidenced by Mr. Parry's statements that he does not understand why this is happening.

Goals	Nursing Interventions	Rationale	Evaluation
Mr. Parry will demonstrate an understanding of the health factors that are contributing to his impotency.	Monitor Mr. Parry's statements about his condition.	In order to determine Mr. Parry's educational needs concerning his condition and treatment options, the nurse needs to determine his current knowledge level.	Mr. Parry verbalizes that his impotency is caused by poor blood circulation to his penis.
	Educate Mr. Parry about how his diabetes and atherosclerosis are contributing to his impotency.	The nurse needs to build upon Mr. Parry's current knowledge level to increase his knowledge of his condition.	

▶ INFERTILITY

Infertility is defined as the inability of a couple to achieve conception after a year of intercourse without birth control measures. Statistics indicate that 10 to 15 percent of all couples in the United States are infertile (Gray, 1992). During the early days of health care, infertility was considered to be a female problem. Subsequent infertility research indicated that approximately 40 percent of infertility is related to a male factor. Some of the causes are preventable or manageable while others are not. The causes of infertility in males include varicoceles, cryptorchidism, impaired sperm, insufficient number of sperm, and hormonal imbalance.

▶ Medical/Surgical Management

▶ Medical

The first step in treating an infertile couple is to obtain a history of sexual practices. In addition, a detailed health history needs to be obtained and physical examination performed. Ask the client what type of undershorts he wears. Tight-fitting undershorts will increase scrotal temperature, resulting in a reduced sperm count. Other activities that can decrease the sperm count are using hot tubs and saunas. Diagnostic tests that may be ordered include the following:

- Semen analysis, including sperm count, motility, and morphology
- Testicular biopsy (done when sperm are absent from the semen) to ascertain the presence of sperm
- Endocrine imbalance testing which measures pituitary, gonadotropin, and testosterone levels
- Male/female interaction studies (Huhner test) to determine motility and number of sperm 2 to 4 hours after intercourse
- Testing of the sex chromosomes

A treatment plan will be formulated based on these diagnostic tests.

▶ Surgical

With a diagnosis of cryptorchidism or varicocele, surgery may be advised (see Structural Disorders).

▶ Pharmacological

If the sperm count or motility is low, testosterone or thyroid extracts may be prescribed.

▶ Diet

Vitamins and a well-balanced diet may be prescribed.

▶ Activity

Rest or moderate exercise may be prescribed. The client will be advised to have intercourse every other day beginning twelve to sixteen days prior to the woman's next menstrual period.

▶ Nursing Process

Assessment

Ask questions to determine the client's knowledge about the condition and treatment options. If surgery is necessary to correct a structural disorder, the nurse will be responsible for postoperative assessment. Ask the client questions to determine his emotional needs, as an infertility diagnosis may cause the client to experience guilt, grief, or a disturbance in self image. Nursing diagnoses, goals, interventions, and evaluation will be based on the assessment findings.

▶ CONTRACEPTION

When choosing a form of contraception, the male client has various options to consider. While weighing the options, safety, ease of use, effectiveness, and cost should be considered. The partner's wishes should also be considered in this decision-making process.

Contraceptive options available to males include abstinence, coitus interruptus, condoms, or voluntary surgical sterilization. Withdrawing the penis from the vagina before ejaculation (**coitus interruptus**) is not a very reliable method because sperm may have already been emitted in the lubricating fluids. Also the man may experience difficulty in controlling the timing of his ejaculation.

Condoms are an inexpensive, readily available form of contraception. A condom is a latex or sheepskin sheath that is slipped over the erect penis before the penis is inserted into the vagina. The condom should be applied by holding it by the tip and unrolling it onto the penis. A space of about one inch should be left for semen at the tip. After ejaculation, the penis should be withdrawn carefully to prevent the condom from slipping off and spilling the contents. The condom should then be discarded, as it is not designed for more than a single use. Condoms are available in a variety of colors, sizes, and other features. The 2 percent failure rate of condoms is probably related more to sporadic use rather than methodology. Other problems associated with condom usage are allergic reactions and reports of reduced sexual pleasure. Positive aspects of condom usage include reducing the risk of STD and HIV exposure. However, sheepskin condoms do not provide protection against HIV.

▶ Medical/Surgical Management

▶ Surgical

When a permanent form of birth control is desired a surgical resection of the vas deferens (**vasectomy**) is done. This simple surgical procedure is usually performed under local anesthesia on an outpatient basis. While occasional failures have been reported, the major disadvantage of a vasectomy is that it is permanent. Reversal of this surgery is expensive and often unsuccessful.

▶ Nursing Process

Because a vasectomy is performed on an outpatient basis, the nurse's role is usually limited to preparation of the client for surgery and postoperative education. The client needs to be educated about follow-up care and possible postoperative complications. He should be encouraged to rest for at least two hours after the surgery, avoid strenuous physical exercise for one week and apply ice to the scrotum for up to four hours postoperatively. Instructions should be given about signs and symptoms of postoperative infection and hemorrhage.

It may take up to six weeks for the semen to be clear of sperm. The client is instructed to return to the clinic for a sperm count after twenty ejaculations. If he is sexually active, during those ejaculations he should use a condom or some other form of contraception. At six months a sperm count should be repeated and then monitored annually thereafter.

▶ **CASE STUDY**

Mr. Able is a seventy-year-old male with a diagnosis of benign prostatic hypertrophy. Prior to his hospital admission for a TURP he has been in good health. He returned from surgery three hours ago with a three-way Foley catheter and continuous bladder irrigation. His vital signs 1 hour ago were as follows: temperature 98.9, apical pulse 68, blood pressure 130/84 and respirations 18. When the nurse enters his room to take another set of vitals, Mr. Able is restless, moaning, has cool, moist skin, and his catheter is not draining properly. His pulse is now 120 and blood pressure is 88/50. The nurse calls the physician to report the change in Mr. Able's condition. The physician orders a STAT hematocrit and a bleeding and clotting time. An increase in the IV fluid drip rate is also ordered. The doctor is planning to arrive at the hospital within the next hour.

The following questions will guide your development of a Nursing Care Plan for the case study.

1. List symptoms/clinical manifestations, other than Mr. Able's, a client may experience following a TURP.

2. List reasons why the doctor has ordered the STAT blood work and the IV changes.

3. List other diagnostic tests that may have been ordered for Mr. Able.

4. Mentally do a head-to-toe or functional assessment on Mr. Able. List subjective and objective data a nurse would want to obtain.

5. Write three individualized nursing diagnoses and goals for Mr. Able.

6. Upon assessing Mr. Able, the doctor decides to inject additional fluid into the balloon that anchors the indwelling catheter and apply increased traction to the catheter. List pertinent nursing actions a nurse would do following these medical interventions:

   • Medications
   • Comfort/rest
   • Cardiac output
   • Intake and output
   • Activity
   • Teaching

7. List resources within the medical center and the local area that could assist Mr. Able with his postoperative recovery.

8. List teaching that Mr. Able will need before his discharge.

9. List at least three successful outcomes for Mr. Able.

SUMMARY

- Benign prostatic hypertrophy is a common disorder in males over age fifty. Early symptoms include hesitancy, decreased force of stream, urinary frequency, and nocturia.
- Male cancers related to the reproductive system, involve the prostate, testes, breast, and penis. Emphasis should be placed on self-examination and regular physical examinations in order to facilitate early diagnosis and treatment
- Common male reproductive system inflammatory disorders include epididymitis, orchitis, and prostatitis. Bilateral epididymitis and orchitis can lead to sterility. Treatment includes antibiotic therapy.
- Male structural disorders include cryptorchidism, hydrocele, spermatocele, varicocele, and torsion of the spermatic cord. Treatment may include surgery.
- Impotence may be caused by emotional or physical factors. Treatment includes counseling, medications, circulatory aids, and surgery.
- Confirmation of male infertility is based on diagnostic tests. These tests will determine the appropriate treatment plan.
- Abstinence, condoms, coitus interruptus, and surgical sterilization are contraception options available to men.

Review Questions

1. Which of the following is the most common site of cancer in the male reproductive system?
   a. breast
   b. testicles
   c. penis
   d. prostate

2. Which of the following factors predisposes males to penile cancer?
   a. alcohol consumption
   b. not being circumcised
   c. advanced age
   d. circumcision

3. Which of the following self-examinations should a young man be taught to do?
   a. rectal
   b. scrotal
   c. prostate
   d. testicular

4. Which of the following complications may occur after a TURP?
   a. water intoxication
   b. difficulty voiding
   c. constipation
   d. hypertension

5. Which of the following methods may be used for clearing obstructed catheter tubing post-TURP?
   a. milking the tubing
   b. changing the catheter
   c. running the irrigation fluid faster
   d. releasing the traction from the catheter

6. Which of the following is a cause of male infertility?
   a. exercise
   b. hypospadias
   c. lack of sleep
   d. frequent hot tub or sauna usage

7. Which of the following is a cause of impotency?
   a. varicocele
   b. heavy exercise
   c. Peyronie's disease
   d. having multiple sexual partners

8. The purpose of post-TURP continuous bladder irrigation is to:
   a. decrease urinary output.
   b. reduce clot formation.
   c. decrease bleeding.
   d. increase urinary output.

9. Which of the following nursing interventions can help alleviate bladder spasms post-TURP?
   a. increasing fluid intake
   b. maintaining traction on the urethral catheter
   c. administering B & O suppositories
   d. apply ice to and elevate the scrotum

10. Which of the following is a method that can be used to assess the client's level of knowledge related to his inflammatory disorder of the reproductive system?
    a. asking the client if he has any questions.
    b. asking the client to describe "safe sex" practices.
    c. asking the client if he has read the pamphlets about his disorder.
    d. asking the client to describe the symptoms of his disorder.

Critical Thinking Questions

1. Discuss the emotional reaction to impotence.

2. Make a teaching plan for a testicular self-examination.

3. Discuss the pros and cons of various treatment methods and their side effects on a client with prostatic cancer.

Medical Terminology

spadias	pertaining to urinary meatus
epi-	over the usual location
epispadias	congenital opening of urethra on dorsum of penis
-cele	pertaining to hernia
varico-	venous herniation
varicocele	enlargement of the veins of the spermatic chord
-itis	pertaining to inflammation
orchio-	pertaining to the testicle or testis
orchitis	inflammation of the testicle
-ectomy	cutting out
orchiectomy	removal of the testis
cysto-	pertaining to bladder
-oscopy	act of examining
cystoscopy	examining the bladder
trans-	across, through
transurethral resection of the prostate	surgical approach through the urethra

transrectal	across or through the rectum
-ur	pertaining to urine
an-	lack of
anuria	lack of urine
dys-	difficult
dysuria	difficult urination
oligo-	little
oliguria	little urine
hem-	blood
hematuria	blood in the urine

News Flash

The Fred Hutchinson Cancer Research Center in Seattle, WA is beginning a major research endeavor to investigate the genetic basis of prostate cancer. PROGRESS (Prostate Cancer Genetic Research Study) will be one of the largest studies ever conducted to examine how genetic makeup predisposes a man and his family to prostate cancer. Previous research findings indicate that men are twice as likely to develop prostate cancer if they have a father, brother, or son with the disease. In addition, these men are more likely to develop cancer at a younger age (de Hart, 1995).

CHAPTER
33

Sexually Transmitted Diseases

Vicki L. Khouli

KEY TERMS

antibiotic-resistant
chancre
exposure
incidence
incubation period
mode of transmission
spirochete
venereal disease
virus

LIST OF DISORDERS

- Chlamydia
- Gonorrhea
- Syphilis
- Herpes Genitalis
- Cytomegalovirus
- Human Papillomavirus
- AIDS
- Trichomoniasis

LEARNING OBJECTIVES

Upon completion of this chapter the learner should be able to:

- Define key terms.
- List the most prevalent STDs, including causative agents.
- Discuss the incidence and reporting requirements for STDs.
- Describe currently used methods of prevention of STDs.
- Describe signs and symptoms, diagnostic aids, and treatment of the most common STDs.
- Utilize the nursing process to plan the care of a client with an STD.
- Demonstrate the ability to teach self-care and reinfection prevention measures to the client with an STD.

▶ *MAKING THE CONNECTION*

Refer to the topics in the following chapters to increase your understanding of sexually transmitted diseases.

- **Chapter 24, Allergies, Immune, and Autoimmune Disorders:** HIV/AIDS, p. 614
- **Chapter 25, HIV Disorders:** Modes of Transmission, p. 621

- **Chapter 31, Female Reproductive Disorders:** Anatomy and Physiology Review, p. 857; Vaginitis, p. 890; Contraception, p. 903; Pelvic Inflammatory Disease, p. 962
- **Chapter 32, Male Reproductive Disorders:** Anatomy and Physiology Review, p. 915; Prostatitis, p. 931; Contraception p. 940

INTRODUCTION

Sexually transmitted diseases (STDs) can be defined as those diseases that are transmitted or passed from one person to another primarily through sexual contact. Another term, which has frequently been used for STDs, is **venereal disease**. Today health care workers prefer the term sexually transmitted disease, which is self-explanatory. Currently the term STD includes the traditional venereal diseases such as, syphilis, gonorrhea, chancroid, granuloma inguinale, and lymphogranuloma venereum, as well as STDs such as chlamydia, herpes genitalis, trichomoniasis and human papillomavirus. AIDS, acquired immunodeficiency syndrome, is not solely a sexually transmitted disease, although sexual activity is one of the primary **modes of transmission** (ways by which a contagious disease is spread) of the disease.

The **incidence** (frequency of disease occurrence) of STDs has been increasing worldwide, with chlamydia and gonorrhea being the most widespread STDs today. Some diseases, such as syphilis, have been described as sexually transmitted diseases for centuries. Currently over 12 million Americans annually are diagnosed with an STD. Chlamydia, for example, affects over 4 million Americans every year, making it more than twice as common as gonorrhea (Erickson, 1994). Syphilis, although less common than either chlamydia or gonorrhea, still affects about twenty people out of every 100,000 in the United States (Hook & Marra, 1992).

The development of antibiotic treatment for STDs in the 1940s caused a dramatic decrease in the prevalence of STDs and for a while it was predicted that STDs would be eradicated completely. But a variety of factors have contributed to the dramatic increase of STDs, especially in the last two decades, such as: casual sex, asymptomatic carriers of the disease, the use of nonbarrier methods of birth control, lack of knowledge of prevention methods of STDs, and inadequate reporting of STDs.

There is no great uniformity in the reporting requirements for STDs. Reporting regulations differ from state to state and from disease to disease. Currently, all states in the United States require that cases of gonorrhea and syphilis be reported to a health officer in that state. Many states also have reporting requirements for diseases such as chancroid and granuloma inguinale. Reporting is not required for STDs such as herpes and trichomoniasis. The Centers for Disease Control and Prevention (CDC) keep statistics on reportable diseases.

Prevention

Public education regarding the causes, methods of transmission, and methods of prevention of STDs is regarded as the most important weapon in the battle against STDs. While many STDs caused by bacterial infection are curable with modern antibiotics, the viruses are not. For example, AIDS generally leads to death within a relatively short period of time. The best option in the management of STDs is still prevention.

Since sexual activity is beginning at earlier ages today, sex education, including information about STDs, is being presented in elementary schools. Many schools have comprehensive education programs already in place to teach about STDs and recommendations to prevent the spread of STDs. Television, especially educational programs, also has been helpful in informing the public that having sex without protection against STDs is dangerous.

Many messages have been disseminated to the general public regarding the best methods of prevention of STDs. The only 100 percent effective method of prevention of STDs is abstinence, (refraining from sexual intercourse or mucous membrane to mucous membrane contact altogether). Couples who are mutually monogamous are also not at risk, unless one of them was previously infected. The popularity of the pill has decreased consistent condom use. Most current methods of birth control are not effective in preventing the transmission of STDs. Only a barrier method, the latex condom, has been effective in preventing the spread of STDs, although even this method only provides safer sex, not totally safe sex.

Another factor that has contributed to the vast increase in STDs in recent years is the increased consumption of alcohol and the use of illegal drugs. Not only is the sharing of needles among intravenous drug abusers a factor in the increased incidence of STDs, but also the lessening of inhibitions that occurs with drug and alcohol abuse. The trading of sex for drugs among drug users has also been presented as a factor in the spread of STDs.

Once the diagnosis of an STD is made, identification of all sexual contacts is also important. Many people are reluctant to be candid regarding sexual activity and sexual contacts, since this is an area of life considered to be extremely private. This is one of the most difficult aspects in dealing with STDs as many of the diseases are totally asymptomatic, especially in women. These asymptomatic partners, who are likely to also become infected with the disease can both transmit the disease to new partners and/or reinfect the treated partner, if they are not identified and treated.

ANATOMY AND PHYSIOLOGY REVIEW

The major systems affected by the sexually transmitted diseases are the reproductive systems, (see Chapters 31 and 32). Males are generally more symptomatic than females and will seek health care more readily since the external genitalia are more visible. The signs and symptoms of the disease are much more readily observed in males. Since in females, the sex organs are internal, they are more likely to suffer complications and increased severity of symptoms by the time the disease is identified. Signs of disease affecting female genitalia are less likely to be readily observed.

In addition to reproductive systems, any area of sexual contact, such as oral and rectal areas, may also exhibit signs and symptoms of the disease process.

COMMON DIAGNOSTIC TESTS

The following is a table of the commonly used diagnostic tests for clients with sexually transmitted diseases.

Test	Explanation/Normal Values	Nursing Responsibilities
EIA or ELISA (enzyme-linked immunoassay) Direct immunofluorescence Microscopic exam of endocervical specimen. Tissue culture—site Men: urethra Women: endocervix	Test for the presence of *Chlamydia trachomatis*. Normal = negative	Explain the specimen collection procedure to client before beginning to collect specimen. Tell client that the cervix (in women) or the urethra (in men) will be swabbed or scraped with a special collection device and that some discomfort may result. Provide special swab with test medium for specimen collection and send to lab as soon as collected.
Men: gram-stained smear of penile discharge (if smear is negative but symptoms strongly positive for gonorrhea, obtain culture of penile discharge) Women: culture of endocervical secretions	Test for presence of *Neisseria gonorrhea*. Normal = negative	Explain collection procedure to client. Provide sterile cotton-tipped swab (for women) or bacteriostatic wire loop (for men), and culture plate or bottle. When culture is applied to medium, take specimen to lab as soon as possible.
VDRL RPR FTA-ABS (Fluorescent Treponemal Antibody-Absorption Test) Reiter test Fluorescent antibody TPI (performed only at CDC in Atlanta)	Blood tests for presence of syphilis. Normal = negative or nonreactive	Explain the test to client, including amount of blood to be drawn. Gather syringes and blood vials to receive specimen.

(continued)

Test	Explanation/Normal Values	Nursing Responsibilities
Tzanck test	Test for presence of herpes genitalis virus. Normal = negative	Explain to client that lesions in the genital area (common sites are endocervix, cervix, vagina and penis) will be cultured, and that the procedure will probably not be painful, but that client must remain still to prevent injury. Provide scalpel blade, glass slide, and stain for collection.
ELISA Western blot	Blood tests used to indicate the presence of HIV. Normal = negative	Explain the procedure of obtaining blood to the client. Make sure that client knows that if first ELISA is positive, a second ELISA will be drawn, before confirmation is done with Western blot.
Physical examination of genital area Dark field examination of wart scrapings	Visual identification of human papillomavirus. Microscopic examination to differentiate genital warts from syphilis condylomata.	Take a careful client history. Examine genital area carefully, and provide scalpel and slide if specimen is to be obtained. Explain procedures thoroughly.
Hanging drop slide Urine specimen	Test to identify presence of *Trichomonas vaginalis*. Normal = negative	Explain to female clients that a specimen of vaginal secretions will be obtained for examination under a microscope. Alternatively, a urine sample may also reveal the presence of *Trichomonas vaginalis* in both women and men. Men may also be asked to provide a semen specimen.

KEY ABBREVIATIONS

The following abbreviations and acronyms are used in this chapter:

AIDS	acquired immunodeficiency syndrome
CDC	Centers for Disease Control and Prevention
CMV	cytomegalovirus
HIV	human immunodeficiency virus
HPV	human papillomavirus
HSV	herpes simplex virus
IUD	intrauterine device
STD	sexually transmitted disease
VDRL	Venereal Disease Research Laboratory

▶ *CHLAMYDIA*

Chlamydia is caused by a spherical bacterial organism known as *Chlamydia trachomatis*. Outside the body, the organism has difficulty surviving, but inside the body, chlamydia reproduces rapidly inside host cells. The mode of transmission in chlamydia must be through intimate body contact, since the organism is so fragile that it cannot survive long when outside of the body.

Approximately 40 percent of all chlamydia cases are asymptomatic. Almost three times more women than men exhibit no symptoms. Chlamydia is known as the "silent STD" for this reason. If left untreated, chlamydial infections cause tissue inflammation, ulceration, and scar tissue formation in both women and men. Asymptomatic salpingitis or pelvic inflammatory disease (PID) can lead to scarring of the delicate fallopian tubes, ectopic pregnancy, or even infertility. Infection during pregnancy can lead to such complications as preterm labor, premature rupture of membranes, and low birthweight babies.

The most common symptoms of chlamydia in men are those of urethritis and epididymitis. Women are likely to have a grayish white mucopurulent vaginal discharge, itching and dysuria, although as many as 70 percent of women will be asymptomatic.

▶ *Medical/Surgical Management*

▶ *Pharmacological*

The Centers for Disease Control and Prevention (CDC) revised the treatment recommendations for chlamydia in 1993 to emphasize the importance of early, aggressive, antimicrobial treatment of suspected cases of chlamydia. The CDC currently recommends treatment with doxycycline (Vibramycin). If compliance with an extended period of drug therapy is thought to be a problem, azithromycin (Zithromax) can be given orally in a single dose. The cost of azithromycin (Zithromax) may be prohibitive, however, since it currently costs about six times more than doxycycline (Vibramycin). Pregnant women may be treated with erythromycin estolate (Ilosone) or amoxicillin trihydrate (Amoxil), but they should be cultured again after treatment is completed to confirm the absence of chlamydial infection. Retesting is not required after treatment with doxycycline or azithromycin, since these medications are so effective against chlamydia. It is important that both sexual partners be treated for chlamydia simultaneously since reinfection is probable if only one partner is treated.

▶ GONORRHEA

Gonorrheal infections are often seen in combination with chlamydia. Gonorrhea is a serious bacterial infection, caused by the gram-negative bacterial organism *Neisseria gonorrhea.* The organism grows well only in the areas of moist mucous membranes, so it is transmitted by direct mucous membrane contact. Mouth-to-mouth kissing does not transmit gonorrhea, but during sexual intercourse a woman has more than a 50 percent chance of becoming infected with the gonorrheal organism. The disease progresses in much the same manner as chlamydia and can cause many of the same complications, such as infertility from salpingitis and PID.

Signs and symptoms of infection may occur within two to six days after **exposure** (contact with an infected person). Again, men are more likely to exhibit signs of the disease, with up to 90 percent exhibiting symptoms such as urethritis with a purulent discharge from the penis. Approximately 50 percent of women are asymptomatic, but the remainder may exhibit signs of abnormal vaginal discharge or abnormal menstrual bleeding, along with the symptoms of painful or burning urination.

If left untreated, gonorrhea may ascend through the cervix and uterus to the upper reproductive tract where it may damage the fragile fallopian tubes. From the tubes, the infection may continue into the peritoneum and the ovaries may also become involved in the disease process. A condition known as PID, pelvic inflammatory disease, may result. Refer to Chapter 31, Female Reproductive Disorders, for more information on PID.

If a women is infected with gonorrhea when she delivers a baby, the infection may be transmitted to the newborn's eyes as it travels through the birth canal. In the United States, all infants are treated with a silver nitrate or an antibiotic opthalmic ointment within an hour or two of birth to prevent the gonorrheal-induced eye infection known as opthalmia neonatorum.

▶ Medical/Surgical Management

Once the presence of gonorrhea has been confirmed by culture, both partners should be treated with a course of antibiotic therapy. One of the problems identified in the fight against gonorrhea is that new, **antibiotic-resistant** strains of gonorrhea have developed in recent years. Penicillin used to be the drug of choice when treating gonorrhea, but since penicillin has been so widely used against many types of infection, some strains of *Neisseria gonorrhea* adapted and are no longer affected by penicillin. The gonococci developed the ability to produce an enzyme, penicillinase, which inactivated the penicillin, no matter what the dosage or length of treatment. The prevalence of the new resistant gonorrhea has led the CDC to recommend treating all cases of gonorrhea as though they were resistant to the traditional drug therapies.

▶ Pharmacological

A variety of antibiotics are effective against gonorrhea. One of the most effective therapies includes a single dose of ciprofloxacin (Cipro), followed by a seven-day course of oral doxycycline (Vibramycin). Because almost half of all clients with gonorrhea also have chlamydia, doxycycline (Vibramycin) is an appropriate choice of drug therapy since it combats both infections effectively. For pregnant clients, or those under 16 years of age, an injection of ceftriaxone sodium (Rocephlin), followed by oral erythromycin estolate (Ilosone) is recommended. Follow-up cultures to determine the success of the course of treatment is recommended when the treatment has been completed.

▶ SYPHILIS

Syphilis, an STD almost eradicated after the discovery of antibiotic therapy in the 1940s, is on the upswing again, especially among urban minority groups. The causative organism of syphilis is a **spirochete**, or spiral-shaped bacterial organism, known as *Treponema pallidum,* first identified in 1905. Transmission of syphilis is either through sexual contact or congenitally (mother to child), since the organism is very fragile and easily destroyed outside of the body. Syphilis is often seen with human immunodeficiency virus infection, just as chlamydia is seen with gonorrhea. Cases of syphilis in the United States have continued to rise in the 1990s to levels of more than 20 cases per 100,000 persons (Hook & Marra, 1992). Concentration of syphilis cases is higher in urban populations, with the states of Florida, California, and New York accounting for more than 50 percent of cases reported to the CDC (Kirchner, 1991).

Syphilis presents in several stages. In the primary

stage of the disease, the **incubation period**, or interval between exposure to syphilis and the appearance of first symptoms, is from ten to ninety days, with the development of **chancre** usually occurring after two to three weeks. A chancre is an clean, painless ulcer, which usually is present at the place where the treponemas entered the body, (see Figures 33-1A and B). There is usually just one chancre present, but multiple chancres have been known to occur. Chancres may occur on the internal genitalia of women (for example, the cervix) and thus not be noticed. The chancre will heal within four to six weeks, either leaving a thin scar or none at all. If not identified and treated at this point, the disease will enter the second stage, usually within six to eight weeks after the chancre has healed. Signs and symptoms of the secondary stage include a classic macular or papular rash, (often beginning on the trunk of the body and spreading to the extremities), low grade fever, malaise, joint aches and pain, and generalized lymph node swelling. Occasionally a wartlike growth known as condylomata lata may be present in the genital area of both men and women. Since this is so close in appearance to the condylomata acuminata of human papillomavirus, it may be confused with genital warts. Since many of these symptoms are also common to many other diseases, syphilis has often been known as "the great imitator."

If not identified and treated at this stage, syphilis will then enter a latent period for a year or two where no symptoms are evident, until it enters the third or tertiary stage. At this point the disease becomes noninfectious, but the client *may* be critically ill. Any organ system may be involved in the destructive, inflammatory changes that are now taking place in the body, but among the most common are CNS system changes,

sometimes known as neurosyphilis. With advanced neurosyphilis, symptoms such as hemiplegia, seizures, blindness, tremors, ataxia, and incontinence may occur. Development of soft tissue tumors is also very common in cases of tertiary syphilis.

▶ Medical/Surgical Management

▶ Pharmacological

Since the time that syphilis was first treated with antibiotic therapy, penicillin has remained the drug of choice, since no cases of resistance to syphilis have been identified. All types of penicillin are effective, but penicillin G benzathine (Bicillin L-A) is often preferred, given in injection form. A single injection of 2.4 million units is usually sufficient treatment for the early stages of syphilis, but late or tertiary stages usually require repeat doses every week for three to four weeks. Antimicrobial therapy will destroy *Treponema pallidum* spirochetes at any stage, but any damage done to body organs is irreversible. If the client has a demonstrated allergy to penicillin, alternative medications may be administered, such as doxycycline (Vibramycin), tetracycline HC (Achromycin V), or erythromycin estolate (Ilosone). For pregnant women who are allergic to penicillin, erythromycin is recommended as the best alternative therapy.

▶ HERPES GENITALIS

Herpes simplex virus produces the characteristic lesions known as "cold sores" in herpes simplex type

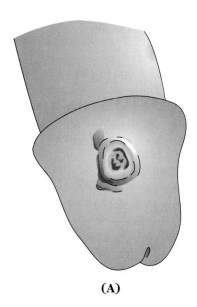

(A)

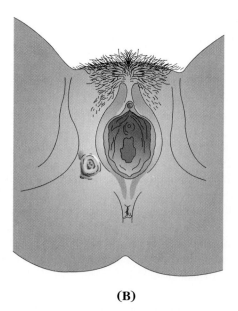

(B)

FIGURE 33-1 The syphilitic chancre usually occurs at the point where the organism enters the body. **(A)** Male; **(B)** Female.

1, or it can produce lesions in the perineal and genital areas in herpes simplex type 2. The infectious virus in both conditions is known as *Herpesvirus hominus*. A **virus** is a minute organism of either DNA or RNA surrounded by a covering of protein and no cell wall; can only be seen with an electron microscope. Herpes simplex virus type 2 (HSV-2), also known as herpes genitalis or genital herpes, was considered to be the sexual scourge of the 1970s, since it was an incurable virus. The advent of AIDS in the 1980s has tended to eclipse herpes, but it is still a disease that requires some lifelong adjustments due to the possibility of frequent recurrences throughout the life span. The number of genital herpes cases is estimated at about 20 million cases in the United States, and is predicted to be growing at a rate of about a million cases a year (Dickason et al., 1993). Genital herpes has been linked to childbirth complications such as spontaneous abortion, premature delivery, and neonatal systemic infection. Genital herpes has also been linked to cervical cancer development.

The incubation period for herpes is from three to seven days, with a primary lesion appearing at the end of that time, usually at the area of contact (see Figure 33-2). Symptoms that may occur just before the appearance of lesions include burning, itching, or tingling sensations in the area of exposure. The lesion usually ulcerates, especially if it is located on mucous membranes. These lesions are painful and may last for many weeks before finally healing. Systemic symptoms are common with the first or primary infection, and include fatigue, malaise, chills, fever, headache, and enlargement of inguinal lymph nodes. Genital lesions generally heal in three to four weeks, and systemic symptoms are less likely to occur in subsequent recurrences. Approximately 75 percent of clients will experience at least one recurrence during their lifetime. Factors that may precipitate a herpes outbreak

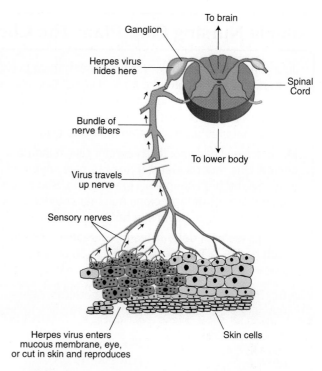

include anxiety, fatigue, sunburn, tight clothing, and fever. Genital herpes is most threatening to the childbearing process and the infant if the primary infection occurs during the pregnancy. Risk to the unborn child is greatly reduced if a secondary outbreak of herpetic lesions occurs during the pregnancy. If the mother has active lesions in the genital area when she goes into labor, a cesarean delivery is generally performed (see Figure 33-3).

▶ *Pharmacological*

There is no known cure for the herpes simplex virus at this time. Treatment has been geared toward alleviating symptoms of the disease. Acyclovir (Zovirax) has been utilized in the treatment of herpes, most often in a topical form applied to the lesions, although it may also be given in oral or intravenous form. Acyclovir (Zovirax) treatment appears to help reduce shedding of the virus and the duration of the lesions in a primary outbreak. It is not effective in preventing recurrences of the herpetic outbreak, or in shortening the duration of those occurrences.

Cleansing the area of the lesions with mild soap and water, hydrogen peroxide or Burow's solution is often helpful in reducing the discomfort of the lesions and decreasing the chance of secondary infections. The area should be blown dry with a hairdryer and then the dry skin may be dusted with a cornstarch powder, which aids in decreasing client discomfort.

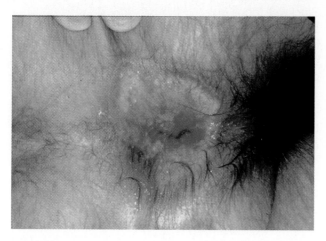

FIGURE 33-2 Chronic mucocutaneous perianal herpes infection. *(Courtesy Centers for Disease Control and Prevention, Atlanta GA 30333).*

Sample Nursing Care Plan: The Client with Herpes Genitalis

Julie Blackwell is a single woman in her middle twenties who has been coming to the clinic for annual Pap smears and birth control for several years. She is a well-nourished, healthy-appearing young woman of medium height. She rescheduled her annual Pap smear to come into the clinic early because she noticed a cluster of small blisters on the inside of her left thigh which also involve the labia majora. She also reports that she has just gotten the flu as evidenced by headache, fever, and general achiness.

Ms. Blackwell has used birth control pills in the past, and reports satisfaction with this method of birth control. She reports that she and her new boyfriend became intimate about two weeks ago, so she wants to renew her birth control pill prescription. She also states that intercourse has been uncomfortble since the appearance of the lesions and that she does not feel comfortable with sexual activity while the lesions are present, since they make her feel "ugly."

Your assessment determines the presence of a cluster of small blisters as well as swollen, tender inguinal lymph nodes. A Tzanck smear test is obtained.

Nursing Diagnoses 1 Sexuality patterns, altered, related to lesions as evidenced by her comment that intercourse has been uncomfortable since the appearance of the lesions.

Goals	Nursing Interventions	Rationale	Evaluation
Ms. Blackwell will express her feelings about potential changes in her sexual behavior before leaving the clinic.	Provide a nonjudgmental atmosphere to encourage Ms. Blackwell to express her feelings about this perceived change in her sexual identity.	This demonstrates the caregiver's positive feelings toward Ms. Blackwell, and any concerns she may have regarding her future sexuality.	Ms. Blackwell states that she is still in shock, but thinks that she will be able to deal with her diagnosis. She also states that she will call back to the clinic in a few days with more questions after she has assimilated some of the information.
	Provide privacy and an uninterrupted amount of time to talk with Ms. Blackwell.	This demonstrates respect for Ms. Blackwell, and conveys reassurance that the caregiver will be comfortable discussing sexuality issues and concerns with her.	
	Provide accurate information to Ms. Blackwell about herpes genitalis, and include literature or videos that she can share with her boyfriend later.	This helps Ms. Blackwell focus on specific, necessary information and encourages her to ask questions.	
	Offer the names of local support groups such as HELP (Herpetics Engaged in Living Productively) or other support persons who will be able to provide information and group support to Ms. Blackwell.	This provides Ms. Blackwell with resources for support once she has returned home and the reality of her diagnosis has set in.	

Nursing Diagnoses 2 Anxiety related to threatened sexual identity as evidenced by her comment that she is not comfortable with sexual activity while the lesions are present since they make her feel "ugly."

Goals	Nursing Interventions	Rationale	Evaluation
Ms. Blackwell will be able to express feelings of anxiety and identify support systems to help her cope with these feelings before leaving the clinic.	Explain any procedures clearly and concisely before performing them. Listen attentively to any concerns or expressions of anxiety that Ms. Blackwell may offer. Include Ms. Blackwell in as many decisions related to her care and follow-up as is possible.	This will help alleviate anxiety. This will allow Ms. Blackwell to identify any anxious behaviors that she may be exhibiting and the source of her anxiety. Involving Ms. Blackwell in decision making regarding her care may reduce her feelings of anxiety and make her feel like she has regained some control.	Ms. Blackwell expresses feelings of anxiety about the diagnosis of herpes. She states that she has a cousin with herpes whom she will use as a resource person. She states that she has a secure relationship with her boyfriend and will talk to him about herpes also. She states that she will continue to call the clinic for any further support or information that she may need.

Nursing Diagnoses 3 Infection, high risk for, related to break in skin integrity as evidenced by the presence of blisters.

Goals	Nursing Interventions	Rationale	Evaluation
Ms. Blackwell's herpes blisters will heal without secondary infection within ten days.	Wear gloves when examining perineal area and when handling exudate from herpes lesions. Teach Ms. Blackwell how to wash hands very thoroughly after using the toilet or handling the area around the herpes lesions. Instruct Ms. Blackwell in the importance of keeping the herpes lesions clean and dry until they heal. Instruct Ms. Blackwell to wear cotton underwear and loose-fitting clothing during occasions of herpes outbreaks.	Gloves prevent secondary infection in herpes blisters from caregiver's hands and offer protection to the caregiver when dealing with wound exudate as part of a standard precautions policy. Handwashing prevents the spread of herpes infection in the genital area to other areas of Ms. Blackwell's body or to another person. Keeping the herpes lesions clean and dry until they heal will help prevent the occurrence of a secondary infection which may delay healing for up to six weeks. These measures will provide for air circulation to promote healing and reduce further local irritation.	Ms. Blackwell has been taught to keep blisters clean and dry and states that she will contact the clinic if the lesions develop any signs of a secondary infection. She makes an appointment to return to the clinic in ten days for a follow-up evaluation.

▶ *CYTOMEGALOVIRUS*

Another virus in the herpes virus family is **cytomegalovirus**, (CMV), which inhabits the salivary glands in humans. Figure 33-4 shows an electron micrograph of CMV. Unlike the more commonly recognized herpes viruses, CMV rarely produces noticeable clinical symptoms.

CMV is primarily transmitted from person to person via contact with body fluids like saliva, urine, and blood. The virus has been identified in semen and cervical mucus, so sexual transmission is a possibility. However, CMV is not usually classified as an STD, since it is felt that other methods of transmission are much more commonly responsible for spread of the disease.

Most people acquire CMV during childhood or adolescence through contact with saliva and respiratory secretions, and by adulthood somewhere between 80 to 100 percent of adults will have developed antibodies to CMV. Most of these people will not notice any symptoms, but occasionally a client will present with complaints of a high fever, accompanied by fatigue and weakness. These symptoms may persist for several weeks, and may lead to a tentative diagnosis of infectious mononucleosis, although the sore throat and swollen lymph nodes of "mono" are not present with CMV.

CMV has been implicated in some complications of pregnancy such as spontaneous abortion or mental retardation of the neonate. Congenital infection of an infant produces cytomegalic inclusion disease that ranges from an asymptomatic condition to a severely debilitating condition that may even result in death. The central nervous system damage to the infant may be profound, although it occurs rarely. CMV can also become a life-threatening illness in a client who has a poorly functioning immune system, such as a victim of AIDS.

There is no antiviral agent specifically utilized for this disorder, since most of the population will not have any symptoms.

▶ *HUMAN PAPILLOMAVIRUS*

Another virus that is sexually transmitted is the human papillomavirus (HPV), which causes genital warts or condylomata acuminata. These genital warts may occur in the urogenital, perineal, or anal areas, and may be either external or internal. The population at risk seems to be teenage girls or young women in their twenties. In the United States, the CDC estimates that there are approximately one million new cases identified every year. Since genital wart infections do

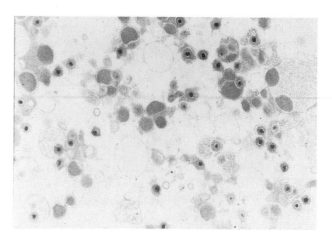

FIGURE 33-4 Electron micrograph of cytomegalovirus. (*Courtesy Centers for Disease Control and Prevention, Atlanta, GA 30333*)

not need to be reported to Federal health officials, no one knows the real prevalence (Schiffman, 1992). The incubation period for genital warts appears to be approximately one to two months, but may be up to six months. Unlike genital herpes, genital warts are usually painless, soft fleshy growths appearing most commonly in the genital area. Sometimes many warts may grow together to form a large cauliflower-shaped growth.

The greatest health threat that HPV poses to a female client is the predisposition to the development of cervical cancer (Lungu, et al., 1992). Although there are over sixty different types pf HPV, only six of those have been associated with the development of cervical cancer. Cigarette smoking has been linked to the development of cancerous cervical changes in women with HPV. Women who have HPV should be advised not to smoke. A diet deficient in vitamins such as folic acid has also been implicated in the development of cancerous cervical changes in women with HPV (Butterworth, et al., 1992). HPV appears to play a role in the development of cervical cancer, along with many other factors. An abnormal Pap test may be the first indication of HPV.

▶ *Medical/Surgical Management*

Since genital warts are caused by a virus, there is no cure for the disease. The focus is on preventing the spread of the disease to sexual partners, and reducing the possibility of cancer. Use of a condom during sexual intercourse is recommended at all times. Exceptions to this rule might be for monogamous couples where the partner with genital warts has had no outbreaks for a number of years. If both partners are infected, condoms are also not required to prevent the spread of warts. Once the genital warts disappear, the disease may lie dormant for many years until there is a recurrence of the outbreak.

▶ Surgical

The warts may be removed under local anesthesia. This is especially recommended if the warts have formed a large fleshy cauliflowerlike growth. Freezing the warts off with cryosurgery, surgical use of extreme cold, is currently the recommendation of choice by the CDC. The warts may also be removed with laser surgery, or cauterized. Whatever treatment is recommended, it must be remembered that the treatment will not cure HPV, but only provide a palliative effect. The warts may recur after any treatment, usually within a period of three to twelve months.

▶ Pharmacological

A topical solution of podophyllium resin (Poddoen) may be applied to the genital warts. It is only recommended for treatment of one or two lesions at a time, since it can be toxic if applied to too large an area at one time. Most people report experiencing a good deal of pain from the treatment. After the solution has been in contact with the genital warts for a period of four to six hours, it is then washed off with soap and water. If not thoroughly washed off, podophyllum may cause chemical burns that heal very slowly and are very painful. This therapy must not be used on a diabetic client, on a client with poor circulation, or a pregnant client..

▶ AIDS

AIDS, or acquired immuno deficiency syndrome, is not truly a sexually transmitted disease, but needs to be discussed briefly here since sexual contact remains one of the primary modes of transmission of this disease. AIDS is the end stage of the disease process caused by the human immunodeficiency virus (see Chapter 25). Similar to the viruses previously discussed in this chapter, AIDS is not curable. Unlike the other viruses, herpes genitalis and genital warts, AIDS is ultimately fatal. AIDS results in a severe disorder of the body's immune system functioning, leading to an inability of the body to fight off disease. The client's failing immune system makes him vulnerable to opportunistic infections, such as *Pneumocystis carinii* pneumonia.

Persons at risk are those who have multiple sexual partners, IV drug users who share needles, and persons with hemophilia. There are three basic modes of transmission—sexual, bloodborne, and from mother to baby either prenatally, during the birth process, or

when breast-feeding. When first identified in 1981, HIV infection was primarily found among homosexual men, but by 1990 the disease was moving into heterosexual populations with great rapidity. By the mid-1990s, cases of AIDS were occurring more frequently among women than among men. The greatest growth in AIDS rates among women occurred in African American and Hispanic women. Teenagers also have one of the fastest growing rates of HIV infection.

▶ Medical/Surgical Management

▶ Medical

Medical management centers around treating the infections and tumors associated with AIDS as they appear. There are a variety of new medications being investigated that may prove helpful in slowing the progress of the disease in the future.

▶ Pharmacological

Many of the drugs used to treat the infections and tumors associated with AIDS are the same ones used to treat other clients with some of the same kinds of conditions. One drug that is specifically geared toward HIV is zidovudine (AZT or Retrovir). This drug interferes with the ability of the virus to transform the cell's RNA into the virus' DNA. Some studies indicate that clients taking zidovudine have prolonged lives, but it is not a cure.

▶ Diet

Attention to diet therapy can be both a preventive and a therapeutic treatment for clients with HIV. The basic diet should be high in kilocalories with adequate high-quality protein. Both the disease process itself and the medications used to treat the disease are very irritating to the gastrointestinal tract.

▶ TRICHOMONIASIS

Trichomoniasis is caused by a parasitic protozoan called *Trichomonas vaginalis*. Trichomoniasis is a very common STD, with an incidence of approximately three million new cases every year. It is seen frequently in combination with gonorrhea. The most common method of transmission is sexual, although the protozoa can survive for a period of time in water so other modes of transmission are possible.

The incubation period after initial exposure to trichomoniasis ranges from approximately one week to one month. About 25 percent of women infected with trichomoniasis will have no symptoms. In these women, the *Trichomonas* organisms may remain dormant in the vagina for years, without becoming an active infection. Precipitating factors that may reduce the normal acidic vaginal pH, and encourage the growth of *Trichomonas* include pregnancy, sexual intercourse, menstruation, or illness. Vulval and vaginal pruritus is the most common symptom. Other symptoms include a vaginal discharge which ranges from a frothy, copious yellow-green mucus to a scanty, watery, whitish discharge. Only 10 percent of women will present with the classic symptoms of a *Trichomonas* infection; severe itching of the vulva, redness, swelling of the vulva, pain on intercourse and urination, urinary frequency and a grayish, malodorous discharge. Males most often present with the same itching and purulent discharge, but may also have urethritis and an accompanying inflammation. In men, *Trichomonas* in the dormant state are usually harbored in the prostate or urethra.

▶ Medical/Surgical Management

▶ Pharmacological

Both partners should be treated with metronidazole (Flagyl) either given orally in a single dose, or for a period of approximately one week. Metronidazole is effective against both protozoal and bacterial infections. If given vaginally, metronidazole (Flagyl) is not as effective. Pregnant women are usually treated after the first trimester to avoid the possibility of birth defects, since metronidazole is known to cross the placenta.

Adverse effects occur in about 10 percent of clients taking metronidazole (Flagyl) and usually affect the gastrointestinal system in the form of nausea, vomiting, diarrhea, and abdominal cramping. CNS effects, such as headache or dizziness, may also be seen. The client must be instructed not to consume alcohol before, during, or after treatment, as severe gastrointestinal distress generally results.

▶ Nursing Process

The following is a general nursing process for the client with an STD.

Assessment

Subjective Data   Data to be gathered from a client who presents with a suspected STD is very similar, regardless of the actual STD. Either the nurse or physician must take a thorough history. A relaxed, nonjudgmental attitude will help to elicit accurate information from the client, since pertinent questioning will deal with very private areas of the client's life. Confidentiality and privacy are extremely important when dealing with both the history and physical examination for STDs. Pertinent information must be gathered regarding the client's sexual orientation (homosexual, heterosexual, bisexual), any prior treatment for an STD and the number of sexual partners that the client has had in the last six months.

Women will be asked about such symptoms as vulval or vaginal itching, vaginal discharge, pain or discomfort, skin rashes or pruritus, and any changes in the menstrual periods or other abnormal bleeding. Men will be questioned regarding the presence of symptoms such as pain or burning on urination, abnormal penile discharges, skin rashes or itching, lesions on external genitalia, or systemic symptoms, such as fatigue, malaise, or sore throat. Both men and women will be questioned regarding urinary frequency or discomfort. Homosexual men need to be questioned regarding rectal symptoms such as abnormal discharge, itching, lesions, or pain on defecation.

Objective Data   The systems that need to be carefully evaluated include the reproductive, gastrointestinal, and integumentary systems. The presence or absence of skin rashes or lesions, abnormal discharges must be determined. Females need a speculum examination of the vagina and cervix to closely observe internal organs for changes consistent with STDs. The rectal area is examined to look for any abnormal discharge, lesions, or tenderness. Inguinal lymph nodes should be palpated to look for signs of infection.

▼ ▼

Possible nursing diagnoses for the client with a STD may include:

Nursing Diagnoses	Goals	Nursing Interventions
▶ *Anxiety related to unknown procedures, embarrassment, or other factors (relates to nearly every client who presents with an STD).*	The client will admit lack of knowledge and embarrassment.	Provide a relaxed, nonjudgmental attitude which will aid in reducing client anxiety. The nurse must examine own attitudes toward STDs and the clients who suffer from them. Listen actively to both the spoken and unspoken concerns of the client.
▶ *Knowledge deficit related to mode of transmission of the STD, prevention methods, and risk for spread of the STD.*	The client will accurately discuss the mode of transmission of an STD and list appropriate measures to avoid reinfection or future infection.	Teach mode of transmission, prevention of further infection, and risk for spread. Take time to make sure that the client has a thorough understanding of all necessary aspects of the disease.
▶ *Noncompliance related to the stigmatizing nature of the disease as well as a lack of understanding of treatment.*	The client will discuss treatment regimen.	Instruct the client regarding the treatment for the disease, including the name of the medication, the action of the medication, how long to use the medication, how to use the medication, and the possible side effects that may arise. Include the consequences of not following through with both the treatment regimen.
▶ *Infection, high risk for, related to incomplete treatment or lack of precautions with untreated, infected partners.*	The client will state the need for having all sexual partners notified and treated. The client will state understanding of the treatment regimen and of the importance of completing treatment. The client will explain appropriate use of latex condoms, including how and when to apply and remove the device.	Discuss the importance of completing treatment regimen. Discuss the need for all sexual partners to be notified and treated. Teach the importance of abstaining from sexual intercourse until the infection is resolved, or of using appropriate measures, such as latex condoms, to prevent reinfection.
▶ *Injury, high risk for, related to noncompliance with treatment.*	The client will have no injury from not completing treatment.	Instruct client on complications arising from not completing treatment regimen.

▶ Evaluation

Each goal must be evaluated to determine how it has been met by the client.

▲ ▲

▶ *CASE STUDY*

Noelle Landers, a seventeen-year-old student, has come to your clinic seeking treatment. Noelle is complaining of pain and burning on urination, as well as pain during intercourse. She states that she is infrequently sexually active with her seventeen-year-old boyfriend, and is also seeking a form of birth control. She has not used any form of birth control in the past and neither has her boyfriend. She also complains of a yellowish vaginal discharge, and has been wearing a panty liner to deal with this. Upon examination, Noelle complains of some abdominal tenderness, but denies that she has had any tenderness prior to this time. Noelle is screened for chlamydia and gonorrhea. She denies having had sex with any other partners, but does admit that she and her boyfriend had a fight and broke up temporarily about a month ago. They went back together about a week later. She does not know if he had any other sexual contacts during their period of separation.

The following questions will guide your development of a Nursing Care Plan for the case study.

1. What other information should be elicited from Noelle?

2. What are the diagnostic tests that Noelle most likely received in the clinic to determine whether she is infected with chlamydia or gonorrhea?

3. What other sexually transmitted diseases will Noelle most likely be tested for in addition to chlamydia and gonorrhea?

4. Write three nursing diagnoses and goals for Noelle.

5. List the medications that Noelle will be most likely to receive to treat a chlamydial infection.

6. List some complications that Noelle may experience if she does not receive treatment for an active chlamydial or gonorrheal infection.

7. What information will you include when you counsel Noelle regarding sexual activity and forms of birth control? (See Chapter 31, Female Reproductive Disorders, for additional information.)

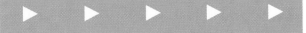
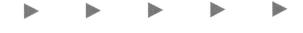

SUMMARY

- Sexually transmitted diseases are among the most common infections occurring in the United States today.
- Despite massive education efforts, the number of new STD cases identified each year continues to grow.
- Early, intensive education regarding STDs is being utilized to help combat the high incidence of STDs, virtually an epidemic among young, urban-dwelling populations.
- Many STDs, such as gonorrhea, syphilis, and chlamydia, are treatable with antibiotics, but many others are caused by viruses and are not curable.
- The only solution to the problem of STDs is prevention.
- Identification of groups at risk for STDs and appropriate prevention teaching are the most effective weapons in the ongoing battle against STDs.

Review Questions

1. When obtaining a health history from a client, the nurse asks the client to report on the presence of which of the following common symptoms of syphilis?
   a. nausea and vomiting
   b. fever, cellulitis, and diarrhea
   c. dysuria and mucopurulent discharge
   d. painless sore or ulcer in the genital area

2. The two most effective medications commonly used to treat chlamydia are:
   a. doxycycline and azithromycin.
   b. penicillin and podophyllum.
   c. erythromycin and acyclovir.
   d. doxycycline and penicillin.

3. The organism responsible for the spread of the sexually transmitted disease, syphilis, is known as a:
   a. bacteria.
   b. spirochete.
   c. virus.
   d. protozoan.

4. When instructing a client with gonorrhea regarding medication, the nurse will be sure to tell him:
   a. to take the medication until it is gone.
   b. to take the medication until symptoms subside.
   c. to take the medication at bedtime.
   d. to avoid sunlight while taking the medication.

5. If a female client with chlamydia fails to complete treatment, complications that may arise in the future include:
   a. fever and headache.
   b. nausea, vomiting, and diarrhea.
   c. infertility and ectopic pregnancy.
   d. urinary retention.

Critical Thinking Questions

1. What would it be like to have syphilis or herpes vaginalis?

2. How would you tell your parents, boyfriend/girlfriend or spouse that you had an STD?

3. Develop a teaching plan for a client with multiple sexual partners. Consider the sensitivity of the information to be shared and the clients' receptivity.

Medical Terminology

cervic-	neck, cervix
cervicitis	inflammation of the cervix
condyl-	condyle, wart
condyloma	wart-like growth
cryo-	cold
cryosurgery	use of extreme cold in surgery
hyster-	uterus, womb
hysterectomy	surgical removal of the uterus
papillo-	nipple-like protuberance or elevation
papilloma	nipple-like growth
papillomavirus	virus producing nipple-like growths
prostato-	prostate
prostatitis	inflammation of the prostate
salpingo-	uterine tube
salpingitis	inflammation of the uterine tubes

News Flash

One of the most important aspects in the fight against the epidemic of sexually transmitted disease has been education. This includes disseminating information on types of available birth control that also protect effectively against STDs. Prior to the advent of such convenient forms of birth control such as oral contraceptives (the "Pill"), injectable contraceptives medroxyprogesterone acetate (Depo-Provera), and the IUD (intrauterine device), the male condom was an effective way to prevent both pregnancy and the transmission of venereal diseases. It became much less frequently used until the appearance of AIDS. Now it is coming back into use again, since AIDS is not only incurable, but is inevitably fatal.

Women suffer greatly from sexually transmitted diseases, often with a greater rate of complications than men due to the asymptomatic nature of STDs in some women. They have been dependent on men to use a condom for greater protection against STDs. Now a female condom has been tested for ease of use and effectiveness. The female condom, a pouch connected by two rings, is effective in protecting against both pregnancy and STD transmission (see Figure 33-5A). It is more effective in protecting against STDs than any of the other barrier methods. One ring fits up against the cervix, much like a diaphragm, while the pouch lines the vaginal walls and connects with the other ring that remains outside the vaginal opening during intercourse (see Figure 33-5D). The inner ring is about 2 inches in diameter, while the outer ring is 2¾ inches in diameter so as to fit firmly against the perineum and vulva. The connecting pouch is approximately 7 inches long. The condom is as easy to apply as a diaphragm and comes prelubricated, with additional lubrication available for increased comfort. As with any method of birth control, it is only effective if used everytime sexual intercourse occurs. The female condom offers greater protection against STDs than other barrier methods.

Hopefully, education and prevention will be the keys to eradicating sexually transmitted diseases in the future. The female condom is only another weapon in the ongoing battle. (*The Female Health Company*, Chicago, IL.)

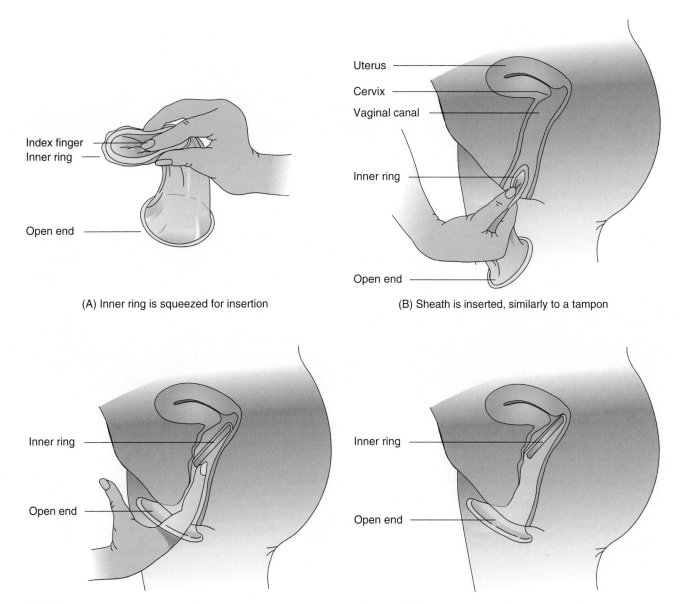

(A) Inner ring is squeezed for insertion

(B) Sheath is inserted, similarly to a tampon

FIGURE 33-5 *Reality,* a female condom, has an inner ring which fits up against the cervix, and an outer ring which provides some protection to the external genitalia. (*Courtesy The Female Health Company, Chicago, IL 60611*)

UNIT 11

Digestion and Elimination

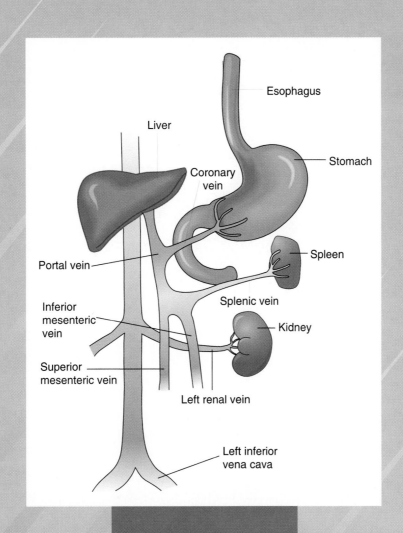

- Esophagus
- Liver
- Coronary vein
- Stomach
- Portal vein
- Spleen
- Splenic vein
- Inferior mesenteric vein
- Kidney
- Superior mesenteric vein
- Left renal vein
- Left inferior vena cava

CHAPTER 34

Digestive Disorders

Leslee R. Sinn

LEARNING OBJECTIVES

Upon completion of this chapter the learner should be able to:
- Define key terms.
- Discuss diagnostic tests associated with the digestive system.
- Discuss components necessary for a complete assessment of the digestive system.
- List medical and surgical management for digestive disorders.
- Describe nursing interventions for digestive disorders.
- Assist with the formulation of nursing care plans for clients with digestive disorders.

▶ *MAKING THE CONNECTION*

Refer to the topics in the following chapters to increase your understanding of digestive disorders:

- **Chapter 8, Health Maintenance:** Dental Caries and Periodontal Disease, p. 131
- **Chapter 10, Nursing Assessment:** Abdominal Assessment, p. 181
- **Chapter 12, Pain Management:** Assessment, p. 211; Subjective, p. 211; Objective, p. 213
- **Chapter 14, Fluid, Electrolyte, and Acid-Base Balances:** Basic Physiology of Body Fluids and Electrolytes, p. 268; Nursing Care of Clients Receiving Fluid and Electrolyte Replacements, p. 286
- **Chapter 15, Oncology Nursing:** Colorectal Cancer, p. 310; Bowel Dysfunctions, p. 316

- **Chapter 16, Caring for the Older Adult:** Common Disorders Related to Aging/ Gastrointestinal System, p. 343
- **Chapter 18, The Dying Process/Hospice:** Care of the Mouth, Eyes and Nose, p. 375; Bowel and Bladder Care, p. 375
- **Chapter 25, HIV Disorders:** Gastrointestinal Manifestations, p. 629; Oral Manifestations, p. 632; Oral Hairy Leukoplakia, p. 633
- **Chapter 36, Ostomies:** Types of Ostomies, p. 1057; Constructions of Stomas, p. 1059; Common Diagnostic Tests, p. 1059; Pathophysiology of Bowel and Bladder, p. 1061; Inflammatory Bowel Disease, p. 1061; Disorders of Ostomies, p. 1069

INTRODUCTION

Disorders and diseases of the digestive system and accessory organs can affect not only the digestive process and nutrient absorption, but the lifestyle of the individual as well.

ANATOMY AND PHYSIOLOGY REVIEW

The digestive system, also known as the gastrointestinal (GI) tract or the alimentary system, is responsible for breaking down the complex food into simple nutrients the body can absorb and convert into energy (see Figure 34-1). This process is known as digestion.

Mouth/Esophagus

Digestion begins in the mouth where the teeth mechanically break food down into smaller pieces by chewing and mixing it with saliva. The chemical breakdown of cooked starches is begun by the enzyme, salivary amylase, in the mouth. The food is then swallowed as a small ball or bolus and transported down the esophagus, a hollow, muscular tube approximately 10 inches long. **Peristalsis**, waves of muscle contractions, pushes the bolus through the esophagus. The cardiac sphincter, also called the lower esophageal sphincter (LES), located at the distal end of the esophagus relaxes and allows the food to pass into the stomach.

Stomach

Further mechanical and chemical breakdown of the food occurs in the stomach, a J-shaped muscular organ located beneath the diaphragm. The stomach secretes gastric juices which contain hydrochloric acid (HCl) and pepsinogen, a nonactive form of the enzyme pepsin. HCl and pepsin are responsible for beginning the breakdown of protein and continuing the breakdown of starches. Starch digestion in the stomach

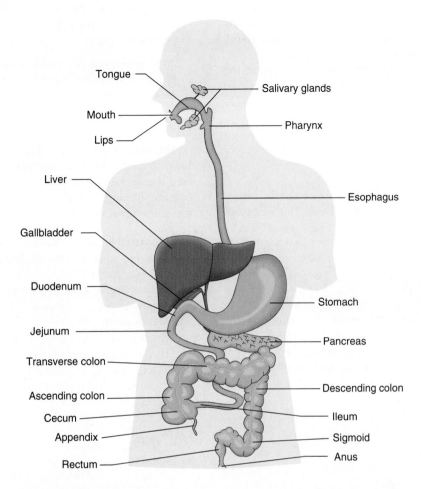

FIGURE 34-1 The digestive system.

gradually stops due to the acid environment. Mucous is secreted to protect the lining of the stomach. The stomach also secretes an intrinsic factor, which is necessary for vitamin B_{12} absorption, and gastrin, which stimulates HCl release.

The peristaltic movement of the stomach mixes the food and enzymes into a semiliquid mass called **chyme**. The chyme will not pass into the small intestine until it is the proper consistency and particles are one millimeter or less. On average, the stomach empties in three to four hours. Carbohydrates are digested most readily followed by proteins with fats taking the longest to pass from the stomach. When the chyme has reached the proper consistency, the pyloric sphincter relaxes releasing a portion of the chyme into the small intestine at a time.

Small Intestine

The small intestine is approximately 20 to 25 feet long and is responsible for absorbing nutrients from the chyme. The small intestine also secretes digestive

enzymes, mucous to protect the mucosa, and hormones to aid in the absorption of nutrients.

The chyme enters the duodenum, the first 10 to 12 inches of the small intestine. The duodenum is responsible for absorbing calcium and iron as well as neutralizing the acids in the chyme. Enzymes from the pancreas and bile from the liver enter the duodenum from the common bile duct by way of the ampulla of vater for the digestion of fats.

The jejunum, the middle of the small intestine is 8 to 10 feet long. It is responsible for absorption of fats, proteins, and carbohydrates. Vitamin B_{12} and bile salts are absorbed in the ileum, which is the distal 12 feet of the small bowel.

Large Intestine

The chyme enters the large intestine, also known as the colon, through the ileocecal valve into the cecum, a small pouch to which the appendix is attached (see Figure 34-1). The colon is approximately 4 to 5 feet long and consists of the ascending or right colon, the transverse colon, the descending or left colon and the sigmoid colon, an S-shaped segment before the rectum. The colon is responsible for absorbing water, electrolytes, and bile salts.

The last 5 inches of the large intestine comprise the rectum. The distal end of the rectum forms the anal canal composed of muscles that control defecation. The opening to the anal canal is called the anus.

Accessory Organs

The digestive system is also comprised of accessory organs that aid in the digestion of food. The accessory organs include the pancreas, liver, and the gallbladder (refer to Figure 34-1).

Pancreas

The pancreas is a fish-shaped glandular organ 6 to 8 inches long extending from the duodenum across the abdomen behind the stomach. The pancreas has both endocrine and exocrine functions. The endocrine functions, which include the production of glucagon and insulin to regulate the blood sugar level, are presented in Chapter 30.

The pancreas produces three main groups of enzymes in pancreatic juice for its exocrine function. The enzymes are:

amylase—converts carbohydrates into glucose
lipase—aids in fat digestion
protease—breaks down protein

Liver

The liver is the largest glandular organ of the body located in the right upper quadrant of the abdomen (see Figure 34-2). The liver is one of the most vascular organs, filtering 1500 cc of blood per minute. Some of the many functions of the liver are:

1. Produces and secretes bile which emulsifies fats
2. Converts glucose into glycogen for storage (**glycogenesis**)
3. Converts glycogen to glucose when blood sugar levels drop (**glycogenolysis**)
4. Metabolizes hormones
5. Breaks down nitrogenous wastes to urea
6. Incorporates amino acids into proteins
7. Filters blood and destroys bacteria present
8. Produces prothrombin and fibrinogen which are necessary for clotting

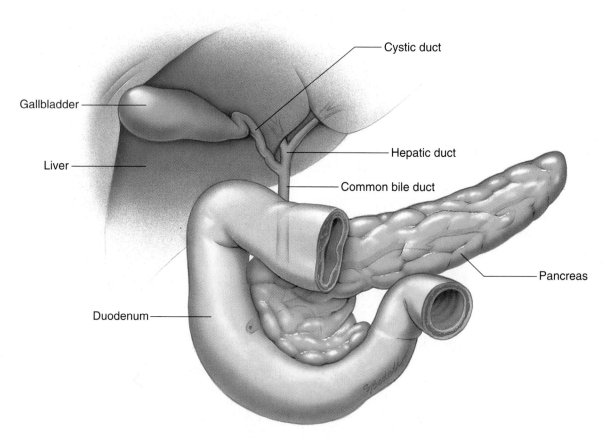

Gallbladder

Liver

Duodenum

Cystic duct

Hepatic duct

Common bile duct

Pancreas

FIGURE 34-2 The biliary tree. Bile travels from the liver to the gallbladder via the hepatic and cystic ducts. The bile is released into the duodenum via the common bile duct.

Table 34-1

CHANGES IN DIGESTIVE SYSTEM WITH AGING		
Common Changes	**Result**	**Implications for Nurses**
Decrease in Peristalsis	Food moves more slowly. Bowel movements more infrequent. Increase in constipation. Feeling full and bloated and may eat less.	Increase fiber and fluid intake. Smaller, frequent meals. Fiber supplements.
Oral Changes	Dentures are common. Food is harder to chew. Eat and drink slower. Taste buds decrease.	Make sure dentures fit. Cut food into small bites. Softer foods may be better tolerated. Some clients may start using more salt and seasonings to compensate for less flavor; monitor salt usage.
Decrease in Enzyme Secretion	Food is harder to digest. Increase in indigestion. Intolerance to some food and seasonings.	Encourage water between meals. Avoid foods that are not tolerated while ensuring adequate nutrient intake.
Decrease in Saliva	Food is more difficult to chew. Swallowing becomes difficult	Encourage fluid intake with meals. Have clients chew food well. Have clients do two swallows with each bite of food. Have client sit up to eat.

9. Manufactures cholesterol
10. Produces heparin
11. Stores vitamin B_{12} and fat soluble vitamins A, D, E, K
12. Detoxifies poisonous substances

Gallbladder

The gallbladder is a pear-shaped sac attached to the undersurface of the liver. The liver produces bile and transports the bile to the gallbladder by way of the hepatic and cystic ducts. The gallbladder stores and concentrates the bile until it is needed in the small intestine. When fats enter the small intestine, the gallbladder releases the bile through the cystic duct into the common bile duct and finally into the small intestine. The cystic duct, hepatic duct, and the pancreatic duct combine to form the common bile duct.

Effects of Aging

As the body ages, several changes may occur in the digestive system (see Table 34-1). It is important to educate clients of these changes and ways they can adapt their lifestyles.

ASSESSMENT

As discussed in Chapter 10, a thorough assessment is necessary to collect data on which to make an accu-

rate nursing diagnosis. For clients complaining of gastrointestinal symptoms, the assessment should include:

1. History of the present complaint including length and frequency of symptoms, when symptoms occur, as well as aggravating factors.
2. Medication history including prescribed and over-the-counter (OTC) medications as well as how effective they are. Clients with GI symptoms frequently self-medicate with antacids, laxatives, suppositories, and enemas.
3. A complete nutritional history; a note should be made of any foods that increase or decrease symptoms. Also, assess if meals aggravate symptoms or if symptoms occur at a specific time period after eating a meal. Note the fiber and fat content of the diet as well as the amount of fluids typically consumed.
4. Psychosocial factors including compliance and noncompliance with health status. Meal patterns should be evaluated: note if the client eats alone, eats large meals at regular intervals, or snacks all day.
5. Physical examination including inspection, auscultation, percussion, and palpation of the abdomen. An evaluation of the client's ability to chew and swallow is also important.
6. Bowel elimination patterns including frequency, consistency, and amounts of bowel movements.
7. Evaluation of diagnostic data including laboratory analysis and radiologic and endoscopic examinations.

COMMON DIAGNOSTIC TESTS

The following is a table of the commonly used diagnostic tests for clients with digestive disorders.

Test	Explanation/Normal Values	Nursing Responsibilities
CBC PT PTT	Refer to Chapter 20, Cardiac Disorders.	
Bilirubin	0.1–1.0 mg/dL Measures bilirubin in the blood. Indicates how the liver is functioning.	Note meds that affect results; steroids, antibiotics, oral hypoglycemics, narcotics as well as others may cause increased levels while barbiturates, caffeine, penicillins and salicylates may cause decreased results. Fasting may be required. Do not shake the tube; protect the tube from light.
Albumin	3.5–5.0 g/dL Protein formed by the liver responsible for maintaining colloidal osmotic pressure. Indicates how the liver is functioning.	Note meds that may affect results; steroids and hormones such as insulin, and growth hormones may increase the results while oral contraceptives and liver toxic drugs may decrease the results.
Globulin	2.3–3.3 g/dL Key for antibody production. Indicates how the liver is functioning.	Note meds that affect results (see Albumin).
Total Protein	6.4–8.3 g/dL Total measure of albumin and globulin.	Note meds that affect results (see Albumin). Instruct client to avoid eating foods high in fat 24 hours before test.
Alkaline Phosphatase	30–85 ImU/mL Enzyme that determines bone/liver disorders.	Fasting may be required.
LDH-5	5–13% of total LDH Enzyme released with liver/muscle injury.	
Gamma-glutamyl Transpeptidase (GGT or GGTP)	Females < 45 years 5–27 U/L Females > 45 years and Males 8–38 U/L Enzyme that detects liver cell dysfunction.	Note meds that interfere with results; alcohol, dilantin and phenobarb may elevate results while oral contraceptives and clofibrate may decrease results. Fast for 8 hours prior to test.
Aspartate Aminotransferase (AST/SGOT)	Enzyme indicates inflammation of heart, liver, skeletal muscle, pancreas, or kidneys. Males 7–21 U/L Females 6–18 U/L	Avoid IM injections; record time/date of any injections. Avoid hemolysis. Hold meds that affect results for 12 hours if possible; several meds such as antihypertensives, cholinergic agents, anticoagulants, digitalis, as well as others, may increase results. Exercise may increase results.
Alanine Aminotransferase (ALT/SGPT)	5–35 U/L Enzyme release with injury to liver.	Note meds that affect results; many medications may increase results including antibiotics, narcotics, oral contraceptives as well as many others.

Test	Explanation/Normal Values	Nursing Responsibilities
Cholesterol	< 200mg/dL Lipid necessary for steroid, bile, and cell membrane production.	Fast 12 to 14 hours with low-fat diet prior to fast. No alcohol 24 hours prior to test. Diet intake 2 weeks prior to test will affect results. Note any meds that may affect results; steroids, phenytoin, diuretics, as well as others, may elevate levels while MAO inhibitors, some antibiotics, lovastatin, and others may decrease levels.
Triglycerides	Males 40–160 mg/dL Females 35–135 mg/dL Form of fat produced in the liver.	Fast 12 to 14 hours prior to test with no alcohol 24 hours before. Diet intake for 2 weeks prior to test affect results.
Amylase	56–190 IU/L Enzyme secreted by the pancreas. Elevation indicates pancreatitis.	Note meds that affect test results; steroids, ASA, alcohol, some narcotics, some diuretics as well as other meds may increase results while citrate, glucose, and oxalates may decrease results.
Carcinoembryonic Antigen (CEA)	< 5 ng/mL Protein present with certain cancers; may indicate return of cancer.	Note if client smokes or has a disease that interferes with results such as hepatitis, cirrhosis, or colitis.
HAA, now called hepatitis B surface antigen (HB$_5$AG)	Negative. A positive result indicates presence of hepatitis or prior exposure.	
Stool O & P	Negative. A positive result indicates infection.	Stool placed in specimen container and taken warm to the laboratory.
Stool Occult Blood (Guaiac) Fecal Occult Blood Test (FOBT) Hemocult	Negative. A positive result indicates blood in the stool that may signify cancer, infection, or hemorrhoids.	Smear of stool placed on a card. Meds such as anticoagulants, ASA, iron preparations, NSAIDs and steroids may cause a false positive result while vitamin C may cause a false negative. Red meat should not be ingested for 3 days prior to test.

RADIOLOGIC TESTS

Test	Explanation/Normal Values	Nursing Responsibilities
Barium Swallow	Exam of pharynx, esophagus, and LES using barium contrast.	NPO 6 to 8 hours prior to test.
UGI with Small Bowel Follow-through	Exam of pharynx, LES, esophagus, stomach, and small intestine using barium contrast.	NPO 6 to 8 hours prior to exam. Procedure can be lengthy; encourage client to take reading material.
Abdominal X-rays	Determines diaphragm position and gas and fluid distribution in the abdomen.	No preparation.
CT Scans	Examines structures, delineates tumors, or growths.	Contrast may be used to enhance images. NPO 4 to 6 hours prior to exam if contrast is used. Client may be required to lie still for up to one hour.
Ultrasound	Use of sound waves to delineate structures.	NPO 8 hours prior to exam.

(continued)

Test	Explanation/Normal Values	Nursing Responsibilities
Barium Enema	Exam of the colon by use of barium contrast.	Bowel cleansing before exam by laxatives and/or enemas. Client may have clear liquids until after the exam.
Gallbladder Series	X-ray visualization of the gallbladder.	Client takes dye tablets the evening before the exam. A low-fat diet or fat-free meal the evening before. Client is NPO except for water after taking the dye.
Esophagogastro-duodenoscopy (EGD)	Exam of the esophagus, stomach and duodenum. Biopsies can be taken. Dilations can be done.	Sedation given. NPO 6 to 8 hours prior to exam.
Endoscopic Retrograde Cholangiopancreatogram (ERCP)	Exam of the CBD, biliary and pancreatic systems following injection of dye. Sphincterotomy, stone crushing, and stone removal can be done.	Sedation given. X-ray used in conjunction. NPO 6 to 8 hours prior to exam. PT, PTT and bleeding time prior to exam. Can last up to 2 hours.
Colonoscopy	Exam of the rectum, colon, cecum, and ileocecal valve.	Sedation given. Bowel cleansing necessary. Clear liquids after cleansing. NPO 6 to 8 hours prior to exam. Client will be gassy & crampy after exam.

OTHER TESTS

Test	Explanation/Normal Values	Nursing Responsibilities
Flexible Sigmoidoscopy	Exam of sigmoid colon and rectum.	Sedation is optional. Enemas prior to exam. Some gas and cramping after exam.
Esophageal Motility Studies (Manometry)	Evaluates muscle contractions and coordination by using a tube with transducers. Used as a diagnostic exam for disorders of the esophagus and LES.	NPO 6 to 8 hours prior to the exam.
Gastric Secretion Analysis	Laboratory analysis of stomach secretions by passing an NG tube into the stomach and aspirating secretions.	NPO 6 to 8 hours prior to procedure.
Liver Biopsy	Tissue sample obtained by inserting a needle into the liver. May be done with ultrasound or CAT scan to guide needle placement. Evaluates cirrhosis, cancer, and hepatitis.	H & H, PT, PTT, and platelets are done prior to the procedure. No NSAIDs including aspirin 1 week prior to procedure. Prep site by scrubbing with a surgical prep solution and draping with a sterile towel. Monitor for signs of hemorrhage post procedure by monitoring vital signs and pain frequently. Have client lie on R side with a towel or bath blanket supporting the biopsy site for two hours. Monitor site for ecchymosis.
Peritoneal Aspiration	Fluid is withdrawn from the abdominal cavity by inserting a needle into the abdomen. The specimen in analyzed for infection or bleeding.	Have client empty bladder prior to procedure. Prep abdomen scrubbing with a surgical prep solution and draping with a sterile drape. Post procedure, dress the site with a sterile dressing and monitor the site for further drainage. Assess vital signs once post procedure.

KEY ABBREVIATIONS

The following abbreviations and acronyms are used in this chapter:

CBD	common bile duct
GI	gastrointestinal
HCl	hydrochloric acid
H&H	hemoglobin and hematocrit
IBD	inflammatory bowel disease
LES	lower esophageal sphincter
LFT	liver function tests
NG	nasogastric
NSAIDs	nonsteroidal antiinflammatory drugs
O & P	ova and parasite
OTC	over the counter
TIPS	transjugular intrahepatic portosystemic shunt
TPN	total parenteral nutrition
UC	ulcerative colitis

▶ DISORDERS OF THE GASTROINTESTINAL TRACT

▶ STOMATITIS

Stomatitis is a painful condition characterized by inflammation and ulcerations in the mouth. Stomatitis can be caused by infections, damage to the mucous membranes by irritants, or by chemotherapy.

▶ Medical/Surgical Management

Cultures may be done to determine if an infectious process is present.

▶ Pharmacological

Because the client's mouth can be sore, topical anesthetics such as xylocaine may be used. Analgesics may also be ordered. If an infection is present, the appropriate medication will be ordered.

▶ Dietary

Dietary restrictions are based on what the client is able to tolerate. Usually bland, soft foods or liquids are tolerated best. As the sores heal, the diet may be advanced as tolerated. It is important to monitor dietary intake as caloric and fluid intake may be poor due to discomfort.

▶ Nursing Process

Assessment

Subjective Data Clients will usually complain of pain in the mouth and difficulty swallowing.

Objective Data Observations will include inflamed mucosa of the mouth with ulcerations frequently present.

▼ ▼

Possible nursing diagnoses for a client with stomatitis may include:

Nursing Diagnoses	Goals	Nursing Interventions
▶ *Pain, acute, related to stomatitis.*	The client will verbalize increase in comfort within 1 hour of initiation of treatment.	Assess the client frequently for discomfort. Administer medications such as topical xylocaine and analgesics as ordered. Allow for rest periods as indicated.
▶ *Nutrition, altered, less than body requirements, related to inadequate caloric and fluid intake.*	The client will be able to maintain caloric intake of 1,500 calories per day by forty-eight hours after initiation of treatment. The client will be able to maintain fluid intake at 2000 cc per day by forty-eight hours after initiation of treatment.	Monitor daily calorie intake and consult with the dietitian to assist with food selection. Administer IV fluids as ordered and monitor I & O.

(continued)

Nursing Diagnoses	Goals	Nursing Interventions
▶ *Oral mucous membranes, altered, related to stomatitis.*	The client will have less inflammation and a decrease in the size of the ulcers by thirty-six hours of initiation of treatment.	Monitor the stomatitis every shift to assess status of condition.
		Provide oral care every 4 hours.
		Administer medications to combat the infection as ordered.

▶ Evaluation

Each goal must be evaluated to determine how it has been met by the client.

▲ ▲

▶ ESOPHAGEAL VARICES

A varix is an enlarged, tortuous vein, or, occasionally an artery. While varices can occur in any part of the digestive system, they occur most frequently in the distal veins of the esophagus. The varices are often associated with cirrhosis of the liver or any other condition that causes chronic obstruction of drainage from the esophageal veins into the portal veins. Swelling of the veins causes the walls to weaken, making them prone to ulceration and bleeding. Anything that causes increased abdominal venous pressure such as sneezing, coughing, vomiting, or the Valsalva maneuver can rupture the varices.

Varices have no symptoms so clients may not be aware of them until they start bleeding. They must be treated, however, to avoid rupture and hemorrhage. Death can ensue rapidly if the hemorrhaging varix is not treated immediately.

▶ Medical/Surgical Management

▶ Medical

The varices may be treated with sclerotherapy, ligation, or balloon tamponade. Sclerotherapy is a procedure in which a caustic substance is injected into the varix. An EGD is performed and a sclerosing agent is injected through a special needle. Several treatments are necessary to cause formation of scar tissue and to stop the bleeding. After the bleeding has stopped and the client has stabilized, the remaining treatments may be done on an outpatient basis.

Complications to sclerotherapy include mediastinal inflammation secondary to extra esophageal injection, perforation, ulceration, stricture secondary to scar formation, and re-bleeding.

Esophageal **ligation**, also called banding, involves placing a rubber band or O-ring on the varix (see Figure 34-3). An EGD is performed to guide the place-

ment of the bands. The complications include rebleeding and stricture formation.

In a case where varices are actively bleeding, a 3 or 4 lumen balloon tamponade, known as a Minnesota or Sengstaken-Blakemore tube is passed into the esophagus. The balloon is then inflated in the esophagus to put direct pressure onto the bleeding varices (see Figure 34-4). The client needs to be kept NPO and the head of the bed elevated 30 to 45 degrees. The balloon is periodically deflated to prevent necrosis of the esophageal tissue. Iced isotonic saline lavages may also be done through the tube.

Complications of the Minnesota tube include perforation of the esophagus from pressure from the balloon and necrosis of the surrounding tissue.

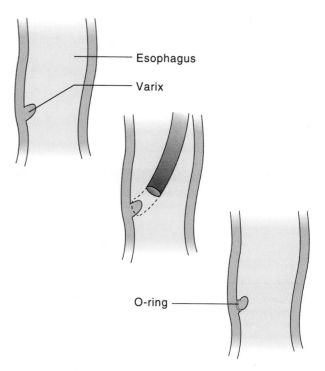

FIGURE 34-3 Banding of an esophageal varix. An O-ring is placed around the varix.

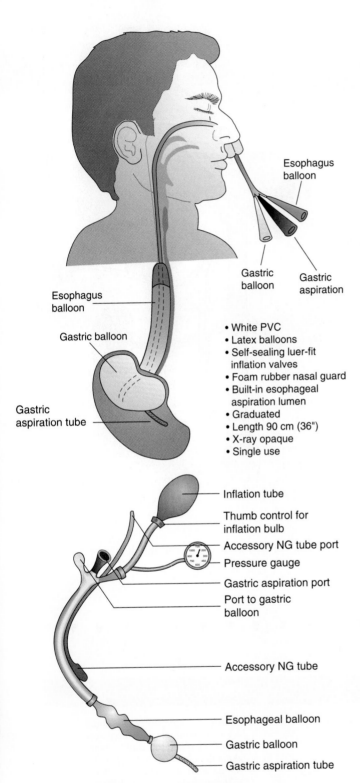

Esophagus balloon

Gastric balloon

Gastric aspiration

Esophagus balloon

Gastric balloon

Gastric aspiration tube

- White PVC
- Latex balloons
- Self-sealing luer-fit inflation valves
- Foam rubber nasal guard
- Built-in esophageal aspiration lumen
- Graduated
- Length 90 cm (36")
- X-ray opaque
- Single use

Inflation tube

Thumb control for inflation bulb

Accessory NG tube port

Pressure gauge

Gastric aspiration port

Port to gastric balloon

Accessory NG tube

Esophageal balloon

Gastric balloon

Gastric aspiration tube

FIGURE 34-4 A Sengstaken-Blakemore tube is inserted into the esophagus, and the esophageal balloon is inflated to compress the bleeding varix. (*Adapted from illustration provided by Bard, Medical Services and Support*)

▶ Surgical

A portosystemic shunt will eventually need to be placed in clients with end-stage liver disease. The shunt will relieve the pressure on the esophageal veins by redirecting blood from the portal vein to the inferior mesenteric vein. Some of the blood bypasses the liver and reenters the circulatory system (see Figure 34-5).

A nonsurgical procedure, transjugular intrahepatic portosystemic shunt (TIPS), may also be performed. With this procedure, the right internal jugular vein is used to place a cannula into the hepatic and portal veins. A connection is made through the liver tissue between the hepatic and portal veins. A stent is placed in the connection. This allows some of the blood to bypass the liver and relieve pressure in the portal vein. This procedure is done in x-ray and is used with clients who are too unstable for surgery. Also refer to Figure 34-11.

▶ Pharmacological

Analgesics may be necessary following sclerotherapy if clients complain of chest discomfort. Clients should avoid NSAIDs and all anticoagulants. IV rehydration as well as blood transfusions may be necessary for clients with active bleeding.

▶ Activity

If varices are bleeding or have recently bled, the client should remain on bed rest. If no active bleeding is present the client may be ambulatory, but should avoid strenuous exercise.

▶ Nursing Process

Assessment

Because varices have no symptoms, clients may not be aware they have them until they start bleeding.

Subjective Data   Assessment would include history of liver disease or alcohol abuse and nausea.

Objective Data   Assessment would include stools positive for **occult blood (guaiac)**; **melena**, a black tarry stool of blood; and **hematemesis**, vomiting blood. Review hemoglobin and hematocrit (H & H) to evaluate anemia and liver profile for elevated bilirubin and globulin levels and a decrease in albumin.

If cirrhosis of the liver is present, **jaundice**, a yellowing of the skin caused when the liver is unable to fully remove bilirubin from the blood, may be present. If the client abuses alcohol, nutritional status is usually poor.

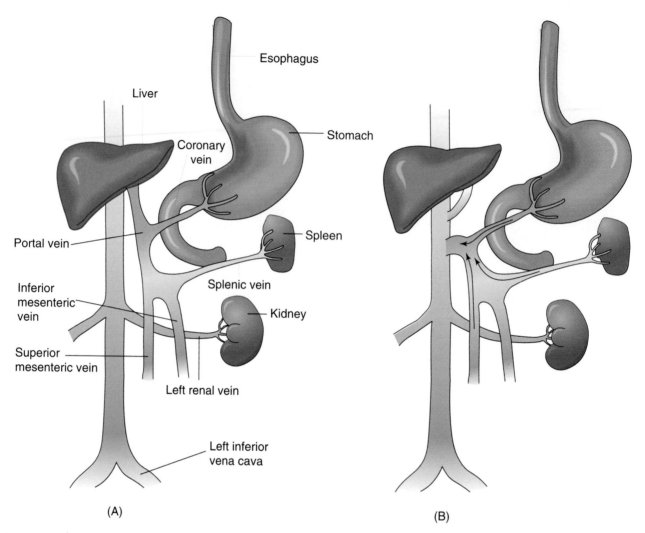

FIGURE 34-5 **(A)** Normal circulation of the liver; **(B)** An example of a portosystemic shunt that may be performed in clients with elevated portal vein pressures resistant to medical management.

▼ ▼

Possible nursing diagnoses for a client with esophageal varices may include:

Nursing Diagnoses	*Goals*	*Nursing Interventions*
▶ *Fluid volume deficit, high risk for, related to esophageal varices (if the varices are not actively bleeding).*	The client will maintain adequate fluid volume.	Monitor vital signs every four hours including orthostatic blood pressures. Orthostatic blood pressure is obtained by taking the blood pressure when the client is lying down and then when standing up. A 20 mmHg difference in blood pressures from lying to standing would indicate a change in fluid volume, possibly indicating varix bleeding.
		Monitor for nausea and dizziness.
		Monitor H & H every four to eight hours as ordered. A decrease in H & H values would indicate bleeding.

Nursing Diagnoses	Goals	Nursing Interventions
▶ *Fluid volume deficit related to bleeding esophageal varices and gastric loss from vomiting.*	The client will maintain a H & H within normal limits.	Monitor H & H.
	The client's blood pressure will be within 20 mmHg of baseline with no orthostatic changes.	Frequently monitor vital signs. Administer IV fluids, electrolyte replacement and blood transfusions as ordered.
▶ *Anxiety (moderate-severe), related to change in health status, threat of death.*	The client will discuss concerns about health status.	Explain all tests and procedures to decrease anxiety. Allow client to express fears and concerns regarding condition.

▶ Evaluation

Each goal must be evaluated to determine how it has been met by the client.

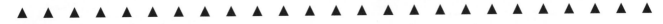

▶ GASTRITIS

Gastritis is an inflammation of the stomach mucosa occurring when the stomach has been exposed to irritating substances such as medications, smoking, food allergens, or toxic chemicals. Another contributing factor to gastritis may be impaired mucosal defenses. Impaired mucosal defenses occur when the epithelial cells of the stomach are not able to secrete adequate quantity or quality of mucous to protect the stomach. The presence of the bacteria *Helicobactor pylori* (*H. pylori*) has also been associated with gastritis.

▶ Medical/Surgical Management

▶ Medical

Diagnosis of gastritis is based on history and symptoms. An UGI or an EGD may be done to help diagnose the condition. If *H. pylori* is suspected, a biopsy is obtained during an EGD and a culture is performed.

▶ Pharmacological

Treatment for gastritis is primarily pharmacological involving antacids and histamine (H₂) receptor antagonists (also call H₂ blockers). Occasionally, a proton pump inhibitor, such as omeprazole (Prilosec) or prostaglandins may be used. If *H. pylori* is present, the use of bismuth preparations to inhibit *H. pylori* growth and antibiotics to eliminate the bacteria may be used. See Table 34-2.

NSAIDs such as ibuprofen (Motrin) and indomethacin (Indocin) have been shown to compromise mucosal defenses and increase acid secretion. Clients who are on NSAIDs chronically, such as clients with arthritis, may need to evaluate if other analgesics would be effective or if a prostaglandin should be taken with the NSAIDs.

▶ Diet

While studies have shown that dietary modifications have little impact on the rate of gastritis healing, some modifications are indicated. Foods that aggravate symptoms should be eliminated. Also, foods that increase acid secretions such as milk, coffee, decaffeinated coffee, tea, colas, and chocolate should be consumed only in small amounts or eliminated if possible. Bedtime eating should be avoided as this increases nocturnal acid secretions.

▶ Lifestyle Changes

Smoking and alcohol aggravate the mucosal lining of the stomach and significantly impair gastritis healing. Smoking and alcohol consumption should be minimal or eliminated if possible.

▶ Nursing Process

Assessment

Subjective Data Clients with gastritis may have no symptoms or may describe epigastric pain or burning, or nausea. They may also complain of certain foods aggravating symptoms.

Objective Data Stools may test positive for blood.

Table 34-2

MEDICATIONS USED FOR ULCERS AND GASTRITIS

Medication	Purpose	Nursing Implications
Antacids aluminum hydroxide (Amphogel) aluminum hydroxide and magnesium hydroxide (Maalox) dihydroxyaluminum sodium carbonate (Rolaids)	Seal impaired mucosa. Neutralize acids	Antacids containing aluminum hydroxide may cause constipation. Antacids containing magnesium hydroxide may cause diarrhea; monitor serum electrolytes; don't give with other meds.
H_2 Receptor Antagonists ranitadine HCl (Zantac) cimetidine (Tagamet)	Decrease gastric acid secretion.	Cannot be taken within 1 hour of antacids.
Proton Pump Inhibitor omeprazale (Prilosec)	Stops gastric acid secretion.	Give with food. Suspend granules in an acid liquid. Takes 4 days to achieve blood level.
Prostaglandins misoprostol (Cytotec)	Decreases gastric acid secretion. Enhances mucosal defenses.	Given when NSAIDs need to be continued.
Bismuth Compounds bismuth subsalicylate (Pepto-Bismol)	Enhances mucosal barriers Inhibits *H. pylori* growth.	Cannot be taken within 1 hour of H_2 blockers.
Antibiotics ampicillin metronidazale (Flagyl)	Eliminates *H. pylori*	Some antibiotics will cause N/V if taken with alcohol. Cannot take with antacids or meals. Clients usually placed on two different antibiotics.

▼ ▼

Possible nursing diagnoses for a client with gastritis may include:

Nursing Diagnoses	Goals	Nursing Interventions
▶ *Pain, related to gastric acid on inflammation.*	The client will experience less pain within seventy-two hours of onset of treatment as identified by pain scale.	Administer medications as ordered. Assess client for improvement of symptoms. Provide diet as ordered. Implement education about lifestyle changes.
▶ *Knowledge deficit, related to condition, therapy, and symptoms of potential complications.*	The client will verbalize understanding of factors related to condition and symptoms of complications and comply with treatment regimen.	Educate regarding medication regimen and lifestyle changes. If the client smokes, provide information on smoking cessation. Discuss dietary modifications.

▶ *Evaluation*

Each goal must be evaluated to determine how it has been met by the client.

▲ ▲

▶ PEPTIC ULCERS

Peptic ulcers are erosions that form in the esophagus, stomach, or duodenum resulting from acid/pepsin imbalance. Gastric ulcers refer to ulcers in the stomach and are correlated to exposure to irritants such as NSAIDs, smoking, alcohol, food allergens, toxic chemicals, *H. pylori* infections, and impaired mucosal defenses. Impaired mucosal defenses occur when the epithelial cells of the stomach are not able to secrete adequate quantity or quality of mucous to protect the stomach.

Clients with gastric ulcers frequently complain of pain one to two hours after eating. Eating may not relieve pain or may even increase pain. Weight loss is common. Risk factors include alcohol use, stress, and NSAID use.

Stress ulcers are a type of gastric ulcer that form when gastritis becomes erosive and starts bleeding. As the name implies, stress ulcers occur in clients whose bodies are experiencing stress, such as clients who have experienced major surgery, trauma, burns, chemotherapy, or radiation therapy. Clients with chronic respiratory disorders may also experience stress ulcers as hypoxia can lead to impaired mucosa. Bleeding may be massive resulting in significant blood loss or can be slow and insidious. Because of the multiple sites of bleeding, stress ulcers may be difficult to manage.

Duodenal ulcers refer to ulcers in the duodenum. Incidents of duodenal ulcers have been correlated to a high secretion of HCl. Clients with duodenal ulcers frequently complain of pain two to four hours after eating. Nocturnal pain may be present, occurring between midnight and 3:00 A.M. Eating frequently relieves symptoms. Weight gain is common. Risk factors include a history of pulmonary disease, cirrhosis, chronic pancreatitis, and/or chronic renal failure.

If an ulcer erodes through a blood vessel, the client may experience a hemorrhage. A perforation occurs if the ulcer erodes through the wall of the stomach or small intestine resulting in gastric or intestinal contents entering the abdominal cavity and causing peritonitis.

Diagnosis of ulcers is based on symptoms, history, and an UGI or an EGD performed to visualize the ulcer. If an *H. pylori* infection is suspected, a biopsy is obtained during an EGD and a culture is performed.

▶ Medical/Surgical Management

▶ Medical

If an ulcer bleeds, an EGD may be performed and the ulcer is either injected with epinephrine to cause vasoconstriction or a special electrical probe is used to cauterize or burn the tissue that is bleeding. A nasogastric (NG) tube may be inserted to remove gastric contents and blood, and iced isotonic saline may be instilled to help cause vasoconstriction and stop the bleeding.

▶ Surgical

If the ulcer continues to bleed or if the ulcer has perforated, the client is taken to surgery and a gastrectomy is performed. When a gastrectomy is performed, the portion of the stomach or duodenum that is perforated is removed and the bowel is reconnected with an anastomosis (see Figure 34-6). A vagotomy may also be performed. A vagotomy is a procedure in which the vagal innervation to the fundus of stomach is removed, thereby decreasing acid production in the stomach.

Complications from gastrectomies include gastric dumping in which the stomach experiences **post prandial** (after eating) rapid gastric emptying. Clients experience abdominal pain, nausea, vomiting, explosive diarrhea, weakness, and dizziness. Clients with gastric dumping have malabsorption of nutrients because the food passes too quickly to permit absorption, thus leading to malnutrition. In addition, many clients with significant symptoms may limit dietary intake to avoid symptoms, compounding the malnutrition and weight loss issues.

Management of gastric dumping include small frequent meals of a high-fiber and high-protein diet, and avoiding simple carbohydrates.

▶ Pharmacological

Treatment of ulcers is primarily pharmacological involving antacids, histamine (H_2) receptor antagonists (also called H_2 blockers), proton pump inhibitor, or prostaglandins. If *H. pylori* is present, the use of bismuth preparations to inhibit its growth and antibiotics to eliminate the bacteria are generally used. Refer to Table 34-2.

NSAIDs such as ibuprofen (Motrin) and indomethacin (Indocin) have been shown to compromise mucosal defenses and increase acid secretion. Clients who are on NSAIDs chronically, such as clients with arthritis, may need to evaluate if other analgesics would be effective or if a prostaglandin should be taken with the NSAIDs.

▶ Diet

While studies have shown that dietary modifications have little impact on the rate of ulcer healing, some modifications are indicated. Foods that aggravate symptoms should be eliminated. Also, foods that increase acid secretions such as milk, coffee, decaffeinated coffee, tea, colas, and chocolate should be consumed only in small amounts or eliminated if pos-

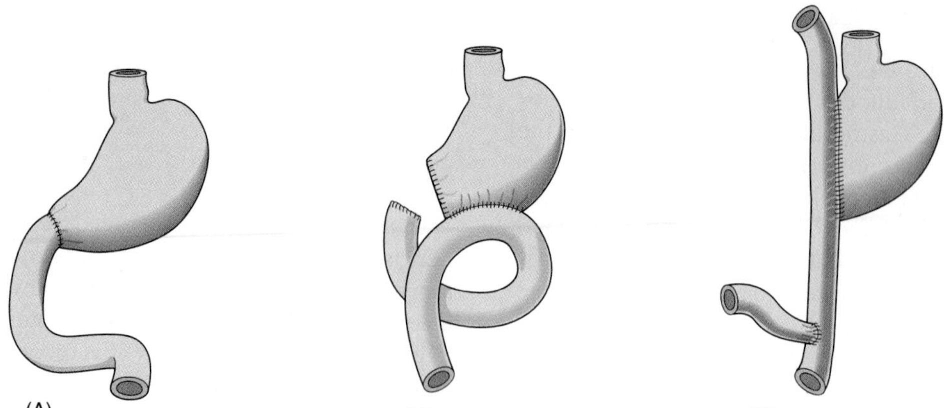

(A)

Bill Roth I
• Gastroduodenal hookup
• Used with vagotomy for duodenal ulcer

(B)

Bill Roth II
• Gastrojejunal hookup
• Used with subtotal gastrectomy

(C)

C-sendes Procedure (Roux-en-Y)
• Esophagogastrojejunostony
• Used in ulcers high in the stomach

FIGURE 34-6 Gastric resections are necessary when an ulcer perforates. The type of gastrectomy depends on the location of the ulcer.

sible. Bedtime eating should also be avoided as this increases nocturnal acid secretions.

▶ Lifestyle Changes

Smoking and alcohol aggravate the mucosal lining of the stomach and duodenum and significantly impair ulcer healing. Smokers also experience a higher recurrence rate. Stress has been shown to increase the rate of peptic ulcers. While the type or severity of stress may not be significant, the client's interpretation of the events as stressful is. Clients need to develop mechanisms for reducing stress such as exercise, biofeedback, and relaxation.

▶ Nursing Process

Assessment

Subjective Data Clients with gastric ulcers may exhibit no symptoms or may describe epigastric pain or burning one to two hours after eating and nausea or bloating. Clients may experience an increase of symptoms when they eat and therefore may decrease dietary intake. When questioned about lifestyle,

NSAID usage, stress, smoking and alcohol use may be discovered.

Clients with duodenal ulcers may exhibit no symptoms or may complain of pain two to four hours after eating. Eating will frequently decrease symptoms so clients will often eat more frequently. When questioned about lifestyle, stress, smoking and alcohol consumption may be discovered. The client may also have a history of pulmonary disease, cirrhosis, chronic pancreatitis, and/or chronic renal failure.

A client who is actively bleeding from an ulcer will experience an acute onset of epigastric pain, shortness of breath, and nausea.

Objective Data Clients with gastric ulcers may show a weight loss and stools may test positive for blood. An H & H may show anemia.

Clients with duodenal ulcers may show a weight gain and stools may test positive for blood. An H & H may show anemia.

The client who is actively bleeding from an ulcer will show signs of shock: pale clammy skin, an elevated pulse rate, and a drop in blood pressure. The client may also have hematemesis. Laboratory tests may show a low H & H. Stools may test positive for blood.

▼ ▼

Possible nursing diagnoses for a client with peptic ulcers may include:

Nursing Diagnoses	Goals	Nursing Interventions
▶ Pain, related to gastric acid on ulcerated mucosa.	The client will experience less pain within seventy-two hours of onset of treatment as identified on pain scale.	Assess clients for improvement of symptoms. Administer medications as ordered. Assess for elevated BP. Provide modified diet as indicated.
▶ Knowledge deficit, related to condition, therapy, and symptoms of complications.	The client will verbalize understanding of factors related to condition and symptoms of complications. Client will comply with treatment regimen.	Identify client's learning style and provide information in a manner compatible with the learning style. Educate regarding medication regime and lifestyle changes. If indicated, provide client with smoking cessation information and stress reduction techniques such as exercise and biofeedback. Include signs and symptoms of possible complications.
▶ Fluid volume deficit, related to bleeding ulcer.	The client will exhibit normal fluid volume as evidenced by stable H & H and blood pressure within 20 mmHg of baseline.	Check vital signs every 4 hours including orthostatic blood pressures. Administer IV fluids, electrolyte replacement, and blood transfusions as ordered. Monitor for dizziness and nausea. Check stool for blood.

▶ Evaluation

Each goal must be evaluated to determine how it has been met by the client.

▲ ▲

▶ APPENDICITIS

Appendicitis is the inflammation of the vermiform appendix, a 10 cm small, slender tube attached to the cecum. The appendix may be inflamed, gangrenous, or ruptured. If the opening to the appendix becomes blocked with feces, the E. coli multiply in the appendix and infection develops with pus formation. If it ruptures, fecal content spills into the abdominal cavity causing peritonitis. Peritonitis may be fatal.

A barium enema or an ultrasound may be ordered and would show inflammation in the appendiceal area.

▶ Medical/Surgical Management

Elderly clients tend to heal slower and are more prone to complications such as pneumonia. Early diagnosis and treatment are necessary for the best client outcome. A white blood count and differential are usually ordered. Most clients will have a WBC above 10,000/mm^3 and neutrophils over 75 percent. Sometimes an appendectomy may be performed along with other abdominal surgeries as a preventive measure.

▶ Surgical

A surgical procedure called an appendectomy is necessary before the appendix ruptures. Appendectomies are the most common emergency surgery and require a hospital stay of two to seven days. If no rupture has occurred, a laparoscopic appendectomy, in which the appendix is removed through a scope, may be done. A laparoscopic appendectomy requires only a small incision and allows the client to be discharged twenty-four hours after the surgery.

▶ Pharmacological

Preoperatively, no analgesics are given so that symptoms will not be masked by the medication. Fluids and electrolytes may need to be replaced prior to surgery. Antibiotics are usually given preoperatively. Postoperatively, analgesics are administered for the relief of incisional discomfort. Antibiotics are usually given postoperatively, especially if a perforation is present.

▶ Diet

Preoperatively, the client is to be NPO. Initially postoperatively, the client is again NPO. If a perforation with peritonitis has occurred, the client will be kept NPO longer and an NG tube will be inserted until bowel sounds have returned. The client is first started on clear liquids and advanced to full liquids and finally, to a regular diet as normal bowel function returns.

▶ Activity

Initially postoperatively, the client is encouraged to turn, cough and deep breathe every 2 hours. The next day, the client should be encouraged to leave bed and

increase ambulation gradually. Activity restrictions will depend on the severity of the appendicitis. Driving, exercise, and lifting will be limited for a few weeks to allow for incisional healing.

▶ Nursing Process

Assessment

Subjective Data   Clients with appendicitis describe abdominal pain, typically located in the right lower quadrant around McBurney's point (halfway between the umbilicus and the right iliac crest). Clients will also complain of anorexia (a loss of appetite) and nausea.

Objective Data   Clients may have vomiting and a fever. Bowel sounds may be diminished or absent. Rebound tenderness, pain that occurs when fingers are pressed into the right lower quadrant and then released suddenly, may also be present. A CBC will be done and WBCs will be elevated above 10,000/mm^3 with neutrophils over 75 percent.

▼ ▼

Possible nursing diagnoses for the client with appendicitis may include:

Nursing Diagnoses	Goals	Nursing Interventions
▶ *Pain, acute, related to appendicitis/appendectomy.*	The client will experience a decrease in pain as evidenced by improved mobility and as identified on pain scale.	Preoperatively, monitor degree of pain. Check abdomen for rigidity. Provide an ice pack to help relieve pain as ordered; never use heat. Postoperatively, give analgesics as ordered and medicate prior to activities such as ambulation. Teach client to use a pillow to splint the incision when coughing. If client is having difficulty passing flatus, administer enemas or a rectal tube as ordered.
▶ *Fluid volume deficit, related to nausea, vomiting and NPO status.*	The client will exhibit normal fluid volume as evidenced by electrolytes within normal range and I & O nearly equal.	Monitor I & O every shift and vital signs every four hours. Monitor skin turgor for signs of dehydration. Administer IV fluids and electrolyte replacement as ordered.
▶ *Skin integrity, impaired, related to the abdominal incision.*	The client will verbalize signs and symptoms of infection and factors that enhance wound healing, by discharge.	Administer antibiotics as ordered. Educate the client that incision may be left open to the air after twenty-four hours and that showers may be taken.

Nursing Diagnoses	Goals	Nursing Interventions
		If adhesive strips are present, leave in place until they no longer cover the incision (approximately ten days to two weeks).
		Educate client regarding signs and symptoms of infection and activity restrictions.

▸ Evaluation

Each goal must be evaluated to determine how it has been met by the client.

▲ ▲

▸ DIVERTICULOSIS AND DIVERTICULITIS

Diverticula are outpouchings or sacs in the wall of the colon. Diverticulosis refers to a condition of the colon in which multiple diverticula are present (see Figure 34-7). The exact cause of diverticulosis is not known. However, a diet low in fiber is felt to contribute to the formation of the pouches. Diverticulosis affects 30 to 40 percent of the elderly population (Cameron, 1995). It is asymptomatic.

Diverticulitis refers to the inflammation of one or more diverticula generally in the sigmoid colon. It is a complication of diverticulosis and is thought to be caused by stool impacted in the diverticula.

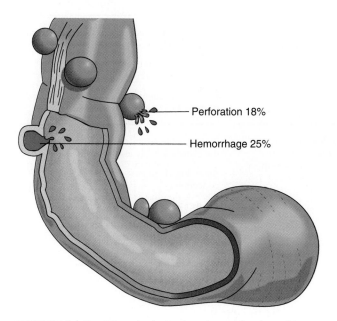

Perforation 18%

Hemorrhage 25%

FIGURE 34-7 Diverticula in the sigmoid colon. Diverticulosis is almost always located in the descending or sigmoid colon.

▸ Medical/Surgical Management

Diverticulosis is typically asymptomatic and needs no intervention. Most cases of diverticulitis are treated with analgesics, antibiotics, bedrest, NPO to rest the bowel, and IV fluid hydration.

A barium enema or abdominal ultrasound is usually ordered when diverticulitis is suspected. A flexible sigmoidoscopy may also be performed.

▸ Surgical

If bleeding or perforation of the diverticula has occurred, or if an abscess has formed, surgery is required to remove the portion of the bowel affected. A colon resection is performed. A colostomy may also be required. If a large amount of inflammation is present, a temporary colostomy may be performed to allow the colon to heal. The colon will be reconnected at a later time. In rare cases, a permanent colostomy may need to be performed. Refer to Chapter 36, Ostomies.

▸ Pharmacological

Clients who have been identified as having diverticulosis are usually placed on fiber supplements or stool softeners. Clients with diverticulitis will be treated with sulfa antibiotics and other antimicrobial agents. Analgesics may also be ordered for discomfort.

▸ Diet

A diet high in fiber is believed to help reduce the occurrence of diverticulosis and to decrease the occurrence of diverticulitis.

Clients experiencing diverticulitis will be NPO to rest the bowel. Once the diverticulitis begins healing, the client will be placed on clear liquids and then advanced to a bland, low residue diet while the diverticulitis heals.

The client will be NPO if surgery is performed until bowel sounds return. The client will then be started on clear liquids, advanced to full liquids as more bowel function returns, and then finally to a regular diet. A high-fiber diet should be encouraged for clients once the diverticulitis episode has resolved.

▶ Activity

For clients experiencing diverticulitis, bed rest is encouraged to allow the bowel to rest. In clients who have had a bowel resection, activity will gradually be progressed postoperatively.

▶ *Nursing Process*

Assessment

Diverticulosis often has no symptoms and, therefore, clients may not be aware they have it.

Subjective Data Clients with diverticulitis will frequently complain of left lower abdominal pain, constipation or diarrhea, bloating, anorexia, and nausea.

Objective Data Assessment would show abdominal distention with tenderness on palpation, decreased bowel sounds, fever, vomiting, and stools may test positive for blood. A CBC will show an elevated WBC and if bleeding is present, a low H & H.

▼ ▼

Possible nursing diagnoses for clients with diverticulosis or diverticulitis may include:

Nursing Diagnoses	Goals	Nursing Interventions
▶ *Pain, acute, related to diverticulitis.*	The client will verbalize a decrease in pain within twenty-four hours after onset of intervention as measured by the pain scale.	Encourage bed rest to decrease metabolic rate. Maintain client as NPO. Administer analgesics and antibiotics as ordered.
▶ *Fluid volume deficit, related to nausea, anorexia, and NPO status.*	The client will demonstrate adequate hydration as evidenced by intake approximately equaling output, moist mucous membranes, and electrolytes within normal limits.	Administer IV fluids and electrolyte replacement as ordered. Monitor I & O every shift. Monitor laboratory reports on electrolytes.
▶ *Infection, high risk for, related to abscess formation or perforation.*	The client will verbalize understanding of signs and symptoms of possible complications.	Monitor vital signs every four hours as well as pain level. Assess abdomen every four hours for increased tenderness and distention. Educate the client to notify staff of chills, shortness of breath, or increasing pain.
▶ *Anxiety, related to possible surgery.*	The client will verbalize fears related to surgery and exhibit decreased anxiety regarding the procedure and follow-up treatment.	Explain all tests and treatments to decrease the client's anxiety level. Allow the client to verbalize fears and concerns. Answer all concerns and questions. If a colostomy is planned, arrange a consult with an enterostomal therapist to help answer concerns.

▶ *Evaluation*

Each goal must be evaluated to determine how it has been met by the client.

▲ ▲

Sample Nursing Care Plan: The Client With Diverticulitis

Mr. W. is a sixty-seven-year-old male admitted to the hospital with abdominal pain that started two days ago. The pain has been increasing in intensity and is now accompanied by nausea and anorexia. A physical assessment includes a temperature 101.7, pulse 96, respirations 24 and a blood pressure of 162/90. Mr. W's abdomen is tender on palpation. Mr. W. is in obvious discomfort and is unable to lie on his back. Mr. W. states he has not been eating any food or drinking adequate fluids for twenty-four hours. Skin turgor is poor. An abdominal ultrasound is ordered and demonstrates diverticulitis. An IV of D5 1/2 NS with 20 mEq KCl, droperidol (Inapsine) IV for nausea, meperidine (Demerol) IM for pain, and IV antibiotics are ordered. Mr. W. is placed on I & O, bed rest with bathroom privileges and is made NPO. Mr. W. states that he does not understand why all this is being done. His first two voidings are 50 cc each and very concentrated (dark gold colored).

Nursing Diagnosis 1 Knowledge deficit, related to diagnosis and treatment regime as evidenced by statement that he does not understand why all this is being done.

Goals	Nursing Interventions	Rationale	Evaluation
Mr. W. will verbalize understanding of treatment plan.	Assess Mr. W.'s knowledge level of diverticulosis/ diverticulitis.	Building on present knowledge helps client relate new information and integrate it into his behavior.	Mr. W. verbalizes understanding of the disease process and treatment regime.
	Assess Mr. W.'s learning style and present information to Mr. W. in a manner compatible with his style.	Presenting information in a learning style compatible with the client's increases understanding and retention.	
	Monitor for signs of pain and fatigue.	Pain and fatigue impair learning.	
	Answer questions and reinforce information.	Following up and clarifying information reinforces the new information learned.	

Nursing Diagnosis 2 Pain, acute, related to diverticulitis as evidenced by tender abdomen.

Goals	Nursing Interventions	Rationale	Evaluation
Mr. W. will verbalize a decrease in pain within twenty-four hours of onset of intervention.	Assess pain utilizing a scale of 1 (no pain) to 10 (extreme pain).	Using the pain scale to assess pain is an objective measure of the client's perceived discomfort and the effectiveness of the analgesics.	Mr. W. demonstrates adequate pain relief as demonstrated by a decrease in pain scale.
	Medicate with analgesics as ordered.	Provides pain relief.	

(continued)

	Encourage Mr. W. to request analgesics when pain is increasing rather than waiting for pain to get intense.	Provides better control of pain.	
	Monitor effectiveness of pain medication by reassessing pain utilizing the pain scale forty-five minutes after the medication.	Provides a measure of analgesic's effectiveness.	

Nursing Diagnosis 3 Fluid volume deficit as evidenced by low urine output and poor skin turgor.

Goals	Nursing Interventions	Rationale	Evaluation
Mr. W. will demonstrate adequate hydration by I & O being nearly equal, normal skin turgor and electrolytes within normal limits by twenty-four hours after onset of intervention.	Monitor I & O every shift. Administer IV fluids as ordered. Assess skin turgor every shift. Monitor laboratory reports for electrolyte levels.	Provides information on the hydration level of Mr. W. Provides information on electrolyte balance.	Mr. W. demonstrates adequate hydration by nearly equal I & O, normal skin turgor, and electrolytes within normal limits.

▶ *INFLAMMATORY BOWEL DISEASE*

Inflammatory bowel disease (IBD) is the term used to describe Crohn's disease and ulcerative colitis (UC). Crohn's disease and UC are diseases characterized by inflammation and ulcerations of the bowel. See Table 34-3.

UC is characterized by mucosal lesions occurring typically in the rectal area and sigmoid colon and progressing throughout the colon. Symptoms include fever, anorexia, weight loss, cramping, spasms, abdominal pain, and bloody diarrhea. Long-term complications include fissures, abscesses, and an increased risk for colorectal cancer. Toxic megacolon, a severe, acute dilation of the colon, may occur in severe cases.

Crohn's disease is characterized by lesions that affect the entire thickness of the bowel and can occur anywhere throughout the colon and small intestine. Symptoms include abdominal pain, diarrhea that usually does not contain blood, fever, anorexia, weight loss, and **steatorrhea** (fat in stools). Electrolyte imbalances, iron deficiency anemia, and amino acid malabsorption may occur when the disease involves the jejunum and the ileum. Long-term complications of

Crohn's include bowel obstructions, fistulas, abscesses, and perforation. The risk for colorectal cancer, while not as high as UC, is still elevated. There is malabsorption of fat and fat-soluble vitamins.

Tests to diagnose Crohn's disease and UC include barium enema with small bowel follow-through, and colonoscopy with biopsies. Early symptoms for Crohn's disease and UC are similar and can make early diagnosis difficult.

▶ *Medical/Surgical Management*

Treatment for Crohn's disease and UC is similar. Crohn's disease, however, is more debilitating since it involves more of the GI tract. UC is more limited, but can still produce significant symptoms.

▶ *Surgical*

In severe cases of UC resistant to medical management, the colon is removed and a colostomy is performed, curing the disease.

Most clients with Crohn's disease need surgery at

some point to repair the structural damage caused by scarring. Intestinal obstructions and perforations may also occur in Crohn's disease necessitating further surgery. Surgical intervention, however, does not cure the disease.

▶ Pharmacological

Treatment for both UC and Crohn's disease includes 5-ASA compounds such as sulfasalazine (Azulfidine) or salicylates such as mesalamine (Rowasa) or olsalazine sodium (Dipentum). If inflammation is severe, corticosteroids may also be administered. Clients may also be placed on antidiarrheal medications. In cases resistant to the 5-ASA compounds and corticosteroids, immunosuppressors may be used. If an infection is present, antibiotics will be administered.

Clients may need IV fluid and electrolyte replacement during severe flare-ups. In the most severe cases, clients may be placed on total parenteral nutrition (TPN) to allow for complete bowel rest and to improve nutritional status.

▶ Diet

Malnutrition is a particular concern in clients with IBD. Because of the severe cramping, pain and diarrhea brought on by foods, these clients typically put themselves on a very restrictive diet that is not nutritionally balanced. Clients with Crohn's disease may also have malabsorption of iron, vitamin B_{12}, amino acids and may develop lactose intolerance.

Nutritional support includes modifying the diet to eliminate foods that exacerbate symptoms while maintaining a balanced diet. High-calorie, high-protein, nutritionally dense supplements may be used.

▶ Stress

While stress has not been shown to exacerbate the symptoms of Crohn's disease or UC, the impact on the client's lifestyle can be significant, especially with Crohn's disease. Support groups can be beneficial. Clients should be encouraged to develop mechanisms to help them cope with the disease process and reduce stress. Exercise, meditation, or biofeedback are often helpful.

▶ Nursing Process

Assessment

Subjective Data   Clients may complain of mild abdominal spasms and cramping which may increase to severe abdominal pain, nausea, and anorexia.

Objective Data   Clients will show abdominal tenderness on palpation, guarding, distention, weight loss, diarrhea, an elevated WBC count, and fever. In clients with Crohn's disease, steatorrhea and iron deficient anemia may be present. In clients with UC, stools may be positive for blood and the H & H may be low. Because Crohn's disease is so debilitating, clients may become depressed.

Table 34-3

CROHN'S DISEASE VS. ULCERATIVE COLITIS		
	Crohn's Disease	**Ulcerative Colitis (UC)**
Involvement	Patchy areas. Can involve small and large intestine.	Starts in lower colon and spreads progressively throughout colon.
Tissue affected	Affects entire thickness of bowel.	Affects mucosal lining of the bowel.
Major complication	Malabsorption	Toxic megacolon
Long-term complications	Intestinal obstruction, fistulas, abscesses, perforations; cancer risk increases with age.	Fissures, abscesses, increased risk for colorectal cancer.
Surgical intervention	Usually needed at some point to repair structural damage. Does not cure or limit the progress of the disease.	Colostomy performed in approximately 20% of cases to remove the colon. Cures the disease.
Cause	Unknown: possibly altered immune state.	Unknown: possibly enteric bacterium *E. coli*
Stools	3 to 4 semisoft/day; rarely blood; steatorrhea mucus.	15 to 20 liquid/day; blood present; no steatorrhea (fat in stool).

▼ ▼

Possible nursing diagnoses for clients with Crohn's disease or UC may include:

Nursing Diagnoses	Goals	Nursing Interventions
▶ *Nutrition, altered, less than body requirements, related to postprandial pain, bowel hypermobility, or decreased absorption.*	The client will demonstrate adequate nutritional status as exhibited by maintaining weight proportionate to height.	Monitor I & O every shift, daily calorie count and daily weight. Administer IV fluid and electrolyte replacement as ordered. Provide high-calorie, high-protein supplements as ordered along with small, frequent meals. Administer TPN, a high-calorie and nutrient-dense IV solution, as ordered. If TPN is administered, closely monitor lab reports for electrolytes and glucose level.
▶ *Fluid volume deficit, high risk for, related to diarrhea and altered intake.*	The client will exhibit adequate hydration as evidenced by electrolytes within normal range, moist mucous membranes, and I & O nearly equal within forty-eight hours of onset of intervention. The frequency and amount of diarrhea will decrease within forty-eight hours of onset of intervention.	Administer 5-ASA compounds, corticosteroids, immunosuppressors, and antidiarrheals as ordered. Monitor I & O every shift. Administer IV fluid and electrolyte rehydration as ordered.
▶ *Powerlessness related to impairment in lifestyle secondary to disease process.*	The client will verbalize a plan to seek support, by discharge.	Provide client with information on national organizations and local support groups. Allow client to verbalize feelings. Arrange social work consult if depression is present.

▶ Evaluation

Each goal must be evaluated to determine how it has been met by the client.

▲ ▲

▶ *INTESTINAL OBSTRUCTION*

An intestinal obstruction, sometimes called an ileus, occurs when the contents cannot pass through the intestine. Obstructions may occur in the large or the small intestine, with most occurring in the ileum. They may be mechanical, neurogenic, or vascular in origin.

A mechanical obstruction may be a partial or complete obstruction caused by a tumor; fecal impaction; hernia; **volvulus**, a twisting of the bowel; **intussusception**, a telescoping of the bowel (see Figure 34-8); or **adhesions**, scar tissue in the abdomen from previous surgeries or disease process such as Crohn's disease.

A neurogenic obstruction, known as a paralytic ileus, occurs when nerve transmission to the bowel is interrupted by trauma, infection, or medications resulting in a portion of the bowel being paralyzed.

A vascular obstruction occurs when blood flow to a portion of the bowel is interrupted as in atherosclerosis and that portion of the bowel becomes necrotic.

When the small intestine becomes obstructed, large amounts of fluid, bacteria and swallowed air build up in the bowel proximal to the obstruction. The normal process of secretion and absorption of the electrolyte-rich fluid is interrupted. Distention and poor absorption occur when water and salts move from the circulatory system to the lumen of the intestine.

An abdominal x-ray and a barium enema or UGI with small bowel follow-through may be ordered when a bowel obstruction is suspected.

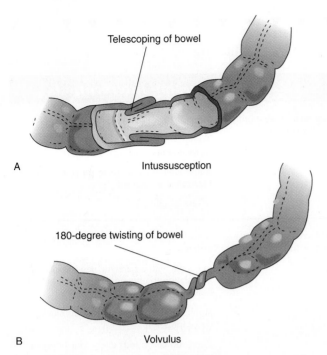

FIGURE 34-8 Bowel obstructions can be caused by **(A)** an intussusception; or **(B)** a volvulus.

▶ Medical/Surgical Management

▶ Medical

Treatment of the obstruction is dependent on the cause and location. Some can be treated medically by inserting an NG tube for decompression (see Figure 34-9), providing IV fluids for rehydration, and treating the cause such as enemas for fecal impaction.

▶ Surgical

Most bowel obstructions require surgery. A bowel resection is performed to remove the portion of the bowel affected by the obstruction.

▶ Pharmacological

Nonnarcotic analgesics are used to avoid the intestinal motility decrease caused by narcotic analgesics. Antibiotics may also be ordered.

▶ Activity

In cases of paralytic ileus, ambulation should be encouraged to help bowel function return. In clients who have had a bowel resection, encourage client to turn, cough, and deep breathe every two hours initially postoperatively. Activity should be progressed the next day.

▶ Nursing Process

Assessment

Subjective Data   Clients will complain of colicky abdominal pain, nausea, constipation, and bloating.

Objective Data   Objective assessment would include abdominal distention and tenderness on palpation. Vomiting will temporarily relieve the abdominal pain. The vomitus may include fecal material.

Laboratory analysis would demonstrate decreased levels of sodium and potassium on electrolytes, elevated BUN, elevated amylase, and elevated H & H due to hemoconcentration.

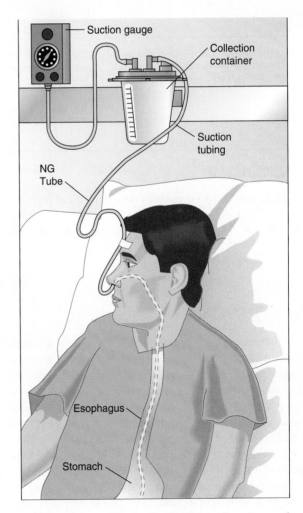

FIGURE 34-9 Nasogastric (NG) suction is used to decompress the abdomen of a client with a bowel obstruction.

▼ ▼

Possible nursing diagnoses for a client with a bowel obstruction may include:

Nursing Diagnoses	Goals	Nursing Interventions
▶ *Fluid volume deficit, related to vomiting, shift in fluids, and NPO status.*	The client will exhibit adequate hydration within forty-eight hours of initiation of treatment as evidenced by moist mucous membranes, electrolytes within normal limits, and I & O approximately equal.	Monitor I & O every shift. Administer IV fluid and electrolyte replacements as ordered. Allow limited ice chips to prevent further electrolyte imbalance. Assess weight daily.
▶ *Pain, acute, related to distention, edema, or ischemia.*	The client will verbalize increased comfort within one hour of analgesic as measured on pain scale.	Administer nonnarcotic analgesics as ordered. In clients with a paralytic ileus, encourage ambulation to encourage return of bowel function. Monitor NG as ordered for abdominal decompression. Check bowel sounds every four hours or more often.
▶ *Knowledge deficit, related to disease process, treatment regimen, and possible surgery.*	The client will verbalize treatment course, possible complications, and possible need for surgery.	Identify client's learning style and present information in a manner compatible with learning style. Client education would include intestinal decompression, need for ambulation, need for good oral care due to fecal drainage, and surgery.

▶ *Evaluation*

Each goal must be evaluated to determine how it has been met by the client.

▲ ▲

▶ *HERNIAS*

A hernia occurs when the wall of a muscle weakens and the intestine protrudes through the muscle wall (see Figure 34-10). Hernias that do not return to the abdominal cavity with rest or with client manipulation and cause complete bowel obstruction are said to be incarcerated. If the blood supply to the hernia is cut off, the hernia is said to be strangulated and requires immediate surgery to restore the blood supply. If this is not done, gangrene will develop and the situation may be fatal.

Several types of hernias exist. A hernia may be umbilical in which a portion of the bowel protrudes through the umbilicus. In children, these generally resolve on their own once the child begins to walk. Umbilical hernias most commonly occur in a multiparous

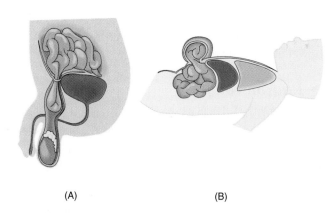

(A)   (B)

FIGURE 34-10 Two types of hernias: **(A)** inguinal; **(B)** umbilical. If the blood flow to the bowel is cut off, the hernia is said to be strangulated.

female or in adults having cirrhosis with **ascites** (fluid in the peritoneal cavity). Due to a high risk for strangulation in adults with umbilical hernias, surgery is usually performed.

Abdominal hernias occur in the midline of the abdomen between the umbilicus and the xyphoid process. Most are asymptomatic with a few causing pain on exertion that resolve with reclining and rest.

Inguinal hernias, the most common hernia, occur in the groin area. Inguinal hernias frequently occur after activities, such as lifting, that increase intraabdominal pressure and subside with relaxation. Pain is located lower than the inguinal hernia. Femoral hernias occur when the intestine pushes into the passageway carrying blood vessels and nerves to the legs, and are more common in women than in men.

Upon evaluation and recommendation of a physician, some hernias can be reduced or pushed back into place. This can be accomplished by having the client recline, applying direct pressure to the hernia and in some cases, having the client exhale to decrease intraabdominal pressure. The nurse should never try to reduce a hernia.

A hiatal hernia occurs when a portion of the stomach protrudes into the mediastinal cavity through the diaphragm. Symptoms of hiatal hernias include indigestion and heartburn, especially after eating a large meal.

▶ Medical/Surgical Management

▶ Medical

Because some hernias have no symptoms or have minimal symptoms, clients may not be aware they have one or simply learn to live with it by reducing it when needed. Clients who are a poor surgical risk may use a truss, a device that applies pressure to the hernia thus keeping it in the abdominal cavity.

▶ Surgical

Hernias can be repaired with a surgery called a herniorrhaphy. The surgery is typically performed on an outpatient basis with clients going home the same day. If the surgery is more complicated because the hernia is incarcerated, the client may stay overnight.

If the hernia is strangulated, surgery is required to restore the blood flow and may even require a bowel resection.

Surgical repair of a hiatal hernia involves reinforcing the esophagus with a portion of the stomach. The surgery is performed laparoscopically with the client remaining in the hospital three to five days postoperatively. Initially, the client will have an NG tube. The NG tube is removed twenty-four to forty-eight hours later and the diet gradually progressed to a soft diet.

▶ Diet

Clients with hiatal hernias may need to modify their dietary patterns to include small frequent meals, avoidance of eating after supper, not lying down for two hours after eating and avoiding aggravating foods.

▶ Nursing Process

Assessment

Subjective Data Clients may complain of pain at the site of the hernia.

Objective Data Assessment may show a bulge through the abdominal wall. If the hernia is strangulated, the client will have the symptoms of a bowel obstruction.

▼ ▼

Possible nursing diagnoses for a client with a hernia may include:

Nursing Diagnoses	Goals	Nursing Interventions
▶ *Pain, acute, related to tissue edema.*	The client will experience less pain within one hour of intervention as measured on the pain scale.	Administer analgesics as ordered.
		Evaluate aggravating activities (i.e., straining to have a bowel movement) and provide information on modification if indicated.
		Educate regarding signs of complications and to notify staff of symptoms.

(continued)

Nursing Diagnoses	Goals	Nursing Interventions
▶ *Tissue perfusion, altered, related to strangulation.*	The client will have minimal tissue necrosis.	Assess abdomen every four hours.
		Insert NG tube to decrease abdominal distention as ordered.
		Prepare client for surgery as ordered. Keep client NPO.
		Administer IV hydration as ordered.

▶ Evaluation

Each goal must be evaluated to determine how it has been met by the client.

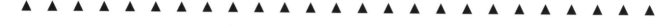

▶ PERITONITIS

Peritonitis is the inflammation of the peritoneum, the membranous covering of the abdomen. Peritonitis is caused by irritating substances such as feces, gastric acids, bacteria, or blood in the abdominal cavity. A ruptured portion of the digestive system such as the appendix, a ruptured tubal pregnancy, or invasion of tumors through the gastric wall can lead to peritonitis. Peritonitis can be a serious, life-threatening condition. Complications following peritonitis include adhesions (scar tissue), ileus, and pneumonia.

▶ Medical/Surgical Management

▶ Surgical

Treatment is primarily surgical with repair of the cause and irrigation of the abdominal cavity with saline and antibiotic solutions. Drains may be left in the abdomen for several days postoperatively to allow any remaining fluid to drain. Since bowel function usually stops due to the irritating substances, an NG tube is placed to decompress the abdomen and relieve nausea.

▶ Pharmacological

Analgesics will be ordered postoperatively for discomfort. If an ileus develops, nonnarcotic analgesics will be ordered. Antibiotics will also be ordered preoperatively and postoperatively.

▶ Diet

Clients will be NPO preoperatively and postoperatively until bowel sounds return. Clients will then be placed on a clear liquid diet and slowly progressed to a regular diet as more bowel function returns.

▶ Activity

Preoperatively, clients will be placed on bed rest. Postoperatively, clients need to be encouraged to turn, cough, and deep breathe. Because clients tend to breathe shallowly with peritoneal inflammation, pulmonary hygiene is important. Activity should be progressed postoperatively as soon as tolerated to increase lung expansion and to encourage bowel function return. Exercise, lifting, and driving will be restricted until the incision heals.

▶ Nursing Process

Assessment

Subjective Data   Clients may describe abdominal pain, nausea, and constipation.

Objective Data   Assessment includes vomiting, absent bowel sound, a tense or distended abdomen with tenderness on palpation, shallow and rapid respirations, weak and rapid pulse, dry mucous membranes, low urine output, fever, and limited mobility because of pain.

Laboratory analysis will include a CBC which will show an elevated WBC. If bleeding is occurring, the H & H will be low. Electrolytes may show low sodium, potassium, and chloride.

▼ ▼

Possible nursing diagnoses for a client with peritonitis may include:

Nursing Diagnoses	Goals	Nursing Interventions
▶ Fluid volume deficit (active loss), related to gastric losses and restricted intake.	The client will maintain hydration as measured by I & O nearly equal and electrolytes within normal limits.	Monitor I & O every shift. Monitor for signs of dehydration: dry mucous membranes, poor skin turgor, and low urine output. Monitor electrolytes. Administer IV rehydration and electrolytes replacement as ordered.
▶ Hyperthermia, related to inflammatory process and dehydration.	The client will maintain temperature within normal limits.	Assess VS including temperature every four hours. Administer antipyretics as ordered; probably rectal suppositories due to NPO status. Monitor for dehydration: decrease in urine output, dry mucous membranes, and poor skin turgor. Provide comfort measures: cool cloth to the head or neck, assist to turn, and a back rub with cooling lotion.
▶ Pain, acute, related to abdominal distention.	The client will have less pain and improved mobility within one hour of analgesics as measured on the pain scale.	Administer analgesics as ordered. Encourage activity such as coughing and deep breathing after analgesics. Monitor NG tube to decompress abdomen. Maintain patency of NG tube. Teach splinting of incision for cough and deep breathing.
▶ Infection, high risk for spread and septicemia, related to traumatized tissues and altered peristalsis.	The client will have infection controlled.	Monitor VS every four hours. Monitor laboratory values for increased WBC. Provide wound care as ordered. Monitor wound and drainage from drains for signs of infection. Assess abdomen every four hours and monitor for increased guarding and tenderness.

▶ Evaluation

Each goal must be evaluated to determine how it has been met by the client.

▲ ▲

▶ HEMORRHOIDS

Hemorrhoids are swollen vascular tissues in the rectal area. The hemorrhoids may be internal or external. Hemorrhoids may be caused by straining with constipation. Sitting on the toilet (reading) for an extended time may also be a cause. Hemorrhoids frequently occur with pregnancy. Hemorrhoids can cause burning, pruritis, and pain with defecation. At times, hemorrhoids can bleed leading to anemia.

▶ Medical/Surgical Management

▶ Medical

Sitz baths or warm compresses for twenty minutes, four times a day often helps decrease swelling.

▶ Surgical

If bleeding continues despite medical intervention, or if discomfort is significant, the hemorrhoids can be surgically removed by a hemorrhoidectomy. If hemorrhoids are external, surgery is performed on an outpatient basis by placing a rubberband around the hemorrhoid allowing it to necrose and fall off on its own. If hemorrhoids are internal, surgery can be done using sclerotherapy, cryotherapy, or laser. This usually requires an overnight stay in the hospital. Hemorrhoids can recur after surgical removal if the cause is not eliminated.

▶ Pharmacological

Treatment includes creams and suppositories to decrease inflammation, some with cortisone to decrease swelling. Fiber supplements and stool softeners may be ordered to keep bowel movements soft.

▶ Diet

Bowel movements can be kept soft with a high-fiber diet of 20 to 30 grams of fiber a day and at least 2500 cc of fluid intake daily.

▶ Nursing Process

Assessment

Subjective Data Clients may complain of rectal burning, pain, and pruritis with bowel movements, constipation and occasionally, bright red bleeding. A dietary history should be obtained to determine fiber and fluid intake.

Objective Data If hemorrhoids are external, they can be visualized during a physical examination. If bleeding is present, laboratory analysis will show a low H & H.

▼ ▼

Possible nursing diagnoses for a client with hemorrhoids may include:

Nursing Diagnoses	Goals	Nursing Interventions
▶ *Pain, acute, related to edema and inflammation of prolapsed varices.*	The client will verbalize a decrease in discomfort within forty-eight hours of initiation of treatment.	Provide sitz baths or warm compresses for twenty minutes, four times a day. Administer creams and suppositories as ordered. Increase fiber and fluids in diet to keep stools soft to avoid straining.
▶ *Knowledge deficit, related to diet, causes of condition, treatment, and potential complications.*	The client will be able to verbalize treatment regime and long-term management of hemorrhoids.	Determine client's learning style and present information in a manner compatible with learning style. Educate client about increasing fiber in diet to 20 to 30 grams per day, increasing fluid intake to 2500 cc per day, causes of hemorrhoids, possible complications such as anemia, and modification of bowel habits (such as not sitting on the toilet for long periods).

▶ Evaluation

Each goal must be evaluated to determine how it has been met by the client.

▲ ▲

▶ CONSTIPATION

Constipation is characterized by hard, infrequent stools that are difficult and painful to pass. Constipation can be caused by tumors, low-fiber diet, some diseases that interfere with the mechanical functioning of the bowel (such as multiple sclerosis) or some medications (such as narcotics, antidepressants, or anti-Parkinson drugs). Because of the aging process, elderly clients will often experience this change in bowel habits.

▶ Medical/Surgical Management

▶ Pharmacological

Fiber supplements and stool softeners may be ordered. Laxatives and enemas may be ordered, but long-term use should be avoided as they interrupt normal bowel function. If constipation is caused by medications the client is taking, the client should discuss with the physician if other options exist such as modifying the dosage or changing the medicine.

▶ Diet

Fiber should be increased to 20 to 30 grams a day. Fluid intake should be increased to 2500 cc a day. Elderly clients may experience constipation and need to be educated to make dietary adjustments to prevent bowel evacuation problems.

▶ Activity

Activity level should be increased if possible as exercise, such as walking, increases motility in the colon.

▶ Nursing Process

▶ Assessment

Subjective Data Clients will complain of infrequent, difficult to pass bowel movements. Dietary assessment of fiber and fluids is usually low. Activity/exercise levels should also be assessed.

Objective Data Bowel movements will be hard-formed.

▼ ▼

Possible nursing diagnoses for a client with constipation may include:

Nursing Diagnoses	Goals	Nursing Interventions
▶ Constipation related to inadequate intake of fiber and fluids.	The client will have soft stools every other day by one week from onset of intervention.	Encourage client to increase fiber in the diet to 20 to 30 grams a day and fluid intake to 2500 cc a day.
		Administer fiber supplements and stool softeners as ordered.
		Determine fluid preferences of the client and always have fluids at the client's bedside within reach.
		Help the client establish a regular schedule for bowel movements, usually thirty minutes after a meal.
▶ Knowledge deficit related to dietary sources of fiber and the importance of adequate fluid intake and exercise.	The client will be able to select a menu high in fiber and fluids utilizing nutrients from the food pyramid within forty-eight hours and verbalize the need for adequate exercise.	Assess client's learning style and present information in a manner compatible with learning style.
		Teach client about foods that are high in fiber (fruits, vegetables, whole grains) as well as the importance of fluid intake.
		Discuss with the client the importance of exercise in maintaining bowel function.

▶ Evaluation

Each goal must be evaluated to determine how it has been met by the client.

▲ ▲

▶ DISORDERS OF THE ACCESSORY ORGANS

▶ CIRRHOSIS

Cirrhosis refers to the chronic, degenerative changes in the structure of the liver that result from the liver repairing itself after chronic inflammation. Causes of cirrhosis include chronic hepatitis, repeated exposure to toxic substances, disease processes (such as sclerosing cholangitis and hemochromatosis), cancer, and chronic alcohol abuse. Alcohol abuse accounts for most cases of cirrhosis.

Because the liver is responsible for so many functions, complications can be significant. Complications include: malnutrition, hypoglycemia, clotting disorders, jaundice, portal hypertension, ascites, hepatic encephalopathy, and hepatorenal syndrome.

Liver dysfunction causes several organ-related complications. Malnutrition results from the liver's inability to absorb fat and fat soluble vitamins, and leads to muscle wasting, weight loss, and fatigue. Hypoglycemia occurs when the liver is unable to perform glycogenolysis efficiently. Clotting disorders result when the liver is not able to produce sufficient amounts of prothrombin and fibrinogen.

Portal hypertension results when blood flow through the cirrhotic liver is inhibited resulting in blood backflowing in the portal vein. Portal hypertension leads to distention of the esophageal veins resulting in esophageal varices.

Because the liver is responsible for metabolizing medications, clients frequently become intolerant to some medications. Jaundice, a yellow discoloration of the skin is usually present. Jaundice occurs when the liver is unable to convert bilirubin, an end product of red blood cell breakdown, into a water soluble form that can be excreted in the bile. The extra bilirubin collects in areas that contain elastin such as the eyes, skin, and nail beds.

When blood flow through the cirrhotic liver is inhibited, blood backs up into the portal system. Congestion of blood in the portal system causes distention of the esophageal, gastric, mesenteric, splenic, and portal veins. The backflow of blood in these vessels increases the pressure in the vessels causing portal hypertension. The distended esophageal veins causes esophageal varices (see the earlier section on esophageal varices in this chapter) and the distended rectal veins results in hemorrhoids. The distended splenic vein causes splenomegaly. Fluid may also accumulate in the pleural cavity in the form of pleural effusions.

Fluid may also accumulate in the peritoneal cavity.

This fluid is called ascites. The cause of ascites is the congestion of blood in the portal system.

Hepatic encephalopathy is a condition in which too much ammonia accumulates in the bloodstream from the liver's inability to filter proteins and protein byproducts. Confusion, lethargy, and/or coma may occur. Symptoms of impending coma are disorientation and asterixis (liver flap), a flapping tremor of the hands. When the client extends the arms and hands in front of the body, the hands rapidly flex and extend.

Hepatorenal syndrome is a complication of cirrhosis in which the client goes into renal failure. Symptoms include oliguria, azotemia, anorexia, fatigue, and weakness.

Cirrhosis is a form of end-stage liver disease for which there is no cure. The process of cirrhosis can be slowed by removing the cause (i.e., abstaining from alcohol), but the damage cannot be reversed. Clients in end-stage liver disease may be evaluated to determine if they qualify for a liver transplant. If they qualify, they will be put on a waiting list until a liver becomes available.

▶ Medical/Surgical Management

▶ Medical

The physician may perform a paracentesis to remove the fluid from the abdomen and relieve pressure on the diaphragm and lungs. A paracentesis is done by making a small incision and inserting a trochar into the abdomen to drain the fluid. Albumin may be infused at the same time to pull excess fluid back into the vascular system.

▶ Surgical

If the client continues to develop ascites after medical treatment, a LeVeen or Denver peritoneal venous shunt may be used. The pressure-regulated shunt is implanted in the peritoneal cavity and threaded through the subcutaneous tissue into the superior vena cava, returning the fluid back to the vascular system. As fluid pressure builds in the peritoneal cavity, a valve opens and drains the fluid into the superior vena cava.

If esophageal varices are present, an EGD with sclerotherapy or banding will be done to prevent hemorrhage. Refer back to Figure 34-3.

If portal hypertension cannot be controlled with medications, a portosystemic shunt or a transjugular intrahepatic portosystemic shunt (TIPS) may be performed. The purpose of the shunt is to redirect the blood flow, thereby relieving the portal hypertension and decreasing the risk of rupturing distended veins in the esophagus (see Figures 34-11A and 34-11B).

▶ Pharmacological

A potassium sparing diuretic, such as spironolactone (Aldactone) is used to decrease ascites and pleural effusion. Lactulose (Cholac) is used to eliminate the ammonia from the blood into the bowel. The lactulose acts as a laxative to cause the body to excrete the stool containing ammonia. Tap water enemas may also be ordered to help the body eliminate the ammonia.

Propranolol hydrochloride (Inderal), an antihypertensive medication, may be ordered to lower portal hypertension. All unnecessary medications should be avoided since the liver cannot metabolize them.

▶ Diet

Clients with cirrhosis are placed on a low-protein diet, usually 40 grams per day. If ascites is present, sodium will also be restricted to 2 grams or less a day to decrease the amount of fluid retained by the body. Fluids may also be restricted to 1000 cc to 2000 cc a day depending on the severity of fluid accumulation.

▶ Activity

If hepatic encephalopathy is present, precautions should be taken to ensure the client's safety, such as elevating bedrails and ambulating only with assistance, especially if the client's gait is unsteady.

Because fatigue is such a common symptom of cirrhosis, the client's tolerance for activity will be diminished. Rest periods should be planned during the day and activities should be scheduled between rests.

▶ Nursing Process

Assessment

Subjective Data Clients will describe fatigue, nausea, anorexia, weakness, and indigestion.

Objective Data Assessment will show ascites, jaundice, enlarged liver and spleen, petechiae (small bruises on the skin), vomiting, weight loss, fever, epistaxis, and decreased breath sounds. Lethargy, confusion, or coma may be present if encephalopathy has occurred.

Laboratory analysis will include a CBC which will demonstrate low WBCs, RBCs, Hgb, and platelets. A liver panel will show an elevated bilirubin, alkaline phosphatase, GGT, ALT, and AST. Albumin will be low. PT, PTT, and clotting times will be delayed.

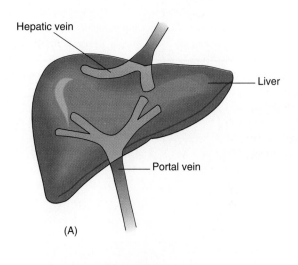

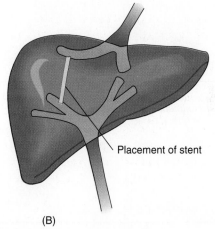

FIGURE 34-11 (A) Blood flow prior to TIPS; **(B)** TIPS is performed in radiology on clients deemed too unstable for the surgery necessary for a portosystemic shunt. A stent is placed to redirect the blood flow.

▼ ▼

Possible nursing diagnoses for a client with cirrhosis may include:

Nursing Diagnoses	Goals	Nursing Interventions
▶ *Thought processes, altered, related to elevated serum ammonia levels and hepatic coma.*	The client will experience less lethargy by forty-eight hours after initiation of treatment, as demonstrated by less time sleeping and improved level of orientation.	Administer tap water enemas and lactulose as ordered to eliminate ammonia-rich stools. An NG tube may be placed to give lactulose if client is comatose. Elevate bedrails to prevent injury. Monitor laboratory reports for ammonia level. As coma lessens, reorient client frequently. Provide low-protein diet.
▶ *Fluid volume, excess, related to ascites.*	The client will have less ascites by discharge.	Weigh daily. Measure abdominal girth daily. Fluid restriction of 1000 to 2000 cc per day depending on the severity of the ascites. Educate client to notify physician of weight gain of 1½ lbs or more in one week. Provide low-sodium diet of 500 to 2000 mg a day depending on the severity of the ascites. Teach client how to measure fluids and calculate sodium in diet. If a paracentesis is done, check vital signs every fifteen minutes during the procedure and after the procedure until the vitals are stable. The amount of fluid removed from the abdomen is measured and sent to the laboratory.
▶ *Skin integrity, impaired, high risk for, related to accumulation of bile salts in skin, poor skin turgor, ascites, and edema.*	The client will not experience skin breakdown while hospitalized.	Provide egg crate mattress. Turn client every two hours. Monitor skin closely for redness and skin breakdown. Apply lotion to skin frequently, especially to pressure areas. Assist with ADLs to promote good hygiene and conserve client's energy.
▶ *Nutrition, altered, less than body requirements, related to inadequate diet, anorexia, or vomiting.*	The client will eat a balanced diet of 1,500 calories a day.	Offer small, high-calorie meals frequently. Assist and encourage client to eat. Offer high nutrient supplements if client is unable to maintain adequate caloric intake. Provide frequent oral hygiene. Observe for changes in mental status that would interfere with caloric intake (i.e., increased lethargy).

▶ Evaluation

Each goal must be evaluated to determine how it has been met by the client.

▲ ▲

► HEPATITIS

Hepatitis is a chronic or acute inflammation of the liver caused by a virus, bacteria, drugs, alcohol abuse, or other toxic substances. There is a diffuse inflammatory reaction with liver cells degenerating and dying. The functions of the liver slow down. Since viral infections are the most common cause of hepatitis, emphasis will be placed on viral hepatitis.

Researchers are still learning about the viruses that cause hepatitis. Five viruses are known to cause hepatitis: A, B, C, D, and E. The viruses are similar and have almost identical signs and symptoms. Incubation period, mode of transmission, and prognosis vary. See Table 34-4 for summary of the viruses.

► Medical/Surgical Management

Treatment is focused on resting the liver and early detection of complications. The liver is rested by modifying the diet so that less bile is needed to digest the food. Treatment is related to the signs and symptoms present and the prevention of transmission.

► Pharmacological

Antiemetics such as hydroxyzine hydrochloride (Atarax) or trimethobenzamide hydrochloride (Tigan) may be given before meals if nausea is present. IV hydration with vitamin C for healing may be ordered. Vitamin B complex may also be ordered to help absorb fat soluble vitamins. Vitamin K may be ordered if clotting time is prolonged. All unnecessary medications, especially sedatives, should be avoided.

Those exposed to hepatitis B by needle puncture or sexual contact should have hepatitis B immunoglobin (HBIG). A vaccine for hepatitis A (HAV) is available and provides protection for up to ten years or more. HAV is recommended for people at risk for exposure to hepatitis A such as homosexuals, IV drug users, travelers to countries with poor sanitation conditions, and laboratory workers who handle live hepatitis A virus.

► Diet

Diet modifications may include decreasing fat intake to decrease the amount of bile needed in the digestive tract. A low-protein diet may be needed if the liver is no longer able to metabolize the protein. Anorexia is a common symptom that can be treated with small, frequent, high calorie meals. Fluids may be restricted if the client is starting to retain fluids. No alcoholic beverages for at least one year or longer if indicated.

► Activity

Bed rest is usually recommended for the first several weeks, generally at home unless the serum bilirubin is > 10 mg/dL or the PT is prolonged. If either occurs, hospitalization is usually recommended.

Once bed rest is no longer necessary, activity should be increased gradually as fatigue will be present for up to several months. Rest periods should be included in the day.

► Nursing Process

Assessment

Subjective Data Symptoms include fatigue, anorexia, photophobia, nausea, headaches, abdominal pain, generalized muscle aches, chills, pruritis, and bloating.

Objective Data The client will have weight loss, hepatomegaly, fever, jaundice, dark amber urine, and clay colored stools.

Laboratory analysis will show an elevated bilirubin, GGT, AST, ALT, LDH, and alkaline phosphatase. Clotting time and PT will be prolonged. Specific hepatitis test will be elevated (see Table 34-4).

▼ ▼

Possible nursing diagnoses for the client with hepatitis may include:

Nursing Diagnoses	Goals	Nursing Interventions
► Knowledge deficit, related to disease process, treatment regime, and mode of transmission.	The client will be able to explain disease process, incubation period, and mode of transmission, by discharge. The client will practice precautions to prevent spread of disease. The client will be able to select a menu using foods from the food guide pyramid maintaining a low-fat, low-protein diet.	Assess client's learning style and present information in a manner compatible with learning style. Educate about disease process and incubation period.

(continued)

Table 34-4

COMPARISON OF DIFFERENT TYPES OF VIRAL HEPATITS					
Hepatitis Virus	**A**	**B**	**C**	**D**	**E**
Other Names	Infectious hepatitis	Serum hepatitis	Post transfusion non-A, non-B hepatitis	Delta virus	Enteric non-A hepatitis
Routes of transmission	Fecal-oral: Spread by feces, saliva, and contaminated food and water.	Parenteral or sexual: Spread by blood and blood products (via transfusion, needle stick or IV drug use); body fluids such as saliva, semen, and vaginal secretions; maternal-fetal contact; and unknown exposures.	Parenteral: Spread by blood and blood products (via transfusion, needle stick, or IV drug use) and unknown exposures.	Appears as a co-infection with hepatitis B; transmitted the same way as hepatitis B.	Fecal-oral: Spread through contaminated water.
Incubation period	15–50 days	45–160 days	14–180 days	15–64 days	15–50 days
Infectivity period	Latter half of incubation period until 1–2 weeks after symptoms start.	Begins before symptoms appear and may continue for client's lifetime if the client becomes a carrier.	Begins before onset of symptoms and may continue for client's lifetime if the client becomes a carrier.	Not known.	Not known.
Diagnostic tests	Anti-HAV igM	HBsAg, HBeAg, anti-HBs, and anti-HBc (numerous other blood tests can also be used)	Anti-HCV	Anti-HDV	No test available
Preventive measures and post-exposure treatment	Standard and enteric precautions indicated; vaccine available; vaccine and immune globulin therapy indicated for postexposure prophylaxis	Standard precautions indicated; vaccine available; vaccine and hepatitis B immune globulin therapy indicated for postexposure prophylaxis; recombinant interferon alfa-2b injections indicated for chronic state	Standard precautions indicated; no vaccine available; recombinant interferon alfa-2b injections indicated for chronic state	Standard precautions indicated; vaccine and hepatitis B immune globulin therapy indicated for postexposure prophylaxis; experimental use of recombinant interferon alfa-2b injections is still being studied	Standard and enteric precautions indicated; no vaccine available; no postexposure prophylaxis available.
Prognosis	Rarely fatal; no carrier state or chronicity; lifelong immunity	High mortality rate; client can become immune or can become chronic carrier; 5–10% of cases progress to chronic hepatitis; chronic hepatitis B associated with liver cancer.	Client can become chronic carrier; 50% of all cases progress to chronic hepatitis, and 20% of chronic cases progress to cirrhosis; possibly associated with liver cancer.	Frequently leads to chronic, active hepatitis and death; client can become carrier, immunity to B gives client immunity to D.	Does not progress to chronic hepatitis but has a 10% mortality rate in pregnant women.

Nursing Diagnoses	Goals	Nursing Interventions
		Teach proper handwashing technique and emphasize importance of washing hands after using the bathroom.
		Emphasize that client cannot donate blood.
		Emphasize importance of follow-up laboratory analysis.
		Instruct in selection of low-fat, low-protein diet.
		For clients with hepatitis A, teach client to disinfect articles contaminated with feces (such as the toilet), not to prepare food for others, and not to share articles such as eating utensils or toothbrushes.
		For clients with hepatitis B teach to avoid sexual contact until they test negative for HBsAg or their partners are immunized with the HBV vaccine.
		For clients with hepatitis C teach that it is unknown whether it can be transmitted through sexual contact, so precautions are recommended until more is known.
▶ Nutrition, altered, less than body requirements, related to inadequate caloric intake, fat intolerance, nausea, and vomiting.	The client will maintain a caloric intake of 2,000 calories/day.	Monitor daily calorie count and monitor I & O every shift.
		Weigh daily.
		Offer small frequent, high-calorie, low-protein diet of 40 gm of protein, low-fat meals.
		Offer the largest meal in the morning as food tends to be tolerated better in the morning.
		Note color and consistency of stools and color of urine.
		Encourage fluid intake of 2500 to 3000 cc daily.
		Administer antiemetic thirty minutes before meals as ordered.
▶ Fatigue, related to decreased energy production and altered body chemistry.	The client will verbalize plan to modify activity, by discharge.	Educate client regarding reasons for fatigue and that fatigue may be present for several months.
		Encourage client to maintain bed rest for several weeks. When resuming normal activity, rest periods should be included until stamina returns.
▶ Pain, related to pruritis resulting from elevated bilirubin level.	The client will verbalize less pain within twenty-four hours of onset of interventions.	Encourage client to wear loose fitting, cotton clothing.
		Educate client to avoid alkaline soaps.
		Encourage client to apply lotion to skin frequently, avoiding lotions that contain alcohol.

▶ Evaluation

Each goal must be evaluated to determine how it has been met by the client.

▲ ▲

▶ *PANCREATITIS*

Pancreatitis is an acute or chronic inflammation of the pancreas caused when pancreatic enzymes digest the lining of the pancreas. In severe cases, the pancreas can hemorrhage resulting in a life-threatening condition. Pancreatitis occurs when obstruction of the pancreatic duct occurs as a result of gallstones, tumors, exposure to chemicals, or injury to the pancreas.

▶ *Medical/Surgical Management*

▶ *Medical*

Treatment is dependent upon the cause of the pancreatitis. If the pancreatitis results from exposure to chemical or alcohol abuse, treatment is primarily medical. An NG tube is inserted to rest the bowel and relieve abdominal distention.

▶ *Surgical*

If the pancreatitis is caused by structural changes such as gallstones, an ERCP with stone removal may be performed. Surgery to relieve the pancreatic duct obstruction may be necessary in cases where tumors or injury are the causes of the pancreatitis.

▶ *Pharmacological*

Insulin may be given if the pancreas is unable to secrete enough to maintain normal blood sugar level. If nausea and vomiting are present, antiemetics may be ordered. Meperidine (Demerol) will be ordered for analgesia as morphine sulfate may cause spasms of the sphincter of Oddi. Atropine sulfate or propantheline bromide (Pro-Banthine) may be ordered to decrease pancreatic activity. Antacids or an H_2 receptor antagonist may be ordered to prevent stress ulcers.

▶ *Diet*

Clients are kept NPO while the serum amylase level is elevated to decrease the demand for digestive enzymes in the bowel. An NG tube may be inserted to decrease pancreatic activity, and to prevent nausea, vomiting, and abdominal distention. As the serum amylase level begins to decrease, clients will be started on clear liquids and slowly advanced to a bland, low-fat, high-protein, high-carbohydrate diet. No coffee or alcohol is allowed.

IV rehydration is necessary while the client is NPO. If the pancreatitis is severe and the client must be NPO for a prolonged period, TPN, a high-calorie, high-nutrient IV solution may be administered.

▶ *Activity*

Clients are frequently placed on bed rest to decrease metabolic rate. Activity can be increase as the serum amylase decreases.

▶ *Nursing Process*

Assessment

Subjective Data Clients will complain of excruciating epigastric pain that radiates to the back. Pain may decrease by leaning forward or lying in a fetal position. Nausea and anorexia are also present.

Objective Data Assessment includes steatorrhea, vomiting, low-grade fever, tachycardia, and jaundice. Laboratory analysis includes an elevated serum amylase followed by an elevated urine amylase and serum lipase a few days later, leukocytosis, and an elevated Hct. Glucose, alkaline phosphatase, and bilirubin may also be elevated.

▼ ▼

Possible nursing diagnoses for a client with pancreatitis may include:

Nursing Diagnoses	Goals	Nursing Interventions
▶ *Pain, acute, related to inflammation and edema of the pancreas.*	The client will verbalize a decrease in pain as evidenced by pain scale by one hour after initiation of interventions.	Monitor NG tube to decompress the abdomen.
		Administer analgesics as ordered and monitor for relief.
		Position client in most comfortable position.
		Assess pain for increasing severity which would indicate worsening pancreatitis.

Nursing Diagnoses	Goals	Nursing Interventions
		Monitor serum amylase, WBCs and H & H for signs or increasing severity of pancreatitis or hemorrhage.
▶ Nutrition, altered, less than body requirements, related to NPO status, nausea, vomiting, and altered ability to digest nutrients.	The client will experience no further weight loss during hospitalization.	Monitor I & O every shift. Weigh daily. Maintain bed rest to decrease the metabolic rate. Insert NG tube to decompress the abdomen as ordered. Administer IV rehydration or TPN as ordered.
▶ Fluid volume deficit, high risk for, related to vomiting, NG tube, or hemorrhage.	The client will maintain adequate hydration as evidenced by I & O nearly equal, electrolytes within normal limits, and moist mucous membranes.	I & O every shift. Administer IV hydration or TPN as ordered. Monitor electrolyte levels and H & H.

▶ Evaluation

Each goal must be evaluated to determine how it has been met by the client.

▲ ▲

▶ CHOLECYSTITIS AND CHOLELITHIASIS

Cholecystitis is an inflammation of the gallbladder. In more than 90 percent of the cases, gallstones are present. Cholelithiasis is the presence of gallstones or **calculi** in the gallbladder. Not all gallstones cause cholecystitis. Some gallstones may pass out of the gallbladder and into the duodenum with the client being unaware of the stones. Sometimes gallstones migrate into the cystic or common bile duct causing an obstruction which, in turn, leads to cholecystitis. The exact cause of the formation of these stones is not known.

These two diseases are more common in multiparous women, age forty-five and older, obese people, those who use birth control pills or control cholesterol with gemfibrozil (Lopid) and people with a history of a disease of the small intestine such as Crohn's disease. Also, clients on sudden weight reduction diets that are low in fat will cause the bile to pool in the gallbladder, increasing the risk for gallstone formation.

Ultrasound of the gallbladder is ordered if gallstones are suspected.

▶ Medical/Surgical Management

In asymptomatic clients, no intervention is necessary.

▶ Medical

If stones are lodged in the common bile duct, an ERCP may be performed. A sphincterotomy, an incision in the ampulla of vater, may be performed to enlarge the opening of the common bile duct. Stones may then be removed or crushed.

▶ Surgical

If the stones are too large or for clients with repeated episode of cholelithiasis, a cholecystectomy, the surgical removal of the gallbladder, may be performed. The cholecystectomy may be performed laparoscopically or by making a large abdominal incision.

Laparoscopic cholecystectomies, while having been performed for less than ten years, have become the surgery of choice for cholelithiasis and cholecystitis. The gallbladder is removed by making four small incisions and extracting the gallbladder through an endoscope. If the cholecystectomy is performed laparoscopically, it is more difficult to perform an exploration of the common bile duct, especially in clients with cholecystitis. An ERCP may need to be performed if stones remain in the CBD. Clients are ready for discharge twenty-four hours after the surgery.

The cholecystectomy can also be performed by making a large abdominal incision. A cholangiogram can be performed easily and therefore this type of procedure is more common in clients with much inflammation of the gallbladder. If damage has occurred to the CBD due to severe inflammation or from a stone, a T-tube will be left in place to allow the bile to drain into a collection bag allowing the CBD to heal. Clients are typically ready for discharge three to seven days after surgery. Exercise, lifting, and driving will be more restricted to allow for incisional healing.

▶ Pharmacological

In acute cholecystitis, analgesics will be ordered to relieve the discomfort. Meperidine (Demerol) is preferred over morphine sulfate as morphine sulfate is believed to increase sphincter spasms. IV hydration may also be ordered if clients are unable to maintain hydration. Antiemetics will also be ordered if nausea and vomiting are present.

In clients who have surgery, analgesics will be ordered after surgery to control discomfort.

▶ Diet

In clients with mild or moderate symptoms, a clear liquid diet to rest the bowel, followed by small frequent meals low in fat may resolve the symptoms.

If clients are to have surgery, they will be NPO before surgery and initially after surgery until bowel sounds return. The client will then be started on clear liquids first and then advanced as tolerated to a regular diet.

▶ Activity

In acute cases of cholecystitis, bed rest is recommended to decrease metabolic rate. If surgery is performed, the client will be encouraged to turn, cough, and deep breathe every two hours initially after surgery. On the day following surgery, assist client out of bed and encourage a gradual increase in activity. Clients who have had a laparoscopic cholecystectomy may be ambulated the evening of surgery. Clients can typically return to previous activity level two weeks after surgery. Clients who have an incision must restrict lifting, driving and exercise until incisional healing is complete, usually four to six weeks.

▶ Nursing Process

Assessment

Subjective Data Clients will describe pain in the right upper quadrant radiating to the right scapular area that occurs two to four hours after a large meal, nausea, flatulence, and indigestion.

Objective Data Assessment may show vomiting, occasionally a fever, jaundice, steatorrhea, clay colored stools and dark amber urine. Laboratory analysis may show elevated alkaline phosphatase and GGT. The WBCs may be elevated on the CBC. The bilirubin may be elevated.

▼ ▼

Possible nursing diagnoses for a client with cholecystitis and cholelithiasis may include:

Nursing Diagnoses	Goals	Nursing Interventions
▶ *Pain, acute, related to inflammation or blocked bile duct.*	The client will experience less pain as evidenced by pain scale within one hour of initiation of treatment.	Keep client NPO or on a clear liquid diet as ordered. Administer analgesics as ordered. Monitor NG tube to decompress the abdomen as ordered. Observe for jaundice and bile flow obstruction.

Nursing Diagnoses	Goals	Nursing Interventions
▶ Breathing pattern, ineffective, related to decreased lung expansion because of pain.	The client will demonstrate appropriate breathing pattern and will not have respiratory complications while hospitalized.	Assist client to cough and deep breathe every two hours. Teach splinting techniques. Turn every two hours and ambulate as soon as indicated. Teach use of incentive spirometer.
▶ Fluid volume deficit, high risk for, related to nausea, NG tube, NPO or bile drainage.	The client will maintain adequate hydration as evidenced by I & O nearly equal and moist mucous membranes.	Monitor I & O every shift including NG drainage and T-tube drainage if present. Administer IV hydration as ordered. Maintain patency of NG tube.

▶ Evaluation

Each goal must be evaluated to determine how it has been met by the client.

▲ ▲

▶ NEOPLASMS OF THE DIGESTIVE SYSTEM

▶ ORAL CANCER

Oral cancer refers to cancers of the lips, tongue, oral cavity, and pharynx. According to the American Cancer Society, the occurrence of oral cancer is several times more frequent in people who use tobacco. The five-year survival rate is low, primarily because the early symptoms are ignored. Symptoms include a sore that does not heal, a sore throat, or difficulty swallowing. On the lips, the cancer may be a growth.

▶ Medical/Surgical Management

▶ Surgical

Treatment is primarily surgical and involves removal of the cancer with excision of tissue and lymph nodes surrounding the cancer. If the cancer is small, the surgical area will be small. If the cancer is large, extensive surgery is performed, removing a large amount of tissue and lymph nodes. In cases of the cancer involving the pharynx, a radical neck dissection is performed, which requires reconstruction of the pharynx. Clients undergoing radical neck dissection frequently have a tracheostomy.

▶ Radiation

In cases where the lesion cannot be surgically removed, radiation or radium implants may be used. High-energy radiation is used to destroy cancer cells. Clients may experience irritated skin, swallowing difficulties, dry mouth, nausea, diarrhea, hair loss, or fatigue. If radiation is done, the client will receive radiation daily for a specified period of time. If radium implants are used, the client will have a radioactive capsule implanted into the area.

▶ Pharmacological

Chemotherapy is not effective against most oral cancers and is, therefore, only used in the most severe cases with metastases. Medications ordered will be based on the client's symptoms. If the client is having side effects from the radiation such as nausea, antiemetics will be ordered.

If a client has surgery, analgesics will be ordered postoperatively. Analgesics may also be ordered if the cancer has progressed and is causing discomfort.

▶ Diet

Because the surgery is in the oral area, nutrition can be difficult to maintain. Depending on the extent of the surgery, clients may have to be on a soft diet or, in some cases, on nutritional supplements to allow the surgical area to heal. Tube feedings, either by a feeding tube or by a gastrostomy tube (a special tube inserted through the abdomen into the stomach) are frequently needed in clients who have undergone a radical neck dissection.

► Activity

If the surgery is minor, no activity restrictions will be necessary. If surgery is extensive, postoperatively, the client will need to turn, cough, and deep breathe. Activity will need to be progressed postoperatively. Clients receiving radiation treatments frequently experience fatigue and must have rest periods scheduled.

► Nursing Process

Assessment

Subjective Data   Clients may complain of a sore throat, difficulty swallowing, or a painful area in the mouth.

Objective Data   Assessment may include a sore or lesion of the lips or in the oral cavity and hoarseness.

▼ ▼

Possible nursing diagnoses for a client with oral cancer may include:

Nursing Diagnoses	Goals	Nursing Interventions
► *Fear, related to diagnosis and long-term prognosis.*	The client will verbalize fear and express plan to cope with diagnosis.	Allow client time alone and with significant others.
		Answer questions.
		Allow client and family to express fears and concerns.
		Encourage contact with support system (i.e., clergy).
		Discuss past experiences with stress and individual responses to those situations.
► *Nutrition, altered, less than body requirements, related to oral surgery or radical neck dissection.*	The client will maintain weight while hospitalized.	Monitor I & O every shift.
		Weigh daily.
		Administer tube feedings and IV rehydration as ordered.
		When indicated, introduce fluids.
		Monitor for aspiration.
► *Body image disturbance, related to disfiguring surgery.*	The client will verbalize feelings regarding surgery and altered body image.	Allow client time to verbalize feelings.
		Discuss options (i.e., plastic surgery or makeup).
		Answer questions.
		Provide information on support groups.

► Evaluation

Each goal must be evaluated to determine how it has been met by the client.

▲ ▲

► COLORECTAL CANCER

Colorectal cancer is the third most common cancer in the United States. Almost all colorectal cancers arise from **polyps**, a growth of tissue that protrudes into the colon. Risk factors for colorectal cancer includes age forty-five or older, history of polyps, family history of polyps and/or colorectal cancer, a history of ulcerative colitis, and a diet high in fat and low in fiber.

Prognosis is very good if caught in the early stages (refer to Figure 34-12). Recommended routine screenings for early detection are in Table 34-5.

Table 34-5

RECOMMENDED SCREENINGS FOR COLORECTAL CANCER		
Risk	**Definition**	**Recommendations**
Average Risk	No personal or family history of colorectal cancer or polyps.	Fecal occult blood testing (FOBT) age 40. Sigmoidoscopy every 3 to 5 years after age 50.
Mild Risk	Blood relative with colorectal cancer.	Begin above testing 5 to 10 years prior to age relative diagnosed or at minimum, the above guidelines.
Moderate Risk	Client with previous colorectal cancer.	Colonoscopy at 6 months, 1 year and 2 years after diagnosis, then every 1 to 3 years.
High Risk	Familial polyposis syndrome.	FOBT age 10 with sigmoidoscopy. Colonoscopy every 1 to 3 years.
Ulcerative Colitis	UC 8 years throughout colon or 14 years in sigmoid colon.	Colonoscopy every 2 years with biopsies.

A colonoscopy or barium enema may demonstrate the disease. A CBC may show anemia if the cancer is bleeding. A CEA may be effective in detecting recurrent cancer, but is not a valid screening test. Signs and symptoms include a change in bowel habits, guaiac positive stools, and abdominal pain.

▶ Medical/Surgical Management

▶ Surgical

Treatment is surgical to remove the cancer. See Table 34-6. In class A tumors, a colonoscopy is performed with a polypectomy, the removal of the polyp. In class B or C tumors, a colon resection will be done (see Figure 34-12). In some cases a colostomy either temporary or permanent, may be performed. In cases of class D tumors, surgery will only be done to relieve symptoms (i.e., bowel obstruction).

Follow-up colonoscopies will need to be done throughout the client's life to monitor for recurrence of the disease.

▶ Pharmacological

In cases of class B, C, and D tumors, chemotherapy will be given following the surgery. Side effects of chemotherapy include nausea, vomiting, weight loss, hair loss, fatigue, and dry skin. Medications to combat some of the side effects of the chemotherapy will be ordered.

Immunotherapy as an adjunct therapy for class C and D tumors may also be ordered to boost the immune system.

▶ Radiation

No significant benefits have been found with the use of radiation on colorectal cancer. However, radiation may be used on metastatic sites in class D tumors.

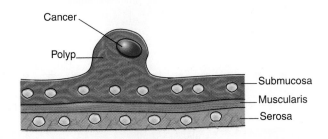

Class A colorectal cancer

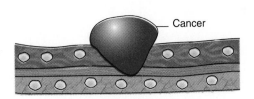

Class B colorectal cancer

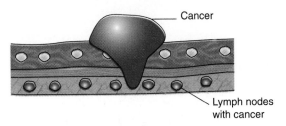

Class C colorectal cancer

FIGURE 34-12 Classes of colorectal cancer.

Table 34-6

COLORECTAL CANCER CLASSIFICATION AND TREATMENT		
Class	**Involvement**	**Treatment**
Class A	Limited to the inner lining of the colon.	Polypectomy during colonoscopy removes cancer.
Class B	Involves from 2 layers to entire thickness of colon wall.	Colon resection, chemotherapy.
Class C	Class B with invasion to lymph nodes.	Colon resection, chemotherapy, and immunotherapy.
Class D	Metastases to other organs (lung and liver most common).	Colon resection as a palliative measure only. Chemotherapy, radiation, and immunotherapy.

▶ Diet

Preoperatively, the client will be NPO. Postoperatively, the client will be NPO and an NG tube will be in place until bowel sounds return. The client will then be started on a clear liquid diet and progressed to a high-fiber, low-fat diet.

▶ Activity

Postoperatively, the client will need to be encouraged to turn, cough, and deep breathe every two hours. The client will be ambulated the next day and activity will need to be progressed.

▶ Nursing Process

Assessment

Subjective Data Clients may complain of a change in bowel habits and possibly abdominal pain.

Objective Data Stools may guaiac positive for blood. An H & H may show anemia.

▼ ▼

Possible nursing diagnoses for a client with colorectal cancer may include:

Nursing Diagnoses	*Goals*	*Nursing Interventions*
▶ *Fear related to diagnosis and long-term prognosis.*	The client will verbalize fear and express plan to cope with diagnosis.	Allow client time alone and with significant others.
		Allow client and family to express fears and concerns.
		Answer questions. Encourage contact with support system (i.e., clergy).
		Discuss past experiences with stress and identify individual responses to those situations.
▶ *Knowledge deficit regarding disease process, treatment options, and follow-up.*	The client will be able to explain disease process, treatment, and follow-up care.	Determine clients learning style and present information in a manner compatible with the learning style.
		Educate client regarding disease process.
		Discuss treatment options.
		Recognize that information may need to be presented more than once.

▶ Evaluation

Each goal must be evaluated to determine how it has been met by the client.

▲ ▲

▶ LIVER CANCER

Primary liver cancer is rare. Most liver tumors are metastatic from other sites in the body. Most cases of primary liver cancer are asymptomatic until later stages. Risk factors for primary liver cancer include a history of cirrhosis, hepatitis B, and exposure to toxic chemicals.

▶ Medical/Surgical Management

A primary liver tumor can be removed surgically if the disease is not extensive. Metastases cannot be surgically removed and are usually treated with chemotherapy and radiation.

▶ EATING DISORDERS

▶ ANOREXIA NERVOSA AND BULIMIA

Anorexia nervosa and bulimia are classified as psychiatric eating disorders. **Anorexia** nervosa is characterized by self-imposed starvation by restricting caloric intake and compulsive exercising (see Figure 34-13). Bulimia, also known as bulimia nervosa, is characterized by periods of binge eating of up to 10,000 calories

at one time followed by self-induced vomiting and other forms of purging such as laxative and diuretic abuse. In bulimia, the client's weight is normal or above normal. In anorexia nervosa, body weight is low and keeps getting lower. Almost all clients with these disorders are female below the age of thirty.

Complications can be serious and include cardiac abnormalities such as bradycardia, hypotension, arrhythmias, CHF, and cardiovascular collapse; oral and esophageal erosions and dental caries from vomiting; renal abnormalities that affect the kidney's ability to filter urine; skin rashes from malnutrition; and bruising from vomiting.

Clients with anorexia tend to be high achievers, perfectionists, have a distorted body image in that they see themselves as fat, and are rigid and ritualistic.

Bulimia occurs more frequently than anorexia with clients experiencing a fear of not being able to stop eating. Clients often experience guilt and depression after a binge.

▶ Medical/Surgical Management

▶ Psychiatric

Treatment is primarily psychiatric involving the client and family and is typically done on an outpatient basis.

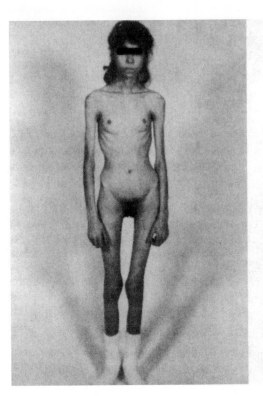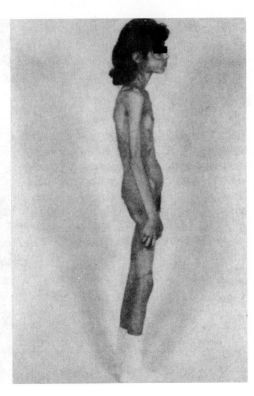

FIGURE 34-13 A client with anorexia nervosa demonstrates severe weight loss with signs of malnutrition. (*Courtesy R.P. Rawlings, S.R. Williams, and C.K. Beck. Mental Health-Psychiatric Nursing, 3rd ed., St. Louis: Mosby-Yearbook, Inc. 1992*)

▶ *Diet*

During severe cases, clients may be admitted for enforced feeding, including the placement of a feeding tube or TPN, IV fluid rehydration, and electrolyte replacement. Clients need to be monitored for refeeding complications such as pancreatitis and gastric dilation. Small quantities are given at first and very gradually the amount is increased.

▶ *Nursing Process*

Assessment

Subjective Data Clients with both anorexia and bulimia may verbalize feelings of helplessness and being out of control, low self-esteem, and overprotective parents. Clients with anorexia may also describe bad dreams and cold intolerance.

Objective Data Assessment of clients with anorexia may show low weight usually lost over a short period of time, reluctance to eat with others, moving food around the plate without eating it, hypotension, heart irregularities, and altered thinking patterns.

Objective assessment of clients with bulimia may show normal weight, tooth erosions and dental caries, puffy face, callused knuckles, broken blood vessels in the eyes and face, reluctance to eat with others, and going to the bathroom immediately after eating.

Laboratory analysis will include a CBC which may show low Hgb, Hct and platelets; electrolytes which may show low sodium, potassium, and chloride; an SMA-22 would show low protein, phosphate, and magnesium; the BUN would be elevated.

▼ ▼

Possible nursing diagnoses for a client with anorexia or bulimia may include:

Nursing Diagnoses	*Goals*	*Nursing Interventions*
▶ *Nutrition, altered, less than body requirements, related to psychological restriction of food intake, excessive activity.*	The client will demonstrate increased consumption of nutrients as evidenced by weight gain daily and improved laboratory values.	Weigh daily. Monitor calorie intake and I & O every shift. Administer IV rehydration, electrolyte replacement, and TPN or tube feedings as ordered. Monitor behavior at and around meal time, such as going to the bathroom right after eating. Monitor exercise patterns.
▶ *Fluid volume deficit, high risk for, related to inadequate intake of liquids, self-induced vomiting, laxative and diuretic use.*	The client's intake and output will be approximately equal, by the second hospital day. The client's electrolytes will be within normal limits, by the third hospital day. The client's fluid intake will be at least 2000 cc per day.	Monitor I & O every shift and bowel movements for diarrhea (a sign of continued laxative abuse). Monitor laboratory reports for electrolyte levels. Administer IV fluid and electrolyte replacement as ordered.
▶ *Coping, ineffective, individual, related to maturational crisis and attempting to control environment.*	The client will verbalize feelings regarding disease process and hospitalization, by the second hospital day. The client will identify current coping strategies, by discharge. The client will identify personal strengths, by discharge.	Provide opportunities for the client to express feelings regarding hospitalization. Encourage client to identify coping mechanisms and strengths. Give positive feedback regarding identified personal strengths.

▶ *Evaluation*

Each goal must be evaluated to determine how it has been met by the client.

▲ ▲

▶ **CASE STUDY**

Ms. R. is a fifty-two-year-old female admitted to the hospital with acute abdominal pain. Ms. R. complains of right upper quadrant pain radiating to the back. She has had prior episodes, usually occurring about two hours after eating. This episode, however, is not resolving. Ms. R. also complains of nausea. Her vital signs are 152/88, pulse 92, and respirations 24 and shallow. Ms. R. is a slightly obese female who states she has recently been dieting to lose weight. Laboratory analysis includes a CBC with slightly elevated WBCs; bilirubin is elevated; and alkaline phosphatase is elevated. An IV is started and Ms. R. is given meperidine (Demerol) IM for pain. Ms. R. has been made NPO. An ultrasound of the gallbladder is ordered.

The following questions will guide your development of a Nursing Care Plan for this case study.

1. List subjective and objective data a nurse would want to obtain about Ms. R.

2. List other risk factors other than those Ms. R. has that would put a client at risk for developing cholecystitis.

3. The gallbladder ultrasound shows stones and an ERCP is ordered. What preparation will Ms. R. need for the procedure?

4. List two nursing diagnoses and goals for Ms. R.

5. The ERCP is successful in removing the CBD stone. The decision is made to perform a laparoscopic cholecystectomy. What teaching will Ms. R. need?

6. Why is meperidine (Demerol) the medication of choice for pain control?

7. List at least three successful outcomes for Ms. R.

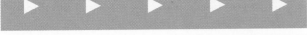

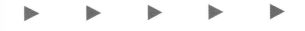

SUMMARY

- The digestive system is a complex system composed of the digestive tract as well as accessory organs.
- Disorders of the GI tract affect the breakdown and absorption of nutrients, breakdown of wastes and byproducts, and the lifestyle of the individual.
- Because the liver is responsible for so many functions in the body, disorders of the liver can affect other systems significantly.
- Peptic ulcers may be either gastric or duodenal. *H. pylori* is a common cause of ulcers and can be treated with antibiotics.
- Diverticulosis is a commonly occurring disorder in the United States and is believed to be caused by a low-fiber diet.

- Inflammatory bowel disease includes both Crohn's disease and ulcerative colitis. IBD can lead to nutritional imbalances, bowel obstructions, alterations in the structure of the intestine, and affected lifestyle.
- Bowel obstructions have multiple causes and can lead to electrolyte imbalances, dehydration, and possibly sepsis.
- Viral hepatitis is a concern for health care professionals at risk for exposure. Standard precautions must be used to prevent the transmission of the virus.
- Colorectal cancer is one of the most preventable forms of cancer if routine screenings are performed.
- Anorexia nervosa and bulimia are psychological disorders affecting mostly women. Severe nutritional imbalances can occur leading to serious effects on the cardiovascular system.

Review Questions

1. A client with a bleeding esophageal varix:
   a. should be encouraged to vomit the blood so as to decrease abdominal distention and pressure.
   b. have an NG tube placed to suction blood from the stomach.
   c. should have the Minnesota tube deflated every four hours.
   d. will not need follow-up once the bleeding has stopped.

2. A client with a perforated duodenal ulcer:
   a. requires an EGD to repair the perforation.
   b. may need to modify his or her diet after surgery.
   c. will have a vagotomy performed.
   d. may experience an increased risk for cholecystitis.

3. Clients with hepatitis C:
   a. should be instructed that all the mechanisms of transmission are not known.
   b. will have a negative HCV if they are a carrier.
   c. should be instructed that recombinant interferon alpha-2b will cure the hepatitis C.
   d. are not contagious until symptoms develop.

4. Changes in the digestive system caused by aging:
   a. are minimal and have little impact on clients.
   b. include an increase in digestive enzymes leading to an increase in the occurrence of ulcers.
   c. require clients to eat larger, fewer meals.
   d. may require the client to swallow two to three times with each bite.

5. Crohn's disease:
   a. can be cured by removing the colon.
   b. usually causes clients to gain weight from the slower metabolism of nutrients.
   c. can be a debilitating disease leading to depression.
   d. is cured as long as the clients remain on 5-ASA compounds.

6. Hernias are a protrusion through the muscle wall and:
   a. can be easily reduced by the nurse applying gentle pressure.
   b. are benign occurrences that do not need any intervention.
   c. can lead to bowel obstructions.
   d. are caused by a lack of exercise.

Critical Thinking Questions

1. What lifestyle changes are needed with a diagnosis of hepatitis A, B, C, and D?

2. Imagine what would it be like to have an NG tube in place?

3. Compare and contrast the symptoms, treatments, and nursing interventions of Crohn's disease and ulcerative colitis.

Medical Terminology

aliment/o-	pertaining to food or nourishment
alimentary canal	the digestive tube from mouth to anus
append/o-	an attachment
appendicitis	inflammation of the appendix
chol/e-	pertaining to bile
cholangiography	radiographic examination of the bile duct
cholecyst/o-	pertaining to the gallbladder
cholecystectomy	excision of a gallbladder
col/o-	pertaining to the colon
colitis	inflammation of the colon
duoden/o-	pertaining to the duodenum
duodenitis	inflammation of the duodenum
esophag/o-	pertaining to the esophagus
esophagalgia	pain in the esophagus
gastr/o-	pertaining to the stomach
gastrostomy	surgical placement of a feeding tube through the abdominal wall into the stomach as a means of providing nutrition
GI	abbreviation for gastrointestinal

hepat/o-	pertaining to the liver
hepatomegaly	an enlarged liver
ile/o-	pertaining to the ileum
ileostomy	an opening into the ileum or terminal portion of the small intestine
jejun/o-	pertaining to the jejunum
jejunostomy	an opening into the jejunal portion of the small intestine
or/o-	pertaining to the mouth
orthopnea	difficulty breathing
rect/o-	pertaining to the rectum.
rectoplasty	plastic surgery on the anus and rectum

News Flash

A breath test to detect the bacteria *H. pylori,* the cause of some ulcers, is currently being researched. The test would mean that clients would no longer have to undergo EGDs to culture the bacteria (*Neergaard, 1996*).

CHAPTER
35
Urinary Disorders

Lois White
with Gyl A. Burkhard
and Beverly F. Hildebrand

LIST OF DISORDERS

LEARNING OBJECTIVES

Upon completion of this chapter the learner should be able to:
- Define key terms.
- Describe the anatomy and physiology of the urinary system.
- Relate diagnostic test results to urinary disorders.
- Discuss the pros and cons of peritoneal dialysis/hemodialysis and kidney transplantation including lifestyle changes for the client receiving dialysis.

- List four drug classifications and two examples of each used in the treatment of urinary disorders.
- State two changes in the urinary system related to the normal aging process.
- Compare and contrast acute and chronic renal failure including nursing care.

- Assist in formulating a nursing care plan for clients with urinary disorders.
- Develop a teaching plan for the client with a urinary disorder.

▶ MAKING THE CONNECTION

Refer to the topics in the following chapters to increase your understanding of urinary disorders.

- **Chapter 8, Health Maintenance:** Urinary Tract Infections, p. 131
- **Chapter 10, Nursing Assessment:** Abdominal Assessment, p. 181
- **Chapter 16, Caring for the Older Adult:** Common Disorders Related to Aging/Urinary System, p. 344
- **Chapter 18, The Dying Process/Hospice:** Bowel and Bladder Care, p. 375
- **Chapter 20, Cardiac Disorders:** Figure 20-3 Grading Edema, p. 451

- **Chapter 31, Female Reproductive Disorders:** Vaginitis, p. 890
- **Chapter 32, Male Reproductive Disorders:** Benign Prostatic Hypertrophy, p. 918; Prostate Cancer, p. 923; Epididymitis, p. 931; Hypospadias and Epispadias, p. 934; Impotence, p. 936
- **Chapter 36, Ostomies:** Types of Ostomies, Urinary, p. 1057; Constructions of Stomas, p. 1059; Pathophysiology of Bowel and Bladder, p. 1061; Disorders of Ostomies, p. 1069

INTRODUCTION

Urology is the study of disorders of the urinary system. The National Kidney Foundation estimates that at least 20 million Americans have kidney or urinary tract related diseases. Disorders of the urinary system may seriously affect an individual's health and, thereby, affect the lives of family members. Clients are treated by a urologist, specialist in urinary tract disorders or a nephrologist, specialist in structure, function, and diseases of the kidney.

According to the National Kidney Foundation, the warning signs of kidney disease are:

- Burning or difficulty during urination
- An increase in the frequency of urination
- Passage of bloody urine
- Puffiness around the eyes, or swelling of the hands and feet
- Pain in the small of the back just below the ribs
- High blood pressure

ANATOMY AND PHYSIOLOGY REVIEW

The urinary system consists of two kidneys, two ureters, (upper urinary tract) a urinary bladder, and a urethra (lower urinary tract) (see Figure 35-1). The kidneys manufacture urine. Urine normally consists of 95 percent water; the nitrogenous waste products of protein which are: urea, uric acid, and creatinine; the excessive electrolytes sodium, calcium, potassium, and phosphates; bile pigments; hormones; and metabolized drugs and toxins. Urine moves steadily by peristalsis through the ureters into the urinary bladder. The urine remains in the urinary bladder until capacity has been reached (about 500 mL) or until a desire to empty the urinary bladder (about 250 mL) is felt. The urine is then expelled from the bladder through the urethra, which is shorter in females than in males. **Micturition**, the process of expelling urine from the urinary bladder, is also known as urinating or voiding.

The kidneys are located beneath the false ribs, in

the **retroperitoneal** space (behind the peritoneum and outside the peritoneal cavity) of the abdominal cavity. The kidneys also assist in acid-base balance, raise blood pressure by secreting the enzyme renin, and produce the hormone erythropoietin which is responsible for **erythropoiesis** (the production of red blood cells and their release by the red bone marrow).

Within the kidneys are microscopic units called nephrons, which are responsible for urine formation. The nephron winds into the cortex and medulla of the kidney. Each nephron includes a renal corpuscle which consists of a glomerulus, a ball-like network of capillaries formed from an arteriole and held within a cuplike Bowman's capsule. The Bowman's capsule is attached to a long, intricate, ultrathin looped and coiled tubular structure called the renal tubule. Continuing on from the glomerulus is an arteriole which forms a capillary network around the tubule. Blood flowing through this system is collected by venioles. The inset in Figure 35-1 illustrates a nephron.

Most of the contents of the blood, except for large molecules and blood cells, are forced out of the blood from the capillaries of the glomerulus and into the Bowman's capsule (glomerulofiltration). This occurs because of the high capillary blood pressure within the glomerulus. The glomerular basement membrane assists with the process of filtration. The material filtered from the blood is called glomerular filtrate which contains water, electrolytes, glucose, various toxic substances, waste products (urea and creatinine), and just about everything else in the blood except large protein molecules and blood cells. As the filtrate passes through the first parts of the tubular structure, various substances such as necessary amounts of electrolytes,

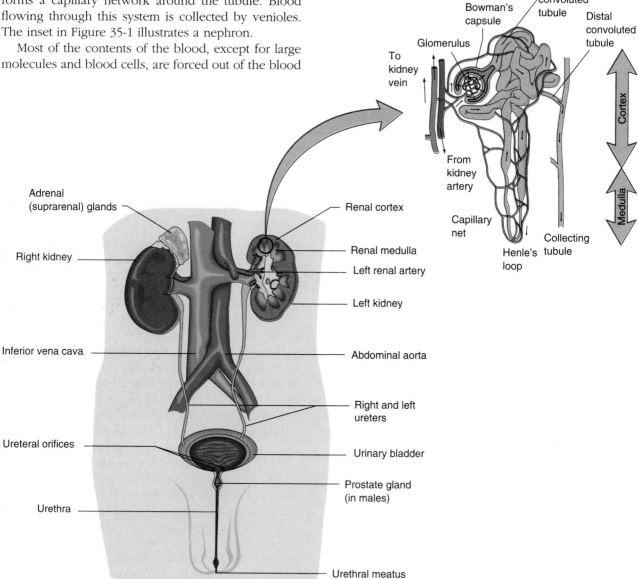

FIGURE 35-1 The urinary system with inset of a nephron.

glucose, and water are reabsorbed (tubular reabsorption) back into the circulatory system through the capillaries or into the interstitial fluid. Tubular secretion then removes certain ions, nitrogen waste products, and drugs from the blood in the capillaries and adds it to the filtrate. The remaining filtrate—water, urea, excess electrolytes, toxic substances and wastes, which constitute urine, continues through the tubules into the collecting duct, which collects urine from many nephrons. The urine passes from the collecting duct into the pelvis of the kidney, then through the ureter into the bladder and out of the body through the urethra.

ASSESSMENT

Assessment of the urinary system is included in the baseline data for all clients. The client may be reluctant to discuss urinary problems. Assist the individual to relax. Ask open-ended questions. Use familiar terms or make sure the client understands the medical terms.

A more in-depth assessment is performed when the client is at high risk for renal disease, because of exposure to nephrotoxins; an altered health state such as diabetes mellitus, pregnancy or hypertension; trauma, dehydration, or fluid retention which can compromise renal function; and those with suspected or active renal disease.

Subjective Data

Ask the client to describe how the symptoms developed and progressed. Is there pain? Is it sharp or a dull ache, constant, or intermittent? Does it radiate to groin, genital area, or leg? Is the pain associated with urination? Have headaches been experienced?

Have the client describe the urine and urination pattern. Is there difficulty starting the stream? Is there urgency, frequency, incontinence, or hematuria? Does the bladder feel empty after voiding? Does the client have pruritis or dry skin?

Objective Data

Assess for edema. If present, ask the client if it is always present or does it disappear during the night? Refer to Figure 20-3 Grading Edema. Monitor I & O and vital signs. Palpate the bladder for retention. Weigh client. Assess mucous membranes for moisture and the skin for dryness and uremic frost. Assess urine for color, clarity, and odor. Assess reports of diagnostic tests.

Changes With Aging

Needham (1993) identifies the following changes in the urinary system due to aging.

1. Nephrons decrease, resulting in decreased filtration and gradual decrease in excretory and reabsorptive functions of renal tubules.
2. Glomerular filtration rate decreases, resulting in decreased renal clearance of drugs.
3. Blood urea nitrogen (BUN) increases 20 percent by age seventy. The creatinine clearance test is a better index than the BUN of renal function in the elderly.
4. Sodium-conserving ability is diminished.
5. Bladder capacity decreases, causing increased frequency of urination and nocturia.
6. Renal function increases when lying down, sometimes causing a need to void shortly after going to bed.
7. Bladder and perineal muscles weaken, resulting in inability to empty the bladder. This results in residual urine and predisposes the elderly to cystitis.
8. Incidence of stress incontinence increases in females.
9. The prostate may enlarge, causing frequency or dribbling in males.

COMMON DIAGNOSTIC TESTS

The following is a table of the commonly used diagnostic tests for clients with problems in the urinary system.

Test	Explanation/Normal Values	Nursing Responsibilities
LABORATORY TESTS		
Urine Tests		
Urinalysis		Explain procedure, purpose, assist with specimen collection if needed.
Color	Clear-amber	Ensure specimen is taken to lab in a timely manner.
Odor	Pleasantly aromatic until left standing; offensive and unpleasant, in kidney infection.	
Albumin (protein)	Negative	
Acetone (ketone)	Negative	
RBCs	2–3/HPF	
WBCs	4–5/HPF	
Bilirubin	Negative	
Glucose	Negative	
Specific gravity	1.005–1.030	
Bacteria	Negative	
Casts	Rare	
pH	4.6–8.0	
Culture and Sensitivity (C & S)	Determines which antibiotics will destroy microorganisms.	Explain procedure. Collect specimen using aseptic technique.
Creatinine Clearance	males 95–135 mL/min females 85–125 mL/min Minimum 10 mL/min to maintain life.	Instruct client about 24 hour urine test. Encourage water intake hourly. Keep urine on ice or in special refrigerator. Drugs affecting results: phenacetin, anabolic steroids, thiazides, ascorbic acid, levodopa, methyldopa (Aldomet), phenolsulfonphthalein (PSP) test.
Blood Tests		
Blood Urea Nitrogen (BUN)	Measures urea, end product of protein metabolism. 5–25 mg/dL	Client NPO for 8 hours preferred. Note client's hydration status. Drugs affecting results: phenothiazines, nephrotoxic drugs, diuretics (hydrochlorthiazide [Hydro-Diuril], ethacrynic acid [Edecrin], furosemide [Lasix]); antibiotics (bacitracin, gentamicin, kanamycin, methicillin, neomycin); antihypertensives (methyldopa [Aldomet], guanethidine [Ismelin]), sulfonamides, propranolol, morphine, lithium carbonate, salicylates.
Serum Creatinine	Specific indicator of renal disease. male 0.6–1.5 mg/dL female 0.6–1.1	Drugs affecting results: amphotericin B, cephalosporins (cepfazolin [Ancef], cephalothin [Keflin]), methicilin, ascorbic acid, barbiturates, lithium carbonate, methyldopa (Aldomet), triamterene (Dyrenium).

Test	Explanation/Normal Values	Nursing Responsibilities
Antistreptolysin O (ASO)	High titer indicates presence of *beta-hemolytic streptococus,* which may cause rheumatic fever or acute glomerulonephritis. Upper limit of normal varies with age, season and geographic area. Adult < 1:100 12–19 years = < 1:200 2–5 years = < 1:100	No food or fluid restriction. Antibiotics give decreased level. Check urine output if ASO elevated. Urine output less than 600 mL/24 hours associated with acute glomerulonephritis.
Serum Electrolytes Sodium Potassium Chloride Calcium Phosphorus	 135–145 mEq/L 3.5–5.0 mEq/L 100–106 mEq/L 4.3–5.3 mEq/L 1.8–2.6 mEq/L	No food or fluid restriction.
Radiographic Tests		
Voiding Cystrourethrography	Bladder filled with dye. X-rays taken to observe bladder filling and emptying. Detects structural abnormalities of the bladder and urethra and reflux into the ureters.	Give enema. Foley catheter inserted and dye injected into bladder and X-rays taken. Catheter removed and client asked to void while more X-rays are taken. Allow client to express feelings, this test may be embarrassing.
Kidney-Ureter-Bladder X-ray (KUB)	Shows abnormalities such as calculi, tumors or change in anatomical position.	Explain procedure. No preparation.
Computed Tomography (CT)	Shows a crosssection of the urinary system for changes in soft tissues.	Explain procedure. Client preparation varies. Check policy.
Magnetic Resonance Imaging (MRI)	Shows soft tissue changes with the use of magnets and computers.	Explain procedure. Remove all metal objects from client. Client may feel claustrophobic and be annoyed by the thumping of the machine.
Intravenous Pyelogram (IVP)	A radiopaque dye is administered IV to detect abnormalities in the urinary tract.	Explain procedure. Client will have a warm feeling during dye injection. Ask client about allergy to iodine or shell fish. Light supper, NPO overnight. Laxative or enema. Schedule before barium studies. Post test, observe for untoward reaction to dye. Encourage fluids for 24 hrs. to eliminate dye.
Renal Angiography	Catheter inserted into femoral artery and threaded to renal artery. Dye injected to show blood vessels in the kidney.	NPO, enema, ask client if allergic to iodine or shellfish. Check vital signs, peripheral pulses. Post test bedrest with leg straight. Monitor vital signs, peripheral pulses, urine output, and puncture site.
Renal Scan	Shows blood flow in the kidneys. Radioactive material, gallium 67, is used.	Check policy on disposal of client's urine for first 24 hours. Pregnant nurses should not care for client during this time because of radiation.

(continued)

Test	Explanation/Normal Values	Nursing Responsibilities
Ultrasound	Sound waves assess the organs for structural abnormalities, tumors or obstructions.	Explain procedure. No preparation.
Urodynamic Tests		
Uroflowmetry	Noninvasive assessment of urination. An electronic device connected to a funneled commode calculates the rate of urine flow, volume voided, and time taken to void.	Explain procedure. Instruct client to void as usual. Leave client alone if possible.
Cystometrogram (CMG)	Measures bladder pressure during filling and emptying. A liquid such as normal saline is injected through a catheter.	Explain procedure. Instruct client to notify tester when sense of fullness is first noticed and when bladder feels full. Client is asked to void and to stop voiding.
Urethra Pressure Profile (UPP)	Assesses functional urethral length and general competency of the urethra and sphincter, at rest or during coughing, straining or voiding. Functional profile length is the length from bladder outlet to point in urethra where urethral pressure equals intravesical pressure. Used in diagnosis of stress or overflow incontinence, or urethral obstruction. Females: bladder outlet through mid-urethra Males: bladder outlet through membranous urethra.	Explain procedure. Often performed when bladder empty and client at rest. May be performed simultaneously with CMG. May be asked to cough or void. Provide privacy, can be embarrassing.
Endoscopic Exam		
Cystoscopy	A cystoscope is passed through urethra into bladder to examine interior of bladder for inflammation, stones, tumors or congenital abnormalities. A biopsy may be performed. Small stones may be removed. Ureteral catheters may be inserted to obtain urine from each kidney. May use topical, spinal or general anesthesia.	Explain procedure. Informed consent signed. Check vital signs. Instruct in deep breathing if having general anesthesia. May have full liquid diet if topical anesthetic is used. Monitor I & O.

KEY ABBREVIATIONS

The following abbreviations and acronyms are used in this chapter:

ARF	acute renal failure	**CRF**	chronic renal failure
ATN	acute tubular necrosis	**EABV**	effective arterial blood volume
AV	arteriovenous	**ESR**	erythrocyte sedimentation rate
BPH	benign prostatic hypertrophy	**ESRD**	end-stage renal disease
CAPD	continuous ambulatory peritoneal dialysis	**ESWL**	extracorporeal shock wave lithotripsy
		UTI	urinary tract infection

ALTERED URINARY ELIMINATION PATTERNS

URINARY RETENTION

A person who is unable to void when there is an urge to void has urinary retention. This creates urinary stasis and increases the possibility of infection. The urine may overflow the bladder's capacity causing incontinence.

There are a variety of causes such as a response to stress; obstruction of the urethra by **calculi** (stones), tumor, or infection; interference with the sphincter muscles during surgery; side effect of medications or perineal trauma.

The client may experience discomfort and anxiety from urinary retention. Frequency of urination, voiding small amounts, and incontinence may also occur. The distended bladder can be palpated above the symphysis.

Treatment may include urinary analgesics and antispasmodics to help the client relax. A urinary catheter may be used to empty the bladder or surgery may be performed to remove any obstruction.

When the client is able to void, a check for residual urine should be done. Immediately after the client voids, catheterization should be performed. The urine left in the bladder, **residual urine**, should be less than 50 mL.

URINARY INCONTINENCE

Urinary incontinence is the uncontrolled loss of urine from the bladder. The incontinence may be a complication of urinary tract problems or neurologic disorders and may be permanent or temporary. Medications such as sedatives, hypnotics, diuretics, anticholinergics, antipsychotics, and alpha antagonists may be associated with incontinence.

Twelve million or more men and women in the United States have some problem with incontinence (Bladder Health Council, 1993). This is not just a physiological problem but also affects the client's emotional, psychological, and social well-being. Incontinence can occur in clients of any age, but is more common in the older adult. It is classified as stress, urge, overflow, total, or nocturnal enuresis.

Stress Incontinence

Stress incontinence is the most common type of incontinence. It is not a disease or a natural, inevitable effect of aging. Anyone can be affected; however, women are more likely to have this condition than men. More than thirty percent of the women with stress incontinence have never discussed it with their physician and more than one in ten women are not aware that help is available (*Stress Incontinence Profiles,* 1995). There is leakage of urine when the person does anything that strains the abdomen such as coughing, laughing, jogging, dancing, sneezing, lifting, making a quick movement, or even walking.

Medical management depends on the underlying cause but it can be treated in 85 to 90 percent of all cases (*Restore Your Active Lifestyle,* 1995). Treatment may include bladder retraining, medicines such as estrogens, conjugated (Premarin Vaginal Cream), or surgery. Surgery may be necessary to restore the support of the pelvic floor muscles or to reconstruct the sphincter. Another possible treatment is having collagen injected into the tissues surrounding the urethra. This closes the urethra enough to prevent urine from leaking out. The procedure is done in a nonsurgical outpatient setting.

The client can be taught pelvic floor exercises (Kegel) to strengthen the muscles thereby preventing or minimizing stress incontinence. Have the client tighten the pelvic floor muscles to stop the flow of urine when urinating and then release the muscles to start the flow of urine again. Once the client can do this, the exercise may be done anytime, anyplace. Practicing the exercise ten times, three or four times a day strengthens the muscles.

Bladder retraining begins with assessing the client's voiding pattern. Encourage the client to void thirty minutes before the projected time of incontinence. Readjust the schedule until the client can stay dry for two hours. Gradually increase the time between voidings until a three to four hour schedule is achieved.

Urge Incontinence

Urge incontinence occurs when a person is unable to suppress the sudden urge to urinate. Sometimes urine may leak without any warning. An irritated bladder is often the cause. Infection or very concentrated urine may irritate the bladder.

Treatment includes clearing up an infection, if present, and encouraging the client to have a fluid intake of 3000 mL/day. This prevents the urine from becoming concentrated. Less fluid does not prevent incontinence but may promote infection.

Overflow Incontinence

When the bladder becomes so full and distended that urine leaks out, it is called overflow incontinence. This occurs when a blocked urethra or bladder weakness prevents normal emptying. The blockage may be an enlarged prostate. The distended bladder cannot contract with enough force to expel a stream of urine. Bladder weakness occurs most often in persons who have diabetes, drink a large quantity of alcohol, and those with decreased nerve function. Bladder retraining may alleviate the situation.

▶ Total Incontinence

When no urine can be retained in the bladder, it is termed total incontinence. The client may be able to manage with an indwelling catheter. A neurologic problem is usually the cause. Surgery to make a temporary or permenent urinary diversion may be required. Refer to Chapter 36, Ostomies.

▶ Nocturnal Enuresis

Incontinence that occurs during sleep is called nocturnal enuresis. Limiting fluid intake after 6 P.M. will help the client remain continent during the night. However, the total fluid intake for the twenty-four hours should remain the same. The bladder should be emptied immediately before going to bed.

▶ INFECTIOUS DISORDERS

▶ CYSTITIS

Cystitis is an inflammation of the urinary bladder. It is classified as a lower urinary tract infection (UTI). It is more common in females because of their short urethra which allows bacteria to ascend through the urethra from the vagina or rectum to the urinary bladder. Also, bacteria from an infected kidney can descend through the ureter into the urinary bladder. The majority of urinary tract infections are caused by *Escherichia coli,* related to urethral catheter use and/or care. A large percentage of these infections are **nosocomial**, that is, acquired in the hospital. Other common causes of cystitis are *Candida albicans,* coitus, prostatitis, and diabetes mellitus.

As women age, pelvic floor muscles relax, leading to a decreased ability to empty the bladder completely. This contributes to stasis of urine and promotion of bacterial growth as in pregnancy or benign prostatic hypertrophy. In men, cystitis usually occurs secondary to another infection such as epididymitis or prostatitis.

Once bacteria enter the bladder, they multiply causing redness and swelling of the wall of the bladder. These changes give rise to urinary frequency, dysuria, pyuria, hematuria, and sometimes burning and urgency with urination. These symptoms increase as the bladder distends with even a small volume of urine.

A clean-catch midstream urinalysis showing a bacteria count greater than 100,000 organisms/mL confirms the diagnosis. The microscopic examination of the urine will also show hematuria and pus.

▶ Medical/Surgical Management

▶ Medical

Treatment of cystitis includes medication and fluids. Recurrence of a urinary tract infection usually occurs when the bacteria are not effectively treated. Obtaining and sending a urine specimen for C & S before the administration of any urinary antimicrobial is necessary to determine the most effective medication. A repeat urinalysis after two or three days on medication will confirm its effectiveness. Chronic lower urinary tract infections are often a factor in the development of pyelonephritis.

▶ Pharmacological

Cystitis treatment entails the use of antimicrobial medication in conjunction with urinary tract analgesics. Cystitis is generally treated with amoxicillin trihydrate (Amoxil), nitrofurantoin (Furadantin), methenamine mandelate (Mandelamine) or sulfonamides: such as sulfisoxazole (Gantrisin) or trimethoprim-sulfamethoxazole (Bactrim or Septra). It is necessary to determine if the client is allergic to sulfonamides or penicillins before administering the medication. The antimicrobial ordered is determined by the results of the urine culture and sensitivity. The length of treatment is related to the type of cystitis, acute or chronic. Some physicians feel that a single dose or short course of antimicrobial therapy may be effective with some acute cases of cystitis. Dysuria related to a burning sensation when voiding can be alleviated with the use of the urinary tract analgesic phenazopyridine hydrochloride (Pyridium) which causes red-orange urine and stains clothing and toilets.

▶ Diet

Fluids are to be encouraged. Clients are usually asked to drink between 3 and 4 liters of noncaffeinated fluid per day. The intake of meats, whole grains, and cranberry juice make the urine more acid, and may discourage the growth of bacteria in the urinary bladder.

▶ Activity

Since cystitis causes frequency of urination, clients on bed rest or those in need of assistance to the bathroom must have the call light answered promptly.

Clients on bed rest are generally not able to empty their bladder completely when using a bedpan. Orders for bathroom privileges or using a commode chair are encouraged. Fear of being incontinent, because the client is unable to get to the bathroom in time, must be prevented.

▶ Nursing Process

Assessment

Subjective Data   The client will usually describe having frequency or urgency of urination or nocturia. This becomes annoying and embarrassing, regardless of age or sex. Burning and pain when voiding are common reasons clients seek medical care. Even clients with an indwelling catheter may complain of dysuria, burning, and frequency. Clients often just do not feel well.

Objective Data   Perineal irritation may be noticed when the client with a catheter pulls on it in hopes of alleviating the bladder pain. The urine will smell foul and appear cloudy. Hematuria may be present. The elderly population in particular, may become anorexic and develop a low grade fever. The urinalysis will indicate the presence of bacteria and the culture and sensitivity will identify the specific microorganism causing the urinary tract infection and the medication to which the pathogen is most sensitive.

▼ ▼

Possible nursing diagnoses for a client with cystitis may include:

Nursing Diagnoses	Goals	Nursing Interventions
▶ Urinary elimination, altered, related to inflammation of the urinary bladder.	The client will return to usual pattern of urinary elimination.	Encourage a large amount of fluid intake, at least 2000 mL each day, especially water and cranberry juice. Administer urinary tract analgesics and antimicrobial medications as ordered. Alert the client, if Pyridium is being taken, that the urine will be red-orange and will stain clothing.
▶ Pain, when voiding, related to inflammation of the urinary bladder.	The client will void without pain and discomfort.	Discuss the importance of taking all medication ordered even after the symptoms are relieved. Teach or reinforce the following preventive measures. Clean the perineum from front to back. If nylon undergarments are worn, they should have a cotton crotch. Wearing tight-fitting jeans and taking long bike rides may be irritating to the perineum. Perfumed perineal products such as menstrual products, douches, powder or bubble bath may also be contributing factors to bladder infections. Spermicidal contraceptive products can be irritating thus encouraging a lower UTI. Advise the client to void more frequently and not keep urine in the bladder. Advise sexually active women to void after sexual intercourse.

(continued)

Nursing Diagnoses	Goals	Nursing Interventions
▶ *Knowledge deficit, related to treatment regimen and prevention of recurrence.*	The client will comply with treatment regimen and practice preventive habits.	Teach the elderly person who uses incontinence control products, such as Attends®, to change the product frequently to prevent cystitis.
		When this client is hospitalized, plan time for frequent ambulation to the bathroom or commode chair.

▶ Evaluation

Each goal must be evaluated to determine how it has been met by the client.

▲ ▲

▶ PYELONEPHRITIS

Pyelonephritis is a bacterial infection of the renal pelvis, tubules, and interstitial tissue of one or both kidneys. This condition is also known as pyelitis or nephropyelitis. Bacteria generally ascend from the urinary bladder, through the ureter and enter the kidney in the area known as the renal pelvis. The bacteria can also enter from the blood and lymph. Pyelonephritis can be secondary to ureterovesical reflux (back flow of urine from the bladder into the ureters) or when urine cannot drain from the pelvis of the kidney because of an obstruction blocking the kidney or ureter. Pyelonephritis may also occur during pregnancy, with prostatitis, when bacteria are introduced during a cystoscopy or catheterization or from trauma of the urinary tract. Pylonephritis can be an acute illness or a chronic condition leading to the development of high blood pressure and/or chronic renal failure.

Escherichia coli is the microorganism most often cultured. The inflamed kidney becomes edematous and the renal blood vessels become congested. Sometimes abscesses form in the kidney. The urine is usually cloudy containing mucus, blood, and pus.

▶ Medical/Surgical Management

▶ Medical

Diagnostic tests which may be ordered include an IVP, a urinalysis with a C & S, CBC, BUN, and creatinine. Urine specimens should be collected prior to the administration of the antimicrobial medication. Medical treatment and care are focused on preventing pyelonephritis from becoming chronic. Follow-up care and treatment may be necessary for up to six months.

▶ Pharmacological

Pyelonephritis is generally treated with sulfonamides, such as trimethoprim-sulfamethoxazole (Bactrim) or the antimicrobial ciprofloxacin hydrochloride (Cipro). Cipro may not be indicated if the client has renal damage. Antipyretics are necessary for fever reduction and analgesics for pain management.

▶ Diet

As with infections in general, the individual's diet should be light during the febrile stage. Fluids must be increased to 3000 mL/day by mouth and supplemented intravenously when indicated.

▶ Activity

The disease process will cause fatigue. Bed rest should be maintained during the acute phase of pyelonephritis. Diversional activities are important while bed rest is ordered. When the client is allowed to be ambulatory, dizziness related to the analgesic medication taken for pain may be a problem.

▶ Nursing Process

Assessment

Subjective Data   In acute pyelonephritis the client is acutely ill with malaise, urgency in urination, pain during voiding and in the flank area. **Renal colic**, severe pain in the kidney, which radiates to the groin, may occur impairing urination. The client may complain of being hot, with or without chills. In chronic pyelonephritis, only a general symptom of nausea may be present. The client may be very anxious that this kidney infection will cause permenent kidney damage.

Objective Data Physical assessment may find the client tender on one or both sides of the lower back. Temperature, pulse, and respiratory rate may all be elevated. The urine is foul smelling and cloudy. The urinalysis results show bacteria and **pyuria** (pus in the urine), and the CBC indicates leukocytosis. The client with chronic disease will have the systemic signs of vomiting, diarrhea, and elevated blood pressure. Some clients with pyelonephritis may be asymptomatic.

▼ ▼

Possible nursing diagnoses for a client with pyelonephritis may include:

Nursing Diagnoses	Goals	Nursing Interventions
▶ Anxiety related to unknown prognosis.	The client will verbalize fears and concerns to family and health care team.	Encourage the client to verbalize fears and concerns. Use active listening and observe for behavioral signs of anxiety. Answer questions honestly.
▶ Pain related to the disease process.	The client will verbalize that pain is relieved.	Administer antimicrobial, analgesic, and antipyretic medications as ordered. Instruct the client on the importance of taking all the antimicrobial medication as prescribed in order to eliminate the bacteria. Explain safety measures for the client to follow after administering an analgesic.
▶ Urine elimination, altered, related to infection and fluid volume excess.	The client will regain normal urinating patterns.	Administer ascorbic acid as prescribed to increase the acidity of the urine. Encourage drinking cranberry juice as acidic urine discourages the growth of microorganisms. Cranberry juice is preferred over other juices such as citrus since they cause an alkaline urine. Monitor intake and output. The intake of fluids is important to maintain function of the urinary system. Evaluate kidney function by measuring and observing urine output and monitoring the results of blood and urine tests.
▶ Knowledge deficit related to disease process, treatment regimen, and prevention.	The client will verbalize understanding of disease process, treatment regimen, and preventive measures.	Teach or reinforce the hygiene measure of cleansing the perineum from front to back and practice this when doing perineal care on any client. Teach the client to refrain from using perfumed perineal products; such as menstrual pads or tampons, or douches; and avoid bubble baths and hot tubs since they can be irritating to the tissues of the genital area. Encourage the client to empty the bladder frequently, to avoid distention. Promote rest periods which aid the healing process.

(continued)

Nursing Diagnoses	Goals	Nursing Interventions
		Inform the client to call the physician immediately if there is a decrease in urine output or signs of infection (elevated temperature, chills, flank pain, urgency, fatigue, nausea, and vomiting).
		Teach client to weigh daily and report sudden weight gain (2 pounds/week) to the physician.
		Emphasize the importance of keeping all appointments with the physician for follow-up care and when signs of infection appear.
		Teach the client the importance of long-term treatment and monitoring for chronic pyelonephritis.

▶ Evaluation

Each goal must be evaluated to determine how it has been met by the client.

▲ ▲

▶ ACUTE GLOMERULONEPHRITIS

Glomerulonephritis is a condition that can affect one or both kidneys. In both acute and chronic disease, the glomerulus within the nephron unit becomes inflamed. It is predominantly a disease of children and young adults when the cause is bacterial. The viral form can affect all ages. The prognosis for most clients is a full recovery; however, some may develop chronic glomerulonephritis. Acute glomerulonephritis during childhood is known as Bright's disease.

Most clients develop symptoms one to three weeks after an upper respiratory infection (tonsillitis or pharyngitis with fever) or skin infection caused most commonly by group A β-*hemolytic streptococcus*. The infection triggers an autoimmune response and the glomeruli are attacked by antibodies at the site of the glomerular basement membrane, resulting in inflammation. Some clients are asymptomatic. Approximately one to two percent of people having acute glomerulonephritis will develop end-stage renal failure.

Immunologic effects on the body are not completely understood. Direct effects on the glomeruli result in the reduced ability of the glomeruli to function. The glomeruli become more permeable, resulting in the loss of red blood cells and protein from the blood. These substances escape from the body in the urine. The inflammatory process causes thickening of the membrane of the glomeruli and potential scarring.

▶ Medical/Surgical Management

▶ Medical

Diagnostic tests on blood and urine as well as x-rays, KUB, will be performed. BUN, serum creatinine, potassium, erythrocyte sedimentation rate (ESR), and antistreptolysin O titer will be elevated. Urinalysis will show protein and red blood cells.

Medical treatment must start as soon as the client is diagnosed in order to restore the kidneys to normal functioning. Management includes drug therapy, diet, and rest. Treatment is correlated with the blood pressure and the results of urine testing for red blood cells and protein. The client is not considered to be free from the disease until the urine tests negative for protein and red blood cells for six months. Prevention of renal complications as well as complications to cardiac and cerebral functioning are the focus of care.

▶ Pharmacological

Prophylactic antimicrobial therapy may be administered. The drug of choice is penicillin. Diuretic and antihypertensive medication, furosemide (Lasix), may be ordered. Corticosteroid, chemotherapeutic drugs such as cyclophosphamide (Cytoxan), and/or immunosuppressive agents such as azathioprine (Imuran) may be ordered to control the inflammatory response.

Plasmapheresis may be indicated if there is no response from other treatments. Between 150 and 400 mL of blood is removed from the client and put in a cell separator. Here the blood is divided into plasma and formed elements. The formed elements are mixed with a plasma replacement and returned to the client through a vein. Another technique filters the client's own plasma to remove a specific disease mediator (antibody) and then returned to the client.

▶ Diet

Fluid retention often requires fluid restriction. The restriction is adjusted according to the client's intake and output record and daily weight. Protein in the client's diet will be regulated according to the BUN and the creatinine blood levels. The kidneys need to rest; however, particularly in children, it may not be necessary to restrict protein. Potassium will need to be replaced if the diuretic promotes its excretion. Strict intake and output are necessary to monitor kidney function.

▶ Activity

Physical and emotional rest are essential. Compliance with bed rest may be difficult, especially for a child or the client who feels well. Bed rest is indicated until the inflammation subsides, urinary flow increases, and as long as the client has hematuria or proteinuria. During this time a strict turning schedule needs to be followed, as skin breakdown is more likely in the presence of edema. Once bed rest restrictions are lifted, the client may feel weakened from the effects of anemia and inactivity.

▶ Nursing Process

Assessment

Subjective Data The health history will likely reveal a recent sore throat, skin infection, flulike symptoms, and a headache. The client describes flank pain as the kidneys become congested. Other symptoms the client may describe are headache, malaise, anorexia, cola-colored "smokey" urine (hematuria), and a marked decrease in the amount of urine (oliguria). Facial edema may have been the first sign noticed, may impair vision, and may cause the client to have negative feelings about body image.

Objective Data Vital signs will generally show an increase in temperature and blood pressure. Facial (periorbital) edema is present. The edema will progress to dependent areas such as the sacral area and the legs. Monitor the location and degree of edema daily. Ascites may also develop. Assess the general condition of the skin and skin integrity. Weigh client to establish a baseline weight. Assess heart and lung sounds for signs of congestive heart failure and pulmonary edema (unusual heart sounds and crackles in the lungs). Neck veins may be distended. Dyspnea on exertion or when recumbent and shortness of breath may be noted. Urine output is decreased and hematuria is present (cola-colored to red).

Monitor results of diagnostic tests: urine for red blood cells and protein (albumin) and blood for BUN, serum creatinine, potassium, ESR, antistreptolysin O titer, and specific gravity, all of which will be elevated.

Possible nursing diagnoses for a client with acute glomerulonephritis may include:

Nursing Diagnoses	Goals	Nursing Interventions
▶ Fear related to potential permanent damage to the kidneys.	The client will communicate fears of kidney damage to the family and the health care personnel.	Since acute glomerulonephritis is treated over a course of several months, provide client and family with ongoing support and understanding. Encourage the client to discuss fears. Explain the importance of protecting the client from other infections. Allow no one with an upper respiratory infection to visit the client. Discuss the importance of compliance with medications, bed rest, and diet to prevent permanent damage to the kidneys.

(continued)

Nursing Diagnoses	Goals	Nursing Interventions
		Emphasize the importance of keeping the follow-up visits to the laboratory for tests and to the physician's office.
		Work together with all members of the health care team to encourage compliance by the client.
		Arrange consultation with social services to assist the client in arranging time off from work and to help the client and family with their financial needs.
▶ *Activity intolerance related to bed rest.*	The client will tolerate activity when bed rest is discontinued.	Incorporate a turning schedule with range of motion exercises in the plan of care for the client.
		Provide mattress devices (eggcrate, Clinitron) to prevent skin breakdown.
		Assist in finding quiet diversional activities of interest to the client, to promote compliance with bed rest such as reading, listening to the radio or tapes, or watching television.
▶ *Fluid volume excess related to decreased urinary output, secondary to renal dysfunction.*	The client will have decreased edema and adequate urinary output.	Fluids will be restricted with specific amounts designated throughout the day. For example, 900 mL of fluids for a day might be divided in the following manner: 7 A.M. to 3 P.M. 600 mL; 3 P.M. to 11 P.M. 200 mL; 11 P.M. to 7 A.M. 100 mL.
		Encourage compliance to the fluid amounts.
		Maintain accurate intake and output records.
		Advise to use low-sodium bottled water in cooking and for the drinking allowance when water supplies are naturally high in sodium or if water is chemically softened.
		Provide oral hygiene several times a day. This is extremely important when water intake is restricted.
		Advise that thirst may be relieved by sucking on hard candy or, if allowed, a few ice chips.
		Provide eye care with normal saline to promote comfort from the periorbital edema.
▶ *Social interaction, impaired, related to changes in body image.*	The client will resume social interaction.	Encourage client to keep in contact with friends and relatives by telephone.
		Encourage keeping appointments with the physician and laboratory.
		Provide eye care with normal saline to promote comfort from the periorbital edema.
▶ *Nutrition, altered, more than body requirements, related to the disease process.*	The client will comply with nutritional restrictions.	Once the client's condition warrants solid foods, provide diet with complex carbohydrates instead of foods with concentrated sugar.

Nursing Diagnoses	Goals	Nursing Interventions
		If hematuria and/or proteinuria are still present, provide a diet with mild to moderate protein restriction to rest the kidney tissue. Protein foods that may be restricted include meats, fish, poultry, eggs, milk products, and whole grains.
		If edema persists, provide low-sodium diet. Processed, canned, or frozen foods will be substituted with foods made with fresh ingredients.
		If a restricted sodium and protein diet are ordered, arrange a dietary consultation to incorporate food preferences, religious and/or cultural needs. Finances may be an issue if the family has to incorporate foods that are not usually part of their budget.
		Teach client to plan menus and to read food labels in order to comply with the dietary restrictions.
		Before discharge, teach client and family about diet, fluids, and activity restrictions and measuring fluid intake and urine output.
		Provide client with guidelines listing reasons to call the physician.

▶ Evaluation

Each goal must be evaluated to determine how it has been met by the client.

▲ ▲

▶ CHRONIC GLOMERULONEPHRITIS

The prognosis for acute glomerulonephritis is often good when treatment is begun early. However, chronic glomerulonephritis generally leads to permanent kidney damage. Those who develop chronic glomerulonephritis may have neither symptoms nor a recent history of an infection. Chronic diseases, such as diabetes mellitus or systemic lupus erythematosus, often mask renal symptoms and the client does not seek medical care until kidney function is impaired. It may take up to thirty years for the signs of renal insufficiency to develop.

Chronic glomerulonephritis is a progressive but slow, destructive process affecting the glomeruli causing loss of kidney function. The kidney will actually decrease in size as glomeruli are destroyed. If end-stage renal disease (ESRD) develops, the client may die quickly.

Nephrons lose their ability to filter nitrogenous wastes from the blood. Protein (albumin) and red blood cells escape into the urine and are present on a urinalysis. Nitrogenous waste remains in the blood and the blood urea nitrogen (BUN) level increases. As glomeruli are destroyed, the serum level of creatinine also increases. BUN and serum creatinine are checked on a regular basis to monitor renal function and to assist with client care management. Serum electrolyte levels are also monitored. Anemia will be evaluated with a CBC.

▶ Medical/Surgical Management

▶ Medical

Medical treatment must begin immediately to limit further destruction of the glomerular tissue. Management includes drug therapy, diet, and bed rest. Exposure of the client to infection of any kind must be avoided. Blood transfusion may be required for severe anemia. The client may need to be transferred to a facility where dialysis and/or kidney transplantation can be performed. Prevention of further renal damage as well as heart or cerebral complications are the focus of care.

▶ *Pharmacological*

Diuretic and antihypertensive medications are ordered. Antimicrobial therapy is generally given prophylactically. Side effects from all medications must be watched and reported to the physician immediately.

▶ *Diet*

Fluid intake is adjusted according to urinary output. Protein allowed in the diet will be regulated according to the BUN and the creatinine blood levels. As these levels increase, protein will be restricted to decrease the nitrogenous wastes. Sodium and potassium restrictions will be determined by the serum electrolyte levels. Carbohydrates are usually increased in the diet to provide adequate energy.

▶ *Activity*

Bed rest is indicated when the client has hematuria or albuminuria.

▶ *Nursing Process*

Assessment

Subjective Data   Clients may complain of a morning headache, pruritis, a decreased ability to concentrate, fatigue, and dyspnea making it difficult to perform ADLs. Facial edema and/or blurring of vision, due to retinal edema, may also be reported by clients.

Objective Data   As chronic glomerulonephritis develops, fluid retention becomes evident leading to shortness of breath, especially at night. Assess vital signs, hypertension is usually present. Lung sounds need to be assessed every shift for crackles, a sign of fluid retention. Weight must be monitored daily, after the baseline weight is obtained. Assess the degree of edema, its location, and if it is pitting or nonpitting. **Anasarca** is generalized edema that appears as the client's condition deteriorates. Assess the skin for color, presence of ecchymosis or rash, dryness, and evidence of scratching. Assess mental functioning, irritability, tremors, ataxia, or slurred speech.

As nephrons lose their ability to concentrate urine, the urine becomes pale and dilute. Intake and output must be closely monitored because initially, polyuria develops giving the client a false sense that recovery will be soon. Monitor the results of blood and urine tests.

▼ ▼

Possible nursing diagnoses for a client with chronic glomerulonephritis may include:

Nursing Diagnoses	Goals	Nursing Interventions
▶ *Urinary elimination, altered, related to the failing kidney function.*	The client will have adequate urine output.	Measure urine output hourly, or every four or eight hours as ordered, to determine kidney function. Parameters will be set by the physician for immediate notification.
		Assess and document the color and consistency of the urine.
		Measure intake to determine compliance with the amount of fluids permitted.
		Weigh client daily at the same time each day, on the same scales and with the same clothes.
▶ *Fluid volume excess related to decreased urinary output.*	The client will have decreased edema.	Assess and describe the location of the edema.
		Administer medications, as ordered, for treatment of the edema.
		Document reactions to the medication.
		Monitor electrolyte values.
		Maintain fluid intake at restricted amount.

Nursing Diagnoses	Goals	Nursing Interventions
▶ Activity intolerance related to progressive weakness.	The client will maintain range of motion.	Turn and position every two hours when the client is in bed. The orthopneic position facilitates respiration. Encourage active ROM or provide passive ROM.
▶ Anxiety related to potential treatment with dialysis.	The client will communicate less anxiety about possible treatment with dialysis.	Assist client to express concerns about possible treatment with dialysis. Arrange for a dialysis nurse to visit client. Home dialysis may be discussed as an option.
▶ Skin integrity, impaired, high risk for, related to immobility and edema.	The client will maintain skin integrity.	Assess skin every time the client is repositioned. Cleanse the skin frequently, especially when crystals of urea form on the skin causing itching and dryness.

▶ Evaluation

Each goal must be evaluated to determine how it has been met by the client.

▲ ▲

▶ OBSTRUCTIVE DISORDERS

▶ UROLITHIASIS

Urolithiasis is a calculus or stone formed in the urinary tract. A calculus (plural–calculi) is a solid mass of mineral salts occurring within a hollow organ such as the renal pelvis, ureters, bladder, or urethra (see Figure 35-2). A urinary calculus can range in size from microscopic to 10 to 20 mm in diameter.

Calculi are formed from minerals that precipitate out of solution and collect within hollow areas. The reason stones form has not yet been identified, but individuals who are immobile, hyperparathyroid, or have recurrent UTIs are predisposed. When a person is immobile for long periods, calcium is pulled from the bones into the blood. The nephrons filter the excess calcium out of the blood into the urine. Calculi can also lodge in and obstruct an indwelling catheter. The size and location of the stone within the urinary system greatly affects the degree of pain and other symptoms present. When the stone is in the kidney, the pain is dull and constant mainly in the back just below the ribs near the spine. Stones in the ureter often cause ureteral colic, an excruciating, intermittent pain that begins in the flank and radiates into the groin, inner thigh, or genitalia. It is caused by spasm of

the ureter as the calculus moves down the ureter. The client often has nausea and vomiting also.

If a calculus becomes lodged any place along the ureter, the urine cannot pass and a condition called hydronephrosis and/or hydroureter occur. The kidney and/or ureter become enlarged with the accumulated urine, as illustrated in Figure 35-3.

Tests to confirm the diagnosis and determine the size and location of the stone include KUB, IVP, cystoscopy, and ultrasound. A BUN and serum creatinine indicate whether the calculus has damaged kidney function. A urinalysis with a culture and a CBC may be ordered to determine if an infection is present. A twenty-four hour urine may be sent to the laboratory to determine if there is abnormal excretion of calcium oxalate, phosphorus, and uric acid.

▶ Medical/Surgical Management

▶ Medical

All urine must be strained whether voided or from an indwelling catheter drainage bag. Urine from a catheter drainage bag must be drained and strained every two to four hours. All strained particles must be saved for the physician or sent to the laboratory.

A very small calculus may be flushed out by peri-

eter. Ultrasound waves directed at the stone break it into small pieces that can be withdrawn through the catheter. The catheter is left in place until the edema subsides, usually one or two days.

A bladder calculus may be crushed with special surgical instruments and the fragments washed out through a catheter. This is called a **litholapaxy**.

Lithotripsy Extracorporeal shock wave **lithotripsy** (ESWL) is a method of crushing a calculus any place in the urinary system. The client is placed in a warm water bath and ultrasonic waves aimed at the stone break the stone into small pieces. An alternate method is to appropriately place a fluid-filled bag on the client's body and aim the ultrasonic waves at the stone through the bag. There is some discomfort and the client may be bruised where the ultrasonic waves hit the body. The urine will be slightly bloody for twenty-four to forty-eight hours and must be strained. The client should drink large amounts of fluids (3000 to 4000 mL/day) unless contraindicated.

▶ *Pharmacological*

Narcotic analgesics are generally prescribed for the severe pain often called renal colic. Antispasmodics such as propantheline bromide (Pro-Banthine) or belladonna preparations may be ordered to relieve ureteral spasms. Antibiotics may be ordered prophylactically.

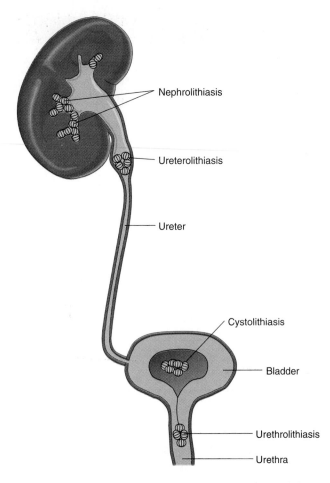

FIGURE 35-2 Common locations of renal calculi formation.

stalsis and fluids. The client is encouraged to drink at least 4000 mL of fluid/day, unless contraindicated by other health problems. This can be a long and painful process and may be more than the client can handle. The urologist may insert a small, pliable catheter into the ureter or urethra to allow temporary drainage of urine around the calculus.

▶ *Surgical*

There are several surgical procedures, depending on the location and size of the calculus, from which the surgeon may choose. These include: cystoscopy, pyelolithotomy, nephrolithotomy, or ureterolithotomy. Figure 35-4 shows several methods of removing a stone.

Another choice is the endoscopic procedure, known as percutaneous nephrolithotomy, in which a small incision is made in the fleshy area on the client's side between the ribs and the hip. A catheter is inserted and an ultrasonic probe is inserted through the cath-

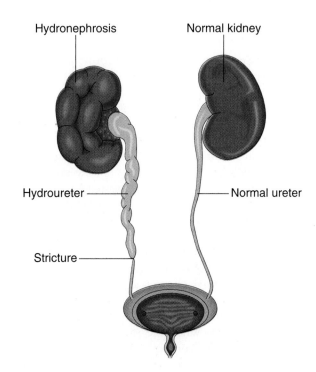

FIGURE 35-3 Hydronephrosis and hydroureter resulting from stone in ureter.

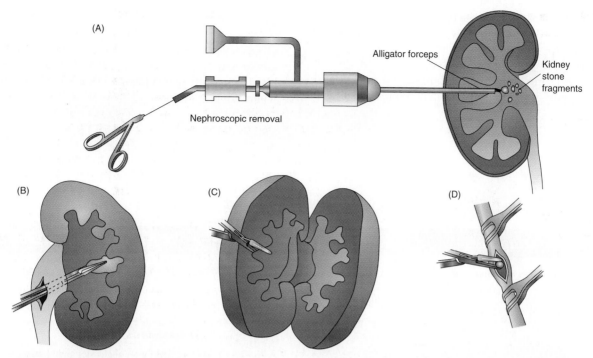

FIGURE 35-4 Methods of removing kidney stones. **(A)** Nephroscopic removal. **(B)** Pyeloleithotomy, removal through renal pelvis. **(C)** Nephrolilthotomy, removal through incision into the kidney. **(D)** Ureterolithotomy, removal through ureter.

Drug therapy is specific to stone composition. Allopurinol (Zyloprim) reduces the serum urate level, thus preventing calcium oxalate stones. Sodium cellulose phosphate (Calcibind) binds with calcium in the bowel and facilitates excretion of calcium. Aluminum hydroxide gel (Amphojel) binds with excess phosphates in the gastrointestinal tract. The phospates are then excreted.

▶ Diet

Individuals who form calcium calculi may need to reduce their intake of dietary calcium, mainly dairy products, to no less than 600 mg/day. When the stones contain uric acid, purine-rich foods (meat, fish, and poultry) should be restricted, and organ meats, anchovies, and sardines avoided. Foods rich in oxalic acid (broccoli, asparagus, chocolate, tea, rhubarb, and spinach) are restricted when oxalate stones form. A deficiency of pyridoxine, thiamin, and magnesium may also contribute to the formation of oxalate stones.

Sometimes an effort is made to change the pH of the urine and thus prevent the formation of calculi. Acid-ash or alkaline-ash diets are used. Acid-ash foods are meats, fish, poultry, eggs, cereals, cranberries, and plums. Alkaline-ash foods are vegetables and all other fruits. These diets are often difficult for the client to maintain.

Drinking large amounts of fluid, at least half of it water, dilutes the urine and helps move any microscopic calculi through the system. Up to 4000 mL/day of fluid is indicated for a client with renal calculi, unless contraindicated by another health problem such as congestive heart failure.

▶ Activity

Exercising regularly helps reduce the formation of calculi, and keeps calculi moving through the urinary tract. Clients on bed rest should have range of motion exercises daily in addition to frequent turning and positioning.

▶ Nursing Process

Assessment

Subjective Data　Some individuals may be asymptomatic until the calculus begins to move or becomes too large. When the stone moves, the client usually describes intractable pain, that is, pain which is not relieved by ordinary measures. Nausea and vomiting are often reported also. The pain is often described as beginning in the flank and radiating down to the groin and inner thigh. Observe for nonverbal client behaviors that indicate pain such as: tossing and turning when in bed, or the inability to sit still when out of bed. If the calculus is not moving, the client may describe symptoms of infection such as lethargy, frequency of urination, dysuria, burning on urination, or feeling very warm. The client may express feelings of frustration related to the inability to complete daily tasks.

Objective Data   Assess for hematuria, vomiting, intake and output, and vital signs. Elevated pulse and blood pressure may indicate pain. Check for stones when urine is strained.

▼ ▼

Possible nursing diagnoses for a client with urolithiasis may include:

Nursing Diagnoses	Goals	Nursing Interventions
▶ Pain related to irritation of the urinary tract and the mobility of calculi.	The client will verbalize there is a reduction in pain.	Develop a pain management plan. Inquire about intensity, location, duration, and alleviating factors of pain. Provide comfort measures and diversional activities. Administer analgesics and antispasmodics as ordered. Observe for nonverbal signs of pain.
▶ Urinary elimination, altered, related to blockage of urine flow by the calculi.	The client will return to normal urine elimination.	Monitor urine for color and amount. Encourage fluids to dilute the urine and flush out the calculi. Assist client to ambulate, if able. Accurately monitor intake and output. If a ureteral catheter is in place, measure and record the urine output from it separately from the urine output from the bladder.
▶ Infection, high risk for, related to obstruction.	The client will have no signs of infection.	Monitor for and report elevated temperature, feeling flushed, or chills. Note if urine is cloudy or malodorous. Encourage fluid intake and keep an accurate intake and output record. Use proper handwashing technique and teach the client to do the same.
▶ Knowledge deficit related to new health problem.	The client will verbalize understanding of the health problem and treatment regimen.	Evaluate the client's readiness to learn and provide information at the client's level of understanding. Teach how to strain urine if no catheter is in place and to keep an accurate intake and output record. Assist client in understanding the reason for drinking large amounts of fluids, prescribed diet restrictions, and the need to be ambulatory. Instruct about the purpose of medications, dosage, schedule, and side effects. Emphasize the need to keep scheduled physician appointments.

▶ *Evaluation*

Each goal must be evaluated to determine how it has been met by the client.

▲ ▲

▶ *URINARY BLADDER TUMORS*

According to the American Cancer Society, the 1994 statistics predicted approximately 51,000 new cases of urinary bladder cancer. As with renal tumors, men are affected more often than women. Bladder cancer occurs most frequently after the age of fifty. In 1994, the American Cancer Society stated approximately 10,000 people died yearly from bladder cancer. The only early warning signs are increased urinary frequency and painless, intermittent hematuria. One risk factor is cigarette smoking. Those individuals who smoke nicotine products have twice the risk of developing bladder cancer than nonsmokers. Other risk factors are working with dyes, rubber, or leather products; caffeine intake and the use of certain artificial sweeteners. Caucasians are at a greater risk of developing this cancer.

Benign papillomas are the most common urinary bladder tumor. Although the papillomas are quite small, they should be treated aggressively as they are considered to be premalignant. Cancer cells develop mainly in the area where the ureters enter the urinary bladder. The primary sites for metastasis are the liver, lungs, or bones. Symptoms resulting from obstruction of the ureters is a frequent reason for the client seeking medical care. Diagnostic studies done usually include a urinalysis, a cystoscopic visualization and biopsy of the lesions, an IVP, and CT scan.

▶ *Medical/Surgical Management*

▶ *Surgical*

Surgical removal of small tumors is generally done with an electrosurgical procedure (**fulguration**) to burn the lesions off the internal bladder wall. Other surgical procedures used are laser surgery, or snaring of the lesion. These procedures are usually performed with cystoscopic visualization. Several times a year, the client who has had bladder lesions should be monitored for recurrence of the lesions. A cytologic examination is done on any lesion(s) noted during a cystoscopic examination.

A cystoscopic examination is performed with either local anesthesia and sedation or general anesthesia. After the procedure, the client's legs may be sore as a lithotomy position is used. Analgesics will be prescribed for use as needed. After a cystoscopic procedure, the client may experience urinary frequency, burning on urination, and the presence of pink-tinged urine.

When the pathology of tissue specimens indicates a need for more extensive surgery, either a partial or total cystectomy may be performed. The surgery may be done in conjunction with radiation therapy or chemotherapy.

A cystectomy is performed for cancer of the bladder (if it appears curable), chronic bladder infections, or where severe trauma has occurred to the urinary bladder. When the urinary bladder is completely removed, a urinary diversion is necessary. Consideration is made for age, extent of the disease, and the prognosis. One option is a bilateral cutaneous ureterostomy, where the ureters are implanted directly into the abdominal wall. Another option is for the ureters to be implanted into a piece of the ileum which is then attached to the abdominal wall as a stoma. This is known as an **ileal** ('wet') **conduit**.

Other methods of urinary diversion are the implantation of the ureters into the sigmoid colon (ureterosigmoidostomy) and the creation of a continent stoma with a pouch of bowel. This urinary diversion is known either as a Kock or Mainz pouch or a Gilchrist ileocecal reservoir depending on which surgical procedure was used. See Chapter 36 for a discussion of these methods of urinary diversion.

▶ *Pharmacological*

One chemotherapy treatment is the instillation of an antineoplastic drug within the urinary bladder. This route is known as **intravesical**. Systemic chemotherapy may also be used for cystectomy clients. Medications to relieve symptoms such as pain and nausea are important for the client's social well-being.

▶ *Diet*

If proctitis (inflammation of the rectum and anus) or diarrhea occurs, a low-residue diet is ordered to facilitate normal bowel elimination.

▶ Activity

When the client is on bed rest, turning and positioning are important to maintain skin integrity as the client may be emaciated due to significant weight loss. Activity should be encouraged as the client's condition warrants. During the intravesical instillation of an antineoplastic drug, the client will have to change positions every fifteen minutes, for a period of several hours, to evenly distribute the chemotherapeutic drug around the urinary bladder.

▶ Nursing Process

Assessment

Subjective Data The client will describe having painless, intermittent hematuria, and changes in voiding patterns. Fatigue may also be mentioned.

Objective Data Weakness will be noted if the client has become anemic from the hematuria. Check urine specimen with a reagent strip for blood. Review results of diagnostic tests. Assess the client's understanding of current health situation.

▼ ▼

Possible nursing diagnoses for a client with urinary bladder tumors may include:

Nursing Diagnoses	Goals	Nursing Interventions
▶ Incontinence, urge, related to decreased bladder capacity.	The client will maintain urinary continence.	Document I & O. Administer medications as ordered. Assign bed close to bathroom or have bedside commode. Assist client to plan regular times to urinate. Limit fluid intake after supper, but maintain adequate total intake.
▶ Anxiety, related to the pending diagnosis.	The client will discuss feelings about the diagnosis.	Make the client and family members feel comfortable. Encourage them to discuss their feelings and ask questions. Answer questions factually and honestly. Initiate teaching preoperatively.
▶ Knowledge deficit related to surgery and treatment regimen.	The client will describe surgical changes and treatment regimen.	If surgical removal of bladder lesions is done as an outpatient procedure, teach the client to observe for pink-tinged urine and to notify the physician if bright red urine is seen. Discuss the use of analgesics as ordered for pain of bladder spasms. Encourage adequate fluid intake. Refer the client with a stoma to the enterostomal therapist for specialized care and teaching. The therapist will assist the client with the appliance and skin care protocol. Monitor the color and integrity of the stoma daily, to ensure that the tissue is receiving adequate circulation. The stoma is normally red and edematous for a time postoperatively. The stoma will remain red in color, but will shrink in size during the healing process.

Nursing Diagnoses	Goals	Nursing Interventions
		If the stoma color changes, notify the physician.
		Refer to a local ostomy group for ongoing support and assistance or to the United Ostomy Association, which provides support and literature.
		Teach the signs and symptoms related to potential problems that should be reported to the physician.
		Encourage the intake of fluids, up to 3000 mL per day, unless contraindicated.
		Teach about the medications to be taken at home.
		Encourage the client to attend all scheduled follow-up visits.
		Assist the client to plan the gradual return to the routines of driving, lifting, sexual activities, and work.
▶ *Urinary elimination, altered, related to surgical procedure.*	The client will maintain adequate urinary elimination.	Accurately monitor urine output as this is the major postoperative concern.
		Assist client to discuss feelings about the altered urinary elimination method.
		Assist the client with a bilateral cutaneous ureterostomy to use leg bags for easier ambulation.
		Change the leg bag tubing back to straight bag drainage to promote uninterrupted sleep.
		Teach the client how to use both kinds of drainage systems.

▶ Evaluation

Each goal must be evaluated to determine how it has been met by the client.

▲ ▲

▶ RENAL TUMORS

In 1994, according to the American Cancer Society, there were approximately 27,000 new cases of kidney cancer. A unilateral renal adenocarcinoma is the most common tumor, and is seen more often in men between the ages of fifty and seventy. Approximately 8,000 people a year die from renal cancer. Renal tumors total about two percent of all cancers. Risk factors include smoking, familial incidence, and preexisting renal disorders.

Intermittent, painless hematuria is often ignored by the client and medical attention is not sought until the malignancy is quite advanced. By this time, the client usually has experienced weight loss, dull flank pain, gross hematuria, and a mass may be palpable in the flank area. Lymph nodes in the area of the kidney, the renal vessels, and/or the inferior vena cava may become involved. The primary sites for metastases are the lungs and bone, resulting in respiratory distress and bone pain. A pathological fracture may be the reason for admission of the client; resulting in the diagnosis of kidney cancer.

▶ Medical/Surgical Management

▶ Medical

An IVP will detect a renal mass. Other diagnostic studies used to evaluate the kidney or the status of other body systems possibly involved are renal sonography or arteriogram, MRI, CT scan, or a needle biopsy. The painless hematuria contributes to a decreased hematocrit. The physician may insert a nephrostomy tube into the renal pelvis of each kidney to evaluate the function of each kidney. Chemotherapy and/or radiation therapy have proved to be of minimal benefit.

▶ *Surgical*

Usually a radical nephrectomy is performed, if the other kidney is healthy and the disease is localized. The surgeon may enter the thoracic as well as the abdominal cavity during this procedure. If the chest is opened, the client will have a closed chest drainage system postoperatively (See Chapter 19, Respiratory Disorders). A nasogastric drainage tube may be in place and attached to suction. Hemorrhage and compromised respiratory effort are the postoperative problems for which to observe.

▶ *Pharmacological*

If the client is receiving radiation therapy treatments, antiemetics or antispasmodics may be ordered. Analgesics are ordered to control pain, facilitate respirations and client activity. An antiemetic will usually be ordered to promote comfort and to encourage eating.

▶ *Diet*

The client having a nephrectomy will have intravenous fluids until food can be tolerated. A well-balanced diet is then ordered. Fluid intake of at least 2000 mL/day is needed to maintain adequate hydration. The use of alcohol should be avoided. If the client is **cachectic** (malnourished or wasting) because of the cancer's pathology, parenteral nutrition may be indicated.

▶ *Activity*

Ambulation is to be encouraged during the client's recovery. Frequent rest periods are also necessary even after discharge.

▶ *Nursing Process*

Assessment

Subjective Data The client will mention having a dull pain in the flank area and noticing blood in the urine intermittently. However, the client often comments that there is no difficulty in urinating. Fatigue and weight loss are also described.

Objective Data Compare weight with usual weight. Assess vital signs and monitor diagnostic test results. Assess lung sounds for possible respiratory distress resulting from metastases. Hematuria may be seen.

▼ ▼

Possible nursing diagnoses for a client with renal tumors may include:

Nursing Diagnoses	*Goals*	*Nursing Interventions*
▶ *Fatigue, related to disease process and treatment.*	The client will understand reason for fatigue and not feel guilty for taking rest periods.	Discuss with client that fatigue is a result of blood loss in the urine and growth of the tumor.
		Since there is increased fatigue following any surgery, plan nursing care so the client will have several periods of uninterrupted rest each day.
▶ *Grieving, anticipatory, related to diagnosis, treatment, and prognosis.*	The client will maintain open communications with family and health care members.	Actively listen to what the client says.
		Encourage the client to express feelings about the diagnosis and treatment.
		Observe for signs of grieving such as crying, denial, anger, or withdrawal.
		Answer questions honestly.
		Assist client in identifying strengths and coping skills.
		Make referrals to other professionals as ordered.

Nursing Diagnoses	Goals	Nursing Interventions
▶ Knowledge deficit, related to limited information of disease process and treatment regimen.	The client will verbalize understanding of information taught.	Inform the client of the assessments to be done: neurological status, lung sounds, the incision, Homans' sign, peripheral pulses, vital signs, and serum electrolyte blood values. Adapt teaching to client's level of knowledge and learning style. Teach the importance of accurate intake and output records. Instruct the client in the proper application of antiembolism stockings, incentive spirometry exercises, and leg exercises. When bowel sounds return, provide clear liquids, progressing to a regular diet as ordered. Encourage the client to eat a well-balanced diet to enhance healing. Have a dietitian consult with the client to manage the proper caloric intake with foods the client enjoys and can tolerate. Instruct the client not to wash off the skin markings if radiation therapy is being used. Teach the name, purpose, dosage, schedule, and side effects of all medications; the importance of drinking plenty of fluids and ambulating as tolerated. Inform the client and family of community resources and support groups. Point out the importance of following the instructions for care when discharged and keeping physician appointments.

▶ *Evaluation*

Each goal must be evaluated to determine how it has been met by the client.

▲ ▲

POLYCYSTIC KIDNEY

Polycystic kidney disease may be inherited or acquired. Multiple grapelike clusters of fluid-filled cysts develop in and greatly enlarge both kidneys. They compress and eventually replace functioning kidney tissue. It has an insidious onset that becomes obvious between 30 and 50 years of age.

Early symptoms include hypertension, polyuria, and urinary tract infections. Flank pain and headache are common. Recurrent hematuria and proteinuria develop. Diagnosis is make by x-ray or sonogram showing the cysts. BUN and creatinine are used to monitor kidney function.

The goal of medical management is to preserve kidney function, prevent infections, and relieve pain. Hypertension is carefully managed with antihyperten-sive medications, diuretics, and fluid and dietary modifications. Eventually, dialysis or renal transplantation may be needed.

▶ RENAL FAILURE

▶ ACUTE RENAL FAILURE (ARF)

The rapid deterioration of renal function with rising blood levels of urea and other nitrogenous wastes (**azotemia**) is termed acute renal failure (ARF). The nephrons also are unable to regulate the fluid and electrolyte or the acid-base balance of the blood. Approximately 5 percent of all hospitalized clients develop acute renal failure with a mortality rate of about

50 percent (Toto, 1992). Predisposing factors include acute glomerular disease; severe, acute kidney infection; decreased cardiac output; trauma or hemorrhage.

There are three major forms depending on the location of the cause: postrenal ARF (disrupted urine flow), prerenal ARF (disrupted blood flow to the kidney), and intrarenal ARF (renal tissue damage). They will be discussed in this order. Both postrenal ARF and prerenal ARF are reversible situations if they are identified early and treatment begun. Undiagnosed postrenal ARF and prerenal ARF lead to intrarenal ARF.

▶ Postrenal ARF

Postrenal ARF is caused by an obstruction and makes up less than 10 percent of all ARF. It should be checked out first when a client has an unexplained decrease in urine output or has anuria. Kidney function can be easily restored by removing the obstruction. Urine volume will vary depending on the location and degree of obstruction. Catheterization, ultrasound, and retrograde pylogram are used to diagnose an obstruction. An obstruction may be caused by renal calculi, blood clots, edema, tumors, urethral strictures, benign prostatic hypertrophy (BPH), or pregnancy. Postrenal failure can be ruled out if there is no obstruction. If an obstruction is confirmed, relief of the obstruction is imperative to minimize renal damage and resolve azotemia. When postrenal failure is prolonged, both blood creatinine and BUN will rise.

▶ Prerenal ARF

Any abnormal decline in kidney perfusion that reduces glomerular perfusion can cause prerenal failure. Fluid volume status does not indicate perfusion. Effective arterial blood volume (EABV) is the amount of fluid in the vascular space that effectively perfuses the kidneys. Even in fluid volume excess situations, such as low cardiac output due to heart failure, the EABV falls causing prerenal failure. The kidney interprets a fall in EABV as fluid volume deficit.

The glomeruli are then unable to filter waste from the blood. The renal tubules are structurally intact, and the kidneys can resume normal functioning if perfusion is restored fairly quickly. Ischemia results from prolonged inadequate perfusion which can cause acute tubular necrosis (ATN).

The client generally has pale, cool skin; orthostatic hypotension; and oliguria. The BUN to creatinine ratio rises from 10:1 to more than 20:1. This rise is because there is greater reabsorption of urea when fluids flow slowly through the tubules. A urinalysis shows a low-sodium level (less than 20 mEq/L), high osmolality (more than 500 mOsm/L), and high specific gravity (more than 1.020). This results because the kidneys are retaining sodium and water in an attempt to correct the perceived fluid volume deficit.

When the client truly has a fluid volume deficit, treatment consists of intravenous fluids and albumin, plasma, or blood to restore the EABV. When the cause is inadequate cardiac output, inotropic agents such as dobutamine hydrochloride (Dobutrex) or amrinone lactate (Inocor) are ordered.

▶ Intrarenal ARF

Tissue damage of the glomeruli and/or tubules causes a loss of renal function known as intrarenal ARF. Glomerulonephritis and ATN are the main reasons for renal tissue damage. The antigen/antibody complexes formed in glomerulonephritis become trapped in the basement membrane where they cause inflammation. The glomeruli then become more permeable so red blood cells and protein are allowed to enter the filtrate and ultimately the urine.

According to Toto (1992), seventy-five percent of all intrarenal failure is caused by ATN, and is the most common cause of nosocomial acute renal failure. ATN is the result of ischemia or toxic insult to the renal tubules. Ischemia may result from untreated prerenal failure or severe hypoxemia. Radiographic contrast dye, pigments (myoglobin and hemoglobin), aminoglycoside and cephalosporin antibiotics, and NSAIDs are all **nephrotoxic** (causes kidney tissue damage) and can cause acute tubular necrosis.

The BUN to creatinine ratio in acute tubular necrosis is usually normal between 10:1 and 15:1; however both the BUN and creatinine are greatly elevated. For example, the BUN may be 70 mg/dL and the creatinine 7 mg/dL. Urine sodium is more than 40 mEq/L, urine osmolality less than 300 mOsm/L, and specific gravity less than 1.010.

There are three phases to the clinical course of ATN: oliguric/nonoliguric, diuretic, and recovery. The first phase is either oliguric or nonoliguric depending on the causative factor.

▶ Oliguric/Nonoliguric Phase

A nonoliguric phase is usually seen when nephrotoxic agents are the causative factor. When adequate urine output is maintained, dialysis is needed less often and the morbidity and mortality rates are lower.

An oliguric phase, which may last one to two weeks, is seen more often when ischemia is the causative factor. Oliguria, less than 400 mL/24 hours, can cause fluid volume overload; electrolyte imbalance, specifically high potassium and phosphorus, and low sodium and calcium; metabolic acidosis; and uremia.

▶ Diuretic Phase

The diuretic phase is seldom seen because early dialysis keeps extracellular fluid volume at a fairly normal level. If it were seen, there would be a tremendous increase in urine output.

▶ Recovery Phase

As renal function begins to improve, the client's urine output returns to normal and serum and urine laboratory test values move closer to normal. There is usually a short period of rapid improvement and then a period (may be several months) of slower improvement. Some clients will have residual renal insufficiency and a few will require long-term dialysis.

▶ Medical/Surgical Management

▶ Medical

Acute renal failure is often reversible and complications can be prevented with early diagnosis and treatment. The goal is to have kidney function stabilized and returned to normal. Problems to be alert for are: fluid volume overload, electrolyte imbalances, metabolic acidosis, high rate of catabolism, uremia, hemotological abnormalities, and infection.

▶ Surgical

The obstructions causing postrenal failure are often removed surgically. The exact procedure will depend on what type of obstruction is present and the location of the obstruction.

▶ Pharmacological

Drugs used in the treatment of acute renal failure include: antihypertensives, diuretics, cardiotonics (inotropics), phosphate-binding antacids, potassium-lowering agents, and electrolyte replacement. It is important to ensure that drugs used are not nephrotoxic. See Table 35-1 for drugs used in acute renal failure.

▶ Diet

Restrictions generally include sodium, potassium, phosphorus, protein, and fluids. Carbohydrates and fats are increased to be sure energy needs are met and protein will be spared as a source of energy. Clients with a high rate of catabolism often require total parenteral nutrition (TPN) to provide adequate nutrition.

▶ Activity

Since the client is often weak and may also be confused, activity is restricted during the initial phase of acute renal failure. As recovery becomes evident, ambulation is begun.

▶ Dialysis

Dialysis is now an early treatment in ATN. Homeostasis is maintained while the cause of ATN is determined and treated. Permanent kidney damage may be averted. See section on dialysis later in this chapter.

▶ Nursing Process

Assessment

Subjective Data The client may have various complaints including diarrhea, nausea, possibly with vomiting; swelling, loss of appetite, headache, increas-

Table 35-1

DRUGS USED IN ACUTE RENAL FAILURE	
Drugs	**Nursing Responsibilities**
Antihypertensives methyldopa (Aldomet) minoxidil (Loniten) clonidine HCl (Catapres) hydralazine HCl (Apresoline)	Monitor BP and pulse, weigh daily, monitor for postural hypotension and K,Na,Cl, and CO_2 levels, I & O.
Diuretics furosemide (Lasix) hydrochlorothiazide (HydroDiuril)	Monitor output, maintain fluid restrictions, weigh daily.
Cardiotonics/inotropics digoxin (Lanoxin) amrinone lactate (Inocor)	Assess apical pulse before giving, report blood level of digoxin, monitor BP & P, monitor blood level of potassium.
Phosphate-binding antacids aluminum hydroxide gel (Amphojel)	Administer with meals, assess for constipation.
Potassium exchange sodium polystyrene sulfonate (Kayexalate)	Monitor serum potassium, assess BP, P, and for constipation.
Electrolyte replacement calcitriol (Rocaltrol) calcifediol (Calderol)	Monitor blood calcium and phosphate levels, report metallic taste.

ing fatigue, and/or a change in mental alertness. Anxiety and fear related to "not knowing" what is happening is often expressed.

Objective Data Physical findings will depend on how far the disease process has progressed. Assess for hypertension, GI bleeding and/or bruising, reduction in urine output, anasarca, poor skin turgor, and dry mucous membranes as vomiting or diarrhea can cause dehydration. In a severe stage, the client may be drowsy, have muscle twitching, and convulsions.

The BUN and serum creatinine will be elevated as are the serum electrolytes potassium and phosphorus. The serum electrolyte calcium will be low. Blood level of red blood cells will decrease as the production of erythropoietin decreases. Leukocyte level will increase in the presence of an infection.

▼ ▼

Possible nursing diagnoses for a client with acute renal failure may include:

Nursing Diagnoses	Goals	Nursing Interventions
▶ *Fluid volume excess related to sodium and water retention.*	The client will maintain a stable fluid volume.	Monitor BUN, creatinine, and serum electrolyte levels.
		Accurately measure urine output, often on an hourly basis. Parameters are often set, for notification of the physician.
		Weigh daily to identify weight gain related to fluid retention. One pound of weight gain is equivalent to 500 mL of retained fluid.
		Assess skin turgor, edema, BP, lung sounds, jugular vein distention, pulse and respiratory rate and quality.
		Provide fluids within the prescribed limits.
▶ *Anxiety related to the disease process.*	The client will verbalize anxieties with the family and health care workers.	Establish rapport with the client.
		Maintain open communications to foster expression of anxieties.
		Listen to the client's concerns.
▶ *Knowledge deficit related to the disease process and treatment regimen.*	The client will verbalize understanding of the disease process and treatment regimen.	Evaluate the client's readiness to learn.
		Provide information at the client's level of understanding.
		Give instructions, both verbally and in writing, related to the prescribed drugs' desired effects, side effects, dosage, and timing.
		Teach the importance of monitoring weight and evaluating fluid intake and urine output.
		Teach asepsis and signs and symptoms of infection.
▶ *Nutrition, altered, less than body requirements, related to anorexia, dietary restrictions, and increased catabolism.*	The client will have stabilized weight within normal limits.	Arrange for a dietary consultation to provide food in keeping with the prescribed restrictions and client preferences including cultural and religious factors.
		Suggest six small meals throughout the day.
		Provide or assist with oral hygiene prior to meals.

▶ Evaluation

Each goal must be evaluated to determine how it has been met by the client.

▲ ▲

Sample Nursing Care Plan: The Client With Acute Renal Failure

Mr. Long, age sixty-five, has had a history of heart trouble for several years. He is admitted because he has urinated very little for two days, he gets dizzy when he gets up from lying down, and he cannot get his shoes on because his feet are "fat." He states that he does not know what is happening to him. Results of laboratory tests are: BUN 90 mg/dL, creatinine 4 mg/dL, urine sodium 15 mEq/L, and urine specific gravity 1.030.

Nursing Diagnosis 1 Fluid volume, excess, related to sodium and water retention as evidenced by "fat feet," urine sodium 15 mEq/L, and urine specific gravity 1.030.

Goals	Nursing Interventions	Rationale	Evaluation
Mr. Long will have reduced fluid volume excess.	Accurately measure and record intake and output.	Provides information about retention of intake.	Mr. Long's feet are no longer "fat." His urine sodium is 18 mEq/L and urine specific gravity is 1.027.
	Weigh Mr. Long daily— same time, scale, clothes.		
	Assess skin turgor, edema, BP, lung sounds for crackles.	Provides information related to presence of fluid in tissue, lungs, or vascular system.	
	Administer inotropics or cardiotonic medications as ordered.	Medications will strengthen heartbeat which will give better perfusion to kidneys.	

Nursing Diagnosis 2 Anxiety related to disease process as evidenced by his statement that he does not know what is happening to him.

Goals	Nursing Interventions	Rationale	Evaluation
Mr. Long will have less anxiety by understanding what is happening to him.	Establish rapport with Mr. Long.	Begins a nurse-client relationship.	Mr. Long says that he feels better knowing what is happening.
	Encourage him to express his fears and anxieties.	Some people need encouragement to express feelings.	
	Provide Mr. Long with information, at his level of understanding, about what is happening to his body, why I & O and weigh daily are important, and what the medications are supposed to do.	Understanding reduces anxieties.	

(continued)

Nursing Diagnosis 3 Urinary elimination, altered, as evidenced by his urinating very little for two days and BUN - Creatinine ratio of 22.5: 1.

Goals	Nursing Interventions	Rationale	Evaluation
Mr. Long will increase amount of urination to 1200 mL/day.	Administer diuretics as ordered.	Diuretics increase water elimination by enhancing the excretion of sodium by the kidneys.	Mr. Long is urinating 1000 mL/day. His BUN is 50 mg/dL and creatinine is 3 mg/dL.
	Accurately measure and record intake and output.	Provides information about movement of fluid through the body.	

▶ CHRONIC RENAL FAILURE (END STAGE RENAL DISEASE [ESRD])

Chronic renal failure is a slow, progressive condition where the kidney's ability to function, ultimately deteriorates. This condition is not reversible. The kidneys have an amazing capability to perform effectively, even though most of the nephrons are destroyed.

Renal erythropoietin decreases causing anemia. Hypertension, acidosis, and glucose intolerance usually are also present. Urea in the blood is extremely elevated. As ESRD progresses, uremia develops.

Kelley (1996) describes three stages of chronic renal failure: reduced renal reserve, renal insufficiency, and end-stage renal disease (ESRD). Symptoms of reduced renal reserve are not apparent until more than 40 percent of the nephrons fail. A prolonged urine concentration test or a decline in glomerular filtration rate (GFR) may be the only evidence of reduced renal reserve. When 75 percent of the nephrons stop functioning, renal insufficiency occurs. BUN and creatinine are above normal, and the client may have nocturia and polyuria. The onset of ESRD occurs when at least 90 percent of the nephrons fail. BUN and creatinine levels rise, polyuria changes to oliguria, and severe fluid and electrolyte imbalances are evident.

When the kidneys become unable to filter blood, an alternate method for filtration is necessary. Lifetime dialysis becomes inevitable unless kidney transplantation is performed and is successful. Life expectancy varies with the initial cause of chronic renal failure and the person's overall health at the time of diagnosis. Each year, according to the National Kidney Foundation, approximately 80,000 people die from kidney disease in this country. There are numerous causes of chronic renal failure. The three leading causes are dia-

betes mellitus, hypertension, and glomerulonephritis. Nephrotoxic drugs, including some over-the-counter drugs, aggravate the situation.

The diagnosis is confirmed when the BUN is at least 50 mg/dL and the serum creatinine level is greater than 5 mg/dL.

▶ Medical/Surgical Management

▶ Medical

Chronic renal failure is a multisystem disease process. See Table 35-2 for effects of chronic renal disease on various body systems. Medical management focuses on preserving the remaining kidney function for as long as possible, and preventing complications. This helps preserve the integrity of the person's life. Fluid retention increases the risk of complications such as edema (ascites), hypertension, and congestive heart failure. Electrolytes are monitored and regulated. Clients and their families face a future filled with frustrations and anxieties. With the help of competent and caring health care providers, the days ahead will become more tolerable.

▶ Pharmacological

Antihypertensives such as methyldopa (Aldomet) and propranolol hydrochloride (Inderal) are used to control hypertension. Diuretics, furosemide (Lasix), are used for treatment of fluid retention; anticonvulsants, phenytoin (Dilantin) to control seizures; antiemetics, prochlorperazine (Compazine); antipruritics, cyproheptadine hydrochloride (Periactin) may also be used. Calcium acetate (Phos-Lo) is used to lower the phosphate level in the blood; however, it can be con-

Table 35-2

CHRONIC RENAL FAILURE EFFECTS ON BODY SYSTEMS

System	Effect
Urinary	Oliguria from renal insufficiency. Azotemia from CRF.
Blood	Anemia from decreased RBC production. Platelet activity decreased, causing bleeding tendency.
Cardiovascular	Hypervolemia and tachycardia from CHF. Hypertension and dysrhythmias from hyperkalemia.
Respiratory	Dyspnea, pulmonary edema from CHF. Hyperventilation from metabolic acidosis. Eventually Kussmaul respirations.
Gastrointestinal	Urea in the blood is converted to ammonia by the mouth, causing uremic halitosis. Hiccoughs, anorexia, and nausea from edema within the gastrointestinal tract.
Skin	Dry skin with pruritis from uremic frost (excretion of urea through the skin with an odor of urine). Pallor with anemia.
Nervous	Lethargy, headaches, confusion, impaired concentration with disorientation, depression, decreased level of consciousness, sleep disturbances, and uremic encephalopathy resulting in seizures and coma.
Sensory	Peripheral neuropathy with numbness and tingling of extremities with complaints of a prickly, crawling feeling in the feet and legs, especially at night.
Reproductive	Decrease in libido. Decreased sperm count. Amenorrhea. Impotence. Delayed puberty.
Musculoskeletal	Joint pain and muscle cramping. Bone demineralization from hypocalcemia.
Immune	Greater chance of infections from immunosuppression. Decrease in antibody production.

stipating. A low renal erythropoietin level causing anemia is often treated with epoetin alpha (Epogen). An iron supplement is used to decrease the anemia-related symptoms. Multivitamins with folic acid are used because dialysis promotes the loss of water-soluble vitamins.

► Diet

Diet restrictions are similar to those in acute renal failure. Sodium, potassium, phosphorus, and protein are restricted. Fluids are also limited. Modifications are made as kidney function deteriorates. With consistent compliance, symptoms decrease resulting in fewer complications. Resources are available for clients to obtain assistance with dietary restrictions. Meal ideas are published in newsletters, like NephroNotes. Long-term dietary compliance is a challenge, as any age group can be affected by chronic renal failure. All the daily activities as well as special events during the year are a continual reminder of the client's dietary restrictions. As with other chronic diseases, those with renal failure need to have all members of their family and their friends encouraging them to adapt to their restrictions. Dietitians can assist the family to incorporate religious and cultural dietary needs. The person with chronic renal failure may also have to incorporate dietary needs for additional diagnoses such as diabetes mellitus and/or coronary artery disease.

With the progression of chronic renal disease, dialysis becomes necessary. Fluid restrictions need to be adhered to and the amount allowed divided throughout the day. The greatest amount of fluid should be allowed during the day, incorporating enough fluids with oral medications. Some fluids should be planned for the evening meal with a small amount to be allowed during the night. For example: days-500 cc, evenings-200 cc, and nights-100 cc. Protein restriction is closely monitored and regulated with the blood albumin level. The development of hyperkalemia will lead to a diet restricted in potassium. Foods high in potassium include dried fruits or dried beans and peas, peanuts, bananas, sweet potatoes, spinach, products with tomatoes, oranges, chocolate, artichokes, avocados, pumpkins, and mushrooms.

► Activity

The client is encouraged to participate in activities of daily living for as long as possible. Safety becomes a significant factor during periods when the client has weakness, fatigue, or mental confusion. Confusion is seen in clients who have uremic encephalopathy. When bed rest is required, turning, ROM, and skin care are important. As symptoms continue to become more severe, the client will need total assistance for all the ADLs.

► *Nursing Process*

Assessment

Subjective Data Inquire about the client's past medical history including the treatments they are currently undergoing for maintenance of their renal disease. Take a complete medication history, including the use of over-the-counter drugs. Description of fatigue, joint pain, severe headaches, nausea, anorexia, some chest pain, intractable singultus (hiccups), decreased libido, menstrual irregularities, and impaired concentration will be given by the client. The client may feel uncomfortable talking directly to the nurse if uremic halitosis is a problem.

Objective Data Assess for changes in the client's neurological status such as reduced alertness and awareness. Kussmaul respirations appear as coma develops. Halitosis with a urine odor and "uremic frost," a white powder on the skin, result from the accumulation of urates.

▼ ▼

Possible nursing diagnoses for a client with ESRD may include:

Nursing Diagnoses	*Goals*	*Nursing Interventions*
► *Fluid volume excess related to compromised renal mechanism.*	The client will understand the importance of prescribed (restricted) fluid amounts.	Monitor daily weight, intake and output (maybe hourly), skin turgor, edema, blood pressure, respirations, lung sounds, and results of serum electrolyte studies.
		Provide prescribed amounts of fluids.
		Teach client to plan nutritional and fluid intake within the prescribed amounts.
		Monitor laboratory reports for serum albumin level.
► *Nutrition, altered, less than body requirements related to dietary restrictions, GI distress, anorexia.*	The client will stabilize weight within normal limits and participate in dietary plan.	Provide or assist with complete mouth care before meals because uremic halitosis leaves a metallic taste in the client's mouth.
		Provide a clean, quiet, odor-free environment for meals.
		Suggest six small meals throughout the day.
		Arrange a consultation with the dietitian to plan alternate ways to prepare foods allowed on the diet.
		Ask the family to bring favorite foods, within the dietary restrictions, from home.
		Encourage self-feeding.
		Administer antiemetics thirty minutes before meals to control nausea.
		Suggest using herbs for flavoring instead of salt or salt substitutes which often contain potassium.
► *Skin integrity, impaired, high risk for, related to pruritis from "uremic frost."*	The client will maintain skin integrity.	Encourage the use of emollients and lotions on the skin.
		Administer antihistamines, as ordered, for the temporary relief of itching.
		Assist the client to change position every two hours.
		Provide an eggcrate mattress or Clinitron bed.

Nursing Diagnoses	Goals	Nursing Interventions
▶ Injury, high risk for, related to neurologic changes.	The client will have no injuries occur.	Document the client's level of consciousness and mental status.
		Provide assistance for client ambulation.
		Protect the client having seizures by padding the bed siderails.
		Administer anticonvulsive and sedative medications as ordered.
		Give instructions slowly and repeat as needed.
▶ Coping, ineffective individual, related to long-term compliance of the treatment regimen.	The client will verbalize feelings and intention to comply with treatment.	Encourage the client to discuss feelings about long-term lifestyle changes.
		Refer client to the local office of the National Kidney Foundation for information about client services and treatments for diseases of the kidney.
		Include the client and family in rehabilitation and discharge planning to ensure compliance. Topics for these sessions include diet, rest, medications, fluid restrictions, intake and output, activities, dialysis required lab tests, and frequent visits to the physician.
		Incorporate into the discharge planning and teaching the client's socioeconomic needs, cultural background, role in the family unit, accessibility to medical care, and anticipated follow-up care.
		Complete referrals prior to discharge in order to lessen client anxiety.
		Consider future needs of a newly diagnosed client with end-stage renal disease and include the availability of dialysis, vocational rehabilitation, home health care, financial assistance with medical needs, and psychological therapy for the client and family.
▶ Fatigue related to anemia.	The client will verbalize feeling less fatigued.	Encourage frequent rest periods throughout the day.
		Keep client's skin clean and dry to promote comfort and rest.
		Administer erythropoeitin medication, iron preparation, and vitamins as ordered.
		Teach about the medications to ensure compliance in taking them.
		Explain to the client and the family to check with the physician before taking any over-the-counter drugs, i.e., products containing aspirin should not be used because they increase the tendency to bleed.

▶ Evaluation

Each goal must be evaluated to determine how it has been met by the client.

▲ ▲

DIALYSIS

As the kidneys continue to deteriorate, nitrogenous waste products accumulate in the circulatory system. These waste products then need to be removed artificially with dialysis. **Dialysis** is a mechanical means of removing nitrogenous waste from the blood by imitating the function of the nephrons. It involves filtration and diffusion of wastes, drugs, and excess electrolytes and/or osmosis of water across a semipermeable membrane into a dialysate solution. The **dialysate**, a solution designed to approximate the normal electrolyte structure of plasma and extracellular fluid, is prescribed specific to the individual client's needs.

There are two types of dialysis, hemodialysis and peritoneal dialysis. These treatments can be obtained throughout the country at dialysis centers or at hospital dialysis units. These centers can also be used by clients when they travel in the United States or abroad.

When the client is referred to a dialysis center, the first impressions are lasting; especially since anxieties will be high. Hemodialysis takes several hours to complete and needs to be done three times a week. Long-term maintenance with either hemodialysis or peritoneal dialysis is aimed toward the prevention of complications associated with ESRD.

Clients who are receiving dialysis need a significant amount of teaching. All clients should have the process thoroughly explained. Other teaching topics are the importance of doctor and laboratory visits, and observations for which the doctor needs to be notified. Clients undergoing dialysis, should wear medic alert tags stating their condition. As a nurse, there is a possibility that you may be employed in a dialysis center or work with dialysis treatment in an acute care or home care setting.

Hemodialysis

Hemodialysis is performed by a machine with an artificial semipermeable membrane used for the filtration of the blood. This machine is often referred to as an artificial kidney. A graft or fistula is surgically prepared to access the clients circulatory system. Figure 35-5 illustrates several ways this can be done. Research and development is improving the quality of graft materials. With each hemodialysis treatment, a catheter is inserted into the graft or fistula. The client's blood is circulated through the semipermeable membrane. Excess fluids are removed by osmosis and by-products of protein metabolism, especially urea and uric acid, as well as creatinine, drugs, and excess electrolytes are removed from the blood by diffusion or filtration. In return, the client receives fluids, electrolytes, and blood products, as necessary. The solution (dialysate) is especially prescribed to meet the client's metabolic needs. Figure 35-6 illustrates a client receiving hemodialysis.

For the entire process, standard precautions must be followed and strict asepsis maintained. The client should be weighed before and after each dialysis session to determine if fluid is being retained. It is important to keep the client comfortable and provide diversional activities during the treatment. Hemodialysis is usually performed three times a week and takes 3 to 6 hours each time.

The graft or fistula site requires strict aseptic care and must be assessed daily for signs of infection: redness, swelling, or drainage. Circulation through the site is assessed by palpation or feeling the area and/or listening with a (Doppler) stethoscope. A thrill should be felt and/or a bruit should be heard. Lack of these may indicate a blood clot, which requires immediate surgical attention. Patency must be documented. Pulses, peripheral to the graft site, must also be assessed.

Blood pressure and blood draws should never be done on the extremity where the graft or fistula is placed. Also, restraints or intravenous solutions should never be applied to or inserted into that extremity. All health care personnel should be made aware of the location of the hemodialysis access site.

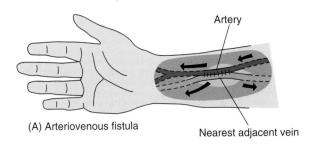

(A) Arteriovenous fistula

Edges of incision in artery and vein are sutured together to form a common opening.

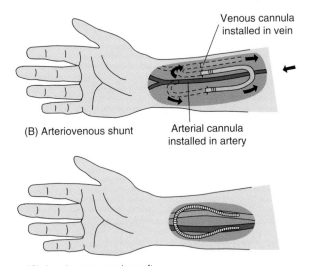

(B) Arteriovenous shunt

(C) Arteriovenous vein graft

Ends of natural or synthetic graft sutured into an artery and a vein.

FIGURE 35-5 Hemodialysis access sites.

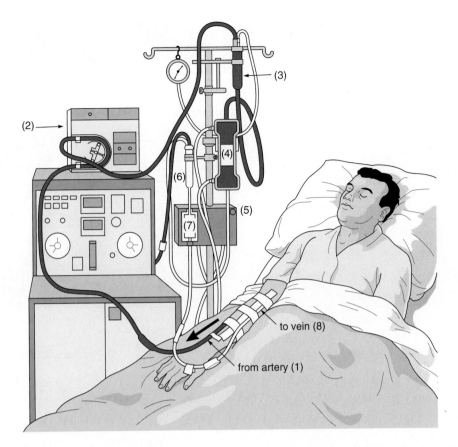

FIGURE 35-6 Hemodialysis. **(1)** Blood leaves the body via an artery. **(2)** Arterial blood passes through the blood pump. **(3)** Blood is filtered to remove any clots. **(4)** Blood passes through the dialyzer. **(5)** Blood passes into the venous blood line. **(6)** Blood is filtered to remove any clots. **(7)** Blood flows through the air detector. **(8)** Blood returns to the client through the venous blood line.

Since most medications are removed during dialysis, they are generally not administered until after the dialysis session. Vancomycin hydrochloride (Vancocin) is not removed during dialysis and so is often used. If the client is hypertensive before dialysis, nifedipine (Procardia) is given because of its fast action.

Possible complications include hemorrhage, infection, and emboli formation. Some factors for the client and family to consider about hemodialysis are the distance they must travel to the dialysis center, the expense, the time involved, and the presence of a permanent arteriovenous (AV) line. Clients can be taught to do their own hemodialysis at a center. Portable units are being developed to make hemodialysis more usable in the client's home. This is a growing trend with home health care.

Peritoneal Dialysis

Peritoneal dialysis uses the peritoneal lining of the abdominal cavity as the membrane through which diffusion and osmosis occur instead of the artificial kidney machine. It is usually performed four times a day seven days a week. A Tenckhoff or a flanged-collar catheter is placed by the physician, under aseptic conditions, into the client's peritoneal space (see Figure 35-7). The client must void just before catheter insertion to prevent accidental puncture of the bladder. As with hemodialysis, the client should be weighed before and after each dialysis session. Bowel sounds should also be checked.

The dialysate, held within a sterile soft container similar to an IV bag, is instilled aseptically through the catheter into the abdominal cavity. To decrease client discomfort, the dialysate should be at body temperature and not instilled too rapidly. Severe pain should not be experienced. The container, still connected to the catheter, is then rolled up and the dialysate remains in the abdominal cavity for a specified length of time. The client is free to ambulate during this time. The container is then unrolled and lowered below the abdominal cavity to allow the dialysate to drain, by gravity, back into the container. The dialysate now contains excess fluids, nitrogenous waste, and other impurities. The outflow of dialysate is inspected for color, sediments and amount. The fluid should be light yellow and clear enough to read the printing on the bag when placed on a white towel. Usually 2 liters of dialysate are exchanged each time. If the outflow does not at least equal the inflow, the client is asked to turn from side to side to increase the outflow.

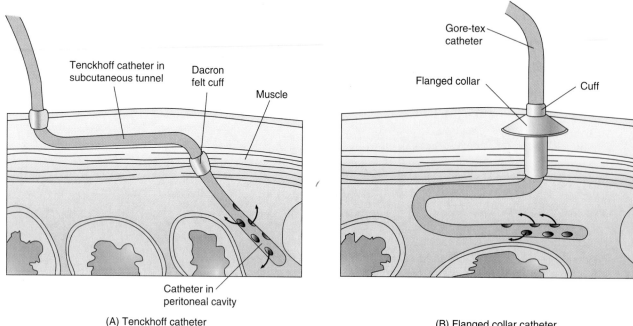

(A) Tenckhoff catheter

(B) Flanged collar catheter

FIGURE 35-7 Peritoneal dialysis catheters.

Peritoneal dialysis may be performed manually by the nurse, client, or family member as just described; by a cycler machine; or by continuous ambulatory peritoneal dialysis (CAPD). The cycler machine automatically completes dialysis after sterile setup and connection. CAPD is performed by the client. After the dialysate is aseptically installed, the empty bag is rolled up under the clothing and the client can go about normal activities. Every six to eight hours, the solution is drained into the bag which is then discarded following standard precaution guidelines. A new bag of dialysate is attached and instilled. This provides continuous dialysis 24 hours/day, 7 days/week. The client's lifestyle is only minimally disrupted. Peritoneal dialysis is less expensive, easier to perform, less stressful for the client, and almost as effective as hemodialysis.

The main complication of peritoneal dialysis is infection. Strict aseptic care of the catheter site is necessary. Standard precautions is essential in caring for the dialysis client. Figure 35-8 shows a peritoneal dialysis set up.

KIDNEY TRANSPLANTATION

According to the National Kidney Foundation, in 1994 there were 11,037 kidney transplants performed. Transplants are either from a live donor (usually a relative), or a cadaver. In 1994, there were 2,663 kidney

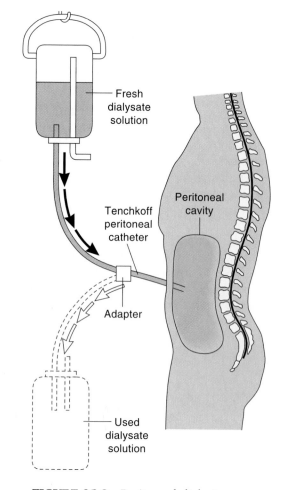

FIGURE 35-8 Peritoneal dialysis.

donations from living persons and 8,374 from cadavers. As of February 1995, there were 27,794 persons on the waiting list for a kidney transplant.

The first kidney transplant was done between identical twins, in 1954, in Boston, Massachusetts. Persons diagnosed with end-stage renal disease and diabetes mellitus have been recipients of pancreas/kidney transplants. As of February 1995, there were 1,116 persons in the United States awaiting this procedure, according to the National Kidney Foundation records.

Prior to being placed on the nationwide donor waiting list, the client with ESRD must be tissue- and blood-typed to determine a compatible donor. Insurance varies with the coverage of this procedure. Lack of funds does not exclude anyone from needed care. Since 1973, an amendment to the Social Security Act allows Medicare to pay 80 percent of the cost for treating ESRD clients, including dialysis and kidney transplantation.

At the time a donor kidney becomes available, the client must be transported to the transplant medical center. The donor kidney can be preserved for thirty-six hours in solution or up to seventy-two hours if it is attached to an irrigating pump with perfusion maintained while en route to the recipient. Through a lower abdominal incision, the surgeon attaches the donor kidney to the client's blood supply. The donor kidney is usually placed in the iliac fossa anterior to the iliac crest. The donor ureter is **anastomosed** (surgical connection of tubular structure) to the client's ureter or surgically implanted into the client's urinary bladder. Generally, the client's nonfunctioning kidney is left in place, to reduce the postoperative risk of hemorrhage. Figure 35-9 illustrates the placement of a transplanted kidney.

After a couple days of bed rest, the client will be allowed increasing activities and if no complications occur, will be discharged in one to three weeks. Routine nursing care includes monitoring urine output, blood tests, vital signs, and level of consciousness. Turning, coughing, and deep breathing are encouraged. The incision is assessed to ensure the wound closures are intact. In addition to these measures, the nurse must assess for rejection.

Organ Rejection

Signs of rejection include generalized edema, tenderness over the graft site, fever, decreased urine output, hematuria, edema (extremities or eyes), weight gain, oliguria or anuria, and/or an increase in feeling tired. The BUN and creatinine will be elevated.

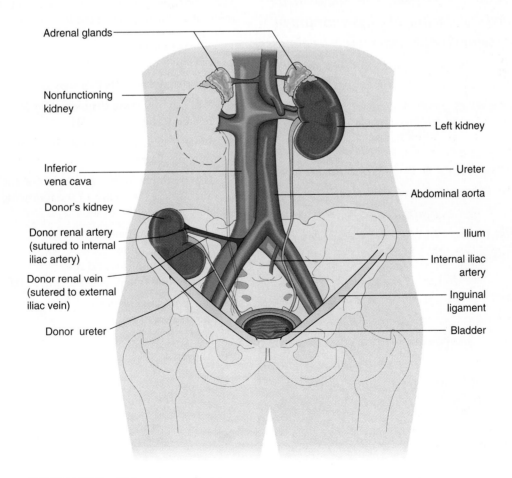

FIGURE 35-9 Kidney transplant.

Immunosuppressive drug therapy is begun to decrease the chance of organ rejection. These drugs include: azathioprine (Imuran), cyclophosphamide (Cytoxan), cyclosporine (Sandimmune), and corticosteroids such as prednisone (Meticorten). The scheduling and dosage of these drugs vary with acceptance of the donor kidney and the side effects exhibited by the client. People continue to survive many years with a kidney transplant and maintain a quality life.

Complications

The greatest complication in renal transplantation is infection. The immunosuppressive therapy to prevent rejection of the kidney increases the risk and masks the usual signs of infection. The client and family must learn how to recognize these signs of infection. There will only be a slight increase in temperature, development of a cough, low back pain, cloudy urine, or wound drainage. The client must always monitor urine output.

With the newly transplanted kidney, the recipient hopes to return to a more normal life. The quality of life improves greatly with more energy and fewer dietary restrictions. Always in the back of the recipient's mind is the fear of organ rejection. The transplanted kidney is foreign tissue and can be rejected by the recipient's body. About thirty percent of cadaver organs are rejected, with significantly fewer live donor organs rejected.

▶ CASE STUDY

Ruth Andrews, fifty-six, is a client in the extended care facility. She has amyotrophic lateral sclerosis (ALS) with muscle weakness that has progressed and involves her legs and arms. A hydraulic lift is used to transfer her out of bed. A student nurse and a classmate enter with the lift to assist Ms. Andrews OOB, when she asks to use the bedpan. As they help her on the bedpan, they recall that the staff nurse gave Ms. Andrews the bedpan about a half hour ago. Returning in a few minutes, they help Ms. Andrews off the bedpan and notice the urine is cloudy with a foul odor. Ms. Andrews is not on I & O; however, they noticed that there is a very small amount of urine. She tells them that she does not know why she is going to the bathroom so often and why her urine smells bad.

The following questions will guide your development of a Nursing Care Plan for the case study.

1. What subjective data should be gathered? What objective data should be gathered?

2. List diagnostic tests that may be ordered.

3. Write two nursing diagnoses for Ms. Andrews, related to her cystitis/UTI.

4. Write a goal related to each of Ms. Andrews' nursing diagnoses.

5. List pertinent nursing actions for the care of Ms. Andrews for each of the following areas as they relate to the cystitis/UTI:

   elimination-bladder
   diet and fluids
   safety, comfort, and rest
   teaching (client and nursing staff)

6. List two classifications of medications used for the treatment of an UTI.

7. List two successful client outcomes for Ms. Andrews.

SUMMARY

- The functions of the urinary system are reflected in their relationship with nearly all the systems in the body.
- Accurate intake and output is imperative for every client with a urinary system disorder.
- Teach proper perineal care, especially to females of all ages, about cleansing from front to back.
- Diet management is important for clients with renal calculi, glomerulonephritis, and renal failure.
- Encourage an adequate intake of fluids for clients unless fluids are restricted.
- Monitor laboratory test results for BUN, creatinine, and electrolytes.
- Level of consciousness, vital signs, lung sounds, and urine characteristics are important to monitor.
- Strict aseptic care is mandatory for dialysis clients.

Review Questions

1. A client states she has had pain when urinating for three days. This would be documented as:
   a. polyuria.
   b. dysuria.
   c. hematuria.
   d. oliguria.

2. A client has been admitted for chronic pyelonephritis. She is jittery and states she is concerned. Which of the following signs would indicate potential kidney damage?
   a. urine output is 100 mL on your shift
   b. blood pressure is decreased with a rapid pulse
   c. blood pressure is elevated with a decreased pulse
   d. BUN and creatinine clearance are within normal limits

3. Georgia Smithson has glomerulonephritis. This condition affects her:
   a. kidney.
   b. ureter.
   c. bladder.
   d. urethra.

4. Mr. Ronald Osborne, seventy-six, has had hematuria for several years and has been diagnosed with cancer of the kidney. His prognosis is poor. He told the nurse that he was too dizzy to go to the bathroom alone. Which of the following shows Mr. Osborne needs further teaching?
   a. putting his bathroom call light on for assistance
   b. holding on to the nurse's arm while walking
   c. refusal to wait for the nurse to lower the siderail
   d. saving his urine to be measured and tested

5. Jake Jones, sixty-four, has had hematuria for several years. He is admitted to your same-day surgical unit scheduled for cystoscopic fulguration. Postoperatively, which of the following would you anticipate?
   a. blood in the urine
   b. an elevated temperature
   c. hypotension
   d. smoky urine

6. Lawrence Denny, twenty-nine, had impetigo two weeks prior to his noting a decrease in urine output and urine that "did not look right." His admission diagnosis is acute glomerulonephritis. He is on intake and output with fluid restriction. Which of the following comments indicates knowledge of his nursing care?
   a. "I had my wife empty my urinal."
   b. "My urine still looks pretty bad."
   c. "I put my call light on so you can empty my urinal."
   d. "My wife helped me out of bed, so I urinated in the bathroom."

7. Gael Dominich is a client with chronic glomerulonephritis. She is discharged home with home health care. As the LP/VN assigned to her case, you are planning Gael's A.M. care. While preparing the bath supplies, she says, "Please do not use any soap. My skin is so dry and flaky." The rationale for this would be:
   a. kidney failure leads to uremia.
   b. the bladder does not concentrate urine.
   c. her blood sugar is elevated.
   d. confusion leads to comments of this nature.

8. Oliguria is best defined as:
   a. scant urine output.
   b. no urine output.
   c. blood in the urine.
   d. excessive urine output.

9. Mr. Tom Surrey, in his fifties, is attending classes to be able to do his own peritoneal dialysis. He states he feels well and is eager to continue to learn. Mr. Surrey asks if washing his hands before the procedure is important. The best response is:

a. "Yes, only if you have not done so today."
b. "Yes, as you want to keep the procedure as clean as possible."
c. "No, since you just went to the bathroom."
d. "No, because all the equipment is sterile."

Critical Thinking Questions

1. What are the pros and cons for peritoneal dialysis, hemodialysis, and kidney transplantation?

2. What can an individual do to prevent urinary disorders?

3. What are the differences between acute and chronic renal failure?

News Flash

Physicians are now able to carefully remove islet cells from a pancreas, grow them in the laboratory, and inject them into the portal system of a recipient. The islet cells become lodged in the liver and begin to secrete insulin.

This is done primarily on clients with diabetes who need a kidney transplant. A kidney transplant will give the client a better life for a period of time, until the diabetes destroys the function of the transplanted kidney. With the injected islet cells eliminating the problem of diabetes, the transplanted kidney will serve the client better for a longer period of time. (*Interview with Geri Carr, Director, National Kidney Foundation of the Texas Coastal Bend. February 20, 1996.*)

Medical Terminology

cyst/o-	bladder
cystitis	inflammation of the bladder
cystectomy	removal of all or part of the bladder
cystoscopy	looking into the bladder
glomerul/o-	glomerulus(i)
glomerulo-nephritis	inflammation of the kidney involving the glomeruli
lith/o-	stone or calculus(i)
urolithiasis	stones in the urinary system
pyel/o-	renal pelvis
pyelonephritis	inflammation of the renal pelvis
ren/o- and nephr/o-	kidney
nephrologist	physician who treats diseases of the kidney
nephrotoxic	toxic or poisonous to the kidney
ureter/o-	ureter
ureterostomy	opening into the ureter
urethr/o-	urethra
urethritis	inflammation of the urethra
-uria	urination or relating to urine
anuria	no urine
dysuria	painful urination
oliguria	scanty urine
urin/o- and Ur/o-	urine
urology	the study of the urinary system
urologist	physician who treats diseases of the urinary system
vesic/o-	bladder
vesicostomy	incision of the bladder

CHAPTER
36
Ostomies

Diana S. Sullivan

LEARNING OBJECTIVES

Upon completion of this chapter the learner should be able to:
• Define key terms.
• Describe expected output from different types of ostomy and care associated with each.
• Recognize realistic goals in the management of ostomy.
• List observations that should be made in the immediate postoperative period.
• List early and late complications related to ostomy surgery.
• Describe different methods of managing an ostomy.
• List principles of colostomy irrigation and steps in the procedure.
• Recognize that altered body image may be a major problem for ostomy clients.

▶ **KEY TERMS**

colostomy
decompress
effluent
fistula
ileostomy
jejunostomy
mucous fistula
ostomy
pouching
stoma
volvulus

▶ *MAKING THE CONNECTION*

Refer to the topics in the following chapters to increase your understanding of ostomies.

- **Chapter 10, Nursing Assessment:** Skin Assessment, p. 178; Abdominal Assessment, p. 181
- **Chapter 14, Fluid, Electrolytes and Acid-Base Balances:** Hypocalcemia, p. 281

- **Chapter 34. Digestive Disorders:** Diverticulitis, p. 983; Ulcerative Colitis, p. 986; Crohn's Disease, p. 986; Peritonitis, p. 992
- **Chapter 35, Urinary Disorders:** Obstructive Disorders, p. 1031; Urolithiasis, p. 1031

INTRODUCTION

The word **ostomy** means to "cut into." This opening may be temporary or permanent. Ostomy is often used interchangeably with **stoma**, such as **colostomy, ileostomy** and gastrojejunostomy. Stoma is the Greek word for mouth and refers to the opening between a cavity and the surface of the body. The prefix used with the word "ostomy" refers to the portion of the gastrointestinal or urinary system brought to the skin surface. For example, "colostomy" refers to the colon opening through the abdominal wall. Figure 36-1 shows an example of a healthy stoma.

Ostomies are done to remove waste to the outside of the body. Ostomies may be created as a permanent or temporary measure. Permanence is determined by the underlying reason for the ostomy surgery. Temporary ostomies are generally done to allow time for the bowel to rest and/or repair itself. Permanent ostomies are generally done when a part of the colon or bladder is removed due to disease processes. Table 36-1 shows types of ostomies.

Ostomy surgery is doubly traumatic for the client. The client not only has a disease process or injury that necessitates the ostomy, but also has to deal with body image changes. These changes are difficult for the client to accept and handle and she needs support and honest acceptance from the nurse during this period of adjustment. Some clients often go through the stages of grief associated with the loss of a body function or

Table 36-1

TYPES OF OSTOMIES		
Ostomy	**Description**	**Output**
Bowel		
Ileostomy	Bringing a portion of the ileum through an opening in the abdomen	Stool is constant and watery
Ascending colostomy	Made from the ascending colon	Stool is semiliquid
Transverse colostomy	Made from the transverse colon	Stool is semiformed
Sigmoid colostomy	Made from the sigmoid colon	Similar to normal bowel movements
Urinary		
Ileo conduit	Stoma made from small piece of ileum, ureters connected to ileum piece.	Urine drips constantly.
Kock or Indiana pouch	Pouch made from piece of ileum or colon to collect urine. Stoma made.	Urine is collected and emptied by catheter several times a day.

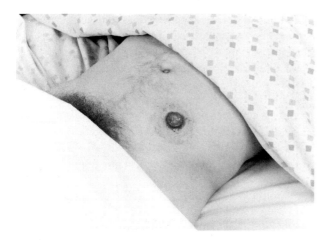

FIGURE 36-1 A healthy stoma.

body part. The nurse must understand this process and help the client work through it. It is also important for the nurse to communicate to the client a positive outlook for recovery. Many clients refuse to even look at the stoma. Clients will in most cases wear a pouch or collecting device on their abdomen to contain the waste material from the bowel or kidneys. This change in body image may raise issues of low self-esteem, and the nurse must be ready to discuss these issues with the client.

In addition to providing emotional support, the nurse must teach the client about care of the ostomy. The nurse should stress to the client that the ostomy will not restrict or prohibit any activity once healing has taken place. Immediately after surgery the client will be under some dietary and lifting restrictions, but these are usually temporary until healing has occurred. The client will need some time and education to cope with the creation of an ostomy.

Support people are available to assist both ostomy clients and nurses in medical centers and around the country. Enterostomal therapists (ET nurses) are also available in most larger institutions to assist with the care of ostomies and with any unusual ostomy problems. The United Ostomy Association (UOA) has chapters worldwide that offer educational programs for volunteers who visit clients either before or after surgery. The client is also invited to attend monthly meetings of the UOA after dismissal from the hospital.

TYPES OF OSTOMIES

There are five main types of ostomies: colostomy, ileostomy, jejunostomy, ileo conduit, and Kock or Indiana Pouch. Each will be discussed in this section.

Colostomy

The colon or large intestine is the final reservoir for the waste of digested food before it leaves the body. The primary function of the colon is to absorb fluid from the liquid waste material that it receives from the small intestine. The waste material exits the body through the rectum as a solid.

Stool consistency depends on the placement of the stoma in the colon. A colostomy (opening from colon through the skin) is named for the part of the colon where it is located. An ascending colostomy takes its name from the ascending colon and would be on the right side of the abdomen. It has a liquid output. A transverse colostomy would be more toward the midline of the abdomen, and the output would be a pasty liquid. A descending colostomy, or sigmoid colostomy, would have solid output. Figure 36-2 shows the different colostomy sites.

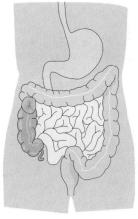
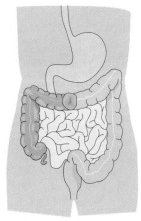
Ascending colostomy   Transverse colostomy

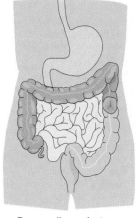
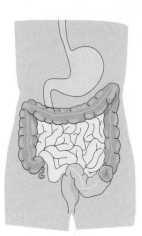
Descending colostomy   Sigmoid colostomy

FIGURE 36-2 Colostomy sites.

Ileostomy

An ostomy made in the small intestine takes its name from the part of the small intestine that is opened. The most common site for an ostomy in the small intestine is the ileum, thus the name ileostomy. The output from an ileostomy is a thin liquid of a usually yellowish-green color. This thin output is called **effluent**. It generally has no odor, and may get thicker in time as the body adapts to the need to retain moisture. Many ileostomies have almost constant effluent output. The Kock continent ileostomy has a pouch made inside the abdomen to hold the effluent until the client is ready to empty the pouch. Figure 36-3 illustrates a Kock continent ileostomy.

Jejunostomy

Jejunostomy is an opening into the jejunum part of the small intestine. It may be done to **decompress** (relieve pressure) the small intestine or, less com-

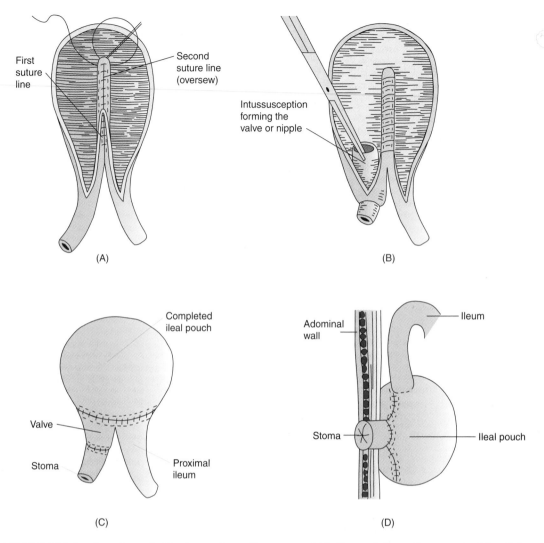

FIGURE 36-3 Creation of a Kock continent ileostomy. **(A)** Flaps of tissue from each side of the suture line are sewn together to form a double suture line. **(B)** A nipple valve is made and its two layers are held in place by many staples and/or sutures. **(C)** Sutures close the ileal reservoir. **(D)** A flush stoma is sutured to the abdominal wall.

monly, to eliminate waste material. Since most of the digestion and absorption of nutrients occurs in the small intestine, a jejunostomy is seldom performed to eliminate waste. When this is done the client is said to have a "short gut." This client would have nutritional deficits such as fluid imbalance (fluid volume deficit), and vitamin deficiencies, such as vitamin B$_{12}$, along with malabsorption due to the loss of part of the small intestine where the absorption of nutrients occurs. Sometimes an ostomy is constructed in the jejunum, and the remaining lower gastrointestinal tract is used to feed the client. A tube inserted into the ostomy is used to drip formula into the remaining intestine (McGinnis & Matson, 1994). This ostomy is called a Roux-en-Y jejunostomy (see Figure 36-4).

Urinary

Stomas may also be created in the urinary system. The most common reason for a urinary system ostomy is removal of the urinary bladder as a result of disease. Two different types of surgical procedures are used to maintain the flow of urine from the kidneys and ureters.

Ileo Conduit

The most common and oldest type of urinary ostomy surgery is the ileo conduit. In this surgery a piece of the ileum (small intestine) is taken out, and the ileum is reconnected. One end of the removed portion of the ileum is closed, while the other end is brought through the abdomen, forming a stoma. The

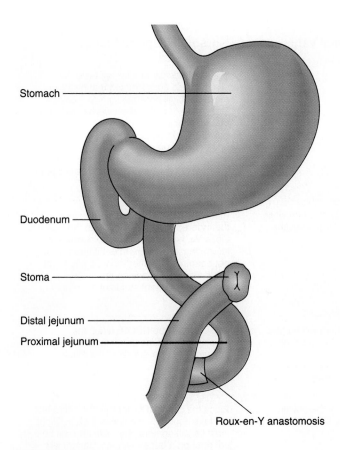

FIGURE 36-4 A Roux-en-Y jejunostomy.

ureters are attached to this section of ileum; urine then passes from the kidneys to the ureters and through this section of ileum to the outside of the body.

Kock or Indiana Pouch

Another urinary system ostomy is the Kock or Indiana Pouch. In this procedure, the surgeon creates a pouch made from part of the ileum and/or the large intestine. The ureters are attached to the pouch where urine collects. A section of the ileum is then used to

connect the pouch to the outside of the body (see Figure 36-5). A catheter is inserted into the pouch several times a day to empty the pouch.

CONSTRUCTIONS OF STOMAS

The construction of the stoma will vary depending on the reason for the surgery and the blood supply of that particular part of the bowel. The name of the type of stoma will be used in the client's chart, indicating what portion of the bowel was used for the stoma construction. The site of the ostomy determines what type of effluent comes from the ostomy. The closer to the rectum the ostomy is the more solid the stool will be.

Direction of Stoma

The terms proximal (close to) and distal (away from) are used in reference to the different parts of the bowel. Proximal refers to that part of the bowel closest to the stomach. The distal part of the bowel is that closest to the rectum.

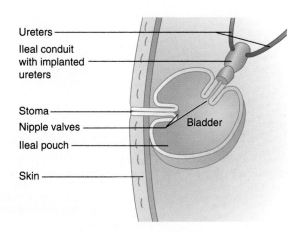

FIGURE 36-5 Urinary Kock pouch.

COMMON DIAGNOSTIC TESTS

The following is a table of the commonly used diagnostic tests for ostomy clients.

Test	Explanation/Normal Values	Nursing Responsibilities
Barium Swallow	The client drinks a glass of barium while x-rays are taken of the esophagus and cardiac sphincter.	Place the client NPO the evening before. Explain the procedure and the time frame for results. Encourage the client to drink fluids and eat fiber after the test. A laxative

(continued)

Test	Explanation/Normal Values	Nursing Responsibilities
		is sometimes given after the test. The client should be instructed that his bowel movement will be white for 1 to 2 days. During the test, the client will be tilted on the x-ray table in various positions. There may be repeated pictures taken at one-half hour intervals as the barium moves through the bowel. Document the client's tolerance of the procedure and passage of the barium.
Barium enema	An enema of barium will be given while x-rays are taken of the large intestine.	Place the client NPO the night before. Give the ordered medication to clean the bowel. Observe the results of the laxatives, and inform the x-ray department if there have not been results. After the test, force oral fluids and give cleansing enema as ordered. Document status of abdomen and stools.
Fistula Gram	Radiopaque dye or barium will be given to drink and x-rays will be taken as the dye or barium passes through the GI tract. The dye will show where the fistula is and how it is connected to the GI tract.	The client will be NPO. Explain the procedure, the time frame for the results, and who will give the client the results.
Computed Tomography (CT Scan)	Produces 3-D pictures of the bowel. A contrast medium may be used for the scan machine.	Place the client NPO. Inform client that test will take about 45 minutes to 1 hour. Client must lie still on hard, flat table and will be put through a large machine. Barium will interfere with the test, so tests using barium should be done after the scan or 4 or more days before.
Magnetic Resonance Imaging (MRI)	Cross section pictures are taken of the abdomen; no x-rays are used. The test can identify blood flow, infection, and tumors. Not recommended for any type of metallic implant, pacemakers or staples. (Uses strong magnetic fields and could displace staples and/or damage pacemakers.)	Client must lie still on a board and be inserted into a machine. Client should be assessed for claustrophobia before the test. Ask if the client has any metallic implants, such as artificial joints, pacemakers, or staples from previous surgery.
Intravenous Pyelogram (IVP)	Infusion of radiopaque dye into a vein, resulting in visualization of the urinary system. The renal pelvis, ureters, and bladder can be seen.	Assess client for allergy to iodine dye. Inform client that the test involves venous access. Client may feel a warm flush when the dye is injected. Assess the client for renal function after the test as the dye is hard on the kidneys. Have client drink lots of fluid to flush the dye out of the kidneys.
Conduitogram	Radiopaque dye may be injected through a catheter into the conduit or piece of ileum to assess by means of x-ray, the length and emptying ability of the conduit, and the presence of stricture or obstruction.	Conduit is a connection between the bladder or pouch and the outside of the body. Explain to the client the x-ray. Assess the client for allergies to iodine-based dye.
Pouchogram	Installation of radiopaque dye into the Kock or Indiana pouch. Done with the continent ostomies to determine the state of healing and size of the pouch created.	Assess the client for allergies to iodine-based dye. Explain the procedure.

KEY ABBREVIATIONS

The following abbreviations and acronyms are used in this chapter:

AARP	American Association of Retired Persons
DRG	diagnosis related group
ECF	extracellular fluid
ET	Enterostomal Therapist (Nurse)
IBD	inflammatory bowel disease
J-P drain	Jackson Pratt drain
UOA	United Ostomy Association

PATHOPHYSIOLOGY OF BOWEL AND BLADDER

Inflammatory Bowel Disease

There are four diseases of the bowel that are commonly and collectively called inflammatory bowel disease (IBD). These diseases are: familial polyposis coli, ulcerative colitis, Crohn's disease, and diverticulitis. Familial polyposis is an inherited condition causing multiple polyps in the colon and rectum. This is usually a disease of adolescence which will result in bowel cancer if left untreated. Treatment is surgical removal of the large intestine.

Ulcerative Colitis

Ulcerative colitis is an inflammatory disease affecting the mucous lining of the colon and rectum. Some clients with acute ulcerative colitis require surgery; others have chronic problems and do not enjoy good health.

Ulcerative colitis usually affects the rectum and extends into the colon, although in many clients the involvement is confined to the rectum and sigmoid. A smaller number of clients have ulcerative colitis affecting the rectum and entire colon (Slater, 1993).

Common symptoms of ulcerative colitis include bleeding, diarrhea, mucous discharge, abdominal discomfort, anorexia, weight loss, anal soreness and pain. Research has shown an increased incidence of colorectal cancer in clients with longstanding ulcerative colitis. This means that clients with ulcerative colitis should have regular colonoscopy examinations. Refer to Chapter 34 for additional information on the management of ulcerative colitis.

Crohn's Disease

Crohn's disease is a chronic inflammatory disease which may involve any portion of the gastrointestinal tract from the mouth to the anus. It often appears to skip areas and typically involves the terminal portion of the ileum, the colon, and the perianal area.

The inflammatory process extends through all the layers of the gastrointestinal tract. Problems include perforation, abscess, and fistula formation, especially in the anal area (Salter, 1993). Clients with Crohn's disease may present with weight loss, anemia, toxicity, and painful colic. Many of the symptoms of Crohn's disease are similar to those of ulcerative colitis. For example, both Crohn's disease and ulcerative colitis are commonly treated with steroids and anti-inflammatory medications, both involve chronic inflammation of the bowel from an unclear etiology, and both may have long periods of remission with episodes of acute inflammation (Doughty, 1994). Refer to Table 34-3 for a comparison of Crohn's disease and ulcerative colitis.

However, an important distinction in treatment is that a client with ulcerative colitis can be cured of the disease with an ileostomy. If operated on, a client with Crohn's disease may have the disease return in another part of the gastrointestinal tract. Therefore, surgery is not the first option for clients with Crohn's disease. Before surgery is considered, anti-inflammatory medication and resting the bowel will be prescribed. The bowel may be "rested" with a clear liquid diet or no oral food, in which case the physician would order hyperalimentation (TPN—Total Parenteral Nutrition) with a central venous catheter. Refer to Chapter 34 for additional information on the management of Crohn's disease.

Diverticulitis

Diverticula are small outpouches that form on the large colon. When these outpouches become inflamed the disorder is called diverticulitis. These small inflamed pouches may become attached to internal organs and break open forming a connection between the colon and the bladder, the skin, or small intestine. When this happens an ostomy is performed to repair or remove the affected colon, and let the body heal. In six to eight weeks after the body and the colon heal the colon may be reattached, thus reversing the ostomy. Refer to Chapter 34 for additional information on the management of diverticulitis.

Trauma

Trauma refers to mechanical or physical injury to a part of the gastrointestinal or urinary tract. There are a variety of ways trauma can affect these structures and lead to the need for an ostomy.

Penetrating injuries are traumas stemming from a variety of causes, such as gunshot or knife wounds to the abdomen, car accidents where a fractured bone penetrates the bowel or bladder, or other causes.

When the bowel is penetrated, surgery is used to create an ostomy or to reanastomose (reattach the two ends of the bowel after cutting out the injured part) the bowel so healing may take place.

Peritonitis is a common consequence of penetrating injuries· of the bowel, due to gastrointestinal contents spilling into the abdominal cavity. The client needs to be closely monitored for signs of infection after a penetrating injury. Signs and symptoms of peritonitis are fever, pain, and rigid abdomen with decreased or absent bowel sounds. Peritonitis may also occur after abdominal surgery, especially if the bowel was operated on or cut into. Refer to Chapter 34 for more information on the management of peritonitis.

Bowel and Urinary Obstruction

There are several conditions that can cause an obstruction or blockage of the gastrointestinal system (GI) or genitourinary system (GU). When a blockage or obstruction occurs, stool or urine cannot pass and the blockage must be removed for normal physiologic functioning to return. Refer to the Chapter 34 for more information on GI and Chapter 35 for GU disorders.

Neoplasms

Neoplasms or growths may be classified as either benign or cancerous. Both are abnormal growths of tissue. When these abnormal tissue growths affect the colon and/or the urinary tract, an ostomy is often done to reestablish the flow of waste material from the colon, small intestine, or kidneys to the outside of the body. If the condition of the client and extent of the tumor warrants, the tumor will be removed surgically. However, at times the client may elect to have an ostomy created to maintain GI or GU function without removal of the tumor or growth.

Volvulus

Volvulus is a twisting of the bowel, in which a loop of bowel twists on itself closing the lumen of the bowel and compromising the blood supply to that area. This condition, at times, will reverse itself without permanent damage to the bowel. However, sometimes surgery will be needed to correct the twisting, and frequently a temporary ostomy will be required to rest and decompress the bowel.

Fistula

A fistula is an abnormal communication (opening) between two or more body structures or spaces. Fistulas may occur internally, in which case the opening is contained inside the body between one internal organ

and another. For example, there may be a fistula between the small intestine and the vagina or between the rectum and vagina. Fistulas can be external, in which case the opening comes through the skin, letting fecal contents spill onto the skin. This is called an external fistula or an enterocutaneous fistula (an opening between the GI tract and the skin). The fistula can cause much pain and trouble for the client. It is best to consult an ET nurse for nursing management of these fistulas.

Fistulas are a devastating complication of surgery and some pathologic conditions. The client with a fistula often suffers from extended hospitalization, pain, risk of sepsis, malnutrition, and emotional distress.

Fistulas may develop with an acute episode of Crohn's disease. The inflamed surface of the bowel wall adheres to adjacent loops of bowel or to adjacent organs such as the bladder, vagina, or abdominal wall (Doughty, 1994). Then, the inflammatory process erodes through the organ walls to form a pathway (fistula) (Doughty, 1994). Any abnormal drainage from the vagina, or bladder, or signs of infection in these areas may indicate fistula formation. Fistula formation is uncommon.

Stones

Renal stones may also cause obstruction of the GU system and can require ostomy surgery. This type of surgery is usually temporary, or until the GU system heals and can be reattached.

Medical/Surgical Management

Surgical

Ostomies are surgically created stomas to relieve either a disease or functional problem in the GI or GU tracts. The surgery usually takes several hours and requires six to eight weeks recovery time. These guidelines may change, however, as new surgical techniques allow instruments and flexible optics entry through smaller openings. Such techniques would be comparable to the current laparoscopic surgery for removal of the gallbladder.

Stoma Construction

The proximal end of the bowel is the functional part of the bowel brought through the abdominal wall during surgery. The end of the bowel is folded back on itself to make a small spout about one-half inch long. The spout is sewn or sutured to the abdomen and peritoneum to create a stoma (see Figure 36-6). When the surgery is finished, a dressing of vaseline gauze is

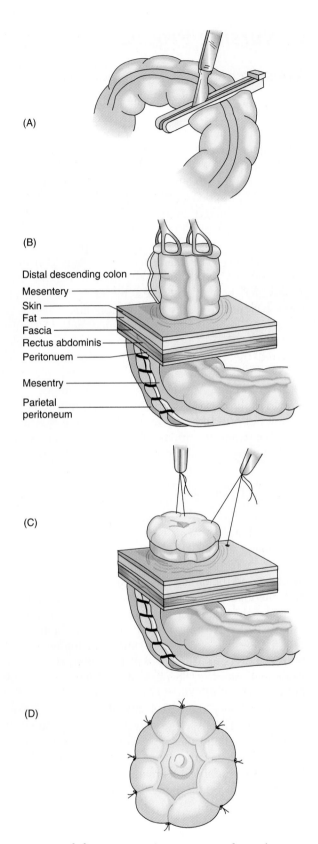

(A)

(B)

Distal descending colon
Mesentery
Skin
Fat
Fascia
Rectus abdominis
Peritonuem

Mesentry

Parietal
peritoneum

(C)

(D)

FIGURE 36-6 Steps in the creation of a colostomy. **(A)** The colon is divided; blood supply is left intact to allow for a 2 cm length of healthy colon to project through the abdominal wall; **(B)** The colon is drawn through the stoma opening; **(C)** The colostomy stoma matures, or heals; **(D)** A mature, healthy stoma.

placed over stomas not expected to function within twenty-four hours (descending or sigmoid colostomy stomas). If the bowel is expected to function within the first twenty-four hours after surgery, such as in an ileostomy or transverse or ascending colostomy, a sterile pouch is placed over the stoma at the end of surgery to contain the effluent.

The part of the bowel that is distal to the stoma may be removed if it is diseased. It may be sutured or stapled shut and left in the abdomen to be reattached at a later date, or a **mucous fistula** (stoma that will secrete mucous) can be made. In cases of rectal disease, the rectum may be removed leaving a drain in the rectal area. Sitting is painful for a while.

Continent Ostomy Procedures

There are some operative procedures that create an artificial colon, or a storage pouch, to hold stool or urine until it can be emptied. These procedures have a variety of names, from the name of the surgeon who first performed them, to the institution that developed and did the first procedure. A continent ostomy has an internal pouch made of large and/or small intestine material to collect either small bowel content (effluent) or urine. This pouch may be constructed in a two- or three-part surgery. The first surgery may end with the client having an ostomy to divert effluent stool or urine, and a pouch made of intestinal material that is not used, so it may heal. In a second and sometimes third surgery the rest of the connections for the continent ostomy to be constructed are completed. The pouch must be kept from stretching out too much, so that sutures or staples are not stretched and/or released. For this reason a catheter is inserted into the pouch to keep it empty and keep the opening from growing closed or collapsing. The tube or catheter will stay in place until the swelling associated with surgery recedes, and then will be inserted frequently at first to empty the pouch. The schedule of pouch-emptying will be prescribed by the surgeon. The time between emptying will gradually be increased to stretch the pouch and allow the client to have a manageable self-care schedule.

Irrigation

Irrigation of the pouch in the first days after surgery will be ordered by the surgeon. The pouch may be irrigated to keep any solid particles of food or mucous or blood clots from obstructing the outlet of the pouch or catheter.

Pharmacological

Laxatives are used preoperatively to clean the bowel and prepare it for surgery. The cleaner the bowel, the less the chance exists for postoperative infection. The following laxatives are used to prepare the bowel for surgery:

- senna (X-Prep): works in six hours and is a stimulant laxative. Would not be given if there are ulcerative lesions in the bowel.
- magnesium citrate (Citro-Mag): works in three to six hours, not given if there are rectal fissures, intestinal obstruction, or renal disease.
- danthron (Dorbane): works in six to twenty-four hours, is safer for cardiac clients, give on empty stomach for best results.
- bisacodyl (Dulcolax): works in six to twelve hours after oral administration, fifteen to sixty minutes after rectal administration. Oral and rectal may be used together for bowel preparation for surgery.

Diet

The client will be NPO after surgery until bowel sounds are heard and flatus has been passed through the stoma. The client may also have a nasogastric tube inserted into the stomach to rest the bowel by removing all gastric secretions until the bowel is functioning again. When flatus is noted in the pouch or bowel sounds are heard, the physician will allow some oral intake. Ostomy clients will start with a clear liquid diet after surgery and gradually be advanced to full liquid, and then regular food as their condition allows. After surgery, the physician will recommend a low residue diet with lots of liquids so as not to irritate the bowel while it is healing. Six to eight weeks after surgery the physician may change the diet to a high-fiber diet with lots of liquid to prevent further bowel disease.

Activity

The ostomy client is encouraged to be up and moving as much as possible without bending or lifting. Increased activity, such as walking, stimulates the bowel to work normally after surgery and should be encouraged.

Preventive Measures

A high-fiber, low-fat diet with plenty of liquids is thought to be a preventive measure for cancer of the bowel. As with all chronic diseases, frequent monitoring by the client's physician is recommended. After the age of forty a yearly rectal examination is recommended with a physical.

▶ Nursing Process

Assessment

Assessment of the ostomy client begins the first time he or she is seen by a health care professional. While many areas should be assessed for any surgical client, this chapter focuses on those that are specific to the ostomy client.

Assessment includes giving the client an opportunity to ask questions and begin coping with a possible altered body image. Before ostomy surgery, the surgeon and the ET nurse talk with the client and explain the reason for the surgery and the possibilities of ostomy surgery. The client may have many concerns and questions that should be answered about the surgery and how it will affect his or her life. If the client has no concerns, a question about what is understood about ostomy surgery may help to clarify what kind of surgery is expected, and how well-prepared the client is. Often, the surgeon may tell the client that ostomy surgery is a possibility, but may not have to be done. The surgeon often cannot tell if enough of the bowel is available to be reattached until the amount of healthy bowel can be seen. If the client does not want to discuss the surgery, that desire should be honored and noted. Some people prefer to wait until they know for sure what is going to be done, instead of coping with possibilities. Frequently, clients may want to see a pouch or other equipment needed for the ostomy. This will depend on their style or method of coping.

Choosing the site or placement of the stoma is an opportunity for the physician or ET nurse to talk with the client and the family. The surgeon or ET nurse will mark the client's abdomen with special skin marking ink the night before or day before surgery. The best place will depend on the type of ostomy being created, the lifestyle of the client, and the contours of the client's abdomen. The site will be within the rectus abdominal muscle. The mark should not be washed off before surgery.

Before surgery, the bowel should be as clean inside as possible. This is done by allowing the client to ingest only a liquid diet for two days before surgery, and by giving laxatives, and/or enemas just before surgery. The number of organisms in the bowel are also often reduced by giving the client antibiotics such as the aminoglycosides (neomycin sulfate or streptomycin sulfate).

▼ ▼

Possible preoperative nursing diagnoses for a client undergoing ostomy surgery may include:

Nursing Diagnoses—Preoperative	Goals	Nursing Interventions
▶ Knowledge deficit, related to lack of information about ostomy surgery and postoperative expectations.	The client will express an understanding of ostomy surgery and postoperative expectations.	Assess how much the client and family know about living with an ostomy, and their readiness to learn.
		Request an ostomy visitor (trained members of the United Ostomy Association or UOA) to visit with the client either in the home or the hospital. They can answer questions about living with an ostomy, tell how they adjusted after surgery, or just demonstrate that there is life after surgery.
		Document all teaching plans. A written plan for each client is important and should be placed in the client's record. This can be a simple checkoff of skills needed to be acquired or a more elaborate plan. Anyone who presents material and/or observes a return demonstration can initial that skill. Teaching plans should begin preoperatively.
		Record the client's readiness to learn and level of education.
▶ Anxiety/fear, related to concerns about surgery and life afterwards.	The client will discuss anxiety and fear with health care professionals and family.	Establish good rapport with the client and family.
		Provide time to discuss concerns about the proposed surgery and life afterwards.
		Offer information and perform nursing care in a professional manner to help reassure the client and family that the staff cares about them.

▶ Evaluation

Each goal must be evaluated to determine how it has been met by the client.

▲ ▲

Assessment Immediate Postoperative

The immediate postoperative concerns are that the client's airway is patent, that the heart and lungs are recovering from the anesthetic, and that pain is managed. This chapter presents postoperative concerns of an ostomy client.

Objective Data   On the client's return from surgery the nurse must assess many areas. Assess the status of the circulatory and respiratory systems first. Next, assess the stoma. Usually, on return from surgery, the client wears a sterile, transparent pouch so the stoma can be seen. Expect a new stoma to be edematous and ranging from deep red to dusky in color. Color is important since it tells the surgeon the status of the

blood supply to the stoma. If blood supply to the stoma is inadequate, the stoma will turn black. The physician should be called if the stoma becomes black. Use a penlight flashlight to assess the color of the stoma.

The size of the stoma is important also. The pouch will make the stoma difficult to measure, but the degree of swelling can be estimated. The swelling or edema will increase at first in response to the injury of bowel tissue. The client needs to be reassured that the stoma will not remain so large, but will shrink for the first six to eight weeks.

Measurement of the stoma, when the pouch is changed, will be aided by the measuring guides contained in packaging material with the ostomy supplies. If a measuring guide is unavailable, trace the edges of the stoma on plastic or paper and measure this with a ruler in centimeters, the length by the width.

Immediately after surgery there may be a small amount of serosanguineous drainage in the pouch. This is normal after surgery. When the pouch is changed and the stoma is cleaned or if the stoma is touched when swollen a small amount of bleeding may occur. The client cannot feel the stoma if it is touched. Reassure the client that the small amount of bleeding is normal.

The time for bowel function of a colostomy depends on where in the colon the ostomy was created. It is important that along with assessing the bowel function and kidney function that the abdomen be assessed for bowel sounds and distention.

A colostomy in the ascending colon will function faster than one in the sigmoid, or descending colon. The time frame for return of bowel function is forty-eight to seventy-two hours. If the surgery was not planned and a bowel prep was not given preoperatively, function may return as soon as twelve to twenty-four hours. By the third day there should be some flatus in the pouch. The pouch will expand with the passage of flatus. This is what most surgeons wait for before the client is started on a diet. There should be no odor associated with bowel function if the pouch is clean, applied correctly, and the clamp is tight.

Ileostomies are expected to function in twelve to twenty-four hours. This is because there is no storage area for the effluent. The effluent will be a thin, yellow-green liquid at first, and will become thicker with time as the bowel adapts to the removal of the large bowel. The pouch will need to be emptied when half full.

Urostomies or ostomies of the urinary tract, will function immediately. Urine production is important to monitor for any postoperative client, as it reflects perfusion of the kidneys and kidney function. Immediately after surgery the urine may be pink- or red-tinged. There will probably be urinary stents (small stiff tubes) in place, coming out through the stoma, to keep the ureters open and allow drainage from the kidneys to the outside. As time passes, the urine will come less from the stents and more through the stoma into the pouch. A careful recording of output from the stents and the pouch is important to determine when the stents may be removed.

▼ ▼

Nursing Diagnoses—Postoperative	*Goals*	*Nursing Interventions*
▶ *Knowledge deficit, related to lack of exposure to information and limited practice in caring for ostomy.*	The client and family will demonstrate the ability to care safely for ostomy.	Interventions will be addressed that relate to the care of the ostomy. The interventions will be listed and explained as they relate to the above nursing diagnosis. There is much to be learned postoperatively, and the client often feels overwhelmed when presented with so much information all at once. That is why an itemized teaching plan broken down into small parts that all health care workers can take part in, will help the client and family master the information.

Pouching

Pouching refers to the placement of a pouch over the ostomy to contain either stool or urine. There are two main objectives with a pouching system. First, to protect the skin around the stoma (peristomal skin); second, to contain the waste product.

The type of pouch used at the client's dismissal should be one that is both functional and easy to apply. There are many types and styles of pouches. An ET nurse will know which type the client will take home. There are basically four types of pouches: a one-piece pouch, a two-piece pouch, an open-ended pouch, and a closed-ended pouch (see Figure 36-7). The most common postoperative pouch is a transpar-ent, one piece, open-ended, one size fits all pouch. For home care, an opaque, two-piece, open-ended pouch with face plate to fit may be more acceptable. The two parts must be the same size to fit together. Washing the hands and maintaining clean technique with each pouch change is important to decrease the chance of infection. Always explain to the client and family what you are doing, and use all opportunities to teach them. The pouch should be changed when it is needed or for teaching purposes. At home the client will change the pouch as needed. Some clients change the pouch every other day, and some every week.

Pouch changing is not difficult, but can seem like a big job to a new ostomy client. With each pouch

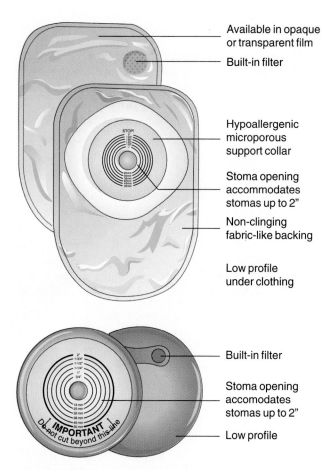

Available in opaque or transparent film

Built-in filter

Hypoallergenic microporous support collar

Stoma opening accommodates stomas up to 2"

Non-clinging fabric-like backing

Low profile under clothing

Built-in filter

Stoma opening accomodates stomas up to 2"

Low profile

FIGURE 36-7 An example of a one-piece pouch. (*Courtesy of Convatec, Skillmah, NJ*)

change, slowly explain what you are doing and why. Assemble your supplies, you will need a pouch with a backing attached or a two-piece pouching system, (one pouch and one wafer), paste or other adhesive, scissors, wipes, (nonsterile gauze works well for new ostomies) a pen or pencil, a measuring guide, gloves, towel, tape, and plastic bag for trash. First, remove the old pouch or covering of the stoma. This will be easier if the pouch is empty. Carefully peel back the adhesive from top to bottom, pressing down on the client's peristomal skin while pulling up on the pouch, or tape and wafer. The pouch may be taken off in one piece even if it is a two-piece pouch. Remember, if the client has just had surgery this may be somewhat painful. It may be a good idea to give the client an analgesic before beginning the procedure.

Place the plastic bag with a towel under the pouch next to the client. Have tissues handy if the ostomy starts to function with the pouch off, as does happen sometimes especially with ileostomies. Urostomies will have a steady trickle of urine from the stoma. For urostomies, roll a sterile 4 × 4 into a tubular shape and place over the stoma touching the stoma. This wicks up the urine to keep the area dry while you work. A cotton ball also will work for a short period of time.

Place the soiled pouch in the plastic bag and cover the stoma with wipes as you work. Be careful to remove the clamp from the old pouch before throwing the pouch away. With the pouch off, assess the surrounding skin and stoma. Check for any redness or irritation from the adhesive or stool that may have been on the skin. Clean effluent or stool from the peristomal skin and stoma with water and gauze if tender, or a washcloth if not tender. If a soap is used, the skin should be rinsed well to remove all residue. Do not use a soap or cleanser that leaves lotion on the skin as this may affect the adhesion of the pouch. Dry the skin well. If the skin is tender, one of the protective films such as "skin prep" by United may be applied. Let the protective film dry before applying the ostomy pouch. Remember that the stoma has many blood vessels and will bleed if scraped, but should stop quickly. The client may need to be reassured that this is normal.

Measure the stoma and transfer the pattern from the stoma measuring to the adhesive skin barrier material on either the pouch or wafer. The adhesive material should be coupled with a skin barrier to protect the skin. Cut out the shape of the stoma, and remove the protective paper backing from the pouch or wafer. This step may be done before removing the soiled pouch if you know the size of the stoma. For a secure fit and added adhesiveness, place a bead of adhesive paste around the edge of the stoma or place on the back of the pouch or wafer. The paste gives a tighter fit and can fill in any irregular surfaces.

Make sure the skin around the stoma is dry and clean, then press the pouch or wafer down over the stoma so it makes good contact with the skin. If the pouch was not attached to the two-piece system before, now attach by pressing down over the ring around the stoma on the wafer. Some wafers and pouches have tape already around the edges. If not, take four pieces of tape and place tape on both the skin barrier and the skin on all four sides of the skin barrier to secure to the skin. Place the clamp on the end of the pouch and you are finished. Place the pouch on toward one side while the client is in bed to make emptying easier. Once the client is up and around the pouch can be put on hanging straight down so the client can empty the pouch into the toilet when in the bathroom. Figure 36-8 reviews the procedure for applying a pouch to a stoma.

Whether the client has tender or thin skin, a preparation to protect the skin is important. There are many on the market which work by putting a thin film over the skin, so when the appliance is pulled off the thin film is taken off—not the client's skin.

The client must also learn how to empty the pouch. The easiest way, once they are out of bed, is to go to the bathroom. The client can sit back on the toilet seat or on a chair facing the toilet. Place the end of the pouch over the toilet, release the clamp, and form a cuff by folding

1. Cut the center hole approximately the same size as the stoma, using the guidelines on the release paper. Do not cut beyond the last line.

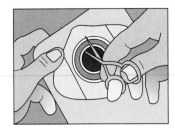

2. Remove the release paper from the picture-frame support adhesive by bending the slit edges sharply backward. Do not remove the release paper from the side edges until later.

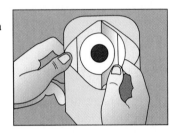

3. When Stomahesive® Paste is indicated, apply a bead of paste to the adhesive side of the skin barrier, around the stomal opening. Allow the paste to set for around 60 seconds prior to applying the pouch to the skin.

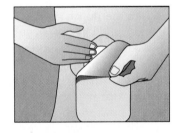

4. Press the disc against the skin, paying particular attention to the area closest to the stoma. Maintain gentle pressure on the disc to improve adhesion. Make sure the picture frame support adhesive is smooth and wrinkle free.

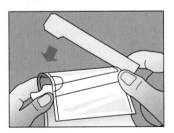

5. To attach the tail closure on drainable pouches, fold the pouch outlet spout over the "knife" edge of the closure only once. Press firmly on the closure, especially at the center, until it snaps and is securely closed.

FIGURE 36-8 How to apply a pouching system. (*Courtesy of Convatec, Skillmah, NJ*)

back the lower edge and then emptying the pouch into the toilet. Clean off the edges, turn the cuff down and apply the clamp. The edges that are exposed and the clamp must be clean to eliminate odor. Some nurses will use peri-bottles or syringes to rinse or clean the pouch after emptying. This is unnecessary, and causes the client to think they must always rinse out the pouch presenting another obstacle to ostomy care.

Activity

Movement is encouraged as soon as the client is awake and can move. Leg exercises will be done first and activity will progress to standing and walking. Activity is important to not only prevent postoperative complications, but also to stimulate the bowel to work again after surgery.

Diet

The client will be NPO for a short time after surgery. Some surgeons keep the client NPO with or without a NG tube until flatus is passed or bowel sounds are heard. Other surgeons allow sips of water and clear liquids right after surgery. Assessment of the abdomen is important to pick up any immobility of the bowel (paralytic ileus) that would complicate the postoperative recovery.

Ostomy Functioning

Once the ostomy has started to function, the color, amount, and consistency of the stool should be noted and documented as with other bowel movements. If the stool is liquid, it should be included as part of the output while the client is on intake and output.

Tubes and Drains

Right after surgery the client will usually have a nasogastric tube (NG) to keep the stomach and small intestine decompressed, thus preventing nausea and vomiting.

The client may have a Jackson-Pratt (JP) drain which looks like a bulb syringe on the end of a long flexible tube. The nurse's responsibility with this closed drainage system is to keep the bulb compressed to maintain the flow of drainage from the incision area. This drain is sutured in place. Drains are used to prevent the pooling of drainage which could be a medium for an infection. The drainage is measured at the end of each shift and recorded as output.

Other drains may be hooked right to a suction machine, such as sump drains. These are used for large areas that are going to drain more than the JP type of drain can handle and/or need irrigation. These drains are usually sutured in place. Take care not to pull on it as this would hurt the client. It is considered good technique to tape the tube to the client or pin it to the gown to prevent pulling on the tube. Emptying the drains is a clean procedure. Apply nonsterile gloves when handling drainage.

With urostomy surgery, stents are used to keep the ureters open. The stents are placed during surgery to allow urine to flow from the kidneys through the ureters which will swell from the surgical injury. The stents will be protruding from the stoma to maintain urine drainage. These drains should be handled with sterile technique to prevent infection, especially when emptying. Urine from these tubes is counted as output and at times kept track of separately from each kidney.

Incision and Wound Care

The surgical incision will be initially covered with a gauze dressing. On the second or third day the dressing is removed and left off. Some surgeons request that the incision be washed with betadine or red antibacterial soap daily to prevent infection.

A perineal resection is the removal of the rectum. This surgery leaves either an open wound packed with gauze, or an incision with a drain of some type. Sitz baths are sometimes ordered for the perineal wound for comfort and cleaning.

Complications—Postoperative

As with any surgery there are complications that may occur. Bleeding or hemorrhage may occur at the incision site or stoma site. If bleeding is unchecked, shock will occur. This is why the client's blood pressure and pulse are checked frequently after surgery.

Infection is always possible when the skin is broken for surgery, or invasive lines are in place. The presence of many microorganisms and people make infection in the acute care setting a real possibility. The risk of infection around the stoma is greater due to the presence of stool around the new suture line.

▶ Teaching Tip

The most important thing a nurse can do for a client with an ostomy is to use good handwashing technique consistently.

Necrosis of the stoma happens when the blood supply to the stoma is cut off. The stoma will turn black and the part without blood supply will slough off, leaving a stoma that is either flat or indented and difficult to pouch. The color of the stoma is checked and documented at least once a shift. The doctor should be notified if necrosis of the stoma is suspected.

Bowel function is checked every shift to monitor for any obstruction or ileus. Bowel function, of course, is very important, and why bowel sounds and abdominal tenderness are checked every four hours.

DISORDERS OF OSTOMIES

Many problems can develop with ostomies. For example, the client may develop a hernia, late obstruction, a recurrent tumor, or experience electrolyte im-

balance or skin excoriation. These and other common difficulties are discussed in this section. Usually, these difficulties occur several weeks or months after surgery.

Hernia Around the Stoma

A hernia is an abnormal outpouching of an organ through the abdominal wall. It is the most frequent complication of an ostomy and is caused when a loop of bowel pushes up through the muscle next to the stoma, and under the skin, creating an outpouching from the abdomen with the stoma in the middle (see Figure 36-9). This results in a stoma that is difficult to pouch. Hernias may be either strangulated or unstrangulated.

Strangulated Hernia

The hernia is considered strangulated if the loop of bowel that is pushed up around the stoma twists on itself and shuts off the lumen of the bowel, creating a bowel obstruction. If the bowel does not unkink, it is an emergency and is corrected surgically.

Unstrangulated Hernia

The hernia is considered unstrangulated when the bowel is not twisted and causes no problem. In this case, if the pouch will stay affixed, the client may choose not to have the hernia repaired.

Late Obstruction

Obstruction of the bowel or ostomy may occur as a complication after surgery. There are two common reasons that the bowel may obstruct after surgery: recurrent tumor and undigested food.

Recurrent Tumor

When the ostomy is created to remove a cancerous tumor, the tumor may recur at the site of the stoma or in a different part of the bowel. This is uncommon; if the tumor does recur, surgery to keep the bowel open

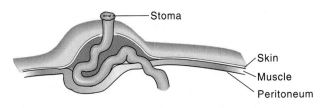

FIGURE 36-9 Hernia of bowel loop.

is generally considered. Removal of the entire tumor is not usually considered at this point, due to the recurrence of the cancer. Surgery at this stage is generally palliative or done for the comfort of the client, not to effect a cure.

Undigested Food

With ileostomies, if clients do not chew their food well, large pieces of food, such as an olive or large piece of meat, may get caught at the opening of the ostomy. Ileostomy clients should be instructed to chew their food well before swallowing.

Prolapse

In prolapse, the bowel will sometimes telescope out, resembling an elephant's trunk. If the bowel continues to work, this is not an emergency. However, the bowel must be put back into the abdomen. The doctor or ET Nurse can try to push the bowel back into the abdomen and hope it stays there (replaceable). If the bowel is nonreplaceable, the doctor is not able to push the bowel back into the abdomen, and the mucosa of the bowel may become injured if left outside of the body. The client usually agrees to surgery to have the prolapse fixed. Prolapse can be frightening for the client and should be discussed in postoperative teaching.

Ileostomy High Output

When the ileum has been injured or damaged by disease it may be too short or not long enough to reabsorb enough effluent to prevent complications, such as electrolyte imbalances. Skin excoriation around the stoma may occur.

Electrolyte Imbalance

A high output ileostomy can cause electrolyte imbalances by loss of large amounts of potassium and protein. The client will have difficulty learning to cope with a pouch that is always filling up and the need to take in enough fluid, protein, and potassium to replace the lost nutrients.

Skin Excoriation

The skin around a high output ostomy is in danger of becoming excoriated if a pouching system that protects the skin cannot be found. Ileostomy effluent contains digestive juices that, if left on the skin, will start to digest the skin, resulting in red, open areas. To prevent this problem, correct pouch fitting that will stay in place is important for these clients.

DISCHARGE TEACHING OF THE OSTOMY CLIENT

Assessment

As the client prepares to go home, it is important to assess the client's or his family's ability to handle the care of the ostomy at home. The client may be still dealing with an altered body image, and not want to look at or touch the stoma. The family may have to help with care and be supportive until the client can assume the care. The client or a family member should change the pouch two times before the client goes home so they feel secure in handling the procedure.

Pouching

Often the most difficult skill for ostomy clients is the ability to pouch the stoma and feel confident that they can handle problems when they are at home. Some clients will be anxious to learn how to apply the pouch, and others will want their husbands, wives, or others to apply the pouch.

Ostomy clients have many choices of different types of available pouches and supplies. The ET nurse or person who sells supplies often can help with selection of the best pouch to fit the client's lifestyle. The type of pouch should be one that the client can use independently.

Colostomy

For colostomies, the client may use either a one- or two-piece pouch with either a closed or open end. If the client has only one bowel movement a day, a closed pouch that is taken off and emptied once a day will be all that is needed. If the client has several stools a day, an open-ended drainable pouch would be best. There are also some pouches with flatus vents that have a charcoal filter in them to vent flatus and reduce odor. They do not always work well, but may improve with advancing technology. If flatus is a problem for the client, eating less flatus-producing foods such as beans, vegetables from the cabbage family, beer, mushrooms, cucumbers, onions, peas, spinach, corn, broccoli, radishes, yeast, dairy products, and carbonated beverages, may help. There are products sold over-the-counter to relieve flatus, such as Gas-X, Delcid, Beano, and others. Flatus does need to be emptied from the pouch when it fills up.

Ileostomies

For ileostomies, the one- or two-piece open-end pouch offers ease in emptying. Since the effluent usually varies from liquid to pasty, the drainage will have to be emptied several times during the day. A pouch that can be drained without taking it off is important. A skin barrier is also necessary for the ileostomy or any ostomy with liquid output.

Urostomy

For urostomies, a one- or two-piece pouch with a drainable spout at the end is best for emptying. There are special skin barriers on the market that will last seven to fourteen days and are designed to be used with liquid drainage such as urine or ileostomy liquid effluent.

The health of the skin around the stoma is important since that is where the pouch is attached. The client should be told to seek help if the skin around the stoma becomes red or sore. The pouch should be changed every three to five days, or as needed.

Men may want to shave the skin where the adhesive for the pouch is applied. The area may be shaved, but always in the direction away from the stoma to avoid cutting the stoma. Remind the client that there are no nerve endings in the stoma for touch, so the client will not know if it is cut or injured.

The urostomy client may want to connect the pouch to bedside drainage at night. This will prevent the pouch from leaking, and the client will not have to get up at night to empty the pouch. Wearing pajama bottoms with the tube down one leg helps keep the client from getting tangled up in the tube. The urine collection container may be placed on the floor inside a wastebasket for stability.

Irrigation

Colostomy irrigation is a means of regulating some colostomies. Irrigation may be used to regulate descending or sigmoid colostomies. Irrigation is also used at times to prepare clients with colostomies for x-ray procedures or other tests on the bowel.

An ileostomy is never irrigated because it is not able to hold any fluid. Irrigation would also be harmful to the small intestine. Urostomies should never be irrigated either.

Colostomies, if they are descending or sigmoid, may be irrigated daily or every other day for control of evacuation. After irrigation, the client may wear a small security pouch or a gauze pad over the stoma the rest of the day. The drawback of irrigation is that it takes about an hour or more to perform. The decision to irrigate is made by the client with the consent of the surgeon after healing has taken place.

Supplies required for colostomy irrigation include an irrigation bag or enema bag with a cone on the end

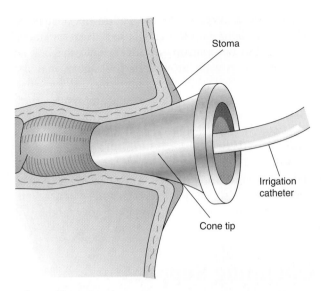

FIGURE 36-10 Cone tip irrigation of the bowel.

of the tubing, a water-soluble lubricant such as KY or Lubrafax, an irrigation sleeve of some type, and gloves. The principle behind a colostomy irrigation is the same as an enema: the fluid stimulates the bowel to evacuate the fluid and accumulated stool. With the colostomy, there is no sphincter to keep the water inside, so as the water is instilled into the colon it comes back out. Warm water is used (85°F to 95°F), and 500 cc to 1000 cc are enough to stimulate the bowel to evacuate. If the irrigation is done for an x-ray prep, the irrigation may have to be repeated until the solution returns clear.

Using the cone on the tip of the tubing prevents the end of the tube from poking into the side of the bowel and injuring the bowel and helps hold the fluid in the bowel (see Figure 36-10). Lubricate the end of the cone with a large amount of lubricating jelly.

The client may be seated on the toilet or lying in bed. Take off the ostomy pouch and apply an irrigation sleeve (see Figure 36-11). Both ends of the irrigation sleeve are open. The wide end goes over the stoma so that the stoma can be reached through the top of the sleeve. The narrow end of the sleeve goes into the toilet or bedpan. Elevate the bag of warm solution to about 18 inches above the bowel, and gently insert the lubricated cone into the bowel. Unclamp the tube and allow the water to run into the bowel. If the client complains of cramping, slow the flow of water or stop and withdraw the cone allowing some of the water to drain out into the toilet or bedpan. Instill the water and remove the cone from the bowel. Close the top of the irrigation sleeve and allow the water and stool to return into the toilet or bedpan.

It may take up to forty-five minutes for all the solution and stool to return. The irrigation sleeve may be left on the client with the end of the irrigation sleeve clamped and brought up and tucked into the belt so the client may walk around or the sleeve may be placed on the bed while the client rests. After forty-five minutes, remove the irrigation sleeve and replace with a regular pouch or dressing.

Document in the client's record how much solution was used, type of solution, how the client tolerated the procedure, the results of the irrigation, and assessment of the abdomen and stoma. Any teaching that was done should also be documented along with the client's acceptance of the ostomy and understanding of the teaching.

Obtaining Supplies

One of the client's first questions will be how to obtain ostomy supplies. There are several mail order suppliers and drug and medical supply stores from which to obtain supplies for clients. The ET nurse

will know where to obtain supplies in the specific area. The AARP has a mail order supply service that is reasonable in price. A supply of ostomy equipment should be sent home with the client.

Support Person

Adjusting to living with an ostomy is often difficult, and the client and family will be grateful for any help offered to them. Upon discharge, the client and family should receive the telephone number of the hospital and unit where treatment was received so they may call if questions arise. The ET nurse will also give her telephone number to the client and family for follow-up questions.

The surgeon is also available for questions and will want to see the client in four to six weeks at the office. Suggest that the client and family write down questions for that visit. Seeing the ET nurse again in four to six weeks is sometimes recommended to check on how the client is doing with ostomy care.

Information about the United Ostomy Association (UOA) should be sent home with the client. Hopefully, a visitor has called on the client or will call on the client at home and invite them to come to a UOA meeting.

Other Concerns

"When will I be able to have intercourse?" is a question that most clients think but may not ask. Information to answer this question should be provided in the discharge teaching. After surgery, intercourse is usually allowed after the four- to six-week checkup. Small pouches that the client could wear during intercourse are available. Pouch covers, and backless or crotchless underwear that can conceal a pouch for intimate moments are also available.

When the client returns home, the diet should be low residue at first until the bowel heals. Following a low-residue diet means avoiding foods high in residue or roughage. Foods high in roughage include raw vegetables, dried fruits, oatmeal, whole grain products, nuts or seeds, meats in casings, wild rice, coconut, and popcorn. These should all be avoided. It is a good idea to introduce new foods one at a time to see how they affect the person's stools. This way the client can tell which foods cause more flatus and/or odor.

Exercise is encouraged after surgery. When the client feels like starting to exercise, the physician should be consulted. As with any exercise program the client should be advised to start slowly. Endurance is built as the client's tolerance permits. Having ostomy surgery is no reason to stop any activity. People with ostomies live full active productive lives.

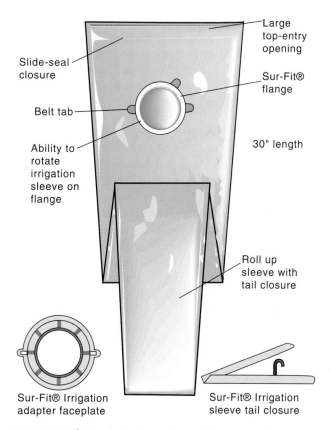

Sur-Fit® Irrigation Sleeve
(two-piece system)

Slide-seal closure

Belt tab

Ability to rotate irrigation sleeve on flange

Large top-entry opening

Sur-Fit® flange

30" length

Roll up sleeve with tail closure

Sur-Fit® Irrigation adapter faceplate

Sur-Fit® Irrigation sleeve tail closure

FIGURE 36-11 Irrigation sleeve. (*Courtesy of Convatec, Skillmah, NJ*)

▶ *CASE STUDY*

Mr. T.J. was admitted to the surgical unit after having an ileostomy with a total colectomy. His entire large intestine was removed due to ulcerative colitis. The incision is covered with a thick gauze surgical dressing; it is dry and intact. The stoma, on the right side of the abdomen, is pouched with an empty, two-piece transparent pouching system. The stoma is red and appears edematous.

Mr. T.J. has an IV of D51/2NS infusing at 125 cc per hour. There is a Jackson-Pratt drain from the lower right abdomen with a small amount of serous drainage in it, and the bulb is compressed. He has a nasogastric tube connected to low, continuous suction. He is drowsy, and responds to his name easily. Mr. T.J.'s vitals are stable; he is comfortable and his family seems supportive.

In the evening, after being medicated for pain, he stands by the side of the bed and marches in place. He is aware of his incision and notices that there is some yellow-green effluent in the pouch on his side. His first response is to make a face and look away.

In the morning Mr. T.J. asks his nurse if the stoma will always be so large. The nurse reassures Mr. T.J. that the stoma will shrink for the first six to eight weeks. As the nurse empties the yellow-green effluent from the ileostomy pouch, she explains the procedure in simple terms. Mr. T.J. looks away and does not seem to pay attention.

The following questions will guide your development of a Nursing Care Plan for the case study.

1. What assessment data in the case study would support the nursing diagnosis of altered body image?

2. Which nursing diagnosis is most important for Mr. T.J. at this time?

3. Develop a short-term goal for Mr. T.J. related to the nursing diagnosis from question 2.

4. List three interventions that you could use in a care plan for Mr. T.J. related to the nursing diagnosis in question 2.

5. Develop outcome criteria for Mr. T.J. that could be used to evaluate your plan of care.

SUMMARY

- An ostomy diverts waste to the outside of the body.
- This surgery is done to remove blockages or repair damage to the gastrointestinal or urinary tract.
- Names of the ostomies are taken from the segment of bowel used to create the stoma.
- Postoperatively, the stoma is checked for color and swelling.
- The stoma has no nerve endings for touch, and may bleed easily when touched.
- Problems specific to ostomy surgery are necrotic stoma, obstruction, hernia, skin excoriation, and inverted stoma.
- Some type of pouching device is necessary after most ostomy surgeries.
- Ostomies are being created with internal pouches made of intestine that are catheterized several times a day to empty.
- The client needs to learn how to change and empty the external pouch or how to catheterize the internal pouch.
- The change in body image is often difficult for the client to deal with.
- Written information on self-care of the ostomy should be provided to the client.
- Give the client names and telephone numbers of whom to call for help. These may include, but are not limited to, the nursing staff, doctor, ET nurse, or/and the United Ostomy Association (UOA).
- Home care may be arranged to help with ostomy teaching.

Review Questions

1. On what would the nurse focus his assessment when a preoperative client is to have an ostomy?

   a. postoperative breathing exercises
   b. the client's knowledge and acceptance of surgery
   c. on the IV fluid and tubing for surgery
   d. vital signs and last bowel movement

2. Postoperatively, an ostomy client's pouch is starting to leak. What is the best action?

   a. Call the ET nurse to come change the pouch.
   b. Change the pouch as fast as possible since the client does not like to see the stoma.
   c. Change the pouch as soon as possible, because the effluent will injure his skin if left very long.
   d. Place a piece of tape over the spot that is leaking and report to the next shift to watch the leak.

3. Which of the following is an appropriate behavioral objective for a client with an urostomy prior to discharge?

   a. Empty the pouch once a day.
   b. Increase intake of orange juice.
   c. Change the appliance without assistance.
   d. Rinse the pouch once a week with water.

4. The ostomy client in room 300 is 5 hours postoperative. Assessment of his stoma reveals it is an edematous dusky to black stoma. What should the nurse do with this information?

   a. Document carefully what the stoma looked like.
   b. Tell the nurse in charge.
   c. Document the appearance of the stoma and tell the charge nurse.
   d. Cover the client back up and check the client in 30 minutes.

5. A client who becomes upset and refuses to eat after the ileostomy appliance leaks should be advised that:

   a. bowel activity will not cease by fasting.
   b. limiting fluid intake will reduce leakage.
   c. elimination can be controlled by irrigation.
   d. unless eating is resumed intravenous feeding will be required.

6. A client with a new ostomy asks her nurse on the first day postoperative day, "Will this stoma be big and red like this forever?" What is the best response?

   a. "I know it looks awful. I'm glad I don't have to live with that."
   b. "I don't know, but I can find out for you."
   c. "The stoma will always be pink to red, but that swelling will go down in six to eight weeks."
   d. "How do you feel about having that stoma on your abdomen?"

7. On the fourth day after surgery, a new ostomy client asks you if he might be able to irrigate his ostomy. He has heard that some people do not have to wear pouches when they irrigate their ostomies. What is the best reply?

   a. "Maybe you will be able to regulate your ostomy by watching your diet."
   b. "Irrigation to manage an ostomy is only done with colostomies, or ostomies that have a storage segment of bowel."
   c. "Irrigation of an ileostomy may be dangerous and would not regulate the ostomy"
   d. "Your doctor will be able to answer that question for you."

8. You are working when an ostomy client who was discharged two weeks ago calls from home to ask what she should do. Her husband went shopping and her pouch is starting to leak. What is the best suggestion?

   a. Wait until her husband gets home; the stores close in two hours.

   b. Use this opportunity to encourage her to change her pouch by herself.

   c. Ask if she would call back tomorrow when the ET nurse is there.

   d. Have her call her home health care nurse for assistance.

Critical Thinking Questions

1. Make a teaching plan for a client with a new ileostomy.

2. Make a teaching plan for a client with a new colostomy.

News Flash

For male clients with bladder cancer, there is a new procedure being used, to create a new bladder that can be attached to the urethra. The longer male urethra with its sphincter is attached to a pouch made from a loop of bowel much like the continent ostomy pouches. (*Conva-Tec, Skillmah, NJ*)

New Products

New products for ostomy care are routinely introduced. One of the latest is a one-piece flushable pouch by Conva-Tec. The pouch fits into a thin flexible sleeve for flushing, so the pouch will not get caught in the plumbing. (*Conva-Tec, Skillmah, NJ*)

UNIT
12

Integration of Body Systems

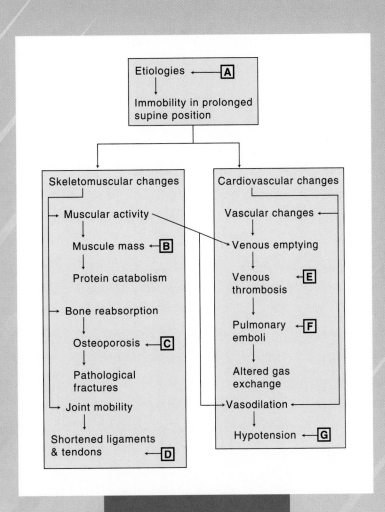

CHAPTER
37

Critical Thinking on Multiple Systems

Gena Duncan

LEARNING OBJECTIVE

Upon completion of this chapter the learner should be able to:
- Experience critical thinking by integrating a condition to several body systems and multiple clinical problems.

▶ MAKING THE CONNECTION

Through careful study of Chapters 1–36 you have sharpened your critical thinking skills and developed a knowledge base to prepare you for the exercises in this chapter. Each critical thinking exercise begins with an index of the body systems relevant to the case study. You may find it useful to refer back to these chapters as you work through the case study.

INTRODUCTION

The format of this chapter is different than that of the other chapters. It is an opportunity to apply critical thinking skills and problem solving techniques to several case studies that encompass more than one body system. Information gleaned from previous chapters will be applied to develop a holistic, integrated view of multiple body systems. An example is diabetes mellitus, a condition with multiple aspects that affect other body systems such as the integumentary, nervous, mus-

culoskeletal, cardiac, vascular, blood, gastrointestinal, urinary, and reproductive systems.

Read the case study, then analyze the relationship of the condition to other body systems. It may be helpful to first outline the condition presented in the case study by making a grid of the pathophysiology, diagnostic studies, signs and symptoms, and nursing interventions. Refer to the grid in answering the questions.

The case study questions can be completed alone, in a study group, or in a classroom setting. Once the case studies have been completed, share the answers and charts with the entire group to enhance the learning experience. Keep in mind that each student or group of students may arrive at the answers or present the answers in a different manner. The process one takes in finding the answer is less important than the opportunity to use critical thinking skills, as long as sound, logical, nursing judgment is used in obtaining an appropriate answer. This is an opportunity to think creatively and freely.

KEY ABBREVIATIONS

The following abbreviations and acronyms are used in this chapter:

AP	apical pulse
BP	blood pressure
DM	diabetes mellitus
IDDM	insulin dependent diabetes mellitus
NIDDM	non-insulin dependent diabetes mellitus
R	respirations

SYSTEMS REVIEWED IN DIABETES MELLITUS EXERCISE

- Vascular (Chapter 21)
- Integumentary (Chapter 23)
- Nervous (Chapter 27)
- Sensory (Chapter 28)
- Endocrine (Chapter 29)
- Male Reproductive (Chapter 32)
- Urinary (Chapter 35)

CRITICAL THINKING EXERCISE WITH DIABETES MELLITUS

Mr. Phillips, a forty-six-year-old insurance salesman, is admitted to the hospital with the diagnosis of insulin dependent diabetes mellitus (IDDM).

- List the etiological risk factors for IDDM.
- Brainstorm subjective and objective data that would be included in the assessment of Mr. Phillips.
- Develop a patho-flow diagram identifying the symptoms Mr. Phillips may have been experiencing on admission and relate the pathophysiology of diabetes mellitus to the symptoms (see the examples of a patho-flow diagram in Figure 37-1 and an interrelationship chart in Figure 37-2).

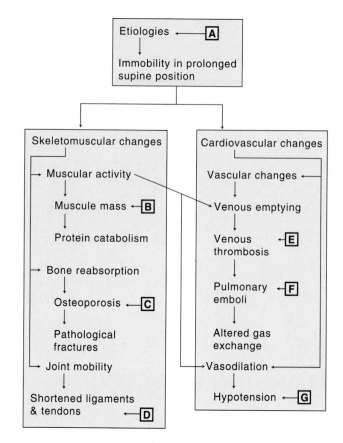

FIGURE 37-1 An example of a patho-flow diagram. Skeletomuscular and cardiovascular changes due to immobility. Complete the following instructions corresponding to the letters located at specific points along the pathophysiological sequence of events. A: List the high-risk conditions that may lead to immobility. B: Name the assessment data at this point. C: List the interventions that would minimize calcium loss. D: Name the outcome criteria associated with effective nursing interventions at this point. E: State the assessment data at this point. F: List the interventions that may prevent the development of this complication. G: List the nursing interventions to minimize this consequence. (*Courtesy of the Journal of Nursing Education*)

- What diagnostic tests could the physician have ordered to confirm the diagnosis of diabetes mellitus?
- Relate the possible results of the diagnostic tests to the pathophysiological cause of the results on the patho-flow diagram.
- If Mr. Phillips had been diagnosed with NIDDM, how would the pathophysiology and nursing care vary?

A couple of days after Mr. Phillips had been diagnosed with DM he said to the nurse, "One of my friends at work said there are a lot of future problems with diabetes. I am concerned about this. What are some of the problems? What can I do not to have these problems?"

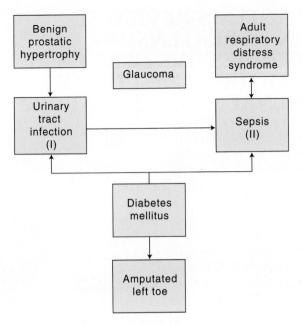

FIGURE 37-2 Interrelationships of conditions and symptoms. (*Courtesy of the Journal of Nursing Education*)

- What would be appropriate responses of the nurse?
- What resources or support groups could Mr. Phillips be referred to in this locale?

The discharge teaching included insulin administration, diet, exercise, foot care, and eye exams.

- What is important to include in the discharge teaching regarding:

  insulin administration
  diet
  exercise
  foot care
  eye exams

- Develop a care plan for Mr. Phillips.

Eight years after Mr. Phillips was diagnosed with DM, he had a routine physical examination. At that time his BP was 174/96. The physician monitored the BP for three weeks and then placed Mr. Phillips on enalapril maleate (Vasotec). His urine had a trace of albumin.

- Physiologically what could be occurring to cause Mr. Phillips to have hypertension, which is a common complication of diabetes?
- How does the action of enalapril maleate (Vasotec) lower the BP?
- What is the rationale for placing Mr. Phillips on enalapril maleate (Vasotec) rather than propranolol hydrochloride (Inderal), verapamil (Calan), or clonidine hydrochloride (Catapres)?

- What other complications could have a circulatory etiology?
- What could be the possible long-term renal complication from diabetes mellitus?
- Explain the pathophysiology of renal complications as they relate to DM. Relate these to the patho-flow diagram previously developed.

One evening, Mr. Phillips was massaging his foot while watching television. He noticed an ulcerated area between his third and fourth toe.

- State possible reasons Mr. Phillips may not have felt pain from the ulcerated area. Relate these to the patho-flow diagram previously developed.

During a yearly physical Mr. Phillips relates difficulty obtaining an erection.

- Explain the rationale for this complication.
- What nursing interventions would be appropriate at this time?

In later years, Mr. Phillips may experience some symptoms from autonomic neuropathies.

- List symptoms that may occur and relate the symptoms to the pathophysiological etiology.

SYSTEMS REVIEWED IN CIRRHOSIS EXERCISE

- Respiratory (Chapter 19)
- Cardiac (Chapter 20)
- Vascular (Chapter 21)
- Blood and Lymph (Chapter 22)
- Integumentary (Chapter 23)
- Musculoskeletal (Chapter 26)
- Nervous (Chapter 27)
- Endocrine (Chapter 29)
- Digestive (Chapter 34)
- Urinary (Chapter 35)

CRITICAL THINKING EXERCISE WITH CIRRHOSIS

Sam Lightfoot, a sixty-year-old male of American Indian descent, was admitted to the hospital with hematemesis. He has a history of alcohol abuse. Sam's wife and two daughters accompany him. Sam is 5′ 10″ tall and weighs 140 lbs. His vital signs are T 98.2, AP 98 and slightly irregular, R 24, BP 152/88. He is lethargic, confused, and jaundiced. When the nurse assessed his lung sounds, she heard pulmonary crackles in all lobes. His abdominal girth measures 44 inches. His wife states he has not gone to the bathroom all morning. He has +3 edema in his feet and ankles. Sam's primary diagnosis is hematemesis with a secondary diagnosis of cirrhosis.

- Brainstorm other subjective and objective data that are important to include in the assessment of Sam Lightfoot.
- Relate the pathophysiology of cirrhosis to the assessed symptoms and other symptoms Sam may have experienced. Develop a patho-flow chart relating the symptoms to the pathological cause.
- List diagnostic tests that would be appropriate for the physician to order for Sam. What abnormal laboratory results would be typical of cirrhosis?
- Relate the possible results of the diagnostic tests to the developed patho-flow chart.
- Besides alcohol abuse, what are some other causes of cirrhosis?
- List complications of cirrhosis caused by chronic alcohol abuse.
- Explain the pathophysiology of portal hypertension as it relates to cirrhosis. Relate these to the patho-flow chart previously developed.
- List diuretics that may be ordered for Sam to decrease the ascites.
- How does the action of lactulose (Cephulac) lower the level of ammonia in the blood?
- What other complications result from portal hypertension?
- Explain the rationale for the complication of pleural effusion.
- Identify possible nursing diagnoses for Sam.
- What nursing interventions would be appropriate at this time?
- Develop a care plan for Sam Lightfoot.
- If Sam's condition improved and he was scheduled for discharge, what is important to include in the discharge teaching regarding:

    bleeding tendencies
    exercise
    weight gain
    skin care

- Explain diet instructions for Sam Lightfoot. Consider cultural influence in the diet instructions.
- List local resources/support groups where Sam and his family could be referred.

Sam's daughter, Mary, says, "I wish Dad would have quit drinking years ago. I was always embarrassed by his behavior when he had too much to drink. His life could have had so much potential."

- What would be appropriate responses of the nurse?

SYSTEMS REVIEWED IN HYPERTENSION, CONGESTIVE HEART FAILURE, AND CHRONIC RENAL FAILURE EXERCISE

- Respiratory (Chapter 19)
- Cardiac (Chapter 20)
- Vascular (Chapter 21)
- Blood and Lymph (Chapter 22)
- Integumentary (Chapter 23)
- Allergies, Immune and Autoimmune (Chapter 24)
- Musculoskeletal (Chapter 26)
- Nervous (Chapter 27)
- Endocrine (Chapter 29)
- Female Reproductive (Chapter 31)
- Digestive (Chapter 34)
- Urinary (Chapter 35)

CRITICAL THINKING EXERCISE WITH HYPERTENSION, CONGESTIVE HEART FAILURE, AND CHRONIC RENAL FAILURE

Trina Brown, a forty-year-old African American female, has had hypertension for twenty years. She has been noncompliant in taking her antihypertensive medications that were prescribed by her physician. She has recently developed symptoms of congestive heart failure and renal failure.

- Brainstorm some reasons for Trina's noncompliance.
- Name some medications that may have been prescribed to treat Trina's hypertension. List the advantage and disadvantage of each medication.
- Using Table 35-2 Chronic Renal Failure Effects on Body Systems, develop a concept map showing the relationship of hypertension to the effects of renal failure on each listed system.
- What is the relationship between hypertension, increased peripheral resistance, cardiac hypertrophy, and congestive heart failure?
- What is the relationship of blood pressure (hypotension and hypertension) and renal failure?
- What is the relationship between the heart's decreasing ability to pump blood through the blood vessels and pulmonary edema?
- Explain the relationship between fluid in the alveoli and dyspnea.

- Physiologically, what is occurring in Trina's body to cause an increased rate of respiration?
- List laboratory results that would indicate that Trina is developing chronic renal failure.
- List symptoms that would indicate Trina is developing chronic renal failure.
- List subjective and objective data for which the nurse would assess for symptoms of chronic renal failure.
- List laboratory results that would indicate that Trina is developing congestive heart failure.
- List symptoms that would indicate Trina is developing congestive heart failure? Give the cause/etiology for each symptom.
- List subjective and objective data for which the nurse would assess for symptoms of congestive heart failure.
- Identify possible nursing diagnoses for Trina.
- List nursing interventions and give rationale for each intervention.

Trina's abdomen is distended and she has lost her appetite for the last two days. She has had hiccups constantly for two hours. She says, "I am so tired of these hiccups. Why am I having them?"

- Explain to Trina the cause for her hiccups.

SUMMARY

Perhaps this may have been the first time facts learned in anatomy and physiology were related to a disease process, or understanding was gained as to the reason clients have particular symptoms with the disease condition. When clients are ill, they rarely have only one disorder, but several inter-related conditions. The purpose of these exercises was to provide an opportunity to think through these situations before they are encountered in a clinical situation. In applying critical thinking skills to the case studies in this chapter, pertinent questions have been asked, clinical situations evaluated and clinical decisions made, much the way it is done in the clinical environment as a student and as a nurse. In working through these questions, analyzing and synthesizing skills were utilized. Perhaps a renewed interest and awe at the complexity of the body was gained upon discovering the inter-relatedness of the body systems. Hopefully, the critical thinking experience is a catalyst to becoming a proficient, critical thinking nurse.

AB index Ankle to brachial arterial blood pressure, obtained by dividing the blood pressure reading in the ankle by the blood pressure reading in the arm.

abortion Termination of pregnancy before the age of fetal viability. May be spontaneous or induced.

abuse Reliance on a substance, but to a lesser degree than dependence. Abstinence does not cause physical withdrawal or psychological craving.

acceptance Acknowledgment that death is inevitable.

accreditation The process of confirming the quality of care provided by an institution or facility by ensuring minimum standards are met.

acculturation The modification of one's cultural values, attitudes and behavior as a result of contact with another culture to become an accepted member of that culture.

acidosis An abnormally high serum hydrogen ion concentration resulting in an arterial blood pH below 7.35.

Acquired Immunodeficiency Syndrome (AIDS) A progressively fatal disease that destroys the immune system and is caused by the human immunodeficiency virus.

acromegaly Gradual marked enlargement and elongation of the bones of the face, jaw, and extremities caused by overproduction of the growth hormone. This chronic disease occurs in middle-aged individuals.

active listening The process of hearing spoken words and noting nonverbal behaviors. Requires energy and concentration.

active transport The movement of substances across cell membranes with the help of chemical energy and specific carrier molecules.

acute pain Pain that has lasted less than six months, usually associated with a specific injury or disease that has caused tissue damage.

addiction An overwhelming preoccupation with obtaining and using a drug for its *psychic* effects. Used interchangeably with dependence.

adhesions A fibrous band of scar tissue that holds structures together and results from trauma or inflammation. Can lead to bowel obstructions in the abdominal cavity.

adjuvant A drug used with another drug to increase or hasten the effect of the other drug.

adult day care The provision of a variety of services in a protective setting for adults who are unable to stay alone, but do not need 24 hour care.

advanced directives Instructions about an individual's health care preferences regarding life sustaining measures that guide family members and health care professionals as to what treatment options should or should not be considered in the event that the individual is unable to decide for herself, i.e. Living Will and Durable Power of Attorney for Health Care.

adventitious Abnormal sounds, including sibilant wheezes (formerly wheezes), sonorous wheezes (formerly rhonchi), crackles (formerly rales) and pleural friction rubs.

adventitious breath sounds Abnormal breath sounds.

advocate A person, such as a nurse or other health care provider, who supports or protects those who cannot support or protect themselves, such as the very young, the very old, those who are debilitated, the mentally incompetent or those under the influence of medications, and those who are uninformed.

affect The outward expression of one's feelings.

agnosia inability to recognize, either by sight or sound, familiar objects such as a hairbrush.

agnostic Individuals who believe that the existence of God cannot be proved or disproved.

agranulocytosis An acute condition causing a severe reduction in the number of granulocytes (basophils, eosinophils, and neutrophils).

Aldrete Score Scoring system developed by J. Antonio Aldrete, MD, MS. to objectively assess the physical status of clients recovering from anesthesia and serve as a basis for dismissal from the postanesthesia care unit (PACU) and ambulatory surgery. (Also known as the Post-Anesthetic Recovery Score)

alkalosis An abnormally low serum hydrogen ion concentration resulting in an arterial blood pH above 7.45.

Allen's test An exam to evaluate the arterial circulation of the hands.

allergen Any substance that causes an allergy.

allergic response A hypersensitivity response to a substance to which an organism has been exposed and has developed antibodies.

allocation of funds The distribution of resources according to a plan.

alopecia Partial or complete baldness or loss of hair. Causes include illness, malnutrition, effects of chemotherapeutic drugs, drug reactions, hormonal imbalances or heredity.

amenorrhea Absence of menstruation. May be primary (when menses never occur) or secondary (when menses have previously occured but have ceased).

amnesia The inability to remember things. Amnesia caused by anesthetic drugs is temporary.

amphiarthrosis Slightly movable joints such as the vertebrae.

amplitude The fullness or quality of each beat of the heart.

analgesia Pain relief without producing anesthesia. Absence of pain in a situation that would normally be painful.

analgesic A substance that relieves pain.

anaphylaxis A systemic reaction to allergens.

anasarca Generalized edema.

anastomose Surgical connection of tubular structures.

androgenic Causing masculinization.

anemia A common hematopoietic disorder in which the client has a decreased number of RBCs and a low hemoglobin level.

aneroid Operating without fluid; utilizing atmospheric pressure instead of a liquid like mercury.

anesthesia The absence of the sensation of pain caused by either the temporary interruption of nerve impulse transmission (regional anesthesia), complete loss of consciousness (general anesthesia), or by disease or injury.

anesthesiologist A person educated and skilled in the delivery of anesthesia who also adds to the knowledge of anesthesia through research or other scholarly pursuits. In the United States this term is used to indicate a licensed physician (MD) who has completed a residency in the field of anesthesia, preferably board certified by the American Board of Anesthesiology or an osteopath (DO) who specializes in anesthesia.

anesthetist General term for a person educated and skilled in the delivery of anesthesia. This term would apply both to Certified Registered Nurse Anesthetists (CRNAs) and Physician Anesthesiologists. In the United States the term anesthetist is most commonly used in reference to a qualified RN, dentist, or a MD who administers anesthetics under the direct supervision of an anesthesiologist or a surgeon.

aneurysm A localized dilation occurring in a weakened section of an artery's medial layer.

angina pectoris Chest pain caused by a narrowing of the coronary arteries.

angioedema Painful, subcutaneous or submucosal swelling of the face, lips, neck, hands, feet, larynx and abdomen often caused by an allergic reaction (also called angioneurotic edema).

angioma Benign vascular tumor involving skin and subcutaneous tissue; most are congenital. Birth marks such as the port wine birthmark (dark red/purple patch) or the strawberry birthmark.

annulus The valvular ring of the heart.

anorexia Loss of appetite.

anosognosia Unawareness of deficits.

antibiotic resistance The ability of bacteria to develop resistance to a previously effective antimicrobial agent.

antibodies Proteins produced by plasma cells in lymph tissue which react with antigens to neutralize or destroy them.

anticipatory grieving Feelings of grief prior to rather than following a loss.

antigens Substances which interact with specific antibodies.

antineoplastic An agent that inhibits the growth and reproduction of malignant cells.

antinuclear antibodies (ANAs) Antibodies that attack the nuclei of cells.

aphasia Inability to communicate. Expressive aphasia is difficulty transforming sound into speech. Receptive aphasia is impairment of the comprehension of the spoken word, that is, the client can physically speak, but incorrectly uses words. Global aphasia is a combination of expressive and receptive aphasia. Often the result of a brain lesion.

areflexia Absence of reflexes.

arteriosclerosis A vascular narrowing and hardening of arteries.

arthrocentesis Procedure done to obtain fluid from a joint using a sterile needle.

arthrodesis Fusion to permanently immobilize a joint.

arthrogram Visualization of a joint by x-ray.

arthroplasty Surgical reconstruction of a joint.

articulation Junction of two or more bones; a joint.

ascites Abnormal accumulation of fluid in the peritoneal cavity containing large amounts of protein and electrolytes. Commonly occurs when the portal vein is obstructed.

asepsis The absence of pathogenic microorganisms.

aseptic technique A collection of principles used to control and/or prevent the transfer of microorganisms from sources within (endogenous) and outside of (exogenous) the client. Used in surgery and other procedures when a sterile field is required.

assault The threat to do something that may cause harm or be unpleasant to another person.

assisted living A combination of housing and services to older persons who require assistance with activities of daily living.

assisted suicide A health professional's deliberate assistance in facilitating a client's death.

asthma Condition characterized by intermittent airway obstruction due to an antigen antibody reaction.

astigmatism Asymmetric focus of light rays on the retina.

ataxia Lack of coordination of voluntary muscle action.

atheists Individuals who do not believe in God or any other deity.

atherosclerosis A fatty deposit on the inner lining, the tunica intima, of vessel walls.

audible wheezes Wheezes which can be heard without the aid of a stethoscope.

aura Peculiar sensation preceding a seizure, may be of taste, smell, sight, hearing, dizziness, or just a "funny feeling."

auscultation To listen for sounds in the body, generally through a stethoscope.

autoimmune disorder Diseases where the immunological response of the body is directed against itself.

autologous From the same organism (person).

automatic implantable cardioverter-defibrillator (AICD) An implantable device that senses a dysrhythmia and automatically sends an electrical shock directly to the heart to defibrillate it.

automatism A mechanical, repetitive motor behavior performed unconsciously.

autonomic dysreflexia A response occurring in quadriplegics or paraplegics with symptoms of hypertension, bradycardia, and seizure activity that can result in a stroke or death. Also autonomic hyperreflexia.

autonomic nervous system The part of the peripheral nervous system consisting of the sympathetic and parasympathetic nervous systems.

autonomy An individual's right of self-determination, independence and freedom.

autopsy Examination of the body after death by a pathologist.

autosomal Pertaining to a condition transmitted by a non-sex chromosome.

azotemia Nitrogenous wastes present in the blood.

bacteria Any of a group of microorganisms capable of causing infectious diseases in humans, plants, or animals. They are classified as spherical, ovoid, rod-shaped or spiral.

bands Immature neutrophils.

bargaining A process used by a dying individual in which the individual enters into an arrangement with God to postpone the inevitable conclusion.

baseline level A lab value that serves as a reference point for future value levels.

battery The unauthorized or unwanted touching of one person by another.

behavioral tolerance Compensatory adjustments of behavior made under the influence of a particular substance.

Bellevue bridge Adhesive strapping used to elevate the scrotum to reduce swelling.

beneficence Within the health care setting, the act of "doing good" for clients who are receiving care.

benign A tumor that is not cancerous and does not spread to other areas of the body.

bereavement A mourning process for what was and what will be as a result of the loss of a loved one.

bioethics Philosophical ethics applied to biology, medicine, nursing, theology, social work, law and other fields that deal with health care. Bioethics involves case law and philosophical ethics.

biologic response modifiers Compounds that fight cancer by stimulating the body's immune system.

biopsy Removal of a small piece of living tissue for microscopic examination.

blastic phase An intensified phase of leukemia that resembles an acute phase in which there is an increased production of WBCs.

bone marrow suppression Decreased function of bone marrow that manufactures erythrocytes, leukocytes and platelets.

borborygmi Loud, rushing sounds produced by the movement of gas in the abdomen.

bradykinesia Slowness of voluntary movement.

breakthrough pain Sudden, acute, temporary pain that is usually precipitated by a treatment, procedure, or unusual activity of the client.

Brodie-Trendelenburg's test An exam to test the ability of the venous valves to hold blood at a certain level in the vein and not allow the blood to retrograde. Also called Trendelenburg's test or retrograde filling test.

bronchial breath sounds Breath sounds that are normally heard over the bronchi, considered abnormal if heard in other sites; tubular, hollow-like sounding breath sounds.

bronchovesicular breath sounds Breath sounds normally heard in the area of the scapula and near the sternum, considered abnormal if heard in other areas; breath sounds are medium in pitch and intensity with an inspiratory and expiratory phase of equal length.

bruxism Grinding teeth during sleep.

buffer systems Chemical or biological mechanisms which promote the absorption or excretion of hydrogen ions to compensate for acid-base imbalances.

cachectic Being in a state of malnutrition and wasting.

cachexia State of malnutrition.

calculus Concentration of mineral salts in the body leading to the formation of a stone. Can occur in the gallbladder, urinary tract or kidneys.

carcinogen Any substance that initiates or promotes the development of cancer.

carcinoma Cancer occurring in epithelial tissue.

cardiac catheterization An exam in which a catheter is passed into the right and/or left side of the heart to determine oxygen levels, cardiac output, and pressures within the heart chambers.

cardiac cycle When an impulse has completely gone through the conduction system of the heart, and the ventricles have contracted.

cardiac output The volume of blood pumped by the left or right ventricle per minute.

cardiac tamponade Collection of fluid in the pericardial sac hindering the functioning of the heart.

carina The point at which the trachea divides into the bronchi.

case management A system designed by insurance companies in an attempt to limit the cost of health care. Prior approval from the insurance company is necessary before a client can be admitted for acute care. A case manager, usually a nurse, evaluates the client to verify the necessity of admission; monitors the care giver; and sets a discharge date.

caseation A process in which the center of the primary tubercle formed in the lungs with TB becomes soft and cheese-like as a result of decreased perfusion.

cauterize To destroy tissue by using electricity to burn an area.

cavitation Process in which a cavity is created in the lung tissue when a primary tubercle liquefies and ruptures.

ceiling effect The dosage beyond which no analgesia occurs.

cellular immunity A type of acquired immunity involving T cell lymphocytes.

central nervous system Consists of the brain and spinal cord.

cephalalgia A headache. Also cephalgia.

cerebral (brain) death The point at which brain cells die as a result of cardiac arrest.

certification A voluntary process that establishes and evaluates standards of care. The process is mandatory for any health care services receiving federal funds.

cerumen A yellowish-brown protective substance, secreted by ceruminous glands, that line the external ear canal and guard against certain bacteria, small insects and traps dust and debris that may damage the inner ear. There are two kinds of cerumen, waxy and dry.

chancre A painless, syphilitic primary ulcer appearing two to three weeks after infection at the site of body contact.

chemoreceptors Receptors found in the aortic and carotid arteries that are sensitive to the level of carbon dioxide in the blood.

chemotherapy Use of drugs to treat illness, especially cancer.

Cheyne-Stokes respirations Breathing characterized by periods of apnea alternating with periods of dyspnea.

chorea Involuntary twitching of extremities or facial muscles.

chronic pain Pain that has lasted longer than the expected healing time. Usually, pain lasting longer than six months.

Chvostek's sign An abnormal spasm of the facial muscles in response to a light tapping of the facial nerve.

chyme Mixture of partially digested food and digestive enzymes.

circulating nurse A RN responsible and accountable for all activities during a surgical procedure through management of personnel, equipment, supplies, the environment, and communication throughout the operation.

closed reduction Reduction of a fracture by external manipulation.

co-dependent A person who is overly affected by other people's behavior and tries to control them.

code of ethics assists members of a professional organization in choosing behaviors that are congruent with the values of the profession. They are those general standards and ideals which members of a group strive to achieve.

coitus interruptus Withdrawing the penis from the vagina before ejaculation.

colostomy An opening that may be created anywhere along the large intestine. Stool exits from that point through an abdominal stoma. A colostomy is performed for inflammatory disease, congenital malformations, cancer, abscesses fistulas obstructions, and perforations.

combination chemotherapy Administering a combination of chemotherapy drugs over a set period of time.

Commission on Accreditation of Rehabilitation Facilities The agency responsible for accrediting comprehensive inpatient rehabilitation programs.

communication The sending and receiving of a message.

competent Being legally qualified to make decisions.

concept A mental picture of abstract phenomenon which serves to organize observation related to that phenomenon. Examples of concepts in nursing are pain, caring, adaptation, grief, homeostasis.

conductive Having the ability to transmit, e.g. sound waves.

confabulation The making up of information to fill in memory gaps.

confidential The process of keeping matters private or secret. For example, information regarding a person's biographical, personal and financial data obtained from working with him or her should be kept private or confidential.

congruent Agreement between two things.

continuing care retirement communities The provision of continuing levels of care as the individual's health care needs change.

contraception Prevention of pregnancy by natural or artificial methods.

contracture Abnormal shortening of muscles usually resulting in a deformity of the part.

cordotomy Surgical ablation of the pain-conducting tracts in the dorsal horn of the spinal cord.

coroner An elected county official who is responsible for determining the cause of a person's death.

costally Relating to the ribs.

crackles Abnormal breath sound that resemble a popping noise, created as air moves through fluid.

crepitus A grating or crackling sensation or sound, caused by the discharge of gas from the intestines.

cretinism Severe congenital hypothyroidism resulting in dwarfism, mental retardation, and puffy facial features among other signs.

critical thinking That mode of thinking—about any subject, content or problem—in which the thinker improves the quality of his or her thinking by skillfully taking charge of the structures inherent in thinking and imposing intellectual standards (or a level of degree of quality) upon them.

cross tolerance A decreased sensitivity to other substances in the same category.

cultural diversity Differences in the beliefs, attitudes, values, and behaviors of individuals from different people groups.

cultural values Values determined by affiliation with a particular cultural group.

culture The integrated pattern of human knowledge, belief and behavior that depends upon man's capacity for learning, and transmitting knowledge to succeeding generations.

curative To heal or restore to health.

cyanosis Bluish discoloration of the skin and mucous membranes caused by an excess of deoxygenated hemoglobin in the blood. Can be observed in lips, nail beds and ear lobes.

cycloplegic Paralysis of the ciliary muscle of the eye.

cystocele Relaxation of the anterior vaginal wall allowing protrusion of the bladder into the vagina.

Cytomegalovirus (CMV) One of the herpes type viruses; inhabits the salivary glands.

dawn phenomenon An early morning glucose elevation in an insulin-dependent diabetic.

death rattle A breathing sound caused by a collection of fluids in the lungs in the period preceding death.

debride To remove dead or damaged tissue or foreign material from a wound.

decompress To relieve pressure in the gastrointestinal tract. A nasogastric tube or other tube inserted into the stomach or intestines is used to relieve the pressure. Pressure develops from bowel obstructions or immobility of the bowel after surgery.

degeneration The gradual deterioration of cells and tissues.

dehiscence A complication of wound healing where there is separation of the wound edges.

dementia A clinical syndrome characterized by decreased intellectual functioning, personality changes and decreased judgment.

denial Disbelief experienced by an individual when presented with information that is too overwhelming to immediately accept.

deontological An ethical theory that views actions as inherently right or wrong, without regard to the end result. Also known as a "duty-oriented" theory, the duty or moral obligation is based on moral absolutes revealed by a higher power, such as God.

dependence Reliance on a substance to such a degree that abstinence will cause functional impairment, and the individual will have physical withdrawal symptoms and/or psychological craving for the substance.

depolarization Neutralization or change in polarity.

depression Altered mood, with a loss of interest in things usually pleasurable. It may be the response of a terminally ill individual to the overwhelming number of losses experienced by the individual.

detoxification The removal of a substance, or the physiological effects of the substance from a person's body.

diabetes mellitus An endocrine disorder of the pancreas; a complex disorder of carbohydrate, fat and protein metabolism that is primarily a result of a relative or complete lack of insulin.

diabetic ketoacidosis (DKA) An acute, life-threatening complication of uncontrolled diabetes mellitus resulting in urinary loss of water, dehydration, electrolyte imbalance, and metabolic acidosis. Also known as diabetic coma.

diabetic nephropathy Renal disease and failure resulting as a long-term complication of diabetes.

diabetic neuropathy Inflammation or degeneration of nerves resulting as a long-term complication of diabetes.

diabetic retinopathy Changes in the small vessels of the retina associated with long term elevated serum glucose level.

dialysate The solution used in dialysis. Designed to approximate the normal electrolyte structure of plasma and extracellular fluid.

dialysis Process of blood moving across a semipermeable membrane to remove toxic materials and to maintain fluid, electrolyte, and acid-base balance.

diaphragmatic Breathing from the diaphragm.

diarthrosis A freely movable joint.

differentiation Acquiring functions different from those of the original.

diffusion The process by which a substance moves from an area of higher concentration to an area of lower concentration

dilatation and curettage (D & C) Surgical dilation of the cervix with instruments and scraping of the endometrial lining. May be performed for a diagnostic or therapeutic purpose.

diplopia Double vision.

discipline A branch of learning, field of study, or occupation requiring specialized knowledge.

disciplined Trained by instruction and exercise; mental faculties trained in habits of order, sobriety, and precision (as in a disciplined mind).

disseminated Scattered over an area, such as throughout the body or an organ.

distal Farthest from the center or trunk.

diverticula Sac-like protrusions of the intestinal wall that result when the mucosa herniates through the bowel wall. Believed to result from a low fiber diet.

dominant group The cultural group exercising the most control over a varied population.

dullness A low-pitched, thud-like sound heard during percussion. A dense organ like the liver will produce dullness. Ascites is another example of dullness.

durable power of attorney for health care An advance directive in which the individual (principal) names another individual to speak for the principal when the principal is unable to do so.

dysarthria Difficult and defective speech due to a dysfunction of the muscles used for speech.

dysarthria Impairment of speech muscles.

dysmenorrhea Painful cramping with the menstrual period, occurs more frequently in clients who have not borne a child.

dyspareunia Difficult or painful intercourse which may be related to structural or physiologic abnormalities.

dysphasia Impairment of speech resulting from damage to the speech center in the brain.

dyspnea Difficulty breathing.

ecchymosis Large, irregular hemorrhagic areas. Ecchymosis is caused by extravasation of blood into surrounding tissues. Also called a bruise.

echocardiogram An ultrasound of the heart.

edema An abnormal accumulation of fluid in the interstitial spaces of the body.

effluent The liquid output from a ileostomy.

ejection fraction A comparison of the volume of blood pumped by the left ventricle to total volume of blood left in the ventricle.

electrolytes Metered or dissolved element or compound that decomposes into ions and can conduct an electric current. Found in body fluids and are essential for normal body functioning.

embolus A mass, such as a blood clot or an air bubble, that circulates in the blood stream.

emotional lability Emotional instability.

empathy The capacity to understand another person's feelings.

empyema The formation of pus within a body cavity, usually refers to a primary infection of the lung.

endocrine The process of a group of cells secreting substances directly into the blood or lymph circulation and effecting another part of the body.

endometriosis Growth of endometrial tissue on structures outside of the uterus, within the pelvic cavity. Often associated as a cause of infertility.

endorphin Substances produced by the central nervous system that act like opioids. Word means "endogenous morphine."

environment The setting in which an individual lives and grows.

Enzyme-linked Immunosorbent Assay (ELISA) The basic screening test currently used to detect antibodies to HIV.

epidural analgesia Analgesics administered outside the dura mater of the spinal cord.

erythema Redness of the skin that may be caused by inflammation of tissues or by sunburn.

erythrocytapheresis A procedure that removes abnormal RBCs and replaces them with healthy RBCs.

erythropoiesis Production of red blood cells.

eschar A dry, dark, leathery scab composed of denatured protein that can result from a chemical or thermal burn, an infection, or an excoriating skin disease.

ethical dilemma A choice between equally undesirable alternatives where right and wrong actions are not clear cut.

ethical principles Common principles that are examined in ethical situations and include: autonomy, nonmaleficence, beneficence, justice, fidelity, and veracity.

ethical rights Rights or privileges based on moral principle and not legally guaranteed. Ethical rights are applied equally to all persons, regardless of income, gender, race, or nationality.

ethics A branch of philosophy originating in Ancient Greece that involves the consideration of what is right and what is wrong, or what causes good and what causes harm. When formalized, ethics are generally organized as systems of appropriate behaviors.

ethics committee A group of professionals from various disciplines that protect client interests, provide staff education in ethical analysis, and policy development for the management of ethical dilemmas.

ethnic group Individuals who share a unique cultural background and subscribe to common patterns of behavior and beliefs.

ethnocentric Individuals who believe in the supremacy of their own ethnic group.

ethnocentrism The belief that one's own cultural beliefs are the most desirable or the best.

eugenics An applied science concerned with improving the hereditary qualities of a species.

euthanasia The act of taking life in order to relieve suffering.

evisceration A complication of wound healing where there is complete separation of wound edges with visceral protrusion.

exacerbation Increase in the symptoms and severity of a disease.

exophthalmos Marked protrusion of the eyeballs resulting from increased orbital volume and caused by a variety of conditions including hyperthyroidism.

expiration The process of the diaphragm moving upward as air is released through the nose/mouth.

exposure An incidence of contact with an infected person or agent.

external respiration The exchange of gases between the atmosphere and the lungs.

extravasation Escape of fluid into the surrounding tissue.

false imprisonment The unlawful restraint of an individual's personal liberty or the unlawful detention of an individual.

fasciculation Involuntary twitching that does not move a joint. May be seen under the skin.

feedback The response from the receiver of a message so that the sender can verify the message.

felony A serious crime, such as drug diversion; conviction of a felony may result in loss of licensure and imprisonment for a year or more.

fibrinolysis The process of breaking fibrin apart.

fibrocystic breast disease Benign overgrowth of the fibrous tissue around the lobes within the breast. Associated with high caffeine intake which keeps hormones triggered to proliferate abnormal tissue growth.

fibroid (leiomyoma) Benign tumor which grows in the serous, mucous, or myometrial layers of the uterus.

fidelity The duty to be faithful to commitments.

filtration The movement of water and solutes from an area of high hydrostatic pressure to one of low hydrostatic pressure.

first assistant An associate of the surgeon, referring physician, or surgical resident who assists the surgeon to retract tissue, aids in the removal of blood and fluids at the operative site, and assists with hemostasis and wound closure.

fistula An abnormal communication between two or more normally disconnected structures or spaces. There are several different types of fistulas. For example, a connection between the intestine and body surface is called a enterocutaneous fistula; enteroenteric or enterocolonic fistulas are connections between two parts of intestines.

flatness A soft, high-pitched, flat sound produced by muscles.

fluid volume deficit A less than normal amount of water and sodium in intracellular and interstitial or intravascular fluids. May be caused by a lack of intake or abnormal loss.

fluid volume excess An excess accumulation of water and sodium in intracellular, interstitial or intravascular fluids.

fracture A break in the continuity of a bone.

fulguration Procedure to destroy tissue with high frequency electric sparks.

functional area Specialized areas of the brain.

functional assessment The process of looking at each individual client through the collection of a nursing history and identification of how that person adjusts, and/or lives within his/her environment.

gastrostomy Surgical placement of a feeding tube through the abdominal wall into the stomach as a means of providing nutrition.

gate control theory A theory proposing that sensory, motivational-affective, and cognitive processes all combine to determine how the person perceives pain.

gatekeeping Guarding professional standards of practice and behavior.

genogram A method of visualizing family members (children, parents, and grandparents) and their specific health problems.

geriatric nursing The specialty practice of caring for older adults.

gerontologic nursing The preferred term for the specialty practice of caring for older adults that reflects an emphasis on healthy aging rather than illness.

gerontology The study of the effects of normal aging and age-related diseases on human beings. A general term used by all health care and social services disciplines.

gestational diabetes Diabetes which develops during pregnancy.

Glasgow Coma Scale An objective, measurable tool for assessing consciousness in clients with head injuries.

glucagon A pancreatic hormone; glucagon stimulates release of glucose from the liver resulting in elevation of serum glucose.

glucose A simple sugar ingested or produced by digestion of many foods; a major source of energy.

glycogenesis The conversion of glucose into glycogen.

glycogenolysis The conversion of glycogen into glucose.

glycosuria The abnormal presence of glucose in the urine.

goiter A pronounced enlargement of the thyroid gland associated with hyperthyroidism, hypothyroidism, or normal levels of thyroid function.

gonorrhea A contagious inflammation of the genital mucous membrane of either sex, caused by the gonococcus bacterium, *Neisseria gonorrhoeae*.

Good Samaritan Law A series of statutes enacted to encourage health care professionals to stop and render assistance in emergency situations.

granulation tissue Delicate connective tissue consisting of fibroblasts, collagen and capillaries. Granulation tissue is soft and pink with fleshy projections visible in the wound base. It is part of the healing process of wounds that are healing by second intention.

greenstick An incomplete fracture.

grief/grieving A natural and normal subjective process of mourning that is experienced with a loss.

gynecology Specialized field of medicine or nursing related to disorders of the female reproductive system, other than those associated with pregnancy.

gynecomastia Abnormal enlargement of one or both breasts in males.

hallucinations Perceiving things that are not present in reality. May be visual, auditory, olfactory or tactile.

health According to the World Health Organization, the state of complete physical, mental and social well-being not merely the absence of disease or infirmity.

Health Care Finance Administration (HCFA) An agency of the federal government that administers the Medicare program.

Health Care Surrogate Law A law enacted by some states that provides a legal means for decision making in the absence of advance directives.

hearing The act or power of receiving sounds.

heart sound A sound heard by auscultating the heart.

hemarthrosis Bleeding into the joints.

hematemesis Vomiting of blood.

hematocrit Percentage of erythrocytes in a given volume of blood.

hematopoiesis Process of blood cell production and development.

hematuria Blood in the urine.

hemiparesis Weakness of one side of the body.

hemiplegia Paralysis of one side of the body.

hemolysis Destruction of red blood cells.

hepatomegaly An enlarged liver.

Herberden's nodes Enlargement of tubercles of last phalanges of fingers.

herpes genitalis A viral infection of the genital and anorectal skin and mucosa with herpes simplex virus type 2; classed as an STD.

hesitancy Difficulty initiating the urinary stream.

histamine A substance released during allergic reactions.

HIV-wasting An unexplained weight loss of more than 10% of body weight associated with either chronic diarrhea or fever in those infected with HIV.

Homan's sign An exam to check for the presence of clots in leg veins. The nurse dorsiflexes the foot. If there is pain in the calf of the leg or behind the knee, it may indicate the presence of a venous clot.

homeostasis A state of balance between the supply and demand of essential substances within the body.

homologous From a donor of the same species.

homonymous hemianopia The loss of vision in half of the visual field with the loss of vision on the same side of both eyes.

hormone A substance produced by an endocrine gland and secreted directly into the blood or lymph circulation to initiate or regulate activity in another part of the body.

hospice A philosophy that believes in palliative (supportive) care for terminally ill individuals.

Human Immunodeficiency Virus (HIV) The retrovirus that causes AIDS.

human leukocyte antigens (HLA) Antigens present in human blood.

Human papillomavirus A virus causing papillomas or warts to develop in humans.

humoral immunity A type of immunity dominated by antibodies.

hypercholesteremia An increased cholesterol level in the blood.

hyperglycemia Elevated serum glucose.

hyperglycemic hyperosmolar nonketotic syndrome (HHNK) An acute complication of NIDDM resulting when there is insufficient insulin to prevent hyperglycemia, but enough insulin to prevent ketoacidosis; life-threatening symptoms of hyperglycemia and oncotic diuresis result.

hyperlipidemia Increased lipids in the blood.

hyperopia Farsightedness.

hypersensitivity An excessive reaction to a stimulus.

hyperthermia A much higher than normal body temperature. The cause can be external, as in heat stroke, or internal as a result of infection. The hypothalamus loses the ability to function at core body temperatures of 106o F or higher.

hypertrophies Increase in muscle mass.

hyperuricemia Increased uric acid blood levels.

hyperventilation Refers to a breathing pattern in which respirations are more rapid and/or deeper than normal.

hypoglycemia Low serum glucose; can occur as a complication of insulin therapy (insulin reaction).

hypothermia A much lower than normal body temperature. A core body temperature below 95o F as result of a prolonged exposure to cold environmental temperatures.

hypovolemia An abnormally low circulating blood volume.

hypoxia Lack of an adequate amount of oxygen.

hysterectomy Surgical removal or excision of the uterus, and/or the uterus, fallopian tubes and ovaries.

iatrogenic Caused by treatment or diagnostic test.

icons Religious paintings, used by the Orthodox church, which depict the Holy Family or a particular saint. These paintings are considered important aids to worship.

idiopathic Occurring without known cause.

ileal conduit Implantation of the ureters into a piece of ileum which is attached to the abdominal wall as a stoma so urine can be removed from the body.

ileostomy An opening into the ileum or terminal portion of the small intestine. Ileostomies may be done for a variety of reasons, including ulcerative colitis, Crohn's disease, familial polyposis, and vascular infarct involving the large bowel.

ileus Intestinal obstruction. Can be mechanical, neurogenic or vascular.

immune response The body's ability to react to substances identified as non-self.

immunity A state of being protected from developing a disease, as a result of previous exposure or injection of agents which stimulate antibody production to the causative agent.

immunotherapy Treatment to enhance immunological functioning.

Impaired colleague A person who is not capable of safely performing his or her duties.

impaired glucose tolerance (IGT) A condition in which serum glucose levels are higher than normal, but lower than those diagnostic of diabetes mellitus.

impaired nurse A nurse under the influence of alcohol or drugs.

incidence The frequency of occurrence of a disease condition over a period of time and in relation to the population in which it is found.

incident report A risk management tool used to describe and report any unusual event which occurs to a patient, visitor, or staff.

incompetent Not legally qualified to make decisions.

incubation period The interval between exposure to an infectious disease and the first appearance of symptoms.

induction doses Initial doses of chemotherapy.

infertility The inability to conceive or carry a pregnancy to full term.

informed consent A legal form signed by a competent client and witnessed by another person, granting permission to have the procedure described by the client's physician and designating understanding of procedure, benefits, risks, possible complications, and alternate treatment options.

inspection To look at; to focus on the appearance of the client's body.

inspiration The process of pulling the diaphragm downward when air is brought in through the nose/mouth.

insulin A hormone produced and secreted by the beta cells in the islets of Langerhans of the pancreas; insulin lowers blood glucose by promotes transport and entry of glucose across the cell membrane.

insulin dependent diabetes mellitus (IDDM) A type of diabetes mellitus characterized by an absolute deficiency of insulin.

interdisciplinary health care team The group of health care professionals responsible for the assessment and planning of care for a client.

internal respiration The exchange of oxygen and carbon dioxide at the cellular level.

intoxication A reversible syndrome, due to the effect of a substance on the central nervous system.

intraoperative A particular time during the surgical experience beginning when the client is transferred to the operating room table and ending upon admission to the postanesthesia care unit.

intrathecal analgesia Analgesics administered into the subarachnoid space.

intravesical Within the urinary bladder.

intussusception The telescoping of one part of the intestine into another.

jaundice A yellowing of the skin, mucous membranes and sclerae of the eyes that occurs when excess bilirubin accumulates in the blood. It is a symptom of several systemic disorders, including liver disease, biliary obstruction and hemolytic anemia.

jejunostomy An opening into the jejunal portion of the small intestine. It may be used to decompress the small intestine or may be used for feeding.

Johnsonian intervention A confrontational approach to a client with a substance problem that lessens the chance of denial and encourages treatment before the client "hits bottom."

joint venturing Two or more agencies joining together to share the planning and executing of a service.

judgment A conclusion based on sound reasoning which can be supported by evidence.

justice Mandates that all persons be treated fairly and impartially, without regards to race, gender, medical diagnosis, marital status, social standing or religious beliefs.

justify To prove or show to be valid.

juvenile rheumatoid arthritis (Still's disease) Rheumatoid arthritis affecting juveniles with onset prior to age 16.

Kaposi's Sarcoma (KS) Multifocal malignant neoplasm, brown or purple, spreads in the skin. Often associated with AIDS.

Kegel exercise An exercise for strengthening the perineal muscles.

keloid An abnormal growth of scar tissue that is elevated, rounded and firm with irregular, clawlike margins. Keloids are more common in young women and black persons.

keratin A tough, fibrous protein produced by cells in the epidermis called keratinocytes. Surface epidermal cells filled with kertin form a protective barrier that repels bacteria and harmful substances.

Kernig's sign A diagnostic test for meningitis. Inability to extend leg when the thigh is flexed against the abdomen.

ketones Acidic byproducts of fat metabolism; excess ketone production occurs in ketoacidosis associated with uncontrolled diabetes mellitus.

ketonuria Abnormal presence of ketones in the urine.

kosher Means clean or fit to be eaten. Refers to dietary restrictions that apply to meats, fish, and dairy products and to the utensils they are prepared and served in.

kyphosis An increased roundness of the thoracic spinal curve.

laryngectomy Surgical opening into the larynx, maybe temporary or permanent.

legal rights Rights that are written in law.

leukemia Cancer occurring in blood-forming tissues.

leukocytosis Increased number of WBCs.

leukopenia Decreased number of WBCs.

liability Legally obligated, responsible for actions or damages.

libel Written words which harm or injure the personal or professional reputation of another person.

licensure A mandatory system of granting licenses according to specified standards. In health care licensure is granted based on education and examination. A process implemented by each state that is designed to assure that health care services meet minimal standards of care.

life review A form of reminiscence in which the client is attempting to achieve integrity.

ligation Application of a band or tie around a structure.

lipodystrophy Atrophy or hypertrophy of the subcutaneous fat.

lipoma A benign tumor consisting of mature fat cells.

liquefaction necrosis Death of tissues, changing to liquid or semi-liquid state. Often descriptive of a primary tubercle.

listening Interpreting the sounds heard and attaching meaning to them.

lithiasis Formation of a calculus (stone).

litholapaxy The crushing of a bladder stone and immediate washing out of the fragments through a catheter.

lithotripsy A method of crushing a calculus any place in the urinary system.

living will An advance directive that validates the individual's wishes when death is expected.

locomotor Pertaining to movement from one place to another

logic The formal principles of a branch of knowledge (such as nursing); interrelation, or connection or sequence, especially when seen by rational analysis to be inevitable, necessary or predictable.

long-term care facility A health care facility that provides services to individuals who are not acutely ill, have continuing health care needs, and cannot function independently at home.

lordosis An exaggeration of the lumbar spine curvature.

loss Being deprived of a loved one or of something of value.

lung stretch receptors Prevents over-expansion of the lungs by monitoring the extent of stretch within the lung tissues.

lymphoma Cancer occurring in lymphatic tissue.

macroallocation The amount of resources available for a particular kind of service.

maintenance therapy Small doses of chemotherapy given every 3-4 weeks to maintain remission.

malignant A cancerous tumor that invades surrounding tissue and spreads to distant areas of the body.

malpractice Negligent acts on the part of a professional; relates to the conduct of a person who is acting in a professional capacity where technical or professional skills are required or expected.

manometry The measurement of pressure in a lumen of the body by the use of transducers.

matrilineal society A society that has a female as its leader.

median survival time Average length of life.

Medicaid A government title program (XIX) that pays for health services for the aged poor, the disabled poor, and low-income families with dependent children.

Medicare An amendment (Title XVIII) to the Social Security Act that helps finance the health care of persons over 65 years and for permanently disabled younger persons who receive social security disability benefits.

Medigap insurance Insurance plans for persons with Medicare that pay for health care costs not covered by Medicare.

melanin The pigment that gives skin its color. Melanin is produced by specialized cells in the epidermis called melanocytes.

melena Stools containing partially broken down blood. Usually black, sticky and tar-like.

menopause Gradual cessation of menstruation related to decreasing hormone levels and altered ovarian function which occurs around 50 years of age.

menorrhagia Refers to an excessively heavy or prolonged menstrual flow.

metastasis Spread of cancer cells to distant areas of the body by way of the lymph system or blood stream.

metrorrhagia Refers to vaginal bleeding between menstrual periods.

microallocation The amount of resources available for a particular person.

microthrombi Very small clots.

micturition The process of urine leaving the urinary bladder, also called urination or voiding.

Minimum Data Set (MDS) An assessment tool developed by the federal government that must be used by all long-term care facilities receiving federal funds.

minority group The smaller in number of two cultural groups.

misdemeanor A less serious crime resulting in fines or probationary status. Imprisonment is rare.

misuse Use of a legal substance for which it was not intended or when the directions are exceeded.

mode of transmission The method or means by which a contagious disease is transferred to another entity.

modulation A central nervous system pathway that selectively inhibits pain transmission by sending signals back down to the dorsal horn of the spinal cord.

mortuary A funeral home.

mucous fistula The distal stoma of the double-barrel stoma or the nonfunctioning stoma of the double-barrel stoma.

Mycobacterium avium complex (MAC) Two closely related mycobacteria, Mycobacterium avium and Mycobacterian intracellalare, that are grouped together to form MAC. The source of exposure is contaminated water, although it has been isolated from soil, dust, sediments and aerosols.

mydriatic Makes pupil of the eye dilate.

myocardial infarction Necrosis (death) of the myocardium caused by an obstruction in a coronary artery.

myopia Nearsightedness.

myxedema The most severe form of hypothyroidism characterized by swelling of the hands, feet, face, or periorbital tissues.

necrosis Death of tissue.

negligence A general term referring to negligent or careless acts on the part of an individual; not exercising reasonable or prudent judgement.

neoplasm Any abnormal growth of new tissue, benign or malignant.

nephrotoxic Substance that causes kidney tissue damage.

neuralgia Nerve pain.

neurogenic shock A hypotensive situation resulting from the loss of sympathetic control of vital functions from the brain. May occur during spinal shock.

neurotransmitters Neurotransmitters are chemical substances that excite, inhibit, or modify the response of another neuron.

nevi Commonly known as birthmarks or moles. Nevi (singular = nevus) are pigmented areas in the skin.

nociceptor Afferent sensory nerves that receive and transmit pain signals.

nocturia Awakening at night to void.

non-insulin dependent diabetes mellitus (NIDDM) A type of diabetes in which clients retain the ability to produce some insulin and may or may not require insulin therapy

nonmaleficence The act of not committing harm; health care providers are required not to harm others intentionally or unintentionally.

nonverbal communication Sending a message without words. Sometimes called body language.

nosocomial Infections acquired from hospitalization.

novenas A period of nine consecutive days during which family and friends gather to pray for the deceased. Practiced by the Mexican Americans.

noxious stimulus Stimulus that triggers harmful electrical activity in the endings of afferent nerve fibers (nociceptors).

nuchal rigidity Pain and rigidity in the neck.

Nursing Practice Act A statute enacted by the legislature of a state that states the legal scope of nursing practice in that state.

nystagmus Constant, repetitive and involuntary movement of the eyeballs in various directions.

occult blood test (Guaiac) Testing for microscopic blood, commonly done on stools.

Joint Commission of Healthcare Organizations (JCAHO) The agency responsible for accreditation of health care facilities.

oligomenorrhea Infrequent menstrual periods or decreased menstrual flow.

Omnibus Budget Reconciliation Act (OBRA) The legal basis for the provision of care in long-term care facilities.

oncology The study of tumors.

open reduction Surgical procedure which enables the surgeon to reduce a fracture under direct visualization.

opinion A personal preference which is not arrived at through reasoning and which is not supported by objective evidence. A subjective belief.

opioid A morphine-like compound that produces bodily effects such as pain relief, sedation, constipation, and respiratory depression.

opisthotonos A complete arching of the body with only the head and feet on the bed.

opportunistic infections Infections in persons with a defective immune system.

orchiectomy Removal of the testis.

orthopnea Difficulty breathing lying down (supine position).

orthostatic hypotension A significant decrease in blood pressure when a person moves from a lying or sitting (supine) position to a standing position with dizziness or light headedness reported.

osmolality The osmotic pressure of a solution expressed in osmols or milliosmols per kilogram of water.

osmosis The movement of a pure solvent, i. e. water, from an area with a low solute concentration through a semipermeable membrane or selectively permeable membrane to an area with a high solute concentration to equalize the concentrations of salt or other solutes.

osteoarthritis A nonsystemic, noninflammatory disorder causing bones to degenerate.

ostomy An opening into.

overview The first observations made usually ascertaining both functional and physical assessment data through a quick inspection.

pain An unpleasant sensory and emotional experience associated with actual or potential tissue damage or described in terms of such. "Whatever the patient says it is, existing whenever the patient says it does." (McCaffery, 1979).

palliative Therapy that relieves symptoms, such as pain, but does not alter the course of disease. Referred to as supportive care.

pallor Abnormal paleness of the skin, seen especially in the face, conjunctiva, nail beds and oral mucous membranes. Anemia is one cause of pallor.

palpation To touch and examine with hands or fingers; to apply pressure to a body part to discover texture, size, and/or location of body parts.

palpitation When a client actually feels the heart beating; a "fluttering" or "pounding" sensation in the chest.

paracentesis Puncture of a cavity for the removal of fluid, usually referring to the abdomen.

paralytic ileus Symptoms of bowel obstruction resulting from the interruption of nerve transmission (paralysis) to the bowel. Occurs from trauma (surgery), infection or medications.

paraplegia Paralysis of lower extremities.

parasthesia Numbness, tingling or prickling sensations.

paroxysmal A symptom that begins and ends abruptly.

paroxysmal nocturnal dyspnea When a person suddenly awakens, is sweating, and having difficulty breathing.

patient-controlled analgesia (PCA) Self-administration of analgesics by the client, usually via a programmable pump.

Patient Self-Determination Act An act legislated by the federal government to provide a legal means for individuals to determine the circumstances in which life-sustaining treatment would or would not be provided to them.

peer assistance program A rehabilitation program which provides an impaired nurse with referrals, professional and peer counseling support group and assistance and monitoring back into nursing.

pelvic inflammatory disease (PID) An ascending pathogenic process which involves the invasion of the pelvic structures by various microorganisms. Symptoms include pelvic pain, foul vaginal discharge, and low grade temperature.

perception The process where neural messages are converted into the subjective experience of awareness.

percussion To place a hand over a body part, tapping the middle finger against different aspects of the body to identify any specific sounds heard.

percutaneous balloon valvuloplasty A balloon is inflated in a stenosed valve and the narrowed valvular space is expanded.

perforation The formation of a hole through a membrane or tissue, i.e., the wall of the stomach or intestine resulting in gastric contents emptying into the peritoneal cavity. The occurence of this produces serious, life-threatening disorder.

perfusion Refers to blood flow through an organ.

pericardial friction rub A short, high-pitched squeak heard as the heart rubs against an inflamed pericardial sac.

pericardiocentesis Removal of fluid from the pericardial sac.

perioperative A term encompassing the preoperative, intraoperative, and postoperative phases of surgery.

peripheral nervous system The cranial nerves, spinal nerves, and the autonomic nervous system.

peripheral resistance Pressure within a vessel that resists the flow of blood such as plaque build up or vasoconstriction.

peristalsis Wave-like movements that occur involuntarily in tubular structures of the body, i.e., the GI tract moves the chyme through the digestive system via peristalsis.

personal values What a person believes to be true and right based upon his or her own unique experiences as a member of society. Personal values are shaped by a person's experiences with family, religion, environment, and culture.

petechiae Pinpoint hemorrhagic spots seen in the dermal or submucosal layers of the skin.

pH Potential hydrogen; numeric value represents the acidity or alkalinity of a solution.

phantom limb pain Sensation of pain in an amputated limb.

phlebitis An inflammation in the wall of a vein without clot formation.

phlebothrombosis The formation of a clot because of blood pooling in the vessel, trauma to the vessel's endothelial lining or a coagulation problem with little or no inflammation in the vessel.

phlebotomy Removal of blood from a vein.

physical assessment A complete appraisal of the body from head-to-toe, incorporating all body functions and actions.

plethysmography Pulse volume recorder.

pleural effusion The collection of exudate within the pleural cavity.

pleural friction rub Low-pitched grating sounds on inspiration and expiration as pleura slide over each other; usually heard with pleurisy.

pleural space Potential space between the visceral and parietal pleura.

Pneumocystis carinii pneumonia (PCP) The most common opportunistic infection associated with advanced HIV, caused by a fungus. The alveoli become honey-combed.

poikilothermy Decreased temperature in an area.

polydipsia Excessive thirst.

polymenorrhea Menstrual periods that are abnormally frequent, generally more than every 21 days.

polymyositis An inflammatory disease involving striated muscle.

polyp Abnormal growth of tissue. May become malignant.

polyphagia Abnormal hunger.

polyuria Increased urination.

post void residual Measurement of urine that remains in the bladder after urination.

post-mortem care The care given immediately after death before the body is moved to the mortuary.

postoperative A particular time during the surgical experience beginning from the end of the surgical procedure until the client is discharged from medical care by the surgeon, not just from the hospital or institution.

postprandial After a meal.

pouch Applying a plastic bag or container to contain waste products or drainage from the body. Such pouches are attached to the body with adhesive and skin barriers.

power of attorney A legal document granting one individual the authority to make decisions for another.

prejudice The strongly held opinion about some topic or group of people that is formed before the facts are known.

premenstrual syndrome (PMS) A collection of symptoms caused by the variation of hormone levels prior to the onset of the menstrual period.

preoperative A particular time during the surgical experience beginning with the client's decision to have surgery, and ending with the transfer of the client to the operating table.

presbycusis Impairment of hearing in older adults often accompanied by the loss of high frequency tones.

presbycusis The impairment of hearing in elderly people, often accompanied by a loss of tone discrimination.

presbyopia Farsightedness, in advanced age, resulting from the loss of elasticity in the lens of the eye. The inability of the lens of the eye to increase its curvature in order to focus on near objects.

prevention Hindering, obstructing or thwarting a disease or illness from occurring.

priapism Prolonged erection that does not occur in response to sexual stimulation.

primary prevention All practices to keep health problems from developing.

primary tubercle Nodule containing tubercle bacilli formed within the lung tissue.

prognathism An abnormal facial configuration in which the jaws project forward.

protozoa Unicellular organisms capable of producing disease in humans.

proxemics Study of the personal and cultural spatial needs of an individual and the interactions within this space.

proximal Nearest center of the body or point of reference. Opposite of distal.

ptosis Drooping upper eyelid.

purpura Reddish-purple patches on the skin indicative of hemorrhage.

pyuria Pus in the urine.

quadriplegia Dysfunction or paralysis of both arms, both legs, and body trunk below the injured spinal area.

racial group A classification of people according to physical characteristics, such as skin pigmentation or facial features.

radiotherapy Treatment of cancer with high-energy radiation.

rapport Relationship of mutual trust and understanding.

rate The number of heart beats/respirations counted during a sixty second time frame (if counting for 30 seconds, multiply the number by 2 and document that number).

reactive depression A response to loss that lasts longer and is more marked than a normal response.

reasoning The use of the elements of thought to solve a problem or settle a question.

reconstructive To rebuild or re-establish.

rectocele Relaxation of the posterior vaginal wall which allows the protrusion of the rectum into the vagina. Associated with difficulty in bowel elimination.

rectus abdominis One of two external abdominal muscles on each side of the spine from the pubic bone to the 5th, 6th, and 7th ribs.

referred pain Pain felt in a point other than its place of origin.

reflective Consideration of some subject matter, idea or purpose with a view to understanding or accepting it or seeing it in its right relationships; introspective contemplation of the contents and qualities of one's own thoughts or experiences.

reflux An abnormal backward flow.

rehabilitation A process designed to assist individuals to reach their optimal level of physical, mental, and psychosocial functioning.

relapse To return to a previous behavior or condition.

religious support system Includes ministers, priests, rabbis, nuns, and lay persons who are able to meet spiritual needs.

remission Decrease or absence of symptoms of a disease.

renal colic Severe pain in the kidney area radiating from the abdomen to groin, often appearing in urolithiasis.

repolarization Diastole, or the recovery phase of the cardiac muscle.

residual urine The urine remaining in the bladder after the individual has urinated.

respiration The process of exchanging oxygen and carbon dioxide.

respite care Care and service that provides a break to caregivers and is utilized for a few hours a week, for an occasional weekend or for longer periods of time.

restraint Any device used to restrict movement. Restraint can be physical or chemical.

resuscitation Procedures implemented to reverse cardiac arrest or respiratory failure.

reticulocytes Immature red blood cells.

retroperitoneal Behind the peritoneum outside the peritoneal cavity.

reverse tolerance When a smaller amount of a substance will elicit the desired psychic effects.

rhinitis Inflammation of the nose and/or nasal passages.

rhizotomy The sectioning of the spinal nerve root as it enters the spinal cord.

rhoncal fremitis A rattle in the throat with vibratory tremors palpated through the chest wall.

rhythm The regularity or irregularity of each heart beat/respiration.

rights A claim or entitlement; rights infer that something is owed to someone. Examples of rights include legal rights (guaranteed by law) and ethical rights (privileges based on moral principles).

rigor mortis A stiffening of the body that occurs after death as a result of chemical changes that occur in the muscle tissues.

rubor Discoloration or redness from inflammation.

sarcoma Cancer occurring in connective tissue.

sclerotherapy A treatment method used with smaller veins or at the same time as vein ligation and stripping that involves injecting a chemical into the vein, causing the vein to become sclerosed (hardened) so blood no longer flows through it.

sclerotic Hardened tissue.

scoliosis A lateral curving deviation of the spine.

Scrub Nurse A RN, LP/VN, or Surgical Technologist providing services under the direction of the circulating nurse, who is qualified by training or experience to prepare and maintain the integrity, safety, and efficiency of the sterile field throughout the operation.

sebum An oily substance secreted by the sebaceous glands of the skin. Sebum lubricates the skin, helping to keep it soft and pliable.

secondary malignancy A second malignant condition that develops after successful treatment of an initial malignancy.

secondary prevention Early detection and intervention, generally before symptoms appear, to reduce the consequences of a health problem.

senescence A complex phenomenon that begins at conception, continues throughout the lifespan and culminates with death.

sensorineural Concerning or pertaining to a sensory nerve; in sensorineural hearing loss, the inner ear or cochlear portion of the eighth cranial nerve may be abnormal or diseased. A tumor, infection, or temporal bone skull fracture may cause destruction of the nerve and result in sensorineural hearing loss.

sexually transmitted disease (STD) A disease acquired as a result of sexual intercourse or sexual contact with an infected individual.

shiva In Judaism, the formal mourning period of 7 days during which time friends visit and comfort the bereaved in their home.

shroud A covering for the body after death.

sibilant wheezes Abnormal breath sounds, high pitched and whistle-like in nature, during inspiration and expiration.

sickled A RBC containing Hgb S becomes crescent-shaped and elongated.

slander Words communicated verbally to a third party which harm or injure the personal or professional reputation of another.

solute A substance dissolved in a solution.

solvent Any liquid capable of dissolving substances.

somatic nervous system The nerves connecting the central nervous system to the skin and skeletal muscles concerned with conscious activities.

somatic pain Pain in body tissue other than viscera.

somogyi effect In response to hypoglycemia, the release of glucose elevating hormones (epinephrine, cortisol, glucose) produces a hyperglycemic state. The hypoglycemia usually occurs during the night, but manifests as an elevated glucose in the morning.

sonorous wheezes A low-pitched snoring sound, louder on expiration. Coughing may alter sound if caused by mucous.

spermatogenesis The production of mature, functional sperm.

sphygmomanometer The calibrated devices used to assess blood pressure, either a mercury or aneroid device is used.

spinal shock The cessation of motor, sensory, autonomic, and reflex impulses below the level of injury. There is flaccid paralysis of all skeletal muscles, loss of spinal reflexes, loss of sensation, and absence of autonomic function below the level of injury.

spiritual care Involves the recognition of spiritual needs and the assistance given toward meeting spiritual needs.

spiritual needs Identified as an individual's need to find meaning and purpose in life, suffering, and death.

spirochete A type of slender, spiral bacteria.

standard A definite level or degree of quality that is proper and adequate for a specific purpose.

standard precautions A set of recommendations published by the CDC in 1996 to protect health care workers and others from infection.

standards of practice Guidelines established to direct nursing care, knowledge and skill level of the health care professional is considered.

staple food The basic food that people eat in their daily diet.

stasis dermatitis An inflammation of the skin due to decreased circulation.

status asthmaticus Persistent, intractable asthma attack.

status epilepticus Acute, prolonged episode of seizure activity lasting at least 30 minutes with or without loss of consciousness.

steatorrhea Bowel movements with a high concentration of fat.

stent A tiny metal tube with holes in it that prevents a vessel from collapsing and keeps the atherosclerotic plaque pressed against the vessel wall. Any material used to hold tissue in place or provide support

stereognosis The ability to recognize an object by feel.

sterile Without microorganisms.

sterile conscience An individual's personal sense of honesty and integrity to adhere to the principles of aseptic technique while admitting and correcting any errors and omissions promptly.

sterile field An area surrounding the client and the surgical site which is free from all microorganisms, created through a process of draping the work area and the client with sterile drapes.

stethoscope Instrument used to listen to body sounds.

stoma The distal end of the gastrointestinal or urinary system brought to the outside of the body and sutured into place.

strabismus The inability of the eyes to focus in the same direction.

stress incontinence A leakage of urine when a person does anything that strains the abdomen, such as coughing, laughing, jogging, dancing, or sneezing.

stroke volume Volume of blood pumped by the ventricle with each contraction.

subacute care Health care designed to provide services for clients who are out of the acute stage of illness but who still require skilled nursing, monitoring, and ongoing treatments.

subluxation A partial separation of an articular surface.

substance A drug, legal or illegal, that may cause physical or mental impairment.

suffocation Obstruction of the airways as a result of choking, drowning, or inhalation of noxious gases.

surfactant Phospholipid present in the lungs which lowers surface tension to prevent the collapse of the airways.

surgeon A licensed doctor of medicine (MD), doctor of osteopathy (DO), oral surgeon, or podiatrist specially trained to have acquired the knowledge, skill, and judgement required to successfully perform the intended surgical procedure and its complications.

synarthrosis An immovable joint.

synergism When two agents work together and produce a greater effect than either could produce alone.

synergy An abnormal pattern of movement seen with increased levels of spasticity that result from an overactive stretch reflex due to central nervous system damage.

synovectomy Excision of the synovial membrane.

synthesiasis A reaction from use of hallucinogens where the individual hears colors and sees sounds.

syphilis An infectious sexually transmitted disease characterized by lesions which may affect any organ. Caused by the spirochete, *Treponema pallidum*.

telangiectasia Permanent dilatation of groups of superficial capillaries and venules. Commonly known as "spider veins."

teleological Derived from the Greek word Telos which means "end." Teleological theory (also known as consequence-oriented theory) states that the "rightfulness" of an action is determined by the end result created from that action. i.e., the end justifies the means.

tenesmus Spasmodic contraction of the anal or bladder sphincter, causing pain and a persistent urge to empty the bowel or baldder.

teratogenic Causing abnormal development of the embryo.

terminal illness An illness that is not curable and is expected to result in death.

tertiary prevention Treating an illness or disease, after symptoms appear, so as to prevent further progression of the illness or disease. Rehabilitation and disability prevention are also included.

tetany A condition characterized by cramps, convulsions, twitching of muscles, and sharp flexion of the wrist and ankle joints associated with a variety of disorders, including hypoparathyroidism.

thallium scan A test in which a radioactive tracer (thallium 201) is injected in an attempt to determine the perfusion of myocardial tissue.

thanatology The study of death and dying.

therapeutic communication Communication that is purposeful and goal directed.

therapeutic touch The practice of touching the body for the purpose of relieving pain or healing; used by cultural healers such as shamans, curanderos, and espiritos.

thoracentesis The puncture of the pleura for the purpose of removing fluid.

thoracically Breathing from the chest or thorax.

thrombectomy Removal of a clot surgically.

thrombocytopenia A decreased number of platelets.

thrombophlebitis The formation of a clot due to an inflammation in the wall of the vessel.

thrombosis The formation of a clot in a vessel.

thrombus A formed clot that remains at the site where it formed.

tinnitus A tinkling or ringing sound in the ear.

tolerance A decreased sensitivity to subsequent doses of the same substance. An increased dose of a substance is needed to produce the same desired effect.

tophi Subcutaneous nodules of urate crystals.

tort A legal wrong committed against the person or property of another.

transcutaneous nerve stimulation (TENS) The process of applying a low-voltage electrical current to the skin through cutaneous electrodes.

transduction Noxious stimulus triggers electrical activity in the endings of afferent nerve fibers (nociceptors).

transesophageal echocardiography (TEE) A diagnostic ultrasonic imaging of the cardiac structures through the esophagus.

transmission The process where the pain impulse travels from the periphery to the brain cortex.

Trousseau's sign A carpal spasm caused by inflating a blood pressure cuff above the client's systolic pressure and leaving it in place for three minutes.

tumescence Swollen or turgid.

tumor markers Substance found in the serum that indicates the possible presence of malignancy.

tympany A loud, high pitched, drumlike quality.

unilateral neglect Failure to recognize or care for one side of the body.

urethrocele Relaxation of the anterior vaginal wall which allows the bladder and/or urethra to protrude into the vagina. Clients may experience urinary frequency and urgency without the presence of burning or dysuria.

urethrostomy Formation of a permanent fistula opening into the urethra.

urticaria The development of pale, nonpermanent wheals on the skin accompanied by itching, redness and swelling (also called hives).

uveitis Any intraocular inflammation, usually involving the iris, ciliary body and choroid, although the retina and cornea may also be involved.

vaginitis An infectious process which occurs in the vagina. May be associated with a variety of pathogenic microorganisms including fungus, protozoa, bacteria, or decreased hormone levels in the vaginal tissues.

vagotomy Removal of the vagus innnervation of the fundus of the stomach.

value system An individual's collection of inner beliefs that guides the way the person acts and helps determine the choices made in life.

values Values are perceptions or ideals that help shape a person's life and provide it with meaning. A person is not born with values; religion, family, societal norms and life experiences help forge a person's value system as he or she matures.

varicosities Visibly prominent, dilated and twisted veins.

vasectomy Surgical resection of the vas deferens.

vasoconstrict A vessel decreases in diameter.

vasodilate A vessel increases in diameter.

vein ligation Tying off an involved section of a vein with suture.

vein stripping Introducing a wire into a vein to strip the walls of the vein.

venereal disease A disease usually acquired as a result of sexual contact; the preferred term currently in use is sexually transmitted disease.

ventilation Movement of gases into and out of the lungs.

veracity A dedication to telling the truth; veracity demands that nurses be truthful to clients and not misleading.

verbal communication Using words to send a message.

vertigo The feeling of moving around in space, or of having objects moving around the person as a result of a disturbance in the equilibrium. Dizziness is sometimes called vertigo.

vesicants An agent that may produce blisters and tissue necrosis.

vesicular breath sounds Soft, low breath sounds heard over the majority of lung tissue.

Virchow's triad Three factors (pooling of blood, vessel trauma and a coagulation problem) that lead to the formation of a clot.

virus A parasitic organism, not visible with usual methods of light microscopy; capable of causing a variety of infectious diseases.

vitiligo De-pigmentation of the skin caused by destruction of melanocytes. Vitiligo appears as milk-white patches on the skin.

volvulus A twisting of the bowel on itself, usually happening in the sigmoid area of the large intestine. The twisting may occlude the bowel.

wellness An optimum state of health where the individual moves toward integration of human functioning, maximizes human potential, takes responsibility for health, has greater self-awareness, self-satisfaction and a wholeness in body, mind and spirit.

Western blot test Detects the presence of anitbodies to specific anitgens. More preceise than ELISA. Used to detect HIV infection.

windowing Cutting a hole in something; often done to a plaster cast to relieve pressure on the skin or a bony area.

withdrawal Ceasing use of a substance to which an individual has dependence. Symptoms vary depending on substance used. May be life threatening.

Yin and Yang The concept of balance. Yin represents the cold and Yang represents the hot. This concept is used to balance meals as food selections have either a yin or yang property. Diseases are also thought to have either a yin or yang property; a cold disease is treated with a hot treatment and a hot disease is treated with a cold treatment.

▶ REFERENCES ▶ ▶ ▶ ▶ ▶ ▶ ▶ ▶ ▶ ▶ ▶ ▶ ▶ ▶ ▶

CHAPTER 1

Baker, C. R. (1996). Reflective learning: A teaching strategy for critical thinking. *Journal of Nursing Education, 35,* 19–22.

Bevis, E. O. (1993). All in all, it was a pretty good funeral. *Journal of Nursing Education, 32,* 101.

Birx, E. (1993). Critical thinking and theory based practice. *Holistic Nursing Practice, 7*(3).

Bowers, B. & McCarthy, D. (1993). Developing analytic thinking skills in early undergraduate education. *Journal of Nursing Education, 32,* 107–113.

Brigham, C. (1993). Nursing education and critical thinking: Interplay of content and thinking. *Holistic Nursing Practice, 7*(3).

Brookfield, S. (1993). On impostership, cultural suicide and owners dangers: How nurses learn critical thinking. *Journal of Continuing Education in Nursing, 24* (5), 179–205.

Duncan, G. (1996). An investigation of learning styles of practical and baccalaureate nursing students. *Journal of Nursing Education, 35,* 40–42.

Ennis, R. H. (1985). A logical basis for measuring critical thinking skills. *Educational Leadership, 43,* 44-48.

Heaslip, P. (1993, September). Intellectual standards: What are they? *Critical Connections* [Newsletter of the Critical Thinking Interest Group, University College of the Cariboo, Kamloops, B.C.]

Heaslip, P. (1994, November). Defining critical thinking. *Dialogue: A Critical Thinking Newsletter for Nurses, 3.*

Kurfiss, J. (1988). *Critical thinking: Theory, research, practice and possibilities.* ASHE-ERIC Higher Education Report No. 2, Washington, DC: Association for the Study of Higher Education.

Miller, M. A. & Malcolm, N. S. (1990). Critical thinking in the nursing curriculum. *Nursing & Health Care, 11,* 66-73.

Norris, S. P. & Ennis, R. H. (1989). *Evaluating critical thinking.* Pacific Grove, CA: Midwest Publication.

Paul, R. (1990). *Critical thinking: What every person needs to survive in a rapidly changing world.* Rohnert Park, CA: Center for Critical Thinking and Moral Critique, Sonoma State University.

Paul, R. & Willsen, J. (1993). *Critical thinking, from an ideal evolves an imperative.* Santa Rosa, CA: The Foundation for Critical Thinking.

White, N. E., Beardslee, N. Q., Peters, D. & Supples, J. M. (1990). Promoting critical thinking skills. *Nurse Educator, 15*(5), 16-19.

Worrell, P. J. (1990). Metacognition: Implications for instruction in nursing education. *Journal of Nursing Education, 29,* 170-175.

CHAPTER 2

Bandman, E. & Bandman, B. (1990). *Nursing ethics through the life span.* Norwalk, CT: Appleton and Lange.

Beare, P. & Myers, J. (1994). *Principles and practices of adult health nursing* (2nd ed.). St. Louis: Mosby-Year Book, Inc.

Becker, B. & Fendler, D. (1994). *Vocational and personal adjustments in practical nursing.* (7th ed.) St. Louis: Mosby.

Bernzweig, E. (1987). *The nurse's liability for malpractice* (4th ed.). New York: McGraw-Hill.

Braun, J. & Lipson, S. (1993). *Toward a restraint-free environment.* Baltimore: Health Professions Press.

Calfee, B. (1995). Going before the board: How to prepare yourself. *Nursing 95, 25* (3), 56–58.

Cazalas, M. (1978). *Nursing and the law* (3rd ed.). Germantown: Aspen Systems Corporation.

Creighton, H. (1986). *Law every nurse should know* (5th ed.). Philadelphia: W. B. Saunders Company.

Curtain, L. (1993). Informed consent: Cautious, calculated candor. *Nursing Management, 24* (4), 18, 20.

Eggland, E. (1995). Charting smarter: Using new mechanisms to organize your paperwork. *Nursing 95, 25* (9), 35–41.

Fiesta, J. (1994). *20 legal pitfalls for nurses to avoid.* Albany: Delmar Publishers Inc.

Green, A. (1995). Are you at risk for disciplinary action? *AJN, 95(7),* 36–42.

Hill, S. & Howlett, H. (1993). *Success in practical nursing: Personal and vocational issues.* Philadelphia: W. B. Saunders

Hughes, T. (1994). Is your colleague chemically dependent? *AJN, 94*(9), 31–35.

Idemoto, B., Daly, B. et al. (1993). Implementing the patient self-determination act, *AJN, 93* (1), 20, 22–25.

Lippman, H. (1992, April). Addicted nurses: Tolerated, tormented, or treated. *RN,* 36–41.

Mandell, M. (1994). Not documented, not done. *Nursing 94, 24* (8), 62–63.

Mayer, T. (1995, April). *Director of nurses' attitudes toward restraint usage in long-term care.* Master's Thesis, Indiana Wesleyan University.

Meyer, C. (1993). "End-of life" care: Patients, choices, nurses' challenges. *AJN, 93*(2), 40–47.

Mitchell, P. & Grippando, G. (1993). *Nursing perspectives and issues* (5th ed.). Albany: Delmar Publishers Inc.

Monahan, F.D., Drake, T., & Neighbors, M. (1994). *Nursing care of adults.* Philadelphia: W. B. Saunders Company.

Sandler, R. L. (1995). Restraining devices. *American Journal of Nursing, 95*(7), 34–35.

Skinner, K. (1993, December). The hazards of chemical dependency among nurses. *The Journal of Practical Nursing,* 8–11.

Taylor, C., Lillis, C., & LeMone, P. (1993). *Fundamentals of nursing: The art and science of nursing care.* Philadelphia: J.B. Lippincott Company.

Walsh, S. M. (1995). Resuscitation decisions: Showing a family the way. *Nursing 95, 25*(8), 50–51.

CHAPTER 3

Aiken, T. D. & Catalano, J. T. (1994). *Legal, ethical and political issues in nursing.* Philadelphia: F. A. Davis Company.

Asch, D. A. (1996). The role of critical care nurses in euthanasia and assisted suicide. *The New England Journal of Medicine, 334* (21), 1374–1379.

Bandman, E. & Bandman, B. (1990). *Nursing ethics through the lifespan.* Norwalk, CT: Appleton and Lange.

Beare, G. & Myers, J. (1994). *Principles and practice of adult health nursing.* St. Louis: Mosby-Year Book, Inc.

Becker, B. & Fendler, D. (1990). *Vocational and personal adjustments in practical nursing.* St. Louis: Mosby-Year Book, Inc.

Beauchamp, T. & McCullough, L. (1984). *Medical ethics: The moral responsibilities of physicians.* Saddle River, NJ: Prentice Hall.

Edge, R. & Groves, J. R. (1994). *The ethics of health care: A guide for clinical practice.* Albany: Delmar Publishers Inc.

Gordon, A.M. & Williams-Browne, K. (1995). Beginnings & beyond, (4th ed.) Albany: Delmar Publishers.

Hamilton, P. (1992). *Realities of contemporary nursing.* Redwood City: Addison-Wesley Nursing.

Hill, S. & Howlett, H. (1988). *Success in practical nursing: Personal and vocational issues.* Philadelphia: W. B. Saunders Company.

McCloskey, J. & Grace, H. (1994). *Current issues in nursing.* St. Louis: Mosby-Year Book, Inc.

Mitchell, P. & Grippando, G. (1993). *Nursing perspectives and issues.* Albany: Delmar Publishers.

O'Neil, A. J. (1995). Ethical decision making and the role of nursing. In Deloughery, G. (Ed.). *Issues and trends in nursing.* St. Louis: Mosby-Year Book, Inc.

Oran, D. P. (1996). Children and adolescents. In Fortinash, K. M. & Holoday-Worret, P. A. (eds.) *Psychiatric-mental health nursing,* 184. St. Louis: Mosby-Year Book, Inc.

Pappas, A. (1994). Ethical issues. In Zerwekh, J. & Claborn, J. (Eds.) *Nursing today: Transitions and trends*. Philadelphia: W. B. Saunders Company.

Piaget, J. (1969). *The theory of stages of cognitive development*. New York: McGraw-Hill.

Proctor, D. (1995). Ethical issues. In Vestal (1995). *Nursing management: Concepts and issues*. Philadelphia: J. B. Lippincott Company.

Quinn, C. & Smith, M. (1987). *The professional commitment: Issues and ethics in nursing*. Philadelphia: W. B. Saunders Company.

Uustal, D. (1993). *Clinical ethics and values: Issues and insights*. East Greenwich, RI: Educational Resources in Healthcare.

Zerwekh, J. & Claborn, J. (1994). *Nursing today: Transition and trends*. Philadelphia: W. B. Saunders Company.

CHAPTER 4

Bandman, E. & Bandman, B. (1995). *Nursing ethics through the lifespan*. Norwalk, CT: Appleton and Lange.

Beauchamp, T. & Childress, J. (1994). *Principles of biomedical ethics (4th ed.)*. New York: Oxford University Press.

Beauchamp, T. & Walters, L. (1994). *Contemporary issues in bioethics*. Belmont, CA: Wadsworth Publishing Company.

Caplan, A. (1994). The ethics of in vitro fertilization. In Beauchamp, T. & Walters, L. (Eds.). *Contemporary Issues in Bioethics*, 216–224.

Caplan, A. (1986). Organ transplants: The cost of success. Mappes, T. & Zembaty, J. (eds.). In *Biomedical ethics (2nd ed.)*. 630–635. New York: McGraw-Hill.

Dubler, N. & Nimmons, D. (1992). *Ethics on call*. New York: Harmony Books.

Erickson, J., Rodney, P. & Starzomski, R. (1995, September). When is it right to die? *The Canadian Nurse*, 29–34.

Friend, T. (1995, September). New directory is first atlas of ourselves. *USA Today*.

Lamm, R. (1994, September/October). Healthcare heresies. *Healthcare Forum Journal*, 45–49.

Latimer, E. & McGregor, J. (1994, October). Euthanasia, physician-assisted suicide and the ethical care of dying patients. *Canadian Medical Association Journal*, 1133—1136.

Macklin, R. (1994). Artificial means of reproduction and our understanding of the family. In Beauchamp, T. & Walters, L. (Eds.). *Contemporary issues in bioethics*, 191–198. Belmont, CA: Wadsworth Publishing Company.

Monagle, J. & Thomasma, D. (1994). *Health care ethics: Critical issues*. Gaithersburg, MD: Aspen Publications.

Quill, T., Cassel, C., Meier, D. (1994). Care of the hopelessly ill: Proposed clinical criteria for physician-assisted suicide. In Monagle, J. & Thomasma, D. (Eds.) *Health care ethics: Critical issues*, 255–260. Gaithersburg, MD: Aspen Publications.

Reilly, P. (1994). Eugenics sterilization in the United States. In Beauchamp, T. & Walters, L. (Eds.). *Contemporary issues in bioethics*, 597–606. Belmont, CA: Wadsworth Publishing Company.

Ruwart, M. (1994, February). To die with dignity. *McCall's*, 90–92, 174.

Siebert, C. (1995, September). The DNA we've been dealt. *The New York Times Magazine*, 51–55, 57, 64.

Soukup, M. (1991, February). Organ donation from the family of a totally brain-dead donor: Professional responsiveness. *Critical Care Nursing Quarterly*, 13(4), 8–18.

VanWeel, H. (1995, September). Euthanasia: Mercy, morals and medicine. *The Canadian Nurse*, 29–34.

Verklan, M. (1993). The ethical use of fetal tissue for transplantation and research. *Journal of Advanced Nursing 18*, 1172–1177.

Williams, J. & Lea, D. (1995). Applying new genetic technologies: Assessment and ethical considerations. *Nurse Practitioner, 20*(7), 16–26.

CHAPTER 5

Anderson, C. (1990). *Patient teaching & communicating in an information age*. Albany: Delmar Publishers Inc.

Bailey, D. & Bailey, D. (1993). *Therapeutic approaches to care of the mentally ill*. Philadelphia: F. A. Davis Company.

Barnsteiner, J. (1996). Newest online journal users: Clinicians. *Reflections, 22*(2), 21.

Barry, P. (1994). *Mental health and mental illness*. Philadelphia: J. B. Lippincott Company.

Brandt, M. (1995, March). Making the CPR vision a reality: Where should you start? *Journal of the American Health Information Management Association, 66*(3), 26–30.

Callanan, M. & Kelley, P. (1992). *Final gifts*. New York: Poseiden Press.

Christensen, B. & Kockrow, E. (Ed.). (1995). *Foundations of nursing*. St. Louis: Mosby-Year Book, Inc.

deWit, S. (1994). *Rambo's nursing skills for clinical practice*. Philadelphia: W. B. Saunders Company.

Dick, R. & Steen, E. (Eds.). (1991). *The computer-based patient record: An essential technology for health care*. Washington, DC: National Academy Press.

Doherty, W. (1992, May/June). Private lives, public values. *Psychology Today, 25*(3), 32–37.

Earnest, V. (1993). *Clinical skills in nursing practice*. Philadelphia: J. B. Lippincott Company.

Fawcett, C. (1993). *Family psychiatric nursing*. St. Louis: Mosby-Year Book, Inc.

Frawley, K. & Asmonga, D. (1996, January). Update on the Medical Records Confidentiality Act. *Journal of the American Health Information Management Association, 67*(1), 12.

Gay, K. (1993). *Getting your message across*. New York: Macmillan Publishing.

Gensing, L. (1990). A formula to avoid miscommunicating. *Nursing 90, 10*(9), 22.

Goldscheider, F. & Waite, L. (1991). *New families, no families?* Berkeley: University of California Press.

Goldsmith, J. (1996). Computers and nurses changing hospital care. *Reflections 22*(2), 8–10.

Hinton, J. (1984). Speaking of death with the dying. In Shneidman, E. S. *Death: Current perspectives* (3rd ed.). 152–161. Palo Alto, CA: Mayfield Publishing.

Jack, L. (1994). Effective communication. In Zerwekh, J. & Claborn, J. (Ed.). *Nursing today: Transition and trends*, 140–170. Philadelphia: W. B. Saunders Company.

Kalman, N. & Waughfield, C. (1992). *Mental health concepts*. Albany: Delmar Publishers Inc.

Kubler-Ross, E. (1978). *To live until we say good-bye*. Englewood Cliffs, NJ: Prentice Hall.

Kubler-Ross, E. (1975). *Death: The final stage of growth*. Englewood Cliffs, NJ: Prentice Hall.

Kubler-Ross, E. (1969). *On death and dying*. New York: MacMillan.

Lindemann, E. (1984). Reactions to one's own fatal illness. In Shneidman, E. S. *Death: Current perspectives*. (3rd ed.). 257–265. Palo Alto, CA: Mayfield Publishing.

Lorton, L. & Legler, J. (1996, April). A telemedicine trial. *Journal of the American Health Information Management Association, 67*(1), 40–42.

Medical Records Institute. (1994). Legality of electronic patient record systems. *Toward an electronic patient record, 2*(7).

Meranda, D. (1995, March). Administrative and security challenges with electronic patient record systems. *Journal of the American Health Information Management Association, 66*(3), 58–60.

Milliken, M. (1993). *Understanding human behavior*. Albany: Delmar Publishers Inc.

Murphy, T. (1990). Improving nurse/doctor communications. *Nursing 90, 10*(8), 144.

Pagano, M. & Ragan, S. (1992). *Communication skills for professional nurses*. Newbury Park, CA: Sage.

Raudsepp, E. (1990). Seven ways to cure communication breakdowns. *Nursing 90, 10*(4), 132.

Ravitch, S. (1996). The Medical Records Confidentiality Act. *For The Record, 8*(9) 8–11.

Roter, D. & Hall, J. (1993). *Doctors talking with patients/patients talking with doctors*. Westport, CT: Auburn House.

Ruben, B. (1992). *Communicating with patients*. Dubuque, IA: Kendall-Hunt.

Sherman, K. (1994). *Communication and image in nursing*. Albany, NY: Delmar Publishers Inc.

Smith, S. (1992). *Communications in nursing*. St. Louis: Mosby-Yearbook, Inc.

Tamparo, C. & Lindh, W. (1992). *Therapeutic communications for allied health professions*. Albany: Delmar Publishers Inc.

CHAPTER 6

Agency for Health Care Policy and Research (June, 1996). Research Activities. [Brochure]. Washington, DC: Author.

Andrews, M. & Boyles, J. (1995). *Transcultural concepts in nursing* (2nd ed.). Philadelphia: J. B. Lippincott Company.

Clark, C. (1996). *Nursing in the community* (2nd ed.). Stamford, CT: Appleton and Lange.

Cultural Diversity in Health Care American Journal of Nursing (video).

Koss-Chioino, J. (1992). *Women as healers, women as patients: Mental health care and traditional healing in Puerto Rico.* Boulder, CO: Westview Press.

Lock, D. (1992). *Increasing multicultural understanding: A comprehensive model.* Newbury Park, CA: Sage.

Merriam Webster's Collegiate Dictionary (10th ed.) (1995). Springfield: Merriam-Webster, Incorporated.

Morley, P. & Wallis, R. (Eds.). (1978). *Culture and curing: Anthropological perspectives on traditional medical beliefs and practices.* Pittsburgh: University of Pittsburgh Press.

Romanucci-Ross, L. (1991). *The anthropology of medicine.* Westport, CT: Greenwood Press.

Specter, R. (1995). *Cultural diversity health and illness* (4th ed.). Norwalk, CT: Appleton & Lange.

Spradley, B. W. & Allender, J. A. (1996). *Community health nursing* (4th ed.). Philadelphia: J. B. Lippincott Company.

Stanhope, M. & Knollmueller, R. (1996). *Handbook of community health and home health nursing* (2nd ed.). St. Louis: Mosby-Year Book, Inc.

U.S. Department of Commerce, Bureau of the Census (1995). *Statistical abstract of the United States, 14.*

U.S. Department of Health and Human Services. (1990). *Healthy people 2000: National health promotion and disease prevention objectives.*

Zola, I. (1966). Culture and symptoms: An analysis of patients presenting complaints. *American Sociological Review, 31,* 615–630.

CHAPTER 7

Andreola, N., Steerfel, L., & O'Sullivan, C. (1993). A different way: A look at alternative therapies. *Nursing Spectrum, 6*(18), 7–9.

Andrews, M. M. (1993). Cultural diversity and community health nursing. In Swanson, J. M. & Albrecht, M. (Ed.), *Community health nursing: Promoting the health of aggregates,* 433–458. Philadelphia: W. B. Saunders Company.

Andrews, M. M. & Bolin, L. (1993). The African American community. In Swanson, J. M. & Albrecht, M. (Ed.), *Community health nursing: Promoting the health of aggregates,* 433–458. Philadelphia: W. B. Saunders Company.

Andrews, M. M. & Hanson, P. (1995). Religion, culture, and nursing. In Andrews, M. M. & Boyle, J. (Eds.). *Transcultural concepts in nursing care.* St. Louis: Mosby-Year Book, Inc.

Bainbridge, W. (1991). Dying east, dying west. *Nursing Standard, 6*(6), 22–23.

Bloch, B. (1993). Nursing care of black patients. In Orque, M. S., Block, B. & Monrroy, L. A. (Eds.). *Ethnic nursing care: A multicultural approach,* 81–113. St. Louis: Mosby-Year Book, Inc.

Boutell, K. A. & Bozett, R. W. (1990, July). Nurses' assessment of patient's spirituality: Continuing education implications. *Journal of Continuing Education in Nursing, 21,* 172–76.

Boyle, J. (1995). Culture and community. In Andrews, M. M. & Boyle, J. (Eds) *Transcultural concepts in nursing care.* St. Louis: Mosby-Year Book, Inc.

Calvillo, E. R. & Flaskerud, J. H. (1991,Winter). Review of literature on culture and pain of adults with focus on Mexican Americans. *Journal of Transcultural Nursing, 2,* 16–23.

Carpenito, L. J. (1997). *Nursing diagnosis: Applications in clinical practice* (7th ed.). Philadelphia: J. B. Lippincott Company.

Cassetta, R. (1993). Emphasizing cultural diversity to improve nursing education. *American Nurse, 25*(8), 6.

Chan, S. (1991). *Asian Americans: An interpretive history.* Boston: Twayne Publishers.

Charnes, L. S. & Moore, P. S. (1992). Meeting patient's spiritual needs: The Jewish perspective. *Holistic Nursing Practice, 6*(3), 64–72.

Conway, F. & Carmona, P. (1990). Cultural complexity: The hidden stressors. *Journal of Advanced Medical-Surgical Nursing, 1*(4), 65–72.

Copp, L. A. (1990, August). The spectrum of suffering. *American Journal of Nursing,* 35–39.

Davis, D. S. (1991). Dealing with real Jewish patients. *Journal of Clinical Ethics, 2*(3), 211–212.

Diaz-Gilbert, M. (1993). Caring for culturally diverse patients. *Nursing 93, 23*(10), 44.

Diaz-Gilbert, M. (1991). *Communicating effectively with Hispanic patients: The complete guide to key vocabulary words and essential and functional phrases in Spanish for direct patient contact.* Haddonfield, NJ: Intercultural Communications Publishing Corp.

Douglas, M. K. (1991). Cultural diversity in the response to pain. In Puntillo, K. A. (Ed.), *Pain in the critically ill.* Rockville, MD: Aspen.

Eleazer, P. G., Hornung, C. A., Egbert, C. B., Egbert, J. R., Eng, C., Hedgepeth, J., McCann, R., Strothers, H., Sapir, M., Wei, M., & Wilson, M. (1996). The relationship between ethnicity and advance directives in a frail older population. *JAGS, 44,* 938–943.

Eliason, M. (1993). Ethics and transcultural nursing care. *Nursing Outlook, 41*(5), 225–228.

English and Spanish: Medical Words and Phrases. (1994). Springhouse, PA: Springhouse Corporation.

Eshleman, J. (1992, November). Death with dignity: Significance of religious beliefs and practices in Hinduism, Buddhism, and Islam. *Today's OR Nurse,* 19–20.

Fish, S. & Shelley, J. (1988). *Spiritual care: The nurse's role.* (3rd ed.). Downers Grove, IL: Inter Varsity Press.

Galanti, G. (1991). *Caring for patients from different cultures.* Philadelphia: University of Pennsylvania Press.

Galanti, G. (1991). *Caring for patients from different cultures: Case studies from American hospitals.* Philadelphia: University of Pennsylvania Press.

Geiger, J. & Davidhizar, R. (1991). *Transcultural Nursing: Assessment and intervention.* St. Louis: C. V. Mosby.

Green, J. (1992). Death with dignity: Jehovah's Witnesses. *Nursing Times, 88*(5), 36–37.

Groode, E. E. (1993, February 15). The cultures of illness. *U.S. News and World Report.*

Grudyknust, W. (1992). *Communicating with strangers: An approach to intercultural communication.* New York: McGraw-Hill.

Iverson, P. (1990). *The Navajos.* New York: Chelsea House Publishers.

Leininger, M. (1978). *Transcultural nursing: Concepts, theories, and practices.* New York: John Wiley & Sons.

Marty, N. M. (1990). Health, medicine, and the faith traditions. In *Healthy People 2000: A Role for America's Religious Communities.* Emory University: The Carter Center and the Park Ridge Center.

McCaffery, M. (1990). Nursing approaches to nonpharmacological pain control. *International Journal of Nursing Studies, 27*(1), 1–5.

McManus, R. J. (1993). Medicine and ethics at the crossroad: A Roman Catholic perspective. *Rhode Island Medicine, 76*(2), 79–81.

Mulaik, J. S., Megenity, J. S., & Cannon, R. B. (1991). Patients' perception of nurses' use of touch. *Western Journal of Nursing Research, 13*(3), 306–323.

Roberson, M. (1993). Defining cultural and ethical differences to adapt to a Chinese patient population. *American Nurse, 25*(8), 6–10.

Robinson, A. (1994). Spirituality and risk: Toward an understanding. *Holistic Nursing Practice, 8*(2), 1–7.

Rourden, B. & Higgs, R. (1992, March). When your patient is a Hmong Refugee. *American Journal of Nursing, 92,* 52–55.

Singelenberg, R. (1990). The blood transfusion taboo of Jehovah's Witnesses: Origins, development and function of a controversial doctrine. *Social Science Medicine, 31*(4), 515–523.

Skolnick, A. (1990). Christian scientist claim healing efficacy equal if not superior to that of medicine. *Journal of the American Medical Association, 264*(11), 1379–1381.

Spector, R. E. (1991). *Cultural diversity in health and illness.* (3rd ed.). New York: Appleton-Century-Crofts.

Villarruel, A. M. & deMontellano, B. O. (1992). Culture and pain: A Mesoamerican perspective. *Advances in Nursing Science, 15*(1), 21–32.

Wenger, A. F. (1991, April-May). Culture specific care and the old order Amish. *Imprint,* 80–85.

West, E. (1993). The cultural bridge model. *Nursing Outlook 41*(5), 229–234.

Yep, J. (1991). An Asian patient: How does culture affect care? *Journal of Christian Nursing 8*(3), 6–8.

CHAPTER 8

Brown, E. (1995, August). An inexpensive and painless alternative to colonoscopy? (coprocytobiology). *Medical Update, 19,* 1.

Carey, B. (1996, July/August). The slumber solution. *Health,* 70–75.

Chase, M. (1996, February 5). Simple handwashing gets new scrutiny for disease control. *The Wall Street Journal,* B1(E&W).

Dixon, B. (1994). *Good health for African Americans.* New York: Random House, Inc.

Don't overdo it: Alcohol paradox. (1996, February 5). *Industry Week, 245*(1), 19.

Eastman, P. (1996, January 17). Task force issues new screening guidelines. *Journal of the National Cancer Institute, 88*(3), 74.

Floyd, P., Mimms, S., & Yelding-Howard, C. (1995). *Personal health: A multicultural approach.* Englewood, CO: Morton Publishing Co.

Gulling, R., Renner, J. & Vargas, F. (1993). *Stay well without going broke.* Lancaster, PA: Starburst Publishers.

Hafen, B. & Hoeger, W. (1994). *Wellness: Guidelines for a healthy lifestyle.* Englewood, CO: Morton Publishing Co.

Health-club hygiene. (1995, November). *Industry Week, 244,* 31.

Hoeger, W. & Hoeger, S. (1995). *Lifetime physical fitness and wellness* (4th ed.). Englewood, CO: Morton Publishing Co.

Hoffman, E. (1995). *Our health, our lives.* New York: Pocket Books.

Ince, S. (1995, June). A bite of the apple. *Harvard Health Letter, 20,* 3.

Inlander, C. & Moran, C. (1994). *77 Ways to beat colds and flu.* New York: Walker Publishing Co., Inc.

Liviton, R. (1995). *Brain Builders.* West Nyack, NY: Parker Publishing Co., Inc.

Lowell, B. (1995). *Body signals.* New York: HarperCollins Publishers, Inc.

Mayell, M. (1995). *52 Simple steps to natural health.* New York: Pocket Books.

Osteoporosis, a silent disease, finds a louder voice. (1995, November-December). *Menopause News, 5,* 1.

Payne, W. & Hahn, D. (1995). *Understanding your health* (4th ed.). St. Louis: Mosby-Year Book, Inc.

Powell, D. (1992). *A year of health hints.* Thorndike, ME: Thorndike Press.

Quaid, K. (1993, September 30). Psychological and ethical considerations in screening for disease. *American Journal of Cardiology, 72,* 64D.

Quench strokes with every sip. (1995, October) *Prevention, 47,* 66.

Reichman, L. & Mangura, B. (1996, February). State-of-the-art tuberculosis prevention. *Chest, 109,* 301.

Robertson, J. (1996). *Peak-performance Living.* New York: HarperCollins Publishers.

Seiger, L., Vanderpool, K., & Barnes, D. (1995). *Fitness and wellness strategies.* Dubuque, IA: Wm. C. Brown Communications, Inc.

Simon, H. (1992). *Staying well.* Boston: Houghton Mifflin Co.

Smith, C. & Maurer, F. (1995). *Community Health Nursing: Theory and Practice.* Philadelphia: W. B. Saunders, Co.

Smith, S. & Lancashire, J. (1995, November-December). Health promotion and disease prevention progress report. *Public Health Reports, 110,* 790.

Social stigma of colon and rectal problems thwarts life-saving cancer screenings. (1995, October). *Executive Health's Good Health Report, 32,* 1.

Sox, H. (1994, June 2). Preventive health services in adults. *The New England Journal of Medicine, 330,* 1589.

U.S. Department of Agriculture, U.S. Department of Health and Human Services. (1995). *Home and Garden Bulletin No. 232* (4th ed.).

U.S. Department of Health and Human Services. (1990). *Healthy People 2000: National health promotion and disease prevention objectives.* Washington, DC: DHHS Publication No. (PHS) 91-50212.

Wash your hands (to help prevent colds). (1996, January). *Consumer Reports on Health, 2*(1).

Weil, A. (1995). *Natural health, natural medicine.* Boston: Houghton Mifflin, Co.

Williams, R. & Williams, V. (1993). *Anger kills.* New York: Random House, Inc.

CHAPTER 9

Alcoholics Anonymous (1990). *Analysis of the 1989 survey of the membership of AA.* New York: Alcoholics Anonymous World Services, Inc.

Alcoholics Anonymous. (1939). *Alcoholics Anonymous.* New York: Alcoholics Anonymous World Services, Inc.

Anderson, N. (1996). Decisions about substance abuse among adolescents in juvenile detention. *Image, 28*(1), 65–70.

Antai-Otong, D. (1995). Helping the alcoholic patient recover. *American Journal of Nursing, 95*(8), 22–29.

Anthenelli, R. & Schucket, M. (1991). Alcohol and cerebral depressants. In *The international handbook of addiction behavior.* Glass, I. (Ed.). New York: Routledge, Chapman and Hall Inc.

Baft, D. & Jenkins, B. (1990). Action Stat!: Alcohol withdrawal syndrome. *Nursing, 20*(10), 33.

Bennett, E. & Woolf, D. (1991). *Substance abuse* (2nd ed.). Albany, NY: Delmar Publishers.

Daley, D., Moss, H., & Campbell, F. (1993). *Dual disorders.* Center City, MN: Hazelden Foundation.

Dubree, D. (1990). Action Stat!: Cocaine overdose. *Nursing, 20*(3), 33.

Gerstein, D. & Harwood, H. (Eds.). (1992). *Treating drug problems.* Vol. 2. Washington, DC: National Academy Press.

Holbrook, J. & McCurdy, H. (1991). Drug screening. In Bennett, E. & Woolf, D. *Substance abuse.* (2nd ed.). Albany, NY: Delmar Publishers.

Hollandsworth, J. (1990). *The physiology of psychological disorders.* New York: Plenum Press.

Janerick, D., Thompson, W., & Varela, L. (1990). Lung cancer and exposure to tobacco smoke in the household. *New England Journal of Medicine, 323,* 632–636.

Jannke, S. (1994). When the mother-to-be drinks. *Childbirth Instructor.* New York: Cradle Publishing Inc.

Johnson, V. (1988). *Intervention: How to help someone who doesn't want help.* New York: New American Library.

Johnson, V. (1973). *I'll quit tomorrow.* New York: Harper & Row.

Johnston, L., O'Malley, P., & Bachman, J. (1991). *Drug use among American high school seniors, college students and young adults 1975–1990.* Rockville, MD: National Institute on Drug Abuse, U.S. Department of Health and Human Services, Alcohol Drug Abuse, and Mental Health Administration.

Kalman, N. & Waugfield, C. (1993). *Mental health concepts* (3rd ed.). Albany, NY: Delmar Publishers.

Kasl, C. (1992). *Many roads, one journey: Moving beyond the twelve steps.* New York: Harper Collins.

Kendig, S. (1995). Women at risk for infection: The woman who is chemically dependent. *Journal of Obstetric, Gynecologic, and Neonatal Nursing, 24*(8), 776–781.

Kinney, J. (1991). *Clinical manual of substance abuse.* St. Louis: Mosby-Year Book, Inc.

Kleber, H. (1994). Opioids detoxification. In Galanter, M. & Kleber, H. *Textbook of substance abuse treatment.* Washington, DC: American Psychiatric Press, Inc.

Landau, E. (1995). *Hooked: Talking about addictions.* Brookfield, CT: The Millbrook Press.

Langone, J. (1995). *Tough choices.* Boston: Little, Brown and Company.

Lippman, H. (1992). Addicted nurses: Tolerated, tormented or treated. *RN, 55*(4), 36.

Marlatt, G. (1992). Substance abuse: Implications of a biopsychosocial model for prevention, treatment and relapse prevention. In Grabowski, J. & Wanden Bos, G. (Eds.). *Psychopharmacology: Basic mechanisms and applied interventions.* Washington, DC: American Psychological Association.

McFarland, R. (1993). *Drugs and your parents* (Rev. ed.). New York: Rosen Publishing Group.

Miller, H. (1990). Addiction in a coworker: Getting past the denial. *American Journal of Nursing, 90*(5), 72.

Naegle, M. (Ed.). (1991). *Substance abuse education in nursing,* Vol. I. New York: National League for Nursing.

Nagy, J. (1992). A comparison of drug use among 8th, 10th, 12th graders. *NIDAs high school senior survey.* Rockville, MD: National Institute on Drug Abuse.

Navarra, T. (1995). Enabling behavior: The tender trap. *American Journal of Nursing, 95*(1), 50–52.

Phelps, G. & Field, P. (1992). Drug testing: clinical and workplace issues. In Fleming, M. & Barry, K. *Addictive disorders*, 125–142. St. Louis: Mosby-Year Book, Inc.

Porterfield, K. (1991). *Coping with codependency*. New York: Rosen Publishing Group, Inc.

Rodriguez, P. (1996, March 18). Potent date-rape drug finding its way into U.S. through Texas. *Corpus Christi Caller Times*. Corpus Christi, TX.

Santomier, J. & Hogan, P. (1991). Health implications of alcohol and other drug use. In Naegle, M. (Ed.). *Substance abuse education in nursing* Vol.1. New York: National League for Nursing.

Seligmann, J., Mason, M., Annin, P., et al. (1992, February 3). The new age of aquarius, *Newsweek*, 66–67.

Septien, A. (1993). *Everything you need to know about codependence*. New York: Rosen Publishing Group.

Woolf, D. (1991). CNS depressants: Alcohol. In Bennett, E. & Woolf, D. *Substance abuse* (2nd ed.). Albany, NY: Delmar Publishers.

Yates, J. & McDanier, J. (1994). Are you losing yourself in codependency? *American Journal of Nursing*, 94(4), 32–36.

Yoshuichi, E. (1992). Fetal alcohol syndrome. *Childbirth Instructor*.

CHAPTER 10

Barkauskas, V. H., Stoltenberg-Allen, K., Baumann, L. C., & Darling-Fisher, C. (1994). *Health and physical assessment*. St. Louis: Mosby-Year Book, Inc.

Bates, B. (1995). *A guide to physical examination and history taking* (6th ed.). Phildelphia: J. B. Lippincott Company.

Bolander, V. B. (1994). *Basic nursing: A psychophysiologic approach* (3rd ed.). Philadelphia: Springhouse.

Bowers, A. C., Thompson, J. M., & Miller, M. (1992). *Clinical manual of health assessment* (4th ed.). St. Louis: Mosby-Year Book, Inc.

Earnest, V. V. (1993). *Clinical skills in nursing practice*. Philadelphia: J. B. Lippincott Company.

Fuller, J. & Schaller-Ayers, J. (1994). *Health assessment: A nursing approach*. Philadelphia: J. B. Lippincott Company.

Gordon, M. (1995). *Manual of nursing diagnoses 95–96* (7th ed.). St. Louis: Mosby-Year Book.

Hood, G. H. & Dincher, J. R. (1992). *Total patient care: Foundations and practice of adult health nursing* (8th ed.). St. Louis: Mosby-Year Book, Inc.

Morton, P. G. (1993). *Health assessment in nursing* (2nd ed.). Philadelphia: Springhouse.

Murray, R. B. & Zentner, J. P. (1993). *Nursing assessment and health promotion* (5th ed.). Norwalk: Appleton & Lange.

Rosdahl, C. (1995). *Textbook of basic nursing* (6th ed.). Philadelphia: J. B. Lippincott Company.

Stiesmeyer, J. K. (1993). Pulmonary assessment: A four step approach. *American Journal of Nursing*, 93(8), 22.

Taylor, C., Lissis, C., & LeMone, P. (1993). *Fundamentals of nursing: The art and science of nursing care* (2nd ed.). Philadelphia: J. B. Lippincott Company.

Weber, J. (1993). *Health assessment* (2nd ed.). Philadelphia: J. B. Lippincott Company.

CHAPTER 11

Abouleish, E., Rawal, N., & Rashad, M. N. (1991). The addition of 0.2 mg subarachnoid morphine to hyperbaric bupivacaine for cesarean delivery: A prospective study of 856 cases. *Regional Anesthesia*, 16, 137–140.

Ben-David, B., Vaida, S., Collins, G., Naum, M., & Gaitini, L. (1994). Transient paraplegia secondary to an epidural catheter. *Anesthesia & Analgesia*, 79, 598-600.

Brockway, M. S., Noble, D. W., Sharwood-Smith, G. H., & McClure, J. H. (1990). Profound respiratory depression after extradural fentanyl. *British Journal of Anaesthesia*, 64, 243–245.

Bromage, P. R. (1993). Nerve injury and paralysis related to spinal and epidural anesthesia. *Regional Anesthesia*, 18, 481–484.

Camann, W. R., Murray, R. S., Mushlin, P. S., & Lambert, D. H. (1990). Effects of oral caffeine on postdural puncture headache: A double-blind, placebo-controlled trial. *Anesthesia & Analgesia*, 70, 181–184.

Carp, H., Singh, P. J., Vadhera, R., & Jayaram, A. (1994). Effects of the serotonin-receptor agonist sumatriptan on postdural puncture headache: Report of six cases. *Anesthesia & Analgesia*, 79, 180–182.

Cohen, D. E., Van Duker, B., Siegel, S., & Keon, T. P. (1993). Common peroneal nerve palsy associated with epidural analgesia. *Anesthesia & Analgesia*, 76, 429–431.

Cousins, M. J. & Mather, L. E. (1984). Intrathecal and epidural administration of opioids. *Anesthesiology*, 61, 276–310.

Dickman, C. A., Shedd, S. A., Spetzler, R. F., Shetter, A. G., & Sonntag, V. K. H. (1990). Spinal epidural hematoma associated with epidural anesthesia: Complications of systemic heparinization in patients receiving peripheral vascular thrombolytic therapy. *Anesthesiology*, 72, 947–950.

Horlocker, T. T., Wedel, D. J., & Offord, K. P. (1990). Does preoperative antiplatelet therapy increase the risk of hemorrhagic complications associated with regional anesthesia? *Anesthesia & Analgesia*, 70, 631–634.

Horlocker, T. T., Wedel, D. J., Schroeder, D. R., Rose, S. H., Elliott, B. A., McGregor, D. G., & Wong, G. Y. (1995). Preoperative antiplatelet therapy does not increase the risk of spinal hematoma associated with regional anesthesia. *Anesthesia & Analgesia*, 80, 303–309.

Kane, R. E. (1981). Neurologic deficits following epidural or spinal anesthesia. *Anesthesia & Analgesia*, 60, 150–161.

Kilbride, J. M., Senagore, A. J., Mazier, W. P., Ferguson, C., & Ufkes, T. (1992). Epidural analgesia. *Gynecology and Obstetrics*, 174, 137–140.

Kroll, D. A., Caplan, R. A., Posner, K., Ward, R. J., & Cheney, F. W. (1990). Nerve injury associated with anesthesia. *Anesthesiology*, 73, 202–207.

Liu, S., Chiu, A. A., Carpenter, R. L., Mulroy, M. F., Allen, H. W., Neal, J. M., & Pollock, J. E. (1995). Fentanyl prolongs lidocaine spinal anesthesia without prolonging recovery. *Anesthesia & Analgesia*, 80, 730–734.

Onishchuk, J. L. & Carlsson, C. (1992). Epidural hematoma associated with epidural anesthesia: Complications of anticoagulant therapy. *Anesthesiology*, 77, 1221–1223.

Phillips, S., Hutchinson, S., & Davidson, T. (1993). Preoperative drinking does not affect gastric contents. *British Journal of Anaesthesia*, 70, 6–9.

Renaud, B., Brichant, J. F., Clergue, F., Chauvin, M., Levron, J. C., & Viars, P. (1988). Ventilatory effects of continuous epidural infusion of fentanyl. *Anesthesia & Analgesia*, 67, 971–975.

Robertson, K., Douglas, M. J., & McMorland, G. H. (1985). Epidural fentanyl, with and without epinephrine for post-Caesarean section analgesia. *Canadian Anaesthesia Society Journal*, 32, 502–505.

Rosen, M. A., Dailey, P. A., & Hughes, S. C. (1988). Epidural sufentanil for postoperative analgesia after cesarean section. *Anesthesiology*, 68, 448–454.

Scott, J. C. & Stanski, D. R. (1987). Decreased fentanyl and alfentanil dose requirements with age: A simultaneous pharmacokinetic and pharmacodynamic evaluation. *Journal of Pharmacology and Experimental Therapeutics*, 240, 159–166.

Selander, D., DhunÄr, K. G., & Lundborg, G. (1977). Peripheral nerve injury due to injection needles used for regional anesthesia. An experimental study of the acute effects of needle point trauma. *Acta Anaesthesiologica Scandinavia*, 21, 182–188.

Soreide, E., Holst-Larsen, H., Reite, K., Mikkelsen, H., Sorejde, J. A., & Steen, P. A. (1993). Effects of giving water 20-450 ml with oral diazepam premedication 1-2 h before operation. *British Journal of Anaesthesia*, 71, 503–506.

Wells, D. G. & Davies, G. (1987). Profound central nervous system depression from epidural fentanyl for extracorporeal shock wave lithotripsy. *Anesthesiology*, 67, 991–992.

Yasuda, N., Lockhart, S. H., & Eger, E. I., II (1991). Kinetics of desflurane, isoflurane, and halothane in humans. *Anesthesiology*, 74, 489–498.

CHAPTER 12

Agency for Health Care Policy and Research. (1992). *Clinical practice guideline: Acute pain management: Operative or medical procedures and Trauma* (AHCPR Publication No. 92–0032). Rockville, MD: U.S. Dept. of Health and Human Services.

Agency for Health Care Policy and Research. (1994). *Clinical practice guideline: Management of cancer pain* (AHCPR Publication No. 94–0592). Rockville, MD: U.S. Dept. of Health and Human Services.

American Pain Society. (1992). *Principles of analgesic use in the treatment of acute and chronic cancer pain* (3rd ed.). Skokie, IL: Author.

Beecher, H. K. (1956). Relationship of significance of wound to pain experienced. *JAMA, 161,* 1609–1613.

Bonica, J. J. (Ed.). (1990). *The management of pain* (2nd ed.). Philadelphia: Lea and Febiger.

Cleeland, C. S., Gonin, R., Hatfield, A. K., Edmonson, J. H., Blum, R. H., Stewart, J. A., & Pandya, K. J. (1994). Pain and its treatment in outpatients with metastatic cancer. *New England Journal of Medicine 330,* 592–596.

Cousins, N. (1979). *Anatomy of an illness as perceived by the patient.* Toronto: Bantam.

Donovan, M., Dillon, P., & McGuire, L. (1987). Incidence and characteristics of pain in a sample of medical-surgical inpatients. *Pain 30,* 69–78.

Fields, H. L. (1987). *Pain.* New York: McGraw-Hill.

Gordon, D. & Ward, S. (1995). Correcting patient misconceptions about pain. *AJN, 95* (7), 43–45.

Liebeskind J. & Melzack, R. (1987). The International Pain Foundation: Meeting a need for education in pain management. *Pain, 30,* 1–2.

McCaffery, M. (1979). *Nursing management of the patient with pain.* (2nd ed.). Philadelphia: J. B. Lippincott Company.

McCaffery, M. & Beebe, A. (1989). *Pain: Clinical manual for nursing practice.* St. Louis: Mosby-Year Book, Inc.

McDevitt, M. J. (1995). A(TENS)tion! *Nursing 95, 25*(12), 46–47.

McGuire, D. B., Yarbro, C. H., & Ferrell, B. R. (1995). *Cancer pain management* (2nd ed.). Boston: Jones and Bartlett.

Melzack, R. (1990). The tragedy of needless pain. *Scientific American, 262*(2), 27–33.

Melzack, R. & Wall, P. D. (1965). Pain mechanisms: A new theory. *Science, 150:* 971–979.

Merskey, H. (1979). IASP subcommittee on taxonomy: Pain terms: A list with definitions and notes on usage. *Pain, 6,* 249.

Paice, J. A. (1991). Unraveling the mystery of pain. *Oncology Nursing Forum, 18,* 843–849.

Porter, J. & Jick, H. (1980). Addiction rare in patients treated with narcotics. *New England Journal of Medicine, 302,* 123.

Streisand, J. B. (1994). OTFC: A new opioid delivery system. *APS Bulletin, 4,* 1.

Whaley, L. & Wong, D. (1987). *Nursing care of infants and children* (3rd ed.). p. 1070. St. Louis: Mosby-Year Book, Inc.

World Health Organization. (1990). Cancer pain relief and palliative care. *Report of a WHO expert committee [World Health Organization Technical Report Series, 804].* Geneva, Switzerland: Author.

World Health Organization. (1986). *Cancer pain relief.* Geneva, Switzerland: Author.

CHAPTER 13

Aldrete, J. (1995). The post-anesthesia recovery score revisited. *Journal of Clinical Anesthesiology, 7*(1), 89–91.

Association of Operating Room Nurses, Inc. (1995). *Standards and recommended practices.* Denver: Author.

Association of Operating Room Nurses. (1995, May) Surgical attire; recommended practices; biological monitors; sterile packages. *AORN Journal, 61*(5).

Atkinson, L. & Fortunato, N. (1996). *Berry & Kohn's operating room technique* (8th ed.). St. Louis: Mosby-Year Book, Inc.

Beare, P. G. & Myers, J. L. (1994). *Principles and practice of adult health nursing* (2nd ed.). St. Louis: Mosby-Year Book, Inc.

Black, J. M. & Matassarin-Jacobs, E. (1993). *Luckmann and Sorensen's medical-surgical nursing: A psychophysiologic approach* (4th ed.). Philadelphia: W. B. Saunders Company.

Bryant, R. A. (Ed.). (1992). *Acute and chronic wounds: Nursing management.* St. Louis: Mosby-Year Book, Inc.

Burden, N. (1993). *Ambulatory surgical nursing.* Philadelphia: W. B. Saunders Company.

Fairchild, S. (1993). *Perioperative nursing: Principles and practice.* Boston: Jones and Bartlett.

Gilchrist, B. (1990). Washing and dressings after surgery. *Journal of the Wound Care Society, 86*(50), 71.

Goodman, K. (1995, September). Transitional diet. *Current topics in nutrition support.* Fort Wayne, IN: Lutheran Hospital of Indiana, Inc.

Goodman, K. (1995, October). Post-op or transitional feeding. *Current topics in nutrition support.* Fort Wayne, IN: Lutheran Hospital of Indiana, Inc.

Ignataviticus, D. D., Workman, M. L., & Mishler, M. A. (1995). *Medical-surgical nursing: A nursing process approach* (2nd ed.). Philadelphia: W. B. Saunders Company.

Lewis, S. M., Collier, I. C., & Heitkemper, M. M. (1996). *Medical-surgical nursing: Assessment and management of clinical problems* (4th ed.). St. Louis: Mosby-Year Book, Inc.

Litwack, K. (1995). *Post anesthesia care nursing* (2nd ed.). St. Louis: Mosby-Year Book, Inc.

Phipps, W. J., Cassmeyer, V. L., Sands, J. K., & Lehman, M. K. (1995). *Medical-surgical nursing: Concepts and clinical practice* (5th ed.). St. Louis: Mosby-Year Book, Inc.

Smeltzer, S. C. & Bare, B. G. (1996). *Brunner and Suddarth's textbook of medical-surgical nursing* (8th ed.). Philadelphia: Lippincott-Raven.

Talabiska, D. G. (1995). Malnutrition in the elderly. *Newlines in Multi-Vitamin Infusion, 4*(2), 1,2,6.

CHAPTER 14

Bove, L. A. (1994). How fluids and electrolytes shift. *Nursing 94, 24* (8), 34–39.

Boyda, E. V. (1994). Knowledge basic to the nursing care of adults with fluid, electrolyte, and acid-base imbalances. In Monohan, F. D., Drake, T. and Neighbors, M. (Eds.). *Nursing care of adults* (37–76). Philadelphia: W. B. Saunders Company.

Carpenito, L. J. (1997). *Nursing diagnosis: Application to clinical practice.* Philadelphia: J. B. Lippincott Company.

Cochran, L. (1995). What you need to know about potassium imbalances. *Nursing 95, 25* (2), 32H, 32J, 32N.

Davis, N. M. (1995). Potassium Perils. *American Journal of Nursing, 95* (3), 14.

Eisenberg, P. G. (1994). Feeding formulas. *RN, 57* (12), 46–52.

Ferrin, M. S. (1996), Restoring electrolyte balance: Magnesium. *RN, 59* (5), 31–34.

Gaedeke, M. K. (1996). *Laboratory and diagnostic handbook.* Menlo Park, CA: Addison-Wesley Publishing Company, Inc.

Jenkins, M. (1995). Racing smart part 1: Dehydration. *220, 1.* 16–20.

Metheny, N. M. (1996). *Fluid and electrolyte balance: Nursing considerations.* Philadelphia: Lippincott-Raven Publishers.

Norris, M. K. (1994). Checking chloride levels. *Nursing 94, 24* (3), 76.

Pagana, K. D. & Pagana, T. J. (1995). *Mosby's diagnostic and laboratory test reference.* St. Louis: Mosby-Year Book, Inc.

Raimer, F. (1994). How to identify electrolyte imbalances on your patient's E.C.G. *Nursing 94, 24* (6), 54–58.

Tasota, F. J. & Wesmiller, S. W. (1994). Assessing A.B.G.s: Maintaining the delicate balance. *Nursing 94, 24* (5), 34–44.

Viall, C. (1995). Taking the mystery out of TPN: Part two. *Nursing 95, 25* (5), 57–59.

Watson, J. & Jaffe, M. S. (1995). *Nurses's manual of laboratory and diagnostic tests.* Philadelphia: F. A. Davis Company.

Weldy, N. J. (1994). Fluids, electrolytes, and acid-base balances. In P. G. Beare & J. L. Myers. (Eds.) *Principles and practice of adult health nursing* (165–212). St. Louis: Mosby-Year Book, Inc.

Winslow, E. H. (1995). We need more calcium. *American Journal of Nursing, 95* (6), 60–61.

CHAPTER 15

Alfaro-LeFevre, R., Blicharz, M., Flynn, A., & Boyer, M. (1992). *Drug Handbook: A nursing process approach.* Redwood, CA: Addison-Wesley, 72–76.

American Cancer Society. (1994). Cancer facts and figures—1994. Atlanta, GA: Author.

Baird, S., Donehower, M., Stalsbroten, V., & Ades, T. (Eds.) (1991). *A cancer source book for nurses* (6th ed.). Atlanta, GA: American Cancer Society.

Belcher, A. (1992). *Cancer nursing*. St. Louis: Mosby-Year Book, Inc.

Camp-Sorrell, D. (1991, April). Controlling adverse effects of chemotherapy. *Nursing 91*, 34–41.

Carrol, D. (1993, September). Managing cancer pain. *Nursing Times, 89*(38), 69–70.

Erickson, J. (1994, November). Update on Hodgkin's Disease. *Nurse Practitioner*, 63–67.

Kohr, J. (1995, April). Measuring your patient's pain. *RN*, 39–40.

Frye, J. (1993). An overview on oncologic emergencies. *Highlights on Antineoplastic Drugs. 11*(1), 2–4.

Hansen, C. (1995, January). Colorectal cancer a preventable disease. *Physician Assistant*, 15–26.

Lewis, S. & Collier, I. (1992). *Medical-surgical nursing: Assessment and management of clinical problems* (3rd ed.). St. Louis: Mosby-Year Book, Inc.

Long, B., Phipps, W., & Cassmeyer, V. (1993). *Medical-surgical nursing process approach* (3rd ed.). 182–227. St. Louis: Mosby-Year Book, Inc.

Lundquist, D. & Stewart, F. M. (1994, October). An update on non-Hodgkin's lymphomas. *Nurse Practioner*, 41–54.

Mandel, J. S., Bond, J. H., et al. (1993). Reducing mortality from colorectal cancer by screening for fecal occult blood. *New England Journal of Medicine, 328* (19), 1365.

McCaffery, M. & Ferrell, B. (1994, July). How to use the new AHCPR cancer pain guidelines. *American Journal of Nursing*, 42–47.

McCarron, E. (1995, June). Supporting the families of cancer patients. *Nursing 95*, 48–51.

Ottery, F. (1994, March/April). Cancer cachexia prevention, early diagnosis and management. *Cancer Practice, 2*(2), 123–131.

Otto, S. (1991). *Oncology nursing*. St. Louis: Mosby-Year Book, Inc.

Porth, C. (1990). *Pathophysiology concepts of altered health states* (3rd ed.), 57–79. Philadelphia: J. B. Lippincott Company.

Robuck, J. & Fleetwood, J. (1993). Nutritional support of the patient with cancer. *Capsules and Comments in Oncology Nursing, 1*(1), 20–30.

Rosdahl, C. (1995). *Textbook of basic nursing*. Philadelphia: J. B. Lippincott Company.

Scherer, J. & Timby, B. (1995). *Introductory medical-surgical nursing* (6th ed.), 145–164. Philadelphia: J. B. Lippincott Company.

Schweid, L. & Werner-McCullough, M. (1994, September). Will you recognize these oncological crisis? *RN*, 23–27.

Smeltzer, S. & Bare, B. (1992). *Burnner and Suddarth's textbook of medical-surgical nursing* (7th ed.). Philadelphia: J. B. Lippincott Company.

Varricchio, C. (1994, July/August). Human and indirect cost of home care. *Nursing Outlook*, 151–157.

Weber, M. (1995, April). Clinical snapshot: Chemotherapy—induced nausea and vomiting. *American Journal of Nursing*.

White, L. & Spitz, M. (1994). Cancer risk and early detection assessment. *Capsules and Comments in Oncology Nursing, 2,*(1), 2–3.

Wood, L. & Gullo, S. (1993). IV Vesicants: How to avoid extravasation. *American Journal of Nursing, 93* (4), 42–46.

Woodward, W. & Thobaben, M. (1994). Special home health care nursing challenges: Patients with cancer. *Home Health Care Nurse, 12*(3), 33–37.

Zwingler, R. (1994). Cancer update 94. *Nursing 94*, 24 (4), 59.

CHAPTER 16

American Association of Retired Persons. (1995). *A Profile of Older Americans*. Washington, DC: Department of Health and Human Services.

Brundage, D. J., et al. (1993). Self-care instruction for clients with COPD. *Rehabilitation Nursing, 18*(5), 321–323.

Cuzzell, J. Z. (1994). Test your wound assessment skills. *American Journal of Nursing, 94*(6), 34–35.

Maslow, A. H. (1970). *Motivation and personality* (2nd ed.). New York: Harper & Row.

Moody, L. E. (1995). Challenges: TB or not TB. *The Nursing Spectrum, 8*(1), 14–16.

Needham, J. F. (1993). *Gerontological nursing—A restorative approach*. Albany, NY: Delmar Publishers.

Needham, J. F. (1995). *Gerontological nursing*. Albany, NY: Delmar Publishers.

Pellino, T. A. (1994). How to manage hip fractures. *American Journal of Nursing, 94*(4), 46–50.

Stolley, J. M. (1994). When your client has Alzheimer's disease. *American Journal of Nursing, 94*(8), 34–41.

Tetlow, K. (1995). Exercise by design. *Contemporary Long Term Care, 18*(3), 38–42.

U.S. Department of Agriculture. (1992). *The food guide pyramid*. Home and Garden Bulletin Number 252.

U.S. Department of Health and Human Services. Agency for Health Care Policy and Research. (1992). *Pressure ulcers in adults: Prediction and prevention. Clinical practice guidelines*. Rockville, MD: U.S. Department of Health and Human Services.

U.S. Department of Health and Human Services. Agency for Health Care Policy and Research. (1992). *Urinary incontinence in adults. Clinical practice guidelines*. Rockville, MD: U.S. Department of Health and Human Services.

U.S. Department of Health and Human Services. Agency for Health Care Policy and Research. (1993). *Cataracts in adults: Management of functional impairment. Clinical practice guidelines*. Rockville, MD: U.S. Department of Health and Human Services.

U.S. Department of Health and Human Services. Agency for Health Care Policy and Research. (1994). *Benign prostatic hyperplasia: Diagnosis and treatment. Clinical practice guidelines*. Rockville, MD: U.S. Department of Health and Human Services.

U.S. Department of Health and Human Services. Agency for Health Care Policy and Research. (1994). *Heart failure: Evaluation and care of clients with left-ventricular systolic dysfunction. Clinical practice guidelines*. Rockville, MD: U.S. Department of Health and Human Services.

Yen, P. K. (1994). Boosting intake when appetite is poor. *Geriatric Nursing, 15*(5), 284.

Yen, P. K. (1994). Preventing disease with vitamins. *Geriatric Nursing, 15*(2), 111–112.

Yen, P. K. (1995). Maximizing calcium intake. *Geriatric Nursing, 16*(2), 92–93.

CHAPTER 17

American Association of Retired Persons. (1995). *A profile of older Americans*. Washington, DC: Department of Health and Human Services.

Abrams, W. B., Beers, M. H., & Berkow, R. (Eds.). (1995). *The Merck manual of geriatrics* (2nd ed.). Whitehouse Station, NJ: Merck Research Laboratories.

Bailis, S. S. (1995). Accreditation: A necessary next step. *Provider, 21*(5), 55–56.

Buckwalter, K. C. (1995). Health care policy 101—what nurses and their clients need to know. *Journal of Gerontological Nursing, 21*(3), 5–6.

Diaz, D. (1995). Geriatric UPDATE 95. *Nursing 95, 25*(3), 62–64.

Fisher, C. (1995). Coming home to assisted living. *Provider, 21*(10), 57–64.

Galarneau, L. (1993). An interdisciplinary approach to mobility and safety education for caregivers and stroke patients. *Rehabilitation Nursing, 18*(6), 395–398.

Glosner, G. W. (1995). How subacute care fills the gap. *Nursing 95, 25*(3), 51.

Gresham, G. E., Duncan, P. W., Stason, W. B., et al. (1995, May). *Post stroke rehabilitation*. Clinical Practice Guideline, No. 16, Rockville, MD: U.S. Department of Health and Human Services. Public Health Service Agency for Health Care Policy and Research. AHCPR Publication No. 95–0062.

Habel, M. (Ed.) (1993). Rehabilitation nursing practice. *The specialty practice of rehabilitation nursing*. Skokie, IL: The Rehabilitation Nursing Foundation of the Association of Rehabilitation Nurses.

Health, Education, and Human Services Division. (1994). *Long-term care reform*. (GA)/HEHS–94–227). Washington DC: U.S. General Accounting Office.

Huey, F. L. (Ed.) (1995). Humpty dumpty: Good egg for rehab? *The Nursing Spectrum, 8*(25), 3.

Lasky, W. F. (1995). Assisted living: A brand new world. *Nursing Homes, 44*(7), 40–41.

Meng, M. E. (1995). Starting an adult day care center. *Provider, 21*(12), 38–40.

Millea, K. (1995). Home health care UPDATE 95. *Nursing 95, 25*(7), 57–59.

Walsh, G. G. (1995). How subacute care fills the gap. *Nursing 95, 25*(3), 51.

Wenckus, E. (1995). Working with an interdisciplinary team. *The Nursing Spectrum, 8*(6), 11–12.

CHAPTER 18

Beckel, J. (1996). Resolving ethical dilemmas in long-term care. *Journal of Gerontological Nursing, 22*(1), 20–26.

Haight, B. & Burggraf, V. (1992). Clinical outlook: Reminiscence and life review: Conducting the processes. *Journal of Gerontological Nursing, 18*(2), 39–42.

Kübler-Ross, E. (1969). *On death and dying*. New York. Macmillan Publishing Co., Inc.

Mitty, E. L., Mathy, M., Rappaport, M., & Ramsey, G. C. (1996). Ethics committees and implementation of the client self-determination act in New York City nursing homes. *Nursing Home Medicine, 4*(1), 21–22, 23–29.

Rhymes, J. A. (1993). Hospice care in the nursing home. *Nursing Home Medicine, 1*(6), 14–16, 22–24.

Taylor, M. A. (1995). Benefits of dehydration in terminally ill clients. *Geriatric Nursing, 16*(6), 271–272.

Taylor, P. B. & Ferszt, G. G. (1994). Letting go of a loved one. *Nursing 94, 24*(1), 55–56.

Ufema, J. (1995). How to help dying clients feel "safe". *Nursing 95, 25*(9), 59.

Ufema, J. (1995). Insights on death and dying. *Nursing 95, 25*(11, 12), 19, 22–23.

CHAPTER 19

Avey, M. A. (1993). TB skin testing: How to do it right. *AJN, 93*(9):42–44.

Borkgren, M. W. & Gronkiewicz. (1995). Update your asthma care: From hospital to home. *AJN, 95*(1):26–34.

Boutotte, J. (1993). T.B.: The second time around and how you can help to control it. *Nursing 93*. May: 42–49.

Centers for Disease Control and Prevention. (1993). *TB facts for health care workers*. (No. 00–5655): 1–7.

deWit, S. (1992). *Keane's essentials of medical-surgical nursing*. (3rd ed.). Philadelphia. W. B. Saunders Company. 386–435.

Grimes, D. E. & Grimes, R. M. (1995). Tuberculosis: what nurses need to know to control the epidemic. *Nursing Outlook, 43*(4): 164–173.

Harkness, G. & Dincher, J. R. (1996). *Medical surgical nursing: Total patient care* (9th ed.). 528–595. St. Louis, MO: Mosby-Year Book, Inc.

Loeb, S., et al. (Eds.). (1991). Diagnostic test implications. Springhouse, PA: Springhouse Corporation.

Prentice, D. & Ahrens, T. (1994). Pulmonary complications of trauma. *Crit Care Nurs Q, 17*(2):24–33.

Ritchie, J. A. & Hagel, C. L. (1994). Asthma: A new look at helium therapy. *RN, 57*(9):18–21.

Robertson, O. (1995, March). Penetrating chest trauma. *Nursing 95*, 33.

Rosdahl, C. B. (1995). *Textbook of basic nursing*. (6th ed.). Philadelphia: J. B. Lippincott Company. 234–241, 1176–1209.

Shaw, T. (1995). The resurgence of tuberculosis: Current issues for nursing. *Nursing Times, 91*(40): 35–37.

Smith, R. N., Fallentine, J., & Kessel, S. (1995, February). Underwater chest drainage: Bringing the facts to the surface. *Nursing 95*, 60–67.

Steismeyer, J. (1993). A four step approach to pulmonary assessment. *AJN, 93*(8):22–31.

Ulrich, S. A., Canale, S. W., & Wendall, S. A. (1994). *Medical-surgical nursing care planning guide*. (3rd ed.). Philadelphia, W. B. Saunders Company. 433–500.

CHAPTER 20

Amin, N. M. (1994). Timely diagnosis and treatment of a great mimic. *Consultant, 3*, 331–343.

Amin, N. M. (1994). The picture is changing: Will you recognize the face? *Consultant, 3*, 319–324.

Arbour, R. (1994). Complete heart block. *Nursing 94*, 8, 33.

Baas, L. & Kretten, C. (1987). Valvular heart disease: Its causes, symptoms, and consequences. *RN, 11*, 30–36.

Beare, P. & Myers, J. L. (1994). *Principles and practice of adult health nursing* (2nd ed.). St. Louis: Mosby-Year Book, Inc.

Beattie, S. (1993). CABG surgery: The second time around. *AJN, 8*, 42–45.

Bove, L. A. (1995). Now! Surgery for heart failure. *RN, 5*, 26–31.

Coronary angiography: Heads up. (1994). *Nursing 94, 12*, 32Q.

Deglin, J. & Vallerand, A. (1995). *Davis's drug guide for nurses* (4th ed.). Philadelphia: F.A. Davis Company.

Goldman, H. (1994). Myocardial infarction—diagnosis and treatment. *Nursing Times, 90* (16), 33–37.

Grab, C. (1992). The cutting alternative to PTCA. *RN, 7*, 22–27.

Hasemeier, C. (1996). Permanent pacemaker: What you need to know to prepare a patient for this intervention. *AJN, 96*(2), 30–31.

Heart and stroke facts: 1996 Statistical supplement. (1996). American Heart Association.

Hicks, S. L. (1994). Standing guard against silent ischemia and infarction. *Nursing 94, 1*, 34–39.

Hole, Jr., J. W. (1993). *Human anatomy and physiology* (6th ed.). Dubuque, IA: Wm. C. Brown Publishers.

Janowski, M. J. (1996). Managing heart failure. *RN, 2*, 34–39.

Lewis, S. & Collier, I. (1992). *Medical-surgical nursing: Assessment and management of clinical problems* (3rd ed.). St. Louis: Mosby-Year Book, Inc.

Linton, A., Matteson, M. A., & Maebius, N. K. (1995). *Introductory nursing care of adults*. Philadelphia: W. B. Saunders Company.

Long, B. C., Phipps, W. J., & Cassmeyer, V. L. (1993). *Medical-surgical nursing: A nursing process approach* (3rd ed.). St. Louis: Mosby-Year Book, Inc.

Pagana, K. D. & Pagana, T. J. (1995). *Mosby's diagnostic and laboratory test reference*. St. Louis: Mosby-Year Book, Inc.

Phipps, W. J., Cassemeyer, V. L., Sands, J. K., & Lehman, M. K. (1995). *Medical-surgical nursing: Concepts and clinical practice* (5th ed.). St. Louis: Mosby-Year Book, Inc.

McDermott, B. & Deglin, J. (1994). *Understanding basic pharmacology: Practical approaches for effective application*. Philadelphia: F. A. Davis Company.

Monahan, F. D., Drake, T., & Neighbors, M. (1994) *Nursing care of adults*. Philadelphia: W. B. Saunders Company.

Olbrych, D. D. (1993). Interpreting C.P.K. and L.D.H. results. *Nursing 93, 1*, 48–49.

Research roundup (1994). *Nursing 94, 12*, 32Q.

Sandler, R. L. (1994). Atrial fibrillation. *AJN, 12*, 26–27.

Scherer, J.C. (1991). *Introductory medical-surgical nursing* (5th ed.). Philadelphia: J.B. Lippincott Company.

Solomon, E. P., Schmidt, R. R., & Adragna, P. J. (1990). *Human anatomy and physiology* (2nd ed.). Philadelphia: Saunders College Publishing.

Sommers, M. (1994). *Concepts and activities: Medical-surgical nursing*. Springhouse, PA: Springhouse Corporation.

Strimike, C. L. (1995). Caring for a client with an intracoronary stent. *AJN, 1*, 40–46.

Swearingen, P. L. (1994). *Manual of medical-surgical nursing care: Nursing interventions and collaborative management* (3rd ed.). St. Louis: Mosby-Year Book, Inc.

Therapy in action: AICD patient handbook. (1995). Guidant Corporation Cardiac Pacemakers.

CHAPTER 21

Beare, P. & Myers, J. L. (1994). *Principles and practice of adult health nursing* (2nd ed.). St. Louis: Mosby-Year Book, Inc.

Bright, L. D. (1995). Deep vein thrombosis. *American Journal of Nursing*, (6), 48-49.

Clinical update 95: Hypertension white-coat warning (1995). *Nursing 95*, (6), 54, Author.

Cuddy, R. (1995). Hypertension: Keeping dangerous blood pressure down. *Nursing 95, (8)*, 34–43.

Davis, E. (1993). The diagnostic puzzle and management challenge of Raynaud's syndrome. *Nurse Practitioner, 18*(3), 18–25.

Deglin, J. & Vallerand, A. (1995). *Davis's drug guide for nurses* (4th ed.). Philadelphia: F. A. Davis Company.

Hickey, A. (1994). Catching deep vein thrombosis in time. *Nursing 94*, (10), 34–42.

Hole, Jr., J. W. (1993). *Human anatomy and physiology* (6th ed.). Dubuque, IA: Wm. C. Brown Publishers.

Linton, A., Matteson, M. A., & Maebius, N. K. (1995). *Introductory nursing care of adults*. Philadelphia: W. B. Saunders Company.

Megerman, J. (1995). Prophylaxis against venous thromboembolism after hip surgery. *JAMA, 273* (4), 287.

Merriam Webster Medical Dictionary. (1995). America on Line Reference Desk.

Monahan, F. D., Drake, T., & Neighbors, M. (1994). *Nursing care of adults*. Philadelphia: W. B. Saunders Company.

Pagana, K. D. & Pagana, T. J. (1995). *Mosby's diagnostic and laboratory test reference* (2nd ed.). St. Louis: Mosby-Year Book, Inc.

Phipps, W. J., Cassmeyer, V. L., Sands, J. K., & Lehman, M. K. (1995). *Medical-surgical nursing: Concepts and clinical practice* (5th ed.). St. Louis: Mosby-Year Book, Inc.

Raimer, F. & Thomas, M. (1995). Clot stoppers. *Nursing 95,* (3), 34–43.

Rowland, R. (Medical Correspondent). (1995, December 20). High blood pressure can lower men's cognitive skills. *Internet CNN Health Briefs.*

Sandler, R. L. (1995). Abdominal aortic aneurysm. *American Journal of Nursing*, (1), 38–39.

Spratto, G.R. & Woods, A.L. (1997) *RN Magazine's NDR-95: Nurse's Drug Reference*. Albany, NY: Delmar Publishers Inc.

Stephenson, J. (1992). The cold facts. *Harvard Health Letter, 17*(3), 1–4.

Swearingen, P. L. (1994). *Manual of medical-surgical nursing care: Nursing interventions and collaborative management* (3rd ed.). St. Louis: Mosby-Year Book, Inc.

Whitaker, L. & Kelleher, A. (1994). Raynaud's syndrome: Diagnosis and treatment. *Journal of Vascular Nursing, 12*(1), 10–13

Williams, N. (1994). Hand arm vibration syndrome. *Occupational Health,* (3), 89–90.

CHAPTER 22

Anderson, K. N. (Ed.). (1994). *Mosby's medical nursing and allied health dictionary* (4th ed.). St. Louis: Mosby-Year Book, Inc.

Beare, P. & Myers, J. L. (1994). *Principles and practice of adult health nursing* (2nd ed.). St. Louis: Mosby-Year Book, Inc.

Black, J. M. & Mastassarin-Jacobs, E. (1993). *Luckman and Sorensen's medical-surgical nursing: A psychophysiologic approach* (4th ed.). Philadelphia: W. B. Saunders Company.

Campbell. K. (1995). Understanding acute and chronic myeloid leukaemia. *Nursing Times, 91*(47), 36–38.

Deglin, J. & Vallerand, A. (1995). *Davis's drug guide for nurses* (4th ed.). Philadelphia: F. A. Davis Company.

Erickson, J. M. (1994). Update on Hodgkin's disease. *Nurse Practitioner, 19*(11), 63–68.

Hole, Jr., J. W. (1993). *Human anatomy and physiology* (6th ed.). Dubuque, IA: Wm. C. Brown Publishers.

Interferon approved for chronic myelogenous leukemia (1996). *RN, 59*(2), 78.

Lewis, S., Collier, I., & Heitkemper, M.M. (1996). *Medical-surgical nursing* (4th ed.). St. Louis: Mosby-Year Book, Inc.

Linton, A., Matteson, M. A., & Maebius, N. K. (1995). *Introductory nursing care of adults*. Philadelphia: W. B. Saunders Company.

Loeb, S. (Ed.) (1993). *Diseases*. Springhouse, PA: Springhouse Publishing.

Lundquist, D. M. & Stewart, F. M. (1994). An update on non–Hodgkin's lymphomas. *Nurse Practitioner, 19*(10), 41–54.

Monahan, F. D., Drake, T., & Neighbors, M. (1994) *Nursing care of adults*. Philadelphia: W. B. Saunders Company.

National Cancer Institute. (1992). *What you need to know about non–Hodgkin's Disease* (2nd ed.) (Brochure). Bethesda, MD: National Cancer Institute.

Pagana, K. D. & Pagana, T. J. (1995). *Mosby's diagnostic and laboratory test reference*. St. Louis: Mosby-Year Book, Inc.

Phipps, W. J., Cassmeyer, V. L., Sands, J. K., & Lehman, M. K. (1995). *Medical-surgical nursing: Concepts and clinical practice* (5th ed.). St. Louis: Mosby-Year Book, Inc.

Scherer, J. C. & Timby, B. K. (1995). *Introductory medical-surgical nursing* (6th ed.). Philadelphia: J. B. Lippincott Company.

Smeltzer, S. C. & Bare, B. G. (1996). *Brunner and Suddarth's textbook of medical-surgical nursing* (8th ed.). Philadelphia: Lippincott-Raven Publishers.

Spraycar, M. (Ed.) (1995). *Stedman's medical dictionary* (26th ed.). Baltimore, MD: Williams and Wilkins.

Swearingen, P. L. (1994). *Manual of medical-surgical nursing care: Nursing interventions and collaborative management* (3rd ed.). St. Louis: Mosby-Year Book, Inc.

Thibodeau, G. A. & Patton, K. T. (1993). *Anatomy and physiology* (2nd ed.) St. Louis: Mosby-Year Book, Inc.

Thomas, C.L. (Ed.). (1993). *Taber's cyclopedic medical dictionary* (17th ed.). Philadelphia: F. A. Davis Company.

Tortora, G. J. & Grabowski, S. (1993). *Principles of anatomy and physiology* (7th ed.). New York: HarperCollins College Publishers.

Tranter, J. (1995). Making sense of blood transfusion. *Nursing Times, (910)* 36, 34–36.

Wasilewski, A. (1995). *Roferon-A (Interferon Alfa-2a, Recombinant) Cleared for Marketing by FDA - First Interferon for Treatment for Chronic Myelogenous Leukemia*. Internet: OncoLink.

CHAPTER 23

Anderson, K., Anderson, L., & Glanze, W. (Eds.) (1994). *Mosby's medical nursing and allied health dictionary,* (4th ed.). St. Louis: Mosby-Year Book, Inc.

Ashburn, M. A. (1995). Burn pain: the management of procedure-related pain. *Journal of Burn Care and Rehabilitation, 16*(3. Pt. 2): Supplement. 365–71.

Beare, P. & Myers, J. L. (1994) *Principles and practice of adult health nursing* (2nd ed.). St. Louis: Mosby-Year Book, Inc.

Calistro, A. M. (1993). Burn care basics and beyond. *RN, 56*(3), 26–32.

Carpenito, L. J. (1997). *Nursing diagnosis: Application to clinical practice* (7th ed.). Philadelphia: J. B. Lippincott Company.

Carroll, P. (1995). Bed selection: help patients rest easy. *RN 58*(5), 44–50

Dennison, P. D. & Black, J. M. (1993). Nursing care of clients with peripheral vascular disorders. In J. M. Black & E. Matassarin-Jacobs (Eds.). *Luckmann and Sorensen's medical-surgical nursing: A psychophysiologic approach* (4th ed.). 1253–1313. Philadelphia: W. B. Saunders Company.

Deters, G. E. (1992). Management of patients with dermatologic problems. In S. C. Smeltzer & B. G. Bare (Eds.). *Brunner and Suddarth's textbook of medical-surgical nursing* (7th ed.). 1445–1500. Philadelphia: J. B. Lippincott Company.

Fowler, A. (1994). Nursing management of a patient with burns. *British Journal of Nursing, 3*(21), 1105–1112.

Frantz, R. A. & Gardner, S. (1994). Clinical concerns: Management of dry skin. *Journal of Gerontological Nursing, 20*(9), 15–18, 45.

Fritsch, D. E. & Yurko, L. C. (1995). Management of persons with burns. In W. J. Phipps, V. L. Cassmeyer, J. K. Sands, & M. K. Lehman (Eds.). *Medical-surgical nursing: Concepts and clinical practice* (5th ed.). 2358–2397. St. Louis: Mosby-Year Book, Inc.

Guay, D. R. P. (1993). An update on plant-related contact dermatitis. *The Journal of Practical Nursing, 43*(4), 24–34.

Hill, M. (1994). Nursing management of adults with skin disorders. In P. G. Beare & J. L. Myers (Eds.). *Principles and practice of adult health nursing* (2nd ed.). 2089–2115. St. Louis: Mosby-Year Book, Inc.

Jackson, L. (1995). Quick response to hypothermia and frostbite. *American Journal of Nursing, 95*(3), 52.

Karch, A. M. (1996). *Lippincott's nursing drug guide*. Philadelphia: J. B. Lippincott Company.

Kornfeld, H. S. (1995). Co-meditation: Guiding patients through the relaxation process. *RN 58*(11), 57–59.

Kovach, T. (1995). The barrier defense: Skin hydration as infection control. *The Journal of Practical Nursing, 45*(1), 13–19.

Morton, O. (1993). Here comes the sun. *Nursing Times, 89*(29), 52–54.

Nicol, N. H. (1993). Nursing care of clients with integumentary disorders. In J. M. Black & E. Matassarin-Jacobs (Eds.). *Luckmann and Sorensen's medical-surgical nursing: A psychophysiologic approach*. (4th ed.). 1955–1982. Philadelphia: W. B. Saunders Company.

Ogden, B. L. (1994). Nursing management of adults with burns. In P. G. Beare & J. L. Myers (Eds.). *Principles and practice of adult health nursing* (2nd ed.). 2117–2142. St. Louis: Mosby-Year Book, Inc.

Penzer, R. (1994). Helping patients cope with psoriasis. *Nursing-Standard, 8*(49), 25–28.

Sabatini, M. M. (1995). Skin cancer: The silent pandemic. *Dermatology Nursing, 7*(1), 45–50.

Seeley, R. R., Stephens, T. D., & Tate, P. (1995) *Anatomy and physiology* (3rd ed.). St. Louis: Mosby-Year Book, Inc.

Seymour, J. (1995). Skin care: Sun protection. *Nursing Times 91*(25), 61, 63.

Weaver, V. (1995) Management of persons with problems of the skin. In W. J. Phipps, V. L. Cassmeyer, J. K. Sands, & M. K. Lehman (Eds.). *Medical-surgical nursing: Concepts and clinical practice* (5th ed.). 2317–2357. St. Louis: Mosby-Year Book, Inc.

CHAPTER 24

Arthur, V. (1994). Nursing care of patients with rheumatoid arthritis. *British Journal of Nursing, 3*(7), 325–327, 329–331.

Bertino, L. S. & Lu, L. C. (1993). The bite of the wolf: Systemic lupus erythematosus. *Rehabilitation Nursing, 16*(3), 173–178.

Carpenito, L. J. (1997). *Nursing diagnosis: Application to clinical practice*. Philadelphia: J. B. Lippincott Company.

Dumas, L. (1992). Arthritis in women: Social considerations in the clinical management of rheumatoid disease. *Journal of Home Health Care Practice, 4*(2), 42–52.

Fritsh, D. E. & Fredrick, D. M. (1993). Exposing latex allergies. *Nursing 93, 23*(8), 46–48.

Hardy, E. M. & Rittenberry, K. (1994). Myasthenia gravis: An overview. *Orthopaedic Nursing, 13*(6), 37–42.

Hausman, K. A. (1995). Interventions for clients with problems of the peripheral nervous system. In D. D. Ignatavicius, M. L. Workman, & M. A. Mishler. (Eds.). *Medical-surgical nursing: A nursing process approach* 1220–1235. Philadelphia: W. B. Saunders Company.

Ignatavicius, D.D. (1995). Interventions for clients with connective tissue disease. In D. B. Ignatavicius, M. L. Workman, & M. A. Mishler. (Eds.). *Medical-surgical nursing: A nursing process approach* 476–491. Philadelphia: W. B. Saunders Company.

Kuper, B. C. & Failla, S. (1994). Shedding new light on lupus. *American Journal of Nursing, 94*(11), 26–32.

Lancaster, L. E. (1992). Immunogenetic basis of tissue and organ transplantation and rejection. *Critical Care Nursing Clinics of North America, 4*(1), 1–24.

Lash, A. A. (1993). Systemic lupus erythematosus part 2: Diagnosis, treatment modalities and nursing management. *Medsurg Nursing, 2*(5), 375–385.

Lash, A. A. (1993). Why so many women? Part 1: Systemic lupus erythematosus. *Medsurg Nursing, 2*(4). 259–264.

Monahan, F.D. (1994). Nursing care of adults with immunodeficiency and hypersensitivity disorders. In F. D. Monohan, T. Drake, & M. Neighbors. (Eds.). *Nursing care of adults* (313–351). Philadelphia: W. B. Saunders Company.

Pagana, K. D. & Pagana, T. J. (1995). *Mosby's diagnostic and laboratory test reference*. St. Louis: Mosby-Year Book, Inc.

Paquette, E.V. (1993). Immunologic System. In J. M. Thompson, G. K. McFarland, J. E. Hirsch, & S. M. Tucker. (Eds.). *Mosby's clinical nursing* 1164–1201. St. Louis: Mosby-Year Book, Inc.

Price, A. & McCarley, P. B. (1994). Physical assessment for patients receiving therapeutic plasma exchange. *American Nephrological Nurses Association Journal, 21*(4), 149–201.

CHAPTER 25

Allen, M. A. & Ownby, K. K. (1991). Tuberculosis: The other epidemic. *Journal of the Association of Nurses in AIDS Care, 2*(4), 9–24.

American Health Consultants (1992). AIDS cases rising fastest in women. *AIDS alert: The monthly update for health professionals, 7*(2), 18–21.

American Medical Association. (1988). HIV blood test counseling. *AMA physician guidelines.*

Anastasi, J. & Lee, V. (1994). HIV-wasting: How to stop the cycle. *AJN, 11,* 18–24.

Anastasi, J. & Thomas, F. (1994). Dealing with HIV related pulmonary infections. *Nursing 94, 24,* 60–64.

Britton, C. B. (1993). The neurology of HIV infection: Clinical, pathogenic, and treatment perspectives. *AIDS, 7,* S218–S223: Supplement 1.

Buchbinder, S., Mann, D., & Louie, L.G. (1993). *Healthy–long term positive: genetic cofactors for delayed HIV disease progression.* Paper presented at the ninth international conference on AIDS, Berlin, Germany.

Centers for Disease Control and Prevention. (1996). Update: Mortality attributable to HIV infection among persons aged 25–44 years—United States, 1994. *Morbidity and Mortality Weekly Report, 45*(6), 10–14.

Centers for Disease Control and Prevention (1996). Continued sexual risk behavior among HIV-seropositive, drug-using men—Atlanta; Washington, D.C.; and San Juan, Puerto Rico, 1993. *Morbidity and Mortality Weekly, 15*(7), 13–15.

Centers for Disease Control and Prevention. (1996). AIDS associated with injecting drug use-United States, 1995. *Morbidity and Mortality Weekly Report, 45*(19), 37–42.

Centers for Disease Control and Prevention. (1995). *Questions and Answers: CDC DRAFT guidelines for HIV counseling and voluntary testing for pregnant women.* CDC HIV/AIDS prevention. 1–5.

Centers for Disease Control and Prevention. (1995). USPHS/IDSA Guidelines for the prevention of opportunistic infections in persons infected with human immunodeficiency virus: A summary. *Morbidity and Mortality Weekly Report, 44*(RR–8), 1–33.

Centers for Disease Control and Prevention. (1994). Guidelines for preventing the transmission of Mycobacterium tuberculosis in health-care facilities, 1994. *Morbidity and Mortality Weekly, 43* (RR–13), 1–132.

Centers for Disease Control and Prevention. (1993). 1993 revised classification system for HIV infection and expanded surveillance case definition for AIDS among adolescents and adults. *MMWR Morbidity and Mortality Weekly, 41*(RR–17):1.

Centers for Disease Control and Prevention. (1992). 1993 revised classification for HIV infection and expanded surveillance case definition for AIDS among adolescents and adults. *Morbidity and Mortality Weekly Report, 41*(9RR–17), 1–19.

Centers for Disease Control and Prevention (1990). Risk for cervical disease in HIV infected women. *Morbidity and Mortality Weekly Report, 39*(47), 846–849.

Centers for Disease Control. (1987). Revision of the CDC surveillance case definition for acquired immunodeficiency syndrome. *Morbidity and Mortality Weekly Report, 36*(Suppl. 1), 1S–5S.

Centers for Disease Control. (1981). Pneumocystis pneumonia–Los Angeles. *Morbidity and Mortality Weekly Report, 30*(21), 250–252.

Cohen, N. & Atwood, J. D. (1994). Women and AIDS: The social constructions of gender and disease. *Family Systems Medicine, 12*(1), 5–20.

Collier, A. C., Coombs, R. W., Schoenfield, D. A., Bassett, R. L., Timpone, J., Baruch, A., Jones, M., Facey, K., Whitacre, C., McAuliffe, V. J., Friedman, H. M., Merigan, T. C., Reichman, R. C., Hooper, C., & Corey, L. (1996). Treatment of human immunodeficiency virus with saquinavir, zidovudine, and zalcitabine. *The New England Journal of Medicine, 334*(16), 1011–1017.

Crowe, S. & Mills, J. (1994). Virus infections of the immune system. In D. B. Stites, A. I. Terr, & T. G. Parslow (Eds.) *Basic and clinical immunology,* (8th ed.). 689–705. Norwalk, CT: Appleton & Lange.

Early HIV Infection Guideline Panel. (1994). *Evaluation and management of early HIV infection: Clinical practice guideline.* (AHCPR Pub. No. 94–0572). Rockville, MD: Public Health Service.

Fegan, C. (1992). Cryptosporidial disease in the adult HIV-infected patient. *Journal of the Association or Nurses in AIDS Care, 3*(4), 11–20.

Finkelstein, D. M., Williams, P.L., Molenberghs, G., Feinberg, J., Powderly, W. G., Kahn, J., Dolin, R., & Cotton, D. (1996). Patterns of opportunistic infections in patients with HIV infection. *Journal of Acquired Immune Deficiency Syndromes and Human Retrovirology, 12,* 38–45.

Flaskerud, J. H. & Ungvarski, P. J. (1995). *HIV/AIDS: A guide to nursing care* (3rd ed.). Philadelphia: W. B. Saunders Company.

Global AIDS News (1994). AIDS cases soar in past year. *Global AIDS News: The Newsletter of the World Health Organization Global Programme on AIDS.* 3, 1–4.

Guyton, A. C. & Hall, J. E. (1996). *Textbook of medical physiology* (9th ed.). Philadelphia: W. B. Saunders Company.

Hoyt, M. J. & Staats, J. A. (1991). Wasting and malnutrition in patients with HIV/AIDS. *Journal of the Association or Nurses in AIDS Care, 2*(3), 16–26.

Kaplan, L. D. (1990). The malignancies associated with AIDS. In M. A. Sande & P. A. Volberding (Eds.). *The medical management of AIDS* (2nd ed.). 339–364. Philadelphia: W. B. Saunders Company.

Lego, S. (1994). *Fear and AIDS/HIV: Empathy and communication.* Albany, NY: Delmar Publishers.

Lindberg, C. E. (1995). Perinatal transmission of HIV: How to counsel women. *Maternal Child Nursing,* 20, 207–212.

Melnick, S. L., Sherer, R., Louis, T. A., Hillman, D., Rodriguez, E. M., Lackman, C., Capps, L., Brown, L. S., Carlyn, M., Korvick, J. A., & Deyton, L. (1994). Survival and disease progression according to gender of patients with HIV infection. *Journal of the American Medical Association, 272*(24), 1915–1921.

Mumu, R. D., Borucki, M. J., Lyons, D. A., & Pollard, R. B. (1991). Evaluation of adult patients infected with HIV. *Physicians Assistant, 15*(1), 23–32.

Mumu, R. D., Lyons, D. A., Borucki, M. J., & Pollard, R. B. (1994). *HIV manual for health care professionals.* Norwalk, CT: Appleton & Lange.

Paar, D. P. (1994). Hepatitis. In R. D. Mumu, M. J. Borucki, D. A. Lyons. & R. B. Pollard, (Eds.) *HIV manual for health care professionals.* Norwalk, CT: Appleton & Lange. 77–86.

Quinn, S. C. (1993). Perspective: AIDS and African American women: The triple burden of race, class, and gender. *Health Education Quarterly, 20*(3), 305–320.

Saag, M. S. (1993). Cryptococcal meningitis. *PAAC–Notes, 5*(1), 34–37.

Saliva test gets FDA approval. (1995). *AJN.* 2, 12: Author.

Singer, M. (1994). AIDS and the health crisis of the U.S. urban poor: The perspective of critical medical anthropology. *Social Science and Medicine, 39*(7), 931–948.

Ungvarski, P. J. (1992). Nursing care of the adult client with AIDS and cytomegalovirus infection. *Journal of the Association or Nurses in AIDS Care, 3*(1), 9–18.

Ungvarski, P. J. (1991). Nursing care of the adult client with infection due to *Pneumocystis carinii. Journal of the Association of Nurses in AIDS Care, 2*(2), 15–28.

Vermund, S. H., Kelley, K. F., Lein, R. S., et al. (1991). High risk of human papilloma virus and cervical squamous intraepithelial lesions among women with symptomatic human immunodeficiency virus infection. *American Journal of Obstetrics and Gynecology* (2), 392–398.

Zurlinden, J. & Verheggen, R. (1994). HIV vaccines: A report from the front. *RN,* 57, 36–40.

CHAPTER 26

Altizer, L. (1995). Total hip arthroplasty. *Orthopaedic Nursing* 4 7–17.

Beare, P. G. & Myers, J. L. (1994). *Principles and practices of adult health nursing* (2nd ed.) St. Louis: Mosby-Year Book, Inc.

Carpenito, L. J. (1995). *Nursing care plans and documentation nursing diagnoses and collaborative problems* (2nd ed.). Philadelphia: J. B. Lippincott Company.

deWit, S. C. (1992). *Kean's essentials of medical surgical nursing.* (3rd ed.). Philadelphia: W. B. Saunders Company.

Donner, C. (1993). Hip dislocation. *American Journal of Nursing* 8, 46.

Engram, B. (1993). *Medical-surgical nursing care plans.* New York: Delmar Publishers, Inc.

Huston, C. J. (1994). Ruptured achilles tendon. *American Journal of Nursing* (12).

Johnson, J., Anderson, C., Barrett, A., Duke, K., & Sharp, D. (1995). Roller traction: Mobilizing patients with acetabular fractures. *Orthopaedic Nursing* 1, 21–24.

Kalb, C. & Cowley, G. (1996, Jan. 29). Hope for damaged joints. *Newsweek,* 55.

Leff, R. L., Kurent, J. E., & Dickoff, D. J. (1994). Polymyositis and dermatomyositis: Meeting the diagnostic challenge. *The Journal of Musculoskeletal Medicine* 4, 57–65.

Linton, A. D., Matteson, M. A., & Maebius, N. K. (1995). *Introductory nursing care of adults.* Philadelphia: W. B. Saunders Company.

Long, B. C., Phipps, W. J., & Cassmeyer, V. L. (1993). *Medical-surgical nursing: A nursing process approach* (3rd ed.) St. Louis: Mosby.

Mac, H. L., Reynolds, M. A., Treston-Aurand, J., & Henke, J. A. (1993). Comparison of autoreinfusion and standard drainage systems in total joint arthroplasty patients. *Orthopaedic Nursing* 3, 19–22.

McConnell, E. A. (1993). Providing cast care. *Nursing 93* (1) 19.

Monahan, F. D., Drake, T., & Neighbors, M. (1994). *Nursing care of adults.* Philadelphia: W. B. Saunders Company.

Mourad, L. A. & Droste, M. M. (1993). *The nursing process in the care of adults with orthopaedic conditions* (3rd ed.). New York: Delmar Publishers Inc.

Pellino, T. (1994). How to manage hip fractures. *American Journal of Nursing* 4, 46–56.

Phipps, W. J., Cassmeyer, V. L., Sands, J. K., & Lehman, M. (1995). *Medical-surgical nursing concepts and clinical practice* (5th ed.). St. Louis: Mosby-Year Book, Inc.

Roshdahl, C. (1995). *Textbook of basic nursing* (6th ed.). Philadelphia: J. B. Lippincott Company.

Rucker, S., Budge, J., & Bailes, B. K. (1994). Perioperative care of patients undergoing spinal stabilization with internal fixation. *Today's Operating Room Nurse* (4), 8–13.

Scherer, J. C. & Timby, B. K. (1995). *Introductory medical surgical nursing* (6th ed.) Philadelphia: J. B. Lippincott Company.

Sipos, D. A. (1995). Carpal tunnel syndrome. *Orthopaedic Nursing* 1, 17–20.

Smeltzer, S. C. & Bare, B. G. (1992). *Brunner and Suddarth's textbook of medical-surgical nursing* (7th ed.). Philadelphia: J. B. Lippincott Company.

Sparks, S. M. & Taylor, C. M. (1993). *Nursing diagnosis reference manual* (2nd ed.) Springhouse, PA: Springhouse Corporation.

Taber, C. W. *Taber's cyclopedic medical dictionary* (17th ed.) Philadelphia: F. A. Davis Company.

Willis, D. (1991). Lyme disease. *The Journal of Neuroscience Nursing* 23, (8).

CHAPTER 27

Anti-inflammatories cut Alzheimer's risk. (1996, March 29). *The Journal Gazette,* p. A7.

Barinaga, M. (1995). Neurotrophic factors enter the clinic. *Science, 264,* 772–774.

Barinaga, M. (1995). Researchers broaden the attack on Parkinson's disease. *Science, 267,* 455–456.

Barr, M. L. & Kiernan, J. A. (1993). *The human nervous system: An anatomical viewpoint* (6th ed.). Philadelphia: J. B. Lippincott Company.

Beare, P. G. & Myers, J. L. (Eds.). (1994). *Principles and practice of adult health nursing* (2nd ed.). St. Louis: Mosby-Year Book, Inc.

Buchanan, L. E. & Nawoczenski, D. A. (1987). *Spinal cord injury: Concepts and management approaches.* Baltimore: Williams and Wilkins.

Carpenito, L. J. (1997). *Handbook of nursing diagnosis* (7th ed.). Philadelphia: J. B. Lippincott Company.

Chipps, E. M., Clanin, N. J., & Campbell, V. G. (1992). *Neurological disorders.* St. Louis: Mosby-Year Book, Inc.

Cochran, I., Flynn, C. A., Goets, G., Potts-Nulty, S. E., Rece, J., & Sensenig, H. (1994). Stroke care: Piecing together the long-term picture. *Nursing 94, 24*(6), 34–41.

Cox, H. C., Hinz, M. D., Lubno, M. A., Newfield, S. A., Ridenour, N. A., Slater, M. M., & Sridaromont, K. (1993). *Clinical applications of nursing diagnosis: Adult, child, women's, mental health, geriatric, and home health considerations.* (2nd ed.). Philadelphia: F. A. Davis Company.

Drucker, T. B. & Zeidman, S.M. (1994). Spinal cord injury: Role of steroid therapy. *Spine, 19,* 2281–2287.

Evans, M. J. (Ed.). (1989). *Neurological-neurosurgical nursing.* Springhouse, PA: Springhouse Corporation.

Fitzgerald, M. A. (1994). *Concepts and activities: Nursing health assessment.* Springhouse, PA: Springhouse Corporation.

Headache Classification Committee of the International Headache Society. (1988). Classification and diagnostic criteria for headache disorders, cranial neuralgias, and facial pain. *Cephalalgia, 8*(7). 9–96: Author.

Hickey, J. V. (1992). *The clinical practice of neurological and neurosurgical nursing* (3rd ed.). Philadelphia: J. B. Lippincott Company.

Huston, C. J. & Boelman, R. (1995). Autonomic dysreflexia. *American Journal of Nursing, 95*(6), 55.

Hyde, T. M. & Weinberger, D. R. (1995). Tourette's syndrome: A model neuropsychiatric disorder. *Journal of American Medical Association, 273,* 498–501.

Kalbach, L. R. (1991). Unilateral neglect: Mechanism and nursing care. *Journal of Neuroscience Nursing, 23,* 25–129.

Laskowski-Jones, L. (1993). Acute SCI: How to minimize. *American Journal of Nursing, 93*(12), 23–31.

Latham, L. (1994). When spinal cord injury complicates med/surg care. *RN, 57*(8), 26–30.

McCance, K. L., Huether, S. E., et al. (1990). *Pathophysiology: The biological basis for disease in adults and children.* St. Louis: Mosby-Year Book, Inc.

Meissner, J. E. (1994). Caring for clients with multiple sclerosis. *Nursing 94,* 24(8), 60–61.

Mitiguy, J. (1991). The brain under attack. *HEADline.* 2–8, 10.

Mitsumoto, H., Ikeda, K., Klinlosz, B., Cedarbaum, J. M., Wong, V., & Lindsay, R. M. (1994). Arrest of motor neuron disease in wobbler mice cotreated with CNTF and BDNF. *Science, 265,* 1107–1110.

Monlus-Swift, C. (1994). Neurological disorders. In P. L. Swearingen (Ed.). *Manual of medical-surgical nursing care: Nursing interventions and collaborative management* (3rd ed.), 181–319. St. Louis: Mosby-Year Book, Inc.

National Spinal Cord Injury Statistical Center. (1990). *Spinal cord injury fact sheet.* Birmingham: University of Alabama at Birmingham. (Supported in part by Grant No. G008535128 from National Institute on Disability and Rehabilitation Research, United States Department of Education.)

National Stroke Association Press Release. (March 13, 1995). *Stroke deaths increase for first time in 35 years.*

New treatment for stroke victims. (1997, January). *The Journal Gazette.*

Reiman, E. M., Caselli, R. J., Yun, L. S., Chen, K., Bandy, D., Minoshima, S., Thibodeau, S. N., & Osborne, D. (1996). Preclinical evidence of Alzheimer's disease in person homozygous for the ε allele for apolipoprotein ε. *New England Journal of Medicine, 334,* 752–758.

Samuels, M. A. (Ed.). (1995). *Manual of neurological therapeutics* (5th ed.). Boston: Little Brown.

Selkoe, D. J. (1992). Aging brain, aging mind. *Scientific American, 267,* (3), 134–142.

Smeltzer, S. C. & Bare, B. G. (Ed.). (1992). *Brunner and Suddarth's textbook of medical surgical nursing* (7th ed.). Philadelphia: J. B. Lippincott.

Thelan, L. A., Davie, J. K., & Urden, L. D. (1990). *Textbook of critical care nursing: Diagnosis and management.* St. Louis: Mosby-Year Book, Inc.

CHAPTER 28

Adair, L. (1992). Touch and the nurse. *Journal of Clinical Nursing, 92*(1), 4–5.

Acute otitis media in adults. (1994). *Emergency Medicine, 26*(6), 44: Author.

A guide to assistive learning devices. (1993). *The Hearing Journal, 46*(2), 23: Author.

Tackling otitis media in adults. (1992). *Emergency Medicine, 24*(2), 67–8: Author.

Baloh, R. W. & Lee, K. (1990). Help for Meniere's disease patients. *Patient Care, 24*(15), 80–4, 89, 92.

Goldenberg, R. A., Brown, M., & Cunningham, S. (1992). Laser stapedotomy: A new method of correcting deafness. *AORN Journal, 55*(3), 759, 761–2, 764.

Goodhill, V. (1992). Evaluation of the aging ear. *Emergency Medicine, 24*(15), 165–6, 169, 173–4.

Maquen, E., Salz, J. J., Neoburn, A. B., (need all authors). (1994). Results of excimer laser photorefractive keratectomy for correction of myopia. *Ophthamology, 101*(9).

Pollen, K. A. (1992). Assessment and management of patients with vision problems and eye disorders. In S. C. Smeltzer & B. G. Bare (Ed.). *Brunner and Suddarth's textbook of medical surgical nursing,* 1543–1614. Philadelphia: J. B. Lippincott Company.

Temple-Mills, B. (1992). Assessment and management of patients with hearing problems and ear disorders. In S. C. Smeltzer & B. G. Bare (Ed.). *Brunner and Suddarth's textbook of medical surgical nursing,* 1591–1614. Philadelphia: J. B. Lippincott Company.

Ruehl, C. & Schremp, P. (1992). Nursing care of the cataract patient: Today's outpatient approach. *Nursing Clinics of North America, 27*(3), 737–743.

Roberts, A. (1994). Smell. *Nursing Times, 90*(6), 37–40.

Roberts, A. (1994). The senses: taste. *Nursing Times, 90*(15), 35–44.

Roberts, A. (1993). The ear and hearing, part 1. *Nursing Times, 89*(45), 10–16.

Roberts, A. (1993). The ear and hearing, part 2. *Nursing Times, 89*(49), 41–44.

Roberts, A. (1993). The ear and hearing, part 3. *Nursing Times, 90*(2), 12–18.

Silverstein, H., Wolfson, R. J., & Rosenberg, S. (1992). Diagnosis and management of hearing loss. *Clinical Symposia, 44*(3), 2–32.

Souder, E. & Yoder, L. (1992). Olfaction: The neglected sense. *Journal of Neuroscience Nursing, 24*(5), 273–279.

Sparks, S. M. & Taylor, C. M. (1995). *Nursing diagnosis reference manual* (3rd ed.). Springhouse, PA: Springhouse Corporation.

Weiss, S. J. (1992). Measurement of the sensory qualities in tactile interaction. *Nursing Research, 41*(2), 82–6.

Woods, S. (1992). Macular degeneration. *Nursing Clinics of North America, 27*(3),761–775.

CHAPTER 29

Anderson, K. N. (Rev. Ed.). (1994). *Mosby's medical, nursing, and allied health* (4th ed.). St. Louis: Mosby-Year Book, Inc.

Angelucci, P. A. (1995). Caring for patients with hypothyroidism. *Nursing, 25*(5), 60–61.

Beare, P. G. & Myers, J. L. (Eds.). (1994). *Principles and practice of adult health nursing* (2nd ed.). St. Louis: Mosby-Year Book, Inc.

Brown, M. J. (Ed.). (1992). *Miller-Keane encyclopedia & dictionary* (5th ed.). Philadelphia: W. B. Saunders Co.

Corsetti, A. & Buhl, B. (1994). Managing thyroid storm. *American Journal of Nursing, 94*(11), 39.

Ignatavicius, D. D., Workman, M. L., & Mishler, M. A. (1995). *Medical-surgical nursing: A nursing process approach* (2nd ed.). Philadelphia: W. B. Saunders Co.

Jaffe, M. S. (1996). *Medical-surgical nursing care plans: Nursing diagnoses & interventions* (3rd ed.). Stamford, CT: Appleton & Lange.

Kee, J. L. & Hayes, E. R. (1993). *Pharmacology: A nursing process approach.* Philadelphia: W. B. Saunders Co.

LeMone, P. & Burke, K. M. (1996). *Medical-surgical nursing: Critical thinking in client care.* New York: Addison-Wesley Nursing.

Lewis, J. A. (Senior Ed.). (1994). *Illustrated manual of nursing practice* (2nd ed.). Springhouse, PA: Springhouse Corp.

Linton, A. D., Matteson, M. A., & Maebius, N. K. (1995). *Introductory nursing care of adults.* Philadelphia: W. B. Saunders Co.

Monahan, F. D., Drake, T., & Neighbors, M. (1994). *Nursing care of adults.* Philadelphia: W. B. Saunders Co.

Norris, J. (Senior Ed.). (1994). *Handbook of medical-surgical nursing.* Springhouse, PA: Springhouse Corp.

Pagana, K. D. & Pagana, T. J. (1995). *Mosby's diagnostic and laboratory test reference* (2nd ed.). St. Louis: Mosby-Year Book, Inc.

Shaw, M. (Senior Ed.). (1995). *Professional handbook of diagnostic tests.* Springhouse, PA: Springhouse Corp.

Siconolfi, L. A. (1994). The forgotten system: Endocrine dysfunction during multiple system organ dysfunction. *Critical Care Nursing Quarterly, 16*(4), 16–26.

Smeltzer, S. C. & Bare, B. G. (1996). *Brunner & Suddarth's textbook of medical-surgical nursing* (8th ed.). Philadelphia: Lippincott-Raven Publishers.

Spratto, G. R. & Woods, A. L. (1996). *RN magazine's NDR–96.* Albany: Delmar Publishers.

Thibodeau, G. A. & Patton, K. T. (1997). *The human body in health & disease* (2nd ed.). St. Louis: Mosby-Year Book, Inc.

Weiss, R. (1994, September 13). Growth hormone provides no extra inches. *Washington (D. C.) Post,* Health Section, p. 7.

Williams, B. R. & Baer, C. L. (1994). *Essentials of clinical pharmacology in nursing* (2nd ed.). Springhouse, PA: Springhouse Corp.

Woodrow, R. (1992). *Essentials of pharmacology for health occupations* (2nd ed.). Albany: Delmar Publishers.

CHAPTER 30

American Diabetes Association. (1996). Nutrition recommendations and principles for people with diabetes mellitus. Position Statement: American Diabetes Association. *Diabetes Care, 19*(1), 16–19.

American Diabetes Association. (1995). American Diabetes Association: Clinical practice recommendations 1995. *Diabetes Care, 18,*(1).

American Diabetes Association. (1994). Nutrition recommendations and principles for people with diabetes mellitus. *Journal of the American Dietetic Association, 94*(5), 504–506.

American Diabetes Association. (1994). *Therapy for diabetes mellitus and related disorders* (2nd ed.). Alexandria, VA.

Barnett, A. (1994). A significant risk. *Nursing Times, 90*(2), 62–64.

Betz, J. L. (1995). Fast-acting human insulin analogs: A promising innovation in diabetes care. *The Diabetes Educator, 21*(3), 195–197.

Brown, S. A. & Hedges, L. V. (1994). Predicting metabolic control in diabetes: A pilot study using meta-analysis to estimate a linear model. *Nursing Research, 43*(6), 362–368.

Budinger, J. M. & Donnelly, S. S. (1994). Nursing care protocols for the kidney/islet cell transplant recipient. *ANNA Journal, 21*(2), 123–128.

Carlisle, B. A. (1993, March). Treatment of diabetes in the elderly. *The Journal of Practical Nursing,* 23–31.

Curry, M. & Weeden, L. Balancing act. *Nursing Times, 9*(89), 50–52.

Diabetes Control and Complications Trial Research Group. (1993). The effect of intensive treatment of diabetes on the development and progression of long-term complications in insulin-dependent diabetes mellitus. *The New England Journal of Medicine, 329,*(14), 977–1036: Author.

Diabetes update. (1993, August). *Nursing 93,* 59–61: Author.

Garrison, M. W. (1993). Identifying and treating common and uncommon infections in the patient with diabetes. *The Diabetes Educator, 19*(6), 522–529.

Geiss, L.S., Herman, W. H., Goldschmid, M.G., DeStefano, F., Eberhardt, M. S., Ford, E. S., German, R. R., Newman, J. M., Olson, D. R., Sepe, S. J., Stevenson, J. M., Vinicor, F., Wetterhall, S. F., & Will, J. C. (1993). CDC surveillance summaries: Surveillance for diabetes mellitus—United States, 1980–1989. *Morbidity and Mortality Weekly Report, 42,* 1–20.

Harley, J. R. (1993, October). Preventing diabetic foot disease. *Nurse Practitioner,* 37–44.

Kerr, C. P. (1995). Improving outcomes in diabetes: A review of the outpatient care of NIDDM patients. *The Journal of Family Practice, 40*(1), 63–75.

Kestel, F. (1994, July). Are you up to date on diabetes medications? *AJN,* 48–52.

Lebovitz, H. A. (1994). *Therapy for diabetes mellitus and related disorders.* (2nd ed.). Alexandria, VA: American Diabetes Association.

LeMone, P. (1994). Responses of the older adult to the effects and management of diabetes mellitus. *MEDSURG Nursing, 3*(2), 122–127.

McCance, K. L. & Huether, S. E. (1994). *Pathophysiology: The biologic basis for disease in adults and children.* (2nd ed.). St. Louis: Mosby-Year Book, Inc.

Oexmann, M. J. (1989). *Total available glucose—a diabetic food system.* New York: William Morrow.

Pagana, K. D. & Pagana, T. J. (1995). *Mosby's diagnostic and laboratory test reference.* (2nd ed.). St. Louis: Mosby-Year Book, Inc.

Reising, D. (1995, February). Acute hyperglycemia. *Nursing 95,* 33–40.

Reising, D. (1995, February). Acute hypoglycemia. *Nursing 95,* 41–48.

Robinsons, M. (1992). Infrared beam for blood glucose monitoring. *Clinical Chemistry, 38*(2), 1618–22.

Schmidt, L. E., Rost, K. M., McGill, J. B., & Santiago, J. V. (1994). The relationship between eating patterns and metabolic control in patients with non-insulin-dependent diabetes mellitus (NIDDM). *The Diabetes Educator, 20*(4), 317–321.

Sheets, C. & James, R. (1991). Older adult. In D. W. Guthrie & R. A. Guthrie (Eds.). *Nursing management of diabetes mellitus.* (3rd ed.). New York: Springer Publishing Company.

Skidmore-Roth, L. (1994). *Mosby's nursing drug reference.* St. Louis: Mosby-Year Book Inc.

Strowig, S. M. (1995, June). Insulin therapy. *RN,* 30–37.

Strowig, S. M. (1993). Initiation and management of insulin pump therapy. *The Diabetes Educator, 19*(1), 50–58.

Tinker, L. F., Heins, J. M., & Holler, H. J. (1994). Commentary and translation: 1994 recommendations for diabetes. *Journal of the American Dietetic Association, 94*(5), 507–511.

U.S. Department of Health and Human Services, National Center for Chronic Disease Control and Prevention, Division of Diabetes Translation (1992). *Diabetes in the United States: A strategy for prevention.* Washington, DC: U.S. Public Health Service.

White, J. R. (1994, March). Update on oral hypoglycemics. *Journal of Practical Nursing,* 24–33.

Williams, S. R. (1994). *Essential of nutrition and diet therapy* (6th ed.) St. Louis: Mosby-Year Book Inc.

CHAPTER 31

Asch, R. (1990). Gamete Intra-fallopian Transfer. *Serona Symposia.* Norwell, MA.

Ball, K. A. (1988). Laser endometrial ablation: Treatment for dysfunctional uterine bleeding. *AORN Journal, 48* (6), 1153, 1155–7, 1159–64.

Baron, R. H. & Walsh, A. (1995). Nine facts everyone should know about breast cancer. *American Journal of Nursing, 95* (7), 29–33.

Brunner, L. & Suddarth, D. (1993) (Ed.) Gynecologic and breast disorders. In *The Manual of Nursing Practice* (6th ed.). 560–603. Philadelphia, PA: J. B. Lippincott Company.

Cant, S. (1992). Infertility: Causes and treatment. *Nursing Standard, 7* (13–14), 28–30.

Chapman, K. (1994). When the prognosis isn't as good. *RN, 57* (7), 55–57.

Corenblum, B. (1993). Amenorrhea: Finding the underlying problem. *Medicine North America,* 16 (9), 713–20.

Curole, D. N. (1992). Evaluation of the infertile couple. *Journal of the American Academy of Physician Assistants, 5* (10), 747–53.

Dest, V. M. & Fisher, S. M. (1994). Breast cancer, dreaded diagnosis, complicated care. *RN, 57* (6), 48–58.

Donaldson, K. E., Briggs, J., & McMaster, D. (1994). RU-486: An alternative to surgical abortion. *JOGNN, 23* (7), 555–9.

Donovan, P. (1995). New nonsurgical abortion method proves to be 90% successful in early trial. *Family Planning Perspectives, 27* (3), 131–2.

Fowler, G. C., Hassalquist, M. B., & Zacur, H. A. (1994). Menstrual irregularities: A focused evaluation. *Patient Care, 28* (7), 155–60, 163–4.

Fox, S. M. & Haney, L. G. (1994). Taxol: New hope for cancer patients. *RN, 57* (11), 33–36.

Frye, B. S. (1993). Abortion. In *AWHONN's Clinical Issues in Perinatal Nursing, 4*(2), 265–271. Philadelphia, PA. J. B. Lippincott Company.

Griffith, C. J. (1995). Premenstrual syndrome: An update. *Journal of the American Academy of Physician Assistants, 8*(4), 31–2, 35–6.

Holm, K., Penckofer, S., & Chandler, P. J. (1995). Deciding on hormone replacement therapy. *AJN, 95*(8), 57–59.

Howes, D. S., Marrazzo, J. M., & Scott, C. (1993). Recognizing pelvic inflammatory disease. *Patient Care,* 27 (11), 186–93, 197–9, 203–4.

Ivey, C. L. (1994). When your patient has ovarian cancer. *RN, 57* (11), 26–32.

Ivey, C. L. & Gordon, S. I. (1994). Breast reconstruction: New image, new hope. *RN, 57* (7), 48–54.

James, C. A. (1992). The nursing role in assisted reproductive technologies. *NAACOGS Clinical Issues in Perinatal and Women's Health Nursing,* 3 (2), 328–34.

Jossens, M. O. & Sweet, R. L. (1993). Pelvic inflammatory disease: Risk factors and microbial etiologies. *JOGNN,* 22 (2), 169–79.

Killion, C. (1994). Pregnancy, a critical time to target STDs. *MCN, 19* (3), 156–161.

Knobf, M. T. & Morra, M. E. (1993). Women and cancer. In *AWHONN's Clinical Issues in Perinatal and Women's Health Nursing, 4*(2), 287–301. Philadelphia, PA. J. B. Lippincott Company.

Lomano, J. M. (1994). A patient's guide to Taxol. *Oncology Nursing Forum,* 21 (9), 1569–72.

Long, B. C. & Glazer, G. (1993). The patient with reproductive problems. In Long, Phipps & Cassmeyer (Ed). *Medical-Surgical Nursing: A Nursing Process Approach,* 1121–1152. St. Louis, MO: Mosby-Year Book, Inc.

Marrs, R. (1990). In vitro fertilization and embryo replacement. *Serono Symposia,* USA.

Mason, E. (1991). Medical causes of abnormal vaginal bleeding. *NAACOGS Clinical Issues in Perinatal and Women's Health Nursing,* 2 (3), 322–7.

Nader, S. (1993). Prostaglandin inhibitors in the management of premenstrual syndrome. *Physician Assistant,* 17 (1), 53–5, 59–61, 107–9.

National Cancer Institute. (1994). *A mammogram could save your life.* (NIH Publication No. 94–3418).

National Cancer Institute. (1993). *Take care of your breasts.* (NIH Publication No. 93–3417).

National Cancer Institute. (1993). *What you need to know about ovarian cancer.* (NIH Publication No. 94–1561).

National Cancer Institute. (1992). *What you need to know about cancer of the uterus.* (NIH Publication No. 93–1562)

National Cancer Institute. (1991). *What you need to know about cancer of the cervix.* (NIH Publication No. 91–2047).

Norwood, S. (1990). Fibrocystic breast disease: An update and review. *JOGNN,* 19 (2), 116–121.

Olshansky, E. F. (1992). Redefining the concepts of success and failure in infertility treatment. *NAACOG Clinical Issues in Perinatal and Women's Health Nursing,* 3 (2), 343–6.

Reid, T. (1994). Treatment for infertility: Counting the cost. *Nursing Times,* 90 (45), 27–8.

Rich, S. E. (1993). Tamoxifen and breast cancer—from palliation to prevention. *Cancer Nursing,* 16 (5), 341–6.

Rickert, B. (1992). Estrogen replacement: Making informed choices. *RN,* 55 (9), 26–32.

Roddy, R. E. (1993). Predisposing factors for pelvic inflammatory disease. *Journal of the Academy of Physician Assistants,* 6 (1), 42–7.

Shaw, K. (1995). Breast cancer and its treatment. *Journal of Practical Nursing,* 45 (1), 21–9.

Shochey, C. (1994). Perimenopause and heavy menstrual flow: Standard treatments and alternative treatment modalities. *Nurse Practitioner: American Journal of Primary Health Care,* 19 (9), 73–5.

Shlafer, M. (1993). *Pharmacology: The Nurse and Drug Therapy,* (2nd ed.) Redwood City, CA: Addison-Wesley.

Smeltzer, S. C. & Bare, B. G. (1992). Management of patients with disorders of the female reproductive system. In *Brunner and Suddarth's Medical-Surgical Nursing* (7th ed.), 1261–1321 Philadelphia, PA: J. B. Lippincott Company.

Soper, D. E. (1994). Pelvic inflammatory disease. *Infectious Disease Clinics of North America,* 8 (4), 821–40.

vanLeeuwen, F. & Benraadt, J. (1994). Risk of endometrial cancer after tamoxifen treatment of breast cancer. *Lancet,* 343 (8896), 448.

Wasaha, S. & Angelopoulos, F. (1996). What every woman should know about menopause. *AJN,* 96 (1), 25–33

White, G. B. (1992). Understanding the ethical issues in infertility nursing practice. *NACCOG Clinical Issues in Perinatal and Women's Health Nursing,* 3 (2), 347–52.

Wilson, B. A. (1993). Tamoxifen for breast cancer therapy: Nursing implications. *MEDSURG Nursing,* 2 (6), 494–5.

CHAPTER 32

Brenner, Z. R. & Krezner, M. E. (1995, April). Update on cryosurgical ablation for prostate cancer. *American Journal of Nursing,* 1995.

Clowers, D. (1995). Personal Communication. *Urodynamics, SCI-Urology.* Erectile Dysfunction Clinic Department of Veterans' Affairs: Seattle, WA.

Cummings, J. M., Parra, R. O., & Boullier, J. A. (1995). Laser prostatectomy: Initial experience and urodynamic follow-up. *Urology,* 45 (3), 414–419.

de Hart, P.M. (1995). Personal communication. Fred Hutchinson Cancer Research Center. Seattle, WA: Researcher.

Gerber, G. S. (1995). Lasers in the treatment of benign prostatic hyperplasia. *Urology,* 45(3), 193–198.

Gray, M. (1992). *Genitourinary disorders.* St. Louis: Mosby-Year Book, Inc.

Hatcher, R. A., Stewart, F., Trussell, J., Kowal, D., Guest, F., Stewart, G. K., & Gates, W. (1992). *Contraceptive technology* (5th ed.). New York: Irvington Publishers.

Heaton, J. R., Morales, A., Adams, M. A., Johnson, B., & Rashidy, R. E. (1995). Recovery of erectile function by the oral administration of apomorphine. *Urology,* 45(3), 200–206.

Kim, J. C., Lunati, F. P., Khan, S. A., & Waltzer, W. C. (1995). T-tube drainage of infected penile corporeal chambers. *Urology,* 45(3), 514–515.

Lepor, H. (1995). Long-term efficacy and safety of terazosin in patients with benign prostatic hyperplasia. *Urology,* 45(3), 406–413.

MacDermott, B. L., Deglin, J. H. (1995). *Understanding basic pharmacology: Practical approaches for effective application.* Philadelphia: F. A. Davis Company.

Marieb, E. N. (1995). *Human anatomy and physiology* (3rd ed.). Redwood City: Benjamin/Cummings Publishing Company.

Martini, F. H. (1995). *Fundamentals of anatomy & physiology* (3rd ed.). Englewood Cliffs, NJ: Prentice Hall.

Morales, A. (1993). Nonsurgical management options in impotence. *Hospital Practices,* 30(3), 55–60.

Speights Jr., V. O., Brawn, P. N., Foster, D. M., Spiekerman, A. M., Kuhl, D., & Riggs, M. W. (1995). Evaluation of age-specific normal ranges for prostate-specific antigen. *Urology,* 45(3), 454–458.

Taber, C. W. (1993). *Taber's cyclopedic medical dictionary* (17th ed.). Philadelphia: F. A. Davis Company.

Twillie, D. A., Eisenberger, M. A., Carducci, M. A., Hseih, W. S., Kim, W. Y., & Simons, J. W. (1995). Interleukin-6: A candidate mediator of human prostate cancer morbidity. *Urology,* 45(3), 542–549.

Van Wynsberghe, D., Noback, C. R., & Carola, R. (1995). *Human anatomy & physiology* (3rd ed.). New York: McGraw-Hill.

Wolcott, J. (March, 1995). Locally refined therapy nipping prostate cancer. *Puget Sound Business Journal,* 18–21.

CHAPTER 33

Addiss, D. G., Vaugn, M. L., Ludka, D., Pfister, J., & Davis, J. P. (1993, January–February). Decreased prevalence of *Chlamydia trachomatis* infection associated with a selective screening program in family planning clinics in Wisconsin. *Sexually Transmitted Diseases 20,* 28.

Ansell, D. A., Hu, T., Straus, M., Cohen, M., & Sherer, R. (1994, March–April). HIV and syphilis seroprevalence among clients with sexually transmitted diseases attending a walk-in clinic at Cook County Hospital. *Sexually Transmitted Diseases 21,* 93.

Avins, A. L., Woods, W. J., Lindan, C. P., Hudes, E. S., Clark, W., & Hulley, S. B. (1994, February 16). HIV infection and risk behaviors among heterosexuals in alcohol treatment programs. *JAMA, 271,* 515.

Burton, A. A., Flynn, J. A., Neumann, T. M., Wilson, C., Quinn, T. A., & Hook, E. W. (1994, May–June). Routine serologic screening for syphilis in hospitalized patients: High prevalence of unsuspected infection in the elderly. *Sexually Transmitted Diseases, 21,* 133.

Butterworth, C. E., Hatch, K., & Macaluso, M. (1992). Folate deficiency and cervical dysplasia. *JAMA, 267*(4), 528–533.

Catotti, D. N., Clarke, P., & Catoe, K. E. (1993, March–April). Herpes revisited: Still a cause of concern. *Sexually Transmitted Diseases, 20,* 77.

Corey, L. (1994, March–April). The current trend in genital herpes: Progress in prevention. *Sexually Transmitted Diseases, 21,* S38.

Dickason, E. J., Silverman, B. L., & Schult, M. O. (1993). *Maternal-infant nursing care* (2nd ed.). St. Louis: Mosby-Year Book, Inc.

Erickson, M. J. (1994, June). Chlamydial infections: Combating the silent threat. *American Journal of Nursing, 94,* 16B.

Ernst, A. A. & Martin, D. H. (1993, March–April) High syphilis rates among cocaine abusers identified in an emergency department. *Sexually Transmitted Diseases, 20,* 66.

Finelli, L., Budd, J., & Spitalny, K. (1993, March–April). Early syphilis: Relationship to sex, drugs, and changes in high risk behavior from 1987–1990. *Sexually Transmitted Diseases, 20,* 89.

Freund, K. M. (1992, February 15). Chlamydial disease in women. *Hospital Practice, 27,* 175.

Garnett, G. P. & Anderson, R. M. (1993, July–August). Contact tracing and the estimation of sexual mixing patterns: The epidemiology of gonococcal infections. *Sexually Transmitted Diseases, 20,* 181.

Hawley, H. B. (1993, August). Gonorrhea: Finding and treating a moving target. *Postgraduate Medicine, 94,* 105.

Herpes simplex virus. (1993, March). *Postgraduate Medicine, 93,* 311: Author.

Hook, E. W. & Marra, C. M. (1992, April 16). Acquired syphilis in adults. *The New England Journal of Medicine, 326,* 1060.

Hook, E. W. (1992, November). Management of syphilis in human immunodeficiency virus-infected patients. *American Journal of Medicine, 93,* 477.

Kirchner, J. T. (1991, September). Syphilis—An STD on the increase. *American Family Physician, 44,* 843.

Klass, P. E., Brown, E. R., & Pelton, S. I. (1994, July). The incidence of prenatal syphilis at the Boston City Hospital: A comparison across four decades. *Pediatrics, 94,* 24.

Lammon, C. B., Foote, A. W., Leli, P. G., Ingle, J., & Adams, M. H. (1995). *Clinical nursing skills.* Philadelphia: W. B. Saunders Company.

Lemp, G. F., Hirozawa, A. M., Givertz, D., Nieri, G. N., Anderson, L., Lindegren, M. L., Janssen, R. S., & Katz, M. (1994, August 10). Seroprevalence of HIV and risk behaviors among young homosexual and bisexual men: The San Francisco/Berkeley Young Men's Survey. *JAMA, 272,* 449.

Libbus, M. K. (1992, September–October). Condoms as a primary prevention in sexually active women. *American Journal of Maternal-Child Nursing, 17,* 256.

Luger, A. (1993, March–April). The origin of syphilis: Clinical and epidemiological considerations on the Columbian theory. *Sexually Transmitted Diseases, 20,* 110.

Lungu, O., Sun, X. W., Felix, J., Richart, R. M., Silverstein, S., & Wright, T. C., Jr. (1992, May 13). Relationship of human papillomavirus type to grade of cervical intraepithelial neoplasia. *JAMA, 267,* 2493.

Majeroni, B. A. (1994, June). Chlamydial cervicitis: complications and new treatment options. *American Family Physician, 49,* 1825.

Mertz, G. J., Benedetti, J., Ashley, R., Selke, S. A., & Corey, L. (1992, February 1). Risk factors for the sexual transmission of genital herpes. *Annals of Internal Medicine, 116,* 197.

Potts, J. F. (1992, January). Chlamydial infection: Screening and management update. *Postgraduate Medicine, 91,* 120.

Research points to drug against genital warts. (1994, May 9). *Cancer Researcher Weekly,* 13: Author.

Schiffman, M. H. (1992, March 18). Recent progress in defining the epidemiology of human papillomavirus infection and cervical neoplasia. *Journal of the National Cancer Institute, 84,* 394.

Sloane, E. (1993). *Biology of women* (3rd ed.). New York: Delmar Publishers, Inc.

Sparks, S. M. & Taylor, C. M. (1993). *Nursing diagnosis reference manual* (2nd ed.). Springhouse, PA: Springhouse

Taylor-Robinson, D. (1994, January 15). Chlamydia trachomatis and sexually transmitted disease: What do we know and what shall we do? *British Medical Journal, 308,* 150.

Touchstone, D. M. & Davis, D. D. (1992, February). Consider chlamydia. *RN, 55,* 32.

White, K. (1992, October 28–November 3). Sterile condition . . . chlamydia. *Nursing Times, 88,* 34.

Workowski, K. A., Lampe, M. F., Wong, K. G., Watts, M. B., & Stamm, W. E. (1993, November 3). Long-term eradication of *Chlamydia trachomatis* genital infection after antimicrobial therapy: Evidence against persistent infection. *JAMA, 270,* 2071.

Zenilman, J. M. (1993, February 28). Gonorrhea: Clinical and public health issues. *Hospital Practice, 28,* 29.

CHAPTER 34

Butler, R. (1994, March). Managing the complications of cirrhosis. *American Journal of Nursing, 94*(3), 46–49.

Cameron, J. L. (1995). *Current surgical therapy.* St. Louis: Mosby-Year Book, Inc.

Carpenito, L. J. (1997). *Nursing diagnosis: Application to clinical practice.* Philadelphia: J. B. Lippincott Company.

Donner, C. (1993, July). Understanding stress ulcers. *American Journal of Nursing, 93*(7), 49.

Hastings, G. E. & Weber, R. J. (1993, February 15). Inflammatory bowel disease: Part I, clinical features and diagnosis. *American Family Physician, 47*(3), 598–608.

Hastings, G. E. & Weber, R. J. (1993, March). Inflammatory bowel disease: Part II, medical and surgical management. *American Family Physician, 47*(4), 811–818.

International Working Party. (1995, February). Terminology of chronic hepatitis. *The American Journal of Gastroenterology, 90,* 181–189: Author.

Jess, L. W. (1993, September). Acute abdominal pain: Revealing the source. *Nursing 93, 23*(10), 34–41.

Lisant, P. & Talotta, D. (1994, May). An overview of viral hepatitis, A through E. *AORN Journal, 59,* 997–1005.

Marx, J. (1993, January). Viral hepatitis: Unscrambling the alphabet. *Nursing 93, 23*(1), 34–41.

McConnell, E. (1994, March). Loosening the grip of intestinal obstruction. *Nursing 94, 24*(3), 34–41

Meissner, J. (1994, July). Caring for patients with ulcerative colitis. *Nursing 94, 24*(7), 54–55.

Neergaard, L. (1996, February 24). Breath test detects bacteria causing ulcers. *Associated Press; Daily Camera.*

Renkes, J. (1993, June). GI endoscopy: Managing the full scope of care. *Nursing 93, 23*(6), 50–55.

Sharp, C. W. & Freeman, C. P. L. (1993, April). The medical complications of anorexia nervosa. *British Journal of Psychiatry, 162,* 452–462.

Sleisenger, M. H. & Fordtran, J. S. (Eds.). (1993). *Gastrointestinal disease: Pathophysiology, diagnosis, management.* Philadelphia: W. B. Saunders Company.

Spiro, C., Grant, E., & Gilley, M. (1994, March). Diverticular disease. *AORN Journal, 59,* 625–634.

Springhouse Corporation. (1991). *Diagnostic testing implications.* Springhouse, PA: Author.

Society of Gastroenterology Nurses and Associates. (1993). *Gastroenterology nursing: A core curriculum.* St. Louis: Mosby-Year Book, Inc.

CHAPTER 35

Anderson, M. A. & Braun, J. V. (1995). *Caring for the elderly client.* Philadelphia: F. A. Davis Company.

Bladder Health Council. (1993). *Answers to your questions about urinary incontinence.* Baltimore: Author.

Brundage, D. (1992). *Renal disorders: Clinical nursing series.* St. Louis: Mosby-Year Book, Inc.

Burke, S. R. (1992). *Human anatomy and physiology in health and disease* (3rd ed.). Albany, NY: Delmar Publishers.

Byers, J. & Goshorn, J. (1995). How to manage diuretic therapy. *AJN 95*(2), 38.

Christensen, B. & Kockrow, E. (1995). *Foundations of nursing* (2nd ed.). St. Louis: Mosby-Year Book, Inc.

Corbett, J. (1992). *Laboratory tests and diagnostic procedures with nursing diagnoses* (3rd ed.). East Norwalk, CT: Appleton & Lange.

Faller, N. & Lawrence, K. (1994). Obtaining a urine specimen from a conduit urostomy. *AJN 94*(1), 37.

Goshorn, J. (1996). Kidney stones. *AJN 96*(9), 40.

Hodgson, B. B., Kizior, R. J., & Kingdon, R. T. (1995). *Nurse's drug handbook* (2nd ed.). Philadelphia: W. B. Saunders Company.

Kee, J. (1991). *Laboratory and diagnostic tests with nursing implications* (3rd ed.). East Norwalk, CT: Appleton & Lange.

Kelly, M. (1996). Chronic renal failure. *AJN 96*(1) 36.

King, B. A. (1994, March). Detecting acute renal failure. *RN, 34*(6).

Lewis, S. M. & Collier, I. C. (1992). *Medical surgical nursing—assessment and management of clinical problems* (3rd ed). St. Louis: Mosby-Year Book, Inc.

National Kidney Foundation-Central New York Chapter.

Needham, J. (1993). *Gerontological nursing: A restorative approach.* Albany, NY: Delmar Publishers.

Palandri, M. K. & Sorrentino, C. R. (1993). *Pocket companion for Luckmann and Sorensen's medical-surgical nursing: A psychophysiologic approach* (4th ed.). Philadelphia: W. B. Saunders Company.

Resnick, B. (1993). Retraining the bladder after catheterization. *AJN 93*(11), 46.

Restore your active lifestyle. (1995). Covington, GA: C.R. Bard, Inc.

Rice, J. & Skelley, E. (1993). *Medications and mathematics for the nurse* (7th ed.). Albany NY: Delmar Publishers.

Rosdahl, C. B. (1995). *Textbook of basic nursing* (6th ed.). Philadelphia: J. B. Lippincott Company.

Scanlon, V. C. & Sanders, T. (1995). *Essentials of anatomy and physiology* (2nd ed.). Philadelphia: F. A. Davis Company.

Scherer, J. C. & Timby, B. K. (1995). *Introductory medical-surgical nursing* (6th ed.). Philadelphia: J. B. Lippincott Company.

Skidmore-Roth, L. (1995). *Nursing drug reference.* St. Louis: Mosby-Year Book, Inc.

Stress incontinence profiles. (1995). Covington, GA: C.R. Bard, Inc.

Swearingen, P. (1994). *Manual of medical-surgical nursing care: Nursing interventions and collaborative management* (3rd ed.). St. Louis: Mosby-Year Book, Inc.

Thayer, D. (1994). How to assess and control urinary incontinence. *AJN 94*(10), 42.

Toto, K. (1992). Acute renal failure: A question of location. *AJN 92*(11), 44–53.

Townsend, C. (1994). *Nutrition and diet therapy* (6th ed.). Albany, NY: Delmar Publishers.

Ulrich, S. P., Canale, S. W., & Wendell, S. A. (1994). *Medical-surgical nursing care planning guides* (3rd ed.). Philadelphia: W. B. Saunders Company.

Walters, N. J., Estridge, B. H., & Reynolds, A. P. (1990). *Basic medical laboratory techniques* (2nd ed.). Albany, NY: Delmar Publishers.

Wood, J. M. & Bosley, C. L. (1995, March). Acute postrenal failure: Reversing the problem. *Nursing 95, 48*(3).

CHAPTER 36

Blablock, B. (1991). Enhancing self-care of the elderly client: Practical teaching tips for ostomy care. *Journal of Enterostomal Therapy Nursing, 18*, 118–121.

Broadwell, D. C. & Jackson, B. S. (Eds.). (1982). *Principles of ostomy care.* St. Louis: Mosby-Year Book, Inc.

Cavas, M. & Makey, S. (1991). The Indiana pouch a continent urinary diversion system. *American Operating Room Nurses, 54*(3), 493–506.

Curry, A. (1991, June). Returning home with confidence discharge planning in stoma care: A conceptual framework. *Professional Nurse,* 536–539.

Doughty, D. B. (1994, July). What you need to know about inflammatory bowel disease. *American Journal of Nursing,* 24–31.

Frost, S. (1991). Managing high output fistulas. *Nursing Standard, 51*(5), 25–27.

Gurganus, E. S. & Morris, E. J. (1991). Pelvic exenteration: The challenge of rehabilitation in a patient with multiple psychosocial problems. *Journal of Enterostomal Therapy, 18*(2), 52–55.

Jansson, J.M. (1991). Dermatologic complications of ostomy care. *Dimensions in Oncology Nursing, 5*(3), 10–13.

Long, L. (1991, October). Ileostomy care overcoming the obstacles. *Nursing 1991,* 73–75.

Madda, M. A. (1991, March). Helping ostomy patients manage medications. *Nursing 1991,* 47–49.

McGinnis, C. & Matson, S. W. (1994, February). How to manage patients with a Roux-en-Y jejunostomy. *American Journal of Nursing,* 43–45.

Meehan, P. A. & Fraher, J. (1995). Gastrointestinal tubes and drains: Nursing management. *Progressions, 7*(3), 3–18.

Paulford-Lecher, N. (1993, September). Teaching your patient stoma care. *Nursing 1993,* 47–49.

Salter, M. (1993). Advances in ileostomy care. *Nursing Standard, 7*(38), 31–36.

Razor, B.R. (1993). Continent uriniary reservoir. *Seminars in Oncology Nursing, 9*(4), 272–285.

Taylor, P. (1994). Beating the taboo sexuality, patient education. *Nursing Times, 90*(13), 51–53.

Thimsen-Whitaker, K. (1991, May-June). Management of loop ileostomy. *Ostomy/Wound Management, 34,* 52–55.

Wilson, R. E. (1992). Patient education sheets. *Ostomy/Wound Management, 38*(4), 45–52.

Wright, A. (1992, January). Routine assessment will identify problems. *Professional Nurse,* 233–236.

CHAPTER 37

Doddato, T. (1995). Advanced practice education for the twenty-first century. *N&HC: Perspectives on Community (16)*5, 266–269.

Duncan, G. (1996). An investigation of learning styles of practical and baccalaureate nursing students. *Journal of Nursing Education, 35*(1), 40–42.

Goodman, L. (1988). Would your assessment spot a hidden alcoholic? *RN, (8),* 56–60.

Irvine, L. M. C. (1995) Can concept mapping be used to promote meaningful learning in nurse education? *Journal of Advanced Nursing, 21,* 1175–1179.

Lewis, S., Collier, I., & Heitkemper, M. M. (1996). *Medical-surgical nursing* (4th ed.). St. Louis: Mosby-Year Book, Inc.

Linton, A., Matteson, M. A., & Maebius, N. K. (1995). *Introductory nursing care of adults.* Philadelphia: W. B. Saunders Company.

Phipps, W. J., Cassmeyer, V.L., Sands, J. K., & Lehman, M. K. (1995). *Medical-surgical nursing: Concepts and clinical practice* (5th ed.). St. Louis: Mosby-Year Book, Inc.

Reynolds, A. (1994). Patho-flow diagramming: A strategy for critical thinking and clinical decision making. *Journal of Nursing Education, 33*(7), 333–336.

Stark, J. (1995). Critical thinking: Taking the road less traveled. *Nursing 95, 11,* 52–56.

INDEX ▶ ▶ ▶ ▶ ▶ ▶ ▶ ▶ ▶ ▶ ▶ ▶ ▶ ▶ ▶ ▶ ▶ ▶ ▶

Page numbers followed by *f* and *t* represent figures and tables respectively.